TEXTBOOK OF
PAEDIATRIC
EMERGENCY
MEDICINE

Commissioning Editor: Michael Parkinson
Project Development Manager: Clive Hewat
Project Manager: Nancy Arnott
Designer: Erik Bigland
Illustration Manager: Gillian Murray
Illustrations by: Ian Ramsden; David Gardner

TEXTBOOK OF PAEDIATRIC EMERGENCY MEDICINE

EDITED BY

Peter Cameron MBBS MD FACEM
Professor of Emergency Medicine, The Alfred Hospital, Prahran, and Monash University, Clayton, Victoria, Australia

George Jelinek MD MBBS Dip DHM FACEM
Professor and Chairman of Emergency Medicine, Sir Charles Gairdner Hospital and University of Western Australia, Hospital Avenue, Nedlands, Western Australia, Australia

Ian Everitt MBBS Dip Anat FRACP FACEM
Emergency Paediatrician, Princess Margaret Hospital for Children, Subiaco, and Joondalup Health Campus, Joondalup, Western Australia, Australia

Gary Browne MD MBBS MSpMed FRACP FACEM
Associate Professor of Paediatric Emergency Medicine, The University of Sydney, The Children's Hospital at Westmead Clinical School, Children's Hospital Institute of Sports Medicine and Department of Emergency Medicine; Visiting Fellow in Sports Medicine and Associate Professor, The University of New South Wales; Head of Academic Emergency Medicine, The Children's Hospital at Westmead, New South Wales, Australia

Jeremy Raftos MBBS FRACP
Director, Paediatric Emergency, Women's and Children's Hospital, Children, Youth and Women's Health Service, North Adelaide, South Australia, Australia

CHURCHILL LIVINGSTONE

ELSEVIER

Edinburgh   London   New York   Oxford   Philadelphia   St Louis   Sydney   Toronto   2006

CHURCHILL
LIVINGSTONE
ELSEVIER

First published 2006

ISBN 0443073481

British Library Cataloguing in Publication Data
A catalogue record for this book is available from the British Library

Library of Congress Cataloging in Publication Data
A catalog record for this book is available from the Library of Congress

ELSEVIER your source for books, journals and multimedia in the health sciences
www.elsevierhealth.com

Working together to grow
libraries in developing countries

www.elsevier.com | www.bookaid.org | www.sabre.org

ELSEVIER   BOOK AID International   Sabre Foundation

The publisher's policy is to use **paper manufactured from sustainable forests**

Printed in Spain

Preface

For emergency physicians working in community hospitals, paediatric presentations are seen as the most challenging. There are very few critically ill children. However, the possibility of missing an early presentation of a potentially life-threatening illness is always present. Children are not always capable of communicating their problems verbally and the parents are inevitably anxious. There are numerous anecdotes of missed diagnoses resulting in catastrophic outcomes. With experience, emergency practitioners develop systematic approaches to overcome these problems. Unfortunately, this is often too late for trainees and clinicians rotating through low-paediatric-volume departments. The reality is that most emergency physicians, even when working in a specialised paediatric centre, will have limited exposure to critically ill children. Regular in-hospital training, courses such as the Advanced Paediatric Life Support (APLS) course, and access to simple reference material are all essential in overcoming this problem.

The purpose of this book is to provide a reference text for medical, nursing and paramedic staff involved in the provision of paediatric emergency care. The book provides a basic approach to the initial care of children with common emergencies whilst giving summary information on more complicated chronic presentations that may present to community hospitals as these conditions are increasingly treated outside the specialist centres. The contributors to the book have been deliberately selected from both specialist paediatric and emergency backgrounds, to ensure a broad perspective.

In Australasia, the United Kingdom, South East Asia and many other regions, paediatric emergency medicine has fallen between specialist training groups with expertise from specialist paediatricians as well as emergency physicians. At times, this relationship has been strained with differing approaches to the management of emergency presentations and training of personnel working in paediatric departments. This is now being improved with joint training programmes and a more collaborative approach. Hopefully this book will help bridge some of the differences between the specialist groups.

This text should be seen as a companion to the *Textbook of Adult Emergency Medicine*, the second edition of which has been published and widely distributed in Australasia, South East Asia and the United Kingdom. It is hoped that a simple straightforward approach to common emergencies will give the reader a method for managing likely emergency presentations. There are frequently many different approaches to managing common medical conditions. Where possible, we have tried to take an evidence-based approach. However, where limited evidence is available we have reverted to consensus amongst the experts in that area. As in most areas of medicine, most of our patient care is dependent on consensus rather than evidence.

For a textbook of this size, an incredible amount of work is necessary to ensure that content is correct and that the project finally comes together within a reasonable time frame. The individual contributors and publication staff at Elsevier should be congratulated. We would also like to thank Ms Mimi Morgan for her considerable patience in co-ordinating this project.

P. C.　　　　　　　　　　2006
G. J.
I. E.
G. B.
J. R.

Contributors

Jason Acworth MBBS FRACP
Deputy Director, Department of
Emergency Medicine, Royal Children's
Hospital, Queensland, Australia

Adrienne Adams MBChB FACEM
Staff Specialist, Emergency Department,
Middlemore Hospital, Otahuhu,
Auckland, New Zealand

Philip Aplin MBBS FACEM
Staff Specialist, Emergency Medicine,
Townsville General Hospital,
Townsville, Queensland, Australia

Franz Babl MBBS MD MPH FRACP
FAAP
Consultant in Emergency Medicine,
Emergency Department, Royal
Children's Hospital, Victoria, Australia

Ruth Barker MBBS FRACP MPH
Staff Specialist, Paediatric Emergency
Department, Mater Children's Hospital,
Brisbane, Queensland, Australia

Roger Barkin MD MPH FAAP FACEP
Vice-President for Paediatric and
Newborn Programs and Vice-President
for Medical Services, HealthONE, USA

Peter Barnett MBBS FRACP
MSc(Epid) FACEM
Deputy Director, Department of
Emergency Medicine, Royal Children's
Hospital, Victoria, Australia

Tom Beattie MB MSc FRCS(Ed)
FFAEM FFSEM DCH
Consultant in Accident and Emergency

Care, Royal Hospital for Sick Children,
Edinburgh, UK

Andrew Berry MBBS FRACP
State Director, NETS (NSW Emergency
Transport Service), New South Wales,
Australia

Robyn Brady DCH MRCPI FRACP
FACEM
Director of Emergency Medical
Training, Paediatric Emergency
Physician, Emergency Department,
Mater Children's Hospital, Brisbane,
Queensland, Australia

Lindsay Bridgford MBBS FACEM
Director of Emergency Services, Albury
Wodonga Integrated Health Services,
Albury Base Hospital, New South Wales,
Australia

Gary Browne MD MBBS MSpMed
FRACP FACEM
Associate Professor of Paediatric
Emergency Medicine, The University of
Sydney, The Children's Hospital at
Westmead Clinical School, Children's
Hospital Institute of Sports Medicine
and Department of Emergency
Medicine; Visiting Fellow in Sports
Medicine & Associate Professor, The
University of New South Wales; Head of
Academic Emergency Medicine, The
Children's Hospital at Westmead, New
South Wales, Australia

Sheila Bryan MBBS FACEM
BSc(Hons) MRACM Dip Ven
Director, Emergency Medicine, Royal

Women's Hospital, Melbourne,
Victoria, Australia

Peter Cameron MBBS MD FACEM
Professor of Emergency Medicine, The
Alfred Hospital, Prahran, and Monash
University, Clayton, Victoria, Australia

Danny Cass MBBS
Director of Trauma, The Children's
Hospital at Westmead, New South
Wales, Australia

Gervase Chaney MBBS FRACP
Paediatrician and Director, Postgraduate
Medical Education, Princess Margaret
Hospital for Children, Western
Australia, Australia

Nicholas Cheng MBBS BSc(Med)
DCH FRACP
Paediatric Emergency Physician,
Emergency Department, The Children's
Hospital at Westmead, New South
Wales, Australia

Raymond Chin MBBS DCH FRACP
Consultant Paediatrician, Paediatric
Emergency – Special interest,
Campbelltown and Camden Hospital,
New South Wales, Australia

Robin Choong MBBS FRACP
FJFICM AIMM
Senior Staff Specialist in Intensive Care,
The Children's Hospital at Westmead,
New South Wales, Australia

Simon Chu MBBS DCH FACEM
Paediatric Emergency Medicine Fellow,

Children's Hospital of Western Ontario, London, Ontario, Canada.

Ron Clark MBBS(Hons) BSc(Hons) PhD FRACP FACEM
Director of Emergency Medicine, Royal Children's Hospital, Herston Road, Herston, Queensland, Australia

Pat Clements BSc(Hons) BSocWk
Social Worker, Department of Emergency Medicine and Paediatric Intensive Care Unit, Royal Children's Hospital, Queensland, Australia

Amanda Jane Cocks MBBS DCH FRACP FACEM FJFICM
Paediatric Emergency Physician, Paediatric Emergency Department, The Women's and Children's Hospital, North Adelaide, South Australia, Australia

David Cooksley MBChB FACEM DRACOG ACCAM
Staff Specialist Emergency Physician, Department of Emergency Medicine, The Townsville Hospital, Queensland, Australia

Elizabeth Cotterell MBBS Dip Paed FRACP
Paediatric Emergency Physician, Emergency Department, Sydney Children's Hospital, New South Wales, Australia

Paul Craven BSc MBBS MRCP FRACP
Staff Specialist in Neonatology, John Hunter Children's Hospital, New South Wales, Australia

Maree Crawford MBBS FRACP
Senior Paediatrician, Child Advocacy Service, Royal Children's Hospital, Queensland, Australia

Nigel Crawford MBBS MPH
Paediatrician, Department of General Paediatrics, University Hospital of Wales, Heath Park, Cardiff, UK

Kieran Cunningham MRCPI DCh DipMedTox FFAEM
Consultant in Emergency Medicine, Sligo General Hospital, Ireland

Sarah Dalton MBBS
Associate Lecturer, School of Women's and Children's Health, University of New South Wales, New South Wales, Australia

Ronald A Dieckmann MD MPH FAAP FACEP
Professor of Clinical Medicine and Pediatrics, University of California, San Francisco; Director of Pediatric Emergency Medicine, San Francisco General Hospital, USA

Linda Durojaiye MBBS BMedSci MRCP FRACP
Paediatric Emergency Physician, Emergency Department, Sydney Children's Hospital, New South Wales, Australia

Daryl Efron MBBS FRACP MD
Consultant Paediatrician, Royal Chidlren's Hospital, Victoria, Australia

Ian Everitt MBBS Dip Anat FRACP FACEM
Emergency Paediatrician, Princess Margaret Hospital for Children, Subiaco and Joondalup Health Campus, Western Australia

Michael Fairley MBBS FRANZP
School of Women's and Children's Health, The University of New South Wales, Sydney, Australia

Bruce Fasher MBBS DRCOG DCH (RCP&S) FRCP(Lond) FRACP
Physician, Emergency Department, The Children's Hospital at Westmead, Sydney, New South Wales, Australia

Peter Francis MBBS FRACP
Emergency Physician, Department of Emergency Medicine, Royal Children's Hospital, Victoria, Australia

Gary Geelhoed MBBS FRACP
Director, Emergency Department, Princess Margaret Hospital for Children, Western Australia, Australia

Padraic Grattan-Smith MBBS(NSW) MRCP(UK) FRACP
Paediatric Neurologist, Sydney Children's Hospital, New South Wales, Australia

Joanne Grindlay MBBS FACEM FRACGP DA(UK) Grad Dip (Rural GP)
Emergency Physician, Department of Emergency Medicine, Royal Children's Hospital, Victoria, Australia

Sonia Grover MBBS MD FRANZCOG
Associate Professor and Director, Department of Gynaecology, Royal Children's Hospital; Gynaecologist, Austin Hospital; Obstetrician and Gynaecologist, Mercy Hospital for Women, Victoria, Australia

Anthony Peter Harrington MBBS(Qld) FRACGP DA RCS(Eng) FACEM
Senior Consultant, Department of Emergency Medicine, Nambour General Hospital, Queensland, Australia

Wayne Hazell MBBS DipObs FACEM
Emergency Physician, Head of Emergency Medicine Education and Research, Middlemore Hospital, South Auckland, New Zealand

Malcolm Higgins MBBS FRACP
Paediatric Emergency Physician, Paediatric Emergency Department, Women's and Children's Hospital, North Adelaide, South Australia

Andrew Holland BSc(Hons) MBBS PhD GradCertEdStudies FRCS FRACS
Associate Professor of Paediatric Surgery and Urology, Department of Academic Surgery, The Children's Hospital at Westmead, New South Wales, Australia

Jason Hort MBBS MRCP FRACP
Staff Specialist, Emergency Department, The Children's Hospital at Westmead, Staff Specialist Paediatrician, Blue Mountains District Anzac Memorial Hospital, New South Wales, Australia

Trevor Jackson MBBS FACEM
Emergency Physician, Sir Charles
Gairdner Hospital and University of
Western Australia, Australia

Andrew Jan MBBS FACEM BA
FAMAC
Director of Emergency Medicine, St
John of God Hospital, Murdoch,
Western Australia, Australia

George Jelinek MD MBBS Dip DHM
FACEM
Professor and Chairman of Emergency
Medicine, Sir Charles Gairdner Hospital
and University of Western Australia,
Nedlands, Australia

Andrew Kemp MBBS FRACP PhD,
Professor of Paediatric Allergy,
The Children's Hospital at Westmead,
New South Wales, Australia

Colin Kikiros MBBS FRACS
Consultant Paediatric Surgeon, Princess
Margaret Hospital for Children, Western
Australia

Judith R. Klein MD FACEP
Assistant Clinical Professor of Medicine,
University of California San Francisco,
Department of Medicine, San Francisco
General Hospital Emergency Services,
California, USA

David Krieser MBBS FRACP
Paediatric Emergency Physician,
Sunshine Hospital, Victoria, Australia

Marian Lee MBBS FACEM DCH
Emergency Physician, Prince of Wales
Hospital, Barker Street, New South
Wales, Australia

Richard S Lennon MBBS
FRACP(Paediatrics) FACEM
Director Emergency Paediatrics, Royal
North Shore Hospital, New South
Wales, Australia

Michelle Lin MD
Assistant Clinical Professor of Medicine,
University of California San Francisco,
San Francisco General Hospital
Emergency Services, California, USA

Kevin Mackway-Jones FRCP FRCS
FFAEM
FAEM Professor of Emergency
Medicine, Manchester Royal Infirmary,
UK

Elly Marillier MBBS FACEM
Clinical Lecturer, Emergency Medicine,
Joondalup Hospital, Western Australia

Jennie Martin MBBS(Hons) DipCH
FACEM
Senior Staff Specialist, Emergency
Medicine, Royal North Shore Hospital,
New South Wales, Australia

Karen McCarthy MBBS FRACP
Paediatrician, Dallas, Texas, USA

Mary McCaskill MBBS BSc(Med)
FACEM Dip Paeds
Medical Head, Emergency Department,
The Children's Hospital at Westmead,
New South Wales, Australia

Terence McGuire MBBS(Qld)
FRCS(Ed) MCH.ORTH(Liv) FRACS
Orthopaedic Surgeon, Mater Children's
Hospital, Queensland, Australia

Patricia McVeagh MBChB FRACP
Visiting Paediatrician, Sydney Children's
Hospital, The Children's Hospital at
Westmead, Tresillian Family Care
Centres, New South Wales, Australia

Helen J Mead MBBS FRACP FACEM
Emergency Physician & Paediatrician,
Emergency Department, Princess
Margaret Hospital for Children; Senior
Clinical Lecturer, School of Paediatrics
& Child Health, University of Western
Australia, Australia

Alastair Meyer BSc(Hons) BMedSci
MBBS FACEM
Director, Department of Emergency
Medicine, Royal Hobart Hospital,
Tasmania, Australia

Owen Miller MBBS BMed(Hons)
FRACP
Senior Staff Specialist, Paediatric
Cardiology, Sydney Children's Hospital,
New South Wales, Australia

Alastair Murray MRCS(A&E)
Specialist Registrar in Emergency
Medicine, Consultant in Emergency
Medicine, St Vincent's University
Hospital, Dublin, Ireland

Yuresh Naidoo MBBS FACEM
Consultant, Joondalup Health Campus,
Joondalup, Western Australia,
Australia

Matt O'Meara MBBS FRACP
Director, Emergency Department,
Sydney Children's Hospital,
New South Wales,
Australia

Ed Oakley MBBS FACEM
Paediatric Emergency Physician and
Director of Emergency Medicine
Training, The Royal Children's
Hospital, Victoria, Australia

Kim Lian Ong MBBS FRCS FHKCEM
FHKAM FAMS
Consultant, Accident and Emergency
Department, Tuen Mun Hospital;
Honorary Associate Professor, Accident
and Emergency Medicine Academic
Unit, Chinese University of Hong
Kong, Accident and Emergency
Department, Tuen Mun Hospital,
Hong Kong

David Orchard MBBS FACD
Paediatric Dermatologist,
Department of Dermatology,
Royal Children's Hospital, Victoria,
Australia

Scott Pearson MBBS FACEM
Staff Specialist, Emergency Medicine,
Christchurch Hospital, New Zealand

Roderic Phillips MBBS FRACP PhD
Paediatric Skin Specialist and Affiliate
Consultant to the Emergency
Department, Royal Children's Hospital
and University of Melbourne, Victoria,
Australia

Robert Pitt MBBS FRACP FACEM
Director, Paediatric Emergency
Medicine, Mater Children's Hospital,
Brisbane, Australia

CONTRIBUTORS

Susan Phin MBBS FRACP
Paediatric Emergency Physician,
The Children's Hospital at Westmead,
New South Wales, Australia

Colin VE Powell MBChB DCH
MRCP(UK) FRACP FRCPCH MD
Consultant Paediatrician and
Assistant Clinical Director for
Integrated Medicine, Department of
General Paediatrics, University Hospital
of Wales, Cardiff, UK

Stephen Priestley MBBS FACEM
Director of Emergency Medicine,
Sunshine Hospital, Victoria, Australia

Michael Ragg MBBS DipObs RACOG
FACEM
Emergency Department, Geelong
Hospital, Geelong, Victoria, Australia

Jeremy Raftos MBBS FRACP
Director, Paediatric Emergency,
Women's and Children's Hospital
Children, Youth and Women's Health
Service, North Adelaide,
South Australia

Fiona Reilly MBBS FACEM
Emergency Physician, Mater Children's
Hospital, Holy Spirit Northside
Hospital, Queensland, Australia

Pam Rosengarten MBBS FACEM
Associate Professor, Director of
Emergency Medicine, Monash Medical
Centre, Victoria, Australia

John Ryan FFAEM FRCSEd(A&E)
DCH DipSportsMed
Consultant in Emergency Medicine,
St Vincent's University Hospital,
Dublin, Ireland

Matt Ryan MBBS FACEM
Emergency Department, Geelong
Hospital, Ryrie Street, Victoria,
Australia

Kam Sinn MBBS FRACP
Emergency Paediatrician and Senior
Specialist, Emergency Department, The
Canberra Hospital, Australian Capital
Territory, Australia

Neil Smith MBChB
Clinical Fellow in Emergency Medicine,
The Children's Hospital at Westmead,
New South Wales, Australia

Mike Starr MBBS FRACP
Paediatrician, Infectious Diseases
Physician, Consultant in Emergency
Medicine, Royal Children's Hospital,
Victoria, Australia

Greg Stevens MBChB FACEM
Staff Specialist, Emergency Department,
Middlemore Hospital, Auckland, New
Zealand

James Tibballs MBBS BMedSc(Hons)
MEd MBA MD FANZCA FJFICM
FACTM
Associate Director, Intensive Care Unit,
Resuscitation Officer, Royal Children's
Hospital, Victoria, Australia

James Tilleard MBBS FACEM
Emergency Physician, Emergency
Department, Nambour Hospital,
Queensland, Australia

Joseph Ting MBBS FACEM BMedSci
Staff Specialist, Department of
Emergency Medicine, Mater Public
Adult Hospital; Clinical Senior Lecturer,
Division of Anaesthesiology and Critical
Care, School of Medicine, Southern
Clinical School, Faculty of Health
Sciences, The University of Queensland,
Australia

Christopher Webber MBBS Dip
RACOG FRACP
Paediatrician and Paediatric Emergency
Physician, Deputy Medical Director,
NETS (NSW Newborn & Paediatric

Emergency Transport Service), New
South Wales, Australia

Julian White MBBS MD FACTM
Consultant Clinical Toxinologist, Head
of Toxinology, Women's & Children's
Hospital, South Australia, Australia

Richard P Widmer BDSc MDSc
FRACDS
Director of Dentistry, The Children's
Hospital at Westmead; Clinical Associate
Professor of Paediatric Dentistry, Faculty
of Health Sciences, University of
Sydney; Visiting Specialist at the
Westmead Centre for Oral Health, New
South Wales, Australia

Barry Wilkins MD MA BChir FRACP
FJFICM FRCPCH MRCP(UK)
DCH(Lond)
Intensive Care Specialist, PICU, The
Children's Hospital at Westmead, New
South Wales, Australia

Gary Williams MBBS FJFICM
Staff Specialist in Paediatric Intensive
Care, Sydney Children's Hospital, New
South Wales, Australia

Frank Willis MBBS DCCH(Edin)
DCH(Glas) FRACP FRCPCH
Paediatrician & Paediatric Nephrologist,
Emergency Department, Princess
Margaret Hospital for Children;
Department of Paediatrics, Fremantle
Hospital, Clinical Senior Lecturer,
School of Paediatrics & Child Health,
University of Western Australia,
Australia

Simon Wood MBBS FACEM
Emergency Physician, Joondalup Health
Campus, Western Australia, Australia

Simon Young MBBS FACEM
Director, Emergency Department, The
Royal Children's Hospital, Victoria,
Australia

Contents

CONTENTS

CONTENTS

CONTENTS

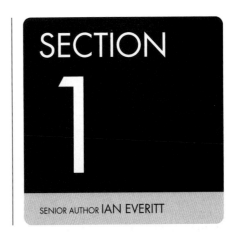
APPROACH TO THE PAEDIATRIC PATIENT

1.1 APPROACH TO THE PAEDIATRIC PATIENT

IAN EVERITT • ANDREW JAN

ESSENTIALS

1 Gaining rapport with the child and the confidence of the parents is the key to assessing children.

2 A child needs to be approached according to chronological and developmental age.

3 Observation is a vital diagnostic tool, which is vastly more important in children than in adult patients.

4 The need for investigations is a balance between an invasive stress on a child and the potential gain of information to aid decision making.

5 Always back up discharge with a concrete action plan and definitive follow up.

6 It is often more important to exclude serious illnesses than make a definitive diagnosis.

7 Addressing parental concerns is an important part of the therapeutic process.

8 Emergency physicians should stay within their comfort zone and when in doubt, consult.

9 A child should be considered potentially sick until one can confidently conclude that he/she is well following a thorough assessment.

INTRODUCTION

Who sees paediatric emergencies?

It is essential that all doctors are familiar with the recognition and management of the seriously ill child. The majority of children presenting to emergency departments are either taken to tertiary paediatric centres or mixed departments that see both adults and children. A small number will arrive, due to close proximity in an emergency, at adult departments where staff may be less familiar with the management of children. Likewise, paediatric emergencies occur remote from emergency departments and may require stabilisation by general practitioners, paramedical staff or laypersons prior to subsequent referral. It is an important role of emergency departments to be an available resource to support the community in the management of paediatric emergencies. This function may occur through advisory, liaison and educative processes.

Some critically ill children will arrive in a more predictable fashion via ambulance and some preparation can occur to plan for their initial treatment. On the other hand, a child in extremis may well be rushed in from a family car, without any prior warning of their arrival. Systems of preparedness for these situations are critical for the immediate assessment and optimal early management of children by emergency department staff (see Chapter 2).

EVOLUTION OF PAEDIATRIC EMERGENCY MEDICINE

In Australia and New Zealand there are currently only nine stand-alone tertiary paediatric emergency departments. Hence, the majority of paediatric patients present initially to mixed departments where approximately 10–30% of attendances are paediatric. This is similar to the UK, Canada and USA. Some of these children will require subsequent referral to a paediatric tertiary centre for ongoing specialist care. The role and functioning of emergency departments has changed dramatically over the past three decades. Paediatric emergency medicine (PEM) has now developed as a speciality. The initial assessment and stabilisation of paediatric patients, which in the past was often deferred to intensive care or anaesthetic colleagues, is now an important role of emergency physicians. In Australasia, the development of PEM as a subspecialty of the College of Paediatrics has seen the establishment of a supervised training scheme by the Paediatric Emergency Medicine Special Interest Group for advanced paediatric trainees. It is hoped that the establishment of a joint training programme overseen by both the Australasian College for Emergency Medicine and the Royal Australian College of Physicians, will see the qualification of further paediatric emergency physicians in the near future. It is paramount that physicians and trainees in both specialist and general emergency departments are well trained and the facilities are appropriate for the resuscitation of critically ill children. Hence, the education and training of emergency physicians in the management of common paediatric emergencies is an important role of both paediatric and emergency colleges. Whether a trainee is seeking a career in a paediatric or a mixed emergency department, experience gained in both environments with exposure to the teaching of both paediatricians and emergency physicians is advantageous. Likewise, a rotation in paediatric intensive care and paediatric anaesthesia provides additional skills in resuscitation, airway management, haemodynamic support and monitoring of critically ill children. The APLS (Advanced

Paediatric Life Support) and ATLS (Advanced Trauma Life Support) or equivalent courses are invaluable additional resources and are requirements to satisfy fellowship qualifications in the training of physicians who will be managing paediatric emergencies.

IDENTIFYING THE POTENTIALLY SICK CHILD

Of the vast number of children attending emergency departments, approximately 2–5% are classified as immediate emergencies (Australasian Triage Scale (ATS) 1 and 2) that require urgent assessment and management.[1] Importantly, children can present with a less urgent triage category, but may rapidly deteriorate from evolving sepsis or airway compromise. The majority of paediatric presentations consist of less emergent problems involving a wide spectrum of injuries and illness. Of this group of paediatric patients there is a subset where the diagnosis is not immediately apparent. Thus, paediatric patients can generally be divided into three broad groups: the obviously well, the obviously sick or the potentially sick child. One of the major tasks for the emergency physician is to identify the 'sick child' from a large undifferentiated group of children who may present as potentially sick. It is by a 'filtering process' via history, examination, observation, investigation and consultation that one identifies the *potentially* sick child (see Fig. 1.1.1). This group of patients includes: those children who have progressed to a severe form of a usually benign illness; those with early, subtle signs of a serious disease; or those who on initial assessment appear unwell, but require investigation to help rule out serious disease. It is often through observation of a child, that one is able to more accurately assess each of these possibilities.[2] With experience, the ability to appreciate a 'sick child' improves, however, a good rule, particularly in the younger child, is, if in doubt, investigate, admit for a longer period of observation or seek the second opinion of a colleague.

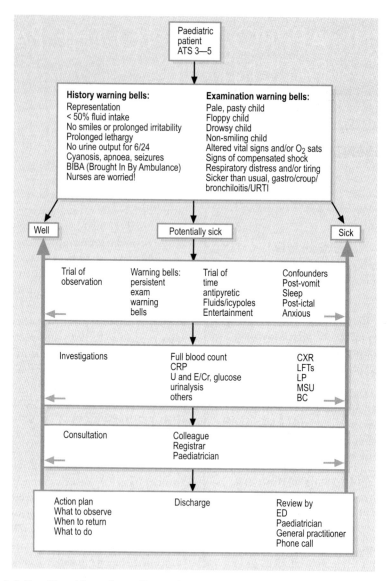

Fig. 1.1.1   Algorithm of paediatric decision making.

CHILDREN WITH FEVER

The concept of occult bacteraemia highlights the difficulties in detecting illness in febrile young children. Bacteraemia can in its most manifest form present as a febrile, pale, pasty, mottled child, centrally warm but with coolish peripheries. Some young children with bacteraemia, however, can appear completely well. Investigations may help identify them with a high white cell count or c-reactive protein (CRP). The problem is not so much that they are sick at that moment of time, but the possibility of the later development of serious bacterial sequelae that necessitates timely treatment. Con-

versely, many bacteraemic children will spontaneously clear the organism without therapy. Therefore, these children remain in the potentially sick category of patients and are obligated to have either admission for observation or discharge with frequent planned reviews for sequelae and a definitive action plan for their parents should the condition change. The evidence for the use of prophylactic antibiotics in these children is controversial. The age of a patient and height of the temperature are useful risk factors to consider in the approach to individual patients. In children less than one month, any fever is significant, whereas older children are more at risk of serious illness with higher temperatures. Likewise, hypothermia can occur in overwhelming sepsis particularly in neonates and infants.

EVOLVING ILLNESS IN CHILDREN

Due to differences in anatomy, physiology, development and psychology, children's diseases are age specific, with serious illness often taking time to evolve.[3] Many children present to an emergency department in the early stage of an illness and making a definitive diagnosis requires time. The clinical status of paediatric patients may also change rapidly. This can occur in response to prior trauma, evolving sepsis, toxin absorption or a seizure and necessitate a change in the initial priority to receive treatment. The younger the child, the greater the potential for rapid deterioration as the early manifestations of a serious illness may be subtle and non-specific. One must be vigilant for the early signs of compensated shock such as tachycardia, decreased capillary refill, mottled skin, cool peripheries, decreased urine output, or drowsiness. Early detection and fluid resuscitation at this point may prevent hypotension in a child with evolving sepsis. Children with severe and deteriorating respiratory illness will manifest fatigue. It is the early recognition of children with serious illness or the potential to deteriorate that is critical to the timely initiation of effective treatment.[2] An important principle in emergency paediatrics is to be proactive. One must be aware of the importance of reviewing a child's response to a given therapy, escalate treatment if required and be vigilant for subtle signs of deterioration.

THE ENVIRONMENT

The physical environment of the emergency department needs to reflect a paediatric milieu with appropriately equipped cubicles for the reception of children accompanied by their carers. Despite the noise inherent in a busy department of sick children, the environment should be as calm and relaxed as possible. Wall or ceiling posters, mobiles, a selection of toys and books are useful to distract younger children from the distress and threat of an unfamiliar hospital environment. Posters of current popular characters such as 'Tele Tubbies', Wiggles or Harry Potter are useful. Not only do these characters make kids feel happy, but their active recognition provides a useful CNS diagnostic tool. A few initial moments gaining a child's confidence with a toy will usually reward the doctor with a more rapid and thorough assessment of the child. Supplies of stickers or bravery certificates are excellent rewards to have on hand for young frightened children who have undergone imaging or blood tests. If possible, in a mixed department, children should be separated from adult patients. Adult patients who are behaviourally disturbed will be distressing for a child and family to see or hear in a nearby cubicle.

Likewise if a child is to undergo a procedure during which he may become distressed, such as intravenous insertion or laceration repair, it is best performed in a closed dedicated procedure room. This will avoid visual or auditory distress to other children and parents. A mounted television/video monitor in this setting can be an excellent distraction during procedures, as an adjunct to analgesia and sedation. For neonates and small infants a radiant heater over the examination bed will aid temperature stability, examination and often the discovery of veins for cannulation.

The paediatric resuscitation area should include wall charts, which refer to emergency algorithms and drug dose guidelines, which can be rapidly referred to during the resuscitation of critically ill children. A white board is handy for pre-sizing and dosing for the imminent arrival of a sick child. Updated clinical guidelines in hard copy and electronic form in the management of common paediatric emergency conditions are a useful resource to be available within the department. Clinical pathways initiated in the emergency department can be useful in ensuring consistency of management from all levels of medical and nursing staff, as well as improving continuity of care in children who require admission to an inpatient unit.

TRIAGE

Paediatric patients arriving in the ED should undergo triage according to standardised Australasian Triage Scale (ATS 1–5) so that they are seen in a prioritised fashion according to acuity. In mixed emergency departments where triage nurses may have had less paediatric experience, there has been a tendency to up-triage paediatric patients.[1] The use of scoring systems for specific conditions or a Triage Observation Tool may be useful in improving the reliability of triage in young children, who may present with non-specific symptomatology.[4] A secondary nursing assessment should occur when the child is admitted to a cubicle with further observations performed at the bedside, so that any change in condition can be detected early and acted on promptly. The senior doctor in the department should immediately be informed of children triaged as ATS 1 or 2 to direct timely management. In times of high workload, children with an ATS 3 may not be definitively assessed within 30 minutes and should have a senior doctor rapidly assess status and initiate therapy, if required.

FAST TRACKING

Some initiation of treatment is appropriate during the triage process, such as the provision of analgesia for pain or an antipyretic in a child symptomatic of fever. It is important that children with pain are given early and appropriate analgesia or have injuries splinted when required. This will facilitate a more comfortable, reliable and expeditious assessment. The use of opiates, when required, will only enhance, rather than detract from the subsequent physician's physical examination.[5] The use of visual analogue scales such as the 'Wong–Baker' faces may assist the assessment of a child's response to analgesia. A process of fast tracking appropriate children with single limb injuries for an X-ray prior to definitive medical review may improve efficiency through the department. Febrile children who present with a rash, not clearly due to a viral exanthema, should be fast tracked to be seen by a senior doctor to consider the possibility of meningococcemia. It is useful to have documented management plans for children who may recurrently present to the department. This includes conditions such as brittle asthma, cyclical vomiting or recalcitrant seizures where a clear plan of management can expedite care by ED staff.

THE PAEDIATRIC APPROACH

The evaluation process of a child in the emergency department involves history, observation, examination and may include relevant investigations.

Each of these components needs to be considered in the formulation of a diagnosis and disposition plan. A child needs to be considered in the context of the family. The assessment of children in the emergency department setting can be both challenging and very rewarding. It is a challenge to modify the clinical approach according to the chronological and developmental level of the individual child. Likewise, treating paediatric patients is a rewarding area of emergency medicine, as children will often respond rapidly to management within the time frame of the ED attendance.

Gaining rapport

Endeavouring to gain initial rapport with a child and the confidence of the parents is the key to assessing children in the ED setting. An unrushed, gentle and caring manner will rapidly settle the fears and anxieties of most children and their parents. This usually allows the examination to proceed in a non-threatening fashion and improves the reliability of clinical signs. It will take time, experience and the observation of colleagues' techniques for every emergency physician to develop their own individual approach to children. A thorough exami-

nation without causing distress to a child is very reassuring to a parent. Many children arrive at an emergency department miserable, in pain, fearful, or with some trepidation of what lies ahead. With a child-friendly approach by all staff, most will leave feeling much better and, hopefully, even having enjoyed the experience.

Age appropriate

The approach to any child in the emergency department is dictated by the child's age and developmental level. It is useful to have a modified approach to suit newborns, infants, toddlers, preschoolers, school children and adolescents. A preverbal or developmentally delayed child won't tell you of pain which has shifted to the right iliac fossa. An unwell 14 month old clinging to mother may actively resist the initial attempts to be examined by a stranger. The absence of familiarity with a family or child that their family doctor may have may further impede the assessment of anxious children. When explaining procedures to children it is important to be age appropriate and above all honest. Never tell a child 'you won't feel a thing!' prior to plunging a cannula through an EMLA anaesthetised cubital fossa. Rather, explain in age-appropriate terms what it may feel like and that it's OK to cry.

Maintaining a child's trust at all times is crucial and will positively influence any subsequent medical contacts the child may have. The demonstration of a procedure on a doll may decrease the anticipatory trepidation in a child.

The assessment of a child should always be carried out in the presence of the parent or carer, unless the child arrives by ambulance or other means without the parent/carer present, and the child's medical needs warrant immediate attention. Otherwise, it is prudent in the non-urgent situation to provide a staff member to support the child and defer the assessment until carers are present.

Development appropriate

Infants particularly benefit from the constant presence of their parent in their visual field in order to avoid stranger distress and are often best examined in the

parent's arms. Neonates can be examined on the examination bed as long as they are kept warm. Toddlers, despite their evolving autonomy will usually be less fretful if examined on a parent's lap. It is a useful sign of illness or other cause, to note when young children do not exhibit these normal stranger anxieties. The preschooler who enjoys a sense of play and imagination can usually be relaxed during an examination or procedure by storytelling or engaging in play with a toy. An anxious early school-aged child may respond to participation in the examination or being asked about school or other more favoured activities. Adolescents on the other hand, need to be approached in a more adult fashion and should be offered confidentiality and the opportunity to choose whether their parents are present.

In the event of an unatonable child resisting any examination, one may have to modify the approach to gain essential clinical findings in a gentle but firm manner. It is unusual, however, for a child to remain 'unexaminable' if appropriate analgesia is given and the child is left for a period of time undisturbed.

Parental involvement

In order to provide emotional support, parents should be encouraged to remain close to their child during any procedures. Parents who appear at risk of vagal syncope are best seated away from the 'viewing of action' but still in their child's earshot for verbal support. Children's behaviour often mirrors that of their parents, so gaining the confidence of the parent will often make an anxious child relax prior to procedures. The use of a confident, calm, caring approach, will be rewarded by a child who will allow a more reliable examination. It is very reassuring to the parents to see that the doctor is experienced in dealing with children and anticipates the expected anxieties and reluctance to examination that a child may have when unwell.

HISTORY

The initial contact with the family should include an introduction of who you are.

The parents should be addressed and the child greeted by name, in an age-appropriate manner. It is important to consider one's approach in terms of the needs of both the child's illness and the parental concerns. The history is generally elicited from the parent or caregiver but it is appropriate, in a verbal child, to augment this information by directly questioning the child.

Critically ill child

Sometimes the normal routine of history, followed by examination will need to be altered in a child who arrives critically ill. The management will need to be expeditious and occur simultaneously with the gathering of pertinent information from the parents. Parents should be given the opportunity to remain at the bedside of their critically ill child undergoing resuscitation, with a dedicated support person.

Parental issues

The clarity of the history given by parents can be affected by parental distress, anxiety or sleep deprivation. One should begin the history in a focused manner according to the presenting complaint. Later it may be useful to explore individual parental anxieties. One of the most important questions to a parent is, 'What is your biggest worry or fear?' Some parents may have specific concerns such as a fear their febrile child has meningococcal disease when community alertness to this condition is heightened. Addressing this concern may occupy most of the doctor's time. The parent of a child who has sustained an accidental scald or injury may be feeling distressed or guilty and sensitivity to this is required. Again addressing guilt will involve much of the doctor's time.

Children-specific issues

In younger children, certain symptoms are less specific. The report of vomiting in an infant may be due to meningitis, pneumonia, tonsillitis or urinary sepsis rather than gastroenteritis. The assessment of wellness or otherwise in infants can be more challenging due to their limited psychomotor activities. Indeed their spectrum of normal behaviours in-

volves sleeping, waking to cry or demand a feed, followed by a return to sleep. Hence, it is important to enquire into their feeding status and sleep/activity pattern as an indicator of compromise due to illness. One carefully needs to clarify what their current intake is compared to their normal breast- or bottle-feeding. An infant who is feeding less than 50% of normal has significant compromise. It is important to note the report of a young febrile child who remains lethargic and fails to smile or interact with parents. In the otherwise well-looking infant, who appears mottled, clarify with parents whether this may be usual for their child. (i.e. physiological cutis marmoratum versus sepsis). In assessing young children with trauma, a thorough history of the timing and mechanism of injury, noting the child's developmental capabilities is paramount to detecting possible non-accidental injuries (see Chapter 18.2 on NAI).

Other useful information to cover in the paediatric patient history is shown in Tables 1.1.1 and 1.1.2.

EXAMINATION

Age appropriate

The examination technique used in paediatric patients depends on the age

and developmental level of the child. The key is to gain the confidence and then the co-operation of the child. Older children are generally compliant, which allows them to be examined in a systematic fashion similar to adult patients. However, younger children usually need to be examined in a less formalised manner, whilst maintaining a high degree of vigilance. The order of the examination

Table 1.1.1 History warning bells
• Child taking less than 50% of normal fluids
• The child with prolonged lethargy
• No urine output for six hours
• Prolonged irritability or inconsolability
• Report of cyanosis, pallor, seizures or significant apnoea
• The child who has not smiled over a period of hours
• Nursing staff feel the child is 'just not right'
• Unplanned re-presentations
• Parental concerns out of proportion to child's illness
• Brought in by ambulance
• History not compatible with injury/ ?non-accidental injury

Table 1.1.2 Important elements of the paediatric history
Presenting complaint
Pregnancy
Perinatal – delivery type, birth weight, need for resuscitation/special care nursery admission
Development – in a CNS problem, compatibility with injury mechanism
Immunisation status
Previous illnesses/surgery/admissions/medications
Allergies
Infectious contacts/recent travel
Family history
Social history – family circumstances may influence a child's disposition
Fasting status if relevant
Feeds – normal bottle or breast feeds for comparison

may need to be adapted according to the individual child's responses. In a reluctant examinee, clinical findings may be achieved by surreptitiously examining through play as the opportunity arises. Much can be ascertained in this situation by careful observation rather than a more threatening 'hands on approach'. Entertaining a young child in a professional manner during examination will generally allow the confounding influence of anxiety to diminish.

Gentle, distraction, painful last

Children are usually reluctant to have any painful area disturbed. Confirming tenderness needs to be gentle and unhurried to minimise any distress. Many young children will respond to age-appropriate verbal banter during the examination, which distracts from the perceived threat of the examining hand. Alternatively, one may need to gently palpate a tender right iliac fossa, whilst using distraction such as the counting of the child's fingers. Sometimes a child may prefer their tender abdomen to be palpated with the examiners hand 'through their own hand'. The examination needs to be adapted to the child's responses, deferring distressing phases until the final moment of examination. Time used initially to gain a child's confidence will make subsequent assessment more rewarding and the clinical signs more reliable. We have all experienced the frustration of trying to assess the abdomen of a screaming or fractious child who demonstrates the pseudo-rigid abdomen! Indeed, the most reliable method of excluding peritonism in a child does not involve any palpation of the abdomen. Asking a child to walk, jump or climb the trolley are useful manoeuvres to help exclude peritoneal irritation.

The examination of ears and throat, tender abdomen or a painful injury, is best left till last in order not to upset a child and make the remaining routine examination difficult. If one detects that a child has an unfortunate fearful memory of a stethoscope or the like, a preliminary auscultation of a child's soft toy and warming the diaphragm will often allow this to subside. Distracters such as a soft

toy placed in the hand may alleviate the examiner from the torture of the curious infant who yanks on the stethoscope tubing during auscultation.

Improvise

The examination of infants and young children is best done in the least threatening position. This is usually best whilst being held securely in the parent's arms or on the knee. If a child is sleeping, the opportunity should be taken to perform auscultation, palpation of a fontanelle/abdomen, which will be altered in the crying state, prior to disturbing the child to wakefulness. A neonate examined supine needs to be kept warm with a blanket or a radiant heater. Hands should be warm. The crying fractious baby may be settled by offering a feed or a pacifier before the examination. The symmetry of normal infant reflexes is a useful screen for any focal motor problem or as a localiser of a painful limb.

Index of suspicion

The routine methods of examination for signs of meningism in children are unreliable. Asking the child to look upwards at an object or down to their umbilicus is a more useful screen to detect nuchal irritation. In children less than two years old, the early signs of meningism are often absent and threshold for cerebrospinal fluid (CSF) examination adapted accordingly. Other significant, but subtle features that may be missed on examination, include persistent tachycardia or tachypnoea that is not clearly related to fever. One needs to be alert to the spectrum of stigmata of non-accidental injuries that may present to the emergency department. (see Chapter 18.2 on NAI)

Respiratory examination

Noisy breathing in children can sometimes be difficult to determine if it is due to airway obstruction of intra- or extrathoracic origin. The localisation of airway obstruction to a particular segment of airway can often be aided by successive auscultation over the nares, mouth, larynx and peripheral airways. Younger children are often easier to auscultate by listening through clothes from behind

whilst being held by the parent. Detection of 'occult' asthma in a child with suggestive symptoms but no wheeze, may be aided by comparing the diminished volume of airflow in expiration compared to inspiration, or alternatively re-auscultation after exercising the child in the ED. Young children with throat discomfort will be reluctant to volunteer a cough, but a gentle tickle of the axilla or palpating the anterior larynx will usually produce a bark to clarify suspicion of croup. Recognising the pattern of respiratory distress in a child from the end of the bed, will often differentiate upper and lower airway obstruction, prior to any auscultation.

Abdominal examination

The abdominal examination needs to always conclude with the nappy area for otherwise occult torsions, hernias, skin problems and for stool examination, if present. The rectal examination in children is not routine and only performed with clear indication. One needs to be cognisant to maintain privacy and dignity, particularly when examining older children and adolescents. The examination of a child with possible sexual abuse is outlined in Chapter 18.1.

ENT last

In preschool age and younger children examination of the ears and throat is best deferred to last. A gentle, but rapid approach is necessary to avail an accurate assessment of the oropharynx, followed by a cuddle from the parent. Despite the potential difficulty, the source of fever will often be overlooked if the throat is inadequately visualised in children. In infants the throat is best examined with the child lying supine with both arms abducted alongside the head to prevent movement. A young child who is fearful of throat examination needs to be held as still as possible for a rapid, 'one gag, one look' approach. This is best performed after explanation, positioning the patient upright on a parent's knee, securing arms beside the trunk with the parent's dominant arm and holding the head straight-ahead with the other. 'Let's count your teeth' is a less threatening signal to most children to open the mouth, rather than mentioning 'the tonsil or throat' words particularly if parents warn you that, 'Nobody has been able to get a look at his throat'. Some children require gently inserting the spatula between clenched teeth to touch the tongue to initiate a gag. Most older children fortunately, will happily volunteer a view of the pharynx.

Following any distressing procedure it is important to acknowledge bravery in a frightened child. Likewise, giving a child an honest, developmentally appropriate explanation of what to expect prior to any procedure such as an IV insertion, is to be encouraged. This is best done immediately prior to the procedure so that an anxious child's fears don't escalate in the intervening period (see Table 1.1.3).

OBSERVATION

Observation is the distant examination of a child that begins prior to introducing oneself to the family, and continues after the examination, whilst one may be writing up notes or between seeing another patient. It also includes the noting of nursing remarks and vital signs recorded in order to obtain additional clues as to the sickness of a child. The trends of nursing observations over time, are useful indicators to detect early signs of disease progression or the response to therapy. This 'ongoing triage', in effect, is particularly important to detect 'evolving illness' that may otherwise remain undetected.

LOOK, prior to examination

Before the 'laying on of hands', much can be gleaned by initially observing a child and parent in the cubicle, from a distance. One's first impressions of a child will often direct a subsequent approach. The child's state of activity and interaction with the environment and parents will often change when a strange doctor approaches. The process of evaluating a child differs from that of an adult by the greater importance of observation.[2] It is important to emphasise the observation of a child to aid diagnosis in the emergency department setting. This is particularly important in evaluating children during their first three years of life. The 'end of bed' observations can be an important indicator for differentiating the potentially sick child.

Observational variables

The general appearance of a child should include noting level of alertness, eye contact, activity, quality of cry, posture, interaction with the environment, irritability, colour, hydration, perfusion, general growth and nutrition, respiratory distress and presence of any unusual smell (e.g. ketotic). The lack of normal resistance to examination or a procedure expected of a child is an important observation to note. The sick child may make none of the resistance expected to examination or venepuncture. Observational variables have been shown to be more predictive of serious disease than historical information in young children.[6] Likewise, clinical examination, considered alone, is a poor predictor of serious illness. Observation of a child needs to be performed as a separate process from the examination and may require a period of time for re-evaluation to detect disease progress. Researchers have used formalised scales such as the McCarthy Observation Scales to aid this assessment in febrile children.[7] In the ED setting, discussion of a child with a colleague can be a rewarding aid to decision making.

A child's posture, undisturbed, can be a useful clue to systemic illness, abnormal neuromuscular function or a painful limb or joint. Children with sepsis or meningitis may be floppy or flaccid. In other cases, the only sign of meningeal irritation may be a child who is holding his neck in a slightly extended position.

Observing breathing

When observing tachypnoea in a child, it is useful to determine whether a child has 'quiet tachypnoea' (breathing fast and quietly) with no evidence of increased work of breathing, such as may occur in conditions of fever, acidosis or cyanotic heart disease. Children with 'noisy tachypnoea' (breathing fast and hard) demonstrate increased work of breathing, due to conditions such as airway obstruction, pneumonia or heart failure.

Confounders

There are several observational confounders that can influence initial decision-making, when children can appear transiently sicker than they really are. There are many times when the ini-

Table 1.1.3 Examination warning bells
The pale, pasty child
The floppy child
The child who appears drowsy
Alteration in vital signs, SaO2
Early signs of compensated shock
The tiring child with respiratory distress
The child who never smiles despite appropriate prompting
The child who looks sicker than the usual child with gastroenteritis/croup/bronchiolitis/URTI
Other specific signs:
Non-blanching rash – petechiae/purpura-sepsis
Bulging or full fontanelle – raised intracranial pressure
Bilious vomiting – bowel obstruction
High pitched cry – meningitis
Grunting – respiratory distress

tially sick-appearing child can pick up and appear well again over a short period of time. This situation usually occurs when the paediatric consultant is called and by the time he or she arrives the child is smiling and running around the department. The vomiting child will often look pale and 'pasty' for up to 20 minutes post vomiting. One-hour post antipyretic the symptomatic febrile child can look like a different child. Children initially emerging from a simple febrile convulsion can look well again in 20 to 30 minutes. A young child's physiological sleep can mimic septic drowsiness or somnolence resulting from head trauma. A fearful child during examination, can escalate the examiner's perception of his illness.

Re-evaluate

This reinforces the power of observation. It allows time for a trial of fluids, reducing fever with an antipyretic, or seeing if a child responds to distraction. Subsequent re-evaluation of the child often allows one to differentiate whether a child is sick or well. The use of observation really allows one to identify the persistence of the initial abnormal examination findings. A child with intussusception may intermittently appear well and observation may be required to observe the clues to prompt the appropriate diagnostic investigation (see Table 1.1.4).

WHEN TO INVESTIGATE

One needs to be judicious with the use of investigations in children in the emergency department. Investigations serve more than one purpose. They help confirm or refute suspicions. Occasionally parents appear to initially want more reassurance than simple clinical assessment and explanation.

Blood tests

Previous medical visits or advice may prompt a parent to feel that reassurance that their child is safe, can only be confirmed by the 'magic of blood tests'. This may be especially so with a young-looking doctor. However, with clinical experience and clear explanation, parents can usually be counselled out of this option, when it is clearly not warranted clinically, by explaining that blood taking is not always straight forward in a chubby toddler and that sometimes two, three or occasionally more attempts are required. The potential psychological stress to the child is not worth the information that will be obtained in this instance. However, on the positive side, blood tests such as a full blood count (FBC) or a CRP may provide reassurance in some uncertain situations. At other times they are useless, for example to exclude meningitis in a child with clinical tonsillitis, as inflammatory markers are already raised.

Investigations may provide extra time for observation and reassurance, however if an investigation is performed, action must follow! The screening of urine in febrile young children is vital to detect occult urinary infection. In children less than two years, dipstick analysis is inaccurate to exclude infection and microscopy must be performed to exclude pyuria. The appropriate techniques for obtaining urine are discussed in Chapter 16.4.

THE PARENTS

Parents who accompany their child to an emergency department are often anxious and fearful regarding the safety of their child. It is important to consider that the parents are entrusting the doctor with the wellbeing of their most cherished and precious possession. The management of the fears and the identification of the needs and expectations of the parents is an important role of the doctor attending to their child. Listening to and addressing the parent's concerns in a sympathetic and unhurried fashion is often the main therapeutic strategy to reassure an anxious parent that a child with a relatively minor illness is safe. Many parents may be sleep deprived due to attending to their sick child and this will influence their ability to convey a lucid history. The time spent at triage or in the waiting area in a busy emergency department can frustrate the most patient parent. This needs to be anticipated and acknowledged at the start of the consultation.

Managing the parents

The emergency department visit may follow previous medical consultation(s) where their concerns may not have been addressed and it is important to explore these. Always acknowledge the parent's fears and anxieties, however medical judgement should allow an objective decision about whether a child is sick or not. An exception to this is the parents of children with a chronic illness or special needs. They are usually correct when they judge that their child is sick. Aggressive and unreasonable carers will

Table 1.1.4   Examination warning bells
Decreased level of alertness, activity, eye contact
Drowsiness or decreased interaction with the environment/parents
Abnormal posture
Abnormal quality of cry
Prolonged irritability or inconsolability
Ongoing pallor
Decreased peripheral perfusion or hydration appearance
Persistence of abnormal recorded vital signs
Respiratory distress/tachypnoea ('quiet' or 'noisy')

- Persistence of examination warning bells
- Confounders – post vomit/seizure, high fever, normal sleep, anxiety

usually respond to a professional, polite and courteous senior doctor. There is usually a reason behind their behaviour that needs to be explored. Even the most anxious parent will usually respond to a thorough assessment of their child followed by an explanation of diagnosis and management. In unplanned second presentations where parents demand admission, it is usually best to admit.

Communication issues

Explanations to parents as a general rule should be appropriate to their level of understanding and education. Provision of handouts or written instructions is useful to reinforce diagnosis and management. Reviewing a parent's understanding of instructions prior to discharge will allow clarification and avoid communication problems. Parents may have fears related to anecdotal advice from family/friends, misinterpretation of media reporting, or other sources, which need to be explored. Gaining the confidence of parents before they leave the department is an essential part of the therapeutic process and has a positive effect on compliance to therapy. It is useful to explain to parents the likely natural history of their child's illness and encourage review should significant deviations from this occur.

MANAGEMENT OF PAEDIATRIC PATIENTS

The urgency of management of children can be graded into the following categories:

- The critically ill child who requires immediate resuscitation and investigations and probable transfer to a tertiary centre.
- The sick child who needs immediate investigation and IV access.
- The child who warrants observation and a trial of fluids or antipyretics in the department. Consider the early placement of Emla® cream if further investigation may subsequently be necessary.
- The child that requires no investigation but whose parents need an explanation of the diagnosis and management.

The management of febrile young children is a large part of emergency paediatric practice. The current approach to those children without a clear focus is controversial and varies between institution and individuals. The two alternative approaches are risk - or test - minimising strategy (see Chapter 9.). Certainly, it is reasonable, in a 3 to 36-month-old child, to be guided by clinical judgement alone with close planned review. If the child appears unwell, a sepsis screen is performed according to symptomatology. Neonates and small infants less than three months, where threshold for investigation is much lower, need to be approached according to departmental guidelines. Undifferentiated febrile children should be reviewed the next day and ongoing, until a definitive diagnosis is made or until the child returns to normal. Parents should be instructed to return to the department if their child deteriorates. The discharge action plan should give clear and understandable instructions on when to return. For example, in the febrile child, this should include: if child becomes more unwell, with decrease in intake to less than 50% normal, no urine output for six hours, or becoming drowsy beyond sleeping. Parents should be alerted to potential complications such as becoming limp, fitting or appearance of a rash, which warrant urgent review.

Turning the corner

Managing children is often about understanding the natural history of the illness and predicting when the child will 'turn the corner'. For example, one needs to be patient with a child who clearly has gastroenteritis who has been vomiting for two hours. Often a child will vomit hourly for eight hours, perhaps once or twice more and then improve. Advising the parents of the likely natural history of a condition and giving a clear action plan can be reassuring.

Decision making

Making decisions in paediatric emergency medicine is a balance of history, examination, intuition, knowing when to trust the parents and maintaining objectivity. If you feel uneasy with your diagnosis regarding a child, respect that feeling and gain support until you do feel comfortable with your decision. There are many strategies to do this:

❶ Consider early consultation with an emergency or paediatric consultant.
❷ Organise early follow up with a paediatrician or general practitioner.
❸ Have a colleague on the floor listen to the story or examine the child.
❹ Phone review the patient's family yourself, later that day or the next morning.
❺ Provide a concrete action discharge plan.
❻ Admit the patient for observation.

When to admit

The decision to admit or discharge a child from the emergency department is easily made when the child requires medical care that is only available in the hospital setting. The receiving ward will need to have appropriate resources for the ongoing management of the child, which should be clarified by discussion with the receiving in-patient unit/paediatrician. Some children may need to be discussed with, and transferred to a tertiary paediatric environment when they require, or have the potential to require, paediatric intensive care facilities or paediatric subspecialty management.

Factors influencing disposition

However, many other factors need to be considered in the disposition decision (see Table 1.1.5). The threshold to admit a child is influenced by the child's age, availability of appropriate follow up, assessment of parent's ability to provide care and ongoing monitoring, the natural history of the illness and likelihood to deteriorate, social factors, comorbidity, distance from hospital, time of day, parental anxiety levels, availability of an early paediatric opinion, and the possibility that a child may be at risk. One needs to assess in a non-judgemental fashion the ability of the parents to carry out any ongoing treatment, and consider admission if there appears to be a need for ongoing support. When in doubt

Table 1.1.5 Factors influencing admission threshold

Age of child
Availability of appropriate follow up/review
Parental ability to provide care and monitoring, social factors
Comorbidity
Distance from hospital
Time of presentation
Parental anxiety levels
To enable a paediatrician opinion
Possible child at risk outside hospital

regarding whether or not to discharge a child, err on the side of caution. It may be prudent to consult, consider a period of observation in the emergency department, or admit the child to hospital.

Continuity of care

It is important for emergency department staff to liaise closely with the admitting paediatrician to provide continuity of care and to ensure ongoing care is expedited in the emergency department. Ongoing management and monitoring of the patient is an important role of medical and nursing staff after this decision has been made, particularly if there is a delay in the transfer process. Any significant change in a child's previous status or treatment needs to be communicated to the appropriate receiving team.

Observation ward

Significant compromise from many childhood illnesses is often transient and will often respond rapidly to interventions commenced in the ED followed by a period of observation. Parents can often be reassured during this period of observation in hospital, that their child has remained well and will respond to management strategies that subsequently can be continued at home. Studies have shown that many children admitted to hospital only require a limited period of subsequent in-patient therapy and are discharged in less than 24 hours.[8] In a tertiary paediatric environment an effective way to manage these

children is by admission to a short-stay observation ward. The ED needs to be appropriately resourced with staff to provide ongoing care and regular review of patients to expedite timely discharge. Conditions suitable for consideration of an observation ward admission will vary with local resources and may include asthma, croup, gastroenteritis, febrile convulsion, presumptive viral illnesses, non-surgical abdominal pain, minor trauma, post sedation recovery or ingestions.[9] In mixed departments, without the facility of a short-stay ward, it is often appropriate to use the paediatric ward to admit patients who would benefit from a period of observation (see Table 1.1.5).

Making a diagnosis

Not every child leaving the emergency department will do so with a specific diagnosis. The unwell febrile child needs to have serious diagnoses such as meningitis considered, before making a diagnosis of viral illness. Many children without a clear diagnosis, can be managed expectantly and safely discharged home with organised review by a local doctor, paediatrician, or return to the department. Giving the parents clear instructions to return should the state of their child not follow an expected course is essential. Children are often seen early in the natural history of their illness and a diagnosis will only become clear with time. It is important to communicate clearly, verbally or in writing, with the doctor who will be following up the child. Close liaison with a local doctor who has referred a patient to the ED is essential. One should always respect the concerns raised by a referring local doctor who usually has the advantage of familiarity with the child and family.

DEVELOPMENTAL MILESTONES

It is important to have an understanding of the major developmental milestones throughout childhood for the provision of care to paediatric patients. These can be rapidly confirmed by examination or parental enquiry. This allows one to use

Table 1.1.6 Normal milestones in first two years of life

Neonate	Lift head, visually fix for period
6 weeks	Smile, follow past midline
4 months	Roll over
6 months	Sit, transfer toy between hands
9 months	Stand holding on, crawl, stranger anxiety
12 months	Walking, single words
18 months	Explorer (trauma/poisons), tantrums, several words
2 years	Combine words, run, jump

an appropriate age-modified approach in the child's evaluation. Some specific behaviours, such as stranger anxiety in a 12 month old, may challenge the assessment, so it is important to adapt the approach to these expected behaviours. Significant deviations from normal warrant consideration of paediatric referral. Useful early milestones are shown in the Table 1.1.6.

GROWTH

It is essential to measure a child's current weight on every ED visit in order to accurately dose any therapeutic drug and to quantify recent weight loss. Where a child is critically unwell and unable to be weighed, estimation can be made via Broselow or other charts. Between the age of one and ten years an estimation of weight is $2 \times (\text{age} + 4)\,\text{kg}$. Standardised percentile growth charts are useful to confirm suspicion of failure to thrive or discrepancy in linear or cranial growth. The trend of growth plotted on a growth chart over time is more important than a single measurement. As a general rule, birth weight doubles by five months, and triples by one year. Newborns are often discharged from hospital in the first few days of life and may present in the first week to an emergency department. Following the expected initial weight loss, term babies should normally regain

Table 1.1.7 Estimated normal growth

Age	Weight (kg)	Height (cm)	Head circumference (cm)
Birth	3.5	50	35
1 year	10	75	47
2 years	13	88	49
> 2 years	+ 2 kg y^{-1}	+ 6 cm y^{-1}	N/A

Table adapted from Fleischer and Ludwig, Textbook of Paediatric Emergency Medicine[10]

Table 1.1.9 Normal vital signs

Age	Weight (kg)	RR (min^{-1})	HR (min^{-1})	sBP (mm Hg)
Birth	3.5	40–60	100–170	50
3 months	6	30–50	100–170	50
6 months	8	30–50	100–170	60
1 year	10	30–40	100–170	65
2 years	13	20–30	100–160	65
4 years	15	20	80–130	70
6 years	20	16	70–115	75
8 years	25	16	70–110	80
10 years	30	16	60–105	85
12 years	40	16	60–100	90
14 years	50	16	60–100	90

Adapted from RCH, Melbourne Clinical Guideline Site[11]

Table 1.1.8 Australian standard vaccination schedule (0–5 years)*

Age	Vaccine
2 months	DTP, OPV, Hib-HepB
4 months	DTP, OPV, Hib-HepB
6 months	DTP, OPV
12 months	MMR, Hib-HepB, MenC
18 months	DTP
2-5 years	MenC
4 years	DTP, OPV, MMR

*This varies between states.

A wall chart in the paediatric resuscitation area is a useful reference as a guide to these parameters. A good rule to remember is any child with a persistent RR > 60 or HR > 160 is definitely abnormal (Table 1.1.9).

their birth weight by the end of the first week. Appropriate neonatal weight gain is an important index of wellness. Head circumference increases by 2 cm in the first three months, 1 cm in the next three months, followed by 0.5 cm per month thereafter (Table 1.1.7).

IMMUNISATION

It is not the role of the emergency department to provide routine immunisations to children. It is useful, however, to clarify a child's immunisation status with regard to the possibility of a particular infection such as epiglottitis, whooping cough or measles. Immunised children can, however, manifest a modified form of these infections. In children who are found to be incompletely or non-immunised, it is opportunistic to provide information regarding the normal vaccination schedule and refer to the local doctor or appropriate community facility for follow up (see Table 1.1.8).

VITAL SIGNS

It is necessary to interpret the vital signs according to the age of a particular child.

REFERENCES

1. Durojaiye L, O'Meara M 2002 A study of triage of paediatric patients in Australia. Emergency Medicine 14: 67–76
2. Luten RC 1988 Recognition of the sick child. Problems in paediatric emergency medicine. Churchill Livingstone, New York, 1–12
3. Browne GJ 2001 Paediatric emergency departments: Old needs, new challenges and future opportunities. Emergency Medicine 13: 409–417
4. Browne GL, Gaudry PL 1997 A triage observation tool improves the reliability of the National Triage Scale in children. Emergency Medicine 9: 283–238
5. Browne GJ, Chong RKC, Gaudry PL, Wilkins BH (eds) 1997 Principles and practice of children's emergency care. McLennan and Petty, Sydney, 1–5
6. Waskerwitz S, Berkelhamer JE 1981 Outpatient bacteremia: Clinical findings in children under two years with initial temperatures of 39.5°C or higher. Journal of Paediatrics 99(2): 231–233
7. McCarthy PL, Sharpe MR et al 1982 Predictive observation scales to identify serious illness in febrile children. Paediatrics 70(5): 802-809
8. Browne G, Penna A 1996 Short stay facilities. The future of efficient paediatric emergency services. Archives of Diseases in Childhood 74: 309–313
9. Scribano PV, Wiley JF, Platt K 2001 Use of an observation unit by a paediatric emergency department for common paediatric illnesses. Paediatric Emergency Care 17(5): 321–323
10. Fleischer GR, Ludwig S 1993 Understanding and meeting the unique needs of children. In: Fleischer GR, Ludwig S (eds) Textbook of Paediatric Emergency Medicine, 3rd edn. Williams and Wilkins, Maryland
11. Royal Childrens Hospital 2003 Clinical practice guidelines resuscitation: Emergency drug and fluid calculator. Melbourne, Australia [http://www.rch.org.au/clinicalguide/cpg.cfm?doc-id=5162]

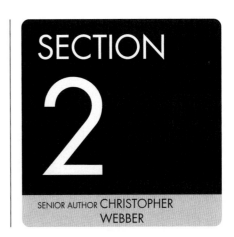

SECTION

2

SENIOR AUTHOR CHRISTOPHER WEBBER

RESUSCITATION

2.1 PAEDIATRIC CARDIOPULMONARY ARREST (CPA)

CHRISTOPHER WEBBER

ESSENTIALS

1 The outcome of cardiopulmonary arrest (CPA) in children, particularly out of hospital, is poor. Arrest survival rates are reported between 0 and 17%, with survivors likely to have a devastating neurological outcome.

2 CPA in children usually results from the development of progressive hypoxia and/or shock, which may be due to myriad causes.

3 The goal is to identify hypoxia and shock early in seriously ill children and instigate appropriate therapy to prevent the progression to cardiac arrest.

4 In contrast to adults the most common arrest rhythm in children is non-VF/VT and is usually either asystole, PEA or EMD.

5 Resuscitation organisations have developed guidelines for paediatric patients to include nuances of the newly-born, infant, young child and older child.

6 Allowing parents to be present and supported during the resuscitation of their child may be associated with a better long-term psychosocial outcome.

7 Unless CPA is associated with drug toxicity or hypothermia, neurologically intact survival is unlikely after 30 minutes of full CPR and several doses of adrenaline.

EPIDEMIOLOGY

Generally, those children who arrive in the emergency department in established cardiac arrest will die or survive with severe neurological disability.[1] Cardiac arrest is, fortunately, an uncommon event in infants and children. As the outcome of cardiopulmonary arrest is poor, the critical focus in caring for unwell or injured children, must be identifying those who are seriously ill and initiating timely therapy to prevent progression to respiratory or cardiac arrest.

Population risk of out-of-hospital cardiac arrest has been estimated to be about two per 10 000 population. The group reviewed included 300 children aged 0–17 years, and comprised 54% being less than one year of age and 76% less than four years. Only 22% of children who had their arrest at home received bystander cardiopulmonary resuscitation (CPR).[2]

AETIOLOGY

The most common causes of cardiac arrest in children are related to the development of hypoxia and/or shock. Shock is the clinical state where there is poor tissue perfusion. Thus, the primary organ systems involved are the respiratory and cardiovascular systems, as well as the central nervous system (CNS). Injury or diseases progressing to failure of these systems may then lead to cardiac arrest. CNS disorders, either with direct dysfunction or due to raised intracranial pressure, may cause respiratory arrest with the resulting hypoxia leading to cardiac arrest. Consequently, the commonest cardiac arrest rhythms in children are asystole, pulseless electrical activity (PEA) and electro-mechanical dissociation (EMD). Commonly preterminal bradyarrhythmias, such as sinus bradycardia, sinus arrest with slow junctional or idioventricular rhythm

and atrioventricular block may precede CPA. Between 10% and 20% of paediatric cardiac arrests out-of-hospital present with ventricular fibrillation (VF).[3] The primary causes of cardiac arrest are heterogeneous and include trauma, sepsis, drug overdose, poisoning, immersion, critical respiratory illness and sudden infant death syndrome (SIDS). This list is by no means complete, and many other conditions may also progress to cardiac arrest.

PATHOPHYSIOLOGY

Significant hypoxic and hypoperfusion insults on the myocardium are the common pathways that may progress to cause cardiac arrest in children. Hence, fluid or blood loss leading to shock if left untreated, will result in myocardial ischaemia and resultant cardiac arrest. Similarly, severe hypoxia, will also result in global myocardial dysfunction and subsequently cardiac arrest. Thus, preventative strategies must identify hypoxia and shock early and instigate appropriate management to improve oxygenation and organ perfusion, thereby preventing progress to cardiac arrest. Poisonings or ingestions may have a direct effect on the heart causing an arrhythmia, coma, with subsequent respiratory arrest and hypoxia.

OUTCOME

Generally, the survival from respiratory arrest alone is much better than from cardiopulmonary arrest. Survival to discharge for children with respiratory arrest (pulse present) is around 75%, and of these up to 88% have a good neurological outcome. Reported survival rates from cardiac arrest in children have varied from 0% to 17%. Overall survival to discharge is about 13%, with 8% survival for out-of-hospital and 24% for in-hospital arrests.[4] 'Survival to discharge' is a very crude marker of 'success' as it does not include a measure of neurological function. Those children who arrive in the emergency department in cardiac arrest will not survive without severe neurological dysfunction, and even then the survival rate is very low; being $\frac{4}{177}$ or 2.3% when data is collated from three different studies.[5] All of these survivors had a devastating neurological outcome.

Unfortunately, the perception of the public and even doctors and nurses, is that the expected survival rate is higher than actual. Lay rescuers, physicians and nurses estimate the survival rate for cardiopulmonary arrest in children as being 63%, 45% and 41% respectively (compared to 53%, 30% and 24% for adult cardiopulmonary arrest).[5] Undoubtedly fictional medical television programs contribute to false bias, and even nonfictional medical programs rarely show death as an outcome.

DIFFERENCES COMPARED TO ADULTS

When comparing children to adults in relation to cardiopulmonary arrest, there are several important differences. The aetiology of the event is usually different. Adults who collapse are more likely to have ventricular fibrillation or pulseless ventricular tachycardia, hence the time to defibrillation is the single greatest determinant of survival. Thus the '*phone first*' principle that applies to adults, is not applicable to most infants and children, in whom the response should be '*phone fast*' (see Chapter 2.2 on BLS).

There are several anatomical and physical differences between children and adults. It is important to consider these differences in relation to the primary event leading to arrest and to the resuscitation techniques subsequently required (see Table 2.1.1).

DEVELOPMENT OF RESUSCITATION GUIDELINES

In 1992 the American Heart Association guidelines for resuscitation were published.

Subsequently representatives of seven resuscitation councils throughout the world, including the Australian Resuscitation Council, formed the International Liaison Committee on Resuscitation (ILCOR). ILCOR advisory statements were produced. A subcommittee on paediatric resuscitation with representation from the American Heart Association and other paediatric representatives from ILCOR (Paediatric Working Group) further developed guidelines for paediatric patients. This group attempted to evaluate the level of evidence for resuscitation recommendations. It was important to attempt to avoid confusion between adult, paediatric and neonatal algorithms and ultimately the *International Guidelines 2000* were published. Subsequently resuscitation courses, like the Advanced Paediatric Life Support (APLS) course have been amended to be consistent with the international recommendations.

ETHICS OF PAEDIATRIC RESUSCITATION

Presence of family

Over recent years, the benefit of allowing the family, mainly parents, into the resuscitation room during active resuscitation has become clearer. This practice has required a behaviour change, and mandates appropriate and professional behaviour and language during resuscitation. Such practice should occur regardless of the presence of any 'outside' witnesses. It is a professional standard that all medical, nursing and other health professionals should aspire to and maintain. It is probably even more important that parents are offered the opportunity to witness the resuscitation, when the outcome is the death of their child.

In hindsight, parents who have witnessed the resuscitation of their child, have valued this opportunity and despite the occasional apparent mayhem, common positive perceptions relate to the efforts made by staff. To achieve a positive (psychosocial) outcome, in relation to the presence of parents during resuscitation, the following issues should be considered:

- Parents being present during the resuscitation of their child should be regarded more as the norm than the exception.
- Parents should not be coerced into being present, but gentle encouragement and explanation by a senior member of staff is usually helpful.
- The senior members of staff engaged in resuscitation should not feel undue pressure as a result of the attendance of parents. Occasionally, however, it may be preferable for the parents to wait outside the immediate resuscitation area during challenging procedures.
- Parents should have a dedicated support person, being a health professional, to remain with them throughout the resuscitation. The support person should ascertain information from medical staff to keep the parents informed of their child's progress and explain procedures to the parents.
- Touching and talking to their child is often important for the parents where this is feasible.
- Parents need to have a quiet room to retreat to, if necessary. Discussion with family should not occur in a busy emergency department corridor.
- Family requests and religious beliefs need to be respected.
- Obligations mandatory by Coronial Law need to be explained with sensitivity.
- The emotional impact on all staff members when a child dies is considerable and this may be compounded by the distress of parents during and following the resuscitation.
- With any resuscitation, particularly those resulting in death, debriefing of staff is essential, as is organising appropriate support and medical follow-up of the parents.

TERMINATION OF RESUSCITATIVE EFFORTS

The decision to cease resuscitation efforts in a child in CPA is influenced by many

Table 2.1.1   Important differences between children and adults

Difference	Implication
AIRWAY	
Prominent occiput tends to cause neck flexion	Neck extension, into a neutral or sniffing position (slight extension), is required to optimise the airway for an infant or child respectively
Mandible is relatively smaller	More difficult intubation
Tongue is relatively larger	Tends to obstruct airway More difficult intubation
Larynx is more cephalad (located almost at base of tongue)	More difficult intubation - tendency for inexperienced operator to insert laryngoscope blade into oesophagus
Epiglottis is proportionally larger and more 'floppy'	Intubation may require straight-bladed laryngoscope to lift epiglottis forward to allow visualisation of vocal cords
Upper airways are more compliant (i.e. distensible)	Tend to collapse during increased work of breathing
BREATHING	
Chest wall more compliant (particularly the newborn infant and more so the preterm infant)	Less efficient ventilation, when increased work of breathing Earlier fatigue
Greater dependence on diaphragm to generate tidal volume	Distended stomach impairs ventilation Importance of venting stomach with gastric tube
CIRCULATION	
Maintains cardiac output and blood pressure by tachycardia initially	Diagnose and treat shock before hypotension develops Hypotension usually indicates late decompensation
GENERAL	
Head has proportionally greater component of body surface area	Loss of body heat during primary event or resuscitation Greater chance of head injury
Compliant chest wall allows transmission of energy to underlying organs, resulting in traumatic damage/rupture, rather than dissipation of energy	Pulmonary, hepatic and splenic injury may occur without overlying rib fractures
Development Language Motor development (fine and gross) Social and cognitive development (including abstract thinking)	Must be considered when interacting with the child and understanding injuries (accidental versus non-accidental)
Parental and staff considerations	Psychosocial issues Presence of family during resuscitation Staff pressure to continue resuscitation Impact on staff from death of child

factors. These include the total arrest time, clinical response to therapy, premorbid state of the child, potential for any reversible factors, likely neurological outcome, information from colleagues who care for a child with long-term medical problems and the parental wishes.

Termination of resuscitation in a newly born baby is likely to be appropriate if the baby remains in cardiorespiratory arrest at 15 minutes. Even after 10 minutes of documented asystole, survival without severe disability is unlikely.

For children in established cardiac arrest the overall outcome is poor. If the child requires adrenaline (epinephrine), and fails to respond to two doses, then survival is unlikely. Generally no longer than 30 minutes of advanced life support resuscitation is required to determine whether discontinuation of resuscitation is appropriate. Recurring/refractory VF or VT, toxic drug exposure or the presence of significant hypothermia in the setting of ice-cold immersion, are situations that may require more prolonged resuscitation efforts (see Chapter 22.2 on immersion). Most children in cardio-respiratory arrest in Australia and New Zealand who are hypothermic, however, have lost body heat due to exposure, without spontaneous circulation after the arrest and therefore this is unlikely to be neuro-protective.

Non-initiation of resuscitative efforts

Resuscitation should not be initiated if there are signs of prolonged death, like rigor mortis or post-mortem lividity. Children who are in a palliative phase of care should have an 'end of life care plan' that includes non-initiation of resuscitation. Children with complex and disabling conditions will occasionally have life-threatening events occur. If prior discussions between parents (and child if appropriate) and physicians have not included limitations of interventions or medical support, then it is difficult to avoid commencing resuscitation. Early and urgent consultation with the child's primary physician would be prudent in these situations. Physicians should not be coerced into undertaking care that they believe is morally wrong or fruitless.

There are specific situations in the newly born baby that may lead to the non-initiation of resuscitation, like extreme prematurity and congenital/chromosomal abnormalities not consistent with long-term survival. This issue is covered in Chapter 2.6 on neonatal resuscitation.

Consent

The philosophy of informed consent should be followed during any treatment, including resuscitation. The patient or their parents/guardian should have an explanation about the management (current and proposed), risks and potential outcomes. This may be limited during resuscitation but is the responsibility of the most senior physician involved with the child's care at the time. The decision to stop resuscitative efforts in the emergency department setting due to a lack of return of spontaneous circulation is a medical decision. It is not a choice that is offered to the parents. The circumstances are completely different to the discussion with parents about 'withdrawal of treatment', which usually occurs in an intensive care unit in a child who is ventilated but has a spontaneous circulation.

Non-accidental injury

It is important that all health care providers involved with children should be aware of their statutory obligations under state or federal law regarding notification of suspicion of non-accidental injury or neglect. Awareness of development of the child, feasibility or compatibility of the history with clinical signs and any delay in presentation should be considered when assessing this possibility. Regardless of the outcome of the resuscitation, if there is a suspicion of abuse or neglect, appropriate notification should be made.

Organ donation

Organ donation is usually a consideration for staff when a child is in an intensive care unit and generally, not in the emergency department. The only situation where it may be contemplated in the ED is when post-mortem organs (like corneas, heart valves) may be retrieved for this purpose. In cases mandating notification of the Coroner, then permission is required prior to any organ harvesting. Liaison with the appropriate local donor co-ordinator is essential. A senior member of staff should have this discussion with the parents and occasionally the parents themselves raise the issue.

If resuscitation has resulted in the return of spontaneous circulation but with likely brain death, then subsequent organ donation may be feasible. The determination of brain death would usually occur in an intensive care unit, as repeated examinations over a period are required. Consultation with and consideration of transfer to a paediatric intensive care unit is required. The focus in the emergency department at this point in time is ongoing care of the child and support of the family.

Death certificates, notification to the coroner and other legal issues

Death in the ED is, by itself, not an indication to notify the death to the coroner. Coroners' Acts vary from state to state and staff must be aware of their statutory obligations. Remember that if a death is to be notified to the Coroner the body then becomes evidence and should be left intact at the termination of resuscitation. Common practices of taking hand/foot prints, locks of hair, removing catheters and tubes must not occur or staff risk being held in contempt of court. Such mementos can be collected following the post-mortem examination. This usually requires liaison with staff in the forensic mortuary.

In the situation where a death does not require notification to the coroner, it must be clarified who can and will complete the death certificate, which includes the cause of death. Consultation with the primary physician involved with the long-term care of a child with chronic illness is obligatory. Medical staff need to be aware of other legal obligations, like the collection of blood alcohol specimens in pedestrian and vehicular accidents, but these would only be collected antemortem by hospital staff. These legal requirements vary between states.

REFERENCES

1. Schindler MB, Bohn D, Cox PN et al 1996 Outcome of out-of-hospital cardiac or respiratory arrest in children. New England Journal of Medicine 335: 1473–1479
2. Sirbaugh PE, Pepe PE, Shook JE, Kimball KT, Goldman MJ, Ward MA, Mann DM 1999 A prospective, population-based study of the demographics, epidemiology, management and outcome of out-of-hospital paediatric cardiopulmonary arrests. Annals of Emergency Medicine 33: 174–184
3. Mogayzel C, Quan L, Graves JR et al 1995 Out-of-hospital ventricular fibrillation in children and adolescents: Causes and outcomes. Annals of Emergency Medicine 149: 210–214
4. Young KD, Seidel JS 1999 Paediatric cardiopulmonary resuscitation: A collective review. Annals of Emergency Medicine 33: 195–205
5. Brown K, Bocock J 2002 Update on paediatric resuscitation. Emergency Medicine Clinics of North America 20(1): 1–26

2.2 BASIC LIFE SUPPORT

JANE COCKS

ESSENTIALS

1 Paediatric cardiopulmonary resuscitation is different to adult resuscitation in many aspects, but the basic principles remain the same:
- Don't panic
- Get help
- Ensure both the patient and you are safe
- Initiate basic life support at the earliest possible moment
- Airway
- Breathing
- Circulation.

2 BLS techniques are modified depending on the child's age and size.

3 In the field, paediatric BLS follows a 'phone fast' response whereas in adult resuscitation it should be a 'phone first' response.

4 Stabilise the cervical spine if the collapse follows any significant trauma.

5 The rate of compressions is 100 per minute for all age groups, except in neonates where it is 120 per minute.

INTRODUCTION

Basic life support (BLS) or basic cardio-pulmonary resuscitation (CPR) is a process by which an individual's basic cardiac and respiratory functions can be restored and maintained through a combination of expired air resuscitation (EAR) and external cardiac compressions (ECC). The provision of BLS sustains the vital functions of the collapsed individual without the need for specialised equipment, minimising the potential hypoxic damage that may occur while advanced life support is being activated.

PAEDIATRIC VERSUS ADULT BASIC LIFE SUPPORT

The aim of basic life support in all age groups is the same and the techniques utilised follow the same general principles, but paediatric BLS differs significantly from adult BLS in some very fundamental ways.

Aetiology of arrests

In adults the most common cause of cardiopulmonary arrest is a sudden, massive cardiac event with little preceding deterioration. Most adults requiring BLS measures are already in a state of full cardiopulmonary arrest, defined as a state of pulseless apnoea.

In children the most common causes of cardiopulmonary arrest are hypoxic and, as a consequence, children generally undergo a period of deterioration with worsening bradycardia preceding the final arrested state. It is therefore important that paediatric BLS is commenced as soon as this bradycardic deterioration is noted and is not withheld until the patient becomes pulseless.

The currently accepted international recommendation for the commencement of external cardiac compressions (ECC) in children of all age groups who are unresponsive with no spontaneous breathing, is a heart rate below 60 beats per minute (bpm).

Anatomy and physiology

The anatomy and physiology of the human body changes markedly with age, progressing from the immature neonatal form to the more adult form of the older child, and these changes are relevant to the provision of BLS at any particular age. The following differences from the adult form are of direct importance in the provision of BLS in children:

- Airway
  Large head (particularly the occiput) and short neck leading to neck flexion
  Large tongue which is predominantly intra-oral. Easily compressible oropharyngeal soft tissues
  Larynx lies more anteriorly and higher (C2–3)
  Cricoid ring is the narrowest part of the airway
  Soft and short trachea
- Breathing
  Increased rate
  More compliant chest wall
  Dependence on diaphragmatic breathing
- Circulation
  Increased rate
  More dependence on heart rate for delivery of adequate circulation
  Small absolute volume of circulating blood
- Metabolism
  Increased metabolic rate
  Increased body surface area (BSA).

BLS TECHNIQUES AND AGE

BLS techniques are modified depending on the child's age and size to ensure that they will be maximally effective. In view of this children are arbitrarily divided into the following internationally accepted age groups:

- Newborn/Neonate: birth to 1 month old
- Infant: less than one year of age
- Small child: age between 1 and 8 years
- Large child: age older than 8 years.

PREPARATION AND EQUIPMENT

Basic CPR requires no extra equipment other than personnel trained in its administration. It is advantageous, how-ever, to have available certain basic equip-ment to assist in the resuscitation process.

- Portable suction and suction catheters, for clearing secretions, improves the ability to achieve and maintain a patent airway.
- An oropharyngeal (Guedel) airway may assist in achieving a patent airway.
- A self-inflating bag and mask, suitable for the size of the patient, improves artificial ventilation and reduces the risk of cross infection.
- Oxygen for ventilation will further reduce the risk of hypoxic injury.

BASIC LIFE SUPPORT SEQUENCE

A 'SAFE' approach

It is extremely important to ensure maxi-mum rescuer and patient safety as a pri-ority on first approaching the collapsed child. To this end, the Advanced Paediatric Life Support course advocates a 'SAFE' approach to collapsed patients. This acro-nym stands for:

- S = **S**hout for help. Call for assistance from surrounding people and request that an ambulance is called, do not leave the patient as immediate resuscitation may be required
- A = **A**pproach with care. Ensure that you are not putting yourself at risk
- F = **F**ree from danger. Remove the patient from immediate danger, if present
- E = **E**valuate the ABCs (airway, breathing, circulation).

The activation of the Emergency Medical Services (EMS) should be performed as early as possible in the sequence of re-suscitation, provided there are adequate numbers of bystanders to allow this to occur without delaying the commence-ment of BLS. Most paediatric arrests will have an underlying hypoxic cause and therefore any delay of BLS will signifi-cantly reduce its effectiveness. This is in stark contrast to adult arrests in which the early activation of EMS is essential to provide rapid access to Advanced Cardiac Life Support measures, which are essen-tial to manage the commonest causes of adult arrests. Hence, in paediatric resusci-tation we adopt a 'phone fast' response whereas in adult resuscitation it should be a 'phone first' response.

Assess responsiveness

Assess the responsiveness of the patient by gently, but firmly stimulating the patient and asking if they are OK. It is important to remember the possibility of cervical spinal injury and, if this is likely, stabilise the cervical spine by placing a hand on the patient's forehead prior to gently shaking their arm.

AIRWAY

Open and maintain the airway

Position yourself at the patient's head, open the mouth and remove any obvious debris. Do not use a blind finger sweep in an infant as this may damage the deli-cate palatal tissues or impact a foreign body, further into the airway. Suction using a large-bore Yankeur catheter is useful for removing vomitus and secretions.

Three manoeuvres will assist in opening and maintaining the airway (see Figs 2.2.1, 2.2.2 and 2.2.3), which is most commonly obstructed by the child's tongue.

1. Head tilt

Place one hand on the patient's forehead and gently tilt the head back. In children the 'sniffing' position is desired as in adult resuscitation. In an infant or neo-nate, a neutral position is required as they have relatively large occiput and are naturally positioned in a sniffing position. A small towel placed under the infant's shoulders, will eliminate the excessive neck flexion caused by the prominent occiput. If there is any possibility of cervical spine injury, the head tilt manoeuvre should be avoided.

2. Chin lift

Placing the fingers of the other hand on the jawbone, lift the chin, taking care not to compress the soft tissues of the floor of the mouth under the jaw.

Fig. 2.2.1 **Chin lift and head position in infants.**

Fig. 2.2.2 **Head tilt and chin lift in children.**

Fig. 2.2.3 **Jaw thrust.**

3. Jaw thrust

Place two or three fingers under the angle of the mandible bilaterally, and lift the jaw upwards. This technique can be performed without head tilt and is indi-cated particularly if the possibility of cervical injury exists.

The patency of the airway can then be assessed by *looking* for chest movement, *listening* for breath sounds and *feeling* for exhaled breath. This assessment is best achieved by placing an ear over the patient's mouth and nose, whilst watching the chest.

Oropharyngeal airway

Insertion of an oropharyngeal airway may assist in maintaining patency of the airway if the above manoeuvres are inadequate. An appropriately sized oropharyngeal airway should reach from the central incisors to the angle of the jaw. In infants and small children, the oropharyngeal airway should be inserted under direct vision 'the right way up', that is it should be inserted concave down in the position in which it will sit in the oropharynx. Gentle depression of the child's tongue with a spatula may help facilitate airway placement. In children older than eight years, oropharyngeal airways should be inserted under direct vision concave up and then rotated through 180 degrees to sit snugly in the oropharynx. Oropharyngeal airways will not be tolerated in conscious or semi-conscious patients because of gagging. If this occurs, the airway should be removed. In this situation a nasopharyngeal airway may be a useful alternative.

Be aware of the risk of cervical spine injury if the collapse is following a motor vehicle accident (MVA) or other form of significant trauma. If this is likely, stabilise the cervical spine by placing one hand on either side of the head and maintaining the head in line with the body at all times. CPR in this case generally requires two operators to perform successfully. If a second operator is not available, attempt to immobilise the cervical spine between sandbags or in a hard cervical collar before proceeding.

BREATHING

Once the airway is opened and patent, if the patient is not spontaneously breathing, deliver two to five slow rescue breaths via expired air resuscitation. Each breath is delivered slowly over 1 to 1.5 seconds duration (inspiratory phase) and up to five may be required to ensure that two effective breaths are delivered.

Expired air resuscitation (EAR) is most commonly performed as mouth-to-mouth but may also be delivered using mouth-to-mouth-and-nose. In the mouth-to-mouth technique, the rescuer seals his or her mouth over the mouth of the patient, pinching off the nose with the free hand, whilst maintaining the patency of the airway with head tilt and chin lift. The mouth-to-mouth-and-nose technique may be necessary for the infant or small child and in that case the rescuer's mouth should seal around the infant's mouth and nose. In the hospital setting the rescue breaths will be delivered utilising bag and mask ventilation (see advanced life support).

Ensure that the degree of chest excursion is frequently reassessed during the EAR. The chest must be seen to rise as if the child was taking a deep breath. Excessive tidal volumes may cause gastric dilatation and regurgitation. If there is no chest movement, the most likely cause is an obstructed airway due to poor positioning of the child's head. Reposition the patient using the above manoeuvres and retry. If there is still no chest movement, there may be a foreign body obstructing the airway, which can be removed with suction or forceps under direct vision (see below).

CIRCULATION

Following the initial five rescue breaths, assess the circulation. Although the pulse check has always been considered the gold standard of circulation assessment, the most recent International Liaison Committee on Resuscitation (ILCOR) recommendations suggest that for non-healthcare professionals, the assessment of pulse has both poor sensitivity and specificity and often delays the decision to commence ECC. The current recommendations, therefore, suggest that lay rescuers assess for 'signs of circulation', specifically the presence of normal breathing, coughing or movement in response to rescue breaths.

Healthcare professionals should check for a pulse as well as assessing for signs of circulation. The pulses that are easiest to feel are the carotid, brachial or femoral pulses and they should be palpated for a period of 10 seconds. The carotid pulse is difficult to feel in small children who have relatively short necks. If there is no pulse or severe bradycardia (heart rate < 60 bpm) with signs of poor perfusion, then ECC on the lower half of the sternum should be commenced.

Chest compressions

The technique of providing ECC varies with the patients' age.

- Infants and neonates require compression with two fingers at a point located by drawing an imaginary line between the nipples and going one fingerbreadth below that level, over the sternum. An alternative technique involves the rescuer encircling the infant's chest with both hands and providing compressions with the thumbs at the same landmark site. This technique is felt to be more effective, but requires two rescuers to provide effective EAR and ECC (Figs 2.2.4 and 2.2.5).
- Small children, between one and eight years of age, require compressions with the heel of one hand, at a point one finger's breadth above the xiphisternum (Fig. 2.2.6).
- Older children, over eight years of age, require compressions with the heel of two hands to achieve effective compressions, at a point two finger breadths above the xiphisternum (Fig. 2.2.7).
- The depth of compression is relative and should be one third to one half of the AP diameter of the chest in all age groups. ECC should be performed on a firm flat surface.

Rate of compressions

The rate of compressions is 100 per minute for all age groups, except in neonates, where it is 120 per minute (see Table 2.2.1). Note that this is the rate or speed of compressions, not the actual number delivered per minute. The actual number of compressions delivered per minute will be less than 100 as there will

Fig. 2.2.4   Infant with two-finger technique of ECC.

Fig. 2.2.5   Infant with two-thumb technique of ECC.

Fig. 2.2.7   Child with two-hand technique of ECC.

Fig. 2.2.6   Child with one-hand technique of ECC.

Table 2.2.1	Rate of ECC and ratio to EAR	
	Rate of ECC	*Ratio of ECC:EAR*
Neonate	120 min⁻¹	3:1
Infant	100 min⁻¹	5:1
Small child	100 min⁻¹	5:1
Large child	100 min⁻¹	15:2

be pauses for the delivery of EAR.

External cardiac compressions should be combined with expired air resuscitation in a ratio of five compressions to one ventilation in infants and small children, independent of the number of rescuers. In the large child or adult the ratio of ECC:EAR should be fifteen compressions to two breaths, independent of the number of operators (see Table 2.2.1).

It is important to check that the chest rises normally when the ventilation is provided to ensure that an effective breath is being delivered. When two rescuers are delivering BLS, the rescuer providing ECC should pause every 5th or 15th compression for the delivery of the breath. Once the airway is secured with intubation, this pause in ECC is no longer required.

Neonates require a combination of ECC:EAR at a ratio of three compressions to every one ventilation and a rate of 120 'events' per minute. This rate aims to achieve approximately 90 compressions and 30 breaths per minute.

Frequent reassessment of the patient is important to assess for return of spontaneous respiration and circulation. Any interruption to basic life support measures during patient assessment should last no longer than 10 seconds after which they should be promptly recommenced to optimise outcome (see Table 2.2.1).

Mechanical devices to provide chest compressions during ECC have been designed and tested only in adults and are not recommended for use in children.

Duration of BLS in the field

Continue BLS for a period of 20 cycles or one minute and then reassess the patient. If there is no return of spontaneous breathing or circulation and the rescuer is alone, he/she should seek help by activating emergency medical services. If the patient is small enough, the rescuer should take the patient with them and attempt to continue BLS whilst seeking help. If the patient is too large to be moved, the rescuer should position the patient appropriately and leave to seek help. Despite many variations in common use today, an optimal recovery position in children has never been identified. BLS should continue until EMS arrives or signs of life return.

PRECAUTIONS AND COMPLICATIONS

Severe iatrogenic injuries are extremely uncommon in children who have undergone CPR, with an incidence of about 3%. The risk of infection to the rescuer from CPR is minimal, with the greatest risk being meningococcus. Standard antibiotic prophylaxis is recommended for any rescuer involved in the resuscitation of the airway of a patient with known or suspected meningococcal infection. There have been no reported cases of transmission of hepatitis B or HIV from mouth-to-mouth ventilation to date. Airway secretions, tears, sweat and vomitus are low-risk fluids, but extra precautions should be taken when contact with blood or other bodily fluids is likely.

RELIEF OF FOREIGN BODY AIRWAY OBSTRUCTION

Presentation

Foreign body airway obstruction (FBAO) in both adults and children is commonly caused by the aspiration of food, but in children it may also occur during play with small objects. In both of these situations, it is likely that a parent or

guardian will be present and the event may have been witnessed. Clinical signs will include the sudden onset of respiratory distress, associated with coughing, gagging and inspiratory stridor. These signs may also be caused by upper airway infections, however the onset is slower and usually associated with other signs of infection, such as fever, lethargy, or coryza.

FBAO MANAGEMENT IN THE RESPONSIVE INFANT OR CHILD

In a child or infant who is responsive with good respiratory effort and forceful coughing, do not interfere with the child's spontaneous efforts. Any attempt to relieve the obstruction in this situation may dislodge the foreign body and worsen the situation by turning partial to complete airway obstruction. Call for help and get the child or infant urgently to an emergency facility.

Attempts to relieve FBAO should only be commenced when the cough becomes ineffective with increasing respiratory distress, or the child becomes unconscious or apnoeic.

FBAO management in the unresponsive infant

A combination of back blows and chest thrusts are utilised to relieve the obstruction. Abdominal thrusts are not recommended for infants because of the lack of protection of the upper abdominal organs by the rib cage and the risk of trauma to these vital structures.

The sequence of response for an unresponsive, apnoeic infant with FBAO is as follows:

❶ Open the airway using chin lift or jaw thrust. Look inside the mouth and remove any visible foreign body. Do not perform a blind finger sweep because of the risk of damaging palatal tissues or pushing a foreign body further into the airway.

❷ Open the airway using chin lift or jaw thrust and attempt up to five rescue breaths. If unsuccessful, reposition and try again.

❸ If rescue breaths are still unsuccessful, perform a sequence of five back blows and five chest thrusts.
- Deliver five back blows with the infant in a prone, head down position lying along the rescuer's forearm with the jaw supported by the rescuer's hand. Using the heel of the other hand between the shoulder blades, deliver five blows with sufficient force to dislodge a foreign body (Fig. 2.2.8).
- If the obstruction is not relieved, turn the baby over and lie him/her along the rescuer's thigh, in a head down supine position. Five chest thrusts are delivered at the same position utilising the same landmarks and technique as for ECC but at a rate of one per second with sufficient force to expel the foreign object (Fig. 2.2.9).

❹ Reopen the airway using chin lift or jaw thrust and remove any visible foreign body and reattempt rescue breaths.

❺ If the obstruction is not relieved, continue the above sequence until the obstruction is relieved or for approximately one minute. If the infant remains unresponsive at one minute, seek help. If the patient is small enough, the rescuer should take the patient with them and attempt to

Fig. 2.2.8 Back blows in an infant.

Fig. 2.2.9   Chest thrusts in an infant.

Fig. 2.2.10   Abdominal thrusts in a standing child.

Fig. 2.2.11   Abdominal thrusts in a supine child.

continue FBAO relief manoeuvres whilst seeking help. If the patient is too large to be moved, the rescuer should position the patient appropriately and leave to seek help. For management in the emergency department setting see inhaled FB. (Chapter 6.2)

FBAO management in the unresponsive child

A combination of abdominal thrusts, back blows and chest thrusts are utilised to relieve the obstruction. The sequence of response for an unresponsive, apnoeic child with FBAO is as for the infant except the rescuer should alternate between chest thrusts and abdominal thrusts with each cycle.

Abdominal thrusts (Heimlich manoeuvre) may be performed with the victim in the upright or supine position.

- With the child in the upright position (standing, sitting or kneeling), the rescuer stands behind the victim and places the fist of one hand on the child's abdomen above the umbilicus and below the xiphisternum. The rescuer's other hand covers the fist and both hands are thrust sharply inwards and upwards in to the abdomen (Fig. 2.2.10).

CONTROVERSIES

❶ Unlike the adult situation, it is unclear whether BLS improves the outcome in children with cardiac arrest.

❷ It is uncertain what the effect on arrest outcome will be of removing the pulse check.

❸ The optimal recovery position for paediatric patients is yet to be determined.

- With the child in the supine position, the rescuer kneels at the child's feet or astride the child's hips. The heel of one hand is placed on the child's abdomen above the umbilicus and below the xiphisternum, the rescuer's other hand covers the first and both hands are thrust sharply inwards and upwards in to the abdomen in the midline (Fig. 2.2.11).
- Abdominal thrusts should be repeated five times unless the foreign body is expelled before then.
- It is important to take care not to touch the xiphisternum or ribs during this manoeuvre due the risk of internal damage.

FURTHER READING

Advanced Life Support Group 2001 Advanced paediatric life support: The practical approach, 3rd edn. BMJ Publishing Group, London
Bush CM, Jones JS, Cohle SD, Johnson H 1996 Paediatric injuries from cardiopulmonary resuscitation. Annals of Emergency Medicine 28(1): 40–44
Hickey RW, Cohen DM, Strausbaugh S, Dietrich AM 1995 Paediatric patients requiring CPR in the pre-hospital setting. Annals of Emergency Medicine 25(4): 495–501
International Guidelines 2000 for Cardiopulmonary Resuscitation and Emergency Cardiovascular Care. Circulation 102(Suppl 1), 22 August

2.3 PAEDIATRIC ADVANCED LIFE SUPPORT (ALS)

JAMES TIBBALLS

ESSENTIALS

1 The causes of cardiopulmonary arrest in infants and children include any cause of hypoxaemia or hypotension or both.

2 Aspects of CPR are different for 'the newly born', infant, small (younger) child and large (older) child.

3 Hypoxaemia should be avoided during attempts at intubation which should be limited to 30 seconds.

4 The approximate endotracheal tube size may be chosen for children over one year by the formula: size (mm) = age (years)/4 + 4.

5 Correct placement of the endotracheal tube in the trachea must be confirmed immediately.

6 One must have a preconceived plan to cope with difficult and failed (impossible) intubation especially when bag-mask ventilation fails.

7 If peripheral intravenous access cannot be rapidly achieved, say within 60 seconds, intraosseous access should be obtained.

8 Lipid-soluble drugs (adrenaline [epinephrine], atropine, lidocaine and naloxone) may be administered via the endotracheal tube.

9 Restoration of intravascular volume should be with isotonic crystalloid solutions (0.9% normal saline or Hartmann's solution) or a colloid in aliquots of 20 mL kg^{-1}.

10 The decision to cease CPR should be based on a number of factors including the duration of resuscitation, response to treatment, pre-arrest status of the patient, remediable factors, likely outcome if ultimately successful, opinions of personnel familiar with the patient and, whenever appropriate, the wishes of the parents.

INTRODUCTION

Definition of ALS

Advanced life support is cardiopulmonary resuscitation (CPR) with use of specific items of equipment available in the hospital or ambulance setting and the use of techniques and skills by specifically trained personnel. It includes the management of critically ill infants and children in pre-cardiorespiratory arrest (CPA), during arrest and post-arrest.

The recommendations for advanced CPR given here are based on publications of several authoritative resuscitation organisations and the International Liaison Committee on Resuscitation (ILCOR)[1–6]. They are intended for use by medical and nursing personnel in hospital and by ambulance personnel in the field.

To add ability to knowledge, it is advisable to undertake a specialised paediatric cardiopulmonary resuscitation course such as the Advanced Paediatric Life Support (APLS) or Paediatric Advanced Life Support (PALS) courses.

Distinctions within the term 'paediatric' are based on combinations of physiology, physical size and age. Some aspects of CPR are different for 'the newly born', infant, small (younger) child and large (older) child. 'Newly-born' refers to the infant at birth or within several hours of birth. The management of the 'newly-born' infant is discussed in Chapter 25. In this section, 'infant' refers to an infant outside the 'newly-born' period up to the age of 12 months. Other terms such as newborn or neonate do not enable that distinction. 'Small/young child' refers to a child of pre-school and early primary school from the age of 1 to 8 years. 'Large/older child' refers to a child of late primary school from the age of 9 up to 14 years. Children older than 14 years may be treated as adults but they do not have the same propensity for ventricular fibrillation as do adults. One guideline[2] regards children of 8 years and over as adults specifically for use of semi-automated external defibrillators (sAED) out-of-hospital.

EPIDEMIOLOGY

The causes of cardiopulmonary arrest in infants and children are many and include any cause of hypoxaemia or hypotension or both. Common causes are trauma (motor vehicle accidents, near drowning, falls, burns, gunshots), drug overdose and poisoning, respiratory illness (asthma, upper airway obstruction, parenchymal diseases), post-operative (especially cardiac), septicaemia and sudden infant death syndrome.

ADVANCED AIRWAY SUPPORT AND VENTILATION

Oxygen

Oxygen should be administered whenever hypoxaemia occurs. The only exception to this rule is when it may cause pulmonary vasodilatation and thereby shunt blood to the lungs away from the systemic circulation as may occur in an infant with a single ventricle, which pumps blood to both circulations. Chronic hypoventilation is not an indication to withhold oxygen therapy during CPR for infants and children.

Numerous devices may be used to supply supplemental oxygen. The choice is dictated by the required inspired oxygen concentration (FiO_2), cost, avoidance of CO_2 rebreathing, imposed airway resistance and tolerance by the patient.

Oxygen catheters

These are easy to use, cheap, do not cause rebreathing and are well-tolerated (permitting eating and drinking) but are limited to supply of up to 40% O_2 because of restriction to gas flow (maximum 4 L min^{-1}) and limitation of gas reservoir (the nasopharynx). Sizes 6, 8 and 10 FG should be available and placed in the same nostril as the nasogastric tube, to limit airway resistance. Size 6 FG is suitable for infants, 8 FG for small children and 10 FG for older children. Excessive flow may desiccate mucosal membranes and cause gastric distension.

Oxygen delivered by nasal cannula (bi-pronged, 'nasal prongs'), which sit at the entrance to the nose or a few centimetres inside, need no humidification and do not cause gastric distension. They may become obstructed by mucus and may obstruct the nose. Flow rates for infants should be regulated by a low-flow meter, graduated 0–2.5 L min^{-1}. Rates of 0.2–4 L min(1 provide 40–70% O_2 to infants 1–10 kg body weight (BW). Improved oxygenation may be caused in part by positive end expiratory pressure (PEEP).

An oxygen catheter placed in the nasopharynx a distance equivalent to that from ala nasi to tragus, provides a small amount of PEEP, and indeed may be used for that purpose. Oxygen concentrations of 30%, 40% and 50% approximately are provided by flows of 45, 80 and 150 mL kg^{-1} min^{-1} respectively[7].

Oxygen masks

Semi-rigid face masks of the Hudson type, can supply approximately 35–70% O_2 at flow rates of 4–15 L min^{-1}. However, they may not be well tolerated by the infant or small child. They may cause rebreathing or fail to deliver the desired FiO_2 especially when peak inspiratory flow rate (PIFR) is high, thus entraining excessive room air. Masks that incorporate a reservoir bag or a venturi may deliver up to 80% O_2 but, likewise, may cause rebreathing if the flow rate does not match PIFR during respiratory distress.

Head boxes and incubators

A clear perspex head box is the best way of administering a high concentration of oxygen to the unintubated infant. Precise oxygen therapy is possible but rebreathing, heat loss and desiccation are potential problems. To avoid rebreathing, a large flow rate (10–12 L min^{-1}) of fresh gas with predetermined oxygen content should be introduced. The practice of introducing a low flow rate of 100% oxygen into a head box (to gain a lesser concentration) may cause hypercarbia. If 100% oxygen is the only compressed gas available, lesser concentrations of oxygen may be attained without rebreathing by using a flow of 100% oxygen and a Venturi device. The relatively large capacity of an incubator precludes the attainment of a high concentration of oxygen, but limited oxygen therapy, up to a maximum of 60%, can be achieved at the cost of very high flow rates.

Self-inflating resuscitation bags

These should not be used to supply oxygen to the spontaneously breathing patient.

BAG-MASK VENTILATION

As soon as practicable, mechanical ventilation with added oxygen should be commenced with either a bag-mask (bag-valve-mask) or via endotracheal intubation. Although intubation is preferred (see below), valuable time should not be wasted in numerous unsuccessful attempts. Initial effective bag-mask ventilation is a necessary prerequisite for successful paediatric CPR but it is a relatively difficult technique to learn and to perform well in emergency circumstances.

Bags of appropriate sizes should be available for infants, small children and large children. A bag of approximately 500 mL volume should be available for newly-born infants and infants. Note that the smallest sized Laerdal bag (240 mL) although termed 'infant', is not suitable for use in term infants and infants less than one year of age[2].

Insertion of an oropharyngeal (Guedel) airway may be necessary to facilitate bag-mask ventilation. Two types of resuscitation devices are available: flow-inflated and self-inflated bags. They can be attached to a mask, laryngeal mask airway (LMA) or endotracheal tube.

Flow-inflated bags

These are designed to give either positive pressure ventilation or to allow a patient to breathe spontaneously. They are exemplified by Jackson-Rees modified Ayre's T-piece. Gas flow must exceed 220 mL kg^{-1} min^{-1} for children and 3 L min^{-1} for infants, to prevent rebreathing during manual ventilation. It is possible to control precisely the concentration of inspired oxygen, which is an advantage, especially for the premature neonate at risk of oxygen-induced retrolental fibroplasia. However, considerable experience is necessary to provide adequate ventilation without barotrauma in the intubated infant. A pressure gauge and a relief valve should be incorporated in the circuit to help prevent barotrauma.

Self-inflated bags

These bags are designed to give positive pressure ventilation. Rebreathing is prevented by one-way duck-bill valves, spring disk/ball valves or diaphragm/leaf valves. The Laerdal bag series (infant, child, adult) typifies these devices. A pressure-relief valve (infant and child size) opens at 35 cm H_2O (3.5 kPa). A pressure monitor can be incorporated in the circuit. Supplemental oxygen is added to the resuscitation bag, with or without attachment of a reservoir bag, whose movement may serve as a visual monitor of tidal volume during spontaneous ventilation when intubated. However, the valve may offer too much resistance for spontaneous ventilation.

These bags should not be used to provide supplemental oxygen to a spontaneously breathing patient with a mask placed near or loosely over the face. With Laerdal and Partner bags, negligible amounts of oxygen (0.1–0.3 L min^{-1}) issues from the patient valve when 5–15 L min^{-1} of oxygen is introduced into bags unconnected to patients[8]. The patient valve is unlikely to open unless the mask is sealed well on the face. Although not recommended, if they are used in this way, it is vital to ensure that the patient valve opens or the reservoir bags deflates in unison with the chest movement.

The delivered oxygen concentration is dependent on the flow rate of oxygen, use of the reservoir bag, and the state of the pressure relief valve (whether open or closed). In the Laerdal series, with use of the reservoir bag and oxygen flow greater than the minute ventilation, 100% oxygen is delivered. Without the reservoir bag the delivered gas is only 50% oxygen, despite oxygen flow rate at twice minute ventilation. At an oxygen flow rate of 10 L min^{-1} to the infant resuscitator bag, the delivered gas is 85–100% oxygen without the use of the reservoir bag.

ENDOTRACHEAL INTUBATION

The trachea should be intubated as soon as practicable but it can be deferred if successful bag-mask ventilation can be given. Intubation has numerous advantages, which include establishment and maintenance of the airway, facilitation of mechanical ventilation with 100% oxygen, minimisation of the risk of pulmonary aspiration, enablement of tracheal suction and provision of a route for the administration of selected drugs. Regurgitation is common during cardiac arrest.

Hypoxaemia should be avoided during attempts at intubation – which should be limited to 30 seconds. If difficulty is experienced, oxygenation should be re-established with bag-mask ventilation before a reattempt at intubation. Initial intubation should be via the oral route, not via the nasal route. The oral route is invariably quicker, is less likely to cause trauma and haemorrhage and the endotracheal tube is more easily exchanged if the first choice is inappropriate. On the other hand, a tube placed nasally can be better affixed to the face and so is less likely to enter a bronchus or be inadvertently dislodged. A nasal tube is preferred subsequently for transport and long-term management. A nasogastric tube should be inserted after intubation to relieve possible gaseous distension of the stomach sustained during bag-mask ventilation.

Correct placement of the endotracheal tube in the trachea must be confirmed immediately. In the hurried conditions of emergency intubation at cardiopulmonary arrest, it is not difficult to mistakenly intubate the oesophagus or to intubate a bronchus. There is no substitute for visualising the passage of the tip of the endotracheal tube through the vocal cords, confirmation of bilateral pulmonary air entry by auscultation in the axillae, continuous observation of rise and fall of the chest on ventilation and maintenance of pink colouration of the patient. In addition, it is recommended that correct placement of the endotracheal tube be confirmed by capnography or CO_2 detection, with the realisation that CO_2 excretion can only occur with effective pulmonary blood flow. This implies that CO_2 detection cannot be expected unless spontaneous cardiac output returns or unless external cardiac compression is effective. Oxygenation should be confirmed with use of a pulse oximeter or measurement of arterial gas tension.

Endotracheal tube size
A size 2.5 mm tube is used for a premature newborn < 1 kg, 3.0 mm for infants 1–3.5 kg, 3.5 mm for infants > 3.5 kg and up to age of six months, size 4 mm for infants seven months to one year (Table 2.3.1). The approximate size may be chosen for children over one year by the formula: size (mm) = age (years)/4 + 4. Tubes one size larger and smaller should be readily available. The correct size should allow a small leak on application of moderate pressure but also enable adequate pulmonary inflation. If the lungs are non-compliant, however, it may be necessary to insert a tube without a leak or insert a cuffed tube.

Depth of tube insertion
The tube is inserted to a specific numerical depth to avoid accidental extubation or endobronchial intubation. Assessment of the depth of insertion during laryngoscopy by noting passage through the vocal cords is not completely reliable since alteration of head position affects depth of tube insertion. The tube depth increases with neck flexion (goes in) and decreases (comes out) during extension. Since intubation is usually performed with the head extended, the tube depth increases when the laryngoscope is removed and the head assumes a position of neutrality or flexion. In a neutral head position, an appropriate depth of insertion measured

Table 2.3.1	Laryngeal mask airways
Sizes are available to suit body weight (kg) of newborns, infants and children	
Size	Weight (kg)
1	< 5
$1\frac{1}{2}$	5-10
2	10-20
$2\frac{1}{2}$	20-30
3	30-50
4	50-70
5	70-100
6	> 100

from the centre of the lips for an oral tube is 9.5 cm for a term newborn, 11.5 cm for a six-month-old infant, 12 cm for a one year old. After one year the depth is given by the formula: depth (cm) = age (years)/2 + 12. An alternative formula for oral tube depth of insertion is: depth (cm) = size (mm) × 3 when an appropriate tube size for age is used. The appropriate depth of insertion for a nasal tube in this age group is: depth (cm) = age (years)/2 + 15. On a chest X-ray taken with the head in neutral position, the tip of the tube should be at the interclavicular line.

LARYNGEAL MASK AIRWAY (LMA)

These have been used for resuscitation by medical, nursing and ambulance personnel trained in their selection and insertion. They may be used to maintain an airway and are a suitable alternative to the use of airway opening manoeuvres and use of oropharyngeal and nasopharyngeal airways. They are useful to establish an airway in the setting of airway obstruction or failed intubation. An intubating LMA serves as a conduit for intubation.

However, the role of LMA in provision of mechanical ventilation remains uncertain. Like bag-mask ventilation, they do not protect the airway from aspiration, which occurs commonly during cardiopulmonary resuscitation. They are a suitable alternative to a face mask as a means to give ventilation before endotracheal intubation[9] and when intubation is difficult[10]. This is a better technique when the operator is unskilled in the use of LMA and intubation[11]. Although insertion of an LMA is easier to learn than endotracheal intubation, training should not replace mastery of bag-mask ventilation. They should not be used in semi-conscious patients or when the gag reflex is present and are not suitable for long-term use or use during transport when endotracheal intubation is far preferable. They are subject to dislodgment during movement and transport. Appropriate sizes according to body weight are given in Table 2.3.2.

MANAGEMENT OF THE DIFFICULT AIRWAY

Unfortunately, unanticipated difficulties with the airway and intubation or failures to follow a prepared plan to cope with difficult and failed intubation continue to cause deaths, irrespective of the degree of skill of the operator.

The airway can be difficult to maintain because of unusual anatomy, injury or illnesses or because of loss of natural maintenance after administration of drugs, which depress consciousness, muscle tone or activity. 'Airway difficulties' refer to maintenance of the airway, bag-mask ventilation and endotracheal intubation. Each situation may rapidly lead to hypoxaemic brain damage and death.

Resuscitators must be well-skilled in the management of the airway and provision of bag-mask ventilation. It is vital to possess good basic resuscitation techniques (see Chapter 2.2 on basic life support (BLS)), to be familiar with equipment, to have skilled assistance and to have appropriate equipment ready-to-hand. They must be familiar with manoeuvres to overcome difficulties with airway maintenance, bag-mask ventilation and intubation. Resuscitators must also have a pre-conceived plan to cope with difficult and failed (impossible) intubation, especially when bag-mask ventilation fails (Fig. 2.3.1).

An obstructed airway may be relieved by simply repositioning of the patient's head and neck, pharyngeal suction, use of an alternative airway-opening manoeuvre, insertion of an oropharyngeal or nasopharyngeal airway and help by an assistant. Persistent obstruction requires urgent endotracheal intubation.

Difficult intubation

With good technique, normally, intubation can be achieved via direct laryngoscopy with a direct line of sight to the glottis. Sometimes 'difficult intubation' is a consequence of anatomical abnormality, trauma or infection but sometimes it is simply the result of unpreparedness or incorrect choice or use of equipment or lack of knowledge of techniques to overcome difficulties.

Anatomical difficulties

Certain conditions imply that intubation will not be easy but it is prudent to inspect the facial and pharyngeal anatomy of every patient before giving sedation or anaesthesia. Common anatomical variants in many conditions, which will disallow a direct line of sight to the larynx are an 'anterior' larynx, prominent upper incisors, a large tongue or a small hypoplastic mandible. Thus Treacher Collins

Table 2.3.2 Endotracheal tube sizes (internal diameter) and orotracheal and nasotracheal depths for infants and children

Age/body weight (kg)	Size (mm)	Oral depth (cm)	Nasal depth (cm)
Newly-born (3.5)	3.0	9.0	11.0–11.5
1–6 months	3.5	9.5–11	12–13
6–12 months	4.0	11.5–12	13–14
2–3 years	4.5	13–13.5	15–16
4–5 years	5.0	14–14.5	17–18
6–7 years	5.5	15–15.5	19
8–9 years	6.0	16–16.5	20
10–11 years	6.5	17–17.5	21
12–13 years	7.0	18–18.5	22
14–16 years	7.5	19	23

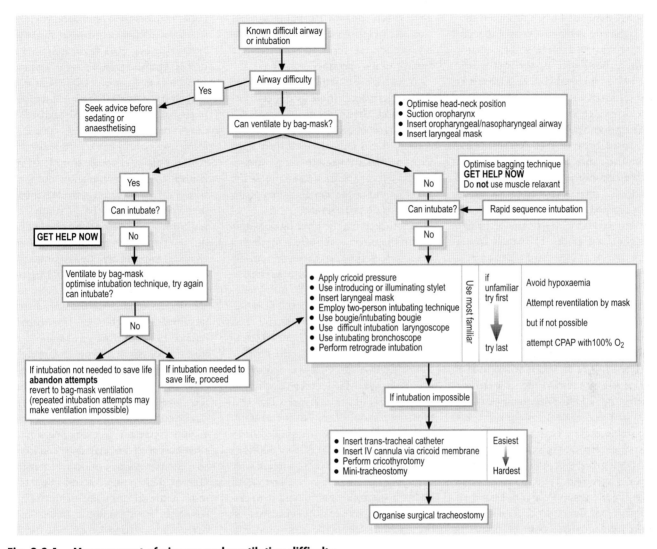

Fig. 2.3.1   Management of airway and ventilation difficulty.

syndrome and Pierre-Robin syndrome (sequence) with mandibular hypoplasia and Beckwith-Wiedmann syndrome with macroglossia are typical conditions in which difficult intubation should be anticipated.

Difficulty with intubation may be unanticipated, but may be predicted with three simple observations. One of these is the relative tongue/pharyngeal size ('Mallampati' test): if the faucial pillars, soft palate and uvula are obscured by the extended tongue on maximum mouth opening, intubation will be difficult. Another predictor is the extent of possible atlanto-occipital extension. If this is less than 35° intubation will be difficult. This corresponds to the angle between the occlusal surface of the upper teeth

and horizontal plane when the head is maximally extended. The third predictor is the amount of mandibular space into which the tongue must be compressed to allow a line of sight to the glottis. This space can be judged by the distance from the thyroid cartilage or hyoid bone to the point of the mandible (thyromental, submental distances) or by the horizontal length of the mandible. In adult-sized patients a thyromental distance of greater than 6 cm and a mandibular length of greater than 9 cm predict easy intubation. Unfortunately, no such distances are known for children and infants.

Thus, the evaluation of intubation difficulty should include pharyngeal examination with extended tongue, inspection of mandibular size or submental space

and examination of atlanto-occipital angle. These special measures should be in addition to routine history of airway management, as would have occurred in previous anaesthesia, inspection of nostrils and history and examination of cardio-respiratory function.

Equipment and technical difficulties

Although Magill's forceps are very useful for directing the tube into the larynx, the use of simple 'tricks' may facilitate intubation. For example, it is important that the patient's head and neck be correctly positioned in the so-called 'sniffing' position (neck flexed, head slightly extended) to offer the best line of sight to the larynx. The blade of a regular laryngoscope is designed to be introduced into the right side of the mouth (not the left) so that when the blade is subsequently centred the tongue is displaced to the left and an unimpeded view of the larynx and sufficient working space is afforded. The tip of a curved bladed laryngoscope (Mackintosh type) is placed in the vallecula (space between base of tongue and epiglottis) whereas the tip of a straight bladed laryngoscope is placed behind the epiglottis. The laryngoscope handle is then elevated upward and away from the operator to lift the tongue out of the line of sight to the glottis. The handle should not be elevated directly upwards or elevated back towards the operator – such actions may not displace the tongue sufficiently and fail to bring the glottis into view, and moreover may damage the upper teeth. The upper teeth should not be used as a leverage point.

The bevel of an endotracheal tube is angled so that it easily enters the trachea when introduced from the right side of the mouth. When introduced from the left side, the tip of the bevel may stick at the laryngeal inlet – but this can be remedied by rotating the tube, thus changing the angle of approach. If the tip of the tube sticks in the anterior larynx, flexion of the neck may direct the tube posteriorly and encourage it to enter the larynx. If the larynx is anterior and difficult or impossible to see, use of an introducing stylet to create a more acute curve at the tube tip may achieve intubation and/or application of posterior cricoid pressure may bring the anterior larynx into view. A tube may be placed 'blindly' into the trachea with or without the use of a stylet or bougie over which a tube can be railroaded. Skilled anticipatory assistance and good suction are essential.

Many other items of equipment are available to assist when intubation proves to be difficult. These include laryngoscopes that have a tip independent of the shaft of the blade, which is used to elevate the epiglottis (e.g. McCoy laryngoscope, Penlon®), or which incorporate a prism to give a view of an anterior larynx (e.g. Belscope®), illuminating stylets and intubating bronchoscopes. Illuminating stylets are malleable and give a 'Jack-o'-lantern'

effect when correctly located in the trachea. All items of equipment are useless unless they are ready-to-hand and are familiar to the operator.

A two-person intubating technique may achieve intubation in difficult circumstances. In this, one person holds the laryngoscope with their left hand and applies cricoid pressure with their right to bring the larynx into view, while a second person applies suction, holds the lower lip out of the way and attempts to pass the endotracheal tube.

Another technique is retrograde intubation (translaryngeal-guided) in which a guide wire is threaded through a needle or intravenous catheter inserted cephalad through the cricothyroid membrane. The end of the wire is retrieved from the oral or nasal cavity, pulled taut and used as a 'tightrope' over which an endotracheal tube is railroaded into the trachea. Alternatively, a string can be tied to the end of the wire which is then drawn from the tracheal puncture. The proximal end of the string can be tied to the Murphy eye of a tube, which is then pulled from below into the trachea. A nasal endotracheal tube can be placed by joining a wire (or string) inserted into the oral cavity via the nasal route and joining it to the wire or string entering the oral cavity via the trachea. Retrograde intubation is a useful technique in cases such as facial trauma, trismus and upper airway masses.

Failed intubation

If endotracheal intubation is impossible when needed, the resuscitationist must be able to oxygenate the patient while preparations are made for tracheostomy or until intubation can somehow be achieved.

Attempts at intubation should not be prolonged, so that hypoxaemia is avoided. Oxygenation should be restored with intermittent bag-mask ventilation. Likewise intubation attempts they should not be overly repetitive because the larynx will be traumatised and this may render bag-mask ventilation, previously possible, now impossible. In situations where intubation is not absolutely needed (i.e. not life-saving) it is prudent to revert to bag-mask ventilation (if that is possible)

rather than persist in intubation attempts, which could ultimately damage the larynx and render bag-mask ventilation impossible. If ventilation is not possible by mask, sometimes application of CPAP with 100% oxygen via an Ayre's T-piece will suffice to maintain oxygenation. Prolonged CPAP cannot be effectively applied with a mask using a self-inflating resuscitator bag.

If the airway is totally obstructed and neither bag-mask ventilation nor intubation can be performed, the situation is desperate. Adequate oxygenation (but not normal ventilation) can be obtained by inserting a trans-tracheal catheter (Mallinckrodt Medical Pty Ltd) otherwise intended for jet-ventilation, or a 14-gauge intravenous cannula percutaneously into the trachea caudad via the cricothyroid membrane (which lies immediately inferior to the thyroid cartilage). To do this, the patient should be lying straight, with the cannula in the midline and angled towards the feet. After removing the needle, the trans-tracheal catheter can be connected directly via its standard $\frac{15}{22}$ mm connector to a bagging circuit. An intravenous cannula can be connected by various ways to a source of oxygen. One of these is direct connection to a resuscitator or a bagging circuit using a connector from a 3.0 mm endotracheal tube. Alternatively, the cannula can be connected to continuous oxygen supply via a three-way intravenous tap (to allow expiration) and a length of plastic tubing. Another option is use of plastic tubing alone that has a side hole cut or a Y-piece inserted, which is intermittently occluded to cause inspiration and unoccluded to allow expiration. With all these techniques care should be taken to allow expiration to avoid barotrauma. Expiration may need to be assisted by lateral chest compression. Ventilation is very difficult but oxygen can be supplied by sustained pressure.

A semi-permanent solution for a totally obstructed airway is cricothyro(s)tomy. To do this the larynx is stabilised throughout the procedure with fingers of one hand while skin over the thyroid-cricoid membrane (between the thyroid and cricoid cartilages) is incised with a scalpel held in the other. Then, bluntly dissect into the trachea with forceps in the mid-line or incise vertically with the scalpel. Insert a small tracheostomy, preferably bevelled, or a small endotracheal tube. Alternatively, perform percutaneous mini-tracheostomy. A formal tracheostomy should be organised while these measures are undertaken.

MONITORING

Vital signs

Routine monitoring of heart rate, respiratory rate and blood pressure are essential for infants and children with critical illness. It is prudent to have ready access to orhave displayed the normal age-related values.

Oximetry

Transcutaneous oximetry (SpO_2) is essential monitoring in critically ill patients. It equates well to arterial haemoglobin oxygen saturation (SaO_2) but not when the SaO_2 is below 70%. Note that an SpO_2 of 90%, although only 10% below normal, represents a partial pressure of oxygen in arterial blood (PaO_2) of 60 mmHg which is 40 mmHg below normal.

End-tidal CO$_2$

End-tidal CO_2 ($P_{et}CO_2$) is recommended after every tracheal intubation and during mechanical ventilation to guard against inadvertent oesophageal intubation and inadvertent extubation, particularly when the intubated patient undergoes transport to, within or between hospitals. Small movements of head and neck, as may occur for example on transfer from one trolley to another or to a bed, may dislodge an endotracheal tube. No CO_2 is excreted unless there is pulmonary blood flow so undetectable CO_2 after intubation basically represents non-tracheal intubation or absence of circulation, or both.

Electrocardiograph (ECG)

The ECG should be displayed with either leads or paddles. Drug therapy or immediate direct current shock is administered according to the existing rhythm. Electrolyte status, especially that of potassium and calcium may be indicated by ECG patterns.

VASCULAR ACCESS

Peripheral venous cannulation

Access to the circulation via a peripheral vein should be attempted immediately on CPA. Any site is acceptable. Visible or palpable peripheral veins are to be found on the dorsum of the hand, wrist, forearm, cubital fossa, chest wall, foot and ankle. In infants, scalp veins are accessible and the umbilical vein can be used up to about a week after birth. The external jugulars are usually distended during CPR and easy to cannulate but this may be impeded by performance of intubation.

Intraosseous access

If peripheral intravenous access cannot be rapidly achieved, say within 60 seconds, intraosseous access should be obtained. This route has been used for patients of all ages. It provides rapid, safe and reliable access to the circulation and serves as an adequate route for any parenteral drug and fluid administration. Syringing via a three-way tap is usually needed. The use of purpose-made intraosseous bone injection needles (e.g. Cook Aus Pty Ltd, 16 g, 3 cm POWCH design) is preferable, although a short lumbar puncture type of needle with an inner trocar may suffice.

The handle of the device needle is held in the palm of the hand while the fingers grip the shaft about a centimetre from the tip. It is inserted perpendicular to the bone surface and a rotary action is used to traverse the cortex. Sudden loss of resistance signifies entry to bone marrow and the needle should stand unsupported. Correct positioning of the needle is confirmed by aspiration of bone marrow (which may be used for biochemical and haematological purposes) but that is not always possible. Bone injection guns (Wais Med Ltd), which fire a needle a pre-set distance according to size of the patient, enable easy intraosseous injection for infants, children and adults.

Although many sites have been used for bone marrow injection, the easiest to identify is the antero-medial surface of the upper or lower tibia. The site of the latter is a few centimetres below the anterior tuberosity and the former a few centimetres above the medial malleolus. Care should be exercised to avoid complications particularly cutaneous extravasation, compartment syndrome of the leg, and osteomyelitis. Contraindications include local trauma and infection.

Central venous cannulation

Cannulation of femoral, subclavian, or internal jugulars or external jugular veins are options. However, central cannulation is difficult in the setting of cardiorespiratory arrest and fraught with potential serious complications such as pneumothorax unless the operator is well practised. This technique is not routinely recommended.

Endotracheal route

Drugs are absorbed into the circulation from the airways. Lipid-soluble drugs (adrenaline [epinephrine], atropine, lidocaine and naloxone) may be administered via the endotracheal tube if either intravenous or intraosseous access is non-existent. Although the optimal doses of these drugs by this route are not known, work in animal models suggests doses should be ten-times the intravenous doses. The drugs should be diluted in normal saline up to 2 mL for infants, 5 mL for small children and 10 mL for large children. It is acceptable and simplest to squirt the drugs from the syringe directly into the endotracheal tube and disperse them throughout the respiratory tree with bagging. Neither sodium bicarbonate nor calcium salts should be administered via the tracheal route because they injure the airways.

Other techniques

Surgical cutdown onto a long saphenous, sapheno-femoral junction or basilic is a valuable skill sometimes required in traumatic exsanguination. Very occasionally, injection into the superior sagittal sinus of an infant may be the only vascular access available. Any pre-existing functioning line can be used provided it does not contain any drug or electrolyte, which may have caused the CPA.

FLUID THERAPY

Circulatory hypovolaemia is expected in trauma, sepsis, dehydration and anaphylactic states. Restoration of intravascular volume should be with isotonic crystalloid solutions (0.9% normal saline or Hartmann's solution) or a colloidal solution such as 4% albumin. There is insufficient evidence to choose between these. Aliquots of 20 mL kg^{-1} intravenously or intraosseously are reasonable volumes to administer in shock states with titration against indices of vascular volume. It is reasonable to administer blood in traumatic haemorrhage if 40–60 mL kg^{-1} has not restored normal blood volume (70–80 mL kg^{-1}). The role of hypertonic solutions are not yet defined for children with hypovolaemic shock, but are in regular use for patients with severe head injury. Dextrose-containing solutions are inadvisable in acute resuscitation unless hypoglycaemia is proven since they may cause osmotic diuresis. Drugs should be flushed into the circulation with boluses of isotonic crystalloid solution.

MANAGEMENT OF PULSELESS ARRESTS

The following discussion assumes that mechanical ventilation with oxygen and external cardiac compression (ECC) have been commenced and continued if an adequate pulse rate is not detectable. The treatment of pulseless arrhythmias (ventricular fibrillation, ventricular tachycardia, asystole, electromechanical dissociation and pulseless electrical activity) are summarised in Figure 2.3.2.

Specific causes of arrhythmias should be treated. For example, calcium channel blockade toxicity is treated with calcium IV or IO (chloride 10% 0.2 mL kg^{-1}, gluconate 10% 0.7 mL kg^{-1}); hyperkalaemia treated with calcium salt, sodium bicarbonate, hyperventilation, insulin and dextrose. All drugs should be flushed into the circulation with a small bolus of isotonic fluid. To prevent inactivation, drugs should not be mixed in the syringe or in infusion lines.

Resuscitation drugs

Adenosine

This endogenous nucleoside is the drug of choice for treatment of SVT if circulation is adequate, otherwise DC shock is the preferred first treatment. It blocks AV node conduction and thus re-entry circuits, which are the usual causes of SVT in infants and children. It has a very short half-life (about ten seconds) in the blood because it is deaminated and inactivated by adenosine deaminase on the surface of red blood cells. Hence, it must be delivered as a rapid bolus. The dose is 100 μg kg^{-1} delivered rapidly intravenously (or intraosseously) and followed by a bolus of normal saline. If ineffective, the dose may be doubled to 200 μg kg^{-1} with the maximum recommended first and second doses as 6 and 12 mg kg^{-1}.

Adrenaline (epinephrine)

Adrenaline is the most frequently used drug in paediatric advanced life support. Its α-adrenergic vasoconstrictive actions are considered its most important by increasing aortic diastolic pressure and coronary perfusion pressure. Its β-adrenergic actions enhance contractility and spontaneous contraction. The usual dose is 10 μg kg^{-1} given intravenously or via the intraosseous route. It should be administered IV/IO every 3–5 minutes at the same dosage when indicated or run as an infusion of 0.05–0.3 μg kg^{-1} min^{-1} (0.3 mg kg^{-1} adrenaline in 50 mL at 1 mL hr^{-1} = 0.1 μg kg^{-1} min^{-1}). Higher bolus doses (up to 200 μg kg^{-1}) or infusions may be administered in refractory asystole and bradyarrhythmic states but there is a risk of severe vasoconstriction, ischaemia, hypertension and onset of ectopy and tachyarrhythmias. If immediate access to the circulation is not available, it can be administered via the endotracheal route at a dosage of 100 μg kg^{-1} but absorption is variable.

Amiodarone

This drug is used to treat a wide variety of atrial and ventricular dysrrhythmias including ectopic atrial tachycardia, junctional ectopic tachycardia (JET), VT and DC-shock resistant VF. It inhibits α- and β-receptors, slows AV nodal conduction, and prolongs the QT interval and QRS duration. It thus may cause *torsade de pointes* VT. The loading dose is 5 mg kg^{-1} infused over several minutes to an hour depending on dysrrhythmia being treated. Repeated doses to a maximum of 15 mg kg^{-1} may be given. Acute side effects are vasodilatation and hypotension and chronic effects are thyroid function disturbance, interstitial pneumonitis, corneal deposits and blue-grey skin discolouration.

Atropine

This parasympatholytic drug is used to treat bradycardia (< 60 min^{-1}) caused by excessive vagal activity or a consequence of atrioventricular block (AV). If inadequate circulation or hypotension are present, severe bradycardia should be treated with adrenaline. Bradycardia caused by hypoxaemia should treated initially with ventilation and oxygen. The dose is 20 μg kg^{-1} (minimum dose 100 μg), which may be repeated after five minutes. Unresponsive bradycardia should be treated with adrenaline.

Calcium

Calcium should not be administered during acute resuscitation unless the cause of collapse is due to hypocalcaemia, hyperkalaemia, calcium channel blocker overdose or hypermagnesaemia. Although intimately involved in myocardial excitation–contraction coupling, it is not useful and possibly harmful, by causing cell death, in the regular treatment of asystole, electromechanical dissociation and ventricular fibrillation. It does not improve outcome. If indicated, the dose is 0.2 mL kg^{-1} of 10% calcium chloride or 0.7 mL kg^{-1} of 10% calcium gluconate and may be repeated after ten minutes according to the serum level if possible.

Glucose

Perturbations of glucose metabolism occur during critical illness. Infants have limited glycogen stores and may sustain hypoglycaemia whereas the stress response may cause hyperglycaemia. Blood levels should be monitored regularly. Hypoglycaemia (< 2.5 mmol kg^{-1}) should be treated with a dextrose infusion of approximately 6–8 mg kg^{-1} min^{-1} or

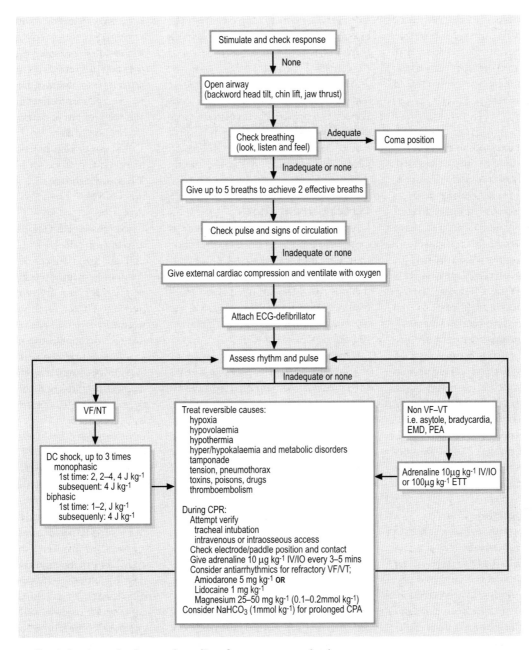

Fig. 2.3.2   Paediatric basic and advanced cardiopulmonary resuscitation.
Key: CPA cardiopulmonary arrest; CPR cardiopulmonary resuscitation; DC direct current; ECG electrocardiograph; EMD electromechanical dissociation; ETT endotracheal tube; IO intraosseus; IV intravenous; J joules; kg kilogram(s); µg microgram(s); mg milligram(s); mmol millimole(s); NAHCO₃ sodium bicarbonate; PEA pulseless electrical activity; VF ventricular fibrillation; VT ventricular tachycardia.

equivalent. Bolus injection may be necessary in which case an appropriate dose is 0.5 g kg^{-1} as provided for example by 5 mL kg^{-1} of 10% or 2 mL kg^{-1} of 25%. Such boluses, however, may cause hyperglycaemia and an acute rise in serum osmolality with osmotic diuresis and harmful rapid changes in brain osmolality.

Hypoglycaemia and hyperglycaemia after brain injury should be avoided.

Lidocaine
This is a sodium channel blocker that decreases automaticity and suppresses ventricular arrhythmias. However, in infants and children it is considered inef-

fective unless dysrrhythmia is associated with focal ischaemia. Although it has been traditionally used for shock-resistant VF and pulseless VT, it has no proven efficacy. If used, the recommended dose is 1 mg kg^{-1} (0.1 mL kg^{-1} of 1%) by rapid injection followed by an infusion of 20–50 µg kg^{-1} min^{-1}. A low infusion dose is recommended if renal or hepatic dysfunction exists. Adverse side effects include myocardial depression with hypotension and central nervous system depression with depression of conscious state and convulsions.

Magnesium

Magnesium inhibits calcium channels and causes a reduction in intracellular calcium thereby causing muscle relaxation, and is used as a bronchodilator in severe asthma. In resuscitation it is used to treat hypomagnesaemia and *Torsades de pointes* VT (q.v.) – a dysrrhythmia associated with prolonged QT interval, which may be congenital (e.g. Jervell–Lange–Nielson and Romano–Ward syndromes) or acquired. The causes of acquired prolonged QT interval are any cause of hypocalcaemia or hypomagnesaemia, drugs (notably tricyclics, phenothiazines, type IA antiarrhythmics such as quinidine and disopyramide, type III antiarrhythmics such as amiodarone and sotalol), central nervous system trauma and myocarditis/ischaemia. The dose of magnesium sulphate is $25–50$ mg kg^{-1} ($0.1–0.2$ mmol kg^{-1}) by intravenous or intraosseous infusion over several minutes.

Sodium bicarbonate

Sodium bicarbonate may be used to counter measured metabolic acidosis in prolonged cardiac arrest but only after hypoventilation has been corrected and preferably only during hyperventilation. Although it can neutralise hydronium ions in the blood it may worsen intracellular acidosis. The product of bicarbonate and hydronium ions is carbonic acid, which freely dissociates to form water and carbon dioxide (CO_2) and, unless hyperventilation is given, the CO_2 may cross into cells where it reforms carbonic acid and librates hydronium ions.

If indicated, an appropriate dose is 1 mmol kg^{-1}. Adverse effects include hypernatraemia and hyperosmolality, hypokalaemia, hypocalcaemia and metabolic alkalosis (which limits oxygen dissociation from haemoglobin). It should not be allowed to mix with catecholamines, which it inactivates, or with calcium salts, which it precipitates. The essential treatment of metabolic acidosis is treatment of the cause.

Vasopressin

The alternative to adrenaline as a vasopressor, vasopressin, has no better survival advantage for adult victims of in-hospital cardiac arrest[12], and has not been adequately investigated for use during CPR for children.

Direct current shock

Unsynchronised DC shock is required as first treatment for ventricular fibrillation (VF) and pulseless ventricular tachycardia (VT). If effective for VF it is called defibrillation. Synchronised DC shock may also be required for pulsatile VT and haemodynamically unstable supraventricular tachycardia (SVT).

Operators of defibrillators should be constantly alert to the possibility of inadvertent electrocution and cardiac arrest of themselves and others by misuse. Paddles should be charged after placement on the patient, not before. Charged paddles should never be carried in one hand and never discharged in the air. If after charging, discharge is not needed, the paddles should be replaced in their storage holders before discharge. It is important that no-one is in contact with the patient or the bed or trolley at the time of discharge.

Defibrillators should have paediatric paddles of cross sectional area $12–20$ cm^2 for use in children < 10 kg. For others, adult-sized paddles ($50–80$ cm^2) are satisfactory provided the paddles do not contact each other. Selectable energy levels should enable delivery of doses $0.5–4$ J kg^{-1}. The closest level to the dose should be selected. One paddle is placed over the mid-axilla opposite the xyphoid or nipple, the other to the right of the upper sternum below the clavicle. Conductive gel (confined to the area beneath the paddles) or gel pads and firm pressure are needed to deliver optimum energy to the heart without causing skin burns. Rescuers should maintain the paddles on the chest and be prepared to deliver a series of three shocks in quick succession, pausing only to verify the rhythm. An antero-posterior position of the paddles (one over cardiac apex, one over left scapula) may be efficacious in refractory arrhythmia. Dextrocardia may be present with congenital heart disease and the position of the paddles should be altered accordingly.

Using a monophasic waveform, the initial dose and mode for VF and pulseless VT is unsynchronised 2 J kg^{-1} progressing to 4 J kg^{-1} if required. The mode and dose for pulsatile VT and SVT is synchronised 0.5 J kg^{-1} initially progressing to 2 J kg^{-1}. The doses of biphasic DC shock for infants and children have not been studied but doses of $1–2$ J kg^{-1} for DC shock for VF and pulseless VT are recommended[6]. In the treatment of refractory arrhythmias, equipment failure or misuse should be excluded.

Although monophasic shock has historically been well accepted for paediatric defibrillation, the optimal dose has never been established. Instead, therapy has been guided by a single study[13], which recommended doses of monophasic shocks of 2 or 4 J kg^{-1}: of 71 defibrillation attempts in 27 children, 91% were successful within 10 watt-seconds (joules) above or below an energy dose of 2 J kg^{-1}. In every case, fibrillation was ultimately terminated by a shock of 4 J kg^{-1} or less.

Faced with no data and a decline in availability of monophasic defibrillators, it is difficult to specify the optimum dose of paediatric biphasic shock. However, a comparative study in adults[14] which used either 150 J biphasic shock or $200–360$ J monophasic shock delivered from semi-automated external defibrillators (sAED), revealed that the lower dose of biphasic shock defibrillated at higher rates than the higher monophasic shocks. By extrapolation from this study, it is suggested that the dose of biphasic shock for children should be $1–2$ J kg^{-1}. This is approximately half the monophasic dose, but higher doses (up to 4 J kg^{-1}) are not likely to be harmful and are more efficacious than equivalent monophasic shocks[6]. This is supported by studies in 'child' and 'infant' animal models in which biphasic shock is more efficacious than the same dose of monophasic shocks[15] and may be delivered in a fixed dose of 50 J by an sAED[16].

The use of monophasic and biphasic semi-automated external defibrillators (sAED) delivering 150–200 J for out-of-hospital use is recommended by the International Liaison Committee on Resuscitation (ILCOR) for children above one year of age, provided that any device has been tested to ensure differentiation of 'shockable' from 'non-shockable' rhythms[5]. However, their use in children less than one year of age is not recommended. Since they cannot reliably distinguish tachycardia in infants their use poses a risk of harmful DC shock. The use of an sAED with adult doses of DC shock for children in hospital is not recommended provided that staff are able to administer weight specific DC shock when indicated within three minutes of cardiorespiratory arrest.

PULSELESS ARRHYTHMIAS (Fig. 2.3.2)

Asystole

Asystole should be treated with adrenaline (epinephrine) 10 µg kg^{-1} intravenously (IV) or intraosseously (IO). If these routes are not available, adrenaline 100 µg kg^{-1} should be administered via endotracheal tube (ETT). Unresponsive asystole should be treated with similar doses (10 µg kg^{-1} IV, IO; 100 µg kg^{-1} ETT) every 3–5 minutes. Higher doses, up to 200 µg kg^{-1} IV or IO may be used but have not altered outcome and predispose to complications (post-arrest myocardial dysfunction, hypertension, tachycardia). In newly born infants, the initial bolus dose is 10–30 µg kg^{-1}. Persistent or recurrent bradyarrhythmia or asystole may require an infusion of adrenaline at 0.05–3 µg kg^{-1} min^{-1}. Doses of < 0.3 µg kg^{-1} min^{-1} are predominantly β-adrenergic, doses > 0.3 µg kg^{-1} min^{-1} are predominantly α-adrenergic. Infuse into a secure large vein. If sinus rhythm cannot be restored, sodium bicarbonate 1 mmol kg^{-1} IV or IO may be helpful but do not allow mixing with

adrenaline since catecholamines are inactivated in alkaline solution. Pacing is not helpful for asystole.

Pulseless electrical activity (PEA) and electromechanical dissociation (EMD)

A normal ECG complex without pulses is called electromechanical dissociation (EMD). If untreated, the ECG deteriorates to an abnormal but still recognisable state when it is called pulseless electrical activity (PEA). Both conditions should be treated as for asystole and their causes ascertained and treated.

Ventricular fibrillation and pulseless ventricular tachycardia

In approximately 10% of paediatric cardiac arrests the initial identified rhythm is ventricular fibrillation (VF) or pulseless ventricular tachycardia (VT). As soon as recognised, VF or pulseless VT should be treated with DC shock. No other treatment takes precedence. If onset is witnessed, a precordial thump may be given but its efficacy has not been proven. The initial monophasic shock is 2 J kg^{-1} increasing up to a maximum of 4 J kg^{-1} in a series of three shocks if the arrhythmia persists. The corresponding doses of biphasic shock are 1–2 J kg^{-1} and 4 J kg^{-1}.

Failure to revert to sinus rhythm should be treated with adrenaline 10 µg kg^{-1} IV or IO or 100 µg kg^{-1} ETT followed by another one to three shocks, if necessary. These shocks should be given at 4 J kg^{-1} monophasic or biphasic after an interval of 30–60 seconds of CPR.

Persistent (refractory) or recurrent VF or VT may be also treated with anti-arrhythmics (amiodarone, lidocaine, magnesium) interspersed with DC shock. Irrespective of other drug therapy, adrenaline should be administered every 3–5 minutes. The dose of amiodarone is 5 mg kg^{-1} IV or IO over several to 60 minutes. It may be repeated to maximum of 15 mg kg^{-1}. The dose of lidocaine is 1 mg kg^{-1} IV or IO bolus followed by an infusion if successful at 20–50 µg kg^{-1} min^{-1}. Amiodarone is more efficacious than lidocaine for DC-

shock resistant VF[17] and pulseless VT[18] and is the preferred drug. Magnesium, 25–50 mg kg^{-1} (0.1–0.2 mmol kg^{-1}) is indicated for polymorphic VT (*Torsades de pointes*).

MANAGEMENT OF SPECIFIC ARRHYTHMIAS

Bradyarrhythmias

In all age groups, bradycardia is defined as a heart rate < 60 min^{-1} or rapidly declining rate with poor perfusion. Sinus bradycardia, sinus arrest with slow junctional or idioventricular rhythm and atrioventricular block are the most common preterminal arrhythmias in paediatric practice. Untreated, bradycardia progresses to asystole. The treatment is reversal of the cause (hypoxaemia, hypotension, acidosis, hypothermia, intracranial hypertension) and, if unresponsive, adrenaline 10 µg kg^{-1} IV or IO or 100 µg kg^{-1} ETT. Bradycardia caused by vagal stimulation should be managed with cessation of the stimulus and/or atropine 20 µg kg^{-1} IV or IO (minimum dose 100 µg). Persistent vagal-mediated bradycardia should be treated with adrenaline 10 µg kg^{-1} IV or IO. If facilities are available, pacing (oesophageal, transcutaneous, transvenous, epicardial) may be effective if sinus node dysfunction or heart block exist.

Tachyarrhythmias (Fig. 2.3.3)

Any heart rate above normal for age should be considered a tachyarrhythmia, particularly if associated with poor circulation and hypotension and if the patient has a history of cardiac disease, has had cardiac surgery or could have been poisoned with cardioactive drugs. Of course, such tachycardia may be the result, rather than the cause of poor circulation, i.e. sinus tachycardia (ST). It is important to determine the type and aetiology of the tachycardia, lest drug or other treatment exacerbate the situation. A history related to the tachycardia and a 12-lead ECG should be analysed carefully. If the diagnosis is not obvious, the

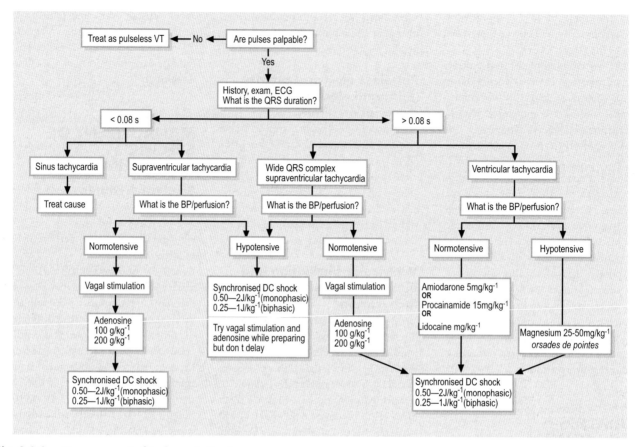

Fig. 2.3.3 Management of tachyarrhythmias.

rate and duration of the QRS are starting points to differentiate sinus tachycardia (ST), ventricular tachycardia (VT), supraventricular tachycardia (SVT) and wide QRS-complex SVT.

Pulsatile ventricular tachycardia

Haemodynamically stable VT may be treated with antiarrhythmic agent such as amiodarone (5 mg kg^{-1} IV over 20–60 minutes) or procainamide (15 mg kg^{-1} IV over 30–60 minutes) or lidocaine (1 mg kg^{-1} IV over 2–4 minutes). Note that both amiodarone and procainamide prolong QT interval and should not be given together. If *Torsades de pointes* (twisting of the peaks) is present, magnesium (25–50 mg kg^{-1}, 0.1–0.2 mmol kg^{-1} IV) may be used. If pulses are present but accompanied by hypotension and poor circulation, cardioversion is needed in which case it should be synchronised at 0.5-2 J kg^{-1} under sedation/anaesthesia.

Supraventricular tachycardia

SVT is the most common spontaneous arrhythmia in childhood and infancy. It may cause life-threatening hypotension. It is usually re-entrant with a rate of 220–300 min^{-1} in infants, usually less in children (approximately 180 min^{-1}). The QRS complex is usually narrow (< 0.08 s) making it difficult sometimes to discern from sinus tachycardia. However, whereas ST is a part of other features of illness, SVT is a singular entity and whereas the rate in ST is variable with activity or stimulation, it is uniform in SVT and often of sudden onset and offset. In both rhythms, a P wave may be discernible.

If haemodynamically stable (adequate perfusion and blood pressure), initial treatment of SVT should be vagal stimulation. For infants and young children, application to the face of a plastic bag filled with iced-water is usually effective. Older children may be treated with carotid sinus massage or perform a Valsalva

manoeuvre – such as blowing through a narrow straw. If unsuccessful, give adenosine 100 µg kg^{-1} IV by rapid bolus (max dose 6 mg), doubling once to 200 µg kg^{-1}. If unsuccessful, give synchronised DC shock (cardioversion) commencing with 0.5 J kg^{-1} progressing if unsuccessful to 2 J kg^{-1}. If SVT is accompanied by haemodynamic instability, proceed to cardioversion (synchronised 0.5–2 J kg^{-1}) immediately, although vagal stimulation or adenosine (IV or IO) may be used provided they do not delay cardioversion. Verapamil should not be used to treat SVT in infants and should be avoided in children because it induces hypotension and cardiac depression.

Wide QRS complex supraventricular tachycardia

SVT with aberrant conduction may cause a wide-complex QRS (> 0.08 s) and thus may resemble VT. If the blood pressure is low or circulation deemed inadequate, the rhythm should be regarded as VT and treated with synchronised DC shock at 0.5 to 2 J kg^{-1}. If pulses are absent, the rhythm should be regarded as pulseless VT and treated accordingly with DC 2–4 J kg^{-1} (monophasic) or 1–2 J kg^{-1} (biphasic).

POST-RESUSCITATION MANAGEMENT

Supportive therapy should be provided until there is recovery of function of vital organs. This may require provision of oxygen therapy, mechanical ventilation, inotropic/vasopressor infusion, renal support, parenteral nutrition and other therapy for several days or longer. Recovery of infants and children is usually slow because cardiorespiratory arrest is often secondary to prolonged global ischaemia or hypoxaemia, which implies that other organs sustain damage before cardiorespiratory arrest. The cause of the CPA should be investigated and treated appropriately, e.g. sepsis or drug overdose. Particular care should be taken to ensure adequate cerebral perfusion with well-oxygenated blood. Hyperventilation is not useful for this purpose.

Survival and neurological outcome is better when deliberate hypothermia is used after cardiac arrest. ILCOR has recommended deliberate hypothermia (32–34°C) for 12–24 hours for adults who remain unconscious with spontaneous circulation after out-of-hospital cardiac arrest when the initial rhythm was ventricular fibrillation, and suggested that for any other rhythm, or cardiac arrest in hospital, such cooling may also be beneficial[4]. Inadvertently hypothermic patients, provided temperature is above 32°C or greater should not be actively warmed and hyperthermia should be aggressively treated. The optimal duration of such requirement, however, is unknown. If deliberate hypothermia is employed, shivering should be prevented with sedation and/or neuromuscular blockade. Seizures should be actively sought and treated with anticonvulsant.

Complications of CPR should be sought especially if secondary deterioration occurs. A chest X-ray should be obtained to check the position of the endotracheal tube, to exclude pneumothorax, lung collapse, contusion or aspiration and to check the cardiac silhouette. An echocardiographic examination is preferable to specifically check contractility and to exclude a pericardial effusion. Measurement of haemoglobin, pH, gas tensions, electrolytes and glucose are important.

CESSATION OF CPR

Long-term outcome from paediatric CPR is poor, but better if arrest is respiratory alone or if CPA occurs in hospital. The decision to cease CPR should be based on a number of factors including the duration of resuscitation, response to treatment, pre-arrest status of the patient, remediable factors, likely outcome if ultimately successful, opinions of personnel familiar with the patient and, whenever appropriate, the wishes of the parents. In general, unless hypothermia or drug toxicity exists, survival to normality is most unlikely if there has been a failure to respond to full CPR after 30 minutes and several doses of adrenaline. In the newly-born infant, discontinuation of treatment is appropriate if CPR does not establish a spontaneous circulation within 15 minutes. Family members should be kept informed, allowed to be present or asked if they want to be present during resuscitation.

POST-RESUSCITATION STAFF MANAGEMENT

Unfortunately, CPA occurring in hospital is often unexpected as when for example a moribund patient arrives unannounced in the emergency department, or a patient's condition deteriorates rapidly on the ward or when a mishap occurs under anaesthesia. These situations test the readiness, training, abilities and skills of individuals and the organisation of the institution. It is prudent to monitor performance with a view to improvement and not ignore the psychological impact that such events have on individuals. Sensitive debriefing sessions may be helpful.

PREVENTION OF CARDIORESPIRATORY ARREST

Outcome of paediatric cardiorespiratory arrest is poor, especially if occurring out-of-hospital. In hospital, it is likewise poor. Of course, hospital personnel should be well-trained and organised to treat unexpected cardiorespiratory arrest, but the far preferable course of action is prevention. Several adult and a paediatric hospital have instituted 'Medical Emergency Team' systems, which can respond rapidly to deterioration in a patient's condition before arrest occurs with consequent reduction in mortality and unplanned admission to intensive care[19-21].

REFERENCES

1. Australian Resuscitation Council 2005 Policy Statements 7.1.2, 7.2, 12.1–12.9. ARC, Melbourne
2. American Heart Association 2000 Guidelines 2000 for cardiopulmonary resuscitation and emergency cardiovascular care. International consensus on science. Circulation (Suppl) 102: I-253–357
3. Advanced Life Support Group 2001 Advanced paediatric life support. BMJ Books, London
4. Nolan JP, Morley PT, Vanden Hoek TL, Hickey RW 2003 Therapeutic hypothermia after cardiac arrest. An advisory statement by the advanced life support task force of the International Liaison Committee on Resuscitation (ILCOR). Resuscitation 57:231–5
5. Samson R, Berg R, Bingham R 2003 Automated external defibrillators for children: An update. An advisory statement by the pediatric advanced life support task force of the international liaison committee on resuscitation (ILCOR). Resuscitation 57:237–43
6. Jacobs I, Tibballs J, Morley P, Dennett J, Wassertheil J, Callanan V, Hall J 2003 Energy levels for biphasic defibrillation. An advisory statement from the Australian Resuscitation Council. Med J Aust 179:451
7. Shann F, Gatchalian S, Hutchinson R 1988 Nasopharyngeal oxygen in children. Lancet 2: 1238–1240
8. Carter BG, Fairbank B, Tibballs J, Hochman M, Osborne J 2005 Oxygen delivery using self-inflating resuscitation bags. Pedi Crit Care Med 6:125–128
9. Stone BJ, Chantler PJ, Baskett PJ 1998 The incidence of regurgitation during cardiopulmonary resuscitation: a comparison between the bag valve mask and laryngeal mask airway. Resuscitation 38: 3–6
10. Benumot JL 1996 Laryngeal mask airway and the ASA difficult airway algorithm. Anesthesiology 84: 686–699
11. Pennant JH, Walker MB 1992 Comparison of the endotracheal tube and laryngeal mask in airway management by paramedical personnel. Anesthesia & Analgesia 74: 531–534

12. Stiell IG, Hebert PC, Wells GA, Vandemheen KL, Tang AS, Higginson LA, Dreyer JF, Clement C, Battram E, Watpool I, Mason S, Klassen T, Weitzman BN 2001 Vasopressin versus epinephrine for inhospital cardiac arrest: A randomised controlled trial. Lancet 358: 105–109
13. Gutgesell HP, Tacker WA, Geddes LA, Davis S, Lie JT, McNamara DG 1976 Energy dose for ventricular defibrillation of children. Pediatrics 58(6): 898–901
14. Schneider T, Martens PR, Paschen H, Kuisma M, Wolcke B, Gliner BE et al 2000 Multicenter, randomized, controlled trial of 150-J biphasic shocks compared with 200- to 360-J monophasic shocks in the resuscitation of out-of-hospital cardiac arrest victims. Optimized Response to Cardiac Arrest (ORCA) Investigators. Circulation 102(15):1780–1787
15. Clark CB, Zhang Y, Davies LR, Karlsson G, Kerber RE 2001 Pediatric transthoracic defibrillation: Biphasic versus monophasic waveforms in an experimental model. Resuscitation 51(2):159–163
16. Tang W, Weil MH, Jorgenson D, Klouche K, Morgan C, Yu T et al 2002 Fixed-energy biphasic waveform defibrillation in a pediatric model of cardiac arrest and resuscitation. Critical Care Medicine 30(12): 2736–2741
17. Dorian P, Cass D, Schwartz B, Cooper R, Gelaznikas R, Barr A 2002 Amiodarone as compared to lidocaine for shock-resistant ventricular fibrillatrion. New England Journal of Medicine 346: 884–890
18. Somberg JC, Bailin SJ, Haffajee CI, Paladino WP, Kerin NZ, Bridges D, Timar S, Molnar J 2002 Amio-aqueous investigators. American Journal of Cardiology 90: 853–859
19. Buist MD, Moore GE, Bernard SA, Waxman BP, Anderson JN, Nguyen TV 2002 Effects of a medical emergency team on reduction of incidence of and mortality from unexpected cardiac arrests in hospital: Preliminary study. British Medical Journal 324: 1–6
20. Salamonson Y, Kariyawasam A, van Heere B, O'Connor C 2001 The evolutionary process of medical emergency team (MET) implementation: Reduction in unanticipated ICU transfers. Resuscitation 49: 135–141
21. Tibbals J, Kinney S, Duke T, Oakley E, Hennessy M 2005 Reduction of paediatric in-patient cardiac arrest and death with a medical emergency team. Preliminary results. Arch Dis Child 2005 (in press)

2.4 SPECIFIC PAEDIATRIC RESUSCITATION

JAMES TIBBALLS

DROWNING

Victims of submersion incidents suffer global hypoxaemia and if arrested, global ischaemia. Associated injuries are aspiration pneumonitis and hypothermia. Aspiration of water and gastric contents is common see Chapter 22.2. In addition, hypothermia (see Chapter 22.4) may be present, but unless the victim was submersed in ice-cold water (< 5°C), this reflects lack of perfusion and is a bad prognostic sign. Hypothermia should be treated but temperature not permitted to rise above 35°C if cardiac arrest has occurred (see Chapter 2.3).

The outcome is often determined by the extent of neurological injury. Bad prognostic indicators are prolonged duration of submersion, lack of bystander CPR, prolonged pre-hospital resuscitation, pulseless arrhythmia on arrival at hospital, fixed dilated pupils, severe acidosis and apnoea. Nonetheless, vigorous resuscitation should be instituted on arrival in hospital of the pulseless victim if not already commenced by ambulance personnel.

Intubation and mechanical ventilation with 100% oxygen should be instituted immediately. Regurgitation of stomach contents should be anticipated and a rapid sequence intubation technique with cricoid pressure should be used. Sedative drugs with cardiovascular depressive actions should not be used or in minimally required doses only. The lung compliance is likely to be poor and it may be necessary to insert a larger-than-usual uncuffed or a cuffed endotracheal tube to obtain adequate lung inflation in the setting of acute respiratory distress syndrome (ARDS). After restoration of cardiac rhythm myocardial contractility should be measured and optimised with inotropic agents.

During resuscitation, the goal is to provide maximum opportunity for cerebral recovery and this is achieved by restoring cerebral perfusion with well oxygenated blood and the avoidance of factors that decrease cerebral perfusion pressure. It is thus vital to restore cardiac output and blood pressure, to oxygenate blood and to avoid factors that would increase intracranial pressure such as venous obstruction. Hypocapnia, hypercapnia, hypoglycaemia and hyperglycaemia should be avoided and convulsions treated.

Any pulseless arrhythmia may be encountered and should be managed along standard lines except that defibrillation should be restricted to three attempts in the presence of hypothermia, and the onset of actions of drugs may be delayed.

There are no important clinical differences between fresh and salt-water immersion. Altered levels of serum electrolytes, especially sodium and potassium, may be detected, but are uncommon and in any case do not influence acute resuscitation.

TOXICOLOGICAL EMERGENCIES

The standard resuscitation protocols may be inadequate in some toxicological emergencies, particularly when poisoning has occurred with cardioactive drugs.

Airway and ventilation management

Problems should not be created by treatment. Gastric lavage should not be undertaken unless the patient has ingested a significant toxin in significant amount within the past hour. Gastric lavage should not be performed in the fully conscious or in the less-than-fully conscious patient, without prior securement of the airway with rapid sequence endotracheal intubation. Likewise, activated charcoal should not be administered by oro/nasogastric tube in a patient who is less-than-fully conscious. The risk of aspiration pneumonitis in these circumstances is significant.

Drug-induced asystole

Infusions of KCl are hazardous. Molar solutions of KCl are in common use in intensive care units especially after cardiac surgery. An inadvertent IV bolus of potassium can cause asystole. Note that a 1 mL bolus of molar KCl (1 mmol) in a 10 kg child will theoretically raise the serum concentration by 2.5 mmol L^{-1}.

Immediately acting treatment (within seconds) is either 10% calcium chloride IV 0.2 mL kg^{-1} (or equivalent) or IV sodium bicarbonate 1 mmol kg^{-1} or both. Calcium antagonises the cardiac effects of potassium on the heart, while the bicarbonate lowers the serum concentration of potassium. Treatment of rapid onset (within minutes) are glucose 0.5 g kg^{-1} IV (e.g. 5 mL kg^{-1} of 10%) plus insulin 0.05 units kg^{-1} or salbutamol 0.25 mg kg^{-1} by aerosol. Slow treatment (within hours) is by resonium, oral or rectal, 0.5–1 g kg^{-1}.

Drug-induced bradycardia

Organophosphate and carbamate poisoning with bradycardia should be treated with atropine – repeated doses of 20–50 μg kg^{-1} every 15 minutes or until secretions are dry and an acceptable heart rate is restored. In organophosphate poisoning (but not carbamate), pralidoxime can reactivate cholinesterase. The dose is 25 mg kg^{-1} IV over 15–30 minutes then 10–20 mg kg^{-1} per hour for 18 hours or more.

Bradycardia induced by β-blocker poisoning is treated with glucagon 7 μg kg^{-1} IV then 2–7 μg kg^{-1} min^{-1}. This is the preferred antidote because it stimulates non-catecholamine cAMP. Isoprenaline 0.05–3 μg kg^{-1} min^{-1} by infusion may be used but it may cause $β_2$-induced hypotension and should not be used if hypotension is pre-existing. Alternatively, an infusion of noradrenalin (norepinephrine) at 0.05–1 μg kg^{-1} min^{-1} may be fused.

Digoxin induced bradycardia may be treated with magnesium IV 25–50 mg kg^{-1} (0.1–0.2 mmol kg^{-1}) or with Digoxin Fab antibody in a dose of 10 vials per 25 of 0.25 mg tablets or per 5 mg elixir ingested. At steady state, the number of vials is calculated as serum digoxin (ng mL^{-1}) × (kg)/100.

Drug-induced tachyarrhythmias

The preferred treatment is a benzodiazepine such as diazepam or midazolam in doses that do not depress CNS function. Other treatments are the ultra-short-acting cardioselective $β_1$ blocker esmolol IV 500 μg kg^{-1} over one minute and then 25–200 μg kg^{-1} min^{-1} by infusion. Treatments such as intravenous adenosine and DC shock are not likely to be effective because the toxic drug effect will be persistent. Calcium channel blockers such as verapamil may cause severe hypotension and should not be given.

Drug-induced hypertension

Hypertension may occur with poisoning by cocaine, amphetamine and similar substances, which cause vasoconstriction, tachycardia and arrhythmias. Benzodiazepines are the preferred treatment. Another alternative is a smooth muscle dilator such as sodium nitroprusside IV 0.5–2 μg kg^{-1} min^{-1}, but its use mandates intra-arterial monitoring. Another choice is phentolamine IV 0.05–0.1 mg kg^{-1} and then an infusion of 5–50 μg kg^{-1} min^{-1}. Propranolol, a non selective β-blocker is contraindicated because it may worsen hypertension when $β_2$-adrenoreceptors are blocked.

Drug-induced ventricular tachycardia and fibrillation

Haemodynamically stable VT can be treated with antiarrhythmic agents. Typical drug causes are tricyclic antidepressants, cocaine and amphetamines. These cause a monomorphic VT by increasing the QRS interval. Treatment should be sodium bicarbonate, especially in cases of tricyclic poisoning. Both components of the sodium bicarbonate contribute to its antidotal effect – the sodium counters the sodium channel blockade effect of the drugs and the alkalosis reduces bio-availability. Induction of respiratory alkalosis is also beneficial. The preferred antidysrrhythmic agent is lidocaine. Phenytoin is no longer recommended. Polymorphic VT (*Torsades de pointes*) of any cause should be treated with magnesium 25–50 mg kg^{-1} IV.

Pulseless VT or VF require DC shock. The use of adrenaline (epinephrine) in this situation should be limited to 10 μg kg^{-1} boluses and higher doses avoided. Propranolol is contraindicated.

Drug-induced shock

Shock may result from drugs that cause depression of myocardial contractility, vasodilatation or loss of intravascular volume, or combinations of these. An extreme rise in peripheral vascular resistance may also lead to myocardial failure. Whenever possible preload, contractility and afterload should be measured.

Preload deficiencies (hypovolaemia) are corrected with volume administration, titrated against blood pressure, right heart filling pressure and against pulmonary artery wedge pressure.

Infusion of dopamine is the preferred inotropic agent in doses of approximately 5–15 μg kg^{-1} min^{-1}, although higher doses may be needed or other inotropic drugs added. If central access is not possible infusion of dobutamine in a similar dose may be given via a peripheral venous access, at least in the short term. Other inotropic agents are infusions of calcium (0.03–0.1 mL kg^{-1} hr^{-1} of 10% $CaCl_2$, i.e. 3–10 mg kg^{-1} hr^{-1}), milrinone (50 μg kg^{-1} loading dose then 0.375–0.75 μg kg^{-1} min^{-1}) and glucagon. It is desirable to measure cardiac output or to assess contractility with echocardiography.

Vasodilatation is treated with an α-adrenergic agent such as noradrenalin (norepinephrine) infusion (0.05–1 μg kg^{-1} min^{-1}) in the higher dose range. Other such agents are phenylephrine (1–5 μg kg^{-1} min^{-1}) and metaraminol (0.05–1 μg kg^{-1} min^{-1}). Vasoconstriction is also obtained with vasopressin infusion (0.002–0.01 units kg^{-1} min^{-1}).

In selected circumstances, cardiac output can be supported with ventricular assist devices, extra-corporeal membrane oxygenation (ECMO) or intra-aortic balloon pumping, although the last named requires intrinsic cardiac rhythm. These techniques are sometimes used in toxicological emergencies in centres that use these techniques for cardiac surgery. They are only indicated when standard supportive measures are insufficient but the situation is recoverable, and organ damage, particularly brain damage, has not occurred. The principal risks with techniques are haemorrhage, infection and mechanical failure.

ENVENOMATION

The main principles of resuscitation, restoration of airway, breathing and circulation apply to victims of envenomation, but with additional special requirements related to the effects of venoms and the treatment of envenomation.

Numerous venomous Australian terrestrial and marine creatures may threaten life (see Chapter 22.1). Snakes, spiders, ticks, jellyfish, octopuses and cone shells inject lethal venoms whereas the venoms of bees, ants and wasps cause anaphylaxis. The number of deaths due to envenomation from 1981 to 1999 was 46 (average 2.6 per year[1]). A similar number of deaths (42) was due to anaphylactic reactions to bee and wasp stings over a similar period from 1979–1996[2].

Death and critical illness is due to: (1) rapid onset neurotoxicity, with respiratory failure and airway obstruction by bulbar palsy; (2) haemorrhage and shock; and (3) renal failure secondary to rhabdomyolysis, disseminated intravascular coagulation, haemorrhage or haemolysis. Rapid cardiovascular collapse within minutes after a snake bite may be due to anaphylaxis to venom, acute vasodilatation or to disseminated intravascular coagulation (DIC)-provoked pulmonary hypertension and cor pulmonale.

Particular resuscitation problems encountered after envenomation include the following.

Respiratory failure and bulbar palsy

Many venoms contains neurotoxins. Respiratory and airway support may be required for a prolonged period. Although paralysis caused by some animals, e.g. blue-ringed octopuses, may be relatively brief lasting perhaps several hours (if support is given), paralysis caused by some snake and funnel-web spider venoms may be lengthy. For example, a child considered to have been bitten by a rough-scaled snake remained ventilator dependent for

10 weeks although antivenom administration in that case was delayed[3].

Coagulopathy and haemorrhage

Snake-bite-induced coagulopathy, and haemorrhage and shock, may be prolonged and may not respond readily to administration of antivenom and clotting factors. Antivenom alone does not *per se* restore normal coagulation. It is prudent to administer clotting factors if normal coagulation is not restored soon after antivenom administration, since serum levels of coagulation factors are not restored by liver function for several hours at least after complete consumption of clotting factors during DIC. In the absence of any ability to measure the serum concentrations of venom components it is difficult to judge how much antivenom is required when the sole effect of venom is coagulopathy. Hitherto recommended neutralisation doses of antivenom have been found inadequate in canine and human plasma models of envenomation and coagulopathy[4,5].

Rhabdomyolysis

Some envenomations cause rhabdomyolysis with implications for renal function, electrolyte disturbances (hyperkalaemia, hypocalcaemia) and muscle weakness. This is expected after envenomation by certain snakes (e.g. tiger snakes, black snakes, beaked sea snake) and funnel-web spiders, particularly if antivenom therapy is inadequate or delayed. Myocardial muscle may be involved.

Cardiac dysrrhythmias

Cardiac dysrrhythmias have been observed after envenomation by some creatures. The venom of funnel-web spiders and of the Irukandji jellyfish cause massive release of endogenous catecholamines, which may be responsible for tachydysrrhythmias and ischaemia. The venom of the box jellyfish can kill rapidly – the exact cause is still unknown but it may be related in part to dysrrhythmia caused by hyperkalaemia secondary to haemolysis.

Hypertension

Severe hypertension may occur after bites

from funnel-web spiders and after stings from Irukandji jellyfish. This is caused by release of endogenous catecholamines. Treatment could be with vasodilators, α- and β-adrenergic blockade. The infusion of magnesium may curtail the effects of Irukandji envenomation[6].

Adverse reactions to antivenom

The treatment of some envenomations by antivenom, may be complicated by reactions to antivenom. Adverse reactions to Australian snake antivenoms occur in approximately 8–13% of cases – which is relatively small compared to some overseas manufactured antivenoms. Nonetheless it is prudent to prevent potential anaphylaxis by premedication with subcutaneous adrenaline (epinephrine) 0.25 mg for an adult, 5–10 µg kg^{-1} for a child.

A prospective, double blind, randomised, placebo-controlled trial of 0.25 mg of subcutaneous adrenaline as premedication for snake antivenom in Sri Lanka found that subcutaneous adrenaline reduced the reaction rate from 43% to 11% ($p = 0.0002$) and reduced the severity of reactions[7]. Thus, although adrenaline has a potential to cause cerebral haemorrhage in a snake-venom-induced coagulopathic state when given intravenously or intramuscularly, but not when given subcutaneously[8], it should be administered. This controversial subject was subject to a systematic review[9], which concluded: 'If clinicians believe local factors do not justify routine adrenaline, then they should test their belief in a randomised trial'. In contrast a randomised, double blind, placebo-controlled trial of promethazine as a premedication for snake antivenom in Brazil[10] did not alter the reaction rate (25% placebo, 24% promethazine) and was thus not beneficial. Moreover, the effects of promethazine, hypotension and CNS obtundation, might exacerbate the illness caused by envenomation. Promethazine is therefore contraindicated as a premedication.

Pressure-immobilisation bandage

Application of a pressure-immobilisation bandage is essential in the early management of selected envenomations. Delay in application or premature removal of a bandage may severely compromise resuscitation. Envenomations by snakes, funnel-web spiders, blue-ringed octopuses, and cone shells all warrant application of a bandage. The venoms of these creatures contain components that cause rapid onset of paralysis. The bandage serves to maintain venom at the bite or sting site and hence prevents venom access to the general circulation and exerting systemic effects.

Unfortunately, application of a bandage is not always performed well or in a timely manner both before and after arrival of the victim at hospital. A critically ill victim should have a bandage applied in the Emergency Department, if one is not already in place on arrival and it should not be removed until antivenom has been administered.

REFERENCES

1. Sutherland SK, Tibballs J 2001 Australian Animal Toxins. Oxford University Press, Melbourne
2. Winkel KD, Bordeaux S, Harrison J, Levick NR 1999 European wasps: An emerging health hazard in Australia. 4th International Hymenopterists Conference. 6–11 January, Canberra
3. Patten BR, Pearn JH, DeBuse P, Burke J, Covacevich J 1985 Prolonged intensive therapy after snake bite. Medical Journal of Australia 142: 467–469
4. Tibballs J, Sutherland SK 1991 The efficacy of antivenom in prevention of cardiovascular depression and coagulopathy induced by brown snake (*Pseudonaja*) species. Anaesthetic Intensive Care 19: 530–534
5. Sprivulis P, Jelinek GA, Marshall L 1996 Efficacy and potency of antivenoms in neutralising the procoagulant effects of Australian snake venoms in dog and human plasma. Anaesthetic Intensive Care 24: 379–381
6. Corkeron MA 2003 Magnesium infusion to treat Irukandji syndrome. Medical Journal of Australia 178: 411
7. Premawardhena AP, de Silva CE, Fonseka MM, Gunatilake SB, de Silva HJ 1999 Low dose subcutaneous adrenaline to prevent acute adverse reactions to antivenom serum in people bitten by snakes: Randomised, placebo-controlled trial. British Medical Journal 318: 1041–1043
8. Tibballs J 1994 Premedication for snake antivenom. Medical Journal of Australia 160: 4–7
9. Nuchpraryoon I, Garner P 2003 Interventions for preventing reactions to snake antivenom. Cochrane Database of Systematic Reviews 1
10. Fan HW, Marcopito LF, Cardoso JL, Franca FO, Malaque CM, Ferrari RA, Theakston RD, Warrell DA 1999 Sequential randomised and double-blind trial of promethazine prophylaxis against early anaphylactic reactions to antivenom for bothrops snake bites. British Medical Journal 318: 1451–1452

2.5 SHOCK

KEVIN MACKWAY-JONES

ESSENTIALS

1 Shock is a syndrome that arises because of acute failure of the circulation. It may result from hypovolaemic, cardiogenic, distributive, obstructive or dissociative causes.

2 The normotensive child may have profound compensated shock.

3 As tachycardia may be a non-specific sign and hypotension occurs late, it is crucial to recognise the early features of shock in a child by assessing indices of peripheral perfusion and alterations of end organ function.

4 The initial management of shock should be volume expansion with a bolus of 20 mL kg^{-1} crystalloid. Further boluses are given according to clinical response. Occasionally, in the exsanguinating child, universal donor blood is indicated.

5 The ongoing management of the shocked child will depend on the specific cause and may include interventions such as: oxygenation, ventilation, glucose administration, cardioversion, broad-spectrum antibiotics, inotropic support, ductus arteriosus manipulation, adrenaline (epinephrine), atropine or surgical intervention.

INTRODUCTION

Shock, in the sense described in this chapter, is a syndrome that arises because of acute failure of the circulation. This acute circulatory failure results in inadequate tissue oxygenation and inability to remove the waste products of metabolism. Shock is a complex construct, having many causes and many expressions. The clinical diagnosis and management of shock is complicated by the fact that many organ systems become involved and because many of the 'signs of shock' actually arise because of the body's attempts at homeostasis rather than because of the underlying process.

The adequacy of circulation (and thereby the adequacy of tissue perfusion) requires proper functioning of the heart, vessels and blood. The heart must pump enough blood to meet peripheral oxygen demand; the vessels that deliver the blood to both the lungs and the other organs must be patent (that is not obstructed), be regulated appropriately at a macro level to ensure delivery of blood at an appropriate pressure to the organs requiring oxygen, and must function appropriately in the periphery so as to allow oxygen diffusion without fluid loss. The blood must have sufficient oxygen carrying capacity and must maintain the ability to allow oxygen exchange. Failure of any aspect of this complicated system will result in inadequate peripheral tissue perfusion and therefore shock.

Conventionally shock is divided into the following five types:

- Hypovolaemic
- Cardiogenic
- Distributive
- Obstructive
- Dissociative.

Hypovolaemic shock arises when there is circulatory volume inadequacy. This classically arises in trauma following haemorrhage or burns but it is also seen following gastrointestinal fluid losses such as diarrhoea and vomiting or volvulus. Cardiogenic shock occurs when the heart fails to pump enough fluid. This can occur because the heart itself is failing secondary to infection, because the heart muscle has been injured (such as in cardiac contusion) or because of a problem with rhythm where the heart is beating too slow or too fast to achieve an adequate cardiac output. In distributive shock, peripheral vascular abnormalities result in failure to appropriately distribute pumped blood. This can be because of infection (as in the septic child), allergic reaction, spinal cord injury or drugs. Obstructive shock arises when there are abnormalities of flow. This can either be because particular vessels themselves are obstructed (such as in pulmonary embolus) or because of extra vascular abnormalities which obstruct the flow of blood (such as tension pneumothorax or cardiac tamponade). Finally, dissociative shock arises when the oxygen carrying capacity of the blood is too low (as in anaemia) or has been reduced as in carbon monoxide poisoning.

DIAGNOSIS AND ASSESSMENT

In all ill children the first need is to recognise the seriousness, or impending seriousness of the condition. This requires a systematic approach to assessment that involves looking at the airway, breathing, circulation, neurological status and exposing the child.

Airway

The ability to speak or cry without stridor indicates a patent airway. The presence of adequate breathing as assessed by looking, listening and feeling for exhaled air also indicates an adequate airway.

Generally, shock affects the airway by reducing conscious level. In acute allergic reaction, airway obstruction (by swelling in the upper airway) and shock due to changes in vascular tone, can both arise as part of the same process.

Breathing

The effort of breathing, efficacy of breathing and effects of inadequate respiration should be examined. Oxygen saturation and respiratory rate should be monitored.

Circulation

This is the crux of shock assessment since homeostatic mechanisms function particularly well in children and compensation for inadequate circulatory function is good. Consequently, in a child it can be difficult to detect circulatory failure until a late stage.

Circulatory assessment should look at both circulatory status and also at the effects of inadequate circulation on other organ systems.

Heart rate and blood pressure are the classical measures of circulatory status but changes in skin perfusion (as shown by capillary refill and by skin pallor or temperature) can be more useful in detecting the early signs of compensated shock.

Heart rate

Tachycardia (relative to age norm) is a key sign of shock. This tachycardia is a homeostatic response to maintaining cardiac output. Bradycardia may occur pre-terminally in the child with overwhelming shock, and untreated will progress to asystole. The peripheral pulses may be weak, thready or absent.

Blood pressure

While it is true that a child with hypotension is shocked it is not true to say that a child that is normotensive is not shocked. This is because maintenance of blood pressure is the key end point of the homeostatic response, and decompensation (and thereby hypotension) occurs late and may be precipitous. The accurate measurement of blood pressure in a distressed child can be a challenge in itself and a judgement as to whether a particular blood pressure is normal or abnormal in a particular age group in any particular circumstances is also challenging. Many widely quoted normal ranges by age are broad – furthermore many of these were derived in the resting out-patient child rather than in the seriously ill or injured child.

Capillary refill

The capillary refill time is measured by applying pressure to the nail bed or other area with visible circulation for some five seconds and then measuring the length of time it takes for the blanching to disappear. A capillary refill time of less than two seconds is normal. A capillary refill time of greater than four seconds is definitely abnormal. Capillary refill between two and four seconds should prompt further consideration of the presence of shock.

Changes in peripheral circulation (which are brought about by an increase in catecholamines) may also show as an increased core to periphery temperature difference (more than 2°C is a sign of poor perfusion) or as a noticeable centripetal temperature gradient. Reduced skin perfusion may result in a mottled, cyanosed, pale appearance and coolness on palpation.

Effects of circulatory inadequacy

Agitation and altered conscious level (that is response to voice or less) are important signs of circulatory inadequacy and the resultant cerebral hypoperfusion. In infants, the manifestations may be more subtle and increased 'irritability' or 'floppiness' or failure to recognise and make eye contact with parents may be the only obvious manifestation.

Increasing respiratory rate is an early sign of inadequate circulation. Latterly, as acidosis ensues, deep sighing respirations occur.

Urine output will decrease with inadequate circulation. If a child has a urine collection device in place then a flow of some 2 mg kg^{-1} h^{-1} in the child under one, and 1 mg kg^{-1} h^{-1} in older children indicates adequate renal perfusion. If there is no urinary collection device then this can be difficult to assess.

Neurological status

As mentioned above, initially agitation and then subsequently depression in conscious level are associated with progressing shock. As in any other case of decreased conscious level a glucose stick test should be performed.

INITIAL MANAGEMENT

The child with shock should be managed in the resuscitation area with monitoring of heart rate, blood pressure, respiratory rate, temperature and oxygen saturation. Urine output should also be monitored as an indicator of response to therapy. The airway and breathing should be managed as in any other case of the seriously ill child. Airway patency should be ensured and high-flow supplemental oxygen delivered. If ventilation is inadequate then this should be supported in the first instance with a bag-valve-mask device. Consideration should then be given to intubation and ventilation through an endotracheal tube if there is no improvement.

Circulation

Once airway and breathing have been managed the next priority is to gain intravascular access. This should be obtained rapidly. An initial assessment to see whether there is a vein available to allow the placement of a short, relatively large, peripheral venous catheter is made. If it is likely that such a catheter can be placed then up to two attempts can be allowed. If these attempts are unsuccessful (or if there is no possibility of placing a venous catheter) then intraosseous access should be gained. In most cases this is done over the medial aspect of the tibia just distal to the knee.

If neither peripheral venous access nor intraosseous access is possible or

desirable, then a Seldinger (guide wire) approach to the femoral vein is probably the next route of choice.

As soon as intravascular access is obtained then blood should be drawn to be tested for haemoglobin, white cell count and platelets together with urea, electrolytes, acid base and lactate level. A blood culture should be taken and a glucose stick test performed to exclude hypoglycaemia.

An initial bolus of 20 mL kg^{-1} of fluid should be given. In most cases the initial fluid will be crystalloid but occasionally universal donor blood may be indicated. There is some controversy as to whether colloid should be administered in cases of sepsis, with proponents arguing that maintenance of oncotic pressure is important in this situation.

If a glucose stick test reveals significant hypoglycaemia then glucose should be administered (5 mL kg^{-1} of 10% dextrose). In such a case hypoglycaemia may be the primary problem but it may also co-exist with other causes of serious illness and resuscitation must therefore be continued if immediate recovery does not ensue with correction of the blood glucose.

If a tachydysrhythmia is identified as a cause of established shock then cardioversion is indicated. This should be undertaken without delay. If the child is alert or otherwise responsive then sedation is usually indicated. If the tachydysrhythmia is supraventricular tachycardia then it may be quicker to give a single bolus of adenosine while preparing for cardioversion.(See Chapter 5.8 on arrythmia.)

If no other cause of shock can be found then it is reasonable to give a broad spectrum antibiotic as part of the initial treatment. A third generation cephalosporin should therefore be given as soon as the blood culture has been taken.

Further management

Once the initial assessment and stabilisation is complete, then it is usually possible to take a more detailed history and undertake a comprehensive examination to try and establish the underlying condition.

The following specific conditions are dealt with in more detail below:

- Hypovolaemia
- Sepsis
- Duct-dependant congenital heart disease
- Heart failure
- Acute severe allergic reaction(anaphylaxis)
- Neurogenic shock.

Hypovolaemia

This diagnosis is usually made because of the presence of trauma, fluid loss from vomiting or diarrhoea or a surgical abdomen.

The further treatment depends on the response to initial fluid bolus. If there are still signs of shock then a second 20 mL kg^{-1} bolus should be given. At this stage a surgical opinion should be sought if an underlying surgical cause is suspected.

It would be most unusual for a child with gastroenteritis to require more than two boluses of crystalloid and, if this is the case, then an alternative diagnosis (such as an underlying intra-abdominal surgical problem or adrenal insufficiency) should be considered.

If the child shows no further signs of shock after two fluid boluses and the underlying diagnosis is gastroenteritis, then it will still be necessary to correct any underlying dehydration and this should be done in the normal manner.

Septic shock

Septic shock arises because of a complex combination of hypovolaemia (relative and absolute), cardiogenic shock (due to myocardial depression) and distributive shock. The underlying cause is, of course, the infection and this should be treated as a matter of urgency. As previously stated, any shocked child in whom there is not an obvious diagnosis should receive broad-spectrum antibiotics as part of the initial management. If a specific diagnosis of septicaemic shock is made and antibiotics have not been given then these broad-spectrum antibiotics (third generation cephalosporins) should be given immediately. Consideration should also be given for a specific prescription of anti-staphylococcal antibiotics such as flucloxacillin and vancomycin if there is evidence of cellulitis or a foreign body, or if the clinical picture is of toxic shock syndrome (high fever, confusion, scarlatinaform rash with desquamation and subcutaneous oedema).

In all cases a further bolus of $20 \, \text{mL} \, \text{kg}^{-1}$ of fluid should be given if there is not rapid restoration of normal circulation following the first bolus. A further fluid bolus should be administered (by IV push) if there is not a good response to the second. It is at this stage that urgent consideration to rapid sequence induction and elective intubation should be given. Many children will develop a degree of pulmonary oedema after the third fluid bolus and oxygenation can only be maintained by positive pressure ventilation (often with the addition of PEEP).

Cardiogenic shock is also a feature of sepsis and this will require specific treatment. Dobutamine at a rate of $10 \, \mu\text{g} \, \text{kg}^{-1} \, \text{min}^{-1}$ should be commenced and adjusted according to the response. Adrenaline (epinephrine) should be considered if there is no response to dobutamine.

Features of raised intracranial pressure due to meningitis can occur during treatment. This is usually presaged by a decrease in conscious level together with abnormal posturing. Early appropriate treatment should be commenced and this will include consideration of diuresis, intubation and ventilation and appropriate positioning of the patient. In this situation, a lumbar puncture is contraindicated.

Duct-dependent congenital heart disease

There are a number of congenital heart defects in which the presence of a patent ductus arteriosus is essential to the maintenance of pulmonary or systemic circulation. These conditions include pulmonary atresia, hypoplastic left heart syndrome and critical aortic stenosis. The ductus usually closes functionally within 24 hours of birth – but may remain patent in the presence of cardiac abnormality.

Babies with critical pulmonary lesions will present within a few days of birth with tachypnoea and apparent breathlessness together with cyanosis, while those with systemic blood flow reduction will present with failure to feed, apparent breathlessness and collapse with poor peripheral circulation. The immediate impression, particularly in the latter group, may well be of severe sepsis.

On examination the babies are in heart failure (usually without a characteristic heart murmur) often with an enlarged liver.

Immediate treatment is to maintain or increase ductus size with an infusion of alprostodil ($0.05 \, \mu\text{g} \, \text{kg}^{-1} \, \text{min}^{-1}$). Immediate transfer to a cardiological centre is indicated. It will usually be necessary to intubate and ventilate these children during transfer.

Heart failure

In babies, heart failure is usually due to structural heart disease, while in older children myocarditis and cardiomyopathy are the commonest underlying diagnoses.

Babies present with breathlessness, feeding problems and failure to thrive and restlessness. In older children more general complaints such as fatigue, anorexia, exercise intolerance and cough are common.

There are signs of increased effort of breathing with increased respiratory rate, recession and positioning. There is an increased heart rate with cool, pale peripheries together with hepatomegaly. On auscultation there may be a gallop rhythm and basal crepitations.

Oxygen should be given in all cases and broad spectrum antibiotics administered if there is any suspicion of sepsis. As discussed earlier, alprostadil should be given if the lesion is duct dependent. In other cases diuretics (furosemide $1–2 \, \text{mg} \, \text{kg}^{-1} \, \text{d}^{-1}$ in 1–3 divided doses initially) should be given urgently. A dobutamine infusion may be indicated to support the failing heart while urgent cardiological advice is sought.

Acute severe allergic reaction (anaphylaxis)

A diagnosis of acute allergic reaction will usually be made because of a history of a previous similar reaction, or because of the presence of typical early symptoms such as itching, facial swelling, urticarial rash, abdominal pain or wheeze.

The initial approach to shock is appropriate administration of fluid boluses. Anaphalactic circulatory shock will usually respond to adrenaline (epinephrine). The recommended dose is $10 \, \mu\text{g} \, \text{kg}^{-1}$ given intramuscularly. Judicious use of $1:100\,000$ adrenaline solution given intravenously in small incremental boluses can also be effective. Over enthusiastic administration of adrenaline in the face of mild allergic reaction or, indeed, in the face of an anxiety attack has resulted in severe dysrhythmias. Caution should therefore be exercised.

If circulatory shock is resistant to the initial bolus of adrenaline then a further intravenous bolus of $20 \, \text{mL} \, \text{kg}^{-1}$ of fluid should be given. At this stage, if the diagnosis is clear, then an infusion of adrenaline at $0.1\text{-}5 \, \mu\text{g} \, \text{kg}^{-1} \, \text{min}^{-1}$ should be commenced.

Neurogenic shock

A child with a spinal injury above T6 will have impaired sympathetic tone below this level once the initial catecholamine release that occurs at the time of injury has ceased to have an effect. The systemic vascular resistance will fall and the reflex tachycardia usually seen as a response to hypovolaemia will not occur. The overall outcome is generalised vasodilatation, bradycardia and loss of temperature control. Systolic blood pressure will fall below 90 mmHg but the skin will appear paradoxically warm and pink.

Initial management is with fluids and a single bolus of $20 \, \text{mL} \, \text{kg}^{-1}$ will usually achieve an acceptable blood pressure. Atropine ($20 \, \mu\text{g} \, \text{kg}^{-1}$) can be given if heart rate falls below 50. Very careful handling is necessary as these children may suffer from postural hypotension if tipped or lifted suddenly. In the early stages fluid management is very important and this may require the insertion of arterial and pulmonary lines. Urinary catheterisation will be necessary as bladder control will be lost.

Concomitant absolute hypovolaemia due to trauma must always be considered as neurogenic shock is invariably caused by trauma in children. Bleeding sources should be actively sought and managed in all children in whom hypotension persists.

FURTHER READING

Alderson P, Bunn F, Lefebvre C, Li Wan Po A, Li L, Roberts I, Schierhout G 2003 Human albumin solution for resuscitation and volume expansion in critically ill patients. Cochrane Injuries Group Cochrane Database of Systematic Reviews 3

Alderson P, Schierhout G, Roberts I, Bunn F 2003 Colloids versus crystalloids for fluid resuscitation in critically ill patients. Cochrane Injuries Group Cochrane Database of Systematic Reviews 3

Bunn F, Alderson P, Hawkins V 2003 Colloid solutions for fluid resuscitation. Cochrane Injuries Group Cochrane Database of Systematic Reviews 3

Dark P, Woodford M, Vail A, Mackway-Jones K, Yates D, Lecky F 2002 Systolic hypertension and the response to blunt trauma in infants and children. Resuscitation 54(3): 245–253

Hartman ME, Angus DC, Clermont G, Kellum JA 2003 Crystalloid solutions for fluid resuscitation in critically ill patients. Cochrane Injuries Group Cochrane Database of Systematic Reviews 3

Kwan I, Bunn F, Roberts I 2003 Timing and volume of fluid administration for patients with bleeding. Cochrane Injuries Group Cochrane Database of Systematic Reviews 3

2.6 NEONATAL RESUSCITATION

GARY WILLIAMS

ESSENTIALS

1 Occasionally deliveries occur in the emergency department when labour cannot be delayed to transfer the patient to a labour ward setting.

2 The emergency department should have available appropriate equipment and guidelines for the resuscitation of the newborn (see Table 2.6.2).

3 The unique physiological events at birth affect the resuscitative interventions in the newborn.

4 Ventilation is the main priority in the resuscitation of the newborn.

5 The heart rate is a reliable indicator of the newborn baby's degree of compromise and response to resuscitation.

6 The easiest way to monitor newborn pulses is by palpation of the umbilicus.

7 Chest compressions are indicated if: (1) absent heart rate; or (2) heart rate < 60 min^{-1} despite adequate assisted ventilations for 30 seconds.

8 Ventilations to achieve approximately 120 'events' per minute.

9 The preferred site of the vascular access during neonatal resuscitation is the umbilical vein.

10 Drugs are rarely required in the resuscitation of the newly born.

11 Volume expansion should be done with crystalloid 10 mL kg^{-1} boluses by slow push.

INTRODUCTION

Epidemiology

Between 5 and 10% of newborns require some assistance to begin breathing at birth and, in developed countries, approximately 1% need intensive resuscitative measures to restore cardiorespiratory function. It has been estimated that birth asphyxia significantly contributes to approximately one in five of the five million neonatal deaths that occur worldwide each year, with the corollary that outcome might be improved for more than one million newborns per year through effective resuscitation at birth.

Neonatal resuscitation is unique in that it is required at a time when the newborn is undergoing a predetermined process of transition from a liquid filled intrauterine environment to spontaneous breathing of room air. There is an accompanying sequence of dramatic alterations in physiology, each of which may be altered and require correction.

There are two important caveats in this process. First, the achievement of lung expansion with an appropriate oxygen-containing gas leading to establishment of a functional residual capacity and adequate spontaneous ventilation is of primary importance. Second, the significance of a vital sign abnormality depends greatly on the time since birth and the time during which effective resuscitation measures have been administered. For instance, bradycardia immediately after birth prior to any resuscitative manoeuvres likely indicates an intrapartum stress. The significance of the same heart rate after one to two minutes of adequate ventilation, suggests a different range of aetiologies and requires a different resuscitative response.

The majority of circumstances where newborn resuscitation will be needed can be predicted, allowing opportunity for preparation of appropriate equipment and personnel. Factors placing the newborn at high risk for neonatal resuscitation include those listed in Table 2.6.1, due to maternal, foetal and intrapartum circumstances.

Aetiology and pathophysiology

The sequence of physiologic changes in the newborn around birth includes:

❶ Cessation of alveolar fluid production and clearance of this fluid from the gas-exchanging part of the airway.

❷ Spontaneous respirations and establishment of functional residual capacity (FRC).

❸ Fall in pulmonary vascular resistance (PVR) (lung expansion, oxygen).

❹ Rise in systemic vascular resistance (SVR) (umbilical artery constriction).

❺ Reversal of flow from left to right across foramen ovale and ductus arteriosis.

❻ Closure of the foramen ovale and ductus arteriosus.

This normal sequence may be interrupted at any point by:

- Inadequate clearance of endogenous lung liquid (precipitous, emergency or operative delivery) or excessive abnormal airway material (blood, mucus, meconium).
- Inadequate respiratory effort (maternal analgesics, CNS injury, sepsis) or excursion (congenital thoracic anomalies).
- Pulmonary disease preventing achievement and maintenance of adequate FRC (parenchymal disease, prematurity, space-occupying lesion) with secondary failure to lower PVR normally and possible intrapulmonary shunting.
- Compromised myocardial function (structural or functional cardiac abnormalities, hypoxia secondary to pulmonary dysfunction).

Interventions should occur in a defined sequence recognising the primary and crucial role of adequate ventilation and be guided by frequent reassessment of other vital signs.

PREPARATION

❶ Summon assistance: if it is anticipated that the infant is at high risk to require ALS resuscitative intervention, more than one experienced person should be mobilised.

❷ Communicate with colleagues to seek available antenatal and intrapartum data.

❸ In the case of extreme prematurity (≤ 24 weeks' gestation) or known congenital anomalies, if time allows, the most senior care provider should seek to discuss with the family their beliefs and desires regarding the extent of resuscitation.

❹ Prepare the environment: a warm, draught-free area with adequate light, radiant heater, prewarmed blankets and a clock.

❺ Prepare required equipment (see Table 2.6.2).

ASSESSMENT AT BIRTH

At birth the infant should be collected in a warm towel, dried and the umbilical cord should be clamped. Gentle stim-

Table 2.6.1 Risk factors for need for neonatal resuscitation

Maternal	Foetal	Intrapartum
Premature or prolonged rupture of membranes	Multiple gestation	Foetal distress
Antepartum haemorrhage	Preterm (< 35 weeks) or post-term	Abnormal presentation
Hypertension	(> 42 weeks) gestation	Prolonged or precipitous labour
Diabetes mellitus	IUGR	Thick staining of amniotic fluid
Substance abuse	Polyhydramnios	Instrumental delivery or emergency caesarean section
Maternal infection or chronic illness	Congenital abnormalities	
Absence of antenatal care		

Table 2.6.2 Equipment and drugs recommended for newborn resuscitation

Equipment	Drugs
Stethoscope	Adrenaline (epinephrine) 1 in 1:10 000 solution.
Suction catheters (6–12 French) and suction	Naloxone hydrochloride 1.0 or 0.4 mg mL^{-1}
8 French feeding tube and 20 ml syringe for gastric decompression	Dextrose 5% or 10%
Face masks	NaHCO$_3$ 4.2% solution
Oropharyngeal (Guedel's) airways	Volume expander (0.9% saline or 4% HSA)
Resuscitation system for PPV	
Laryngoscope with straight blade	
ET tubes 2.5 to 4 mm internal diameter	
ET stylets	
Tape for ETT and IV fixation	
Cannulae, syringes and UV catheterisation equipment	

Table 2.6.3	Apgar score		
Score	0	1	2
Heart rate	Absent	Less than 100	Greater than 100
Respiratory effort	Absent	Irregular	Crying
Muscle tone	Limp	Some flexion	Active motion
Reflex irritability	Absent	Grimace	Grimace and cough
Colour	Blue, pale	Acrocyanosis	Pink all over

ulation may be provided (rubbing the back, flicking soles of feet if required) and an assessment of initial cry, respiratory effort, heart rate, colour and tone should be made virtually simultaneously (see Table 2.6.3).

VENTILATION

The initial assessment is an evaluation of the presence and quality of respirations.

- If respirations are adequate, the heart rate is then evaluated.
- If respirations are shallow or slow, a brief period of stimulation may be provided.
- If the infant has not established adequate breathing by 30 seconds, face mask rescue breaths should be administered and if this is not successful with breathing established by two minutes endotracheal intubation should be performed.
- There should be no delay in commencing rescue breaths if the infant is born with, or develops evidence of, asphyxia with signs of flaccidity, pallor and/or bradycardia (heart rate less than 60 min^{-1}).

Artificial ventilation

Various bag and mask systems are available for neonatal resuscitation but detailed studies have shown that many are ineffective, probably because pressure limitation (either by leak or pop off valve) prevents inflation pressure being maintained long enough to deliver an adequate inflation. Consensus view is that a reservoir volume of at least 500 mL is required to achieve the required initial long inflation times. It is suggested in fact that the invariable success of rescue breathing at birth is because the FRC is established by an induced inspiratory ef-

fort via Head's paradoxical reflex (inspiratory effort induced by any lung inflation). The corollary is that face mask rescue breathing is unlikely to be effective in the severely asphyxiated infant.

Regardless of these issues, it is generally accepted that higher inflation pressures (> 30 cm H$_2$O water) and longer inflation times (> 1.5 s) may be required for the first several ($\approx$ 5) breaths. Visible chest wall movement and audible breath sounds are the best indicators of adequate ventilation. Ventilations should be administered at a rate of 40–60 min^{-1} and after 30 seconds of effective ventilation, the heart rate should be evaluated.

HEART RATE

Assessment of the heart rate can be done by palpating the umbilical stump, brachial or femoral pulse or auscultation of the apical heart sounds.

- The heart rate is a reliable indicator of the baby's degree of compromise and response to resuscitation. It should be assessed at least every 30 seconds in the first two minutes if necessary, until the baby's required level of support is established.
- If the heart rate is less than 60 min^{-1} despite adequate assisted ventilation, compressions are required. When the heart rate is greater than 100 min^{-1}, only ventilation is continued. If the heart rate is between these two points, the level of intervention should be increased or decreased depending on the serial change in the heart rate.
- If the heart rate is not rising after 30 seconds of effective ventilation combined with chest compressions, then adrenaline (epinephrine) should be administered.

- Once a bradycardic heart rate has increased above 60 min^{-1} and is rising, cardiac compressions may be discontinued.

Compression technique

If required, compressions should be instituted using the two-hand-encircling technique (preferred if greater than one rescuer) or two finger technique (if only one rescuer). The lower third of the sternum (just below an imaginary intermammary line) should be depressed one third of the depth of the chest. These should be coordinated with ventilations (to avoid simultaneous delivery) in a ratio of 3:1 with about 90 compressions and 30 breaths each minute. The xiphoid portion of the sternum should not be compressed because such compression may damage the neonate's liver.

COLOUR

Once the heart rate has been evaluated, the infant's colour should be assessed by examining the trunk and mucosae.

- Peripheral cyanosis (acrocyanosis) is common in the first few minutes after birth and is not pathological.
- Central cyanosis reflects inadequate oxygenation and may be pulmonary or cardiac in origin. If present despite adequate ventilation and a heart rate greater than 100 beats per minute, 100% oxygen should be administered until the cause of the cyanosis is known.
- Pallor is suggestive of a decreased cardiac output and may be due to myocardial dysfunction, severe anaemia, hypovolaemia, hypothermia or acidosis.

MUSCLE TONE AND REFLEX IRRITABILITY

These physical signs are valuable composite reflections of the adequacy of cerebral perfusion and oxygenation. As such, they constitute two of the five components of the Apgar score (see Table 2.6.3) used to assess a newborn's condition after birth.

MEDICATIONS

Medications are rarely required during neonatal resuscitation. A recent study suggested medications were required in only 0.12% of all births with severe foetal acidosis or ventilatory problems responsible for the need. This reaffirms the primary and critical importance of achieving optimal ventilation before resorting to medications in neonatal resuscitation.

Vascular access

Adrenaline (epinephrine) may be administered by intravenous (IV), intraosseous (IO) or endotracheal (ET) routes. If perfusion is adequate naloxone hydrochloride may be given via the intramuscular (IM) route as well as possibly by the ET route. The other drugs and volume expansion, detailed below, will require emergency vascular access. Once vascular access is achieved, if the child remains in arrest, an adrenaline dose should be immediately administered via the IV route.

The preferred site of the vascular access during neonatal resuscitation is the umbilical vein, the larger thin walled single vessel (in comparison to the paired thicker walled arteries), which appears when the umbilical cord is trimmed 1 cm above the skin. A 3.5 or 5 French catheter flushed with saline should be inserted only until a good blood return is achieved (usually to a depth of 1 to 4 cm below the skin). Peripheral veins on extremities or scalp may be attempted or alternatively an intraosseous cannula may be placed on the medial aspect of the tibia just below the tibial tuberosity, if umbilical or other direct venous access is not readily obtainable.

Adrenaline (epinephrine)

Adrenaline is administered with the aim of producing α-adrenergic mediated vasoconstriction, an increase in coronary perfusion pressure and myocardial blood flow. Adrenaline is indicated if the heart rate remains less than 60 beats per minute after a minimum of 30 seconds of adequate ventilation and 30 seconds of combined ventilation and chest compressions. The recommended IV or ET dose is 0.1–0.3 mL kg^{-1} of a 1:10 000 solution (10-30 µg kg^{-1}) repeated every three to five minutes as indicated. ET delivery should be followed by 1 mL of normal saline and several good inflations to achieve optimal delivery to the pulmonary vascular bed. Most infant animal experimental dosing data supporting adrenaline's efficacy has been obtained in VF models and as such its value may not be directly applicable to the apparent preterminal bradyarrhythmia in an asphyxiated newborn with markedly elevated $P\text{CO}_2$.

Through the early 1990s some experimental and human data showed that higher doses of adrenaline (100 µg kg^{-1}) were capable of achieving higher plasma adrenaline levels as well as greater myocardial and cerebral blood flow. However, several subsequent adult and paediatric studies showed no ultimate clinical benefit in survival or neurological outcome with a significant risk of adverse effects from the higher dose (myocardial dysfunction or necrosis, hyperadrenergic states, reduced cerebral cortical blood flow). Specifically, there is an increase in potential risk of intraventricular haemorrhages (IVH) in preterm infants. For these reasons, the currently recommended initial IV dose is 10 µg kg^{-1} in neonates.

The endotracheal route is likely to be the most accessible route for initial doses of adrenaline. Again, there is a paucity of both experimental as well as human data regarding dosage and efficacy of ET adrenaline in neonates. There is data to suggest a slower onset with a more prolonged and variable effect at higher dosages. For these reasons the dose recommended is 10–30 µg kg^{-1} every 3–5 minutes during arrest.

Bicarbonate

Although correcting acidosis that has occurred during cardiac arrest to improve both myocardial function and adrenaline's effectiveness makes theoretic sense, there is little supportive experimental data. The vast majority of adult studies have found either no difference or that bicarbonate had deleterious effects on myocardial performance. There are no neonatal animal or human studies specifically examining this question. Bicarbonate administration has multiple possible adverse effects (metabolic alkalosis compromising peripheral tissue oxygen delivery, paradoxical intracellular hypercarbic acidosis). Pertinent to neonates are studies demonstrating large increases in plasma osmolality and reductions in cerebral blood flow, both of which may increase the risk of IVH in newborns. Therefore, bicarbonate administration is only recommended during prolonged arrests, unresponsive to other therapy after establishment of adequate ventilation and perfusion. The dose is 1–2 mEq kg^{-1} of 4.2% solution by slow IV push over at least two minutes.

NALOXONE

Naloxone is a narcotic antagonist, recommended for the neonate who exhibits respiratory depression secondary to narcotics given to the mother within four hours of delivery. Obviously, prompt institution of adequate ventilation is the first priority in such a situation and naloxone is not recommended for newborns whose mothers are suspected narcotic abusers as abrupt withdrawal may be precipitated. Following IV administration, onset of action occurs in 1–2 minutes and is variable in duration. The recommended IV dose is 0.1 mg kg^{-1}. Since the duration of action of narcotics may exceed that of naloxone, continued surveillance and repeat administration are often required. Naloxone may be administered IM with some adult data suggesting slower onset and more prolonged duration of action via this route. There are no studies examining the ET route of administration in the neonate.

Dextrose

Hypoglycaemia is a potential problem for all stressed and asphyxiated babies and should be treated by using a slow bolus of 5 mL kg^{-1} of 10% Dextrose IV.

Volume expansion

If hypovolaemia is present because of known or suspected blood loss or loss of vascular tone following asphyxia, volume expansion may be appropriate. Isotonic non-dextrose containing crystalloid (normal saline or Ringer's lactate) 10 mL kg^{-1} intravenously over 5–10 minutes is recommended. Group O negative packed red cells may be indicated for replacement of large volume blood loss. Albumin-containing solutions are used less frequently because of limited availability, risk of infectious disease and an observed association with increased mortality. A recent randomised controlled comparison of albumin versus normal saline for hypotension in premature newborns showed that those who received albumin required significantly more volume expander to maintain normal blood pressure and had a higher mean percentage weight gain in the first 48 hours after birth.

SPECIFIC RESUSCITATION SITUATIONS

Premature neonate
Preterm newborns have an increased likelihood of respiratory depression requiring assisted ventilation at birth. This occurs because of diminished lung compliance, weak respiratory muscles and immature respiratory drive and may make it difficult to establish and maintain an adequate FRC. For these reasons, infants born at or before 32 weeks gestation should receive face mask resuscitation by 30 seconds and be intubated at 60 seconds after birth if the onset of adequate spontaneous respirations is delayed. Also, because preterm infants often have low body fat and a high BSA to mass ratio, they are more difficult to keep warm and therefore at increased risk of cold stress. Rapid boluses of volume expander and use of hyperosmolar solutions may produce large fluctuations in blood pressure or osmolarity and therefore are not recommended.

Meconium aspiration
Approximately one in 20 infants born through meconium stained amniotic fluid (MSAF) will develop meconium aspiration syndrome (MAS) due to aspiration into the distal airways either in utero or with the initial breaths following birth. However, of these 25–50% will require mechanical ventilation and 5% will die.

Although the evidence supporting the practice is somewhat conflicting, it is recommended that infants delivered through MSAF undergo intrapartum suctioning of the oro and nasopharynx once the head is delivered, prior to delivery of chest or shoulders. If the baby born through MSAF *is not* vigorous after delivery (depressed respirations, muscle tone or heart rate less than 100 min^{-1}) direct intratracheal suctioning (using continuous suction directly applied to the tracheal tube as it is withdrawn) should be performed. If meconium is recovered, the procedure should be repeated (if the heart rate is greater than 60 min^{-1}) before proceeding with resuscitation.

Congenital heart disease
Central cyanosis at birth apparently unresponsive to 100% oxygen particularly in a vigorous baby with adequate spontaneous respiratory effort and minimal respiratory distress may indicate duct-dependent cyanotic congenital heart disease (primarily right heart obstructive lesions, transposition of the great vessels and anomalous pulmonary venous return with complete atrial admixture). The major differential diagnoses are primary pulmonary hypertension or major pulmonary structural abnormalities (e.g. congenital diaphragmatic hernia). In such a circumstance ventilatory support requirement should be dictated by degree of respiratory distress with a target Pa_{CO_2} of 35–40 mmHg.

Detailed cardiac auscultation should be attempted thought there may be no abnormal murmurs audible and simultaneous pre- and post-ductal oximetry measurements should be performed. If a cyanotic cardiac abnormality is strongly suspected, documentation of preductal Pa_{O_2} after breathing 100% oxygen for several minutes (hyperoxia test) will give the best indication of the presence and size of a significant intracardiac right to left shunt. (See Chapter 5.1 on cyanosis.) An urgent bedside echocardiogram, if available, is indicated to delineate the cardiac anatomy. Where this is not available, one should consult with the local tertiary neonatal unit. If a diagnosis of a duct-dependant cyanotic cardiac lesion

is confirmed on echocardiogram, IV alprostadil (PGE$_1$) 25–50 ng kg^{-1} min^{-1} will restore and maintain ductal patency until definitive decisions regarding surgical correction can be made. The main side effects of this medication are flushing, fever and possibly apnoea if respiratory support is not already in place.

Alternatively, babies with duct-dependent systemic circulation usually due to some structural problem with left ventricular outflow (e.g. critical aortic stenosis, severe coarctation, hypoplastic left heart syndrome) may present in the first few days of life with heart failure and poor peripheral perfusion triggered by ductal closure. The most reliable physical signs of heart failure are tachycardia, tachypnoea and hepatomegaly. If shock is present (poor pulse volume, pallor, altered conscious state) respiratory support and fluid volume expansion may be required to restore the circulation. Subsequently, alprostadil or inotrope infusion and continuing judicious fluid administration may be required. The most important steps in restoring systemic circulation in this situation are artificial ventilation to normocapnia, together with re-establishing and maintaining ductal patency. (See Chapter 5.4 on cardiology.)

POST-RESUSCITATION STABILISATION

Post-resuscitation stabilisation should be directed towards preventing any ongoing or repeated primary insults (primarily to the brain) as well as limiting any secondary injury and organising a stable transfer to an appropriate neonatal unit.

- Artificial ventilation should be continued if required to maintain normocapnia (CO$_2$ 35–40 mmHg).
- Oxygenation should be optimised (aim for Pa_{O_2} usually 60–90 mmHg, although this target may be set higher in the face of documented pulmonary hypertension).
- ET tube migration or obstruction should be vigorously avoided.
- With regard to control of body temperature (see hypothermia in the Controversies section below).

- Blood pressure should be monitored meticulously and hypotension treated promptly with fluid resuscitation or inotropes as required.
- Close monitoring of body weight, fluid balance, electrolytes, calcium and magnesium is indicated.
- Evidence of hypoxic insult to major organs other than the brain should be sought (urinalysis, serum creatinine, LFTs, serum troponin level, coagulation parameters).
- Both hyper- and hypoglycaemia may aggravate injury following hypoxic ischaemic insult and therefore normoglycaemia should be targeted.

- There is no evidence in neonatal post-resuscitation cerebral care for hypertonic or osmotic agents to treat or minimise cerebral oedema. The same applies to glucocorticoids and prophylactic anticonvulsant treatment. While the early use of barbiturates in the reduction of seizures, neuronal metabolic demands and excitatory amino acid production is theoretically sound, there is no solid data on which to support their use in this prophylactic way following a perinatal insult.
- Liaison with and transfer to an NICU should be organised as soon as possible with clear documentation of the resuscitation interventions required and responses achieved to this point.
- The parents should also be kept well informed of the infant's condition and efforts made for them to have contact with the baby.

PROGNOSIS

Giving a prediction of outcome at an early stage may be difficult but the most reliable early predictors of adverse outcome are the disturbance of the clinical examination (i.e. degree of encephalopa-

CONTROVERSIES

❶ *Air or O₂ for newborn resuscitation.* Traditionally, 100% oxygen has been used for neonatal resuscitation, but recent animal studies and human trials have confirmed that ventilation with room air is equally successful in neonatal resuscitation. Use of air may even have advantages (reduced oxidative stress, less delay in onset of spontaneous respirations). A recent guideline review has recommended removal of a statement that 'brief hyperoxia during resuscitation is not harmful'. Despite this evolving data in favour of room air, there may still be situations in which 100% oxygen is advantageous (pulmonary hypertension, diffusion abnormalities, alterations in cerebral blood flow). Further research is required to answer the question of whether room air or O₂ is the preferable default. Regardless, the data do suggest that oxygen use in a neonatal resuscitation should be individualised in that the dose should be tailored to clinical response and monitored by the prompt use of pulse oximetry.

❷ *Hypothermia.* Traditionally, post-resuscitation care has involved heat-loss prevention or even external warming on the basis that recovery from acidosis will be facilitated by this procedure. However, recent animal studies have clearly shown that early modest cerebral hypothermia (32–34°C) can modulate hypoxic ischaemic injury. Studies in human neonates remain limited, though evidence of safety has been published recently. Multicentre trials in human neonates to examine efficacy as well as optimal depth of temperature and window of opportunity are underway. At present cerebral hypothermia can not be recommended as part of post-resuscitation care until there is better scientific evidence. However, hyperthermia should definitely be avoided as there is very strong evidence that this is deleterious.

❸ *Ethics of resuscitation.* The decision to withdraw or withhold resuscitation from extremely premature newborns or those with severe congenital abnormalities, requires clear communication with the family and accurate clinical data. It is difficult to issue consensus guidelines on such issues, as multiple factors enter into these decisions. However, overall there is general agreement that overly aggressive treatment is to be discouraged.

- Recent studies demonstrate extremely poor survival rates for infants less than 23 weeks gestation (< 1%) with a better but still poor rate if the infant had been admitted to the NICU (5%). Mortality is less at 23, 24 and 25 completed weeks (11%, 26% and 44% survival in one large recent study). However, severe disability in childhood is present in 20 to 30% of survivors at these gestations and some disability can be expected in 50%. Prognosis is probably better predicted by gestational age (if accurately known) rather than weight, though both factors have a role and gender is also important (lower mortality/morbidity in females).
- Non-initiation of resuscitation in the delivery room is appropriate for infants with confirmed gestation less than 23 weeks or birth weight less than 400 gm, anencephaly or confirmed trisomy 13 or 18. Options include a trial of resuscitation, non-initiation or discontinuation after further assessment. It is important to remember that initiation of resuscitation in such cases does not mandate continued support.
- International guidelines state that discontinuation of resuscitative efforts may be appropriate if resuscitation of an infant with cardiorespiratory arrest does not result in spontaneous circulation in 15 minutes (i.e. Apgar score 0 at 15 minutes). Recent data suggests that this recommendation may be applied at 10 minutes.

thy) and electroencephalographic assessment. A sustained low-voltage EEG or discontinuous activity on an EEG within six hours of birth are strongly predictive of death or significant adverse neurologic sequelae.

REFERENCES AND FURTHER READING

Boyle RJ and Mcintosh N 2001 Ethical considerations in neonatal resuscitation: clinical and research issues. Seminars in Neonatology 6: 261–269

Kattwinkel J, Niermeyer S, Nadkarni V, et al. 1999 ILCOR advisory statement: resuscitation of the newly born infant: an advisory statement from the pediatric working group of the International Liaison Committee on Resuscitation. Circulation 99: 1927–1938

Niermeyer S, Van Reempts P, Kattwinkel J, et al. 2001 Resuscitation of Newborns. Annals of Emergency Medicine 37(4): S110–S125

Perlman JM, Risser R 1995 Cardiopulmonary resuscitation in the delivery room. Arch Pediatric Adolescent Medicine 149: 20–24

Saugstad OD 2001 Resuscitation of newborn infants with room air or oxygen. Seminars in Neonatology 6: 233–239

So KW, Fok TF, Ng PC, et al 1997 Randomised controlled trial of colloid or crystalloid in hypotensive preterm infants. Archives of Diseases in Childhood 76: F43–46

Wood NS, Marlow N, Costeloe K, et al. 2000 Neurologic and developmental disability after extremely preterm birth. New England Journal of Medicine 343(6): 378–384

Wu TJ and Carlo WA 2002 Neonatal resuscitation guidelines 2000: framework for practice. Journal of Maternal-Fetal and Neonatal Medicine 11: 4–10

SECTION

3

SENIOR AUTHOR DANNY CASS

TRAUMA IN CHILDREN

3.1 INTRODUCTION TO PAEDIATRIC TRAUMA

DANNY CASS

ESSENTIALS

1 Trauma is the prime cause of death and serious injury throughout childhood.

2 Prevention strategies have resulted in most of the improvement in mortality due to childhood injuries.

3 The advent of trauma teams has led to great improvement in paediatric injury care.

4 Delayed management of airway obstruction or hypovolaemia are the two most common contributors to preventable paediatric deaths in trauma.

5 The initial assessment of the seriously injured child should follow a structured approach so that life-threatening problems are rapidly identified and managed simultaneously.

6 It is important to provide early psychological support to other family members who arrive with the child with major injuries.

7 The team leader needs to co-ordinate the resuscitation of the child multi-system trauma, so that patient care is at all times expeditious and tailored to the specific and prioritised needs of the child.

PREVALENCE

Overall trauma is the number three cause of mortality (6%) and serious morbidity. However, trauma is the number one cause of death and disability between the ages 1 and 44. Therefore it is the prime cause of death and serious injury throughout childhood – rendering it the most important health issue in children and adolescents. In most Western societies road trauma contributes about half (50%) of all serious injuries and deaths, with drowning incidents contributing up to 25%. The third major cause is burns and the remainder include a range of miscellaneous causes. In most series, child abuse contributes less than 10% of all child deaths.

This chapter concentrates on those aspects of trauma management that are different in children. Overall paediatric surgeons and paediatricians have taken a holistic view of trauma and have been heavily involved in aspects of prevention, succinct treatment and rehabilitation.

PREVENTION

Over the last decades, Australia has done well in reducing the death rate from approximately 11.5 deaths per hundred thousand to about 8.5[1] (World Health Organization). However, while the death rate has been almost halved, it is still double that of some of the best OECD countries. Most developed countries have significantly reduced injury death rates. Unfortunately this is not the case in underdeveloped countries. While we have achieved much through prevention strategies there is still more to be done.

Prevention has involved the work of many individuals ranging from legislators (seat belts, baby capsules, cycle helmets) through to educators and implementation groups such as 'Kidsafe'. Generally the community has been supportive of the minor inconveniences that accompany improvements in child safety.

Future progress will depend on campaigns refreshing the messages, as every few years there is a new generation of young parents and it cannot be assumed that a good campaign three to five years previously will suffice. There needs to be ongoing activity. We also need to be aware that we are promoting healthy, safe activities. This does not equate to safety above all other considerations. Our children should not be sitting in front of televisions and computer games and never going outside because that is perceived as being dangerous. Rather, by a scholarly approach we should be able to further identify problem areas that are key factors in the causation of road trauma, drowning, house fires and sporting injuries. Our children should be safely riding their cycles rather than believing that cycling is unsafe. This will require much more work by all levels of community as individuals, councils and governments. We do need to take account of children's needs for activity in playgrounds, skateboard areas, walkways and cycle paths in order to plan prevention strategies.

SUCCINCT TREATMENT (SALVAGE)

The advent of trauma teams and trauma systems in hospitals that receive paediatric patients has led to great improvements in paediatric injury care. It is estimated that there may have been a 20% decrease in mortality as a result of these systems. Prevention strategies have still resulted in most of the improvement in mortality.

Hospitals now have trauma teams ready to receive the child. This may occur by forward notification by EMS. Trauma team activation should occur on notification when a child is at high risk of life-threatening injury according to prediction by determined clinical and mechanism parameters (Table 3.1.1).

The trauma team should include a team leader, airway doctor, procedure doctor, and nursing staff from within the emergency department. Activation may involve alerting appropriate colleagues from

Table 3.1.1 Major trauma predictors at high risk of life-threatening injury	
Clinical parameters Glasgow Coma score < 13 Systolic BP < 90 Respiratory rate < 10 or > 30 **Injury** Penetrating injury to chest, abdomen, head, neck and groin Significant injury to two or more body areas Severe injury to head, neck or trunk Two or more proximal long bone fractures Burns of > 15% or to face or airway	**Mechanism** High impact trauma Fall from significant height Crash speed > 60 kph Ejection of child from MVA Rollover MVA Death of same-car occupant Pedestrian/cyclist struck at > 30 kph

Source: Adapted from Cameron P 2004 Textbook of adult emergency medicine, 2nd ed.

radiology, anaesthetics, intensive care and surgical specialities according to local resources and protocols in order to expedite emergent care. The activation process needs to be adapted to the varying local resources of the individual department, which will vary between institutions.

Regular trauma meetings to review cases or videotape evaluation of resuscitation can provide education with lessons learnt on 'how to do things better'. As major paediatric trauma is relatively uncommon, mock paediatric resuscitation scenarios can provide the emergency department staff with an opportunity to improve preparedness. There is now a good body of international literature available to keep the trauma team up to date with the optimal care of paediatric trauma victims. The use of a trauma proforma sheet may be useful for the documentation of the assessment and resuscitation of children with major injuries (see Table 3.1.1).

Clinicians often worry about managing children with major trauma and wonder how much they should treat them as an adult and how much they should take note of their differences. In adults it is well established that the *A, B, C, D, E primary survey* approach is the correct paradigm. In managing paediatric trauma clinicians sometimes get confused. They have a vague memory that 'children are different'. They are not sure therefore whether to clearly follow the A, B, C, D, E or a different approach.

The best way to remember the acute management of trauma in children is to remember the a, b, c, d, e as lower case.

That is, the sequence is exactly the same as in adults but there are additional nuances in children to optimise their care. However, more children suffer or die in the acute management of trauma by clinicians panicking and not following the A, B, C, D, E approach rather than doctors not being completely familiar with these nuances (see primary survey below). Delayed management of airway obstruction or hypovolaemia are the two most common contributors to preventable paediatric deaths in trauma. One should refer to Chapter 2 for a detailed discussion of BLS and ALS techniques in children that are applicable in trauma.

The worst response is to panic and freeze. In this situation a child may be left un-intubated, where in an adult patient intubation would be performed as a reflex decision. A child should not be left with face mask oxygen when they clearly have a Glasgow Coma Scale (GCS) of less than eight, and in an adult there would have been a rapid movement towards intubation. Similarly, intravenous lines can be difficult to insert in the shocked paediatric patient, and children may receive delayed fluid resuscitation if intraosseous access is not considered as an alternative where indicated. The supportive management of the child's family is a further important consideration in the emergency setting.

PRIMARY SURVEY

The initial assessment of the seriously injured child should follow a structured

approach so that life-threatening problems are rapidly identified and managed simultaneously. This approach is based on the prioritised principles as outlined in the teaching dictums of courses such as the Advanced Paediatric Life Support (APLS) and Advanced Trauma Life Support (ATLS) groups, which are invaluable for practitioners who deal with paediatric trauma victims.

The approach includes initially the primary survey with securing of (A) airway, (B) breathing and (C) circulation, and immediate management of life threat. The stabilization of the cervical spine occurs concurrently with airway management. Following this rapid initial stabilisation, a brief neurological assessment of the child should occur (D) and complete exposure of the patient for otherwise occult signs of injury and a prompt to consider environmental relevance such as hypothermia in a child (E).

In the team approach, the management should 'occur horizontally', with simultaneous attention to these priorities by designated members of the team, overseen by the team leader. The role of the primary survey is therefore to detect and treat abnormal physiology immediately in order to prevent potential secondary insults due to hypoxia or hypovolaemia. A secondary survey follows with a head to toe, front and back examination of the child.

PAEDIATRIC DIFFERENCES

A: Airway AND cervical spine control

In the setting of trauma, A refers to securing of the child's airway with concurrent attention to the possibility of an unstable cervical injury. The cervical spine should be immobilised using an appropriate sized hard collar, sandbags, tape and a spinal board where appropriate. It may be helpful in an infant to place a small towel under the space in the shoulder region caused by 'the elevation off the bed' by the prominent occiput at this age. As discussed in the ALS section in Chapter 2, the characteristics of the paediatric airway make it more vulnerable to obstruction. This can be exacerbated by the necessary supine positioning of the child on the resuscitation trolley. Due to comparatively higher oxygen demands and less reserve, a child will manifest hypoxic decompensation earlier than adults. This reinforces the increased importance of airway management in achieving adequate ventilation. The airway-opening manoeuvre in trauma patients should be by the jaw thrust technique to maintain cervical spine immobilisation. Suctioning of any oro-pharyngeal soiling from blood, vomit, teeth or other foreign bodies may be necessary. Adjuncts such as the placement of an oro-pharyngeal airway may be required. In children, these should be placed into the oral cavity directly, using gentle depression of the tongue with a spatula to allow for atraumatic positioning. Naso-pharyngeal airways are not recommended due to the potential presence of cribriform plate fractures, and trauma to the turbinates may cause bleeding that may further complicate airway patency.

The indications for intubation in children with major trauma are no different than those in adults. Thus, definitive airway intervention should occur in the child who is apnoeic (usually coma related), has persistent airway obstruction despite the above manoeuvres, is requiring bag-mask ventilation to achieve oxygenation, has respiratory insufficiency from major chest injury, has significant ongoing bleeding due to facial trauma compromising the airway or has high risk of subsequent compromise such as from an airway burn.

The technique of intubation should be rapid sequence with cricoid pressure. The control of the cervical spine during intubation should occur by manual immobilisation by a dedicated assistant. The patient should have continuous monitoring, pre-oxygenation and difficult airway adjuncts available, if required. The choice and dosage of the sedation agent (thiopental, midazolam, or fentanyl, for example) may be individualised according to factors such as the level of coma, cardiovascular status of the child and the presence of other injuries. A rapidly and short acting muscle relaxant such as suxamethonium usually provides the most optimal intubation conditions, despite the potential for transient increase in intra-cranial and intraocular pressures with fasciculation. Children less than two years of age are prone to significant bradycardia on laryngoscopy, which may be blunted by the administration of atropine, prior to intubation. Confirmation of correct ETT placement should occur according to the methods described in Chapter 2. One needs to be prepared for the possibility of the difficult airway or failed intubation and have a planned algorithm to deal with this possibility (see Chapter 2.3 on ALS). It is not the failed intubation that causes the problem, but the lack of a plan of action to alternatively oxygenate the patient in this situation, whilst summoning assistance.

B: Breathing AND high-flow oxygen

All children with severe trauma should receive high-flow oxygen (10–15 L min^{-1}) by a reservoir face mask, independent of the need determined by saturation monitoring. Inadequate spontaneous ventilation is supported by bag and mask assistance. As discussed above, if this need is ongoing, intubation is required. At this stage, a rapid screen for life threats, such as a tension pneumothorax, should occur. This may require immediate decompression by needle aspiration for the child in extremis and a subsequent formal chest drain, as described in the section on chest trauma. The possibility of developing tension due to a pneumothorax should be borne in mind as one of the potential precipitants of rapid deterioration following initiation of positive pressure ventilation.

C: Circulation AND stop haemorrhage

It is important to be aware that a child may be profoundly shocked from blood loss resulting from trauma well before the occurrence of hypotension. A child will respond to hypovolaemia by tachycardia and increase in peripheral vascular resistance. Therefore, the assessment of circulation status needs to be focused on the heart rate, pulse volume and the parameters of skin perfusion such as capillary refill time, colour and temperature. Perfusion inadequacy should be proactively corrected with volume resuscitation, rather than waiting for hypotension as an indicator for the need for filling. Hypotension occurs late due to cardiac decompensation and indicates that a child is nearing collapse. Likewise, bradycardia is often a prelude to imminent arrest. The persistence of tachycardia in the child with trauma should prompt concern and evaluation for occult ongoing blood loss.

The child with major trauma requires urgent intravenous access with the largest practical cannulae into visible or palpable peripheral veins. In the shocked child, cephalic, femoral or great saphenous veins are usually the most accessible. Where vascular cannulation is unsuccessful, after 60–90 seconds, the child who requires immediate fluids or drugs to facilitate intubation, should have a rapid intraosseous needle placed as described in Chapter 23.11. This is clearly the second line method that should be used in children without hesitation, rather than cutdown techniques that may be applicable in adults. In certain circumstances, such as the small child backed over by a motor vehicle with obvious major abdominal, pelvic or lower limb trauma it may be prudent to use additional alternative access into a vein that drains into the SVC (e.g. external jugular or subclavian). In this rare situation, lower limb intraosseous infused volume may not access the circulation effectively due to the injury's disruption of the normal continuity of the intraosseous and intravascular spaces.

The fluid resuscitation should initially be with crystalloid or colloid titrated to clinical response. Boluses of 20 mL kg^{-1} should be given using pressure infusion. In the hypotensive child who arrives in extremis the early use of uncross-matched O negative blood may be indicated. Otherwise, after two boluses of crystalloid or equivalent has been infused, ongoing hypovolaemia should be with cross-matched blood replacement. Whole blood or packed cells should be given in boluses of 20 and 10 mL kg^{-1} respectively. Fluids should be warmed in order to reduce the incidence of hypothermic stress complicating the resuscitation. The child with ongoing cardiovascular instability needs urgent surgical intervention.

Part of the circulation phase of management includes therapy to limit ongoing blood losses from external or fracture sites by direct pressure or splinting. This is of vital importance as a child's blood volume is only 80 mL kg^{-1} and small ongoing losses will contribute to the haemodynamic instability.

Although in major trauma the most likely cause of shock is blood loss, one needs to consider other possible contributors such as myocardial injury, pericardial tamponade, spinal shock or tension pneumothorax.

D: Disability

The most rapid way to assess a child's conscious level in the primary survey is by using the AVPU scale (see Table 3.2.2).

A child who scores a non-purposeful P or U correlates with a GCS of eight or less and requires intubation and ventilation. The brief neurological assessment during the primary survey is completed by checking equality of pupil size and reactivity to light.

E: Exposure and environment

The child should be undressed fully to allow examination of the entire body in order to detect all external stigmata of injury. Once this is completed, the child should then be covered by warm blankets. The potential for hypothermia can also be decreased by the use of radiant heaters and warm resuscitation fluids.

OTHER ISSUES DURING INITIAL STABILISATION

1. Early analgesia

Children who have significant pain or distress need to have prompt provision of analgesia as soon as intravenous access is obtained. This is usually best achieved by titrating intravenous morphine in doses of 0.1–0.2 mg kg^{-1} to effect. Adequate analgesia allows a more rapid and reliable clinical assessment.

2. Continuous monitoring

This should include heart rate, blood pressure, respiratory rate, oxygen saturations and clinical assessment of perfusion.

3. Support of family members

It is important to provide early psychological support to other family members who arrive with the child with major injuries. This should occur via a senior member of the team assisted by a nurse or social worker who is dedicated to this role. Non-comatose children are often fearful and distressed and it is useful to have the parents available to provide comfort to them.

SECONDARY SURVEY

The secondary survey follows when initial resuscitation has stabilised the child from immediate life threats. Continuous monitoring of vital signs and neurological status is paramount, as any deterioration should prompt immediate discontinuing of this phase of the assessment and return to the primary survey. The secondary survey should include:

❶ **History** – from ambulance staff, parents and child where possible.
A: Allergies
M: Medications
P: Past history
L: Last ate
E: Event – in order to clarify mechanism of trauma and potential for injury.

❷ **Head to toe, front and back examination** – the child should have a methodical and thorough clinical examination to identify all injuries. The head, face, neck, chest, abdomen, pelvis, spine and extremities (see orthopaedic trauma below) need to be examined. A more formal neurological assessment using a paediatric Glasgow coma score. The spinal immobilisation needs to be maintained until clinical or radiological clearance, in cases where this is possible. During this phase, placement of an oro-gastric tube may occur if gastric decompression is indicated. A urinary catheter (with the standard precautions of a potential urethral injury) is indicated in the unconscious child or where the accurate measurement of urine flow is required.

❸ **Investigations** – the appropriate bloods should be sent on initial intravenous access, along with a bedside glucose measurement. In the multiply injured child, initial radiological films should include a resuscitation room CXR, lateral cervical spine and pelvis. A 12-lead ECG should be done where a child has sustained significant trauma to the chest.

Definitive care and disposition

After the secondary survey and reassessment of the child's physiological response to resuscitation, the next step is to prioritise injuries to determine the need and timing of further imaging or any surgical intervention. The general rule is if the child remains hypotensive despite a $\frac{1}{2}$ blood volume resuscitation over the first 1 to 4 hours, the child needs surgery. Persistent fluid and blood resuscitation can quickly cause a coagulapathic state. It may be necessary to involve multiple surgical specialists depending on the child's injuries and the approach will vary according to local resources. The team leader needs to co-ordinate these inputs so that patient care is at all times expeditious and tailored to the specific and prioritised needs of the child. In the non-paediatric tertiary environment, early liaison with appropriate colleagues from a trauma centre with the capacity for definitive care of a child with major injuries, will help determine the most appropriate means for the individual child optimally to reach definitive care. Transfer of a child to definitive care is discussed in Chapter 27.

Care in paediatric hospitals often results in a lower rate of non-therapeutic laparotomies. The skill of the paediatric surgical trauma team is often in deciding when not to operate. Repeated examinations often identify the child who is continuing to bleed and highlight the child who may have a hollow viscus injury. Patterns of injury, such as with seat-belt bruises, are often recognised and are able to be put in the context of the child's overall physiology. The optimal care of an injured child is in a paediatric institution where there is familiarity with children and a sufficient volume of work to maintain that. The care of the child throughout the hospital stay should include other important considerations such as early physiotherapy to stop limb contractures, early involvement of the rehabilitation team and schooling.

ORTHOPAEDIC TRAUMA

A discussion of specific injuries and their management is dealt with in detail in Chapter 24.

Bony injuries are common in children who have multiple trauma. Once the child is stable, the secondary survey must include assessment of all limbs, clavicles, as well as ribs, pelvis and spine. The splinting of long-bone fractures before moving the patient from the resuscitation room is important, even in the face of other serious injuries. This avoids ongoing pain and blood loss as well as further soft tissue injury to the limb.

A careful tertiary survey the following day may reveal minor bony injuries, which were not detected during the initial resuscitation phase. These injuries need to be immobilised and, if necessary, a plan made for reduction as soon as the general condition of the child allows. Once the life-threatening injuries heal, a missed displaced bony injury is a major problem for the child in the longer term.

Isolated orthopaedic trauma is one of the most common types of trauma presenting to an Emergency Department. Review of history and mechanism of injury and an overall examination is needed to exclude concurrent injury. The possibility of a non-accidental injury must also always be considered. The time of last oral intake should be documented and the child should receive nil orally until the management plan is established.

In order to avoid causing further pain to a child, much of the examination of the fracture area can be done by observation.

- Lack of spontaneous movement gives a clue to the location of a painful injury.
- Deformity or angulation, swelling and bruising, or breach of the overlying skin suggests an open fracture.

- Gently eliciting localised areas of tenderness helps direct the most efficient use of radiology to identify the site of injury. It is best to exclude non-tender regions first. A co-operative child can point to the area of maximal tenderness, whereas in a younger child the parent may be able to indicate which areas cause the child to be apprehensive.
- The function and range of motion of surrounding joints should always be checked.
- Vascular complications can be assessed by colour, perfusion and pulses of the distal limb. As pain often limits motor function, neurological assessment to test sensory components is important.
- Compartment syndrome should be looked for when a displaced fracture has significant associated swelling. In children the volar surface of the forearm is frequently the site involved. Pain on passive stretch of involved muscles is the hallmark. Distal pulses may be preserved. Neurological dysfunction often develops.

Pain relief involves first immobilising the limb with a sling, a temporary backslab or seating the child in a wheelchair or bed. The need for medication for pain relief can then be assessed. Analgesia is required before radiological investigation, so that any limb movement necessary to take the appropriate films is less distressing for the child.

Plaster immobilisation in the Emergency Department should generally involve using a backslab technique, rather than a circumferential plaster because of the potential for early limb swelling. The slab should be of sufficient strength to keep the fracture stable. Plaster of Paris strips usually require 12 layers for the upper limb and 20 layers for the lower limb. For displaced fractures an initial temporary plaster slab can reduce movement and therefore pain at the fracture site during the X-ray. The soft padding can be used to line the plaster slab, rather than winding it around the limb to reduce movement on application.

The reduction of any displaced fractures should be done with appropriate analgesia, anaesthesia and sedation, which should be administered by a second doctor. Often this is best achieved with a general anaesthetic where there is significant need for manipulation or fracture instability. The reduction of any fracture in children should be done by a doctor with the appropriate training and experience, so that multiple attempts and further injury are avoided. Complicated fractures and those in which the reduction will be hard to maintain require additional expertise.

Appropriate orthopaedic follow-up of even minor fractures in children is vital. Within 5–7 days the swelling will have subsided, the back slab will not hold the fracture, which may lose position. At that stage a circumferential plaster can usually be used. Because the child frequently falls, a change in fracture position can easily occur. A repeat X-ray at review is necessary to determine if the fracture has maintained position.

REHABILITATION

Rehabilitation should start from the time of admission and there should be early involvement of the appropriate teams. There have been major improvements in the diagnosis and care of cervical spine injuries and management of severe head injuries. There needs to be continuing work on the outcome of minor head injuries and the debilitating long-term consequences of serious long bone fractures.

Finally, the child's social situation and their own propensity to partake in risky behaviour needs to be assessed, as there is some evidence that children with injuries tend to have further future injuries. Careful assessments of the child's social history may allow appropriate interventions.

REFERENCES

1. A League Table of Child Deaths by Injury in Rich Nations. Innocenti Report Card Issue No. 2, February 2001. United Nations Children's Fund.

TRAUMA IN CHILDREN

3.2 PAEDIATRIC NEUROTRAUMA

DAVID COOKSLEY

ESSENTIALS

1 Neurotrauma is the leading cause of morbidity and mortality in paediatric trauma.

2 The prevention of secondary brain injury is the primary focus of acute medical intervention in the emergency department.

3 A careful history and examination is important to assess the significance of the injury and determine the need for further investigation or admission.

4 Head injury alone rarely causes shock, but infants and small children may become hypovolaemic due to blood loss associated with large intracranial bleeds.

5 Any child with a GCS ≤ 14, clinical evidence of a skull fracture or penetrating skull injury should have an emergent cerebral CT scan.

6 The prime role of resuscitation is to rapidly identify and correct hypoxia and hypotension in children with severe TBI, as they are significant contributors to secondary brain injury.

7 Rapid sequence oral intubation with in-line stabilisation of the cervical spine is the preferred technique for securing airway control in the head-injured child.

8 Children sent home from the emergency department following a head injury must be discharged to the care of a responsible adult who is given clear discharge instructions and a written head-injury sheet containing advice on when to seek review.

9 The family of the child with a significant head injury requires appropriate support and explanation as an important facet of care whilst in the emergency department.

INTRODUCTION

Paediatric neurotrauma is a common presenting problem in emergency medicine practice, the vast majority of cases being a result of blunt head trauma. This chapter will deal principally with paediatric head injury or, more correctly, traumatic brain injury (TBI), and spinal cord injury. Spinal injury is also covered in Chapter 24.3.

EPIDEMIOLOGY

TBI covers a spectrum of injury from trivial to lethal. It is the leading cause of morbidity and mortality in paediatric trauma.[4] The number of children admitted to hospital in a recent study indicated an annual rate in Australia of 232 per 100 000 for those aged 0–4 years, 158 per 100 000 for those aged 5–9 years and 203 per 100 000 for those aged 10–14 years.[1] These figures are higher than the overall, age standardised, annual rate of between 140 and 150 per 100 000 population.[1,2] It is important to remember that these figures only reflect hospital admissions and the true incidence of TBI in the community is much higher.[3]

In Australia the most common cause of TBI is falls, followed by motor vehicle related accidents.[1] A much smaller percentage result from being struck by objects, crushed, assaulted (non-accidental injury) and other miscellaneous causes. Males consistently outnumber females with most studies reporting approximately a 2:1 ratio for all age groups. These results are comparable to those found in overseas studies.[14–16,18,19,23,26,31]

The overall incidence of spinal cord injury in Australia for children aged 0 to 14 years is unknown.[75,76] The age standardised incidence in the 15 + year old population is 14 per million of population per year with a male to female ratio averaging 4:1, but peaking at 9:1 in the 15–24 year age group.[76]

Preventive strategies have made the most impact on the improved outcomes of paediatric trauma over the past two decades.

PATHOPHYSIOLOGY

TBI, like spinal injury, can be divided into primary and secondary trauma. Primary trauma occurs during the initial impact and only preventive measures such as using protective equipment (e.g. helmets and seatbelts), better engineering (e.g. safer roads), education and legislation can alter the extent of this injury. Secondary trauma or insult occurs when post-traumatic acute phase response and mediators, or subsequent physiologic insults, such as hypoxia, hypotension and increased intracranial pressure, occur and cause further damage to the already traumatised tissues or structures. The prevention of secondary injury, particularly due to cerebral hypoxia and reduced cerebral perfusion, is the primary focus of acute medical intervention.

Children have unique anatomical, physiological and developmental differences when compared to adults. They have a large head to body ratio leading to a high centre of gravity (falls) and to the head being the primary 'target' for trauma. The skull is thinner and more plastic and thus transmits rather than attenuates impact.[4,40] Skull fractures are therefore more common in children and equally brain injury can occur without an associated skull fracture.[13,14,24,25,32]

In children the dura is more closely adherent to the skull compared to adults making extradural haematomas less common in children, particularly in infants.[17,40] Unfused sutures and an open fontanelle can expand to accommodate intracranial haemorrhage or cerebral oedema.[17] Some authors have thought children to be more prone to 'malignant cerebral swelling' that can cause rapid and sometimes fatal deterioration even after minor TBI.[10,14,19] However, this view has recently been questioned and swelling may be no more common in children than in adults.[43]

Physiologically, children have a lower systolic and mean arterial blood pressure, which implies a lower cerebral perfusion pressure (CPP). This, in turn, may cause problems with maintaining adequate cerebral perfusion if they have raised intracranial pressure. Infants and small children may become hypovolaemic with large intracranial bleeds. This is not seen in larger children or adults.[4]

Cerebral blood flow is often very low and may approach ischaemic levels following more severe TBI.[57] This may be related to a low brain metabolic rate in comatose patients, increased intracerebral pressure and vasospasm. Autoregulation of cerebral blood flow (CBF) may be lost following TBI, and in this setting CPP largely determines CBF. This underscores the importance of maintaining an adequate CPP in the head-injured patient, especially those with more severe injuries.

Head injury, as opposed to TBI, may be described as extra-axial or intra-axial. Extra-axial injury refers to pathology outside the brain parenchyma.[40,41] Extra-axial structures include the skull, structures between the skull and brain and the ventricular spaces within the brain. Common extra-axial lesions include skull fractures and extradural, subdural, subarachnoid and intraventricular haemorrhages. Extra-dural haemorrhage occurs, as its name implies, outside the dura. Medical literature often refers to this as 'epidural haemorrhage' but in Australasia the term 'epidural' is generally used only to describe lesions outside the dura of the spinal cord. Intra-axial injuries are true TBIs and include contusion, laceration, haemorrhage and diffuse axonal injury (DAI). The later is a product of rotational-shearing forces occurring within the brain during head trauma. DAI may result in considerable disability with little to see on radiological investigation.[40]

CLASSIFICATION

The generally accepted method of classifying severity of TBI is by using the Glasgow Coma Scale (GCS), although other measures such as duration of unconsciousness or amnesia are sometimes used. The GCS was first described for adults in 1974 and scores three variables: eye opening, verbal response and motor response (see 'examination' and Table 3.2.1).[5] It has proved to be a very useful tool in rating severity of TBI and prognosis.[7]

The problem with using the GCS on young children, particularly those aged less than two years, is that the best verbal response is limited by their language development. In an attempt to overcome this difficulty, modified GCSs have been proposed, including the so-called Child Coma Scale (CCS).[6,14] It is important to note that, unlike the GCS, the CCS has never been properly validated and many studies of head injury in children deliberately exclude those aged less than two years.

TBI is usually divided into three categories: mild, moderate and severe.

Mild TBI (GCS 14 to 15)

Mild TBI, sometimes termed 'minor' TBI, was originally defined as head trauma patients with a GCS from 13 to 15 (and/or varying periods of LOC and amnesia).[9] The problem with this definition is that patients with GCS 13 have a significantly higher risk of intracranial injury, with subsequent risks for deterioration and neurosurgery, than patients with a GCS of 14 or 15. They more properly belong in the moderate head injury group.[19,21]

The original definition of GCS 13 to 15 continues to be used in international and Australasian literature but the recognised definition of mild TBI in Australasia is GCS of 14 or 15.[10] Some authors believe that even this is too liberal and the definition of mild TBI should be restricted to patients with a GCS of 15.[21,28]

Approximately 80% of children with TBI will fall into this category.[34] The reported incidence of intracranial haemorrhage (ICH) varies between 4 and 7% in children with GCS 15, and increases to

Table 3.2.1	Adult and child Glasgow Coma Scores (GCS)	
Score	Adult	Child
Eye opening		
4	Spontaneous	
3	To speech only	Same
2	To pain only	
1	No response	
Verbal		
5	Orientated in person, place and time	Happy/smiles/interacts normally
4	Confused	Crying but consolable
3	Inappropriate but intelligible speech	Inconsistently consolable
2	Incomprehensible sounds	Inconsolable and/or irritable
1	No response	No response
Motor		
6	Obeys commands	
5	Localises painful stimulus	
4	Withdraws to painful stimulus	Same
3	Flexor posturing to painful stimulus	
2	Extensor posturing to painful stimulus	
1	No response	

approximately 10% in children with GCS 14.[14,15,19,22] The overall mortality in this group is reported to be as high as 2%.[19] These figures may be subject to significant selection bias.

The terms 'minimal' or 'trivial' TBI are sometimes used to describe a subgroup of mild TBI who meet the following criteria: GCS 15, normal neurological examination and no signs of a skull fracture.[15,26,28] Transient LOC or amnesia does not exclude patients from this subgroup.

Moderate TBI (GCS 9 to 13)

Approximately 18% of children with TBI fall into this category.[34] The incidence of ICH and overall mortality in this group of children is uncertain (almost all research focuses on either mild or severe TBI).

Severe TBI (GCS 8 or less)

Approximately 2% of children with TBI fall into this category.[34] Patients in this category are, by definition, comatose. Overall mortality in this group is between 30 and 40%.[36]

ASSESSMENT

History

Careful history and examination is important when assessing the significance of the injury and determining the need for further investigation or admission.

Initial assessment and treatment may need to occur simultaneously. Ensuring an adequate airway, breathing and circulation with resuscitation as required is the first priority. The best approach is to undertake a 'primary survey' with correction of life threats, followed by a 'detailed history plus secondary survey' as for any other trauma patient. Spinal precautions using immobilisation must be maintained until clinical or radiological clearance of the spine has been completed.

Assessment of the child may be extremely difficult, if not impossible, if the child is distressed with pain or is cerebrally irritated. The early use of simple analgesia such as paracetamol 20 mg kg^{-1}, codeine 0.5 mg kg^{-1}, or a very small dose of parenteral narcotic such as morphine 0.05 mg kg^{-1} intravenously may make assessment and management much easier. Concern about masking changes in neurological function should not prevent the use of adequate analgesia for children who are distressed by pain.

The following information is relevant and should be ascertained if possible:

- Time and mechanism of the injury
- Any loss of consciousness or period of altered level of consciousness and its duration
- Any post-trauma seizure-type activity
- Any post-injury vomiting
- Any headache or other neurological symptoms such as diplopia, weakness or altered sensation
- Any retro- or anterograde amnesia
- Progression of any symptoms and signs from the time of injury
- Details of pre-hospital care assessment and therapies.

The possibility of non-accidental injury (NAI) must always be considered in children with skull fractures or intracranial injuries. Be particularly vigilant with children aged < 2 years, when a parent or carer has delayed seeking medical care or the stated mechanism is not in keeping with degree of injury observed.[32]

Past history that is particularly relevant in the context of neurotrauma is:

- Previous head or spinal injury
- Congenital CNS problems
- CNS surgery (such as the insertion of a VP shunt)
- Bleeding diatheses such as haemophilia or thrombocytopenia
- Psychomotor or developmental problems, such as autism, that make assessment particularly difficult.

It is important to remember:

- Medications, and other ingestants that may influence assessment of a head injury including possible illicit drugs or medications and chemicals to which a young child may have gained access at home
- Allergies
- Immunisation status
- Last food or fluid intake.

Examination

Check vital signs, including bedside blood sugar level, to immediately exclude:

- Hypoxia ($SaO_2 \leq 90\%$ or PaO_2 ≤ 60 mmHg)
- Hypotension (SBP $\leq$ 5th percentile for age or SBP < 90 mmHg)
- Hypoglycaemia (BSL < 3.0 mmol L^{-1}).

These reversible factors may be contributing to the child's altered level of consciousness and also cause secondary brain injury. Determine the child's weight early, either by measurement or inference, as it is necessary for calculating drug and fluid requirements.

Glasgow Coma Scale (GCS)

This should be used to define the child's level of consciousness and to monitor any change over time. Serial neurological observations should be performed regularly to monitor for deterioration or improvement in the child's conscious state. Once a child's GCS is normal and stable, the frequency of neurological observations can be decreased. It is important to note that the GCS is intended to score global function not focal deficit. When using the GCS to classify the severity of TBI, the best post-resuscitation score should be used.

If a painful stimulus is needed to test motor function, apply pressure to the supra-orbital margin to test for localisation of pain. This is superior to a 'sternal rub'. To test for withdrawal or abnormal flexion/extension, use a pen or pencil to apply pressure to finger-nail or toe-nail beds. Abnormal flexion is usually termed 'decorticate posturing' and abnormal extension termed 'decerebrate posturing' although this was discouraged in the original description of the GCS as it implied a specific physio-anatomic correlation.[5] The best score should be recorded after testing all four limbs and any discrepancy between limbs should be recorded separately.[5]

It should also be noted that it may not be possible to score verbal or motor function in some patients, for example those who are intubated (verbal score) or have a high-level spinal cord injury or limb injuries (motor score).

Table 3.2.1 allows comparison of the GCS and the CCS used by Hahn et al and others.[14,20] The CCS has never been properly validated and assessment of verbal response is somewhat subjective, particularly in children aged less than six months.[6]

A rapid assessment of a child's neurological disturbance can also be made using the AVPU scale, which denotes the child's response to stimuli (see Table 3.2.2). The child who demonstrates a non-purposeful response to pain (withdrawal, flexor or extensor responses) has a level of consciousness consistent with a GCS of < 9 and the unresponsive child, a GCS of 3.

Assess the child carefully for signs of trauma to the head, neck and thoracolumbar spine. A skull vault fracture may be suggested by scalp haematoma, crepitus or palpable depression. A basilar skull fracture should be suspected in the presence of 'racoon eyes', Battle's sign (bruising around the mastoid process), haemotympanum or CSF rhinorrhea/otorrhea. Any sign of trauma above the clavicles increases the likelihood of intracranial pathology being detected on CT scanning.[30]

A careful examination of the cranial nerves and peripheral nervous system should follow to assess for any localising signs. If spinal cord injury is suspected the sensory level of injury (dermatome) should be defined, not forgetting to check for intact perianal sensation and normal anal tone. Hypotensive bradycardia, altered perspiration below the level of the lesion, priapism and urinary retention all signify autonomic dysfunction, which may occur with spinal injury. Any sensory or motor function below the level of injury implies that the cord lesion is incomplete and denotes a better prognosis.

Table 3.2.2	AVPU scale	
A	**A**lert	
V	Responds to **V**oice	
P	Responds to **P**ain	Purposeful Non-purposeful
U	**U**nresponsive	

Pupil size, equality and reactivity, particularly in the unconscious child should be checked and recorded. A dilated pupil is defined as > 4 mm diameter, asymmetry as > 1 mm difference between pupil size and non-reactivity as < 1 mm movement when a bright light is used to test the reflex.[8] The pupillary size and reaction may be also altered by direct trauma to the globe. Fundoscopy has been regarded as an important part of the initial examination[28] but its usefulness, apart from checking for retinal haemorrhages in suspected cases of 'shaken baby syndrome', has been challenged.[33] Whenever possible, neurological examination should include an assessment of gait.

INVESTIGATIONS

Bedside
Blood sugar level
This is better thought of as a 'vital sign' than a bedside investigation, particularly in the context of an altered mental state or focal neurological deficit. It should be measured at the same time as HR, BP, RR and SaO_2.

12 lead ECG
This should be performed in the child who has associated chest trauma and considered in any patient with moderate or severe head injury, as catecholamine release from TBI can cause myocardial injury.

Laboratory
In patients with mild TBI laboratory investigations are not indicated unless there is known or suspected coexistent pathology such as haemophilia or thrombocytopenia.

In patients with moderate or severe TBI the following should be checked:

- Haemoglobin level and platelet count
- Coagulation profile including fibrin degradation products (FDPs). Tissue thromboplastin released from the brain can cause coagulopathy and disseminated intravascular coagulation, the presence of which denotes a poor prognosis[11,12]
- Electrolytes. These serve as baseline during fluid resuscitation and subsequent monitoring for hyponatraemia. Transient hypokalaemia is a well-recognised consequence of TBI and may occur even in mild cases.[13] It usually resolves spontaneously after several hours and no treatment is required
- Arterial blood gases should be considered depending upon clinical situation. In ventilated patients arterial blood gases (ABGs) should be used to confirm that the end tidal CO_2 ($ETCO_2$) accurately reflects $PaCO_2$.

Radiological
Skull X-rays
Before the widespread availability of CT scanning, skull X-rays were often used to decide which children should be observed in hospital or have a cerebral CT scan.[13,20] While it is acknowledged that children with a skull X-ray demonstrating a fracture have a higher incidence of ICH compared to those without a fracture, many children without fractures also have an ICH.[14,19,20,24,25] To compound this problem, the reported sensitivity and specificity of skull X-rays in detecting a fracture is reported to be as low as 21% and 53% respectively.[29] Also, emergency department staff nowadays often have little or no experience of interpreting skull X-rays and may be more likely to misinterpret sutures or vascular markings as fractures and visa versa.

However plain films may still have a role in helping to risk stratify very young children (age < 2) with head trauma who can be difficult to keep still for CT scanning without sedation or general anaesthetic and in those whom possible NAI is suspected.[27] Skull X-rays may also be useful in screening for depressed skull fractures or penetrating skull injury, particularly in environments where CT scanning is not readily available.

Cervical and thoracolumbar spine X-rays
These should be obtained for any child with suspected cervical or thoracolumbar trauma, or evidence of spinal cord injury, and those in whom the spine cannot be

cleared clinically. Young children (age < 10 years) are more prone to high cervical spine injuries whereas older children, like adults, are more prone to lower cervical spine injuries.[77] Spinal cord injury without radiological abnormality (SCIWORA) was thought to be principally a paediatric phenomenon but is in fact seen much more often in adults.[78]

A low threshold should be held for CT scanning any child with high clinical suspicion of spinal injury or possible radiological abnormality on plain film.

Computed tomography (CT) scan

In cases of TBI, CT scan is the modality of choice for imaging the skull for fractures and brain for acute haemorrhage, oedema, mass effect, pneumocephalus and hydrocephalus.[39,40] It is rapid, inexpensive and can accommodate a wide range of life support and monitoring equipment. Any child with a GCS ≤ 14, clinical evidence of a skull fracture or penetrating skull injury should have an emergent cerebral CT scan (Table 3.2.3; see also 'mild TBI'). The child needs to be accompanied by appropriate staff and monitoring equipment to the CT scan environment to continue optimal monitoring and rapidly manage any potential complications.

The CT is also used as the initial investigation of choice to further evaluate suspected spinal injury although it cannot exclude ligamentous injury and it provides limited information on injury to the spinal cord itself.[79,81]

Magnetic resonance imaging (MRI)

MRI is superior to CT scanning for detecting oedema, contusion and diffuse axonal injury in cases of TBI.[40] It is also superior to CT scanning for visualising the posterior fossa and brainstem. It is the investigation of choice for spinal cord injury and the actual patterns of haemorrhage and oedema within the cord carry prognostic significance.[79,80] MRI imaging of ligamentous tissues can be used to investigate possible spine instability. However, clinical correlation with MRI findings in 'mild' cases is still lacking.[80]

MANAGEMENT

1. Mild TBI (GCS 14, 15)

The management of mild TBI is controversial. The debate primarily focuses on the question of whether or not children in this group can be risk stratified and managed clinically without further investigation, or whether they need to have a cerebral CT scan regardless of clinical findings. Concern stems from the observation that even children with a GCS of 15 and a normal neurological examination can harbour clinically significant intracranial pathology with attendant risks for subsequent deterioration and death. One study of 429 children with mild TBI found that 16% of the children with GCS 15 and no LOC had significant IC injury.[35] Of these, 1.4% required neurosurgery and 2% died.

On the other hand, CT scanning involves a significant radiation dose of 2 mSv for the child (according to the UK National Radiological Protection Board, 2 mSv radiation exposure is the equivalent of one year of natural background radiation and carries a risk of 1:10 000 for developing a malignancy – for comparison a CXR gives a radiation dose of 0.03 mSv). Also, if very young, the child may require sedation or a general anaesthetic with their attendant risks of apnoea, hypoxia, aspiration and prolonged sedation.[32] In addition, the cost of scanning all children with head trauma would be considerable.

The observation has been made that the greatest benefit in treating patients with TBI is not with aggressive management of the severely injured, but in preventing deterioration and complications in those with mild or moderate injuries who appear to be at low risk.[32]

Risk factors for IC injury or deterioration, such as LOC, amnesia, headache, vomiting, seizures and focal neurological deficit have been studied in an attempt to identify those children with mild TBI who do not require a CT scan.[19,22,25,30,31,35,37,38,41,42,44] The presence of any of these risk factors increases the likelihood of intracranial pathology and it is important to note that a child can have all of them and still have a GCS of 15. In order to be widely accepted, risk stratification on clinical grounds alone would have to be close to 100% sensitive at detecting clinically significant IC pathology. Prospective studies evaluating such clinical decision rules for children are still to be completed.

The risk of developing clinically significant IC pathology following the initial trauma decreases over time. Although current Australasian guidelines for children suffering mild TBI suggest discharge after four hours of observation if the child has a GCS of 15 and is asymptomatic,[10] a large study of over 28 000 children admitted to hospital following head injury demonstrated that six hours of post-injury observation was required to identify all children who were likely to deteriorate.[45]

It has been estimated that a child with trivial head injury, who has no LOC and who is completely well (i.e. none of the

---

Table 3.2.3   Indications for CT scan

- GCS < 15
- Focal neurological deficit
- Signs of skull fracture or penetrating skull injury

STRONGLY CONSIDER IF ...
- Persistent vomiting
- History of LOC*
- Post-traumatic seizure (delayed)
- Post-traumatic amnesia
- Moderate to severe headache
- Underlying bleeding risk

*The duration LOC does not correlate well with the risk of intracranial pathology and anything greater than transient LOC (i.e. > 1 min) should be considered significant.[28,32]

above mentioned symptoms or signs) has a less than 1:5000 chance of significant IC pathology and can be discharged to the care of a responsible adult without further investigation.[28]

Based upon current knowledge, the management and disposition algorithm shown in Figure 3.2.1 is suggested.

2. Moderate and Severe TBI

These groups will be considered together. It should be noted that the best GCS after resuscitation is used for classification of the TBI, and that a child with a GCS ≤ 8 is, by definition, comatose. The priorities of management include maintenance of the airway, oxygenation and cerebral perfusion.

Airway control, oxygenation and ventilation

It is important to rapidly identify and correct hypoxia as this is a significant contributor to secondary brain injury.[46–49] Supplemental oxygen should be applied in order to maximise oxygen delivery to any ischaemic tissue and the child's SaO_2 should be monitored.

Children who are not protecting their airway or maintaining adequate ventilation should be intubated and ventilated. In general, this would include any child with a GCS ≤ 8. In-line stabilisation of the cervical spine during rapid sequence oral intubation should occur to prevent potential secondary spinal injury. Rarely, the agitated or combative child with a higher GCS may require intubation in order to facilitate imaging or to stabilise a potentially at risk cervical spine until it can be cleared.

Pharmacologic adjuncts to intubation should be used as required. However, care is required to avoid transient hypotension as this worsens neurologic outcome (see below). Lidocaine 1.5 mg kg^{-1} may be given two to three minutes prior to intubation in order to blunt the rise in ICP that occurs with pharyngo-laryngeal stimulation.[50] This offers a theoretical benefit but has not been shown to alter outcome.

The endotracheal tube should be securely fastened to the child's face with tape rather that using the standard 'tie around the neck'. This avoids the risk of impairing cerebral venous drainage and causing a consequent rise in ICP. Hard collars may also constrict the neck and therefore interfere with venous drainage, particularly when fitted incorrectly.

An oro-gastric tube should be passed to decompress the stomach. The naso–gastric route should be avoided as inadvertent intracranial placement can occur if the child has a basal skull fracture.

SaO_2 and PaO_2 are not good indicators of adequate ventilation and continuous $ETCO_2$ monitoring should occur if the child is ventilated. The child should be ventilated to maintain an $ETCO_2$ in the low–normal range (i.e. aiming for an $ETCO_2$ of 35 mmHg). Hypercarbia secondary to inadequate ventilation may result in cerebral vasodilation and secondary increase in ICP. Hypocarbia causes cerebral vasoconstriction and therefore decreases ICP, but increases the risk of causing or exacerbating cerebral hypoperfusion with secondary ischaemia.[51] Routine 'prophylactic hyperventilation' in adults has been shown to worsen outcome[52] and presumably does so in children. Therefore hyperventilation to a $PaCO_2$ of 25 mmHg should be reserved for the child who is rapidly deteriorating with signs of increased intracranial pressure or cerebral herniation, such as new onset pupil asymmetry or rapidly decreasing GCS.

Circulation

Hypotension is the single most significant factor contributing to secondary

Fig. 3.2.1   Suggested management algorithm for mild TBI.

brain insult.[46,48] Hypotension is defined as an SBP <90 mmHg in adults and a SBP <5th percentile for age in children.[46-49,53] One or more episodes of hypotension from time of injury through resuscitation at least doubles mortality and significantly increases morbidity.[46,48,53-55]

Despite studies focusing upon SBP, the true objective in the patient with TBI is to maintain an adequate CPP. This is the difference between mean arterial pressure (MAP) and intracranial pressure (ICP) [i.e. CPP = MAP − ICP]. The normal ICP is 0–10 mmHg and an ICP of 20 mmHg is generally regarded as the threshold for initiating specific therapy to reduce it. The optimal CPP is uncertain but consensus opinion recommends ≥70 mmHg.[56] In the pre-hospital and emergency department settings, the ICP is unknown so treatment is purely empirical. It is reasonable to aim for a MAP of ≥90 mmHg that would maintain a CPP ≥70 mmHg (i.e. allowing for ICPs up to 20 mmHg).

Initial resuscitation should be with dextrose-free isotonic solutions such as 0.9% saline or compound sodium lactate (Hartmann's) solution, although the use of hypertonic saline may be considered (see below). In the hypotensive patient, give a 20 mL kg^{-1} bolus (if using an isotonic crystalloid) and monitor the response. Repeat if the patient remains hypotensive. After a total of 40 mL kg^{-1} volume resuscitation, consideration should be given to the use of vasopressor support to maintain adequate MAP for cerebral perfusion. In the setting of hypovolaemia due to acute blood loss, ongoing resuscitation fluid will require blood product replacement.

Hypertonic saline

Hypertonic saline solutions have been used for initial resuscitation, as maintenance fluid and as specific treatment for raised ICP. In addition to rapidly restoring circulating volume, increasing blood pressure and reducing ICP, these solutions appear to have important and beneficial immuno-modulatory and neuro-chemical effects that may reduce secondary brain injury.[58,59]

A suggested regimen for the use of 3% saline for either initial resuscitation or to rapidly decrease ICP is to give a 5 mL kg^{-1} bolus, repeated if necessary according to patient response. It would appear that rapid changes in serum sodium concentration do not cause complications such as central pontine myelinolysis in humans, and most studies do not place an upper limit on serum sodium concentration.[58,59,60]

However, there have been no controlled trials demonstrating improved outcomes with hypertonic saline.

Mannitol

Mannitol has been used as both a resuscitation fluid (plasma expander) and as therapy for acute deterioration secondary to increasing ICP. Boluses of 0.25 g kg^{-1} to 1 g kg^{-1} body weight have been used successfully for short-term reduction of ICP and may be repeated every 4 to 6 hours.[61] Mannitol acts as an osmotic diuretic and can lead to subsequent problems with hypovolaemia and acute renal failure via acute tubular necrosis, particularly if serum osmolarity rises above 320 mOsmol L^{-1}. A loop diuretic such as furosemide is sometimes used in addition to mannitol for treatment of acute rises in ICP. A urinary catheter is essential in any patient receiving mannitol or diuretics.

Positioning

The child's head should be kept in the midline to avoid jugular venous compression. Venous drainage is improved if the head of the bed is elevated 15–30 degrees with resultant decrease in ICP. However, CPP is also reduced by this manoeuvre and there may be no net benefit unless ICP monitoring is in place and CCP adjusted as required.

Prophylactic anti-seizure therapy

Seizures that occur within seven days of a TBI are termed early post-traumatic seizures (EPTS) and those thereafter are late post-traumatic seizures (LPTS).[62] The overall incidence of seizures in children with TBI is probably between 5 and 15% but rises with increasing severity of TBI, occurring up to 40% of the time in those

with a GCS ≤8.[48,62-64] Greater than 95% of PTS are early and approximately 80% of these occur within the first 24 hours.

Seizures may cause or exacerbate secondary brain injury by increasing cerebral metabolic demands, increasing intracerebral pressure and by causing or exacerbating cerebral hypoxia.[63,64]

The incidence of EPTS can be reduced by the use of prophylactic anticonvulsants such as phenytoin. Their use is recommended[66,67] in those with:

- GCS < 10
- Seizure within 24 hours of injury
- Depressed skull fracture or penetrating head wound
- Subdural, extradural or intracerebral haematomas
- Cortical contusion.

It should be noted, however, that reduced EPTS does not translate into reduced mortality[65,67] and it remains to be seen whether or not an overall improved level of functioning occurs in those survivors given prophylactic anticonvulsant therapy. It should also be noted that prophylactic anticonvulsants do not alter the incidence of LPTS and their routine use after seven days is not recommended.[67]

The management of active seizures should be with benzodiazepines and should follow the guidelines discussed in Chapter 8.3.

Antibiotics

Intravenous antibiotic prophylaxis with flucloxacillin 25 mg kg^{-1} six-hourly should be given for compound skull fractures or fractures in communication with sinuses.

Steroids

Various steroids have been used in an attempt to improve outcome from TBI. To date no statistically significant improvements or detriment have been found, although research is still continuing in this area.[68-71]

Thermoregulation: prophylactic hypothermia and prevention of hyperthermia

Mild hypothermia (32–35°C) is known to decrease ICP and, in animal models, has been shown to be neuro-protective.[59,72,73] Outcomes in humans have been conflicting and mild hypo-thermia may increase complications such as sepsis, pneumonia and bleeding in the TBI patient.[59] Research is ongoing in this area and prophylactic hypothermia cannot be recommended at this stage.

Hyperthermia is associated with a worse outcome in children with severe TBI.[74] It is not known if actively cooling the patient alters outcome and further research needs to be conducted in this area. In the mean-time it would seem reasonable to attempt to cool a febrile brain-injured child.

SPINAL CORD INJURY

There is a great paucity of research into the optimal management of acute spinal cord injury in children. Therefore there is in-sufficient data to support diagnostic or treatment standards.[81] However, the prin-ciples of management of acute spinal cord injury are considered to be no different from TBI. The focus of therapy is to pre-vent secondary injury. Attention should be paid to the maintenance of strict spinal immobilisation, adequate oxygenation, ventilation, blood pressure and good sup-portive care as per moderate–severe TBI.

The use of high-dose steroids in acute spinal injury is controversial.[82,83] The issue is further complicated in the paediatric population by the fact that children < 13 years were excluded from the major trials of steroids for spinal cord injury.[81] If steroids are used they should be administered within eight hours of injury. Practice currently varies between insti-tutions. The recommended dosing sched-ule is: methylprednisolone 30 mg kg^{-1} bolus over 15 minutes followed by a 45-minute break, then 5.4 mg kg^{-1} hr^{-1} continuous infusion for 23 hours.[10]

SUPPORTIVE CARE

Immobilisation of children at risk of spinal injury is difficult when they are non-cooperative and needs to include the body as well as the head. Involvement of parents or carers and calming of the child are important adjuncts. Pressure area care should occur for all patients who are immobilised. Children who arrive in the emergency department on 'spinal boards' should be moved off them as soon as practical as they cause pressure areas to develop rapidly.

Hard collars should be checked for correct fit and potential pressure areas. They should be changed to padded collars such as Aspen® or Philadelphia® collars if immobilisation is needed for an extended period.

A urinary catheter should be placed in children who require volume resusci-tation, mannitol or diuretics, or who are unable to communicate their need to micturate because of TBI, or who have a spinal cord injury.

The child's temperature should be monitored and inadvertent cooling avoided (see comments on thermoregu-lation above). Children have a larger body surface to weight ratio than adults and are therefore more prone to heat loss with associated risk of hypothermia.

The child's analgesic requirements should be regularly reviewed and anal-gesia titrated as required. Small doses of parenteral narcotic given intravenously are best.

Attention should be given to eye pro-tection in children who are sedated. This is to prevent desiccation of, or accidental trauma to, the globe. The eyelids should be taped shut or an ocular lubricant used, particularly in those children who are ventilated.

FAMILY CONSIDERATIONS

There are considerable immediate stresses during the initial stabilisation phases on the parents and family of the child who has sustained neuro-trauma. The family require appropriate support and expla-nation whilst in the emergency depart-ment. If possible, it is useful to provide a dedicated staff member to be with the child's family. This person may be an experienced nurse or social worker. The family should be kept well informed of the child's status and its proposed man-agement by a designated senior medical member of the resuscitation team. Con-sideration should be given to allowing parents into the resuscitation room to be with their child (see Chapter 2.1). Explanations to the parents should be as jargon free as possible and convey the facts in language that is appropriate to the recipient. Premature or vague con-clusions of prognosis should be avoided until all relevant assessments and inves-tigations have been made. Consent for procedures should be obtained whenever possible.

DISPOSITION

The disposition for children with mild TBI has been outlined above. Children sent home from the emergency department fol-lowing a head injury must be discharged to the care of a responsible adult who is given clear discharge instructions and a written head-injury sheet containing advice on when to seek review. Simple analgesics such as paracetamol can be used for mild headache, which should be ex-pected to be short-lived. Any child with a suspected NAI should be admitted to hospital for safety and further evaluation.

All children with moderate or severe TBI or spinal cord injury should be transferred to a paediatric high depen-dency or intensive care unit for admission under the care of a neurosurgeon. The inter-hospital transfer of the child needs appropriately skilled staff and monitoring to deal with any potential complications en route.

REFERENCES

1. O'Connor P 2002 Hospitalisation due to traumatic brain injury, Australia 1997–98. Australian Institute of Health and Welfare
2. Khan F, Baguley I, Cameron D 2003 Rehabilitation after traumatic brain injury. Medical Journal of Australia 178(6): 290–295
3. Anderson V, Catroppa C, Morse S et al 2001 Outcome from mild head injury in young children: A prospective study. Journal of Clinical Experimental Neuropsychology 23(6): 705–717
4. Inaba A, Seward P 1991 An approach to paediatric trauma. Emergency Medical Clinics of North America 9(3): 523–548

5. Teasdale G, Jennett B 1974 Assessment of coma and impaired consciousness. Lancet July: 81–83
6. Simpson D, Reilly P 1982 Paediatric Coma Scale. Lancet August: 450
7. Traumatic Brain Injury Guidelines Taskforce 2000 Glasgow Coma Scale score. Journal of Neurotrauma17(6/7): 563–570
8. Traumatic Brain Injury Guidelines Taskforce 2000 Pupillary diameter and light reflex. Journal of Neurotrauma 17(6/7): 583–590
9. Mild Traumatic Brain Injury Committee of the Head Injury Interdisciplinary Special Interest Group of the American Congress of Rehabilitation Medicine 1993 Definition of mild traumatic brain injury. Journal of Head Trauma Rehabilitation 8(3): 86–87
10. Neurological Society of Australasia and Royal Australasian College of Surgeons 2002 The Management of Acute Neurotrauma in Rural and Remote Locations, 2nd ed
11. Vavilala M, Dunbar P, Rivara F et al 2001 Coagulopathy predicts poor outcome following head injury in children less than 16 years of age. Journal of Neurosurgical Anaesthetics 13(1): 13–18
12. Keller M, Fendya D, Weber T 2001 Glasgow Coma Scale predicts coagulopathy in paediatric trauma patients. Seminars in Paediatric Surgery 10(1): 12–16
13. Lazar L, Erez I, Gutermacher M et al 1997 Brain concussion produces transient hypokalaemia in children. Journal of Paediatric Surgery 32(1): 88–90
14. Hahn Y, McLone D 1993 Risk factors in the outcome of children with minor head injury. Paediatric Neurosurgery 19: 135–142
15. Davis R, Mullen N, Makela M et al 1994 Cranial computed tomography scans in children after minimal head injury with loss of consciousness. Annals of Emergency Medicine 24(4): 640–645
16. Mitchell K, Fallat M, Raque G et al 1994 Evaluation of minor head injury in children. Journal of Paediatric Surgery 29(7): 851–854
17. Moura dos Santos A, Plese J, Ciquini O Jr et al 1994 Extradural hematomas in children. Paediatric Neurosurgery 21: 50–54
18. Davis R, Hughes M, Gubler D et al 1995 The use of cranial CT scans in the triage of paediatric patients with mild head injury. Paediatrics 95(3): 345–349
19. Keskil I, Baykaner M, Ceviker N et al 1995 Assessment of mortality associated with mild head injury in the paediatric age group. Childs Nervous System 11: 467–473
20. Hahn Y, Chyung C, Bartherl M et al 1988 Head injuries in children under 36 months of age. Demography and outcome. Childs Nervous System 4: 34–40
21. Culotta V, Sementilli M, Gerold K et al 1996 Clinicopathological heterogeneity in the classification of mild head injury. Neurosurgery 38(2): 245–250
22. Schunk J, Rodgerson J, Woodward G 1996 The utility of head computed tomographic scanning in paediatric patients with normal neurologic examination in the emergency department. Paediatric Emergency Care 12(3): 160–165
23. Beattie T 1997 Minor head injury. Archives of Diseases in Childhood 77: 82–85
24. Lloyd D, Carty H, Patterson M et al 1997 Predictive value of skull radiography for intracranial injury in children with blunt head injury. Lancet 349: 821–824
25. Quayle K, Jaffe D, Kuppermann N et al 1997 Diagnostic testing for acute head injury in children: When are head computed tomography and skull X-rays indicated? Paediatrics 99: e11
26. Roddy S, Cohn S, Moller B et al 1998 Minimal head trauma in children revisited: Is routine hospitalisation required? Paediatrics 101(4): 575–577
27. Gruskin K, Schutzman S 1999 Head trauma in children younger than 2 years: Are there predictors for complications? Archives of Paediatric and Adolescent Medicine 153(1): 15–20

28. Committee on quality improvement, American Academy of Paediatrics 1999 The management of minor closed head injury in children. Paediatrics 104(6): 1407–1415
29. Homer C, Kleinman L 1999 Technical report: Minor head injury in children. Paediatrics 104(6): 1380
30. Haydel M, Preston C, Mills T et al 2000 Indications for computed tomography in patients with minor head injury. New England Journal of Medicine 343(2): 100–105
31. Mandera M, Wencel T, Bazowski et al 2000 How should we manage children after mild head injury? Children Nervous System 16: 156–160
32. Schutzman S, Greenes D 2001 Paediatric minor head trauma. Annals of Emergency Medicine 37(1): 65–64
33. Smally A 2001 Management of minor closed head injury in children. Paediatrics 107(5): 1231
34. Murgio A, Patrick P, Andrade F et al 2001 International study of emergency department care for paediatric traumatic brain injury and the role of CT scanning. Children Nervous System 17: 257–262
35. Simon B, Letourmeau P, Vitorino E et al 2001 Paediatric minor head trauma: Indications for computed tomographic scanning revisited. Journal of Trauma 51(2): 231–238
36. Johnson D, Krishnamurthy S 1998 Severe paediatric head injury: Myth, magic, and actual fact. Paediatric Neurosurgery 28: 167–172
37. Ng S, Toh E, Sherrington C 2002 Clinical predictors of abnormal computed tomography scans in paediatric head injury. Journal of Paediatric Children Health 38: 388–392
38. Batchelor J, McGuiness A 2002 A meta-analysis of GCS 15 head injured patients with loss of consciousness or post traumatic amnesia. Emergency Medicine Journal 19: 515–519
39. Schwartz D, Reisdorff E 2000 Emergency Radiology. McGraw-Hill, USA
40. Poussaint T, Moeller K 2002 Imaging of paediatric head trauma. Neuro-imaging Clinics of North America 12: 271–294
41. Ratan S, Pandey R, Ratan J 2001 Association among duration of unconsciousness, Glasgow Coma Scale, and cranial computed tomography abnormalities in head injured children. Clinical Paediatrics July: 375–378
42. Ramundo M, McKnight T, Kempf J et al 1995 Clinical predictors of computed tomographic abnormalities following paediatric traumatic brain injury. Paediatric Emergency Care 11(1): 1–4
43. Lang D, Teasdale G, MacPherson P et al 1994 Diffuse brain swelling after head injury: More often malignant in adults than children? Journal of Neurosurgery 80: 675–680
44. Dahl-Grove D, Chande V, Barnoski A 1995 Closed head injuries in children: Is hospital admission always necessary? Paediatric Emergency Care 11(2): 86–88
45. Sainsbury C, Sibert J 1984 How long do we need to observe head injuries in hospital? Archives of Diseases in Childhood 59: 856–959
46. Pigula F, Wald S, Shackford S et al 1993 The effect of hypotension and hypoxia on children with severe head injuries. Journal of Paediatric Surgery 28(3): 310–316
47. Chiaretti A, De Benedictis R, Della Corte F et al 2002 The impact of initial management on the outcome of children with severe head injury. Childs Nervous System 18: 54–60
48. Chiaretti A, Piastra M, Pulitano S et al 2002 Prognostic factors and outcome of children with severe head injury: An 8 year experience. Childs Nervous System 18: 129–136
49. Ong L, Selladurai B, Dhillon M et al 1996 The prognostic value of the Glasgow Coma Scale, hypoxia and computerised tomography in outcome prediction of paediatric head injury. Paediatric Neurosurgery 24: 285–291
50. Hamill J, Bedford R, Weaver D et al 1981 Lidocaine before endotracheal intubation:

Intravenous or laryngotracheal. Anesthesiology 55: 578–581
51. Skippen P, Seear M, Poskitt K et al 1997 Effect of hyperventilation on regional cerebral blood flow in head-injured children. Critical Care Medicine 25(8): 1402–1409
52. Traumatic Brain Injury Guidelines Taskforce 2000 Hyperventilation. Journal of Neurotrauma 17(6/7): 513–520
53. Traumatic Brain Injury Guidelines Taskforce 2000 Hypotension. Journal of Neurotrauma 17(6/7): 591–595
54. Winchell R, Simons R, Hoyt D 1996 Transient systolic hypotension. A serious problem in the management of head injury. Archives of Surgery 131: 533–539
55. Kokoska E, Smith G, Pittman T et al 1998 Early hypotension worsens neurological outcome in paediatric patients with moderately severe head trauma. Journal of Paediatric Surgery 33(2): 333–338
56. Traumatic Brain Injury Guidelines Taskforce 2000 Resuscitation of blood pressure and oxygenation. Journal of Neurotrauma 17(6/7): 471–478
57. Traumatic Brain Injury Guidelines Taskforce 2000 Guidelines for cerebral perfusion. Journal of Neurotrauma 17(6/7): 507–511
58. Doyle J, Davis D, Hoyt D 2001 The use of hypertonic saline in the treatment of traumatic brain injury. Journal of Trauma 50(2): 367–383
59. Bayr H, Clark R, Kochanek P 2003 Promising strategies to minimise secondary brain injury after head trauma. Critical Care Medicine 31(1): S112–S117
60. Peterson B, Khanna S, Fisher B et al 2000 Prolonged hypernatremia controls elevated intracranial pressure in head-injured paediatric patients. Critical Care Medicine 28(4): 1136–1143
61. Traumatic Brain Injury Guidelines Taskforce 2000 Use of mannitol. Journal of Neurotrauma 17(6/7): 521–523
62. Ong L, Dhillon M, Selladurai B et al 1996 Early post-traumatic seizures in children: Clinical and radiological aspects of injury. Journal of Paediatric Children's Health 32: 173–176
63. Ratan S, Kulshreshtha R, Pandey R 1999 Predictors of posttraumatic convulsions in head injured children. Paediatric Neurosurgery 30: 127–131
64. Chiaretti A, Benedictis R, Polidori G et al 2000 Early post-traumatic seizures in children with head injury. Childs Nervous System 16: 862–866
65. Haltiner A, Newell D, Temkin N et al 1999 Side effects and mortality associated with use of phenytoin for early posttraumatic seizure prophylaxis. Journal of Neurosurgery 91: 588–592
66. Temkin N, Dikmen S, Anderson G et al 1999 Valproate therapy for prevention of posttraumatic seizures: A randomised trial. Journal of Neurosurgery 91: 593–600
67. Traumatic Brain Injury Guidelines Taskforce 2000 Role of antiseizure prophylaxis following head injury. Journal of Neurotrauma 17(6/7): 549–553
68. Traumatic Brain Injury Guidelines Taskforce 2000 Role of steroids. Journal of Neurotrauma 17(6/7): 531–534
69. Bazarian J 2002 Corticosteroids for traumatic brain injury. Annals of Emergency Medicine 40(5): 515–517
70. Alderson P, Roberts I 2003 Corticosteroids for traumatic brain injury. Cochrane Database of Systematic Reviews 1
71. Roberts I 2003 Aminosteroids for acute traumatic brain injury. Cochrane Database of Systematic Reviews 1
72. Tokutomi T, Morimoto K, Miyagi T et al 2003 Optimal temperature for the management of severe traumatic brain injury: Effect of hypothermia on intracranial pressure, systemic and intracranial haemodynamics, and metabolism. Neurosurgery 52(1): 102–112

73. Gadkary C, Alderson P, Signorini D 2003 Therapeutic hypothermia for head injury. Cochrane Database of Systematic Reviews 1
74. Natale J, Joseph J, Helfaer M et al 2000 Early hyperthermia after traumatic brain injury in children: Risk factors, influence on length of stay, and effect on short-term neurologic status. Critical Care Medicine 28(7): 2608–2615
75. Research Centre for Injury Studies 1998 Spinal cord injury, Australia 1995/6. Australian Injury Prevention Bulletin 18
76. O'Connor 2001 December Spinal cord injury, Australia, 1999-00. Australian Institute of Health and Welfare

77. Eleraky M, Theordore N, Adams M et al 2000 Paediatric cervical spine injuries: Report of 102 cases and review of the literature. Journal of Neurosurgery (Spine 1) 92: 12–17
78. Hendey G, Wolfson A, Mower W et al 2002 Spinal cord injury without radiographic abnormality: Results of the national emergency X-ray utilization study in blunt cervical trauma. Journal of Trauma 53(1): 1–4
79. Sledge J, Dain A, Hyman J 2001 Use of magnetic resonance imaging in evaluating injuries to the paediatric thoracolumbar spine. Journal of Paediatric Orthopaedics 21(3): 288–293

80. Frank J, Lim C, Flynn J et al 2002 The efficacy of magnetic resonance imaging in paediatric cervical spine clearance. Spine 27(11): 1176–1179
81. Hadley M 2002 Management of paediatric cervical spine and spinal cord injuries. Neurosurgery 50(3): S85–S99
82. Hurlbert R 2001 The role of steroids in acute spinal cord injury: An evidence-based analysis. Spine 26(24 Supplement): S39–S46
83. Canadian Association of Emergency Physician Position Statement 2003 Steroids in acute spinal cord injury. www.caep.ca [Revised 22 January 2003]

3.3 THORACIC INJURIES IN CHILDHOOD

PHIL APLIN

ESSENTIALS

1 Thoracic injuries in children are common, are usually due to blunt trauma and are often associated with other injuries.

2 The pathophysiological differences in children depend principally on their age and size. These must be appreciated in order to optimise outcome.

3 The most common injuries are pulmonary contusions, rib fractures, pneumothoraces and haemothoraces. These can usually be managed by a combination of adequate oxygenation, IV fluids, thoracostomy tube drainage and analgesia.

4 Injuries to the aorta and diaphragm may be clinically occult and CXR findings are often non-specifically abnormal. Further diagnostic evaluation is always indicated in suspect cases.

5 Surgical intervention is indicated in cases of massive haemothorax, cardiac tamponade, major airway and oesophageal injury, as well as in aortic and diaphragmatic injuries.

6 ED thoracotomy is principally indicated in cases of penetrating chest trauma and an arrest or pre-arrest presentation.

INTRODUCTION[1-3]

Thoracic injuries in childhood are second only to head injuries as a cause of mortality. Isolated chest injuries have a mortality of around 5% but this increases substantially when combined with head and/or abdominal injury to between 25 and 40%. Injuries to the great vessels and aorta, bronchi, lung lacerations and cardiac tamponade are the chest injuries most likely to cause early death. Small children provide a small target particularly in blunt trauma, so multiple injuries should be expected. Between 70 and 80% of children with chest injuries have associated injuries of the head, abdomen or limbs.

The common mechanisms of injury vary with the age of the child. Overall, the majority (60–80%) are due to blunt trauma and are motor vehicle related. In infants and toddlers common mechanisms include:

- Injured passengers in MVAs
- Pedestrians struck or run over by a car (commonly in the driveway of the family home)
- Falls (from stairs, balconies etc).

Child abuse predominantly occurs in this age group and should be considered in all cases of trauma in children less than three years of age. School-age children are involved in MVAs as passengers, pedestrians or on bicycles. Accidents involving falls from bicycles, skateboards and other sport-related trauma are common. In teenagers, the incidence of personal/interpersonal violence increases dramatically and associated with this the incidence of penetrating trauma and self-harm. Inexperienced teenage drivers are at increased risk for MVAs.

There are a number of anatomical and physiological features of small children that must be appreciated when managing paediatric chest trauma. These are summarised in Table 3.3.1.

INITIAL MANAGEMENT[4]

Initial management follows the usual priorities. After ensuring airway patency, breathing should be assessed. High-flow oxygen should be applied. Signs of respiratory compromise and tension pneumothorax should be managed by needle decompression prior to CXR followed by chest tube insertion. A large haemothorax may compromise ventilation as well as

Table 3.3.1   Important pathophysiologic differences between children and adults in chest trauma

- Small target – multiple injuries common
- Narrow airway – prone to obstruction
- Anterior larynx – difficult intubation
- Increased surface area – increased risk of hypothermia
- Increased oxygen consumption, diaphragmatic breathing, low functional residual capacity – prone to hypoxia
- Increased pliability of ribs – decreased incidence of rib fractures
- Response to blood loss – hypotension is a late sign of shock
- Developmental considerations - paediatric coma scoring

Table 3.3.2   Indications for operative intervention in chest trauma

- Great vessel injury
- Pericardial tamponade
- Large haemothoraces
- Tracheobronchial injuries
- Oesophageal injury
- Diaphragmatic lacerations
- Open pneumothorax with major chest wall defect
- Penetrating chest trauma that crosses the mediastinum

Once stabilised thoracic CT scan may be indicated to further delineate the extent of pulmonary injury, evaluate the great vessels and detect pneumothoraces.
Analgesia should be initiated early in appropriate doses.

circulation requiring early chest tube placement and fluid resuscitation, whilst an oro–gastric tube (OGT) should be placed early to decompress the stomach as gastric distension may compromise ventilation. Mechanical ventilation should be instituted for signs of ongoing respiratory distress/respiratory failure not relieved by optimisation of oxygen delivery, chest tube insertion, closure of open chest wounds and OGT placement. Ongoing signs of circulatory compromise without evidence of blood loss should raise the possibility of cardiac tamponade and myocardial contusion in a child with chest injuries. A portable CXR should be the first radiological test ordered. FAST (focused abdominal scan in trauma) scanning should occur early in the resuscitation of a child, where available, and imaging of the pericardium always be included to detect haemopericardium. Drainage of the pericardium may occasionally be performed in the ED in an unstable patient if operative

intervention is not immediately available. Other indications for operative intervention are listed in Table 3.3.2.

CHEST WALL INJURY[5]

Rib fractures

The elasticity and flexibility of the younger child's chest wall leads to a lower incidence of rib fractures. Significant underlying intrathoracic injury can occur in the absence of rib fractures. In the 0 to 3 year age group rib fractures should raise the concern of abuse, in one study $\frac{2}{3}$ of 0–3 year olds with rib fractures were victims of abuse, and a careful assessment of all aspects of the clinical presentation is mandatory. Radiological findings suggestive of abuse include: multiple fractures, fractures of varying ages and bilateral fractures. A bone scan is a more accurate test in the setting of potential abuse.

Rib fractures in children are a marker of potential severe associated injuries. Multiple rib fractures (> 1) increase the risk severe intrathoracic injury, multiple injuries and mortality. Fracture of the first rib requires significant force mandating a high degree of suspicion of associated injuries to the great vessels and the trachea.

Flail chest injuries are rare in children and clearly indicate serious injury with reduced ventilatory effectiveness and associated lung contusions contributing to the significant potential for respiratory failure. Assisted ventilation is indicated for those with respiratory failure despite optimal non-invasive ventilation and analgesia or associated injuries, particularly to the head.

Management of rib fractures involves analgesia, treatment of associated intrathoracic injuries, assessment and ongoing

monitoring of the child's respiratory status and further evaluation for complications that may arise. Analgesia is important to reduce the pain with breathing and the consequences of hypoventilation, poor cough and immobility such as atelectasis and secondary infection. Adequate analgesia is best titrated intravenously in the ED.

PULMONARY INJURY[6,7]

Contusion

In children it is important to appreciate that significant lung injury can occur in the absence of rib fractures or other external signs of chest wall injury. Pulmonary contusion most commonly results from blunt injury and requires significant force. Pathological findings are intra-alveolar haemorrhage, consolidation and oedema causing V/Q mismatch, reduced lung compliance and subsequent hypoxaemia. CXR findings of increased pulmonary opacity are usually present in the ED but may evolve over time. CT scanning of the thorax may reveal contusion that is not evident on the initial plain films. Approximately half of the CXRs showing pulmonary contusion show other abnormalities, most commonly fractured ribs and pneumo/haemothoraces.

Management of pulmonary contusion involves:

❶ Maintenance of oxygenation. Supplemental O_2 is initially delivered by high flow mask (10–15 L min^{-1}). Persisting hypoxaemia requires non-invasive or invasive ventilatory support depending on severity and associated injuries.
❷ Pain relief should be provided as indicated.
❸ Excessive intravenous fluids should be avoided.
❹ Respiratory physiotherapy is useful.

Both ARDS and pneumonia may complicate pulmonary contusion.

Pneumothorax[3,8]

Traumatic pneumothoraces vary in their size and clinical significance. They occur in about $\frac{1}{3}$ of children with significant thoracic trauma and $\frac{2}{3}$ have associated injury. All pneumothoraces should be considered as having the potential to cause cardiorespiratory compromise. The clinical signs of pneumothorax (PTX) vary from nothing to decreased air entry, hyperresonance and subcutaneous emphysema.

A small asymptomatic pneumothorax may not be visible on a supine CXR. Subtle signs include increased radiolucency on the ipsilateral side and a deep sulcus sign. They are commonly revealed on CT scan of the chest and/or abdomen. The significance and hence management of these small pneumothoraces is debated. A small uncomplicated PTX in a stable patient with isolated chest trauma, who is not likely to require positive pressure ventilation or prolonged transport (particularly aeromedical), can be considered for observation, high-flow O_2 and analgesia in a HDU setting. Most other traumatic pneumothoraces require insertion of a chest drain.

Tension pneumothorax

This is a clinical condition resulting from increasing intrathoracic pressure, lung collapse and mediastinal shift with subsequent decreased venous return and cardiovascular collapse. The diagnosis is clinical and treatment should precede radiology in clear-cut cases. Signs are of ↓AE, hyperresonance and hyperexpansion plus ↓ movement of the affected side. The signs of tracheal deviation and elevation of the JVP maybe difficult to detect in children who have short necks. JVP elevation may also be absent if there is associated hypovolaemia. Patients are always tachypnoeic with respiratory distress and tachycardia, but hypotension is a late sign if solely due to a tension PTX. Immediate needle decompression with a 16G cannula inserted into the 2nd intercostal space in the mid clavicular line should occur whilst preparing for a formal intercostal tube insertion via a lateral approach.

However, hypotension and/or hypoxaemia may have other causes in the traumatised child. The differential diagnosis of a tension PTX includes: haemorrhage; pericardial tamponade; haemothorax (which may cause tension); pulmonary contusion; and air embolism. Common benign causes that may occasionally be confused with a tension PTX are intubation of the right mainstem bronchus and gastric distension. Endotracheal tubes must be inserted the appropriate distance (age/2 + 12 cm) and movement of the child's neck minimised. This is particularly so in small children where neck flexion (tube pulled out) or extension (tube down the [R] main bronchus) may result in the malposition of the ETT. An oro-gastric tube should be placed early.

Open pneumothoraces may occur with penetrating chest trauma. Respiratory compromise relates to the effects of the PTX, underlying lung injury and a sucking chest wound if the defect is large enough. If the diameter of the chest wound is approximately $\frac{2}{3}$ or greater that of the trachea air will preferentially be sucked into the chest on inspiration leading to acute severe respiratory compromise. Management requires urgent wound coverage on three sides only with an occlusive dressing, to prevent the development of an iatrogenic tension PTX, and chest tube placement away from the wound. Once the chest drain is in place the wound can be sealed and arrangements made for definitive surgical care. Significant ongoing respiratory distress is an indication for mechanical ventilation.

Pulmonary lacerations[4]

Pulmonary lacerations are principally caused by penetrating injuries but can occur with blunt mechanisms especially associated with rib fractures. They usually result in a haemothorax (sometimes massive) or PTX and rarely can be complicated by air embolism. Air embolism typically occurs after the initiation of positive pressure ventilation and causes sudden haemodynamic deterioration ± focal neurological signs. Development of a tension PTX, pericardial tamponade or massive haemothorax are the main differentials.

In the setting of deterioration after initiation of ventilation, by far the most likely cause is the development of tension PTX, which should be managed as above. In the rare event of air embolism, if suspected, management includes 100% oxygen, and reduction of the ventilation pressures. Emergency thoracotomy with clamping of the hilum on the affected side and aspiration of ventricular air has occasionally been life saving.

Haemothorax[8,9]

Clinically relevant haemothoraces occur in about 15% of cases of blunt chest trauma. The source of bleeding is most commonly from lacerations to the lung, intercostal or internal mammary vessels or occasionally from mediastinal vessel injury (often fatal). Each hemithorax can hold up to 40% of a child's blood volume.

The clinical presentation is of varying degrees of hypovolaemia and respiratory compromise depending on the amount of blood lost into the chest, associated pneumothorax and the development of increased intrathoracic pressure. Chest examination reveals reduced air entry and dullness to percussion ± signs of tension. Management is via a chest drain. Drainage of massive haemothoraces may precipitate further bleeding as the tamponade effect is removed.

Ongoing blood loss via the drain, haemodynamic response to resuscitation, mechanism of injury (blunt vs. penetrating) and associated injuries (especially head) are used by cardiothoracic surgeons in determining the need for thoracotomy.

Indications for thoracotomy include:

- Initial drainage exceeding > 15 mL kg^{-1} of estimated blood volume
- Continued bleeding greater than 1–2 mL kg^{-1} h^{-1}
- Increasing bleeding
- Significant residual haemothorax post drainage.

Management involves oxygenation and ventilatory support if indicated, urgent chest tube placement of the appropriate size via the lateral approach directed posteriorly and volume resuscitation. The concept of hypovolaemic resuscitation in uncontrolled traumatic haemorrhage has not been evaluated in children.

However, it is important to consider early surgical intervention in any patient who is haemodynamically compromised due to haemorrhage or showing signs of on-going bleeding.

Longer-term complications of haemo-thoraces include haematoma organis-ation with secondary lung entrapment and empyema formation. Prophylactic antibiotics are indicated when chest tubes are placed for penetrating trauma. The literature suggests a reduced infec-tion rate even in previously closed trau-matic haemothoraces requiring drainage.

TRACHEOBRONCHIAL INJURIES[9]

These uncommon injuries may occur with penetrating or severe blunt trauma and have a high mortality if not recog-nised and treated rapidly. In blunt trauma intrathoracic airway injuries usually occur near the origin of the main stem bronchi. Typically they present with respiratory distress and signs of subcuta-neous (SC) emphysema and a tension PTX. Haemoptysis also occurs. Urgent chest tube placement is required and shows a large ongoing air leak and failure of lung expansion on CXR. At this point an airway injury is usually considered. A second chest tube should be placed and urgent cardiothoracic surgical consul-tation obtained. Once stabilised a CT scan may be helpful in further injury delineation and assessing lung inflation as massive SC emphysema can make CXR interpretation very difficult. Bronchoscopy is useful as a diagnostic modality in suspected tracheobronchial injury and operative intervention is often required.

MEDIASTINAL INJURY[4,8,9]

Aortic transection

Aortic rupture is a rare event in young children but the incidence increases with adolescents involved in high speed MVAs. About 80% occur at the aortic isthmus just distal to the origin of the left subclavian artery. Most are rapidly fatal at the scene. Diagnosis in hospital depends on clinical suspicion based on

Table 3.3.3 CXR signs of aortic injury

- Widened mediastinum (mediastinum to chest ratio > 0.25)
- Loss or abnormal contour of aortic knob
- Depression of left mainstem bronchus
- Deviation of the trachea to the right
- Deviation of the oesophagus (NG or OG tube) to the right
- Left pleural cap
- Left haemothorax
- Upper rib fractures

mechanism of injury, physical signs (often absent) and CXR findings. CXR in cases of aortic rupture are usually abnor-mal but findings are non-specific (see Table 3.3.3) and the suspicion of aortic injury on clinical or radiological grounds requires further diagnostic imaging.

In young children the normal thymic contour may give the impression of a widened mediastinum. Further imaging may include CT angiography, aortogram or transoesophageal echocardiography depending on availability, expertise and local practices. Absence of a mediastinal haematoma on CT angiography has been used to exclude aortic injury. The evidence for this approach in children is lacking.

Management in confirmed cases is surgical. β-blockers may be commenced preoperatively in haemodynamically stable patients to reduce vessel wall stress.

CARDIAC INJURIES[10]

As with aortic injury clinically significant cardiac injury from blunt trauma in chil-dren is uncommon and is usually associ-ated with other intrathoracic injuries. Pericardial tamponade can certainly occur with blunt trauma, though it is more common in penetrating injuries (see below). Myocardial contusion may mani-fest as an arrhythmia or otherwise unex-plained tachycardia and/or hypotension. Valvular injury and septal defects are also reported. Diagnosis suffers from the lack of a gold standard and the questionable clinical relevance of test results. Most of the evidence comes from adult trauma patients. A normal ECG has a high nega-tive predictive value for the occurrence of clinically significant complications in

suspected myocardial contusion. Evidence for the value of cardiac markers is lacking. Echocardiography is a very useful mo-dality in assessing suspected clinically sig-nificant myocardial contusion such as the presence of unexplained hypotension, tachycardia or new murmurs.

In the absence of ECG abnormalities, hypotension or new murmurs, ongoing ECG monitoring is not required.

Commotio cordis[11,12]

The phenomenon of sudden cardiac arrest following a localised blow to the chest is well documented in children. In these cases autopsy fails to identify myocardial contusion, structural cardiac abnormality, conduction system or coronary artery pathology. The proposed theory is that a blow to the chest during the vulnerable phase of the electrical cycle induces VF/VT. Protective chest guards are recommended in at-risk sports.

Penetrating cardiac trauma[13]

In children this occurs predominantly in the adolescent age group. Cardiac lacer-ations may lead to rapid exsanguination or pericardial tamponade. Any penetrating chest or upper abdominal wounds have the potential to injure the heart. Clinical signs of tamponade include tachycardia and elevation of the JVP (in the absence of hypovolaemia), with subsequent hypo-tension and cardiac arrest with pulseless electrical activity. The CXR is typically normal in the absence of associated mediastinal or lung injury. Echocardio-graphy has excellent accuracy in the detection of pericardial blood and can be done rapidly in the ED. Management requires urgent cardiothoracic surgical involvement. A conscious patient with a perfusing blood pressure requires urgent surgery. A rapidly deteriorating patient in the ED requires needle pericardio-centesis if there is any surgical delay. Cardiac arrest with vital signs present at the scene and a short transit time to hos-pital or arrest in the ED is an indication for ED thoracotomy or pericardiocen-tesis depending on the skills of personnel available. Pericardiocentesis is performed using a long 16 or 18G over the needle cannula via the subxiphoid approach at a

35 degree angle to the skin and aiming at the left shoulder with ECG monitoring. Ultrasound control may assist where available. Aspiration of 10–20 mL may result in significant clinical improvements. The needle should be removed but the catheter remain in place for repeat aspirations. Failure to aspirate blood does not exclude tamponade as the cannula may miss the pericardium or the pericardial blood may have clotted.

DIAPHRAGMATIC INJURY[8,9,14]

Diaphragmatic injury is another uncommon paediatric injury, but it is important nonetheless, as if undiagnosed, complications eventually will arise, though this may take years. Left-sided injury is more common than right-sided in blunt trauma and associated intra-abdominal injury is common.

Upper abdominal penetrating trauma that injures intrathoracic structures (and visa versa) must also have caused diaphragmatic injury and requires repair. Diagnosis is difficult unless CXR reveals clear signs of herniated stomach or bowel or the NG tube curling up into the thorax. More commonly the CXR is non-specifically abnormal with findings of an abnormal diaphragmatic contour ± lower zone opacity. Often the diagnosis is made at laparatomy or laparoscopy for associated injuries. Barium studies are normal if bowel contents are not herniated. CT scanning may miss small tears whilst MRI has greater accuracy. Suspected occult diaphragmatic lacerations in penetrating trauma can be investigated by laparoscopy/thoracoscopy or open operation.

Oesophageal injury[4]

This is essentially only seen in penetrating trauma and in these cases a high index of suspicion is required as missed injuries cause inevitable serious morbidity and mortality. On initial CXR a finding of mediastinal air is an early clue. Over subsequent hours an evolving sepsis with left plural effusion and mediastinitis ensue. Conscious patients able to verbalise complain of chest and epigastric pain but this is difficult to interpret in the setting of other chest injuries. Suspicion of an oesophageal injury must be followed by a gastrograffin study, oesophagoscopy or both. If positive, broad spectrum antibiotics and urgent surgery are required.

ED THORACOTOMY[13]

The only definite indication for thoracotomy in the ED is in the scenario of penetrating chest trauma with loss of vital signs shortly before arrival in the ED or during ED resuscitation, with the purpose of pericardial drainage, repairing penetrating injury to the heart or controlling bleeding from the hilum or lung. Open cardiac massage can also be performed as well as cross-clamping of the aorta. The universally poor outcome of blunt trauma patients who arrive at the ED with no vital signs/signs of life argues strongly against performing ED thoractomy in these patients. Blunt thoracic trauma patients who deteriorate in the ED despite full resuscitation may occasionally survive following ED thoracotomy but in general these very unstable patients should go to the operating theatre if possible.

REFERENCES

1. Peclet MH, Newman KD, Eichelberger MR et al 1990 Thoracic trauma in children: An indicator of increased mortality. Journal of Paediatric Surgery 25: 961–965
2. Black TL, Snyder CL, Miller JP et al 1996 Significance of chest trauma in children. Southern Medical Journal 89: 494–496
3. Nakayama DK, Ramenofsky ML, Rowe MI 1989 Chest injuries in children. Annals of Surgery 210: 770–775
4. Fleisher GR, Ludwig S 2000 Textbook of paediatric emergency medicine, 4th edn. Lipincott Williams and Wilkins, Philadelphia 1341–1360
5. Garcia VF, Gotschall CS, Eichelberger MR et al 1990 Rib fractures in children: A marker of severe trauma. Journal of Trauma 30: 695–700
6. Bonadio WA, Hellmich T 1989 Post-traumatic pulmonary contusion in children. Annals of Emergency Medicine 18: 1050–1052
7. Allen GS, Cox CS, Moore FA et al 1997 Pulmonary contusion: Are children different? Journal of American College of Surgeons 185: 229–233
8. Bliss D, Silen M 2002 Paediatric thoracic trauma. Critical Care Medicine 30: 1–13
9. Wesson DE 1998 Thoracic injuries. In O'Neill JA (ed) Paediatric surgery, 5th edn. Mosby, St Louis, 245–260
10. Dowd MD, Krug S 1996 Pediatric blunt cardiac injury: Epidemiology, clinical features and diagnosis. Journal of Trauma 40: 1–12
11. Cantor RM, Leaming JM 1998 Evaluation and management of pediatric major trauma. Emergency Medicine Clinics of North America 16: 229–256
12. Maron BJ 1995 Blunt impact to the chest leading to sudden cardiac death from cardiac arrest during sports activities. New England Journal of Medicine 333: 337–342
13. Polhgeers A, Ruddy RM 1995 An update on pediatric trauma. Emergency Medicine Clinics of North America 12: 267–287
14. Jackimczyk K 1993 Blunt chest trauma. Emergency Medicine Clinics of North America 11: 81–91

3.4 ABDOMINAL AND PELVIC TRAUMA

SCOTT PEARSON

ESSENTIALS

1 Children may have significant internal injury with little evidence of external trauma. The abdominal viscera are less well protected by the musculature and rib cage.

2 Meticulous assessment and reassessment will detect subtle abdominal injuries and a change in physiological status due to blood loss.

3 Persistent tachycardia may be the only clue of intra-abdominal haemorrhage in the child without other overt source of bleeding.

4 Unrecognised abdominal trauma is an important cause of preventable trauma deaths in children.

5 Selective non-operative management of solid visceral injuries is common but requires institutional support and may necessitate transfer of the child to a regional centre.

6 Pelvic fractures are a marker of severe injury, and there is a strong association with head, abdominal, and chest trauma.

7 The treatment of children with significant abdominal or pelvic trauma requires a planned team approach and early liaison with a paediatric surgeon and paediatric tertiary centre.

8 CT scan is the investigation of choice in stable children with abdominal trauma in consultation with a paediatric surgeon.

INTRODUCTION

Well over 90% of abdominal injuries in children are the result of blunt trauma. While penetrating injuries are increasing in incidence in the adolescent population, this remains an unusual phenomenon in most Australasian communities. When they do occur, there is a higher likelihood of injury to hollow viscera. Abdominal injuries resulting from blunt trauma commonly affect the solid organs, particularly the liver and spleen. Overall mortality is generally < 5%, but obviously this depends on injury mechanism.[1] In children with multi-trauma, the subtle early clinical findings of intra-abdominal injury may be masked by change in conscious state, and chest and limb injuries, and requires repeated abdominal examination.

There are unique characteristics of children that predispose them to intra-abdominal injuries. The rib cage does not extend as far distally as in the adult, the ribs are more compliant, and the abdominal wall and musculature frequently thinner and less protective. Consequently, the upper abdominal viscera are more at risk of injury, and relatively minor forces can be transmitted, resulting in a serious disrupting injury.[2]

The bladder is not as well protected by the bony pelvis as in the adult, increasing the risk of bladder injury in lower abdominal trauma. Gaseous distension of the stomach from air swallowing during crying or bag–valve–mask ventilation occurs rapidly and can impair ventilation.[3] Likewise, acute gastric dilatation or a large bladder can also seriously impede one's clinical assessment of the abdomen. It is worth noting that the very compliant body of the child is capable of absorbing considerable amounts of kinetic energy without external signs, yet be associated with significant internal derangement.[2]

Early surgical involvement in treating children with abdominal injury is vital to care in the emergency department. The child with multiple injuries requires senior experienced clinicians involved in decision making during the resuscitation. Because such a patient will invariably mean several specialties may be involved, a trauma team approach, with clear leadership of the resuscitation, is imperative.

HISTORY

Obtaining details of the exact mechanism of injury cannot be over-emphasised. This will often give a clue to the potential injury pattern. Information can be obtained from possible or actual witnesses, ambulance officers, family, friends, or care-givers. One member of the trauma team should be delegated to obtain this information, so that primary survey can occur simultaneously.

Mechanisms of injury in children include pedestrians struck by motor vehicles, falls, occupants of motor vehicles involved in crashes, bicycle-related injuries, contact sports, assaults, and abuse. Information such as the aspect of the child when struck and likely speed of vehicles is useful in predicting injury patterns. Likewise, factors such as the use of restraint devices, type used, and wearing of a bicycle helmet, where appropriate, are helpful in defining the resulting injuries. Lap belts can be associated with rib and lumbar spine fractures, and upper abdominal organ injuries. With a fall mechanism, the events leading to the fall, and fall height and surface are all pertinent information that can usually be obtained rapidly. Handlebar injuries may cause serious blunt intra-abdominal injuries. The resultant injuries to pancreas and duodenum can be subtle and delay diagnosis. Hence the threshold for observation or imaging may need to be varied accordingly in children presenting with this mechanism of injury.

Small children are particularly at risk of being unsighted and backed over in driveways, and receive major internal injuries. The recognition of abuse as a causal mechanism in younger children and infants is important to consider in paediatric patients with abdominal trauma. There may be minimal signs of external injury, and the reported history may suggest a minor incompatible mechanism or no history of injury at all. The emergency physician needs to maintain an index of suspicion in the infant who presents in shock or with an altered level of consciousness (see Chapter 3.2).

Other information, such as medications, allergies, and significant past history, should be obtained.

EXAMINATION

Primary survey will focus on the ABCs and may result in early interventions such as intubation or treatment of shock. The examination of the abdomen is usually delayed until the secondary survey. Where endotracheal intubation has already occurred, this invariably involves chemical sedation and paralysis. The information obtained by palpation of the abdomen in this situation is somewhat limited, and these children will require a CT scan of the abdomen where there is a possibility of intra-abdominal injury.

Vital signs are essential, particularly the respiratory rate, pulse rate, non-invasive blood pressure, and oxygen saturations. Attention should be given to the child's peripheral perfusion to detect hypovolaemia and treat prior to the occurrence of hypotension. The blood pressure needs to be measured with an appropriately sized cuff for the child's habitus. The width of the cuff should be approximately two-thirds of the length of the upper arm. Automated blood pressure machines, while useful in freeing staff to attend to other aspects of care, can be unreliable when hypotension exists and can result in delays in obtaining these recordings. Single vital sign recordings are of limited use, but it is the progression of recordings and the monitoring of perfusion that more accurately reflect volaemic state. In the critically ill child, pulse and blood pressure should be measured at 3–5-minute intervals.

The use of the terms *unstable* and *stable* is discouraged when conveying information regarding the child's status to colleagues. They are non-specific and are defined differently by individual practitioners. It is more useful, when relaying the circulatory status of a child, to convey the vital signs, progression over time, and response to fluid to indicate volaemic state. Other parameters, such as capillary refill time, have some limitations but can add to the assessment.

In children with less severe trauma, the technique of abdominal examination is important to reliably exclude significant intra-abdominal injury clinically. Where physical examination is to be relied on as the major indicator of abdominal injury, it should ideally be performed regularly by the same observer. With serial examination and vigilance to vital signs, changes are detected early and appropriate management implemented. The aim of the abdomen examination is to exclude any physical signs, such as tenderness, rebound, guarding, or rigidity, which will require evaluation by a CT scan.

Pain from injuries and other distress will all add to the difficulty of abdominal assessment. Judicious and early use of parenteral opiates is safe, will decrease a child's distress, and will allow a more accurate clinical assessment. Abdominal examination must be performed by gentle palpation with warm hands. There should be a brief but careful visual assessment of the abdominal wall for the distribution of any penetrating wounds, bruising, or marks (e.g. seat belt or handlebar).

Gastric dilatation may greatly impede examination as well as impair ventilation. Insertion of a nasogastric tube will help facilitate examination by decompressing the stomach, while also reducing the risk of aspiration and improving diaphragmatic excursion. Aspiration of blood from the nasogastric tube usually signifies the presence of a significant intra-abdominal injury. A persistently distended abdomen after nasogastric tube insertion may signify intra-abdominal bleeding.

Eliciting rebound tenderness should be modified in young children because, when positive, it invariably causes pain and distress for the child. This can make further assessment more difficult. The same information can usually be obtained by gentle palpation with occasional use of percussion tenderness. This technique is acceptable in children with minor trauma who have careful re-examination. Auscultation of the abdomen has limited usefulness. Rectal and vaginal examinations are rarely indicated in the child with minor abdominal trauma and then should be performed once, usually under a general anaesthetic. Indications for rectal examination include:

- assessment of rectal tone if possibility of spinal injury
- checking for gastrointestinal blood and prostate position.

In the child with only minor injuries, the way the child moves around the emergency trolley or walks can be a useful screening tool as to whether intra-abdominal injury exists.

INVESTIGATIONS

Pathology

Blood should be taken for group and hold, full blood examination (FBE), liver function tests, amylase, and blood glucose.

Elevated liver transaminase levels are a reliable indicator of hepatic injury. Both aspartate aminotransferase (AST) and alanine aminotransferase (ALT) rise soon after the hepatic injury and are usually raised at the time of initial evaluation in the emergency department. In the context of pancreatic injury, serum amylase often rises, but the initial amylase may be normal with increasing values over 3 days.[4]

Focused assessment by sonography for trauma (FAST)

Ultrasound has been promoted as a quick and effective initial screening tool in the evaluation of the abdomen in the traumatised child.[5–8] Ultrasound in this setting is aimed at the detection of free fluid in the peritoneal cavity. No attempt is made during this rapid assessment to identify solid visceral injury. This examination takes between 3 and 5 minutes, and can be achieved at the bedside in the resuscitation area. While there is much supportive literature for this modality,[5–7] there is also some cautionary research.[8] Detractors cite concerns of low sensitivities in the detection of free fluid; however, several studies have documented sensitivities from 89 to 100%. Providing the limitations of FAST are appreciated, it remains an invaluable tool, particularly in the assessment of the multiply injured child. Identification of free fluid in the stable child with normal vital signs should be followed by CT examination. The detection of free fluid in the child with deteriorating vital signs supports the decision for operative treatment. FAST ultrasound is operator-dependent and should be performed only by clinicians with appropriate training and credentialing.

CT Scan

This is the investigation of choice in stable children with abdominal trauma in consultation with a paediatric surgeon. With the evolution and common acceptance of non-operative management of blunt abdominal injuries, diagnostic imaging is an essential component of the assessment process of the injured child. CT has emerged as the gold standard.[9] It will identify free intra-abdominal fluid, solid visceral injury and the injury configuration, and loops of bowel, and will demonstrate free peritoneal gas. The retroperitoneum is well visualised. CT examination should be performed after the administration of intravenous contrast. This enables better visualisation, although in situations of renal hypoperfusion renal failure can be precipitated, and allergy to the contrast is a rare but potentially serious problem.

The use of oral contrast is more controversial. Some authors suggest oral contrast is essential, particularly to optimise the ability to detect evidence of hollow viscus injury.[1] Oral contrast will assist identification of bowel on CT but, in the presence of ileus, the contrast may reach only the proximal portion of the gastrointestinal tract. There are also issues of administration of oral contrast to an injured (often supine) child, risks

of emesis and aspiration, and delayed CT. There is little place for oral contrast in the resuscitative phase.

Formal ultrasound

Formal ultrasound has been supplanted in many institutions by FAST. A detailed upper and lower abdominal ultrasound examination takes longer to perform and is more observer-dependent than CT examination. Abdominal distension caused by ileus and luminal distension, and the presence of abdominal tenderness in the child, can make ultrasound examination more difficult. Hence there is little role for ultrasound in the definitive diagnosis of abdominal trauma, except when CT scan is unavailable. There is no advantage over CT, apart from availability.

Diagnostic peritoneal lavage (DPL)

The indications for DPL in children are rare. The decision to perform this should be made by the paediatric surgeon caring for the child. The procedure is technically more challenging in children, and intra-peritoneal organs and retroperitoneal structures can easily be injured. The child with stable vital signs and abdominal tenderness will be evaluated by repeated clinical examination, CT, or ultrasound. The child who has deteriorating vital signs, and no response or only transient response to fluid therapy represents more of a dilemma. Decisions must be made with the paediatric surgeon in attendance. If there is no evidence of bleeding elsewhere, then the decision for laparotomy may be clear. In the situation of associated pelvic injury, DPL – unreliable in this situation – may be useful in determining rapidly whether laparotomy or angiography and embolisation is the preferred option. This is an uncommon situation in the paediatric setting. FAST ultrasound, in experienced hands, can deliver the same information and has superseded DPL in this situation (when available). In the child with free fluid on CT, but no evidence of solid visceral injury, and a mechanism consistent with hollow viscus injury, DPL may have a place. Once again, this is the domain of the paediatric surgeon, as lavage fluid

can be irritating for the peritoneum for 48 hours and make reassessment by clinical examination or CT difficult.[10]

GENERAL MANAGEMENT

The assessment begins with primary survey and any life-saving interventions, while historical details are obtained simultaneously. Oxygen should be administered and vital signs monitored regularly. Vascular access is obtained early and appropriate blood samples for blood cross-matching, haematology, and biochemistry. Where there is delay in obtaining venous access, intraosseous access remains an effective method of resuscitation. Trauma series films of chest, pelvis, and lateral cervical spine should be obtained, when indicated, during the resuscitation. Views of thoracic and lumbar spine may also be required if indicated on mechanism or clinical findings.

The abdominal examination is usually reserved until the secondary survey. Attention should be exercised to ensure that the child is warm to prevent the development of hypothermia during resuscitation.

Fluid therapy should begin with 20 ml kg^{-1} of warmed crystalloid (normal saline) and repeated if required. If further fluid therapy is required after two crystalloid boluses, blood should be used in volumes of 10 ml kg^{-1}. The rapidity of blood loss may rarely dictate the use of O-negative or group-specific blood rather than wait for full cross-matched blood.

Early consideration of gastric decompression with a nasogastric tube will assist abdominal assessment and aid ventilation. The insertion of a urinary catheter may be necessary, depending on the requirement to aid haemodynamic monitoring of fluid resuscitation and to detect haematuria. Perineal haematoma and blood at the external urethral meatus are contraindications to routine catheter insertion and mandate retrograde urethrogram or cystogram to assess the urethral integrity. In this situation, the opinion of surgical colleagues should be sought.

FAST ultrasound, when available, can be performed, often within the first

20 minutes of the patient's arrival, and may or may not show evidence of free fluid. Ongoing management is usually dictated by the haemodynamic response of the child to fluid resuscitation. CT examination is ideal but may not be possible in a very small number of exsanguinating children with deteriorating vital signs despite fluid resuscitation. In this situation, decision making requires early surgical consultation regarding urgent laparotomy.

SURGICAL ISSUES

Selective non-operative management of solid visceral injury in children is now well established. It is clear that bleeding from an injured spleen, liver, or kidney is generally self-limiting.[11] Success rates in excess of 90% with non-operative care mean that operative management is an exceptional event at many institutions. Pancreatic injuries, however, usually result in a higher incidence of operative intervention. Operative management is the rule for hollow viscus injuries. Some injuries, such as duodenal haematoma without evidence of perforation, may be managed without surgery. The decision about operative versus conservative is made by the surgeon who will have ongoing care of the child. Obviously, this decision is strongly influenced by clear details regarding progression of vital signs, response to fluid therapy, and associated injuries. A non-operative approach must take place in an institution with an available surgeon with a commitment to the injured child and dedicated paediatric intensive care or high-dependency facility.[11] This may necessitate the transfer of the child to a regional centre.

PENETRATING TRAUMA

Penetrating abdominal injury in a child usually requires exploration by laparoscopy or laparotomy. Because the abdominal wall is often thinner than in adults, penetration into the peritoneal cavity occurs more readily. A careful assessment, including a log roll for back examination, to exclude other injuries is necessary. Gunshot wounds should be explored in theatre. The approach to initial resuscitation is identical to that for blunt trauma. An erect chest X-ray or lateral decubitus film will help to identify the presence of free air.

PELVIC FRACTURES

A child who sustains a fractured pelvis has been exposed to severe trauma. These are uncommon injuries in children, occurring at half the frequency as in adults.[12] There are several major differences in the bony pelvis between the child and adolescent or the adult. There is greater elasticity in the sacroiliac joints and pubic symphysis, and plasticity of the bone, in the paediatric pelvis, therefore greater amounts of kinetic energy must be involved to cause fracture. Avulsion fractures occur in children and adolescents because cartilage is weaker than bone. This occurs at the physis. Greater laxity of the joints in the paediatric pelvis means that single fractures occur more commonly, as opposed to the adult pelvis, where there is the double-break concept. Fractures occurring through epiphyseal and apophyseal growth centres may result in growth arrest, leg length discrepancy, and deformity. Children also have increased capacity for remodelling because of the immature bony pelvis.[13]

The common mechanisms for pelvic fracture are motor vehicle accidents and motor vehicle–pedestrian collisions, followed by falls.[13,14]

There are several classification systems for pelvic fractures. None are ideal. Torode and Zeig described four groups of pelvic fracture but failed to include isolated acetabular fractures.[15] This has been modified by Silber et al,[13] and this represents a useful classification by mechanism of injury and description (Table 3.4.1).

Associated injuries increase in frequency with the increasing severity of fracture type. Other skeletal injuries are common, followed by head, abdominal, and pulmonary injuries. In one large series, 19% of the total group had visceral injures. Therefore, when a pelvic fracture is identified on initial X-ray, a thorough search for other injuries must be undertaken. The management of those other injuries would usually take priority over the pelvic fracture management.

Bladder injury, while more common than in the adult, is an infrequent association. In a review of 166 children with pelvic fractures, there was one urethral disruption and two bladder contusions.[13] There is a strong association of these injuries with straddle-type mechanism. Children commonly receive 'fall astride' injuries related to playground equipment or while riding bicycles.

In Silber's series, 97% of children were treated non-operatively.[13] The majority of these injuries (63%) were type 3 fractures. The remainder were type 2 (17%)

Table 3.4.1 Classification of paediatric pelvic fractures

Type	Mechanism	Description
1	Avulsion	Separation through or adjacent to an apophysis
2	Lateral compression	Iliac wing fractures
3	Anteroposterior compression (usually)	Simple ring fractures: • isolated pubic rami fractures • disruption of the pubis symphysis without disruption of the sacroiliac joint • isolated acetabular fractures
4	Anteroposterior compression (usually)	Ring disruption fractures: • fracture (or diastasis) of both anterior and posterior structures • pelvic fracture with an acetabular fracture • straddle fracture: bilateral superior and inferior pubic rami fractures

Originally described by Torode and Zeig[15] and modified by Silber et al.[12]

and type 4 fractures (17%). In this series, six children died; all these deaths were due to associated injuries. The mortality rate from paediatric pelvic fractures is consistently less than 6% in recent studies.[12] In a study comparing paediatric and adult fractures, the mortality rate for children was 5.7% compared with 17.5 % in the adult group.[12] Vascular injury and exsanguination in children is rare, in contrast to in adults. This is thought to be due to the greater skeletal flexibility and the greater ability of paediatric arteries to constrict after injury.

In those children in whom blood loss is significant, early involvement of an orthopaedic surgeon and interventional radiologist is essential to optimise management. External fixation and angiography have both been used successfully, particularly in adolescent children.

DISPOSITION

Almost all children with a significant abdominal or pelvic injury will require admission from the emergency department. The nature and severity of the injuries and intended management will determine the most appropriate location for this to occur. Surgical colleagues involved in the ongoing care of the child will need input into this decision.

Younger children who have experienced a significant mechanism of injury (e.g. fall from great height, high-velocity motor vehicle crashes, pedestrian hit, or run over by motor vehicle) but who are apparently injury-free or have only minor injuries should also be admitted for observation (for 12–24 hours). Abdominal injuries in young children may initially have minimal or subtle signs, which

CONTROVERSIES

❶ The necessity to use double contrast for CT abdominal examinations. IV contrast is required, but the need for oral contrast is unclear.

❷ Defining the haemodynamically unstable child. When in doubt, discuss the child with an emergency or surgical colleague. Children can be profoundly hypovolaemic with normal vital signs or only a mild tachycardia. Ongoing fluid requirements and indices of peripheral perfusion are important indicators of volaemic status.

❸ The acceptance of FAST ultrasound. While there are strong advocates, the place of this modality in the paediatric trauma patient is less well defined than in the adult population. In the future, it is likely that FAST ultrasound will become an integral part of the early assessment of the paediatric patient with blunt abdominal trauma.

become more apparent after observation and serial examination. Because of the plasticity of the paediatric skeleton, significant internal derangement can occur without obvious external evidence of trauma.

In the older child, however, it may be appropriate to discharge the patient who is injury-free or has only minor injuries. This should occur after several assessments while in the emergency department and with arrangements for follow-up with a medical practitioner within 24 hours.

Parents should be instructed to return earlier should a child's symptoms change. In general, children with ongoing abdominal pain after trauma should not be discharged, regardless of negative imaging results.

REFERENCES

1. Stafford PW, Blinman TA, Nance ML 2002 Practical points in evaluation and resuscitation of the injured child. Surgical Clinics of North America 82: 273–301
2. Tepas JJ 2003 Paediatric trauma. In: Moore EE, Mattox KL, Feliciano DV (eds) Trauma, 4th edn. McGraw-Hill Education, New York, 1075–1098
3. Rouse TM, Eichelberger MR 1992 Trends in pediatric trauma management. Surgical Clinics of North America 72: 1347–1364
4. Sjovall A, Hirsh K 1997 Blunt abdominal trauma in children: Risks of nonoperative treatment. Journal of Pediatric Surgery 32: 1169–1174
5. Akgur FM, Aktug T, Olguner M et al 1997 Prospective study investigating routine usage of ultrasonography as the initial diagnostic modality for the evaluation of children sustaining blunt abdominal trauma. Journal of Trauma 42: 626–628
6. Thourani VH, Pettitt BJ, Schmidt JA et al 1998 Validation of surgeon-performed emergency abdominal ultrasonography in pediatric trauma patients. Journal of Pediatric Surgery 33: 322–328
7. Corbett SW, Andrews HG, Baker EM et al 2000 ED evaluation of the pediatric trauma patient by ultrasonography. American Journal of Emergency Medicine 18: 244–249
8. Coley BD, Mutabagani KH, Martin LC et al 2000 Focused abdominal sonography for trauma (FAST) in children with blunt trauma. Journal of Trauma 48: 902–906
9. Tepas JJ 1993 Blunt abdominal trauma in children. Current Opinion in Pediatrics 5: 317
10. Advanced Life Support Group 2001 Advanced Paediatric Life Support Manual, 3rd edn. BMJ Books, London
11. American College of Surgeons Committee on Trauma 1997 Advanced Trauma Life Support Student Manual, 6th edn. ACS, Chicago
12. Ismail N, Bellemare JF, Mollitt DL et al 1996 Death from pelvic fracture: Children are different. Journal of Pediatric Surgery 31: 82–85
13. Silber JS, Flynn JM, Koffler KM et al 2001 Analysis of the cause, classification and associated injuries of 166 consecutive pediatric pelvic fractures. Journal of Pediatric Surgery 21: 446–450
14. McIntyre RC, Bensard DD, Moore EE et al 1993 Pelvic fracture geometry predicts risk of life threatening haemorrhage in children. Journal of Trauma 35: 423–429
15. Torode I, Zeig D 1985 Pelvic fractures in children. Journal of Pediatric Surgery 5: 76–84

3.5 BURNS

PETER BARNETT

ESSENTIALS

1 Burns are one of the leading causes of death in children in Australia.

2 In the emergency department setting, the definitive assessment of the 'depth' of the burn may be difficult, as the appearance can evolve during the first 24 hours.

3 The calculated amount of fluid (burn-deficient plus maintenance) to be replaced in 24 hours is only a guide and should be adjusted according to the child's haemodynamic response.

4 Children with major or complicated burns should be treated in a paediatric burns unit.

5 One needs to consider non-accidental injury if the presentation is delayed or if the history given is inconsistent with the burn sustained.

6 Electrical injuries are more commonly seen in two age groups: toddlers within the home setting and male adolescents involved in risk-taking behaviour. High-voltage exposures have a more serious outcome, as they are more likely to be associated with injury to internal structures.

INTRODUCTION

Burns sustained by children are a common presentation to emergency departments and often cause significant distress to both the child and the parents. Burns are one of the leading causes of death in children in Australia. The mortality is increased in younger children. Deaths are generally related to flame burns, which may be complicated by inhalation of smoke and other toxic gases (e.g. in house fires). Early fatalities are related to respiratory complications, whereas late deaths are usually related to infection. The use of early debridement and skin grafting has led to an increased survival rate in patients who would have previously died because of infection.

Most burns are fortunately less serious, resulting mainly from scalds caused by hot liquids. This commonly occurs in pre–school-aged children due to their inquisitive nature precipitating accidents in the home. Flame burns occur in older children often experimenting with inflammables. Chemical and electrical burns are uncommon. One must be alert to the possibility of burns presenting as a manifestation of non-accidental injury in a young child.

Several preventive strategies can help decrease the risk and degree of burns sustained, especially with thermal burns. Lowering the temperature of hot water heaters to a maximum of 50°C significantly increases the contact time needed to produce deep or full-thickness burns. Flame-resistant clothing and smoke detectors in homes have saved many lives. Spill-proof mugs, guards around wood fire stoves, and child-resistant taps have all been shown to prevent burns. Further prevention strategies will have a far bigger impact on burns than advances in burn management.

PATHOPHYSIOLOGY

The skin is the largest organ in the body, and its functions include:

- preventing heat loss to the environment, thus regulating the body's temperature
- preserving body fluids by preventing water loss from the body
- acting as a barrier to infective organisms.

Therefore children with extensive burns have difficulty retaining fluid and regulating temperature, and are at risk of infection.

The skin is composed of two main layers.

❶ Epidermis: composed of stratified squamous epithelium, which is largely non-viable. It acts as the barrier to infectious agents as well as preventing fluid loss from the body.

❷ Dermis: contains the epithelial adnexal structures, for example hair follicles, sweat glands, and neural receptors for pain and pressure. It also contains blood vessels, which contribute to temperature regulation of the body via radiant heat loss.

After a burn, injury to the deeper specialised epithelial cells prompts a change into stratified squamous epithelium. These cells proliferate, gradually covering the burn with a non-epithelial barrier. Therefore, if the dermal structures are damaged, skin grafting is the only means to cover the skin. When these deeper layers are involved, scarring results and contractures may occur.

The depth of the burn will depend on the temperature of the substance in contact with the skin, the length of time the substance is in contact with the skin, and the extent of subsequent cooling of the burned skin area. Hypothermia due to cooling occurs quickly in children due to their higher surface area to weight ratio, compared with in adults. Also, children have thinner skin, which leads to deeper burns for a given contact temperature and duration.

CLASSIFICATION

Burns are generally classified into superficial, partial thickness, or full thickness. Previous nomenclature (first, second, and third degree) has been replaced to give a more accurate description of the burn. In the emergency department setting, the definitive assessment of the 'depth' of the burn may be difficult, as the appearance can evolve during the first 24 hours. Likewise, often the burn is not uniform in depth, and it may take time for it to become clear on the depth and therefore the definitive management. Superficial and partial-thickness burns are the most common burns seen in children.

Superficial

Superficial burns generally involve only the epidermal layer. These are commonly seen resulting from sunburn or minor scalds. Blistering does not occur immediately but may over the next few days. The pain and swelling generally last only a few days. The skin is erythematous and blanches normally. The epidermis will often peel within 3–7 days and is completely healed by 7–10 days without scarring.

Partial thickness

Partial-thickness burns occur when the whole epidermis is involved and part of the dermis. The more the dermis is involved, the increased scarring that will occur with healing.

Superficial partial-thickness burns involve the papillary layer of the dermis and are characterised by erythema with blistering. The blisters may remain intact and later burst due to an external pressure. The skin underlying the blister has a pink or red colour and moist appearance. These burns are extremely painful, as the nerve endings are exposed. The deeper the burn, the slower the healing process. Generally, superficial partial-thickness burns heal in 2–3 weeks.

Deep partial-thickness burns involve the reticular layer of the dermis. They may be less painful than their more superficial counterpart, due to oedema lessening the exposure of the nerve endings. They are a paler colour with a speckled appearance due to thrombosed superficial vessels. The skin is non-blanching. It may initially be difficult to distinguish between full- and deep partial-thickness burns. Deep partial-thickness burns generally heal after 3–6 weeks.

Scarring is common, and skin grafting is sometimes necessary.

Full thickness

Full-thickness burns generally occur after flame burns or after prolonged contact with a hot surface. Other causes include hot oil, prolonged immersion, or chemical burns. They involve the epidermis and all the dermis, including epidermal appendages. They have either a dry, hard, white, leathery appearance or may be black in colour. They usually have no sensation because the nerve endings have been destroyed, and pain is due to more superficial burns on the edge of the full-thickness burn. Full-thickness burns are able to heal only from skin regrowth from the edge of the burn, which causes scarring. Therefore most will require skin grafting.

All significant burns will become colonised with bacteria. Heat causes coagulation of tissue, which leads to oedema and non-viable skin. This will potentially become a rich source of nourishment for bacteria. Adequate debridement is required to reduce the risk of infection. Infection will increase the depth of skin damage and thus the degree of scarring.

The location of the burn is also important regarding potential scarring, contracture, and caring for the acute burn. Facial, hand, foot, and perineal burns may be difficult to dress. Hence the part of the body involved by the burn will influence whether in-patient or specialist care is required.

HISTORY

The history is generally obtained from the parent to clarify events. Ambulance officers may have important additional information. It is important to know the substance and estimated temperature of the substance that caused the burn (e.g. hot cup of tea, cooking oil, flame), and the duration of contact with skin (e.g. was the patient clothed at the time, in what, and for how long?).

With flame burns, was the patient trapped in an enclosed space, therefore at risk of inhalation problems, or was there any loss of consciousness? These features may suggest inhalation issues such as carbon monoxide poisoning. The historical information may determine the potential for associated injuries resulting from falls or explosions.

One needs to consider non-accidental injury if the presentation is delayed or where the history given is inconsistent with the burn sustained. Past medical history and immunisation status, particularly for tetanus, should also be obtained (see Chapter 1.1).

EXAMINATION

Note that children who are distressed may require the provision of immediate appropriate analgesia at the outset to aid examination.

Primary survey

The initial assessment of the child should be directed to the presence of any features to suggest potential airway involvement. These include singed nasal hairs or eyebrow hairs, oral or facial burns, coughing up carbonaceous sputum, barking cough, altered voice, stridor, wheeze, or respiratory distress. Airway compromise (upper or lower) may have an insidious onset, so frequent re-examination of the child is vital during the first 12–24 hours. If stridor or hoarse voice is present, this indicates upper airway involvement, and early intubation is required prior to evolving oedema causing total airway obstruction. Delayed intubation in this setting can be increasingly hazardous due to distortion of the normal laryngeal anatomy. Scalds to the face rarely cause airway compromise.

The circulation status should be assessed next. Hypovolaemia resulting from third-space fluid loss will not occur for a few hours after a severe burn. Therefore, if early-onset cardiovascular instability is present, then an alternative explanation, such as bleeding, should be sought. The peripheral perfusion of limbs should be assessed where circumferential burns are apparent. Comparing the pulse wave forms of various digits on the limb using a saturation oximeter may assist this in questionable instances.

Evaluation of burn area

The extent and depth of the burn should be assessed after the patient has been stabilised. This is usually done from a body chart (see Fig. 3.51, p. 87), which can be useful to aid documentation of the burns. This chart is used because the surface area involved will alter depending on the age of the child and the parts of the body the burn is located. A simple method, using the palmar surface of the child's hand, can also be used to estimate the area of burn. This correlates to approximately 1% of the child's total surface area. The adult formula using the 'rule of nines' can be used in adolescents older than 15 years.

INVESTIGATIONS

Patients who require intravenous resuscitation should have a baseline full blood count, electrolytes, creatinine and urea, and blood group and hold performed. In severe burns, replacement with blood, protein, and electrolyte may be necessary. Carboxyhaemoglobin levels should be obtained in patients with inhalation burns and extrapolated to the time of injury. A level of > 15% on arrival in emergency suggests significant smoke inhalation. Urine output should be monitored in severe burns, both to guide adequacy of resuscitation and also to screen for presence of myoglobin.

Oxygen saturation monitoring and arterial blood gases (when indicated) will aid clinical assessment of respiratory involvement. A chest X-ray should also be obtained if inhalation burns are suspected. However, inhalation burns will often evolve over time, and the initial film can be normal. The early appearance of X-ray changes generally indicates a more severe pulmonary injury.

MANAGEMENT

Pre-hospital

The main aims of pre-hospital care are stabilising ABCs, preventing ongoing burn injury, provision of analgesia, covering the area involved, and rapid transfer to an emergency department.

The first priority in any burn is to assess and stabilise the airway and breathing. Oxygen should be administered where there is suspected carbon monoxide poisoning with inhalation burns. Circulation is generally not a problem in the first hour after a major burn, and rapid transport to hospital should occur. If transfer time is greater than 1 hour, and the burn is greater than 20%, then intravenous fluid replacement should begin en route where possible.

The burns should be covered with water-soaked sterile cloth. Excessive cooling of major burns will cause hypothermia and worsen the patient's outcome. Recently sustained minor burns should be cooled under running water. This acts to minimise the extent of the burn and also affords some pain relief.

Analgesia is generally required early, and a single dose of parenteral narcotic (e.g. morphine 1–2 mg kg^{-1} IM) is a good choice in burns less than 20%. Greater than 20%, then intravenous access should be obtained and morphine titrated to the patient's pain.

If electrical injury has been sustained, then cardiac monitoring should occur during transfer. Patients with chemical burns should undergo extensive washing of the affected area before transport.

Emergency department

The initial priority should focus on stabilisation of airway, breathing, and circulation, with concurrent provision of analgesia. If airway burns are suspected, then early intubation should be considered, as previously discussed. Patients with obvious stridor due to upper airway compromise require urgent intubation. Supplemental oxygen should be instituted and oxygen saturation monitored.

Other potential indications for ventilation in major burns include:

- Extensive burns (> 60–70%) to decrease the patient's work of breathing.
- Full-thickness circumferential chest burns, which may compromise chest expansion.

- Severe inhalational lung injury causing pulmonary oedema and hypoxaemia. Inhalation burns will generally get worse in the first 12–24 hours, and ventilation may be needed during any of this time frame. Early consultation with paediatric intensive care colleagues in these instances is appropriate.

Assessment of circulation includes pulse rate, blood pressure, and peripheral perfusion of limbs. The fluid losses due to the burn itself do not cause early circulatory failure, and other contributing injuries should be sought in the patient with early shock. It is also important to note the time the patient is evaluated, relative to the time of the burn. Children who have delay (e.g. a few hours) in presentation may arrive with circulatory compromise from skin fluid losses.

Intravenous access should be placed in all children with burns body surface area (BSA) of > 20%. Fluid resuscitation rates should be calculated using the time of the burn, not the time of presenting to the emergency department (see *Fluid resuscitation* below). Peripheral venous access, preferably through non-burnt skin, is preferred over central venous access for the initial resuscitation. Monitoring of urinary output (via urinary catheter, weighing nappies) is important in determining the adequacy of fluid replacement. A nasogastric tube should also be inserted in children with severe burns, as gastric dilatation can occur, leading to respiratory compromise.

Analgesia should be given early, during the stabilisation of the A, B, and C. In severe burns, a morphine infusion should be started after adequate initial intravenous analgesia has been titrated. Large doses of narcotics are sometimes needed in severe burns to control the patient's pain. Using intramuscular morphine is less reliable, due to variable absorption, in patients in shock or with burns > 20%.

A careful secondary survey should then be undertaken, looking at the extent, depth, and anatomical relevance of the burns. It is important to determine if there are any circumferential burns to limbs and chest. In superficial or partial-thickness burns, careful monitoring of circulation or ventilatory compromise is required. In full-thickness circumferential burns, an urgent escharotomy may be required to restore circulation to the limb or allow for adequate ventilation. A paediatric burn specialist should be consulted in this situation.

The secondary survey should also include careful examination for any other injuries requiring attention (e.g. head, neck, chest, limbs, pelvis, intra-abdominal). Burns to the face should also include examination, with fluorescein staining of the eyes to check for corneal involvement.

Fluid resuscitation

Fluid resuscitation should be calculated based on the weight of the child and the total surface area of the burn. Several formulas are used to calculate the resuscitation fluid requirement in the first 24 hours. The Parkland formula (BSA affected % × weight (kg) × 4) gives the number of millilitres of *resuscitation fluid* to be given over the first 24 hours. Half the fluid is given in the first 8 hours and the remainder in the subsequent 16 hours. The 24-hour period should begin from the time of the injury. Thus if a patient has received very little fluid in transfer, and it is 4 hours since initial burn, then the fluid calculated should be given over the next 20 hours, and half the calculated fluid given in the first 4 hours.

In addition, *maintenance fluid* for the 24-hour period should also be given. This is calculated as 100 mL kg^{-1} for 0–10 kg, 50 mL kg^{-1} for 11–20 kg, and 25 mL kg^{-1} for > 20 kg. Thus a 30-kg child's maintenance = 1000 + 500 + 250 = 1750 mL over 24 hours. It is also important to monitor ongoing losses (urinary output, respiratory loss, etc.).

The calculated amount of fluid (burn deficient plus maintenance) to be replaced in 24 hours is only a guide and should be adjusted according to the haemodynamic response. Patients need to be maintained in a positive fluid balance for the first 24–48 hours. The adequacy of fluid replacement is monitored by urine output and clinical parameters of perfusion. In children, 0.5–1 mL kg^{-1}

per hour is the recommended urine output and should be monitored by a urinary catheter in severe burns. A central venous catheter is generally not required in the emergency department phase of management.

The type of fluid used varies between burn specialists, and it is best to be familiar with the preference of the local paediatric burns unit. In the shocked child, a 20 mL kg^{-1} bolus of normal saline should be given. This can be repeated if necessary to restore peripheral circulation. Ongoing replacement is generally with crystalloid in the first 24 hours, as colloid will leak through the burnt capillaries, causing worsening oedema. After 24 hours, then colloid is used as part of the replacement fluids in the intensive care setting. When calculating the initial fluid requirements, it is important to subtract the bolus fluids given from this amount.

Additional fluids may be required in severe electrical burns causing muscle damage, as myoglobin may cause renal failure secondary to renal tubular deposition, and therefore maintaining adequate glomerular filtration is very important.

Management of burns

(Table 3.5.1)
Major burns
These patients should be treated in a specialised burns unit. Covering the burn with a sterile dressing is required prior to transfer. Specific dressing type is best decided after discussion with the receiving unit. Within the burn centre, patients are generally dressed with topical silver sulphadiazine (SSD) cream that should be changed each day. At each change, the wound should be cleaned with warm

water and debrided to remove any avascular tissue (which may lead to infection). The burns are covered with a non-stick dressing over the SSD cream (e.g. Melolin), and then wrapped in crepe bandages to prevent contamination of the burn. The face and perineum are generally left open and covered with a water-based gel. SSD should not be used on the face, as the patient may spread it into their eyes.

Minor burns
Partial-thickness burns < 20% or full-thickness burns < 5–10% can often be managed on an outpatient basis and reviewed in a burn clinic.

There are several ways to dress wounds in the emergency department. Burns with intact blisters, unless over a joint surface, should be left intact initially. The intact skin acts as a barrier to bacteria, and the skin underneath can heal. After 7–10 days, the intact blisters should be removed and the need for grafting assessed. If unclear at this stage, then they should be redressed and assessed in a further 7 days. If the burn has ruptured blisters (i.e. partial thickness), the dead tissue should be removed. This is generally very easy to do but requires adequate analgesia. Nitrous oxide inhalation is an effective method of pain relief for these short procedures.

The methods of dressing burns will vary according to local practice. Traditionally, after debridement, wounds were covered with an SSD cream, and gauze and crepe applied over the top. This dressing needed to be changed at least daily, which required visits to a local doctor and usually painful dressing changes. It is also difficult to remove all

Table 3.5.1 Admission criteria for paediatric burns unit

Require admission
- partial-thickness burns > 20% BSA
- full-thickness burns > 5–10% BSA
- smoke inhalation suspected
- child abuse suspected

Consider admission
- burn to hands, feet, face, perineum, or joints
- burns < 20% BSA and other concerns – age < 12 months
- comorbidity
- other injuries

the SSD, and it may accumulate on the skin, leading to an 'SSDoma'. SSD should not be used on the face.

A better method of treatment is to apply an antibiotic ointment–impregnated gauze layer (e.g. Bactigras) or a silver-impregnated gauze. This acts like a skin graft and will stick to the burnt surface. Gauze and crepe are then placed over this layer. As with any burn, fluid will exude from the burn and pass through the layer of Bactigras and into the gauze. This outer dressing should be left on for 5–7 days and only changed before this if there is excessive discharge.

At 5–7 days, the outer two layers (gauze and crepe) are changed but the Bactigras is left on the burn site. As the burn heals over the next 1–2 weeks, the Bactigras will lift off. It is important not to take the Bactigras off if it has not separated from the skin, as this will remove the new granulation tissue that has formed. The obvious advantage of this method is there is no need for daily dressing changes, and the burn itself is cleaner. Silver-impregnated gauze is generally left on for a longer period of time.

Superficial burns

For small superficial burns, a clear plastic dressing (e.g. Tegaderm) can be placed over the burn to provide protection and left on until it also falls off. The disadvantage of this type of dressing is that fluid from the burn tends to collect under the dressing, is a rich source of 'food' for bacteria, and can lead to infection. Tegaderm is better applied after a few days, when the exudate from the burn has ceased.

A more porous adherent dressing, such as Fixomul, is better when exudate is going to occur, as it will allow some egress of fluid to occur. A covering dressing of gauze and crepe is needed for the first few days. Removal of this type of dressing is problematic. Olive oil must be applied to the Fixomul several hours before the dressing can be removed, otherwise pulling the dressing off will lead to removal of the new granulation tissue.

Superficial burns rarely become infected, but infection should be suspected if the patient:

- has unexplained fever, or
- has evolving pain, redness, and tenderness.

Foul discharge from the burn does not always indicate that infection is present. In this case, the dressing should be changed earlier and the burn inspected, as antibiotics may not be indicated. As the skin heals under a dressing, it will become pruritic, which may require an antihistamine or cooling of the dressing (particularly in hot weather).

Superficial burns on the face should be managed non-dressed, and cleaned two or three times a day with warm water. Solugel can be applied to the face or it can be left completely non-dressed. As a burn on the face starts to dry up, application of Vitamin E cream or mild lanolin ointment or cream can be used to aid in healing by softening the skin. The burn should also be protected from the sun, as sunburn of a burn area will cause increased pigmentation to the skin.

Tetanus prophylaxis is important in major burns or minor burns (which are contaminated). Antibiotics should be used only when a definite infection is present. Prophylactic use of antibiotics is not beneficial.

Pain management for minor burns is generally achieved by the dressing itself. Covering the burn decreases the pain substantially. Generally, paracetamol with or without codeine should be sufficient during the first 24 hours.

Patients with burns involving hands, feet, or face should be referred to a burn specialist for ongoing management.

ELECTRICAL BURNS

Introduction

These are infrequent presentations to emergency departments but have unique problems. Electrical injuries are more commonly seen in two age groups: toddlers within the home setting and male adolescents involved in risk-taking behaviour.

Young children generally sustain electrical burns from low-voltage (< 1000 V) or household currents (240 V). These may be due to frayed electrical cords or children inserting metal objects into power sockets. Mouth burns may occur when small children chew on power cords. In most states in Australia, safety switches are installed in all new houses, cutting the current when overloaded, thus preventing many severe electrical burns. These low-voltage exposures rarely result in significant internal injury, and most children are asymptomatic apart from distress from the cutaneous burn.

High-voltage (> 1000 V) injuries are seen most often in adolescent males as a consequence of risk-taking behaviour (e.g. climbing electrical poles, train surfing). These high-voltage exposures obviously have a more serious outcome, as they are more likely to be associated with injury to internal structures.

Clinical effects

Electrical currents preferentially flow along low-resistance tissues such as blood vessels, nerves, and muscles, rather than the skin. There is generally an entrance and exit burn in non–water-related current injuries, with increased tissue damage at these sites. The internal injury to deeper structures results from current passing through low-resistance structures and is more severe in the extremities. Wet or moist skin increases current flow dramatically by decreasing the tissue resistance.

Clinical manifestations will vary according to the voltage exposure and may range from trivial to cardiac arrest.

Skin

- Entry and exit burns: well-demarcated pale areas with charred centre.
- Arc burns: heat produced can cause extensive tissue injury.
- Flame burns: due to ignition of clothing.

Burns to the mouth (often full thickness) caused by toddlers chewing or sucking on power cords can lead to severe scarring and contractures. These will require specialist referral. Bleeding from the labial artery may occur 1–2 weeks after the initial burn, when the eschar separates.

Cardiac

Arrhythmias:

- Low voltage: sinus tachycardia, atrial fibrillation, ventricular fibrillation. Myocardial injury is uncommon.
- High voltage: asystole.

Muscular

- Prolonged tetany of musculature: apnoea, fractures and dislocations.
- Muscle necrosis and rhabdomyolysis.

Neurological

- Acute: altered mental state; seizures; headache; speech, motor, or sensory disturbances.
- Delayed: spinal cord injury, memory and mood disturbance.

Renal

- Renal failure secondary to myoglobinuria.

Other

- Eyes: cataracts.
- Gastrointestinal tract: ulceration, perforation.
- Trauma following associated falls.

Management

Assessment of the child's A, B, and C is the initial priority with electrical exposure, followed by examining for skin burns and potential internal injuries. A baseline 12-lead ECG should be done (unless a trivial exposure), and cardiac monitoring only continued if the initial ECG is abnormal or the child is symptomatic (e.g. chest pain or impaired conscious state). A search for an entrance and exit wound should occur to determine the potential for deeper burns. Analgesia should be provided for the burn or muscle pain. Potential complications and associated injuries are treated on their merit.

Specific issues

Burns

All electrical burns warrant review by a burn specialist.

Fluids

Calculating fluid requirements for significant electrical burns is underestimated using the Parkland formula, as most of the damage is internal. Therefore fluid requirements are significantly more than estimated, and one should aim to maintain a urine output of 2 ml kg^{-1} per hour.

Myoglobinuria

Muscle involvement leads to myoglobinuria, which may cause renal failure. A forced diuresis with diuretics and/or alkalinisation will help to prevent renal failure.

Compartment injury

A compartment syndrome may occur also due to oedema and burn of the affected muscles. Fasciotomy may be necessary, with debridement of non-viable muscle.

Disposition

Admission

- Any high-voltage injury.
- Any child with evidence of cardiac or neurological abnormality.
- Other associated complications requiring in-patient management.

Discharge

- Asymptomatic child with low-voltage injury with normal ECG.

CHEMICAL BURNS

There are wide ranges of chemical agents where accidental exposure to children can cause burns. They are generally either acid or alkali. Acid burns cause coagulation of the skin, which seems to limit the depth of penetration. Alkali burns cause liquefaction and thus result in a deeper injury. Caustic chemicals tend to give deeper burns than thermal injury, as there is generally a long duration of contact. Oedema tends to occur more quickly in chemical burns, which may cause a deeper burn to appear more superficial.

Treatment

Copious irrigation of the burn is the mainstay of treatment. Sufficient analgesia and topical anaesthesia is required to achieve this in a child. This can be achieved simply with water. Flushing of the burn should continue for at least 10–15 minutes and sometimes longer. Determination of wound pH via litmus paper may guide the duration of irrigation. If chemicals are introduced into the eye, then irrigation should continue until pH is neutral. This usually requires topical anaesthetic to the eye prior to flushing the eye with saline. A Morgan lens is a good method of flushing eyes, as this requires less cooperation from the patient. Fluorescein staining of the eye should then determine the extent of the burn. Chemical burns to the eye require urgent ophthalmological referral. The treatment of a dermal chemical burn after decontamination should be the same as for any other burn.

Some chemicals may cause system toxicity from absorption through the burned skin, and these should be managed accordingly.

FURTHER READING

Henry DB, Foster RL 2000 Burn pain management in children. Pediatric Clinics of North America 47(3): 681–698

Herndon DN, Rutan RL, Rutan TC 1993 Management of the pediatric patient with burns. Journal of Burn Care and Rehabilitation 14: 38

Hight DW, Bakalar HR, Lloyd JR 1979 Inflicted burns in children: Recognition and treatment. Journal of the American Medical Association 242: 517–520

Hunt JL, Sato RM, Baxter CR 1980 Acute electric burns: Current diagnostic and therapeutic approaches to management. Archives of Surgery 115: 434–438

Pruitt BA Jr, McManus AT, Kim SH et al 1998 Burn wound infections: Current status. World Journal of Surgery 22(2): 135–145

Rose JK, Herndon DN 1997 Advances in the treatment of burn patients. Burns 23(Suppl 1): S19–S26

Smith ML 2000 Pediatric burns: Management of thermal, electrical, and chemical burns and burn-like dermatologic conditions. Pediatric Annals 29(6): 367–383

Walker AR 1996 Emergency department management of house fire burns and carbon monoxide poisoning in children. Current Opinions in Pediatrics 8: 239–242

Wyatt D, McGowan DN, Najarian MP 1990 Comparison of a hydrocolloid dressing and silver sulfadiazine cream in the outpatient management of second-degree burns. Journal of Trauma 30: 857–865

A

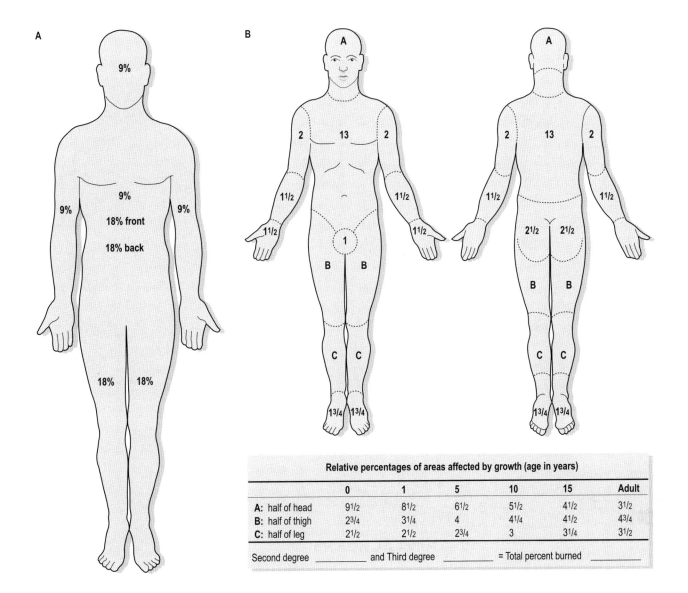

B

Relative percentages of areas affected by growth (age in years)						
	0	1	5	10	15	Adult
A: half of head	9 1/2	8 1/2	6 1/2	5 1/2	4 1/2	3 1/2
B: half of thigh	2 3/4	3 1/4	4	4 1/4	4 1/2	4 3/4
C: half of leg	2 1/2	2 1/2	2 3/4	3	3 1/4	3 1/2

Second degree _____ and Third degree _____ = Total percent burned _____

Fig. 3.5.1

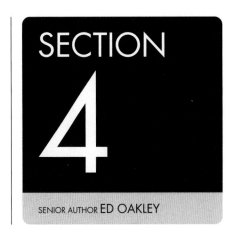

WOUND MANAGEMENT

4.1 WOUND MANAGEMENT

ED OAKLEY

ESSENTIALS

1 Goals of management of wounds are to avoid infection, minimise discomfort, facilitate healing and minimise scar formation.

2 In children management will often require sedation, adequate local anaesthesia and analgesia.

3 Meticulous wound care and repair should ensure the best possible outcome and functional result.

4 The care of the patient as a whole should be the first management priority.

5 The comprehension level and the co-operation gained from the child influence wound examination and the information gained.

6 Distraction techniques, adequate topical anaesthesia and appropriate use of sedation can all aid in wound assessment in children.

7 Examination of function, sensation and circulation distal to the wound is best performed prior to exploration of the wound and prior to regional anaesthesia.

8 In the child less than 5 years old observation of posture, symmetry and general movement is required.

9 If presence of a foreign body is expected radiological investigation is advised.

10 Sedation should only be undertaken by personnel experienced in its use, able to manage the complications of airway compromise, oxygen desaturation and respiratory depression.

11 Surgical debridement of non-viable tissue is vital to prevent wound infection or delayed wound healing.

12 The technique chosen for wound closure depends on the type and position of the wound.

13 Tissue adhesives are for external use only and should not be placed within wounds or used on mucous membranes.

14 All patients should be provided with written information on care of their wound.

15 Trauma to the distal fingers is often associated with nail-bed injury. An underlying fracture of the distal phalanx should be assessed with radiographs.

16 In general, sutures are removed earlier in children than in adults.

17 Non-accidental injury should be considered especially when the history and injury are inconsistent.

INTRODUCTION

Lacerations account for up to $\frac{1}{3}$ of paediatric emergency presentations, boys represent $\frac{2}{3}$ of these presentations, and 40% of all lacerations involve a fall. The scalp and face account for more than 50% of all lacerations, and about $\frac{1}{3}$ occur on the hands. The goals of management of these wounds are to avoid infection, minimise discomfort, facilitate healing and minimise scar formation. Meticulous attention to wound care and repair should ensure the best possible outcome and functional result. In children this will often require sedation in addition to adequate local anaesthesia and analgesia. It must be remembered that universal precautions should always be followed when assessing or managing any wound. Gloves (preferably sterile), drapes and eye protection are mandatory.

Anatomy of the skin

Skin is composed of two layers – dermis and epidermis. The epidermis acts as a protective layer for the dermis, preventing infection and desiccation. It is avascular and relies on diffusion of nutrients from the dermis. The dermis is rich in collagen and thus provides most of the tensile strength of the skin. It has a rich network of nutrient vessels and capillaries. The subcutaneous fat is composed of loose connective and adipose tissues.

Pathophysiology of wound healing

The stages of wound healing are coagulation, inflammation, proliferation and maturation. Wound healing is a sequential process that begins immediately after tissue injury. Coagulation is initiated by platelet aggregation then by fibrin clot formation. This supplies haemostasis and allows accumulation of neutrophils and monocytes, which herald the inflammatory phase. The inflammatory phase provides phagocytosis of bacteria, other organisms and foreign matter or dead tissue in the wound. The macrophages release factors that stimulate proliferation of local fibroblasts in the dermis. These provide a collagen network and stimulate new vessel growth. This phase is characterised by pink granulation tissue and wound contraction. A warm moist environment that is supplied either by dressings or scab formation aids this process. Collagen synthesis reaches its peak towards the end of the first week of healing. Remodelling continues to occur for up to 12 months, thus the scar will usually fade and contract over the first 2 to 3 months and the final appearance may not be obvious for up to 6 months post injury.

A number of factors affect the healing of a wound. Adequate nutrition (including vitamins C and A, which are required for collagen formation) is essential. Corticosteroids and immunosuppressive drugs interfere with cellular proliferation and immunity, and anticoagulants inhibit clot formation and initial wound stabilisation. Infection interferes with collagen synthesis and will delay wound healing and cause an increase in scar tissue formation.

Tensile forces of the surrounding skin affect the healing and scar formation of a wound. The most cosmetically pleasing outcome occurs when the long axis of the wound is in the direction of maximum skin tension – along Langer's Lines of skin tension. Wounds that have long axis perpendicular to the lines of skin tension will heal with greater scarring, but there is significant inter-child variability. Dynamic skin tension caused by joint movement also impairs wound healing and causes increased scar formation, and immobilisation of joints while the laceration heals will minimise this effect.

Wound infection

Wound infection is relatively uncommon, occurring in about 5% of all lacerations. In general a wound in a child is less likely to become infected than a similar wound in an adult. Identified risk factors for infection include severe wound contamination, inadequate wound cleansing, inadequate debridement of dead tissue (especially in crush injuries), use of subcutaneous sutures, larger laceration (> 5 cm) and site of injury. Specific sites identified as infection risks include axillae, perineum or groin, and feet. In general limb wounds are at increased risk compared to head and neck wounds.

CLASSIFICATION OF WOUNDS

Lacerations

Lacerations are the most common type of wound seen in the paediatric age group. The edges are usually ragged, if the wound penetrates into the dermal capillaries it will bleed and if it extends into the subcutaneous tissue it will gape. Lacerations can be caused by tension on the skin (usually seen in areas with significant subcutaneous tissue) or by compression of the skin between an object and bone. There is always damage done to surrounding tissues and healing is therefore delayed. Compression injuries usually have more surrounding tissue damage and thus tend to heal more slowly.

Incised wounds

A sharp object such as a knife blade or glass shard makes an incised wound. The wound has margins that are clearly defined and there is little or no surrounding tissue damage. These wounds heal faster than lacerations and, in general, have a lower incidence of infection.

Abrasions

Abrasions are caused by sheering forces on the surface of the skin. The upper layers of the epidermis and sometimes dermis are scraped away. The depth of injury usually varies throughout the wound. If the epidermis alone is involved there is no bleeding, but a transudation of fluid. If the dermis is involved the wound will bleed and there is said to be an increased incidence of infection and foreign body retention.

EVALUATION OF THE PATIENT WITH A LACERATION

The care of the patient as a whole should be the first management priority. The airway, breathing and circulation should be assessed and treated as appropriate and a thorough secondary survey undertaken in most patients to exclude or allow management of serious injuries as well as detecting other minor injuries.

History

In evaluating a wound the mechanism of trauma (cut, crush, fall, bite, burn) and the time of injury are important as they may alter the management of the wound. Crush and bite injuries characteristically cause significantly more surrounding tissue damage and thus are more likely to have delayed healing or infection. When possible determine the cleanliness of the inflicting object, the amount of blood loss, the presence of a foreign-body sensation, and the motor function and sensation distal to the affected area. The location of the wound should be noted and the possibility of injury to other structures explored.

The health status of the patient should be explored especially with regard to chronic illnesses that may impact on wound healing – such as diabetes mellitus, obesity, malnutrition, chronic renal impairment, cyanotic congenital heart disease, chronic respiratory illness, tumours, and bleeding disorders. Immunisation history should be obtained and further tetanus vaccination guided by the recommendations of the National Health and Medical Research Council (see Table 4.1.1). Current medications are important for both drug interactions with antibiotics that may be prescribed and for medications that may interfere with wound healing – such as immunosuppressive drugs and corticosteroids. A history of allergies must be determined prior to use of cleansing agents, dressings and tapes and prescription of medication. A history of latex allergy should be specifically sought. In wounds that require management under general

Table 4.1.1   Tetanus prophylaxis in wound management

History of tetanus vaccination	Time since last dose	Type of wound	DTP, DT, Td or Tetanus toxoid† (as appropriate)	Tetanus immunoglobulin*
≥ 3 doses	< 5 years	All wounds	NO	NO
≥ 3 doses	5–10 years	Clean, minor wounds	NO	NO
≥ 3 doses	5–10 years	All other wounds	YES	NO
≥ 3 doses	> 10 years	All wounds	YES	NO
< 3 doses or uncertain	–	Clean, minor wounds	YES	NO
< 3 doses or uncertain	–	All other wounds	YES	YES

*Recommended dose for TIG is 250 IU to be given as soon as possible after the injury, if > 24 hours has elapsed since the injury 500 IU should be given.
†Tetanus toxoid vaccine should only be used if diphtheria toxoid is contraindicated.
DTP, diphtheria-tetanus-acellular pertussis vaccine; DT, adsorbed diphtheria-tetanus vaccine (paediatric formulation – for < 7 years old); Td, adsorbed diphtheria-tetanus vaccine (adult formulation – for ≥ 7 years old)

anaesthesia or sedation a history of when the child last ate or drank is important. Non-accidental injury should be considered especially when the history and injury are inconsistent.

Examination

Once assessment and management of more serious injuries has occurred the patient should be assessed for the current severity of any chronic illness, and appropriate management initiated.

The co-operation able to be gained and comprehension level of the child influence wound examination and the information gained. Distraction techniques, adequate topical anaesthesia and appropriate use of sedation can all aid in wound assessment. A calm unhurried friendly approach, involving the parents, will maximise the chances of co-operation. Examination of the wound should be done with optimal lighting and with bleeding minimised. Examination of function, sensation and circulation distal to the wound is best performed prior to exploration of the wound and prior to regional anaesthesia.

Functional assessment requires the movement of all joints distal to the wound. In an older child each joint is examined individually on command and the strength documented. In the child less than 5 years old, observation of posture, symmetry and general movement is required. In wounds to the flexor tendons of the hand close attention

should be paid to the resting position of the fingers (partial flexion). The finding of extension of one finger at rest and the failure of the finger to flex at play or after application of a noxious stimulus confirms the tendon injury.

Injury to nerves is classically assessed with two-point discrimination and this should be possible in older children. Using a paperclip bent so that its ends are separated 4–8 mm is useful in this process. In upper limb injuries formal assessment of the median, ulna and radial nerves is required. In children less than 5 years old this approach needs to be modified. Noxious stimulus applied to the fingers will illicit sensation but risks losing patient confidence. Another method of determining intact innervation is to look for sweating of the fingers. Since autonomic response includes sweating, denervated fingers do not sweat. An ophthalmoscope can be used to examine for sweat beads or the cleaned body of a pen can be run over the fingers with less resistance in the denervated, thus dry, segment. Arterial circulation is assessed by palpation of peripheral pulses, capillary return distal to the injury, and skin colour and temperature.

Assessment of the wound should include site, size, depth, nature of the edges, cleanliness, and presence of foreign bodies. The wound should be explored to determine the depth and involvement of any underlying tissues including vessels, nerves, tendons, ligaments, muscles,

joints, bones and specialised tissues (especially ducts and glands). Bones adjacent to the wound should be palpated for deformity or crepitus and the wound searched for foreign bodies (including the sound of glass on the metal forceps). This assessment and exploration should take place after appropriate anaesthesia of the wound and any required sedation.

Investigation

If presence of a foreign body is expected radiological investigation is advised. In wounds caused by glass all but superficial wounds should be investigated with plain soft tissue X-ray of the region to exclude a glass foreign body. Most glass foreign bodies more than 2–3 mm in size should be visible. If a radiolucent foreign body is suspected, ultrasound can be useful to both confirm the presence of the foreign body and provide a guide to its depth and location in the wound. Other investigations should be determined by the findings of possible injuries to adjacent structures, such as bony X-rays for fractures.

TREATMENT OF WOUNDS

Wound anaesthesia

Analgesia and sedation are discussed in more detail in Chapter 20. Anaesthesia is required to adequately examine and then treat most wounds. Often, in children, analgesia and sedation will also be necessary, depending on the location of the wound, the involvement of underlying structures, and the age and anxiety of the child.

The options for anaesthesia include topical anaesthesia, local infiltration, regional anaesthesia, dissociative anaesthesia, or general anaesthesia.

Topical anaesthetics include ALA (adrenaline, lidocaine and amethocaine) – commonly known as LET (lidocaine, epinephrine and tetracaine) in North America, or EMLA cream (eutectic mixture of local anaesthetics) – manufactured by AstraZeneca. ALA is highly effective on facial and head wounds but less so on limb wounds. It has replaced TAC (tetracaine, adrenaline and cocaine) in most institutions. Due to the vasoconstricting properties of adrenaline (epinephrine) these anaesthetics should not be used in areas of end arteries (fingers, nose, lips, ears, genitalia). EMLA has been shown to be safe and effective when applied to limb wounds. Topical anaesthetics should be applied in the wound either as a liquid dripped onto cotton wool placed in the wound or as a methyl cellulose gel. The wound is then covered with an occlusive impermeable dressing and adequate anaesthesia is usually obtained within 30 minutes.

Local infiltration is the classical method of anaesthetising a wound. The anaesthetic is injected into the wound margins. Pain of injection can be minimised by using warmed anaesthetic, buffering the drug with sodium bicarbonate (mix 10 mL of 1% lidocaine with 1 mL of 8.4% sodium bicarbonate), infiltrating slowly, using the lowest concentration possible, and using needles sized 25 gauge or smaller. The most commonly used local anaesthetic is lidocaine 1 or 2% with or without adrenaline (epinephrine) 1:100 000. The onset of action is rapid with duration of action of 30 minutes to 1 hour. Addition of adrenaline (epinephrine) is useful to prolong the duration of action and help minimise bleeding, however adrenaline (epinephrine) should be avoided in regions of end arteries (fingers, nose, lips, ears, genitalia), and its use may increase the risk of infection. The safe dose of plain lidocaine is 3 mg kg^{-1} or 6 mg kg^{-1} for lidocaine mixed with adrenaline (epinephrine).

Regional anaesthesia is useful for facial, hand and foot lacerations where nerves are readily accessible near bony landmarks. A regional nerve block involves anaesthetising the nerve or nerves that supply a specific anatomic region. Regional anaesthesia is especially useful for large lacerations and lacerations where local infiltration causes distortion of tissue anatomy. Regional anaesthesia is especially useful for anaesthetising digits. Lidocaine or bupivacaine hydrochloride 0.5%, which have duration of action of 3 to 6 hours, are the most commonly used agents. The safe dose of bupivacaine is 2 mg kg^{-1}.

Sedation is often required when treating lacerations in children. Options for sedation include benzodiazepines – such as midazolam or diazepam, fentanyl, nitrous oxide or ketamine. Sedation should only be undertaken by personnel experienced in its use and able to manage the complications of airway compromise, oxygen desaturation and respiratory depression. Adequate equipment to deal with these complications should also be available. Some form of physical restraint may also be necessary to prevent excessive movement during repair, however, the aim must be to provide adequate analgesia and anxiolysis.

Wound preparation and cleansing

Hair near the wound should only be removed if it interferes with the meticulous closure of the wound. If hair removal is desired the hair should be clipped, not shaved, as shaving disrupts hair follicles and increases the incidence of wound infection. Eyebrow hair should not be removed because this may lead to abnormal or delayed regrowth.

The surrounding skin and wound edges should be thoroughly cleaned. This should be undertaken in a manner and with a substance that provides adequate antisepsis without tissue damage or impairing wound defence mechanisms. A solution such as aqueous povidone-iodine or aqueous chlorhexidene applied with gauze or cotton wool should be used. Care should be taken to minimise the amount of cleanser to penetrate the wound to minimise damage to wound defences increasing the risk of infection.

Surgical debridement of crushed or non-viable tissue is vital to prevent wound infection or delayed wound healing. However, as little tissue should be debrided as possible. Manual removal with forceps of large particles of foreign material should also be meticulously undertaken. When a heavily contaminated wound contains specialised tissues such as tendons or nerves, consultation is recommended.

Once the wound is adequately anaesthetised it should be thoroughly cleaned. Irrigation is the method of choice for removing dirt and bacteria from wounds. Saline (0.9%) is the irrigation solution of choice, as it causes no tissue damage. The ability of irrigation to decontaminate a wound is directly related to pressure of the irrigating stream, the size of the particles to be removed, and the volume of irrigant. At least 100 to 200 mL per 2 cm of laceration are required. The fluid should be injected from a 30 to 60 mL syringe via an 18 to 20 gauge cannula. Higher pressures should be avoided as they may cause tissue damage and increase the incidence of wound infection. The volume and pressure of irrigation should be modified as necessary according to the location and cause of the wound. High-pressure irrigation does not enhance the dissemination of bacteria into soft tissue wounds, but excessive use can cause local tissue oedema enhancing risk of infection. Use of a device to minimise splashing of the irrigant is desirable and wearing of gloves, goggles and gown mandatory.

Antibiotic prophylaxis

The use of prophylactic antibiotics in wound care is controversial. Decontamination with appropriate irrigation techniques is more beneficial than the use of prophylactic antibiotics. When indicated (see Table 4.1.2) antibiotics should be given as soon as possible. The initial dose should be given intravenously and be relatively large to provide rapid reliable high tissue concentrations. The first dose should be given before wound closure to ensure an effective concentration of antibiotic in the wound tissue fluid at the time of wound closure. When choosing an antibiotic the likely causative organisms should be born in mind. The organisms contaminating the wound and the commensal organisms found in that region of the body. In general bites and wounds in regions with high bacterial counts (hands, feet, groin) should be treated with antibiotics to cover *Staphylococcus epidermidis*, *S. aureus* and *Streptococcus* sp. Specific circumstances also need to be born in mind. Patients at risk of endocarditis should have all wounds treated with antibiotics to cover *S. aureus* and *S. epidermidis*. Ampicillin/amoxicillin is the currently recommended

drug in Australia. However, in communities where the incidence of penicillin resistance is high a cephalosporin and an aminoglycoside are recommended.

Wounds associated with fractures, tendon or muscle involvement should be considered for prophylaxis, as should large wounds, wounds with significant devitalised tissue such as crush injuries and stellate lacerations. Wounds contaminated with faeces should be treated with coverage of coliforms and anaerobic bacteria. Wounds in children with a compromised immune system should all be considered for treatment. Wounds with closure delayed more than 12 hours should also be considered high risk for infection. Treatment should be for 3 to 5 days with a penicillinase-resistant antibiotic such as a first generation cephalosporin or amoxicillin-clavulanic acid (co-amoxiclav).

WOUND CLOSURE

The aim of wound closure is to reduce discomfort, aid healing and produce the best cosmetic result possible. The technique chosen for wound closure depends on the type of wound. Most wounds in children can be managed with primary closure, as the risk of infection is relatively low. Infected, heavily contaminated wounds and wounds resulting form high-energy projectiles are best managed by delayed primary closure, with initial cleansing and packing then closure 3 to 5 days later, once the risk of infection has decreased. Wounds with

delayed presentation (>24 hours), or those contaminated with saliva or faeces should also be considered for delayed closure. Some wounds, such as puncture wounds or contaminated wounds in areas of poor perfusion should not be closed but allowed to heal by secondary intention. Once it is decided to close the wound a technique that allows apposition of the wound edges that is secure and accurate and holds the wound edges in apposition until the strength of the wound is sufficient should be chosen. With improved technology the options for wound closure are growing. Those presently available included sutures, staples, tissue adhesives and tapes.

Sutures
Suturing is the traditional method of wound closure. Sutures are divided into two classes on the basis of their degradation properties. Absorbable sutures degrade rapidly in vivo, and lose their tensile strength within 60 days. Sutures that degrade more slowly are classified as non-absorbable (see Table 4.1.3 for individual suture material characteristics).

Absorbable sutures are made from either collagen or synthetic polymers. Gut sutures are manufactured from the submucosa of ovine or bovine intestines. The collagen is then treated to strengthen the material and increase resistance to tissue degradation (plain gut). Coating with chromium trioxide provides more resistance to absorption (chromic gut). These suture materials have a somewhat unpredictable absorption. Synthetic

---

Table 4.1.2 Indications for antibiotic prophylaxis in wounds
Wound Characteristics:
High risk anatomic site (hands, forefoot, groin, axilla)
Devitalised tissue
Extensive surrounding soft tissue injury
Stellate lacerations
Contaminated with body fluids or organic matter or dirt
Large lacerations (> 5 cm)
Closure delayed (> 12 hours)
High risk for endocarditis:
Prosthetic heart valves
Patent ductus arteriosis
Tetralogy of Fallot
Ventricular septal defects
Coarctation of the aorta
Immunocompromised children

Table 4.1.3   Characteristics of common suture materials

Suture material	Ease of handling	Tensile strength	Degradation (d)*	Tissue reactivity	Infection potential
Non-absorbable					
Nylon (Ethilon®, Dafilon®)	Average	Good	–	Low	Very low
Polypropylene (Prolene®)	Poor	Very good	–	Very low	Low
Silk	Good	Poor	–	High	High
Absorbable					
Chromic gut	Average	Average	10–14	High	High
Surgical gut	Poor	Average	5–7	High	High
Polyglactin (Vicryl®)	Average	Good	30	Low	Low
Polyglycolic acid (Dexon®)	Good	Good	30	Low	Low
Polydioxanone (PDS)	Average	Very good	45–50	Very low	Low

*Time to loss of 50% of tensile strength.

absorbable sutures have improved strength and delayed and more reliable absorption characteristics. Absorbable sutures are used for closing deep layers of a laceration and can be used for skin closure – especially where removing sutures in a young child may be difficult.

Non-absorbable sutures are made from either natural (silk, cotton, linen) or synthetic (nylon, Dacron®) fibres. They can also be classified according to their physical characteristics. Monofilament sutures are made from a single filament (nylon, Prolene®), and sutures containing multiple fibres are called multifilament (silk, cotton, nylon). Of these sutures only nylon is available in both types of filament. Non-absorbable sutures are used to close fascial layers (where healing is slow) and for skin closure.

Sutures come in varying sizes. The size of the suture to be used depends on the wound location and the tensile strength of the tissue to be sutured. Heavy sutures such as 4–0 or 5–0 should be used in the limbs and trunk, and should also be used on mucous membranes and subcutaneous tissue. Heaviest sutures such as 3–0 should be used on thick skin (such as the sole of the foot) or over large joints. Small sutures such as 6–0 should be used on tissues with light tensions such as facial skin and subcutaneous tissue.

Needles

Needles come in varying sizes and shapes also. Needles are describes by the arc of curvature the needle possesses, and the shape of the needle itself. The most commonly used for skin closure is the $\frac{3}{8}$ circle (135°) needle or the $\frac{1}{2}$ circle (180°) needle (see Fig. 4.1.1). For closure of fascial layers $\frac{1}{2}$ circumference needles are usually used. Needles that have two circumferences of curvature (compound needles) are able to be passed through the tissue with less rotation of the forearm. Needles come with different shapes as well as curvatures (see Fig. 4.1.1). A reverse cutting needle is the most common type used for skin closure. The needle cuts an inverted triangle and the suture sits on the base of the triangle decreasing the likelihood of cutting out.

A conventional cutting needle cuts a triangle into the skin and the suture sits in the apex of the triangle. For fascia a taper point needle is used. The cross-section of these needles is a circle that is tapered to a point. It does not cut but pushes the tissues aside causing less tissue damage and reducing the chance of the stitch cutting out. For deep tissues that are stronger (such as tendon) a tapercut, or combination needle is used - it has a tapered body, but the point is a reverse cutting edge.

Needles are grasped with a needle holder. The swage of the needle – the region where the needle is hollowed out to join with the suture – is the weakest point and grasping the needle in this region should be avoided. The needle should be grasped in the body one half or two thirds of the distance from the tip of the needle.

Suturing techniques

For closure of a wound with sutures a number of instruments are needed to maintain a sterile field and to allow manipulation of the tissues and needle (see Table 4.1.4). Finer instruments should be available for facial laceration repair.

Sutures should be placed to allow apposition of all injured layers of the skin. Proper suture placement should result in slight eversion of the wound edges, avoiding a depression of the scar when contraction takes place during wound healing. To ensure eversion of skin edges the skin suture must be placed so that an equal amount of tissue is included on each side of the wound, and so that the needle bite includes a broad base (Figs 4.1.2 and 4.1.3). This is accomplished by lifting the wound edge as the needle is passed through the skin on each side, maximising the deep tissues included in the suture.

Most wounds sutured in the ED are closed with interrupted skin sutures. Synthetic non-absorbable sutures are most commonly used. However, rapidly

Table 4.1.4 Example of instruments required for a simple suture tray
1 × Needle holder (Halsey or Hegar)
1 × Toothed dissecting forceps
1 × Curved artery/mosquito forceps
1 × Straight artery/mosquito forceps
1 × Suture scissors
1 × IV scissors
1 × Scalpel handle (e.g. No. 3)
2 × Huck towels
2 × Small bowls or trays

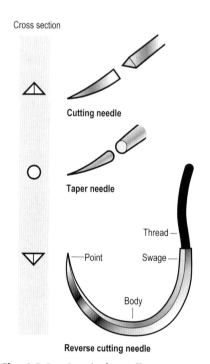

Fig. 4.1.1 Surgical needle characteristics and types. (From an original drawing by Elaine Wheildon)

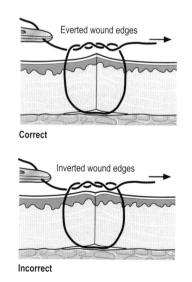

Fig. 4.1.2 Normal suture. Suturing technique for wound edge eversion.

WOUND MANAGEMENT

absorbable sutures can be used to close the skin in children, avoiding the discomfort of suture removal. To place a simple interrupted suture the needle is held so the tip enters the skin at a right angle, and the hand rotated to ensure the needle remains at right angles to the skin throughout its passage, this aids in maximising the deep tissues captured in the bite. The stitch should be secured

Fig. 4.1.3 Deep sutures. (A) The buried subcutaneous suture; (B) the horizontal dermal stitch.

with an instrument tie and the knots secured to one side of the wound to minimise inflammation to the healing tissue. The initial throw should include two wraps of the suture material around the needle holder, subsequent throws should be wrapped once. The knot should be tied just tight enough to appose the skin edges. Tying the knot too tightly will cause a reduction in the blood supply to the wound edges and increase the risk of infection and poor cosmetic outcome. Synthetic sutures with poor handling should have 4 or 5 throws per knot.

The more sutures placed per centimetre the finer the control over the wound edge. For facial lacerations the skin sutures should be placed approximately 3 mm apart and enter the skin about 3 mm from the wound edge. For other areas of the body sutures should be placed 4 to 5 mm apart and should pierce the skin about 5 mm from the wound edge. The number of sutures used to close a wound should be the minimal number that allows a desired cosmetic outcome. In general, the better the blood supply, the closer together sutures can be placed.

There are generally two methods for closing a laceration, either suturing from one end to the other, or placing sutures that serially bisect the wound. A small linear wound is easily sutured from end to end, and long wounds without good landmarks on either side are most easily closed by placing the first stitch in the middle and then serially subdividing the wound. In wounds with definite landmarks such as palmar skin creases or the vermillion border of the lip the first

suture should be placed to align these landmarks.

Deep sutures should be placed where there are multiple layers of tissue involved and the skin sutures would be under tension. They are placed to reapproximate the dermal layers of the skin and remove skin tension, thus improving cosmetic outcome. Placing deep sutures inserts a foreign body into the wound and increases the risk of wound infection so they should only be placed when necessary and the minimum number necessary used. For this reason, deep sutures should be avoided in the hands and feet. Deep sutures placed close to the skin are sometimes extruded through the wound. To place a deep suture the needle is placed at the depth of the wound and removed at a more superficial level. The needle is then placed at the same superficial level on the opposite side of the wound and exits deeply so the knot is tied deeply in the wound (see Fig. 4.1.3).

Special suturing techniques

A variety of special suturing techniques are available with the sole purpose of aiding the provision of skin apposition with everted wound edges. The vertical mattress suture is useful in regions with minimal subcutaneous tissue where the edges are difficult to maintain in eversion. The technique is begun the same way as a simple skin suture, but after the suture loop is made the skin is re-entered 1 to 2 mm from the wound edge and then tied (see Fig. 4.1.4). The horizontal mattress suture reinforces the subcutaneous tissue and relieves skin tension, but does not provide wound edge approximation

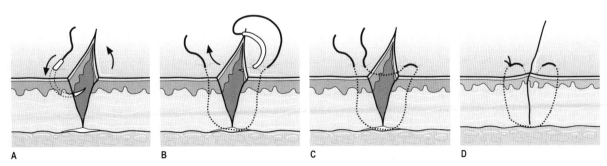

Fig. 4.1.4 The vertical mattress suture technique is useful to evert wound edges with a natural tendency to roll inwards despite correctly placed simple sutures. (From an original drawing by Elaine Wheildon)

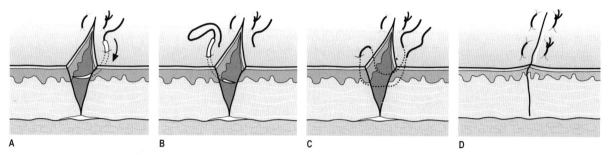

Fig. 4.1.5   The horizontal mattress suture redistributes tension and everts wound edges. (From an original drawing by Elaine Wheildon)

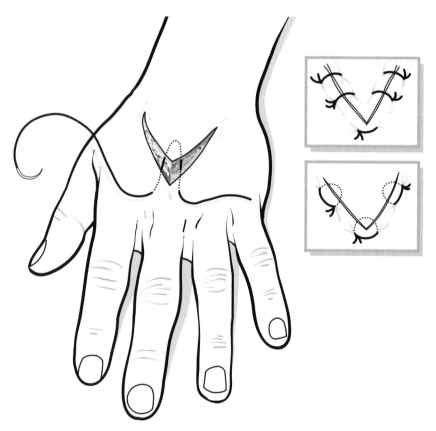

Fig. 4.1.6   Closure of a flap requires an initial suture of the apex, after which either simple or horizontal mattress sutures may be used. (From an original drawing by Elaine Wheildon)

as well as the vertical mattress suture (see Fig. 4.1.5). The modified or half-buried horizontal mattress suture (or corner stitch) is the method of choice for closing a flap. It relieves tissue tension and avoids vascular compromise when approximating the tip of the flap (see Fig. 4.1.6).

A continuous suture can be used to close the laceration. It is faster to place than interrupted sutures, removal of su-tures is easier and faster, and the tension is spread evenly along the wound. The continuous suture can be percutaneous or subcutaneous and made with absorb-able or non-absorbable suture material. The disadvantages are that if one part of the suture breaks the integrity of the whole wound is lost, and if the wound becomes infected the whole wound needs to be opened to drain the pus. To place a percutaneous running stitch an interrupted suture is placed at one end of the wound and only the free end of the suture is cut. Suturing is continued along the wound in a coil pattern ensuring that the needle passes perpendicularly across the wound with each pass. The loop is tightened after each pass and the last stitch placed beyond the end of the laceration. The stitch is tied using the last loop as the tail.

Correction of dog ears

A dog ear is the term given to a conical pucker of redundant skin that may develop at the ends of the wound during suturing. It is avoided by suturing the wound from the middle by sequentially bisecting the wound. Dog ears can be removed in many ways the simplest of which is the overlap excision technique. The redundant skin is pulled across the wound from one side and excised along the line of the wound. Redundant skin from the opposite side is pulled across the wound and also excised along the line of the wound. The wound is then closed (see Fig. 4.1.7).

Staples

Stainless steel staples can be applied more rapidly than sutures, and they are associated with a lower rate of foreign body reaction and infection. Staples are generally considered especially useful for lacerations of the scalp, trunk, and limbs. However, they do not allow such meticulous wound apposition as sutures, and are slightly more painful to remove. They should not be used on the face or in any other wound where cosmetic out-come is a high priority.

Fig. 4.1.7   Dog ear. Direct overlap excision technique. (From an original drawing by Elaine Wheildon)

Tissue adhesives

Tissue adhesives have now been in use for several decades. The basis of the adhesive is a cyanoacrylate polymer. The cyanoacrylate polymerise in the presence of hydroxyl ions – found in water or blood – allowing them to bind to the skin. Tissue adhesives are for external use only and should not be placed within wounds or used on mucous membranes.

It is in the repair of lacerations to young children that tissue adhesives have become most popular. They are easy and relatively painless to apply and provide a cosmetic result that is as good as suturing, with no risk of causing suture marks. No removal is required, as they slough off in 7 to 10 days. They are, however, not suitable for use in all wounds. If the laceration cannot be approximated and the wound edges brought together with minimal tension then tissue adhesive is not appropriate. Care should be taken not to apply too much tissue glue and to avoid placement over currently bleeding wounds as the polymerisation is exothermic and the patient will notice a heat sensation. Also, contact with excess blood causes polymerisation above the skin limiting the tensile strength of wound-edge closure.

The tissue glue is applied over the surface of the wound once its edges have been approximated by digital pressure. A thin layer of glue is applied across the wound and the wound held approximated for about 30 seconds. Care is taken not to allow glue to spill into eyes or orifices, and to avoid fixing forceps or gloves to the patient. The cyanoacrylates also act as their own dressing providing moist wound healing conditions under the glue, and have a degree of intrinsic antimicrobial activity. Careful attention to wound cleansing is still needed to avoid wound infections. In general, they are less expensive than sutures or staples and are strongly preferred by patients and families. A comparison of the various methods of wound closure is found in Table 4.1.5.

Skin tapes

Skin tapes can be used to close small wounds with low tensile forces. They cannot be used over areas of motion such as over joints. Wound haemostasis is vital as the tapes will not stick to wet skin. Application of an adhesive agent to the skin adjacent to the wound is necessary to provide adequate adhesion of the tapes. These adhesive agents (e.g. Tinc benz®) are toxic to tissues and cause pain, so great care should be taken not to spill them into the wound. Tapes are not suitable for use in small children as they frequently pull them off. Tapes are a useful adjunct to wound closure, for example after suture removal or tissue adhesive application to decrease tension on the wound.

POST-WOUND-CLOSURE CARE

All patients should be provided with written information on care of their wound. Parents and children must understand the importance of ongoing wound care and be provided with instructions about follow up.

Dressing and suture removal

After the wound has been sutured it should be covered with a non-adherent

Table 4.1.5	Characteristics of wound closure techniques	
Technique	Advantages	Disadvantages
Suture	Greatest tensile strength Meticulous closure	Requires removal Painful Slow application Costly Slow to apply Increased tissue reaction
Staples	Rapid application Low cost Low tissue reactivity	Less meticulous closure Discomfort of removal
Tissue adhesives	Painless Rapid application No removal needed Low cost No risk of needle stick	Lower tensile strength Not for use over joints
Surgical tapes	Least reactive Rapid application Patient comfort No risk of needle stick Low cost	Low tensile strength Difficulty maintaining adhesion Requires use of toxic adjuncts

occlusive or semi-occlusive dressing to protect the wound from bacterial invasion and provide a moist healing environment and speed wound healing. Ideally the dressing is left intact until suture removal. The dressing should only be removed if it becomes saturated or there is a risk of infection and inspection is warranted. If the wound is not covered with a waterproof dressing the dressing can be removed every few days for showering. Non-absorbable sutures should be removed at the appropriate time, depending on the location of the injury. Removal of the sutures too early risks dehiscence, leaving sutures too long increases tissue reaction and the risk of cross-hatching and wound infection (see Table 4.1.6). In general, sutures are removed earlier in children than in adults. Wounds closed with tissue adhesive should not be covered with an occlusive dressing, as the extra moisture will more rapidly decrease the ability of the glue to maintain wound edge apposition. The wound should be kept dry for three days, after which the patients may shower but should avoid bathing and swimming. Wounds closed with skin tapes should be kept dry to prevent premature removal.

Immobilisation and drains

Wounds that cross joints or are in areas of highly mobile skin should be immobilised. The joint should be splinted in the position of function for 7 to 10 days. Plaster of Paris can be used to make a cheap and easily applied splint, or a bulky dressing can be used to limit motion and prevent the child tampering with the wound.

Table 4.1.6	Timing of suture removal
Wound location	Time of removal (days)
Face	4
Scalp	5
Upper limbs, trunk	7–10
Lower limbs	8–10
Over joints	10–14

In general, drains should not be used in wound that have been closed as they promote wound infection. If a wound is considered at high risk for infection delayed primary closure should be undertaken rather that closure and drainage.

TREATMENT OF SELECTED INJURIES

Abrasions

In abrasions the underlying tissues are relatively uninjured, providing a degree of protection against infection. Cleansing the abrasion is important to flush away bacteria and remove particulate matter, which should be removed to prevent infection or tattooing. Large abrasions or those heavily contaminated may need cleaning under general anaesthesia. After adequate cleansing and debridement the wound should be covered with a non-adherent occlusive or semi-occlusive dressing. A moist environment enhances healing, and the environment under a scab is ideal. However, wounds without extensive scab formation are more comfortable, so a dressing provides the moist environment. Children with large or deep abrasions should be reviewed in 2 to 3 days to check the wound. Ongoing review should be once or twice weekly.

Eyelid lacerations

A thorough eye examination needs to be performed for all eyelid lacerations. Attention should be given to the possibility of a ruptured globe (eccentric pupil) or trauma to the globe (hyphaema, dislocated lens or retinal detachment). Visual acuity should be measured and documented. Any wound that penetrates the tarsal plate or the inner canthus requires specialist attention, as do wounds involving the lid margins. Any wound that cannot be adequately assessed (e.g. in a young child) should be referred for evaluation under anaesthesia.

Superficial wounds of the eyelid are relatively easily repaired with 6–0 fast absorbing gut with sutures placed close to the wound edge. Care must be taken not to suture into the tarsal plate or other deep structures.

Lip lacerations

Inspection of the teeth and oral mucosa is mandatory in all lip lacerations. Tooth injuries should be documented and referred for management where necessary, missing teeth warrant investigation to ensure they have not been inhaled or imbedded in the soft tissues of the mouth. Ideal anaesthesia is via nerve block of the mental or alveolar nerves for the lower lip or the infra-orbital nerve for the upper lip. Alternatives include sedation and direct infiltration, with or without application of methylene blue to the margins of the vermillion border.

Wounds that involve the vermillion border (the junction of the dry oral mucosa and the facial skin) must be exactly realigned to achieve acceptable cosmetic results. A 6–0 suture should be used with the first suture placed to exactly reappose the vermillion border. Further sutures should close the skin and the dry mucosal surface of the lip with the wet mucosal surface only closed if it is gaping significantly.

Deep or through and through lacerations of the lip require deep sutures to repair the orbicularis oris muscle, if this is the case, an absorbable 6-0 suture should be used. The deep sutures should be placed after the initial suture is placed at the vermillion border and before tying that stitch.

Tongue lacerations

Most tongue lacerations can be left to heal without intervention with good results. Large lacerations involving the free edge of the tongue should be repaired to avoid healing with a notch, interfering with the function of the tongue. Large flaps and lacerations that continue to bleed should also be repaired. Care should be taken when repairing these injuries because of the risk of airway compromise, especially considering moderate to deep sedation is likely to be necessary.

The tongue should be maintained in position by a gentle pull using a towel clip or 4–0 suture placed through the tip. Interrupted 4–0 absorbable sutures should be placed using full thickness bites to include both mucosal surfaces and the lingual muscle in each stitch. Multiple knots should be used to secure the sutures and the parents warned that while the tongue is anaesthetised the child may bite through the stitch.

Fingertip amputation

Young children tend to injure their fingertips in doors and windows. Most of the injuries in young children are contused lacerations of or partial amputations and complete amputation is less common. Older children are more prone to injury with knives or tools. Fractures are less common in the older age group. These wounds should be evaluated for tissue loss and with radiography for bony injury.

If the amputated fragment has been retained and involves any of the nailbed some surgeons will reimplant as a graft with approximately 50% chance of the graft taking. If the tissue is not retained or is small, and there is no bone on view, it is most appropriate to allow the wound to heal by secondary intention. Fingertips allowed to heal naturally have greater length and better sensory outcome than those treated with grafts. These wounds should be covered with a non-adherent occlusive or semi-occlusive dressing to allow moist wound healing after thorough cleaning and debridement as needed. Follow up should be maintained until the wound is healed.

Injuries involving just the fingertip but not the nail heal very well. Injuries involving the nailbed or nail, but sparing bone, heal well. Those that involve the nailbed, nail and distal phalanx heal less well. Any injury with bone on view should be referred for specialist care.

Nailbed lacerations

Trauma to the distal fingers is often associated with nailbed injury. An underlying fracture of the distal phalanx should be assessed with radiographs. Unrepaired nailbed lacerations can permanently disfigure the growth of the new nail from the matrix.

If the nail is lacerated, completely avulsed, or only loosely attached the nail bed must be explored. This can be done under local anaesthesia with a ring block of the digital nerves or under general anaesthesia. The nail must be removed and the nailbed repaired with 5–0 or 6–0 absorbable suture material. The space between the nailbed and nailfold must be packed with xeroform gauze or the nail replaced to prevent adhesions. If a fracture is present antibiotics should be given. If the nail is partially avulsed only and is tightly adherent to the nailbed it is reasonable to leave this intact as it will adequately splint and maintain apposition of any nailbed injury.

Subungual haematoma

A subungual haematoma is a collection of blood between the nail and nailbed. It is most commonly seen with blunt fingertip injuries and may be associated with a fracture of the distal phalanx. Drainage of the haematoma usually provides symptomatic relief and should be undertaken whenever the haematoma is causing pain. Generally no local anaesthesia is required to drain the haematoma with cautery or needle burring using a 19-gauge needle. If there is an underlying fracture antibiotics should be administered. There is no size of haematoma that requires nail removal for inspection of the nailbed.

Puncture wounds to the foot

Puncture wounds to the foot carry a high risk of infection and retained foreign body. All puncture wounds should be assessed for retained foreign body with radiography, and ultrasound for radiolucent foreign bodies. Anaesthesia with local infiltration or a posterior tibial nerve block is needed. The wound should be soaked to remove any scab on the surface, debrided and irrigated. The wound should be left open once any foreign material has been removed. The wound should be cleaned with an antibacterial solution (such as Betadine®) and dressed with a non-adherent dressing. Close review is important to detect infection early. Prophylactic antibiotics have not been shown to prevent infection and may predispose to *Pseudomonas* infection.

Bites
Animal bites
Animal bites are a common presenting problem for the ED. Dog and cat bites account for virtually all bites seen in the ED with dog bites being about six-times more common. Rodents and other animals account for less than 1 to 2% of bites.

Dog-bite injuries tend to be relatively large, relatively superficial crush injuries, which are seen most commonly on the face, neck and scalp in children. The overall infection rate for dog bites is about 10%, with facial wound infection rates of about 5%. Dog-bite wounds are infected with multiple organisms on all occasions, with both aerobic and anaerobic bacteria. It is reasonable to cleanse and close most dog bites with antibiotic prophylaxis provided only to wounds that are high risk for infection (see Tables 4.1.7 and 4.1.8).

Cat bites on the other hand are typically puncture wounds with less surrounding tissue injury. They have bacteria inoculated deep into the wound, which is difficult to explore, irrigate or debride. The risk of infection is significantly higher than in dog bite – at least twice as likely – because of the puncture type wound, the most common location of the bite being

Table 4.1.7	Wound infection risk factors	
	High risk	*Low risk*
Biting species	Cat	Dog
	Human	Rodent
Location of wound	Hand	Face
	Over a joint	Scalp
	Below knee	Mucosa
	Through and through oral	
Wound type	Puncture	Large
	Extensive crush	Superficial
	Old	Recent

the hand, and the high incidence (about 80%) of *Pasteurella multocida* found in cats' mouths. *P. multocida* is a facultative, anaerobic Gram-negative rod that often results in rapidly progressive cellulitis. It is sensitive to the penicillins and variably sensitive to macrolides and first-generation cephalosporins. All these drugs have been documented as adequately treating infections of *P. multocida*, but treatment failures have been documented for erythromycin and first-generation cephalosporins. It is recommended that all cat bites receive prophylactic antibiotics (see Table 4.1.7).

Human bites

Most human bites are probably at no more risk of infection than ordinary lacerations and they are not considered to carry a high risk of HIV transmission. However, the clenched-fist injury (or fight bite), which commonly causes a ragged laceration over the fourth or fifth metacarpophalangeal joint is at high risk of infection. These latter wounds should all receive prophylactic antibiotics, as should human bites (including self-inflicted bites) that have high-risk properties (see Tables 4.1.7 and 4.1.8.).

Table 4.1.8   Management of bite wounds

Species	Suturing	Antibiotics
Dog	Yes	High-risk wound type only
Cat	Face only	All
Rodent	Yes	No
Human – hand bites	No	Yes
Human – other bites	Yes	High risk only

CONTROVERSIES

❶ Subcutaneous sutures close deep wound dead space reducing fluid collection and infection, deep sutures of themselves can cause infection by acting as a foreign body.

❷ Dressings for all wounds is changing to promote moist wound healing, this speeds rate of healing and improves wound comfort.

❸ A number of topical anaesthetic creams are being used in extremity wounds despite not being licensed for this use.

❹ Wound drains are not indicated in the management of wounds in the ED, and delayed primary closure is a preferred technique.

❺ Debridement should remove as little tissue as possible to maximise cosmetic outcome.

❻ Prophylactic antibiotics, while intended to prevent infection, have been shown in some wounds to increase the risk of infection with unusual organisms.

SECTION

5

SENIOR AUTHORS MATT O'MEARA
OWEN MILLER

CARDIOVASCULAR

5.1 CYANOTIC HEART DISEASE AND TETRALOGY OF FALLOT SPELLS

ROBIN CHOONG

ESSENTIALS

1 Cyanosis is dependent on haematocrit and oxygen saturation.

2 Cyanosis is caused by arterial oxygen desaturation or increased capillary oxygen extraction.

3 The hyperoxia test helps differentiate cardiac from other causes of cyanosis:
- Measure SpO_2 in room air or low FiO_2;
- Remeasure SpO_2 in 100% O_2;
- If SpO_2 remains low consider a fixed intracardiac shunt (cyanotic congenital heart defect);
- If SpO_2 increases consider other causes, e.g. lung disease.

4 If a cardiac cause is suspected check the pulses, blood pressure, ECG, and chest X-ray. Consult with a neonatologist, paediatrician or cardiologist early.

5 Cyanosis may be due to a duct-dependent lesion. A prostaglandin infusion may be advised following consultation.

Tetralogy spells

1 Cyanosis is variable and depends on the amount of pulmonary blood flow and right-to-left shunting.

2 Hypercyanotic spells treatment:
- 'Knee-chest position' or over parent's shoulder with knees bent;
- Supplemental oxygen;
- Sedation: intravenous or subcutaneous morphine, 0.1 mg kg^{-1};
- Intravascular volume expansion.

3 In prolonged cyanosis consider a vasoconstrictor.

4 For prevention of spells propranolol (0.5–1 mg kg^{-1} po qid).

5 A Blalock–Taussig shunt may be used for palliation before corrective surgery.

INTRODUCTION

Cyanosis is a bluish discolouration of skin and mucous membranes due to excessive concentration of reduced haemoglobin in the blood.[1] Cyanosis is evident when deoxygenated haemoglobin in the cutaneous veins reaches approximately 5 g dL^{-1}.[2] Deoxygenated haemoglobin may occur either from arterial blood desaturation or increased oxygen extraction by peripheral tissue. Central cyanosis is produced as a result of arterial desaturation, i.e. aortic blood carrying deoxygenated haemoglobin. Isolated peripheral cyanosis may result from excessive deoxy-haemoglobin caused by extensive oxygen extraction.[1] Haemoglobin level affects the presence of cyanosis. Cyanosis is detected at a higher oxygen saturation in children with polycythaemia and is more difficult to detect in children with severe anaemia. Causes of cyanosis are listed in Table 5.1.1.

CYANOTIC CONGENITAL HEART DISEASE

Cyanotic congenital heart disease generally presents in the neonatal period. In the newborn, mild cyanosis (mild hypoxia $SaO_2 > 85\%$) may be difficult to detect.[5] Other confounding factors may be acrocyanosis (a normal finding, which may last 72 hours), polycythaemia (giving the appearance of cyanosis) and dark skin (cyanosis is more difficult to detect). Cyanosis is better appreciated in natural light than in artificial light.

Arterial oxygen saturation should always be assessed with pulse oximetry when considering cyanosis in the newborn. The hyperoxia test may help distinguish cyanosis caused by cyanotic heart defects from other defects.[2–4,8]

Hyperoxia test:
- Measure SpO_2 in room air or low FiO_2
- Remeasure SpO_2 after 15 minutes in 100% O_2
- If SpO_2 remains low consider fixed intracardiac shunt (cyanotic congenital heart defect)
- If SpO_2 increases consider other causes, e.g. lung disease.

CLINICAL FEATURES[2,7]

A comprehensive cardiac and respiratory examination is essential in any cyanosed child. The key features are:

- Pulses – rate, rhythm, volume
- Blood pressure – all four limbs if the pulse volume is abnormal
- Precordial impulse – heaves, thrills

Table 5.1.1   Causes of cyanosis[2-7]
Differential diagnosis
Arterial oxygen desaturation (central cyanosis [$PO_2 < 50$ mmHg]) 1. Airway • Airway obstruction 2. Breathing • Lung disease • Central nervous system depression (e.g. coma) • Respiratory muscle weakness • Reduced respiratory drive (e.g. morbid obesity) 3. Circulation • Intracardiac right-to-left shunt (e.g. cyanotic congenital heart disease, pulmonary hypertension) • Intrapulmonary shunt (e.g. pulmonary atrioventricular fistula)
Increased capillary oxygen extraction (peripheral cyanosis) 1. Circulatory shock, e.g. sepsis 2. Congestive heart failure 3. Environmental, e.g. cold 4. Acrocyanosis of the newborn (autonomic – may last 72 hours)
Abnormal haemoglobin (not related to level of oxygenation) 1. Methaemoglobinaemia ($PO_2 > 50$ mmHg but low O_2 saturation)

- Auscultation – abnormalities of P_2, murmurs
- Pre-and post-ductal oximetry if there is differential cyanosis.

INVESTIGATIONS

Investigations are directed at likely causes after history and clinical examination. They may include arterial blood gas, serum electrolytes, glucose levels, full blood count, haematocrit, and cultures.

The CXR can be very useful and should be examined carefully for heart size (normal cardiothoracic ratio in AP film is < 0.6), oligaemic lung field with decreased pulmonary blood flow, e.g. tetralogy of Fallot, or pulmonary venous congestion with an obstructive lesion, e.g. totally anomalous pulmonary venous drainage (TAPVD), cor triatriatum.

MANAGEMENT

The presentation of cyanosis in an infant or child mandates urgent review by a neonatologist, paediatrician or paediatric cardiologist. Echocardiography may be necessary urgently.

An important issue in the management of cyanosis in the newborn period

is recognising the duct-dependent lesion. A duct-dependent lesion is one that results from the ductus arteriosus remaining patent so that blood flow is delivered to both the pulmonary and systemic circuits:

- Pulmonary atresia/critical pulmonary stenosis. The ductus shunts right-to-left to ensure adequate pulmonary blood flow.
- Coarctation of the aorta/critical aortic stenosis/interrupted aortic arch. The ductus shunts right-to-left to ensure adequate systemic blood flow.
- Transposition of the great arteries. Mixing is required usually at atrial, ductus and ventricular levels.

If a duct-dependent lesion is considered consult a paediatric cardiologist before starting an intravenous infusion of prostaglandin E_2. Important side effects are respiratory depression and fever.

Chronic cyanosis stimulates a reactive polycythaemia that increases the oxygen-carrying capacity. When haematocrit reaches 65% or more, a large increase in blood viscosity occurs.

Hyperviscosity and coagulopathy often occur and in patients with a right-to-left intracardiac shunt may result in stroke and brain abscess.

TETRALOGY SPELLS

INTRODUCTION[2-10]

Hypercyanotic, hypoxic or cyanotic spells occur in young infants with tetralogy of Fallot. These occur most commonly under 6 months of age and may be precipitated by agitation from any cause. The cause is likely to be multifactorial including a component of dynamic infundibular obstruction. The net result is an imbalance of pulmonary to systemic blood flow.

Tetralogy of Fallot consists of anterior deviation of the outlet septum leading to the characteristic morphologic features of:

❶ Subpulmonary infundibular stenosis ± pulmonary valve stenosis ± hypoplastic pulmonary arteries.
❷ Subaortic perimembranous ventricular septal defect (VSD).
❸ Aortic root overriding the crest of septum and VSD.
❹ Secondary right ventricular hypertrophy.

Clinical features include:

- Intense cyanosis
- Hyperpnoea and acidosis
- Quieter and shorter ejection murmur (compared to before the spell)
- Irritability, lethargy, loss of consciousness, seizures, death.

Triggers include dehydration, exertion and emotional distress. The child may have a history of previous squatting. Spells are usually self-limiting though sequelae include hypoxic-ischaemic encephalopathy and death. Spells are less common since the advent of early systemic-pulmonary shunts or early corrective surgery.

INVESTIGATIONS

Investigations include laboratory testing and imaging as follows.

Laboratory
Blood gas analysis – usually shows acidosis with hypoxia.

ECG

The ECG in tetralogy of Fallot usually shows:

- Right ventricular hypertrophy in the unipolar and standard leads
- Right axis deviation ($+120°$ to $+150°$)
- Dominant R wave in the right and a dominant S in the left precordial leads
- Right atrial hypertrophy
- Normal PR interval and QRS duration
- Tall, peaked T waves
- Reversal of the RS ratio.

Chest X-ray

The classic *coeur en sabot* or boot-shaped cardiac silhouette is caused by the elevation of the apex due to right ventricular hypertrophy, combined with a concavity in the area of the main pulmonary artery. A right-sided aorta is present in 25% of tetralogy patients.

Echocardiography

An echocardiogram will accurately confirm tetralogy of Fallot but is not useful in acute management of spells.

TREATMENT[2–6, 8–13]

❶ If possible, the child should be in a quiet, calm environment.

❷ The knee-chest or squatting position is preferred as it increases afterload thus decreasing R to L shunting.

❸ Supplemental high-flow oxygen ($6–8$ L min^{-1} of 100% oxygen) should be provided.

❹ Monitoring includes continuous ECG monitoring, pulse oximetry, and non-invasive BP.

❺ Morphine ($0.1–0.2$ mg kg^{-1} IV or SC) should be used to treat hyperpnoea and decrease systemic catecholamines.

❻ Consider a small fluid volume challenge ($5–10$ mL kg^{-1}) to increase preload and reduce dynamic outflow obstruction.

❼ Propranolol ($0.05–0.2$ mg kg^{-1} slow IV push over 10 minutes, repeat once every 15 minutes) can be used to block β-receptors in the infundibulum, thereby lessening RV outflow obstruction. Other β-blockers may be useful.

❽ Phenylephrine (phenylephrine, $5–10$ µg kg^{-1} IV [maximum dose = 10 mg]) increases afterload thereby decreasing R to L shunt. Alternatives include metaraminol (0.01 mg kg^{-1} IV) or methoxamine (0.1 mg kg^{-1} IV).

❾ Consider NaHCO$_3$ ($1–2$ mmol L^{-1} IV) for correction of acidosis.

❿ Check temperature and blood glucose. Correct hypoglycaemia and hypothermia.

DISPOSITION

Organise hospital admission and paediatric cardiology consultation.

Failure to respond to the above treatment mandates intubation, ventilation and deep sedation or general anaesthesia and intensive care admission. Emergency surgery is rarely indicated.

REFERENCES

1. Anderson DM 1994 Dorland's Illustrated Medical Dictionary. WB Saunders, Philadelphia
2. Park MK 1996 Pathophysiology of cyanotic congenital heart defects. In: Park MY (ed) Pediatric Cardiology for Practitioners, 3rd edn. Mosby-Year Book, St Louis
3. Abelson WH, Garth Smith R 1987 Residents handbook of pediatrics, 7th edn. The Hospital for Sick Children, Toronto, Canada, BC Decker Inc, Toronto
4. Guzman MF, Hedley Brown A, Been M, Cook S, Wren C, Richens D 1989 Manual of cardiorespiratory critical care. Butterworth, Sevenoaks, Kent
5. Kilham H, Isaacs D 1999 The New Children's Hospital Handbook. RAHC, Westmead
6. Browne GJ, Choong RKC, Gaudry PL, Wilkins BH 1997 Principles and practice of children's emergency care. MacLennan & Petty, Sydney
7. Emmanouilides GC, Riemenschneider TA, Allen HD, Gutgesell HP (eds) 1995 Moss and Adams' heart disease in infants, children, and adolescents: Including the fetus and young adult, 5th edn. Williams & Wilkins, Baltimore, MD
8. Nichols, Cameron, Greely et al 1995 Critical heart disease in infants and children. Mosby-Year Book, St Louis
9. Zuberbuhler JR 1995 Tetralogy of Fallot. In: Emmanouilides GC, Riemenschneider TA, Allen HD, Gutgesell HP (eds) Moss and Adams' heart disease in infants, children, and adolescents: Including the fetus and young adult, 5th edn. Williams & Wilkins, Baltimore, MD
10. Park MK 1996 Tetralogy of Fallot. In: Pediatric cardiology for practitioners, 3rd edn. Mosby-Year Book, St Louis
11. van Roekens CN, Zuckerberg AL 1995 Emergency management of hypercyanotic crises in tetralogy of Fallot. Annals of Emergency Medicine 25(2): 256–258
12. Baele PL, Rennotte MT, Veyckemans FA 1991 External compression of the abdominal aorta reversing tetralogy of Fallot cyanotic crisis. Anaesthesiology 75(1): 146–149
13. Nussbaum J, Zane EA, Thys DM 1989 Esmolol for the treatment of hypercyanotic spells in infants with tetralogy of Fallot. Journal of Cardiothoracic Anaesthesiology 3(2): 200–202

FURTHER READING

Archer N, Burch M 1998 Paediatric cardiology: An introduction. Chapman & Hall Medical, London
Emmanouilides GC, Riemenschneider TA, Allen HD, Gutgesell HP (eds) 1995 Moss and Adams' heart disease in infants, children, and adolescents: Including the fetus and young adult, 5th edn. Williams & Wilkins, Baltimore, MD
Nadas AS 1992 Tetralogy of Fallot. In: Nadas paediatric cardiology. Hanley & Belfus, Philadelphia
Nichols, Cameron, Greely et al 1995 Critical heart disease in infants and children. Mosby-Year Book, St Louis
Park MY 1996 Pediatric cardiology for practitioners, 3rd edn. Mosby-Year Book, St Louis
van Roekens CN, Zuckerberg AL 1995 Emergency management of hypercyanotic crises in tetralogy of Fallot. Annals of Emergency Medicine 25(2): 256–258

CARDIOVASCULAR

5

5.2 HEART FAILURE

ROBIN CHOONG

ESSENTIALS

1 Congestive heart failure (CHF) is a clinical syndrome and may result from:
- Excessive work load caused by increased pressure or volume, usually increased pulmonary blood flow, and/or
- Normal workload faced by a damaged myocardium.

2 Clinical signs may include tachycardia, tachypnoea, increased work of breathing, sweatiness, cardiomegaly and hepatomegaly. In addition infants may have failure to thrive, recurrent lower respiratory tract infections and respiratory distress.

3 In older children, new onset heart failure may be less overtly symptomatic. Malaise, decrease in the level of daily activity, abdominal pain, nausea, anorexia and weight loss may be present.

4 Current medications used in heart failure include diuretics, digoxin and angiotensin-converting enzyme inhibitors.

CAUSES OF CONGESTIVE HEART FAILURE[1-3]

Most cases of congestive heart failure in childhood result from congenital heart defects.

❶ Left-to-right shunts with increased pulmonary blood flow, e.g. VSD, AVSD, PDA.
❷ Acute left heart obstruction, e.g. aortic stenosis, coarctation of the aorta, interrupted aortic arch, hypoplastic left heart syndrome.

A smaller number of cases may be from:

❸ Primary myocardial dysfunction, e.g. myocarditis, cardiomyopathy, anomalous left coronary artery.
❹ Other causes, e.g. anaemia, metabolic, toxic, dysrhythmia.

Age-based

The causes of congestive heart failure change with age. Congenital heart defects generally present in the first days or months of life. Acquired cardiac disease may occur at any age.

First days of life

Asphyxia, left heart obstruction, metabolic, sepsis.

One day to one week of age

Left heart obstruction in duct-dependent lesions, e.g. aortic stenosis, coarctation of the aorta.

Large left-to-right shunt lesions, e.g. large VSD, AVSD, truncus arteriosus.

First month

Large left-to-right shunt, e.g. large VSD, AVSD, truncus arteriosus.

First three months

Large left-to-right shunt, e.g. large VSD, AVSD, truncus arteriosus.

Metabolic disease.

Acquired heart disease may occur at any age due to:

- Inflammatory/infective, e.g. viral myocarditis, Kawasaki disease, pleuropericarditis, rheumatic fever
- Metabolic genetic, e.g. inherited cardiomyopathy
- Dysrhythmia, e.g. sustained SVT, VT
- Severe anaemia.

CLINICAL MANIFESTATIONS AND INVESTIGATIONS[1-3]

Presentation

Infants may present with problems related to feeding such as sweatiness, tachypnoea, reduced volume of feeds leading to failure to thrive. Respiratory problems, such as cough, recurrent respiratory infections, tachypnoea and increased work of breathing are prominent. Lower respiratory tract infection may have features in common with CCF. Cardiac failure should be considered in atypical, persistent or recurrent cases.

General features

- Tachycardia – due to fixed stroke volume.
- Tachypnoea – due to decreased compliance with increased lung water.
- Gallop rhythm, weak pulse.
- Failure to thrive – from decreased energy intake, increased energy expenditure.
- Cardiomegaly – may be due to left heart obstruction with left-to-right shunt or left ventricular dysfunction.
- Sweaty (cold sweat) – prominent with feeding.
- Fatigue/lethargy.
- Hepatomegaly – not specific to right heart failure, may occur with any aetiology.

Investigations

- Chest X-ray
  Cardiomegaly (in an AP film the normal cardiothoracic ratio is < 0.6)
  Pulmonary plethora in left-to-right shunt
  Pulmonary venous congestion in left heart obstruction/left ventricular dysfunction. Radiologic features include reticulogranular pattern, fluid in lung fissures, pleural effusions, pulmonary oedema.

- ECG
  Assess rhythm, myocarditis (voltages), ischaemia (ST-T wave).

Referral

The diagnosis of cardiac failure in an infant or child mandates urgent review by a paediatrician or paediatric cardiologist. Echocardiography will usually be performed following the consultation.

MANAGEMENT[1-3,5-14]

Current medications used in heart failure include diuretics, digoxin and angiotensin-converting enzyme inhibitors.

Acute management

❶ Resuscitate with ventilatory support if required.

❷ If desaturated consider supplemental oxygen. Caveat: large left-to-right shunt lesions (e.g. truncus arteriosus) may worsen with high FiO_2. Consult early in these cases.

❸ Fluid restriction and diuretic therapy.

❹ Infants with left heart obstruction may present with cardiorespiratory failure when the ductus arteriosus closes. Prostaglandin infusion may reopen the ductus and assist systemic perfusion.

Diuretics

❶ Acutely: furosemide 1 mg kg^{-1} dose^{-1} IM or IV (anticipate hypokalaemia).

❷ Chronically: furosemide 1–3 mg kg^{-1} day^{-1} in divided doses, with spironolactone, 1 mg kg^{-1} dose^{-1} po q12h. Beware potassium sparing effect of ACE inhibitors.

Digoxin

- Severe congestive heart failure treated with initial IV administration. Early failure in less distressed infants can be treated orally. All patients should have oral therapy as soon as possible. IV dosage is only 70–80% of amount used orally.

- The total digitalizing dose (Premature: 20 micrograms/kg; infant: 30–40 micrograms/kg; over 2 yr: 30 micrograms/kg) may be given as $\frac{1}{2}$ stat, $\frac{1}{4}$ in 6–12 hr, and $\frac{1}{4}$ in another 12–18 hr.

- Maintenance dose (IV, oral) is micrograms/kg 12 hrly. If heart failure is not severe, then may stat with maintenance dose only.

- Digoxin is contraindicated in complete heart block, pericardial tamponade, hypertrophic cardiomyopathy and other outflow tract obstructions. reduce dose in renal failure.

- Monitor with ECG and serum digoxin level (keep below 2.5 nmol/L [2.0 ng/L]).

Angiotensin-converting enzyme inhibitors

Angiotensin-converting enzyme inhibitors (ACEi) are used in heart failure due to large left-to-right shunts and heart failure caused by ventricular failure. Oral captopril (0.1–1 mg/kg/dose 8 hrly) or lisinopril (0.1 mg/kg daily, increasing to 0.2–0.4 mg/kg daily over 4–6 weeks) may be used.

β-blockers

β-blockers have a role in paediatric heart failure though doses are extrapolated from adult data. However, their role in children with heart failure remains to be fully defined.

FUTURE RESEARCH

The completion of prospective, randomised trials in children will provide much needed information for guiding rational treatment of paediatric heart failure. Especially the evaluation of chronic therapy (e.g. β-blockers), early introduction of ACE inhibitors and more accurate metabolic/genetic diagnosis of cardiomyopathy.

REFERENCES

1. Park MK 1996 Congestive heart failure. In: Park MY (ed) Pediatric cardiology for practitioners, 3rd edn. Mosby-Year Book, St Louis
2. Talner NS 1995 Heart failure. In: Emmanouilides GC, Riemenschneider TA, Allen HD, Gutgesell HP (eds): Moss and Adams' heart disease in infants, children, and adolescents: Including the fetus and young adult, 5th edn. Williams & Wilkins, Baltimore, MD
3. Abelson WH, Garth Smith R 1987 Residents handbook of pediatrics, 7th edn. The Hospital for Sick Children, Toronto, Canada, BC Decker Inc, Toronto
4. Guzman MF, Hedley Brown A, Been M, Cook S, Wren C, Richens D 1989 Manual of cardiorespiratory critical care. Butterworth, Sevenoaks, Kent
5. Chang AC, Hanley FL, Wernovsky G, Wessel DL 1998 Pediatric cardiac intensive care. Williams & Wilkins, Baltimore, MD
6. Shaddy RE 2001 Optimizing treatment for chronic congestive heart failure in children. Critical Care Medicine 29(Suppl): S237–S240
7. Schwartz SM, Duffy JY, Pearl JM, Nelson DP 2001 Cellular and molecular aspects of myocardial dysfunction. Critical Care Medicine 29(Suppl): S214–S219
8. Clark BJ, IIIrd 2000 Treatment of heart failure in infants and children. Heart Disease 2(5): 354–361
9. Buchhorn R, Hammersen A, Bartmus D, Bursch J 2001 The pathogenesis of heart failure in infants with congenital heart disease. Cardiology in the Young 11(5): 498–504
10. Kay JD, Colan SD, Graham TP Jr 2001 Congestive heart failure in pediatric patients. American Heart Journal 142(5): 923–928
11. Wernovsky G, Hoffman TM 2001 Pediatric heart failure management: Solving the puzzle. Critical Care Medicine 29(10 Suppl): S212–S213
12. Shaddy RE 2001 Beta-adrenergic receptor blockers as therapy in pediatric chronic heart failure. Minerva Pediatric 53(4): 297–304
13. Shekerdemian L 2001 Nonpharmacologic treatment of acute heart failure. Current Opinions in Paediatrics 13(3): 240–246

FURTHER READING

Allen HD, Gutgesell HP, Clark EB et al 2001 Moss and Adams' heart disease in infants, children and adolescents, 6th edn. Lippincott Williams and Wilkins, Philadelphia
Archer N, Burch M 1998 Paediatric cardiology. An introduction. Chapman & Hall Medical, London
Park MK 1996 Congestive heart failure. In: Park MY (ed) Pediatric cardiology for practitioners, 3rd edn. Mosby-Year Book, St Louis

5.3 SYNCOPE

LINDA DUROJAIYE

ESSENTIALS

1 The most common cause of syncope in children is vasovagal.

2 A careful and detailed history will usually enable the diagnosis of vasovagal syncope to be established with confidence.

3 The main differential diagnoses of syncope in childhood include cardiovascular causes, seizures, migraines, hypoglycaemia, drugs, and psychogenic events.

4 A 12-lead ECG should be done for all children at the initial presentation with syncope.

5 Any child in whom a cardiac cause of syncope is either suspected or diagnosed should be referred to a cardiologist.

INTRODUCTION

Syncope is the term used to describe any event of sudden and transient loss of consciousness and postural tone.

The range of incidences of syncope occurring in childhood is described as being from 0.1–50%, with peak incidences occurring amongst toddlers and adolescents. The most common events seen in the paediatric setting are episodes of vasovagal syncope. Differentiating the common, benign vasovagal event from rare differential diagnoses is essential to the appropriate management of children who present with syncope.

By contrast, in the adult population syncope is the cause of 1–3% of all ED attendances, and malignant cardiac arrhythmias are commonly the underlying cause.

AETIOLOGY

The final common pathway that leads to all episodes of syncope is a sudden decrease in delivery of metabolic substrates, namely oxygen and glucose, to the brain.

In childhood and adolescence the major cause of syncope is transient autonomic dysfunction. In toddlers such episodes usually manifest as either blue breath-holding spells or 'reflex anoxic seizures' (also called 'pallid breath-holding spells'). The mechanism for the cyanosis in blue breath-holding spells is poorly understood. The precipitant for reflex anoxic seizures may be a noxious stimulus causing reflex asystole, which leads to an anoxic seizure.

In older children and in adolescents such episodes most commonly present as episodes of vasovagal syncope. A combination of hypotension and profound bradycardia, or either bradycardia or hypotension alone leads to cerebral hypoxia. Complete understanding of the underlying mechanisms is lacking. Other terms used to describe these episodes include neurocardiogenic syncope, vasodepressor syncope or neurally mediated syncope.

The differential diagnoses of syncope in childhood include cardiovascular causes, seizures, migraines, hypoglycaemia, drugs, and psychogenic events. These are listed in more detail in Table 5.3.1. It should be noted that situational syncope (syncope that occurs during micturition, swallowing cold liquids, defecation or coughing), and carotid sinus sensitivity are rare in the paediatric population. Mitral valve prolapse has not been conclusively proven to be a cause of syncope.

CLINICAL

History

A careful and detailed history will usually enable the correct diagnosis of the most common cause of childhood syncope, vasovagal syncope, to be established with confidence. Any unusual features of the history should raise suspicion of an alternate diagnosis.

A complete history should include the following:

- A description of the event by a witness if possible. Ask specifically about duration of loss of consciousness, seizure activity, incontinence of urine, pallor or cyanosis, and post-ictal drowsiness or confusion.
- Any antecedent events such as sudden emotion or pain, anxiety, fasting, intercurrent illness, blood loss, or a warm environment.
- Activity and posture at the time of the event.
- Prodromal symptoms such as nausea, sweating, visual or auditory changes, an aura, perioral paraesthesia and carpopedal spasm, palpitations, dyspnoea or chest pain.
- Relevant medical history including previous episodes of syncope, cardiac disease, epilepsy, diabetes, drug use and past sexual activity.
- Family history of sudden collapse or death, cardiac disease, epilepsy, syncope and metabolic disease.

Vasovagal syncope

The typical history of vasovagal syncope is that the episode occurs whilst standing or sitting upright. There may or may not be a stressful antecedent event (this occurs less commonly in frequent recurrent vasovagal syncope). There is a prodrome of nausea, dizziness, visual disturbance and a sensation of warmth, followed by a period of loss of tone and consciousness. Witnesses will describe marked pallor. Seizure activity is unusual, but brief tonic-clonic activity or stiffening is possible. Urinary incontinence may also occur. Recovery to a normal level of consciousness is usually prompt once in the supine position. Children who recognise the prodrome may avoid a syncopal episode by

Table 5.3.1   Causes of childhood syncope

Abnormality of circulation	Vasovagal syncope Reflex anoxic seizures Blue breath-holding attacks Cerebral syncope Acute volume depletion Chronic hypovolaemia Orthostatic hypotension Pregnancy

Cardiac causes	• Tachyarrythmias
	   Supraventricular tachyarrhythmias
	   Wolff–Parkinson–White syndrome
	   Ventricular tachycardia
	   Ventricular fibrillation
	• Conduction disturbances
	   Long QT interval
	   Atrio-ventricular block
	   Sinus node disease
	• Left ventricular outflow tract obstruction
	   Valvular aortic stenosis
	   Coarctation of the aorta
	   Idiopathic hypertrophic subaortic stenosis
	• Right ventricular outflow tract obstruction
	   Pulmonary stenosis
	   Tetralogy of Fallot
	   Primary pulmonary hypertension
	   Eisenmenger's syndrome
	   Large pulmonary embolism
	• Dilated cardiomyopathy
	   Myocarditis
	   Idiopathic
	   Coronary artery anomalies
	• Pericarditis with tamponade
	• Vertebro-basilar insufficiency

Central nervous system disorders	Seizure Migraine
Hypoglycaemia	
Hypoxia	
Drugs and poisons (no QT prolongation)	Antihypertensive drugs Antiarrhythmics Carbon monoxide poisoning Volatile nitrites Others
Psychogenic	Hyperventilation Hysteria Malingering Munchausen's by proxy Panic disorder

assuming the lying position. The child may have a headache, or be fatigued for minutes to hours after the event.

Cardiac syncope

A cardiac cause of syncope should be suspected in a patient with a history of congenital heart disease or with a family history of sudden death. Cardiac events are more likely to cause episodes of syncope that occur with no warning, with associated chest pain, during exercise, whilst sitting or supine, or in association with palpitations (though palpitations are frequently described by individuals with vasovagal syncope, and with hyperventilation).

Long QT syndrome is an ECG diagnosis that is associated with episodes of syncope or seizures caused by episodes of paroxysmal ventricular tachycardia (often *Torsades de Pointes*). It may result in sudden death. Syncopal episodes in patients with this diagnosis may be precipitated by exercise or a startle, or may be spontaneous. The condition may be congenital or acquired. The ECG in sinus rhythm reveals a prolonged QT interval. The QT prolongation may be minimal, and a high index of suspicion is needed to make the diagnosis. The QT interval is calculated with Bazett's formula:

$$QTc = \frac{QT}{\sqrt{RR}}$$

where QTc is the corrected QT interval (normal < 0.44 seconds), QT is the QT interval in seconds, and RR is the RR interval in seconds.

Reflex anoxic seizures and blue breath-holding spells

Blue breath-holding spells are usually associated with a prolonged episode of crying after which the child has a prolonged forced expiration and apnoea, and becomes cyanosed. This may be followed by a brief period of loss of consciousness, with a rapid recovery to full normal activity. They occur in children between the ages of one to five years, with a peak incidence at the age of two years. They are more common than reflex anoxic seizures.

Reflex anoxic seizures occur when an infant is suddenly startled (for example by an injury). The infant is seen to give one or two cries, quietens and then becomes pale. There is then an abrupt loss of consciousness, during which the infant may have brief tonic posturing and upward eye deviation. Tonic-clonic movements may occur. Episodes usually last less than one minute, and are immediately followed by normal consciousness and posture.

Of these children, 85% have no further episodes after the age of five years, though 17% may get recurrence of syncopal episodes later in life. There is no increased tendency in these children to develop epilepsy, and there are no associated abnormalities found on electroencephalogram (EEG) testing.

Hypovolaemic states

There will usually be a history suggestive of fluid or blood loss and obvious signs of shock may be present. Orthostatic hypotension and tachycardia may be the only positive clinical signs. These tend to occur immediately, as distinct from the changes seen in vasovagal syncope, which occur after more prolonged orthostatic stress.

Seizures

It may be difficult to differentiate seizures from vasovagal episodes, as they may both be associated with brief convulsions as well as a loss of consciousness. A history of significant post-event disorientation is helpful in differentiating seizures from other causes of syncope. Seizures are also more likely to be associated with cyanosis, tongue biting, and a more prolonged period of loss of consciousness.

Hysterical syncope

Hysterical syncope is a diagnosis to be made once all other possible causes have been excluded, but clues strongly suggestive of the diagnosis are often witnessed during the event. The child will have no hypotension, bradycardia or pallor, and fluttering of half-closed eyelids may be seen.

Hyperventilation syncope

Syncope due to hyperventilation may be associated with a prodrome of light-headedness and blurred vision. It is not as commonly seen as other symptoms associated with hyperventilation, such as feelings of anxiety, breathlessness and perioral paraesthesiae or carpopedal spasm.

EXAMINATION

A structured approach to the clinical examination of all children presenting with syncope is essential to ensure that all relevant findings are elucidated.

- The airway must be examined, and the work of breathing noted.
- The peripheral pulse rate, rhythm and character must be noted, and the orthostatic blood pressure recorded (this is abnormal if there is a decrease in systolic blood pressure of more than 20 mmHg between measurements taken in the supine and

sitting or standing position). Cardiac auscultation and a 12-lead ECG should be performed on all patients.
- The level of consciousness, posture and mental state of the child should be noted, and pupils and fundi should be examined.
- The child's temperature should be recorded.
- The history and the initial assessment should direct further examination of the child. In addition to searching for clues to the cause of the syncope, it is important to examine the patient for any injuries sustained during the event.

INVESTIGATIONS

Clinical Investigations within the ED

A 12-lead ECG should be done for all children at the initial presentation with syncope. The primary aim is the exclusion of a prolonged QT interval, and of any arrhythmia or other abnormality of conduction.

A blood sugar level is an appropriate investigation for the child with a history of fasting, or with a family history of metabolic disease.

A βHCG is indicated in fertile and sexually active adolescent females.

Other investigations are usually unnecessary, and if done should be appropriate to the clinical history and examination findings for the child.

Further investigations performed in the ED may include:

- Cardiac monitoring and pulse oximetry for any child in whom the history is suggestive of an arrhythmia, or who remains unwell.
- Blood haemoglobin concentration where a history suggestive of significant blood loss or anaemia is obtained.
- Serum electrolytes, urea and creatinine, and urinary specific gravity where a diagnosis of dehydration is suspected.
- A chest X-ray where a structural cardiac abnormality is suspected.
- Urine drug screen for patients with a history or examination that suggests

intoxication with a specific substance. This is not a useful investigation when done routinely.

Any abnormality found in these investigations should then direct further investigation and referral.

Out patient investigations of syncope

Consider referral and further investigation for any child with an atypical history or abnormal examination, or with severe or frequent vasovagal syncope (Table 5.3.2).

Any child in whom a cardiac cause of syncope is either suspected or diagnosed must be referred to a cardiologist. It may be appropriate to arrange secondary investigations such as an echocardiogram or Holter monitoring prior to discharge from the ED. It should be noted that Holter monitoring is often unhelpful as symptoms rarely occur whilst the patient is monitored. Some children may go on to have electrophysiological studies, exercise stress tests or cardiac angiography.

Where a history obtained suggests that the child has had a seizure, an electroencephalogram (EEG) should be arranged in consultation with the neurologist or paediatrician to whom they are referred.

Head-upright tilt-table testing may be done in children with frequent, recurrent syncope, and in those children in whom a cause for syncope is not certain. Protocols for the test vary, but the three requirements are that the child has a period of supine rest before tilting and is then tilted at a defined angle for a period of time. The most common positive response seen is a combination of hypotension and bradycardia prior to syncope or near syncope. Other positive responses

Table 5.3.2 Indications for referral and further investigation of a child with syncope
- Atypical history
- Abnormal cardiovascular or central nervous system examination
- Suspect cardiovascular cause
- Suspect seizure
- Recurrent and problematic vasovagal syncope

Table 5.4.1 Normal respiratory rates, BP and heart rates

Age	Respiratory rate (breaths per minute)	Systolic blood pressure (mmHg)	Heart rate (beats per minute)
< 1	30–40	70–90	110–160
1-2	25–35	80–95	100–150
2-5	25–30	80–100	95–140
5-12	20–25	90–110	80–120
> 12	15–20	100–120	60–100

Auscultation of the heart starts with listening for the heart sounds, especially splitting of the second heart sound. In children splitting is usually only audible during inspiration at the upper left border of the sternum. The absence of variation between inspiration and expiration (fixed splitting) occurs in atrial septal defects. Third heart sounds are heard in 20% of normal children. Listen for clicks in early systole (in aortic and pulmonary stenosis).

Murmurs should be assessed with regard to their:

- Timing – systolic, diastolic or continuous.
- Localisation – the point of maximum intensity.
- Loudness – increasing loudness from grades 1 to 6.
- Character – ejection, pansystolic, early/mid/late diastolic.
- Radiation – audible in areas away from precordium.

Auscultation of the chest should note air entry and presence or absence of crackles.

Abdominal palpation should pay particular attention to the liver span, edge and presence of pulsation.

At the completion of the cardiovascular examination one should be able to determine whether the child is cyanosed or not and whether the child has cardiac failure. The pulses, blood pressure and precordial findings assist with the assessment of the type of cardiac problem, even if a specific diagnosis is not possible. A chest X-ray and electrocardiograph may assist.

Chest X-ray

Key features to assess on the chest X-ray are:

- Patient name and date.
- Cardiac position (dextrocardia, situs inversus).
- Quality of the film – centring, penetration, degree of inspiration.
- Cardiothoracic ratio (usually less than 50% but up to 60% in AP films in neonates).
- Cardiac contour – especially size of pulmonary artery and position of the aorta.
- Lung fields – vascularity.

In acyanotic heart disease with left-to-right shunting there may be increased pulmonary vascularity.

In cyanotic heart disease increased pulmonary vascularity occurs in truncus arteriosus, totally anomalous pulmonary venous drainage (TAPVD) and transposition on the great arteries (TGA). Decreased pulmonary vascularity occurs with pulmonary atresia, tricuspid atresia, Ebstein's anomaly, tetralogy of Fallot and critical pulmonary stenosis.

Electrocardiography

The rate, rhythm and axis should be assessed.

Normal QRS axis varies with age. At birth, the range is from $+60°$ to $+180°$, at 1 year $1°$ to $100°$, at 10 years $1°$ to $130°$.

Systematically look at the P waves, PR interval, QRS complexes, ST interval and T waves.

Atrial enlargement:
- Right atrial enlargement – peaked P wave with height of > 2.5 mm
- Left atrial enlargement – P wave > 0.08 s, may also be plateaued or notched.

Ventricular enlargement:

Right ventricular hypertrophy
- R greater than S in V1 after 1 year
- T wave upright in V1 after 1 week
- SV6 greater than 15 mm at 1 week, 10 mm at 6 months, 5 mm at 1 year.

Left ventricular hypertrophy
- SV1 + rV6 greater than 30 mm to 1 year
- SV1 + rV6 greater than 40 mm after 1 year.

THE CHILD WITH AN ASYMPTOMATIC MURMUR

Murmurs may be heard in around half of normal school-aged children and are heard even more frequently in infants. Many murmurs are innocent and can be recognised by their specific characteristics. Innocent murmurs occur when there is normal or increased blood flow through a normal heart and vessels. Recognising common innocent murmurs enables exclusion of organic heart disease and the need for unnecessary investigation and referral.

There are four characteristic types of innocent murmurs

❶ Vibratory murmur.
❷ Pulmonary flow murmur.
❸ Carotid bruit.
❹ Venous hum.

The *vibratory murmur* (Still's murmur) is a short mid-systolic murmur best heard at the left sternal border or between the apex and the left sternal border. The murmur is of medium frequency and has a slight musical or vibratory character. It is often softer when the child stands or extends the neck and is louder when lying supine.

The *pulmonary flow murmur* is a soft blowing murmur maximal in intensity in the pulmonary area. Murmurs in this location are common in young children, but are often difficult to differentiate from an atrial septal defect or pulmonary stenosis, so may require assessment by a specialist.

A *carotid bruit* produces a rough ejection systolic murmur of medium frequency heard over the base of the neck, but is much softer below the clavicle.

A *venous hum* causes a high-pitched, blowing continuous murmur over the neck or sterno-clavicular junctions. It disappears when the child lies flat or when the neck veins are gently compressed.

DISPOSITION

Referral for specialist consultation is indicated for a child with a murmur who has:

- Symptoms that may indicate cardiac disease (e.g. breathlessness, cyanosis, chest pain)
- Abnormalities of the heart sounds (e.g. fixed splitting of the second heart sound)
- A murmur that cannot be confidently identified as innocent
- A murmur with an associated thrill (grade 4 intensity or greater).

INVESTIGATIONS

Electrocardiography (ECG) and chest X-ray are readily available, but are poor screening tests for children with asymptomatic murmurs.

The ECG is unlikely to disclose any unsuspected heart disease, but may assist in reaching the specific diagnosis when there is underlying pathology.[1] Recent studies have demonstrated that electrocardiography abnormalities are common in athletic children.[2]

Similarly, screening asymptomatic children with a heart murmur chest X-ray is limited by poor sensitivity, specificity and reproducibility.[3] Performing ECG and chest X-ray for children with murmurs has been shown to be more often misleading than helpful for paediatricians and cardiologists.[4]

Clinical assessment by a paediatrician or cardiologist correctly identifies almost all murmurs as innocent or needing further investigation. Echocardiography is not necessary in children identified by a specialist as having an innocent murmur.[1]

COMMON HEART DEFECTS IN INFANCY AND CHILDHOOD

Heart disease in children may present with the presence of an abnormal murmur, the development of symptoms or signs of congestive cardiac failure or central cyanosis. Defects are broadly divided into those that are cyanotic and those that are not. Examples of cyanotic defects include the tetralogy of Fallot and transposition of the great arteries.

Acyanotic defects

These make up about 75% of all congenital heart defects. They include those associated with isolated left-to-right shunts such as ventricular septal defect (VSD), atrial septal defect (ASD), persistent ductus arteriosus (PDA) and those without shunting such as aortic stenosis (AS) pulmonary stenosis (PS) and coarctation of the aorta.

Ventricular septal defect (VSD)

VSDs make up 30% of all cardiac defects. The defect may be small or large and involve the membranous or muscular parts of the septum.

Clinical presentation depends on the amount of left-to-right shunting. A murmur may be noted incidentally on examination or congestive cardiac failure may develop in infants with larger defects and more shunting.

The characteristic clinical features of a VSD are a loud, harsh, high-pitched systolic murmur at the left sternal border, often associated with a thrill. The heart sounds are normal. Larger VSDs may cause a parasternal heave, a displaced apex beat, a softer systolic murmur and a diastolic murmur due to increased flow through the mitral valve. An infant with a large VSD will fail to thrive and become tachypnoeic and sweaty with feeds.

The chest X-ray with small VSDs is normal. With larger defects there may be cardiomegaly and pulmonary plethora. The ECG often has features of biventricular hypertrophy.

Many small VSDs become smaller or close spontaneously. In untreated cases complications of pulmonary hypertension and aortic valve prolapse may develop. Early surgical closure is indicated in cases where congestive cardiac failure develops in infancy or if pulmonary hypertension is present. Repair at a later age may be required if the defect fails to close or aortic valve prolapse develops.

Persistent ductus arteriosus (PDA)

The ductus arteriosus, connecting the pulmonary trunk with the aorta, usually closes in the newborn period. It may remain open in premature infants or if the ductus is congenitally abnormal.

The clinical features depend on the size of the ductus. The only sign of a small ductus may be a continuous 'machinery' murmur at the upper left sternal edge. The diastolic component is often soft, creating the impression of a systolic murmur. With a large ductus the pulses may be bounding, the apex displaced and a mid-diastolic murmur audible due to increased flow across the mitral valve. An infant with a large PDA will fail to thrive, be tachypnoeic and may develop recurrent chest infections.

In small defects the ECG and chest X-ray are normal. Larger PDAs cause cardiomegaly, pulmonary plethora and left ventricular hypertrophy.

Premature infants with PDA may be successfully treated with indometacin. Early closure in indicated in symptomatic term infants and premature infants following unsuccessful medical treatment of a PDA. Closure may be delayed in an asymptomatic infant with a small ductus. Closure with catheter may replace the traditional closure by ligation.

Atrial septal defect (ASD)

ASDs are most commonly situated in the region of the fossa ovale and are called secundum ASDs.

Isolated ASDs cause an ejection systolic murmur in the pulmonary area, due to increased flow through the pulmonary valve. A soft mid-diastolic murmur may be heard at the lower sternum due to increased flow through the tricuspid valve. The pulmonary component of the second heart sound is delayed, causing wide fixed splitting.

Symptoms are mild. There may be mild effects on growth and exercise tolerance. Adults with unrecognised or unrepaired ASD may develop atrial arrhythmias and dyspnoea.

Chest X-ray shows increased cardiac size with pulmonary plethora. ECG shows partial right bundle branch block.

Closure is recommended for all cases with a significant shunt. Closure by catheter-delivered device is suitable in selected cases.

Atrioventricular septal defect

This group includes defects low on the atrial septum, abutting on the atrioventricular valves and may also involve the ventricular septum.

Defects involving the atrial septum and atrioventricular valves are known as ostium primum ASDs. The AV valves are usually abnormal, particularly the left AV (mitral) valve, which is cleft. Children with minor mitral regurgitation present with features like a secundum ASD. Infants with severe mitral regurgitation present with congestive cardiac failure.

When a significant ventricular defect coexists (complete atrioventricular septal defect) infants present with features like a large VSD with congestive cardiac failure in early months. This is the commonest defect associated with Down's syndrome.

The chest X-ray shows marked cardiomegaly and pulmonary plethora. ECG shows left axis deviation and partial right bundle branch block.

Surgical repair is required to repair the defects in the atrial and ventricular septa and atrioventricular valves.

Pulmonary stenosis (PS)

PS is the commonest obstructive malformation. The pulmonary valve is abnormal with thickened leaflets and partially fused commissures. The valve may be bicuspid.

The right ventricular outflow tract may be narrowed at other sites including in-

fundibular stenosis, supravalvular stenosis and branch pulmonary stenosis.

Usually pulmonary stenosis is evident as an asymptomatic murmur. Moderate stenosis may lead to dyspnoea and angina with exercise and cardiac failure. More severe cases may present in infancy with cyanosis due to right-to-left shunting through a patent foramen ovale or ASD.

There is an ejection systolic murmur maximal in the pulmonary area, which radiates to the back. A thrill may be present. The pulmonary component of the second heart sound is soft. An ejection click in early systole can be heard at the left sternal border with valvular stenosis.

The chest X-ray may show a bump on the upper left heart border from post-stenotic dilatation of the pulmonary artery. The ECG shows right ventricular hypertrophy in more severe cases.

Most cases can be treated with balloon dilatation.

Aortic stenosis (AS)

In aortic stenosis the aortic valve is abnormal with thickened leaflets and fused commissures. The valve is often bicuspid.

Left ventricular outflow tract obstruction may also occur due to hypertrophic subaortic stenosis and supravalvular aortic stenosis.

Most children present with an incidentally found murmur. Symptoms increase with age to include syncope, angina and dyspnoea on exertion and sudden death. Infants with critical aortic stenosis may present with severe cardiac failure.

The murmur is ejection systolic, maximal at the right sternal edge and radiates to the carotids. A thrill may be felt over the carotids, in the sternal notch or aortic area. An ejection click indicates valvular stenosis and is best heard at the apex. In more severe cases a forceful apical impulse may be present and the pulse pressure narrowed.

The ECG shows left ventricular hypertrophy in more severe cases.

Treatment options are open valvotomy or balloon aortic valvuloplasty but this may worsen aortic incompetence.

Coarctation of the aorta

There is a discrete narrowing of the aorta, near the site of the ductus arteriosus.

There may be associated intracardiac anomalies including bicuspid aortic valve, aortic stenosis, VSD and mitral valve abnormalities.

Coarctation may present in early weeks of life with cardiac failure. Milder cases may only become evident with hypertension, a murmur or reduced femoral pulses in later years.

Physical findings are reduced volume femoral pulses. Delay of the femoral pulse compared to the brachial is evident only in later childhood after collateral vessels develop. The upper limb blood pressure may be elevated and a discrepancy occurs between upper and lower limb blood pressures of over 20 mmHg.

In infants with cardiac failure the chest X-ray will show cardiomegaly with pulmonary congestion. In later years the X-ray may show rib notching due to enlarged intercostal collateral vessels.

Infants with coarctation of the aorta develop cardiac failure from closure of the ductus arteriosus. In addition to supportive treatment, infusion of prostaglandin E1 may help maintain patency of the ductus. Surgical repair is urgently required. Patients with milder degrees of coarctation require monitoring for development of hypertension.

Hypoplastic left heart

Some infants with severe aortic stenosis or coarctation of the aorta have associated gross hypoplasia of the left ventricle. Aortic and mitral valve atresia may also be present.

Infants with hypoplastic left heart present with shock in the first few days of life.

Resuscitation and infusion of prostaglandin E_1 (alprostadil) may help support. Treatment options include palliation and heart transplantation, although donors are rare.

Cyanotic cardiac defects

Cyanotic defects account for about one quarter of all congenital heart malformations.

There are three main types of defects – cyanotic defects with reduced pulmonary blood flow (e.g. tetralogy of Fallot), cyanotic defects with bidirectional shunting (e.g. truncus arteriosus) and cyanosis with separation of pulmonary and systemic circulations (e.g. transposition of the great arteries).

Tetralogy of Fallot

The four components of tetralogy of Fallot are pulmonary stenosis, ventricular septal defect, right ventricular hypertrophy and overriding aorta. The pulmonary stenosis is caused by infundibular muscular obstruction, often with valvular hypoplasia and commissural fusion, resulting in elevated right ventricular pressure. Although right and left ventricular pressures are similar, the resistance to ejection into the pulmonary circulation results in right-to-left shunting across the VSD into the aorta.

Cyanosis if often mild at birth and increases during infancy. Cyanosis is usually more obvious with crying or exertion. Hypercyanotic spells due to reduced pulmonary blood flow may occur and are characterised by marked pallor or cyanosis with respiratory distress, particularly after exercise. Children may have reduced exercise tolerance and squat on the ground. This manoeuvre increases systemic vascular resistance to reduce right-to-left shunting.

A systolic murmur due to infundibular stenosis is maximal at the left sternal edge and pulmonary area, radiating through to the back. The second heart sound is often loud and single as the sound of pulmonary valve closure is inaudible.

In untreated cases cyanosis gradually increases, resulting in decreased exercise tolerance, clubbing and growth retardation. Polycythaemia and thromboembolic complications may occur as well as endocarditis.

The chest X-ray shows a normal-sized heart with reduced pulmonary vascularity. The heart shape is severe cases has uptilting of the apex, resulting in a 'boot-shaped' heart. ECG shows right ventricular hypertrophy.

Total surgical repair may be possible in infancy if the pulmonary valve and vessels are suitable. If not, palliation to increase pulmonary blood flow can be achieved with a synthetic shunt between aorta and pulmonary artery (modified Blalock-Taussig shunt).

Persistent truncus arteriosus

In this rare defect a single artery arises from the heart and branches into pulmonary artery and aorta. The truncal valve sits across a large VSD and receives blood from both ventricles.

Cyanosis is mild and congestive heart failure appears in the newborn. Systolic and diastolic murmurs are usually heard from flow through the truncal valve, which is often incompetent.

The chest X-ray shows cardiomegaly and pulmonary plethora. The ECG is often normal for age.

Surgical correction involves separating the pulmonary artery from the truncus, connecting it to the right ventricle with a valved conduit and closing the VSD.

Transposition of the great arteries

In this condition the aorta and pulmonary arteries arise from the incorrect ventricles. Deoxygenated systemic blood is directed through the right side of the heart and back into the aorta. Oxygenated blood from the pulmonary veins is directed through the left side of the heart and back into the pulmonary circulation. Survival is possible only if there are flows between each independent circuit through a foramen ovale, ductus arteriosus or septal defect.

Cyanosis is marked from birth. There may be a forceful right ventricular impulse but often no murmur. Metabolic acidosis may develop due to tissue hypoxia.

The chest X-ray shows a normal or slightly enlarged heart with increased pulmonary vascular markings. The abnormal arrangement of the great vessels gives the appearance of an 'egg on its side'. The ECG is normal or may show T-wave changes.

An urgent balloon atrial septostomy may be performed to increase interatrial shunting. Surgical correction with an 'arterial switch' operation is usually performed in early infancy. This also involves transferring the coronary arteries to the new aorta. An alternative is an intra-atrial patch ('atrial switch') to redirect blood flow at an atrial level (Mustard or Senning procedure).

Long-term complications of congenital heart disease

Bacterial endocarditis remains a risk with many congenital cardiac defects, especially palliated cyanotic congenital heart defects. Antibiotic prophylaxis should be carried out for procedures (see Chapter 5.6).

Arrhythmias may develop in children with congenital heart defects, particularly Ebstein's anomaly of the tricuspid valve, mitral valve prolapse, and after repair of transposition of the great arteries with atrial switch and repair of tetralogy of Fallot (see Chapter 5.8).

Many patients who have undergone total corrective surgery for left-to-right shunts such as ASD, VSD, PDA will have few if any haemodynamic problems.

Children with repaired coarctation of the aorta may develop hypertension and restenosis. Late problems include coronary artery disease, congestive cardiac failure and ruptured aortic aneurysms.

Aortic stenosis often progresses with age. A gradient over 50 mmHg increases the risk of arrhythmias, syncope, sudden death, endocarditis and angina.

Patients with untreated VSD or atrioventricular septal defect may develop Eisenmenger syndrome with associated cyanosis and polycythaemia. Patients with palliated cyanotic congenital heart defects and patients with Eisenmenger syndrome should avoid situations in which dehydration may occur and lead to increased viscosity and risk of stroke. During illnesses such as gastroenteritis diuretics may need to be decreased or temporarily discontinued. High altitude, airline travel and sudden exposure to changes in environmental temperatures should also be avoided.

REFERENCES

1. Smythe J, Teixeira O, Vlad P et al 1990 Initial evaluation of heart murmurs: Are laboratory tests necessary? Paediatrics 86: 497–500
2. Sharma S, Whyte G, Elliott P et al 1999 Electrocardiographic changes in 1000 highly trained

junior elite athletes. British Journal of Sports Medicine 33: 319–324
3. Birkebaek NH, Hansen LK, Elle B et al 1999 Chest roentgenogram in the evaluation of heart defects in asymptomatic infants and children with a cardiac murmur: Reproducibility and accuracy. Paediatrics 103: e15
4. Rajkumar K, Weisse M, Rosas A et al 1999 Comparative study of clinical evaluation of heart murmurs by general paediatricians and paediatric cardiologists. Clinical Paediatrics 38: 511–518

FURTHER READING

Allen HD, Gutgesell HP, Clark EB et al 2001 Moss and Adams' heart disease in infants, children and adolescents, 6th edn. Lippincott Williams and Wilkins, Philadelphia
APLS 2001 The practical approach, 3rd edn. BMJ Books, London
Harris W, Choong R, Timms B 1992 Examination paediatrics. McLennan & Petty, Sydney
Jordan SC, Scott O 1989 Heart disease in pediatrics, 3rd edn. Butterworth, Cambridge
Wilkinson J 2003 Common heart defects and disease in infancy and childhood. In: Robinson DM, Beck SW, Robertson DM (eds) Practical paediatrics, 5th edn. Churchill Livingstone, Sydney

5.5 ACUTE RHEUMATIC FEVER

SARAH DALTON

Essentials

1 Acute rheumatic fever (ARF) is a disease of connective tissue inflammation that may follow two to four weeks after a Group A streptococcal throat infection.

2 Diagnosis is based on the presence of carditis, arthritis, skin and neuropsychiatric sequelae.

3 The major complication of recurrent disease is progressive destruction of cardiac valves leading to rheumatic heart disease.

4 Treatment is comprised of eliminating streptococci, controlling joint pain and managing carditis, heart failure and chorea.

5 Antibiotic prophylaxis to prevent further attacks of ARF and episodes of infective endocarditis is mandatory.

INTRODUCTION

Acute rheumatic fever is an acute inflammatory disease that may follow group A β-haemolytic streptococcal infection. It primarily affects connective tissue causing carditis, arthritis and chorea and may follow a remitting and relapsing course for several years after the primary episode.

Long-term complications of recurrent disease include progressive cardiac damage, which is associated with significant morbidity and mortality in the adult population.

Epidemiology

Rheumatic heart disease is steadily decreasing in the developed world in association with improved standard of living and the availability of penicillin. Amongst developing countries prevalence is variable, with one of the highest prevalences worldwide found in the Pacific region. In Australian Aboriginal communities the incidence of acute rheumatic fever is up to 200 times that of non-aboriginals, and the prevalence of rheumatic heart disease almost eight times greater. A family history of ARF is common. This is in part due to a genetic predisposition and may also be explained by recent suggestions of a link between pyoderma and acute rheumatic fever.

Pathophysiology

The exact pathogenesis of acute rheumatic fever remains unclear. It is postulated that certain virulent strains of Gram-positive Group A β-haemolytic streptococci (*Streptococcus pyogenes*) invade the pharynx, leading to the production of anti-streptococcal antibodies, which cross-react with host connective tissue.

History

Acute rheumatic fever usually presents in school-age children but may present at any age. A history of pharyngitis several weeks previously is found in 70% of older children, but younger children are less likely to recall a sore throat. Typically, rheumatic fever presents with up to a week of high fevers, followed by several weeks of milder temperatures. At this time a rash, erythema marginatum, may be present. Specific symptoms of rheumatic fever include migratory joint pain, chorea, or neuropsychiatric manifestations such as abrupt personality change or poor attention span. If carditis has occurred there may be symptoms of congestive heart failure. Non-specific symptoms such as weight loss, fatigue, pallor, headache and abdominal pain may also be present.

Examination

The diagnosis of acute rheumatic fever relies upon satisfying the Jones criteria (see Table 5.5.1). To make the diagnosis, two major or one major plus two minor criteria must be present. Evidence of recent Group A *Streptococcus* infection,

Table 5.5.1 Jones criteria for diagnosis of ARF

Major criteria
1. Carditis
2. Polyarthritis
3. Chorea
4. Subcutaneous nodules
5. Erythema marginatum

Minor criteria
1. Fever
2. Arthralgia
3. Prolonged PR interval on ECG
4. Elevated acute phase reactants, e.g. ESR and CRP

CARDIOVASCULAR

5

pharyngitis must be demonstrated in all cases.

Group A *Streptococcus* documentation

- Positive throat culture or rapid streptococcal antigen test.
- Elevated or rising streptococcal antibodies.

There are three exceptions to the Jones criteria, where each of the following conditions may warrant diagnosis without fulfilling standard criteria.

❶ *Indolent carditis.* This may present late, typically after previous symptoms of rheumatic fever were undiagnosed and when laboratory investigations for Group A *Streptococcus* have normalised.

❷ *Chorea.* Movement disturbance can also occur late in the course of disease and may be the only manifestation of illness.

❸ *Past history of rheumatic fever.* Newly unwell patients with a history of acute rheumatic fever and evidence of recent Group A *Streptococcus* infection are very likely to have a recurrence of rheumatic fever. As new carditis may be difficult to substantiate clinically in these patients, the presence of one major or several minor criteria may suffice for diagnosis.

CARDITIS

A pancarditis, manifested as endocarditis, myocarditis or pericarditis, occurs in nearly 50% of cases of acute rheumatic fever. Clinical diagnosis is based on the identification of a new or changing murmur. This must be distinguished from an innocent murmur in a febrile child to avoid over diagnosis. The mitral valve is most commonly affected, followed by the aortic valve. Echocardiography has increased the recognition of carditis, which may be clinically undetectable in up to one half of cases. It has been suggested that echocardiographic criteria replace existing Jones criteria for carditis, but this has not been universally accepted. Myocarditis may be associated with rhythm disturbance,

such as first degree heart block or other conduction disturbance. A sinus tachycardia out of proportion to fever may be present. Signs of pericarditis (chest pain, rub and ECG changes) or congestive heart failure may also be present. With recurrent rheumatic fever progressive valve damage may occur, leading to chronic valve deformities and rheumatic heart disease.

POLYARTHRITIS

The most common and earliest manifestation of rheumatic fever is polyarthritis or arthralgia. In up to one third of cases it may be the single presenting problem. Generally large joints are involved, beginning in the lower extremities. The pain may be migratory and typically there is a marked response to aspirin. In most cases pain resolves within a week and virtually never results in permanent joint deformity.

SKIN

Erythema marginatum

Erythema marginatum is a distinctive feature of rheumatic fever, but is only found in approximately 10% of patients. Lesions usually begin as small, pink, non-pruritic macules or papules on the trunk or limbs. The lesions gradually spread to develop a raised pink serpiginous edge with central clearing and remain late into the course of illness.

Subcutaneous nodules

Subcutaneous nodules are becoming an uncommon manifestation of rheumatic fever. They are firm, non-tender nodules found over the extensor surface of the elbow, metacarpo-phalangeal joints, knees, and ankles. Up to three or four can appear in the first weeks of illness and they may remain for up to a month.

NEUROPSYCHIATRIC SEQUELAE

Sydenham's chorea

Chorea occurs in up to 30% of patients with rheumatic fever, and is postulated to be due to cross-reactivity between anti-

streptococcal antibodies and basal ganglia neurones. It presents with jerky, purposeless movement of limbs, speech impairment, involuntary grimacing or emotional lability, which may arise several months after the original Group A *Streptococcus* infection. Movements may be asymmetric and usually disappear during sleep. Generally symptoms improve in 1–2 weeks and resolve completely over 2–3 months, although the course can be variable.

PANDAS

Paediatric autoimmune neuropsychiatric disorders associated with streptococcal infections (PANDAS) is a recently identified phenomenon that describes a relapsing, remitting symptom complex characterised by major depressive disorder, tic disorder, attention deficit hyperactivity disorder and obsessive-compulsive symptoms. It may occur either at the time of rheumatic fever or several months later and, like chorea, is thought to be secondary to antibody cross-reactivity in the basal ganglia.

INVESTIGATIONS

Laboratory

Although throat cultures are usually negative by the time of rheumatic fever, an attempt to isolate the organism prior to antibiotic treatment should be made. A better diagnostic tool is anti-streptococcal antibodies, which rise in the first four weeks post-infection, plateau at three to six months, and normalise after six to twelve months. These tests have a sensitivity over 90% when both anti-streptolysin O antibodies and anti-deoxyribonuclease B antibodies are used. Sensitivity can be further increased with the addition of anti-streptokinase antibodies. Acute phase reactants such as the erythrocyte sedimentation rate and C-reactive protein are also highly sensitive, but non-specific, tests.

ECG

An ECG should be performed to demonstrate pericarditis and first-degree heart block.

Imaging

To further evaluate ventricular and valvular morphology and function both a chest X-ray and echocardiography are indicated.

Differential diagnosis

Each clinical manifestation of rheumatic fever is associated with multiple alternative diagnoses, hence the need for strict diagnostic criteria. Differential diagnoses deserve special attention where isolated symptoms may suffice for diagnosis of rheumatic fever. Sydenham's chorea is a diagnosis of exclusion after eliminating other causes of movement disorder such as drug toxicity, SLE, and Wilson's disease. Erythema marginatum is not specific for rheumatic fever, also being found in sepsis, glomerulonephritis and some drug reactions. Subcutaneous nodules are also seen in rheumatoid arthritis. Several systemic inflammatory conditions such as SLE and juvenile arthritis may fulfil all Jones criteria and must be excluded.

TREATMENT

Acute management

Children who present with features of ARF should be admitted to hospital under a paediatrician for further evaluation and management. There are four priorities in the management of acute rheumatic fever.

1. Group A *Streptococcus* eradication

Once identified, Group A *Streptococcus* must be eliminated to prevent ongoing antibody formation. The Australian Antibiotic Guidelines recommend phenoxymethylpenicillin 10 mg kg^{-1} up to 500 mg po q12h for 10 days. In poorly compliant patients or those intolerant of oral therapy, use benzathine penicillin 900 mg im, as a single dose for patients over 20 kg. Roxithromycin may be substituted in cases of penicillin sensitivity.

2. Control of pain and inflammation

High-dose aspirin, 80–100 mg kg^{-1} day^{-1}, is indicated for control of pain and inflam-

mation. It should not be commenced prior to definitive diagnosis, as discriminating clinical manifestations may be masked. Aspirin should be continued until resolution of inflammatory symptoms.

3. Treatment of carditis and control of heart failure

Prednisone may be indicated for moderate to severe carditis, but its use is controversial. Recommended dosage is 2 mg kg^{-1} day^{-1} continued for 2–4 weeks. Anti-failure medication or corrective valve surgery may be required depending on the clinical situation.

4. Management of chorea

A variety of antipsychotics and antiepileptics have been used to control Sydenham's chorea. Haloperidol is commonly recommended, but its use is not universal and management should be undertaken with specialist consultation.

PREVENTION AND PROPHYLAXIS

Continuous anti-streptococcal prophylaxis is recommended in all patients with a documented history of rheumatic fever to prevent recurrence with subsequent Group A *Streptococcus* infections. The Australian Cardiovascular Guidelines recommend benzathine penicillin 900 mg im monthly in all age groups. Oral phenoxymethylpenicillin 250 mg q12h may be used but is associated with poorer compliance and efficacy. In cases of penicillin sensitivity alternatives include oral erythromycin. Duration of therapy should be a minimum of five years, preferably until 21 years old in those without carditis, a minimum of ten years, preferably until 35 years of age in those with mild/moderate carditis and life-long for those with severe carditis or severe residual valve disease. Recent studies suggest third-weekly rather than fourth-weekly prophylaxis is associated with fewer episodes of recurrent rheumatic fever. This regimen should be considered in high-risk patients.

Endocarditis prophylaxis is mandatory for all those with residual valve

disease (see Chapter 5.6 on infective endocarditis).

Prognosis

Acute rheumatic fever resolves in most patients by three months. Complete spontaneous healing of valvulitis occurs in up to 80% of cases receiving prophylactic antibiotic therapy. Recurrent episodes of rheumatic fever are more common in younger patients and usually occur within five years. Prognostic indicators for chronic valve disease include total number of rheumatic fever episodes and time delay between onset of Group A *Streptococcus* and antibiotics in each instance. Of all patients with initial mitral valve insufficiency, up to 30% may have evidence of rheumatic heart disease at follow-up. This figure increases substantially where aortic valve involvement, congestive heart failure or pericarditis was present at diagnosis.

FURTHER READING

Australian Antibiotic Guidelines, Version 11 2000 Therapeutic Guidelines Limited

Australian Cardiovascular Guidelines, Version 3 1999 Therapeutic Guidelines Limited

Carapetis JR, Currie BJ 1996 Pyoderma and rheumatic fever. The Lancet 347(9010): 1271–1272

Chin TK, Worley C, Li D 2003 Rheumatic fever. E-medicine [http://www.emedicine.com/ped/topic2006.htm]

Currie BJ, Brewster DR 2002 Rheumatic fever in Aboriginal children. Journal of Paediatrics and Child Health 38(3): 223–225

Guidelines for the diagnosis of rheumatic fever. Jones criteria 1992 update. Journal of American Medical Association 268: 2069–2073

Manyemba J, Mayosi BM 2002 Penicillin for secondary prevention of rheumatic fever. Cochrane Databases of Systematic Reviews 3: CD002227

Steer AC, Carapetis JR, Nolan TM, Shann F 2002 Systematic review of rheumatic heart disease prevalence in children in developing countries: The role of environmental factors. Journal of Paediatrics and Child Health 38(3): 229–234

Stollerman GH 1997 Rheumatic fever. Seminar. The Lancet 349(9056): 935–942

Wilson NJ, Neutze JM 1995 Echocardiographic diagnosis of subclinical carditis in acute rheumatic fever. International Journal of Cardiology 50: 1–6.

5.6 INFECTIVE ENDOCARDITIS

SARAH DALTON

Essentials

1 Infective endocarditis is the microbial infection of cardiac endothelium.

2 Risk factors include congenital heart disease, central venous access, intravenous drug use and immunodeficiency.

3 Diagnosis is based on the presence of positive blood cultures with evidence of carditis, peripheral embolisation and immunological phenomena.

4 Acute management includes elimination of causative organisms and treatment of associated complications such as congestive heart failure.

5 Long-term chemoprophylaxis is recommended for procedures likely to result in bacteraemia in at-risk patients.

INTRODUCTION

Infective endocarditis (IE) is the microbial infection of the endothelial lining of the heart. Infection may be bacterial or fungal, and may arise in both structurally normal and abnormal hearts. Presentation can be acute or subacute and the long-term morbidity and mortality is high, despite recent advances in the management of the disease.

EPIDEMIOLOGY

Over the last decade the incidence of IE has increased owing to the improved survival of children with congenital heart disease and an increase in patients with central venous catheters. Up to 75% of children with bacterial endocarditis are known to have pre-existing cardiac abnormalities, most commonly ventricular septal defect and tetralogy of Fallot. Other risk factors include acquired valve disease, e.g. rheumatic heart disease, intravenous drug use, immunodeficiency and previous bacterial endocarditis.

PATHOPHYSIOLOGY

Turbulent cardiac blood flow due to or caused by stenotic valves or abnormal connections between cardiac chambers can damage endothelium and lead to overlying thrombus formation. Transient bacteraemia may infect the thrombus and a vegetation is formed. Bacteraemia can arise spontaneously or may complicate a focal infection or invasive procedure. The local effects of IE vegetations include valvular insufficiency, valvular obstruction, and perivalvular extension leading to the formation of intracardiac fistulae and conduction system abnormalities. Extracardiac manifestations are the result of peripheral embolisation of thrombus material with subsequent infarction or infection of involved tissue. Mycotic aneurysms are secondary to bacterial embolisation causing infection and distension of the arterial wall and are most common in intracranial arteries.

MICROBIOLOGY

Streptococcus viridans and *Staphylococcus aureus* are the most frequently encountered organisms in children with IE. Less common aetiological agents include enterococci, *Staphylococcus epidermidis* and the Gram-negative HACEK bacilli – *Haemophilus, Actinobacillus, Cardiobacterium, Eikenella* and *Kingella* species. Fungal species such as *Candida* and *Aspergillus* may cause IE in neonates, immunocompromised patients and those with long-term central venous lines. Other agents such as *Coxiella, Pneumococcus* and *Listeria* are rare causes of endocarditis.

HISTORY

Patients with acute infective endocarditis are often readily identified by their presentation with systemic toxicity and high fever of short duration. The clinical presentation of subacute endocarditis is more variable and usually consists of non-specific symptoms including fever, anorexia, malaise, cough, headache and arthralgia. Given the subtlety of symptoms and signs, a high degree of suspicion is required to identify patients with subacute disease. Any patient with unexplained prolonged fever, new neurological deficit or other embolic phenomena should be evaluated for endocarditis. Systemic embolisation occurs in up to 50% of patients with IE, and is most frequently seen in the first 2–4 weeks post-diagnosis. Embolic events may lead to infarction and haemorrhage or peripheral abscess formation in the brain, lungs, kidneys, spleen, bone and extremities. Peripheral embolisation is often absent in acute endocarditis and right-sided heart disease, making their diagnosis more difficult. Endocarditis may also be associated with cardiac failure secondary to acute valvular insufficiency or obstruction, fistulous tract formation or prosthetic dehiscence.

EXAMINATION

The physical signs of endocarditis are subtle in many patients. Valvitis may be detected by the presence of a new or changing murmur, but this can be difficult to distinguish from an innocent murmur or from the murmur of a pre-existing cardiac abnormality. Other findings include associated congestive heart failure or evidence of peripheral embolisation. Peripheral stigmata include Osler nodes (tender, red nodules of finger pulps), Janeway lesions (non-painful, haemorrhagic areas of palms or soles) and splinter and subungual haemorrhages. These stigmata, which develop late in the course of disease, are unusual in children. Roth spots (retinal haemorrhages with a pale centre) are occasionally seen on fundoscopy. Neurological deficit arises in 30–40% of patients from embolic infarcts, abscesses or intracerebral haemorrhage. Associated findings include splenomegaly in up to 30% of patients, and new onset clubbing may occur. Immune-mediated glomerulonephritis may result in haematuria, proteinuria and renal impairment.

Clinical diagnosis is based on the Duke Clinical Criteria for Diagnosis of Infective Endocarditis (see below).

Duke clinical criteria for diagnosis of infective endocarditis
Major criteria

- Two positive blood cultures of a typical organism for IE > 12 hours apart.
- Mobile echodense intracardiac mass depicted on echocardiogram.
- Periannular abscess depicted on echocardiogram.
- New partial dehiscence of prosthetic valve depicted on echocardiogram.
- New valvular regurgitation depicted on echocardiogram.

Minor criteria

- Predisposing factor – history of IV drug use or congenital heart disease.
- Fever > 38°C.
- Vascular phenomena – arterial emboli, pulmonary infarcts, mycotic aneurysm, intracranial haemorrhage, conjunctival haemorrhage, Janeway lesions.
- Immunologic phenomena – glomerulonephritis, Osler nodes, Roth spots, positive rheumatoid factor.
- Positive blood cultures or echocardiographic findings not meeting above criteria.

These criteria outline three diagnostic categories: definite endocarditis, possible endocarditis and rejected cases. For a definite clinical diagnosis 2 major, 1 major and 3 minor or 5 minor criteria must be present. Possible endocarditis is defined by the presence of 1 major or 3 minor criteria. Rejected cases are those where manifestations are explained by a clear alternate diagnosis or resolve after antibiotic therapy for less than four days.

INVESTIGATIONS
Laboratory

The most definitive test for bacterial endocarditis is the culture of a known causative organism from more than one blood culture. In all cases of suspected endocarditis three sets of blood cultures should be collected from different peripheral sites prior to antibiotic administration. Cultures do not need to be timed with spikes of fever, as the bacteraemia is constant. In up to 10% of all cases of IE cultures remain negative, usually where organisms are highly fastidious or non-bacterial, or where the microbiological techniques are inadequate. It is necessary to notify the laboratory in cases of possible IE so that blood is cultured for longer periods on an enriched medium. Other non-specific inflammatory markers such as peripheral white cell count, CRP, ESR and rheumatoid factor may be increased. Normocytic anaemia is another common finding.

Imaging

The initial investigation of possible endocarditis should include an electrocardiogram (ECG) and chest X-ray (CXR) but findings are non-specific. A CXR may reveal evidence of cardiac or pulmonary complications but is not diagnostic of infective endocarditis. Transthoracic echocardiography is the most definitive investigation. It yields excellent images in paediatric patients and is used to identify vegetations and to assess for complications of IE.

Sensitivity and specificity can both be increased by performing transoesophageal echocardiography (TOE), which is the investigation of choice in children where transthoracic images are inadequate or difficult to obtain, but may require general anaesthesia.

DIFFERENTIAL DIAGNOSIS

The presentation of IE is similar to a multitude of systemic inflammatory conditions. The presence of positive blood cultures often distinguishes the diagnosis, but in presentations suggestive of IE where blood cultures remain negative, further consideration must be given to other diagnoses. Rheumatic fever, Kawasaki disease, systemic lupus erythematosus and leukaemia may present similarly to infective endocarditis, hence the need for rigorous diagnostic criteria.

TREATMENT
Medical

The medical management of IE includes the elimination of causative microorganisms and the treatment of complications such as congestive heart failure. The bacterial infection of vegetations is relatively protected and must be completely eradicated with prolonged parenteral therapy. As the aetiological agent is not known at the time of presentation for most cases of suspected endocarditis, empiric antibiotic therapy should be commenced. The Australian Antibiotic Guidelines recommend benzyl penicillin (60 mg k^{g-1}, max. 3 g) and flucloxacillin (50 mg kg^{-1}, max. 2 g) intravenously every four hours with daily intravenous gentamicin (5 mg kg^{-1}, max. 160 mg), to be adjusted when organisms and microbial sensitivities are known. The duration of parenteral therapy is usually 4–6 weeks, modified by the aetiological agent and response to therapy. Monitoring of drug levels and consultation with microbiologists should be undertaken to optimise therapy.

Surgical

The need for surgical management of IE is largely dictated by the severity of complications and their response to medical management. Perivalvular abscesses,

CARDIOVASCULAR

5

obstructive vegetations, cardiac fistulae and prosthetic dehiscence cannot usually be corrected by medical therapy alone and may indicate the need for surgical intervention. Other indications include persistent bacteraemia, recurrent embolisation, and some cases of fungal endocarditis.

PROGNOSIS

The overall mortality of IE remains approximately 25% despite recent advances in antimicrobial treatment. Morbidity is also significant, with up to 60% of confirmed cases developing significant complications. One important prognostic indicator is the aetiological agent, and poor prognosis is associated with *Staphylococcus aureus* infection and fungal disease. Severe cardiac failure, prolonged clinical symptoms and poor response to antibiotics are also linked to increased morbidity and mortality.

PREVENTION

Antibiotic prophylaxis for bacterial endocarditis is currently recommended internationally but has not been conclusively shown to reduce the morbidity and mortality of the disease. Prophylaxis is advised depending on the underlying cardiac condition and the risk of the proposed procedure. The Australian Cardiovascular Guidelines recommend prophylactic antibiotic cover for these conditions (see Table 5.6.1).

The nature of chemoprophylaxis is dependant on the procedure being performed. In general, the Cardiovascular Guidelines suggest dental and upper respiratory tract procedures be managed with amoxicillin 50 mg kg^{-1} orally as a single dose one hour before the procedure. This can be substituted with cefalexin or clindamycin in the penicillin-sensitive patient. For genitourinary and gastrointestinal procedures gentamicin (2 mg kg^{-1} IV) and ampicillin (50 mg kg^{-1} IV) are used just before the procedure, followed by ampicillin (25 mg kg^{-1} po) six hours later. Table 5.6.2 shows selected examples of procedures requiring endocarditis chemoprophylaxis.

Antibacterial prophylaxis should be individually tailored to suit patient hypersensitivities and co-existing medications. Current therapeutic guidelines should be consulted to optimise management in each case.

FURTHER READING

Australian Antibiotic Guidelines, Version 11 2000. Victorian Postgraduate Medical Foundation Therapeutic Guidelines Limited, Melbourne

Australian Cardiovascular Guidelines, Version 3 1999. Victorian Postgraduate Medical Foundation Therapeutic Guidelines Limited, Melbourne

Bayer S et al 1998 Diagnosis and management of infective endocarditis and its complications. AHA scientific statement. Circulation 98: 2936–2948

Behrman RK, Kliegman R, Jenson HB 1996 Nelson textbook of paediatrics, 16th edn. WB Saunders, Philadelphia, PA

Dajani AS et al 1997 Prevention of bacterial endocarditis: Recommendations by the American Heart Association. Journal of American Medical Association 277: 1794–1801

Milazzo AS, Li JS 2001 Bacterial endocarditis in infants and children. Paediatric Infectious Disease Journal 20(8): 799–801

Reyes G, Wiewall-Winkelmann J, Bailey DM 2002 Endocarditis, bacterial [http://www.emedicine.com/ped/topic2511.htm]

Table 5.6.1   Australian Cardiovascular Guidelines on IE prophylaxis

Prophylaxis recommended	Prophylaxis not recommended
Most congenital heart disease	Isolated secundum ASD
Surgically constructed systemic-pulmonary shunts	Complete surgical or device closure of ASD, VSD, or PDA (> 6 months post-repair)
Prosthetic valves	Pacemakers and implanted defibrillators
All acquired valvular heart disease	Previous rheumatic fever or Kawasaki disease without valve dysfunction
Mitral valve prolapse with regurgitation	Mitral valve prolapse without regurgitation
Hypertrophic cardiomyopathy	Physiological or functional murmurs
Previous endocarditis	

Table 5.6.2   Australian Cardiovascular Guidelines on IE prophylaxis related to procedures

Prophylaxis recommended	Prophylaxis not recommended
Dental • Any procedure causing bleeding of the gingiva, mucosa or bone	• Local anaesthetic injection • Fluoride treatment • Orthodontic appliance placement and adjustment
Respiratory tract • Rigid bronchoscopy	• Flexible bronchoscopy • Endotracheal tube insertion
Genitourinary tract • Cystoscopy • Catheterisation associated with UTI	• Catheterisation without UTI
Gastrointestinal tract • Surgical operations involving intestinal mucosa	• Transoesophageal echocardiography • Percutaneous endoscopic gastrostomy
Other procedures Incision and drainage of local abscess • Procedures through surgically prepared skin	

5.7 KAWASAKI DISEASE

DARYL EFRON

ESSENTIALS

1 Kawasaki disease is an uncommon ED presentation, but should be considered in any child with an unexplained prolonged fever, particularly in the presence of a rash and red eyes.

2 The diagnosis is *clinical* with presence of fever and four out of five other criteria.

3 Diagnostic criteria can appear sequentially and may not all be present at the same time, which can make early diagnosis difficult.

4 Patients with 'atypical Kawasaki disease' are being increasingly recognised in which full criteria are not met but the patient has coronary artery abnormalities. These are often infants.

5 Any child with suspected Kawasaki disease should be treated immediately, regardless of the duration of symptoms.

6 Intravenous immunoglobulin (single dose of 2 g kg^{-1}) significantly reduces the risk of coronary artery abnormalities, especially if given in first ten days of illness.

INTRODUCTION

Kawasaki disease (KD) is an acute, self-limiting vasculitic illness predominantly affecting infants and young children. It is now a leading cause of acquired heart disease in children in Western countries. The diagnosis is made clinically, and effective treatment is available to reduce the likelihood of potentially fatal coronary vasculitis. KD was first described in 1967 as 'mucocutaneous lymph node syndrome' in a series of 50 Japanese children.[1] Although it is most common in Japanese and Korean children (annual incidence 90–150/100 000 children younger than five years), it occurs in all ethnic groups, with an annual incidence in the United States of approximately 10/100 000 children younger than five years. The majority of cases (85%) occur in children aged less than five years of age. It is 1.5 times more common in boys than girls.[2]

Many features of KD suggest an infectious aetiology. These include: seasonal variation (peak in winter/spring); occasional outbreaks; 10-fold higher risk in siblings than in the general population; rarity in young infants (suggesting protection from maternally acquired antibody); low recurrence rate (4%, which suggests acquired immunity); as well as the resemblance of the clinical presentation to other self-limiting infectious diseases, such as measles, adenovirus infection and staphylococcal toxic shock syndrome. However, despite much investigation of a variety of viral and bacterial pathogens, there is as yet no good evidence to implicate any known organism in KD. The ethnic variation suggests a genetic predisposition.

There is debate as to whether the inflammatory response in KD is initiated by a conventional antigen or a superantigen, and there are some immunologic features to support both hypotheses. Unreplicated reports of increased expression of specific T-cell receptor V β-regions suggests toxin activation, whereas infiltration of paratracheal and vascular tissue with reactive clonal IgA plasma cells suggests entry of a conventional antigen via the respiratory route.[3]

PATHOPHYSIOLOGY

The pathophysiology of KD involves vasculitis of medium-sized vessels including coronary, renal, hepatic and splanchnic arteries, beginning in both adventitial and intimal surfaces and proceeding toward the media. Coronary changes occur in approximately 20% of untreated patients. Immune activation involving cytokines and growth factors leads to inflammation and aneurysm formation, with the risk of thrombosis. The process evolves for a long period after the acute illness. In the majority of patients with echocardiographically-demonstrable coronary artery lesions, the vessels remodel and have a normal appearance within a year or so. However there is evidence of subtle long-term changes in coronary artery function, the clinical significance of which remain unclear.[4] The risk of early adult coronary artery disease in these patients is unknown.

A diffuse inflammatory process of a variety of tissues has been found in autopsy specimens including lymph nodes, liver and gall-bladder.[2] Endothelial changes are prominent, with hyperplasia, necrosis and thrombosis. Myocardial abnormalities include hypertrophy of myocytes and fibrosis.

CLINICAL FEATURES

KD should be considered in the differential diagnosis of all infants and young children with a fever, rash and red eyes, as well as those with a prolonged fever without an alternative explanation. The diagnostic criteria are outlined in Table 5.7.1.

The diagnosis can be made earlier than day 5 if other features are present. This is important, as there is evidence that earlier administration of IVIG is associated with a shorter illness and reduced risk of coronary disease.[5]

The fever is often associated with irritability, which responds poorly to paracetamol. Over 90% of patients develop a rash, which can take any of a number of forms – scarlatiniform, morbilliform, or maculopapular. It often has the appearance of a viral eruption or allergic reaction,

Table 5.7.1   Diagnostic criteria for Kawasaki disease

- Fever (at least 5 days)

Plus four of the following five features:
- Bilateral conjunctival infection
- Enanthem – dry, cracked lips; oropharyngeal erythema; strawberry tongue
- Exanthem – polymorphous
- Peripheral changes – erythema (palms and soles), oedema (hands and feet), desquamation (2nd to 3rd week)
- Cervical adenopathy

but can appear urticarial. Petechiae are sometimes seen, as are micropustules. The red eyes demonstrate characteristic sparing of the avascular perilimbic region, giving the appearance of a halo around the cornea. There is not usually an exudate. The changes may resolve rapidly, such that this important feature may be present only on history rather than being present when the child is examined. The cervical nodes are commonly unilateral and in the anterior chain. Generalised lymphadenopathy and splenomegaly are absent. The subacute phase occurs from 2–4 weeks with resolution of fever. Desquamation (periungual) of fingers and toes may occur during this time.

KD is a multisystem disease with many and varied clinical manifestations. In addition to those in the diagnostic criteria, common features include marked irritability, diarrhoea, cough, arthralgia/arthritis, urethritis with sterile pyuria, otitis media, mild hepatic dysfunction, hydrops of the gallbladder and aseptic meningitis.

Cases of 'atypical KD' are being increasingly recognised in which full criteria are not met, but the patient has coronary artery abnormalities. This is more common in young infants, resulting in delayed diagnosis and therapy.[6] Given that infants under six months appear to be at increased risk of developing coronary abnormalities,[6] a lower threshold for treatment is probably indicated in this group. Diagnosis is also more likely to be delayed in older children, in whom less classical manifestations such as gastrointestinal and joint symptoms often predominate.[7]

DIFFERENTIAL DIAGNOSIS

Depending on which features are present, a broad differential diagnosis needs to be considered in cases of possible KD. These include viral infections (e.g. measles, adenovirus, enterovirus), streptococcal and staphylococcal toxic-mediated illness (scarlet fever, toxic shock syndrome), drug allergy (including Stevens–Johnson syndrome), inflammatory bowel disease, connective tissue disease and malignancy.

COMPLICATIONS

The major concern with KD is coronary artery disease. Younger children, especially under 12 months of age, are at highest risk. Changes seen include dilatation (ectasia) and discrete aneurysms. The dilatation commonly resolves, however, as discussed above, the vessels may remain functionally abnormal long term. Fibrosis may lead to stenosis with risk of ischaemia, and thrombosis of coronary aneurysms can cause myocardial infarction and sudden death. Rarely myocarditis can occur causing congestive cardiac failure or arrhythmias.

INVESTIGATIONS

Any child who presents with possible features of KD should be discussed with a paediatrician.

There is no definitive diagnostic test for KD. Investigation is directed toward excluding alternative diagnoses, as well as gathering supporting evidence for the diagnosis of KD. At least one set of blood cultures should be taken, and cultures of urine, CSF and other sites may be indicated. Serological testing for Group A *Streptococcus*, and for specific viruses such as measles may be helpful. In KD, the peripheral white cell count and inflammatory markers are generally significantly raised. The ESR may continue to rise as the child improves clinically. A marked thrombocytosis is commonly seen in the second to third week of the illness. Pyuria, due to sterile urethritis, is often found on a voided sample (not on SPA or catheter). Serum gamma GT is commonly elevated.

Echocardiography should be undertaken as soon the diagnosis of KD is suspected. The American Heart Association guidelines suggest repeat echocardiograms at 2 weeks (time of maximal aneurysm formation), 6 weeks and 12 months (looking for late sequelae). If abnormalities are demonstrated on echocardiography, closer cardiological follow-up may be required depending on the lesion. A 12-lead ECG is most often normal but may show dysrythmias, change in PR or QT intervals or non-specific ST changes.

TREATMENT

Treatment of KD is directed towards reducing the inflammation as rapidly as possible. The clinical markers of response to therapy are the temperature and patient's general well-being, supported by the white cell count and CRP.

Intravenous immunoglobulin (IVIG) therapy has been demonstrated to induce resolution of fever as well as significantly reduce the risk of coronary artery abnormalities (from around 20% to around 3–5%) if given within the first ten days of the illness.[8] The precise mechanism of action of IVIG is unknown. Theories include saturation blockade of Fc receptors or direct antibody activity against an unidentified causative pathogen or toxin. The optimal dose is 2 g kg^{-1} day^{-1} as a single infusion over 10–12 hours. There is some evidence that IVIG is also effective if given beyond ten days,[9] however treatment as early as possible is optimal.[5] If the fever does not resolve after the first dose of IVIG (approximately 10% of cases), a second dose is indicated.

In the 1980s, high-dose aspirin was shown to decrease the incidence of coronary artery involvement in KD.[10] The current role of aspirin in KD is difficult to determine as it has been used in combination with IVIG in the major trials. Many centres use high-dose aspirin (80–100 mg kg^{-1} day^{-1} in 3–4 divided doses, for anti-inflammatory effect) initially, and switch to low-dose (3–5 mg kg^{-1} day^{-1}, antiplatelet effect) after the patient's fever resolves. Low-dose aspirin is continued for 6–8 weeks, and then stopped if there is no coronary involvement. In patients treated with IVIG, concomitant use of high-dose aspirin initially results in shorter duration of fever and hospitalisation than low-dose, but the incidence of coronary artery aneurysm appears to be independent of aspirin dose.[11]

Pulses of methylprednisolone (30 mg kg^{-1}) have been used in cases unresponsive to two doses of IVIG.[12] The role of steroids in KD is a subject of continuing research.

Long-term antiplatelet therapy may be indicated in patients with coronary artery abnormalities following acute KD. New antiplatelet agents are under investigation.[13] There have been reports of the use of thrombolytic agents in patients with KD with thrombus seen within coronary aneurysms.[14] Anticoagulation with warfarin is required for patients with 'giant' (≥ 8 mm) or multiple aneurysms, and surgical intervention (e.g. angioplasty, bypass grafting) is occasionally necessary.

PROGNOSIS

Mortality is less than 1%, being highest in those less than 12 months old. Outcome is excellent in the absence of coronary artery involvement and if the child receives treatment in the first ten days of illness.

REFERENCES

1. Kawasaki T 1967 Paediatric acute mucocutaneous lymph node syndrome: Clinical observation of 50 cases. Arerugi [Japan Journal of Allergy] 16: 178–222 (in Japanese)
2. Burns JC 2001 Kawasaki disease. Advances in Paediatrics 48: 157–177
3. Meissner HC, Leung DYM 2000 Superantigens, conventional antigens and the etiology of Kawasaki syndrome. Paediatric Infectious Diseases Journal 19: 91–94
4. Freeman AF, Shulman ST 2001 Recent developments in Kawasaki disease. Current Opinions in Infectious Disease 14: 357–361
5. Tse S, Silverman E, McCrindle B, Yeung R 2002 Early treatment with intravenous immunoglobulin in patients with Kawasaki disease. Journal of Paediatrics 140: 450–455
6. Rosenfeld EA, Corydon KE, Shulman ST 1995 Kawasaki disease in infants less than one year of age. Journal of Paediatrics 126: 524–529
7. Stockneim JA, Innocentini N, Shulman ST 2000 Kawasaki disease in older children and adolescents. Journal of Paediatrics 137: 250–252
8. Newburger JW, Takahashi M, Beiser AS et al 1991 A single intravenous infusion of gamma globulin as compared with four infusions in the treatment of acute Kawasaki syndrome. New England Journal of Medicine 324: 1633–1639
9. Marasini M, Pongiglione G, Gazzolo D et al 1991 Late intravenous gamma globulin treatment in infants and children with Kawasaki disease and coronary artery abnormalities. American Journal of Cardiology 68: 796–797
10. Koren G, Rose V, Lavi S et al 1985 Probable efficacy of high-dose salicylates in reducing coronary artery involvement in Kawasaki disease. Journal American Medical Association 254: 767–769
11. Terai M, Shulman ST 1997 Prevalence of coronary artery abnormalities in Kawasaki disease is highly dependent on gamma globulin dose but independent of salicylate dose. Journal of Paediatrics 131: 888–893
12. Wright DA, Newburger JW, Baker A et al 1996 Treatment of immune globulin-resistant Kawasaki disease with pulsed doses of corticosteroids. Journal of Paediatrics 128: 146–149
13. Williams RV, Minich LL, Tani LY 2001 Pharmacological therapy for patients with Kawasaki disease. Paediatric Drugs 3: 649–660
14. Tsubata S, Ichida F, Haramichi Y et al 1995 Successful thrombolytic therapy using tissue-type plasminogen activator in Kawasaki disease. Paediatric Cardiology 16: 186–189

CONTROVERSIES

❶ The immunological mechanism of the inflammatory response in KD is the subject of continuing research – there is some evidence to support a conventional antigen, but other evidence suggests a superantigen.

❷ The optimal dose of aspirin in the acute febrile phase is uncertain.

❸ The role of steroids in KD is debated.

❹ The clinical significance of subtle long-term changes in coronary artery function in some patients who have had KD remains unknown.

5.8 PAEDIATRIC ARRHYTHMIAS

GARY WILLIAMS

INTRODUCTION

Identification and management of the paediatric patient with a cardiac arrhythmia in the ED requires an initial focus on and, if required, attention to the patient's haemodynamic stability followed by a team approach to diagnose and treat the arrhythmia if necessary. Although arrhythmias occur less frequently in acutely ill infants and children compared to adults, vigilance is required as a correct acute assessment and management of the arrhythmia will have significant long-term consequences.

The primary aim of this initial assessment and resuscitation phase in an unstable patient is to recognise and treat arrhythmias that are compromising cardiac output using the safest means possible so that longer-term management decisions can be made in consultation with a paediatric cardiologist.

NORMAL CONDUCTION SYSTEM

The normal heartbeat is initiated by an impulse which originates from the sinoatrial (SA) node located in the wall of the right atrium near the superior vena cava junction. The impulse is then propagated via conducting cells that form a specialised system throughout the heart. Initially the impulse travels across the atria and via transatrial internodal pathways that converge on the atrioventricular (AV) node. The impulse proceeds down the bundle of His to the right and left bundle branches; the impulse then finally spreads throughout the Purkinje fibres to depolarise the ventricular muscle. The conducting cells of this specialised system have a rapid conduction velocity to rapidly propagate the electrical impulse throughout the heart. The various parts of this conduction system are also capable of spontaneous depolarisation and impulse generation under abnormal conditions.

The SA node is normally the dominant (fastest) cardiac pacemaker but this can change if sinus node dysfunction occurs or if other parts of the conduction system develop increased automaticity. As stated above, the SA node is located near the junction of the SVC and the right atrium. The SA node is innervated by both sympathetic and parasympathetic nerve endings. Parasympathetic tone predominates during rest. Children are known to have relatively greater parasympathetic tone than adults and are also known to have developmental and age-dependent differences in action potential amplitude and conduction speed. Accordingly there

are age-dependent normal values for resting heart rate as well as PR interval and QRS duration in addition to many other electrophysiology parameters (see Table 5.8.1).

Depolarisation initiated in the SA node spreads rapidly through the internodal pathways to converge on the AV node. Usually the atria and ventricles are electrically separated from one another by a ring of fibrous tissue at the atrioventricular junction (the annulus fibrosis). Accordingly, in usual circumstances, the impulse must pass to the His bundle via the AV node. The AV node is located in the inferomedial wall of the right atrium near the insertion of the septal leaflet of the tricuspid valve. Conduction through the AV node is slow to allow completion of atrial systole (and ventricular diastole). This delay (and therefore potentially the completeness of ventricular filling) can be reduced during sympathetic stimulation.

After leaving the AV node the impulse travels along the bundle of His for 1–2 cm along the postero-inferior margin of the membranous portion of the interventricular septum before dividing into the right and left bundle branches. These extensions of the conducting system spread

subendocardially across the ventricular chambers to the base of the papillary muscles. The left bundle separates into two distinct fascicles (anterior and posterior). From these specialised fibres the impulse spreads from endocardium to epicardium throughout the right and left ventricles.

Abnormally situated embryonic remnants of conducting tissue can persist as accessory tracts. These are most commonly found around the AV node and are capable of conducting electrical activity between the atria and ventricles thus bypassing the AV node. These remnants are the anatomical substrate for re-entrant tachyarrhythmias.

THE CARDIAC ACTION POTENTIAL

The cardiac action potential is divided into five phases: 0, 1, 2, 3, 4.

Phase 0 is depolarisation due to voltage gated opening of sodium channels with sodium rushing into the cell. There is an intense entry of sodium for a brief period resulting in depolarisation of the entire cell as well as cell-to-cell propagation.

Phase 1 is a phase of partial repolarisation due to several factors but including chloride entry into and possibly potassium egress from the cell.

Phase 2 is the plateau phase thought to be important in co-ordinated and sustained ventricular contraction. During this phase there is a slow inward calcium current and slow inward sodium current balanced by a gradually increasing outward potassium movement.

Phase 3 is repolarisation and it occurs by inactivation or closure of the slow calcium and sodium channels and then a voltage gated progressive opening of potassium channels leading to outward potassium ion movement and a progressively more negative membrane potential. Also during this phase, the fast sodium channels are reactivated and the cell is primed for further depolarisation.

During phase 4, an energy-dependent membrane Na K ATPase removes the sodium and restores the potassium to the cell. Most myocardial cells maintain a

Table 5.8.1 Normal resting heart rates, PR intervals and QRS durations in children				
Age	Heart rate mean	Range	PR interval (ms)	QRS duration (ms)
<1 d	119	94–145	70–120	50–84
1–7 d	133	100–175	70–120	40–79
7–30 d	163	115–190	70–120	40–73
1–3 mo	154	124–190	70–130	50–80
3–6 mo	140	111–179	70–130	60–80
6–12 mo	140	112–177	80–130	50–80
1–3 y	126	98–163	80–150	50–80
3–5 y	98	65–132	90–150	60–84
5–8 y	96	70–115	100–160	50–80
8–12 y	79	55–107	100–170	50–84
12–16 y	75	55–102	110–160	40–80

Source: Adapted from Liebman 1982.

constant level of depolarisation during this phase but Purkinje or conducting cells, by way of reduced outward potassium flow and some inward sodium flow, achieve slow depolarisation until the AP threshold is reached. These conducting cells have a briefer action potential of lower amplitude thought to be mediated more predominantly by slow calcium flux.

Vaughan Williams antiarrhythmia drug classification

Antiarrhythmic drugs are classified into five classes in the Vaughan Williams classification by the mechanism or channel that they most reliably affect during in vitro studies. It has to be remembered, however, that there is considerable overlap as far as certain drugs are concerned.

Class 1 drugs block the fast inward sodium channels and thereby increase the refractory period. This class is further subdivided into:

1a. Those that prolong action potential duration (e.g. quinidine);

1b. Do not change or shorten action potential duration (e.g. lidocaine); or

1c. Produce some mild action potential prolongation (e.g. flecainide).

It is fair to say that these are infrequently used in paediatrics though lidocaine is still an option in the ventricular fibrillation protocol and flecainide may sometimes be used in supraventricular tachyarrhythmias.

Class 2 agents are β-blockers, which act by a combination of β-antagonism and a quinidine-like membrane stabilising effect. There is a slowing of conduction velocity, prolonging of action potential duration and reducing of automaticity. Their main clinical use is in treating supraventricular tachyarrhythmias (SVT, atrial fibrillation, atrial flutter) by increasing the refractory period of the AV node. Propanalol or atenolol may be used but in acute situations many clinicians favour esmolol, a very short-acting parenteral β-1-antagonist (half life nine minutes), which can be useful in SVT and possibly VT.

Class 3 drugs act primarily as potassium channel blockers and basically prolong the phase 3 repolarisation phase, thereby causing a prolongation of the action potential and increase in the effective refractory period. This class of drug is particularly useful in ventricular tachyarrhythmias and includes amiodarone and sotalol.

Amiodarone is one of these antiarrhythmics with a plethora of effects in that it is primarily class 3 (i.e. potassium channel blocker) but also has sodium channel blocking, β-antagonism and calcium channel blocking effects. Oral amiodarone has unusual pharmacokinetics with clinical effect only apparent after several days of treatment and a half life of 3–15 weeks. Side effects are frequent and serious (corneal photosensitivity, hyper- or hypothyroidism, pulmonary fibrosis and pro-arrhythmia). Intravenous amiodarone is used in the acute management of postoperative tachyarrhythmias (usually JET). In the adult ventricular fibrillation protocol, a randomised comparison between amiodarone and lidocaine found a greater chance of successful resuscitation (but not survival) with amiodarone. Therefore some authorities have recommended amiodarone as the agent of choice to help effect defibrillation after adrenaline (epinephrine). In haemodynamically stable VT the agent of choice is probably sotalol unless there is impaired ventricular function (EF < 40%, signs of congestive heart failure) when amiodarone is recommended. In unstable or polymorphic VT the recommended agent depends a little on the initial trace. If it looks like *torsade de pointes* with the trace oscillating around the baseline (or in polymorphic VT with a normal QT interval) the clear recommendation is IV magnesium. If it is not *torsade-like* and the QT interval can be determined and is not prolonged, amiodarone is a second-line agent to β-blockers. If the QT interval is prolonged, then IV magnesium, followed if necessary by lidocaine, would be the recommended approach.

Sotalol is classified as a class 3 drug, although it is a non-selective β-blocker with additional class 3 properties. It therefore combines the β-blocking effect on the SA and AV nodes with prolongation of AP duration and lengthening of refractory period elsewhere in the heart. It is valuable acutely and long term in preventing SVT of all sorts and is the agent of choice in monomorphic stable VT with apparent normal ventricular function. Like amiodarone, it does increase the QT interval and is therefore pro-arrhythmic as well as having the other risks of hypotension and bradycardia, presumably resulting from its β-blocking effects.

Class 4 agents are calcium channel blockers and the prototype remains verapamil, which has wide-ranging effects on shortening the plateau phase and reducing contractility, but is primarily used in the adult setting because of its reduction of conduction velocity in the AV node, thereby controlling the ventricular response rate to SVT, atrial flutter or atrial fibrillation. Even in that use it is still used as a second line agent to adenosine for SVT termination in adults provided there is good LV function. However, because of serious bradycardia, hypotension and cardiac arrest in infants it is not used in children. Instead, β-blockers are used in Wolf-Parkinson-White syndrome and digoxin in non-WPW patients.

Finally, class 5 agents are a miscellaneous class and include adenosine and digoxin. Adenosine is an endogenous purine nucleoside with a very rapid half life (less than five seconds). It acts by depressing slow calcium channels and enhancing potassium conduction. Its main effects are to depress sinus node and AV node activity with a shortening of atrial refractoriness. Because of its effect in blocking AV nodal activity, adenosine is superbly suited to block re-entry phenomena, the most frequent cause of SVT in children. Series show that adenosine will terminate 90-100% of SVTs but the arrhythmia will re-initiate in approximately 25%. Other atrial tachycardias like multifocal atrial tachycardia, atrial flutter or atrial fibrillation will almost always be resistant to adenosine. Adenosine is given in increasing doses from 50–200 μg kg^{-1} every two minutes using a two-syringe technique so that it can be flushed rapidly into the circulation. Side effects can be facial flushing, bronchospasm or sinus arrest. Adenosine is essentially very safe although there is a single case report of ventricular fibrillation occurring after a dose of adenosine in a neonate with a concealed WPW syndrome previously treated with digoxin.

Although adenosine is unlikely to be controlling in supraventricular tachycardias other than re-entrant SVT, the acute injection of adenosine may transiently slow AV nodal activity and allow the flutter wave or P wave morphology to be assessed. This may be very valuable in diagnosing the specific rhythm. In a haemodynamically stable wide complex tachycardia of uncertain origin the differential diagnosis is primarily between VT and SVT with aberrant conduction. Adenosine administration might be discussed as a way of making this distinction (i.e. effective in the latter but not in the former). In the adult literature unless SVT origin is strongly suspected, this practice is discouraged because of the potential for brief hypotension, and accelerated accessory pathway conduction following adenosine injection.

Digoxin is still very commonly used parenterally, acutely and as a maintenance medication primarily to slow AV conduction and decrease the ventricular response to atrial dysrhythmia like flutter or fibrillation. It will rate control and sometimes convert supraventricular tachyarrhythmias. There is an important caveat with digoxin, that it may shorten accessory pathway refractoriness and increase the resulting ventricular response. Therefore, it should not be used in accessory pathway dysrhythmias like WPW syndrome. Remember that virtually any arrhythmia can arise from intoxication with digoxin. This risk is greater with hypokalaemia and the acute treatment is intravenous *Digitalis* antibody.

PATHOGENESIS OF ARRHYTHMIAS

Bradyarrhythmias

Two mechanisms are responsible for bradyarrhythmias:

❶ Some form of sinus node dysfunction.
❷ Conduction system block.

Tachyarrhythmias

There are three fundamental mechanisms proposed for the generation of tachyarrhythmias:

❶ Re-entry.
❷ Enhanced automaticity.
❸ After depolarisations (triggered arrhythmias).

1. Re-entry

Re-entry is said to exist when a closed loop of specialised conducting tissue allows an electrical impulse to travel in a circular fashion and permits atrial or ventricular electrical activation with each pass around the circuit. Re-entry may occur on a large (macro) or small (micro) scale. Atrial flutter and ventricular fibrillation are examples of micro re-entry; paroxysmal supraventricular tachycardia is an example of macro re-entry.

Macro re-entry usually involves the participation of an accessory conduction pathway. Accessory pathway conduction characteristics vary widely among patients. The accessory pathway in some patients conducts antegrade during sinus rhythm whereas in others it conducts only retrograde during tachycardia. When anterograde conduction is possible down the accessory pathway the standard ECG will show pre-excitation with a short PR interval and wide QRS including an initial delta wave resulting from the pre-excitation of the ventricle from the sinus impulse conducting through the accessory pathway before the impulse has passed through the normal conducting system. Patients with WPW can have not only orthodromic but also (rarely) antidromic tachycardia involving retrograde conduction up the usual atrioventricular route or via an alternative accessory connection.

Supraventricular tachycardia is the most common sustained tachyarrhythmia in children and almost always has a re-entry mechanism. Most commonly, particularly in children younger than 12 years of age this re-entry is caused by an accessory atrioventricular connection (resulting in atrioventricular (or AV) re-entrant tachycardia). In adolescents AV node re-entry is the mechanism in up to one third of patients. Previously we believed that this

was due to a re-entry circuit within the compact AV node but a newer concept involves tissue, most likely atrial muscle, more than several millimetres outside the compact atrioventricular node.

The commonest mode of accessory connection-mediated re-entry tachycardia is orthodromic tachycardia with the circular movement of the electrical impulse going antegrade through the atrioventricular node and then retrograde up the accessory connection.

2. Enhanced automaticity

The primary pacemaker cells of the SA and AV nodes usually demonstrate spontaneous depolarisation as well as having somewhat slower action potential propagation. The cells of the conduction system have more rapid action potential propagation but are also capable of spontaneous action potential generation if the opportunity arises. These cells are, however, normally overridden and kept refractory by the dominant (faster) pacemaker of the SA node. Under certain adverse physiologic conditions (e.g. hypokalaemia, hypoxia) the threshold for spontaneous automaticity for these conducting cells may be altered. This potentially creates a situation of enhanced automaticity and secondary enhanced pacemakers. One example of a tachycardia due to enhanced automaticity is multifocal atrial tachycardia.

3. After depolarisations

After depolarisations are due to oscillations of the membrane potential during repolarisation that has reached the threshold membrane potential and triggered a second complete depolarisation. This process may become self-perpetuating. *Torsade de pointes* is the classic example of such a triggered arrhythmia.

GENERAL PRINCIPLES FOR ARRHYTHMIA MANAGEMENT

❶ Direct primary attention to assessment and correction of ABCs.
❷ If patient has an acute arrhythmia with haemodynamic compromise

(e.g. shock or loss of consciousness), assess whether the rhythm is fast and/or disorganised or slow and/or irregular. If the rhythm is fast or disorganised cardioversion or defibrillation should take priority. If slow and/or irregular, cardiopulmonary resuscitation should commence.

❸ Obtain venous access and draw blood for biochemistry, specifically Na, K, Ca, Mg and BSL.

❹ Record a 12-lead ECG as soon as possible.

Bradyarrhythmias

Normal heart rate varies as a function of age. Pathological bradyarrhythmia may present as fatigue, light-headedness or syncope in an otherwise well child or inappropriate absence of tachycardia in a critically unwell child under stress.

Sinus bradycardia

Sinus bradycardias can be caused in children by:

- Parasympathetic stimulation (e.g. suctioning)
- Metabolic disturbances (e.g. hypoxia, asphyxia, hypothermia)
- Poisoning (e.g. β-blocker, calcium channel blocker)
- Raised intracranial pressure
- Surgical injury to the sinoatrial node (e.g. following Mustard or Senning procedures for transposition, Fontan, closure of ASD or correction of TAPVD)
- Cardiomyopathy.

Sinus node dysfunction

Sinus node dysfunction may manifest as sinus pauses (a transient interruption of normal sinus mechanism), sinus exit block (abnormal propagation), either of which may occur with or without an associated escape rhythm and may evolve to sinus arrest.

Management

❶ Treatment is required if an adequate cardiac output is not being maintained.

❷ If possible remove the cause (i.e. suction catheter).

❸ Ensure adequate ventilation.

❹ If life threatening, commence compressions and administer atropine 20 µg kg^{-1} IV or ET (minimum dose 100 µg).

❺ If this is ineffective, or bradycardia recurs, use β-adrenergic agonist or adrenaline (epinephrine) bolus. Commence adrenaline (epinephrine) or isopreterenol by infusion while urgent preparations made for temporary cardiac pacing.

Conduction disturbances
Atrioventricular block

This involves delayed or incomplete conduction through the AV node. Causes include a congenital form (maternal systemic lupus erythematosus) and an acquired form. Acquired AV block occurs in poisoning, metabolic disturbances, myocarditis, rheumatic fever, Lyme disease, fibrosis in the area of the conduction system associated with previous cardiac surgery (particularly VSD or AVSD closure, tetralogy repair or aortic valve replacement) and inferior myocardial infarction.

First degree AV block Is present when the PR interval is longer than usual for age (see Table 5.8.1) but normal sinus rhythm and 1:1 AV conduction is maintained. This is a normal feature of the ECG of endocardial cushion defects. It may occur in a normal heart during parasympathetic stimulation or digoxin treatment and usually does not require treatment.

Second degree Mobitz type I AV block (Wenckebach) Is characterised by progressive prolongation of the PR interval, culminating in a single non-conducted beat. This usually is a benign normal variant but may represent a temporary pathological prolongation of the atrioventricular node refractory period.

Second degree Mobitz type II AV block Manifests as a regular intermittent failure of P wave conduction while the PR interval remains constant. This is more likely attributable to a block within the His conduction system and as such has

greater potential to progress to complete (3rd degree) atrioventricular block.

Third degree atrioventricular block (or complete heart block) Represents complete failure of atrial depolarisation to propagate to the ventricle. Anatomically the block may occur at atrioventricular node or at infranodal level. ECG will show complete dissociation of P waves and QRS complex. A narrow QRS junctional escape rhythm implies a nodal block whereas a widened slower QRS escape rhythm suggests an infranodal site for the block.

Clinical features Patient may be asymptomatic but will usually demonstrate an inadequate cardiac output particularly in episodes of atrioventricular block associated with slower heart rate. In third degree AV block, cannon 'A' waves are visible in the neck and a slow cardiac rhythm with variable first heart sound is present on auscultation.

Management Emergency treatment is only required if cardiac output is inadequate. Optimise ventilation and initiate β-agonist by infusion while organising temporary external/transvenous cardiac pacing. This is definitely indicated in symptomatic children with Mobitz type II second degree AV block and 3rd degree AV block.

Bundle branch block

Bundle branch block patterns are unusual in paediatrics but occur when impaired conduction is present in the specialised intraventricular conduction tissue resulting in delayed right or left ventricular depolarisation and a resulting broad aberrant QRS complex. *RBBB* (wide QRS with rSR pattern in right ventricular leads) may be a normal variant but also occurs in congenital heart disease (especially involving RVH), cor pulmonale and acute pulmonary embolism. *LBBB* (wide QRS with RR pattern in left chest leads) is associated with LV strain or hypertrophy or operated congenital heart disease.

Tachyarrhythmias

There is a wide range of tachyarrhythmias. Immediate diagnosis and management is best based on the width of the QRS complex when compared to age-based normal values.

Wide complex tachyarrhythmia

The differential diagnosis of a wide or broad complex tachycardia (i.e. QRS duration greater than normal for age, usually > 0.08 seconds) is between:

❶ Ventricular tachycardia.
❷ SVT with intraventricular aberrant conduction (e.g. pre-existing bundle branch block).
❸ Atypical or antidromic SVT (where during the tachycardia antegrade conduction occurs down the fast accessory pathway and retrograde component goes via the atrioventricular node).
❹ Atrially originated arrhythmias conducted via an accessory connection to the ventricular muscle.

Ventricular tachycardia in children usually presents as a wide complex rhythm between 120 to 220 per minute. There is usually AV dissociation but retrograde VA conduction may occur. It may be mono- or polymorphic, sustained or non-sustained. Causes include metabolic abnormalities, poisoning, myocarditis, cardiomyopathy, ventriculotomy, ventricular tumours and congenital or acquired long QT syndrome.

Most children with VT will be symptomatic with lethargy, symptoms of pulmonary congestion, poor circulation and possibly palpitations.

The other three differential diagnoses outlined above are unusual causes of a wide complex tachycardia in children. The most important differential to think about is SVT with aberrant conduction, because it should respond to vagal manoeuvres or adenosine administration. A previous electrocardiogram is of great value in determining the presence of an accessory pathway or a pre-existing bundle branch block in that these features point to SVT with aberrant conduction. Classically, VT is a wide complex tachycardia with a left access deviation and more frequently a left bundle branch

block pattern, whereas a right bundle branch block pattern (with rSR in V_1) is more commonly seen in SVT. Again, the P wave morphology is crucial and if P waves can be distinguished, the loss of a one-to-one relationship between P wave and QRS complex is highly suggestive of VT. Sometimes, however, in VT there still may be a one-to-one ventriculo–atrial relationship. The presence of fusion beats indicating an ectopic focus below the level of the AV node is also strongly suggestive of VT.

If there is strong evidence supporting a supraventricular origin and preserved LV function, vagal manoeuvres and/or adenosine administration can be tried. The caveat is that in doing this, there is a small but important potential for hypotension and accelerated accessory pathway conduction from the adenosine administration that has been responsible for conversion of SVT to VT or even worse on occasions.

If there are no pointers towards a supraventricular origin or the above manoeuvres are unrewarding the diagnosis is most likely VT.

If the patient is severely compromised, direct current cardioversion is clearly indicated. It is debated whether this is better synchronous or asynchronous. The simplest approach is to start with the former.

If the patient has reasonable perfusion, the recommended drug depends on the appearance of the VT. If the VT is monomorphic and the patient has preserved LV function, intravenous sotalol is the agent of choice with amiodarone as a second-line agent. Amiodarone is definitely the drug of choice if LV function is impaired. If the rhythm is polymorphic, there should be some further assessment of the trace. If the trace is *torsade*-like with complexes that vary in height and appear to twist around the baseline intravenous magnesium is clearly recommended. If the QT interval is prolonged, IV magnesium followed probably by IV lidocaine is recommended. If the QT interval can be seen not to be prolonged, β-blockade is the primary approach with amiodarone again the agent of choice if LV function is impaired.

Narrow complex tachyarrhythmia

A narrow complex tachycardia is defined as one with a QRS duration normal for age (approximately ≤ 0.08 seconds). The narrow QRS complex almost always indicates that these tachyarrhythmias are supraventricular.

Supraventricular tachycardia refers to a family of tachyarrhythmias requiring the atrium, AV node or both for their perpetuation. SVT accounts for 90% of all significant tachyarrhythmias in children. It is most useful to subclassify these tachyarrhythmias on the basis of site of origin and mechanism into primary atrial tachycardias (including MAT, atrial fibrillation and atrial flutter), atrio-ventricular reciprocating, AV nodal re-entry and junctional ectopic tachycardia. Primary atrial and junctional ectopic tachycardias will be dealt with later. Atrio-ventricular reciprocating and nodal re-entry tachycardias are the commonest forms of SVT in childhood.

Atrio-ventricular reciprocating tachycardia   Occurs due to the presence of an accessory conduction pathway setting up a re-entry circuit. In the commonest variety (*orthodromic reciprocating*), the impulse travels antegrade via the AV node to the ventricles (as usual) and then retrograde via the accessory pathway back to the atria. If the accessory pathway is capable of conducting antegrade, *antidromic reciprocating* tachycardia can occur with the impulse travelling in the opposite direction, i.e. forward down accessory pathway, returning retrograde via AV node.

AV nodal re-entrant tachycardia   In this tachyarrhythmia the two conduction pathways are thought to be within or adjacent to the AV node. Beyond 5 years of age, this becomes the most common form of SVT. Classically, the P wave is buried within the QRS complex on ECG. In AV nodal re-entrant tachycardia for long-term prophylaxis therapy digoxin is the preferred agent. However, β-blockers may be considered in resistant cases, either alone or in combination with digoxin.

The crucial step in distinguishing between the above mentioned atrial, atrioventricular or nodal tachycardias is an identification of the P wave and its relationship to the QRS complex. This is sometimes best done with a 12-lead electrocardiogram with the paper run at 50 mm s^{-1}. Atrially driven tachycardias will have a P wave preceding each QRS. If the P wave is upright in inferior leads, the origin of the tachycardia is high in the atrium whereas the P wave axis will be negative in inferior leads if there is atrioventricular nodal re-entry or a low atrial ectopic focus. The P wave is usually absent in junctional ectopic tachyarrhythmia or VT. An abnormal P wave morphology usually indicates an origin other than the sinus node and several morphologies will indicate multifocal atrial tachycardia (or MAT). If the P wave follows the QRS complex, the differential diagnosis involves atrioventricular nodal re-entry tachyarrhythmia and ventricular tachycardia. If the P waves are dissociated from the QRS complexes, the diagnoses are most likely junctional ectopic tachycardia or VT.

Regardless of these diagnostic considerations, the approach is essentially the same. If the patient is acutely compromised, basic life support followed by attempted DC cardioversion with 0.5–1 J kg^{-1} of DC shock (under sedation if possible) and with continuous ECG monitoring is recommended. IV adenosine is an alternative if this is immediately available. If the patient has adequate perfusion, consider vagal manoeuvres/eliciting of diving reflex, administer adenosine in increasing doses as above.

The importance of a continuous 12-lead electrocardiogram during this process cannot be over emphasised. This is because just a few beats of sinus rhythm before reversion back to the tachyarrhythmia might well shed considerable light on the diagnosis. If the arrhythmia is resistant to adenosine, the next step is probably use of a β-blocker with digoxin being an alternative for maintenance (see below for caveats re digoxin in WPW).

Failure of adenosine to convert such a tachyarrhythmia makes unusual diagnoses more likely. For multiple atrial ectopic foci, sotalol is effective but probably only as a bridge to radiofrequency ablation. For JET the agent of choice is amiodarone. In atrial fibrillation/flutter, rate control can be achieved using digoxin but usually elective cardioversion is required to terminate the arrhythmia. In post-surgical cases recurrence is common and sotalol probably has the strongest demonstrated efficacy in reducing recurrences (and controlling ventricular rate) if they occur, though only as a bridge to possible cryoablation.

Wolf–Parkinson–White syndrome

WPW is present when the accessory atrioventricular connection allows ventricular pre-excitation by rapid antegrade conduction of the normal sinus impulse, thereby avoiding the normal delay in the AV node. This is present in 22–73% of cases of paediatric SVT and produces a shortened PR interval and slurred upstroke on the QRS complex (delta waves). It produces usually orthodromic reciprocating atrio-ventricular tachycardia but in a small proportion of cases (approximately 10%) an antidromic reciprocating tachycardia can occur.

If WPW is known to be present (by past history or presence of delta waves on a non-tachyarrhythmia ECG) β-blockers (propanolol or atenolol) are the agents of first choice (slow conduction through AV node with little, if any, effect on accessory pathways). Digoxin has traditionally been the drug of choice for prophylaxis against SVT in WPW but has pro-arrhythmia risks, particularly in antidromic reciprocating tachycardia (decreases accessory pathway refractory period, thereby facilitating accessory connection conductance of atrial arrhythmias), and should therefore be avoided. Sotalol combines β-blocker and class-3 antiarrhythmic actions and is effective and safe in resistant SVT. There is also some evidence supporting a role for flecainide (class 1C agent) or amiodarone (class 3 agent) as maintenance treatments in resistant cases.

Atrial flutter

Atrial flutter is an atrial tachycardia that probably propagates via an intra-atrial re-entrant pathway. It is uncommon but can occur in infancy, when it is usually not associated with structural heart disease. Beyond infancy 95% of atrial flutter is associated with structural heart disease (Mustard/Senning operation for TGA, Fontan, repaired TAPVR).

Clinical features Palpitations, cardiac failure or asymptomatic, dependent on rate of ventricular response.

ECG Characteristic saw-tooth flutter wave at 300 beats per minute, best seen in II, III and a VF with 2:1 or 3:1 AV block.

Management Infants without structural heart disease will usually respond to low energy (0.5 J kg^{-1}) DC cardioversion, repeated after digoxin loading if initially unsuccessful. Atrial flutter is more resistant in the older patient who will usually have associated structural cardiac disease. Amiodarone or class 1A agents have been shown to be effective. Radiofrequency catheter ablation may be valuable as a more definitive therapy.

Atrial fibrillation

Unlike in adults, atrial fibrillation is a relatively rare tachyarrhythmia in infants and children.

Clinical features Irregular, rapid palpitations with cardiac failure if a rapid ventricular response is present.

ECG Absence of discrete P waves with an irregularly irregular narrow, rapid ventricular complex.

Aetiology
- Atrial distension or scars
- Rheumatic heart disease
- Hyperthyroidism
- Hypocalcaemia
- Poisoning
- Intrathoracic pathology.

Management Should focus on removing the aetiologic cause if possible. Therapy is directed toward controlling the ventricular rate (primarily using digoxin or β-blockade to slow AV nodal conduction). Synchronised DC cardioversion is

CONTROVERSIES

❶ Requirement for ongoing prophylactic antiarrhythmic therapy with paroxysmal supraventricular tachycardia in infants when the natural history of this condition suggests fewer attacks with age beyond 12 months.

❷ Applicability and safety of automated external defibrillators for use in young children.

❸ Safety of amiodarone and its replacement of lidocaine as antiarrhythmic agent of first choice in children with shock-resistant ventricular fibrillation.

❹ Expanding role for vasopressin in asystole or shock-resistant ventricular fibrillation either alone or in combination with adrenaline (epinephrine).

effective in conversion of atrial fibrillation to sinus rhythm but because of the embolic risk, the procedure is avoided in children with long-standing atrial fibrillation, cardiac failure and/or enlarged atria.

Ventricular fibrillation

In confirmed ventricular fibrillation, the first priority is rapid defibrillation. Basic life support should be initiated while a defibrillator is sought. Conducting pads or conductive gel should be placed on the chest in the left 5th intercostal space mid axillary line and second intercostal space to the right of the sternum being careful that gel areas are not contiguous to avoid shorting of current. The paddles are applied, charged on the chest, 'stand clear' is called, and the operator verifies that this direction has been followed by other staff. Then 2 J kg^{-1} of current is discharged in asynchronous mode. If persistence of VF is verified this process is repeated in rapid succession at 2 J kg^{-1} and then 4 J kg^{-1} then access to the circulation is sought. Adrenaline (epinephrine) is then administered. After a further 30–60 seconds of CPR a 4th shock is given and if the patient remains in VF, amiodarone 5 mg kg^{-1} by rapid IV bolus is the antiarrhythmic of choice. This is then followed by further attempts at defibrillation while CPR is continued. Lidocaine is a second choice agent, magnesium is recommended.

FURTHER READING

Alexander ME, Berul CI 2000 Ventricular arrhythmias: When to worry. Paediatric Cardiology 21(6): 532–541

Anonymous 2000 Guidelines for cardiopulmonary resuscitation and emergency cardiovascular care. Part 10: Pediatric advanced life support. The American Heart Association in collaboration with the International Liaison Committee on Resuscitation. Circulation (Supplement I) 8(I 291): I342

Bink-Boelkens MTE 2000 Pharmacologic management of arrhythmias. Paediatric Cardiology 21(6): 508–515

Kudenchuk PJ, Cobb LA, Copass MK et al 1999 Amiodarone for resuscitation after out-of-hospital cardiac arrest due to ventricular fibrillation. The New England Journal of Medicine 341(12): 871–878

Kugler JD, Danford DA 1996 Management of infants, children and adolescents with paroxysmal supraventricular tachycardia. Journal of Paediatrics 129(3): 324–338

Liebman J 1982 Tables of normal standards. In Liebman J, Plonsey R, Gillette PC (eds) Pediatric electrocardiography, 1st edn. Williams & Wilkins, Baltimore, 82–133

Luedtke SA, Kuhn RJ, McCaffrey FM 1997 Pharmacologic management of supraventricular tachycardias in children. Part 1, WPW and AV nodal re-entry. The Annals of Pharmacotherapy 31: 1227–1243

Luedtke SA, Kuhn RJ, McCaffrey FM 1997 Pharmacologic management of supraventricular tachycardias in children. Part 2, Atrial flutter, atrial fibrillation and junctional and atrial ectopic tachycardia. The Annals of Pharmacotherapy 31: 1347–1359

McKee MR 2004 Amiodarone – an 'old' drug with new recommendations. Current Opinion in Paediatrics 15: 193–199

Perry JC, Fenrich AL, Hulse JE et al 1996 Pediatric use of intravenous amiodarone: Efficacy and safety in critically ill patients from a multicenter protocol. Journal of American College of Cardiology 27(5): 1246–1250

Pfammatter JP, Paul T 1997 New antiarrhythmic drugs in pediatric use: Sotalol. Paediatric Cardiology 18: 28–34

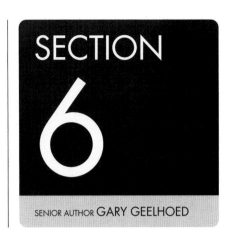

RESPIRATORY

6.1 UPPER RESPIRATORY TRACT INFECTIONS

PETER BARNETT

ESSENTIALS

1 Over 90% of childhood URTIs are viral and do not require antibiotics.

2 Upper respiratory tract infections are common and normal children may have 6 to 8 URTIs per year.

3 In the child with presumed URTI who has significant constitutional symptomatology, one needs to consider alternative diagnoses.

4 Symptomatic nasal obstruction in infants should be treated with saline drops and gentle bulb aspiration.

5 The likelihood of bacterial infection is age related and tonsillitis in children under four years is usually viral in aetiology.

6 Stomatitis in children is usually caused by herpes simplex or coxsackie virus and symptomatic treatment to aid fluid intake is all that is required.

7 Tonsillitis is a feature of EBV, thus always examine for node enlargement and organomegaly.

INTRODUCTION

Infections involving the upper respiratory tract are the commonest infections seen in children and the most frequent reason for presenting to EDs. These infections may involve anatomical structures including the nasopharynx, mouth, ear and upper airway. Specific diagnosis needs to be made to decide whether antibiotic treatment is necessary.

NASOPHARYNGITIS

INTRODUCTION

Nasopharyngitis or the common cold is a viral illness of the upper respiratory tract. This is commonly called an upper respiratory tract infection (URTI) even though it only affects part of upper respiratory tract. A URTI is usually caused by rhino and corona viruses, but during the winter season, parainfluenza and respiratory syncytial virus (RSV) are also common. It is important to note that other viral/bacterial infections may begin with URTI symptoms and progress to involve the lower respiratory tract, e.g. influenza, *Bordetella pertussis*, adenoviruses. If symptoms are persistent, an open mind regarding alternative diagnoses is required. It would seem that all colds lasting more than ten days have sinusitis. In their first six years children generally have between six to eight URTIs per year and infections are more frequent in those attending day care. The breast feeding of babies may offer some protection.

HISTORY

This illness is characterised by mild to moderate fever, blocked or runny nose, sneezing, mild cough (generally dry in the first few days) with an irritating sore throat. Infants may also become restless and irritable. Nasal congestion may interfere with feeding in infants under six months due to mechanical obstruction. Over the first few days the watery nasal discharge will become thicker and more mucopurulent. Nasal obstruction leads to mouth breathing and increased throat discomfort. The characteristic of the cough may change, in becoming moist after a few days. Sputum production occurs but in small children is generally swallowed rather than expectorated. Generally the child is not particularly unwell. If a child has significant constitutional symptoms, one needs to consider alternative diagnoses such as lower respiratory infection or influenza. Other family members may have or be recovering from cold symptoms.

EXAMINATION

Examination reveals a well child with nasal discharge, which may cause obstruction. Mucopurulent discharge does not indicate a bacterial cause. The tympanic membranes maybe slightly dull or pink in appearance but with no evidence of fluid in the middle ear. The throat may be red but not associated with exudate or cervical lymphadenopathy. The chest is clear to auscultation, although there may be transmitted upper airway sounds, originating from the nasal passages.

INVESTIGATIONS

There is no indication for investigations in a child with common cold.

TREATMENT

Therapy is supportive, combined with explanation and providing a management plan for parents. Parents need to ensure the child has adequate rest and fluids to maintain hydration. Nasal congestion/obstruction in infants may be improved with saline drops (1 teaspoon salt in 1 cup boiled water and allowed to cool or commercial saline spray) into the nares intermittently. In addition, aspiration of mucus using a bulb suction device may be helpful.

The routine use of oral decongestants is generally unhelpful and may cause side effects. In children symptomatic of nasal obstruction, topical decongestants may be used if saline and aspiration are not helpful. They should be used judiciously and never longer than three days to avoid rebound nasal mucosal swelling.

There is no indication for antibiotics in this setting. Pharyngitis or tonsillitis associated with a URTI is viral in nature and will not respond to antibiotics. The inappropriate use of antibiotics in these patients may be a contributory factor to antibiotic resistance. Herbal remedies such as echinacea, vitamin C, or zinc have not been shown to treat URTIs. There maybe a role for these medications in prevention but the data is not conclusive.

An explanation to parents of the expected natural history may decrease the likelihood of inappropriate seeking of antibiotics. One should encourage early review should their child's course deviate from that expected. Paracetamol is indicated if a child is symptomatic of fever or to diminish the discomfort of a sore throat. The use of over-the-counter cold preparations has not been shown to alter outcome.

STOMATITIS

INTRODUCTION

Children with stomatitis often present to emergency due to difficulties in drinking. In children it is most commonly caused by herpes simplex virus (gingivo-stomatitis) or coxsackie virus (hand, foot and mouth). These viral infections cause vesicular lesions, which may involve the buccal mucosa, gingiva, tongue, palate and the pharynx. Fungal infection with *Candida albicans* (thrush) may be seen in neonates or immunosuppressed children. Aphthous ulcers are uncommon in children but are often recurrent.

HISTORY

Primary herpes simplex produces a severe gingivo-stomatitis involving most of the mouth and characteristically has a few lesions on the outer lip area. Fever is prominent and can last for 7–10 days. The associated mouth pain can result in intolerance of saliva, decreased oral intake and subsequent dehydration. Oral herpes can be spread to the digits in patients who suck their fingers leading to a herpetic whitlow.

EXAMINATION

Children may be distressed by mouth pain and have a high fever. Hydration should be assessed. Herpes causes multiple shallow ulcers of the oral mucosa and associated gingival inflammation. Coxsackie tends to cause fewer ulcers in the mouth, more on the palatal mucosa and is less likely to cause gingivitis. It is classically associated with vesicular lesions on the hands, feet and buttocks. Oral thrush presents with characteristic white plaques on the buccal mucosa and tongue. Clinical confusion may arise in the baby who has recently taken milk, which may give a similar appearance. Differentiation can be made by trying to scrape off the plaques which either causes bleeding or they are unable to be removed.

INVESTIGATION

Diagnosis is clinical and usually requires no investigations. Immunofluorescence for herpes simplex may be required for isolation purposes or in the immunosuppressed.

TREATMENT

Viral stomatitis is self-limiting and symptomatic treatment to reduce pain and allow eating and drinking is the mainstay of therapy. Topical anaesthetic treatment such as Xylocaine® viscous or gel 2% applied sparingly to the lesions, half an hour prior to drinking, may be beneficial. In addition, oral analgesics such as paracetamol ± codeine should also be used. Icy poles, cool drinks or a soft diet may also be an effective way to achieve an adequate fluid intake. The child with severe stomatitis, who is dehydrated, may require admission for intravenous fluids. Aciclovir has been used to hasten the resolution in immunocompromised patients, but it has not been proven to be effective in normal patients admitted to hospital for hydration.

Treatment for oral thrush is either topical antifungal gel or oral drops four times a day for ten to fourteen days. Drops should be applied after a feed and inserted onto the buccal mucosa not into the general oral cavity. Systemic antifungals are only indicated in immunocompromised patients.

PHARYNGITIS/TONSILLITIS

INTRODUCTION

Pharyngitis/tonsillitis is a common infection involving the throat including the tonsils. In children, particularly in the first four years, a viral aetiology is most likely. Viruses that can cause pharyngitis include adenovirus, enterovirus, para/influenza, or Epstein–Barr virus.

Group A *Streptococcus* is the most common bacterial infection of the throat, but only accounts for up to 20% of tonsillopharyngitis. The incidence is age related and is uncommon in children under four years of age. Twenty percent of children are colonised by Group A *Streptococcus*, hence, a positive throat swab may be incidental in a child with an acute viral infection. The clinical dilemma is distinguishing viral from bacterial infections and therefore the need for antibiotics.

HISTORY

The presentation can vary according to the age of the child. Older children may complain of sore throat, headache, dysphagia or have referred abdominal pain. Younger children may present with less localising symptomatology with fever, decreased oral intake and clinging to parents. Patients presenting with associated coryzal symptoms and cough are unlikely to have a bacterial cause for their pharyngitis.

EXAMINATION

The clinical distinction between bacterial and viral is difficult (see Table 6.1.1). Group A *Streptococcus* is most likely in the child with fever, swollen tender cervical nodes, isolated sore throat and florid exudative tonsillopharyngitis. Viral tonsillitis may indeed have an exudative appearance. Associated conjunctivitis may suggest an adenoviral pharyngoconjunctivitis. The presence of ulcers on the pharynx suggests a viral aetiology of the pharyngitis, such as enterovirus. The presence of a scarlatiniform rash (red, sandpaper-textured skin) or a strawberry tongue is supportive of streptococcal infection. Epstein–Barr virus (infectious mononucleosis) is common in adolescents and can have a similar pharyngeal appearance to bacterial infection, except that the patient may have a general swelling of the neck and face, due to marked cervical adenopathy. They may also have enlargement of the spleen and liver, but this is more common in younger children. (See Table 6.1.1.)

INVESTIGATIONS

The use of throat swabs in the ED remains controversial due to the *Streptococcus* A colonisation that occurs in up to 20% of children. One approach is, if Group A *Streptococcus* pharyngitis is suspected, then a throat swab should be taken. A rapid strep test is very specific for *Streptococcus* A infection, but not very sensitive. If a rapid strep test is negative, then a culture should be sent. If using a culture, then there is the option to either treat the patient at the time of consultation and cease the antibiotics if the swab is negative or wait until the swab is positive to treat the patient. If one suspects EBV, an FBE or monospot test may be helpful, although the early monospot (within one week of onset of symptoms) can be falsely negative.

TREATMENT

Treatment of confirmed Group A streptococcal infection with antibiotics will decrease the length of symptoms approximately by one day (four vs. five days) and decreases the likelihood of rheumatic fever. Oral penicillin is the drug of choice, either 250 mg bd (age < 10 y) or 500 mg bd (age >10 y) given for ten days. A long-acting parenteral penicillin (benzathine) is also effective in children who are refusing oral medication.

Most children with a sore throat have a viral infection and do not require antibiotics. Symptomatic relief using paracetamol or soluble aspirin or salt-water gargles may be helpful. Topical anaesthetic can also decrease the throat pain. Ensuring adequate hydration improves patient's general well being. In those unable to drink and who are dehydrated, admission may be required. Children with severe tonsillomegaly and neck swelling from EBV can develop airway obstruction and may benefit from a short course of steroids.

FURTHER READING

Bisno AL, Berber MA, Gwaltney JM, Kaplan EL, Schwartz RCH 1997 Diagnosis and management of Group A streptococcal pharyngitis: A practice guideline. Clinical Infectious Disease 25: 574–583

Dowell SF, Marcy SM, Phillips WR, Gerber MA, Schwartz B 1998 Principles of judicious use of antimicrobial agents for paediatric upper respiratory tract infections. Paediatrics 101(1): 163–165

Dowell SF, Phillips WR, Schwartz B 1998 Appropriate use of antibiotics for URIs in children: Part II. Cough pharyngitis and the common cold. American Family Physician 58(6): 1335–1342

Hay AD, Wilson AD 2002 The natural history of acute cough in children aged 0–4 years in primary care: A systematic review. British Journal of General Practice 52(478): 401–409

Korppi M 1997 Recurrent respiratory infections in children: A practical approach for clinical work. Paediatric Pulmonology – Supplement 16: 144–145

Peat JK, Keena V, Harakeh Z, Marks G 2001 Parental smoking and respiratory tract infections in children. Paediatric Respiratory Reviews 2(3): 207–213

West JV 2002 Acute upper airways infections. British Medical Bulletin 61: 215–230

Table 6.1.1	Features of viral and bacterial tonsillitis
Viral	Bacterial
Age < 4 years	Age > 4 years
Associated cough, coryza, conjunctivitis, diarrhoea	Tender jugulo-digastric adenopathy
Features to suggest EBV strawberry tongue	Toxic appearance, scarlatiniform rash, *Marked* exudative tonsillitis

6.2 INHALED FOREIGN BODY

PETER BARNETT

ESSENTIALS

1 The presentation of a child with airway obstruction due to an inhaled foreign body to an emergency department can be life-threatening and requires rapid assessment.

2 One needs to have a prepared approach, which differentiates the situation of total from partial obstruction.

3 One needs to be cautious to avoid the potential to convert partial upper airway obstruction to complete obstruction by unnecessary interventions.

4 Many children who were initially symptomatic, may be asymptomatic by the time they are seen in the emergency department and have minimal clinical findings.

5 The majority of objects are radiolucent and the radiological findings are those secondary to the physical presence in the airway.

6 Indication for bronchoscopy should be based on history, examination and radiological investigations. When in doubt, consult a paediatric respiratory physician.

INTRODUCTION

Foreign body (FB) aspiration usually occurs in children less than three years of age. Foreign bodies may lodge at any place along the airway from the hypopharynx to the segmental bronchus. Upper airway obstruction due to foreign bodies causes several deaths in Australia each year. The reason toddlers are more prone to aspiration is due to their general inquisitive nature, the presence of small food or non-food objects in the general home environment and their inability to efficiently grind food objects (due to lack of molar teeth).

The most common inhaled foreign bodies are food materials (e.g. peanuts, carrot or apple pieces) and small pieces of toys. Inhaled foreign bodies are rarely radio-opaque, therefore, often not visible on a plain X-ray. Foreign bodies in the upper airway, account for only 5–10% of all inhaled objects, but have a higher mortality and morbidity.

UPPER AIRWAY FOREIGN BODIES

HISTORY

The presentation of a child with upper airway obstruction due to an inhaled foreign body can be life threatening and require rapid assessment. One needs to have a prepared approach, which differentiates the situation of total from partial obstruction. These children present with acute onset of upper airway obstruction – partial or total. There is no preceding history suggesting an infective cause such as croup or epiglottitis. Occasionally, the aspiration incident is witnessed as a choking episode, but often not, and a child is only discovered with breathing difficulty.

EXAMINATION

A foreign body in the upper airway presents with acute signs of obstruction and respiratory distress. The signs reflect the degree of airway obstruction. In life-threatening cases there may be respiratory arrest with apnoea and cyanosis. Less urgent cases may have stridor, wheeze, cough and abnormal voice or cry. The child may be intolerant of saliva.

INVESTIGATIONS

In a stable child with partial obstruction, a soft tissue XR may be useful to localise the foreign body, if radio-opaque.

This is best performed in the ED so that the airway is monitored.

TREATMENT

Total obstruction

Untreated, *total* airway obstruction will rapidly lead to hypoxic loss of consciousness and cardiorespiratory arrest. In the child presenting with complete obstruction, basic life support should be commenced (see Chapter 2.4 on resuscitation). The performance of back blows and chest thrusts to dislodge the foreign body should be followed by attempted ventilation with bag and mask. In older children the Heimlich manoeuvre should be used. If these methods are unable to remove the foreign body and allow ventilation, then direct visualisation of the larynx and Magill forceps extraction of the foreign body should occur. In the unlikely event of a foreign body visualised below the cords, suctioning may expedite its removal or, if not possible, advancing the object past the carina may allow ventilation as a temporising measure.

Partial obstruction

The approach to the child with partial airway obstruction, but who is able to ventilate to maintain adequate oxygenation needs to be cautious. One needs to avoid the potential to convert the situation to one of complete obstruction by unnecessary interventions. It is best to leave the child undisturbed and as comfortable as possible. Small children are best kept in a parent's arms. Oxygen should be administered if required and tolerated. Causing distress and crying will usually worsen the degree of airway obstruction. This child needs to be carefully transferred from the ED to an appropriate environment where the object can be safely removed with anaesthetic, endoscopic and surgical facilities available. DO NOT attempt to remove the object by the methods mentioned above as this may convert the partial obstruction to complete obstruction.

LOWER AIRWAY FOREIGN BODY

HISTORY

The majority (70%) of patients presenting with an inhaled foreign body have a clear history to suggest an inhalation. However, up to 30% have a delayed presentation and no history of foreign body aspiration.

Patients generally present with sudden onset of coughing and choking, occasionally associated with a brief period of cyanosis. After the initial coughing episode, the child may have an audible wheeze and/or a persistent dry cough. Depending on the size of the foreign body the symptoms may be mild. Foreign bodies tend to lodge in the right main stem bronchus more than the left, which has a more acute deviation from the lumen of the trachea. A patient may also suddenly deteriorate as the foreign body is coughed from one bronchus to the other causing increasing degree of lower airway obstruction. Likewise, many children who were initially symptomatic, may be asymptomatic by the time they are seen in the ED.

EXAMINATION

Examination usually reveals a well child with mild to moderate respiratory distress. The patient may have a cough. One may be able to detect hyperinflation of one side of the chest due to gas trapping. Auscultation may reveal diminished air entry on one side compared to the other. There may be wheeze heard only on the side of the lower airway obstruction.

Table 6.2.1 Indications for bronchoscopy if two of the following:
History
• Coughing and choking episode and cyanosis or persistent cough after choking episode
Examination
• Unilateral wheeze or unilateral decreased air entry
Investigations
• Hyperinflation on expiration chest X-ray or subsegmental atelectasis or positive fluoroscopy

However, in some cases the inhaled object will be occult and the chest examination may be completely normal. A high index of suspicion is required, particularly if the history is suggestive.

INVESTIGATIONS

The initial investigation of the child with suspected inhaled foreign body should include a plain chest X-ray. The majority of objects are radiolucent and the radiological findings are those secondary to the physical presence in the airway. This may be normal or may show signs of hyperinflation.

Inspiratory and expiratory X-rays are helpful. If there is air trapping, then the affected lung or part of the lung remains inflated in expiration. There may be segmental or lobar collapse distal to the foreign body. Fluoroscopy, if available, shows decreased movement of the diaphragm on the affected side.

If the presentation has been delayed then the chest X-ray may show air trapping as above or signs of resorption atelectasis distal to the foreign body. Persistent changes on X-ray or recurrent pneumonia in the same place may signal an occult foreign body.

TREATMENT

Initially, the patient's airway and breathing should be assessed and oxygen given if required. Referral for bronchoscopy is the definitive treatment for confirmed or suspicious cases. Indications for bronchoscopy should be based on history, examination and radiological investigations (see Table 6.2.1).

Patients should then be referred to an appropriate service, which can perform a rigid bronchoscopy to remove the foreign body. When in doubt, consult with a paediatric respiratory consultant.

Children who have had a minor choking episode but no ongoing symptoms or signs and a normal XR can be discharged. Parents need to be instructed to return should any relevant symptoms evolve (wheeze, persistent dry cough, etc.).

PREVENTION

• Children under three years should be protected from access to toys with small parts or foods requiring molar function, as they are potential inhalation risks.

FURTHER READING

Lau KF, Jayaram R, Fitzgerald DA 2001 Diagnosing inhaled foreign bodies in children. Medical Journal of Australia 174(4): 194–196

Messner AH 1998 Pitfalls in the diagnosis or aerodigestive tract foreign bodies. Clinical Paediatrics 37(6): 359–365

Reilly J, Thompson J, MacArthur C, Pransky S, Beste D, Smith M, Gray S, Manning S, Walter M, Derkay C, Muntz H, Friedman E, Meyer CM, Seibert R, Riding K, Cuyler J, Todd W, Smith R 1997 Paediatric aerodigestive foreign body injuries are complications related to timeliness of diagnosis. Laryngoscope 107(1): 17–20

Rovin JD, Rodgers BM 2000 Paediatric foreign body aspiration. Paediatrics in review 21(3): 86–90

6.3 ACUTE ASTHMA

COLIN V. E. POWELL

ESSENTIALS

1 Acute asthma is one of the commonest paediatric presentations to an emergency department.

2 It is important to understand the patterns of asthma in children – infrequent episodic, frequent episodic, and persistent.

3 There are three major groups of factors contributing to 'high risk' asthma in children: previous severe asthma, management issues and psychological factors.

4 The most important parameters in the assessment of the severity of childhood asthma are the general appearance/mental state and work of breathing.

5 Life-threatening asthma is characterised by: silent chest, cyanosis, poor respiratory effort, exhaustion and altered mental state.

6 The main therapies for paediatric asthma include oxygen, inhaled bronchodilators and steroids modified according to severity.

7 Discharged patients should be given a clear asthma action plan and have appropriate follow-up organised.

8 There are many areas of contention regarding the management of asthma in children and the recommended guidelines vary between countries. One should be familiar with the local paediatric guidelines.

INTRODUCTION

The National Asthma Campaign for Australia updated its 1998 guidelines in 2002[1]. However there are other best practice guidelines[2,27] and national guidelines[3-5] and these are important resources for cross-reference and comparison to highlight the controversies.

Acute asthma is one of the commonest reasons for presentation to an ED and admission to a hospital and in many cases admissions to hospital may be preventable[6] if managed effectively by the family and medical team involved with a child's care. There are still great gaps between best practice guidelines and what actually happens in practice.[15,28]

HISTORY

Consider acute asthma when a child presents with signs of increase work of breathing, widespread wheezing and shortness of breath. There are other causes to consider such as mycoplasma pneumonia, aspiration, inhaled foreign body, allergy and cardiac failure (see Table 6.3.2). In the setting of a child with a previous history of asthma or where asthma seems the most likely diagnosis, one can rapidly perform a primary assessment of severity and institute the initial treatment at the outset of history taking. It is important to understand the patterns of asthma in children – infrequent episodic, frequent episodic and persistent.[1] The pattern of asthma determines the need for preventive therapy. When a child is discharged from the ED or ward, consideration of the child's preventative treatment is essential.

Infrequent episodic asthma

Infrequent episodic asthma (IEA) is the most common pattern, accounting for 70 to 75% of children with asthma. In this pattern, children have isolated episodes of asthma lasting from 1–2 days up to 1–2 weeks, usually triggered by an upper respiratory tract infection (URTI) or an environmental allergen. The episodes are usually more than 6–8 weeks apart and these children are asymptomatic in the interval periods. They require management of the individual episode only and regular preventive therapy is unnecessary. Within this group there is a wide range of severity. Most are mild, but this group accounts for up to 60% of paediatric hospital admissions for asthma.[1]

Frequent episodic asthma

Frequent episodic asthma (FEA) accounts for approximately 20% of childhood asthma. This pattern is similar to IEA but the interval between episodes is shorter, less than 6–8 weeks, and the children have only minimal symptoms such as exercise-induced wheeze in the interval period. These children may benefit from regular preventive therapy with sodium cromoglicate, nedocromil sodium, leukotriene antagonist or low-dose (not greater than 400 μg d^{-1}) inhaled corticosteroids. Commonly these children are troubled through the winter months only and may require preventive treatment for that part of the year.[1]

Persistent asthma

Persistent asthma (PA) accounts for 5–10% of childhood asthma. These children can have acute episodes like the categories above, but they also have symptoms on most days in the interval periods. These symptoms commonly include: sleep disturbance due to wheeze or cough, early morning chest tightness, exercise intolerance and spontaneous wheeze. There is a wide range of severity in this group of patients. Some children have mild symptoms four to five days per week, readily controlled with low-dose preventive therapy. Others have frequent severe symptoms and abnormal lung function requiring intensive therapy.[1]

Table 6.3.1   Severity of asthma

Symptoms	Mild	Moderate	Severe and life-threatening*
Altered consciousness	No	No	Agitated *Confused/drowsy*
Accessory muscle use/recession	No	Minimal	Moderate *Severe*
Oximetry on presentation (SaO$_2$)	>94%	94–90%	<90%
Talks in	Sentences	Phrases	Words *Unable to speak*
Pulsus paradoxus	Not palpable	May be palpable	Palpable
Pulse rate	<100	100–200	>200
Central cyanosis	Absent	Absent	Likely to be present
Wheeze intensity	Variable	Moderate-loud	Often quiet
Peak expiratory flow	>60%	40–60%	<40% *Unable to perform*
FEV1 (% predicted)	>60%	40–60%	<40% *Unable to perform*
Arterial blood gases	Test not necessary	If initial response is poor	If initial response is poor *Yes*

*Life-threatening asthma is characterised by[3]:
- Silent chest
- Cyanosis
- Poor respiratory effort
- Hypotension
- Exhaustion
- Confusion
- Coma.

Acute episode

Mortality from acute asthma is fortunately rare. Confidential enquires into deaths from asthma suggests that there are three major factors contributing to the death.

1. The severity of the disease. Most children who die from asthma have persistent asthma. However, a minority of children who die have only mild to moderate disease.[3,7,8] Previous near fatal asthma, previous admission in the last year, previous admission to PICU, heavy use of β$_2$-agonists, and repeat attendances at the ED are all factors associated with risk of a severe attack, near fatal asthma or death.[3]

2. Medical management. Inadequate treatment with steroids, heavy or increasing use of β$_2$-agonists, inadequate monitoring of the asthma, under use of written asthma plans and delay in seeking help, have all been associated with deaths from asthma.[3,7,8]

3. Psychological factors. Non-adherence to therapy, poorly perceived symptoms, failure to attend clinics, conflict between child and parent or medical staff, and family dysfunction are all risk factors associated with risk of death from asthma.[3,9]

A child should be considered as 'high risk' when attending the ED with an acute exacerbation of asthma when there is a combination of features of previous severe asthma and one or more adverse psychological factors.

EXAMINATION

The most important parameters in the assessment of the severity of acute child-

Table 6.3.2   Differential diagnosis of asthma

Acute	Chronic
Bronchiolitis, mycoplasma	Cystic fibrosis
Allergy	Cilial dyskinesia
Aspiration	Immune deficiency
Heart failure	Bronchiectasis
Foreign body	Airway abnormalities

hood asthma are general appearance/ mental state and work of breathing (accessory muscle use, recession), as indicated in Table 6.3.2. Initial SaO$_2$ in air, heart rate and ability to talk are helpful but less reliable additional features. Wheeze intensity, pulsus paradoxus, and peak expiratory flow rate are not reliable.[2] Clinical signs of acute asthma correlate poorly with the severity of the asthma attack and none of the signs in isolation are predictive of severity.[3] Classification of an acute attack, using the NAC Australian guidelines[1] is as follows:

INVESTIGATIONS

A chest X-ray is not generally required in children with asthma, unless one has suspicion of an alternative diagnosis or complication (air leak or atelectasis). Arterial blood gas and spirometry are rarely required in the assessment of acute asthma in children.

DIFFERENTIAL DIAGNOSIS

During an acute episode of wheezing, asymmetry on auscultation is often found due to mucous plugging, but may warrant consideration of a foreign body. Other causes of acute wheezing in children include bronchiolitis, mycoplasma, aspiration, allergy or heart failure. Chronically wheezy children may have a diagnosis other than asthma such as cystic fibrosis, cilial dyskinesia, immune dysfunction, developmental/congenital abnormality, upper airway problems or bronchiectasis. There may be clues in the family or perinatal history or the symptoms and signs, which may suggest an alternative diagnosis to asthma.[3]

TREATMENT

Mild

- Salbutamol by pMDI/spacer (see below) – once and review after 20 minutes.
- Ensure device/technique appropriate.
- Good response – discharge on β_2-agonist as needed. Poor response – treat as moderate.
- Oral prednisolone (1 mg kg^{-1} d^{-1} for 1–3 days) if on prophylaxis or episode has persisted over several days.
- Provide written advice/action plan on what to do if symptoms worsen.

- Consider overall control and family's knowledge. Arrange follow-up as appropriate (see discharge pack).

Moderate

- Give oxygen if O_2 saturation is < 92%. Need for O_2 should be reassessed.
- Salbutamol by pMDI/spacer (see below) or nebuliser – three doses, 20 minutely. Review 10–20 minutes after 3rd dose to decide on admission or discharge.
- Oral prednisolone (1 mg kg^{-1} d^{-1} for 3 days).
- The few children of moderate severity who can go home must be discussed with the senior doctor and should not leave ED until review at least one hour after their last spacer treatment.
- Arrange home treatment and follow-up as above.

Severe

- Oxygen.
- Salbutamol by pMDI/spacer (see below) or nebuliser – three doses 20 minutely. Review on-going requirements 10–20 minutes after 3rd dose – if improving reduce frequency, if no change continue 20 minutely, if deteriorating at any stage treat as life threatening.
- Ipratropium (see below) by pMDI/spacer or nebuliser – three doses 20 minutely in first hour.
- Oral prednisolone (1 mg kg^{-1} d^{-1}). If vomiting give intravenous methylprednisolone, 1 mg kg^{-1} or hydrocortisone 4 mg k^{g-1} IV six-hourly.
- Involve senior staff.
- Arrange admission after initial assessment and stabilisation.

Life threatening

- Oxygen. Continuous cardiac and saturation monitoring.
- Continuous nebulised salbutamol (0.5% undiluted).
- Nebulised ipratropium 250 µg – three doses 20 minutely in first hour.
- Methylprednisolone, 1 mg kg^{-1} or hydrocortisone, 4 mg kg^{-1} IV six-hourly.

- *If deteriorating* give intravenous salbutamol. Initial bolus 5 µg kg^{-1} over 10 minutes then by infusion at 1–5 µg kg^{-1} min^{-1}.
- If poor response to IV salbutamol, *consider* aminophylline 10 mg kg^{-1} IV, maximum dose 250 mg over 60 minutes. If currently taking oral theophylline, do not give IV aminophylline in ED – take serum level. Following loading dose, give continuous infusion (1–9 years: 1.1 mg kg^{-1} h^{-1}, 10 + years: 0.7 mg kg^{-1} h^{-1}; commence in ED if there will be > 2 h before transfer to ward).
- Involve senior staff and liaise with local PICU.
- Where *intubation* is indicated, ketamine is the induction agent of choice due to its bronchodilator action.

DISPOSITION

Indications for admission include: severe or life-threatening asthma, children who require oxygen or if the child requires inhaled bronchodilators more frequently than three-hourly. The decision can be influenced by other factors such as previous life-threatening episodes, sudden and labile attacks, current steroid use, bronchodilator use prior to presentation, compliance to therapy, social circumstances and distance from hospital. A period of monitoring may be necessary to determine the safety of discharge in borderline cases.

Each child should have a written action plan on discharge from the ED. The child's inhaler technique should be observed before discharge. Advise parents to seek medical review should their child's condition deteriorate or if there is no significant improvement within 48 hours. At discharge all patients should have an out-patient appointment or appropriate follow-up arranged with the local doctor or paediatrician. Parents should be informed of other sources of information about asthma such as the Asthma Foundation. The concept of an asthma discharge pack is useful to ensure all aspects of discharge are considered. Adult data suggest that self-monitoring, regular review and written action plans can improve outcomes.[10] Two paediatric studies suggest that an intensive nurse-led discharge concentrating on education, written action plans and inhaler technique, appropriate follow up with discharge prescription for steroids can reduce readmissions and following morbidity.[11,12] A child should be ready for discharge when it is considered that they can be stable on 3–4 hour inhaled bronchodilators.[13] This is often a subjective decision.

Discharge pack

1. Review need for preventative treatment

Consider preventative treatment if there are wheezing attacks less than six weeks apart, the attacks are becoming more frequent and severe or there are increasing interval symptoms. Options for initial preventative treatment for frequent episodic asthma are cromoglicate, nedocromil, and inhaled steroids. If a child has persistent asthma use inhaled steroids.

2. Check inhaler technique

Emergency attendance or admission should provide the patient and family with the opportunity to use a spacer device and pMDI. Make sure that the child and family can use the device adequately and know the importance of using it for all preventative therapy and treatment for significant exacerbations.

3. Family education

On discharge from the ED or ward it is important that families understand the immediate management of their child's asthma. It is not appropriate to educate them on all aspects of asthma during an acute episode. This is best reserved for a visit to an out-patient clinic or local doctor, at a time remote from the acute episode when a reasonable amount of time can be allocated and it is more likely that the information will be understood and retained.

4. Prescription

A prescription for all medications should be provided at the time of discharge.

5. Follow-up

All patients should have a clear follow-up plan. For some it will be appropriate that they visit their local doctor for an early review, particularly if their condition deteriorates or fails to improve significantly with 48 hours. Children with first diagnosis, frequent or persistent asthma, warrant a specialist review and should have appropriate follow-up arranged with a paediatrician within 4–6 weeks. This visit will be used for medical review and, most importantly, appropriate education about asthma management.

6. Written action plan

All patients should have an individual written action plan and the discharging doctor should spend time going over the plan with the family.

7. Communicate with the local doctor

For every emergency attendance there should be communication with the patient's local doctor. The local doctor should receive a copy of the action plan.

PROGNOSIS

Those with episodic asthma tend to improve throughout childhood, with asthma resolving by their adult years in approximately two-thirds. Those who continue to wheeze tend to have very mild asthma and maintain normal lung function. On the other hand, those with persistent asthma in childhood are more likely to continue to wheeze in their adult years (about two-thirds) with some impairment of lung function. Available evidence suggests that treatment does not influence the natural history of childhood asthma.[1]

PREVENTION

There are two areas of prevention: primary prevention – attempts to stop the development of asthma, and secondary prevention – interventions to try to reduce the impact of the disease. These should be considered, but the data are mostly inconclusive and confusing.

Areas of potential primary prevention are allergen avoidance during pregnancy or early infancy, breast feeding, modified infant milk formulae, pre- and probiotic use, immunotherapy and avoiding pollutants (e.g. cigarette smoke). However, the only evidenced-based recommendations in this area are that:

- Breast-feeding should be encouraged as this will reduce the likelihood of developing asthma particularly in families with an atopic history.[3]
- Parents and parents-to-be should be advised not to smoke as maternal smoking, particularly, both antenatally and postnatally, is associated with increased risk of infant wheeze.[3]

In children with asthma a number of non-pharmacological methods of secondary prevention are debated, for example allergen avoidance, house dust mite control measures, avoiding smoking and air pollution, antioxidant and mineral supplementation, fish oils and fatty acids use, breathing exercises, chemotherapy and immunotherapy. Recent evidence-based recommendations are that:

- In committed families, house dust mite avoidance by use of bed covers, removal of carpets and soft toys, dehumidification and high temperature washing of bed linen may reduce morbidity from asthma.[3]
- Maternal smoking during pregnancy has an effect on lung development and infants whose mothers smoke are four-times more likely to develop wheezy illness during the first year of life. Thus environmental tobacco smoke should be avoided.[3]

If an organized discharge from hospital is completed as per recommendations (above), then this is more likely to prevent readmission or representation and reduce morbidity. A number of preventable factors associated with admission have been identified and these issues should be addressed at discharge: adherence issues, prophylactic treatment, action-plan use and advice to prevent delay in seeking medical advice.[6]

CONTROVERSIES

There are many areas of contention regarding the management of asthma, where there is inadequate data to make an evidenced-based guideline and consensus statement has to be the only level of recommendation.

❶ Bronchodilator aerosol delivery

Pressurised metered dose inhalers (pMDI) and spacers are an effective way of delivering inhalation medication to treat mild to moderate and probably severe attacks of asthma.[21] Successful implementation[22,23] and sustained use of spacers after change over from nebulisers by families discharged from hospital has been demonstrated.[24] There are fewer side effects, such as tachycardia, vomiting and hypoxia, compared to when a drug is given via a nebuliser.[21] There is still debate as to the cost in different countries and whether the pMDI/spacer combination use in adult acute asthma is as effective as nebulisers.[21] The pMDI/spacer combination is used less frequently in adult patients.[15]

Various doses are suggested for salbutamol pMDI/spacer dosing:

- 6 or 12 puffs every 20 minutes for the first hour and then titrate depending on response[1,2]
- 2–4 puffs every 20–30 minutes according to clinical response with an increase of two puffs every two minutes up to 10 puffs for more severe[3]
- 4–8 puffs every 20 minutes for four hours then every 1–4 hours as needed[5]
- 10 puffs every 15 minutes[4]
- 4 puffs if less than 20 kg, 1–2 hourly or 8 puffs, 1-2 hourly, if > 20 kg.[27]

It probably does not make much difference what doses are given – if there is a response, cut down the dose, if there is no response increase it!

Nebulised doses are similar between 2.5–5 mg of salbutamol per nebuliser every 20 minutes.[1–5,27] There is little evidence for any benefit for continuous nebulised treatment compared to frequent intermittent doses of treatment[3] although NAC Australia suggest using continuous treatment for life-threatening asthma.[1] The nebulised terbutaline dose is 10 mg dose^{-1} in the BTS guidelines.[3]

❷ Ipratropium bromide

Repeated doses of ipratropium bromide, during the first one to two hours of presentation are associated with improved outcomes.[14] It is recommended for children with severe and life-threatening attacks[1–5] but often overused in children with moderate and mild attacks.[15] It is not clear whether there are any benefits from continued use after the attack has shown response to treatment. Although doses of inhaled ipratropium bromide are recommended for use with a metered dose inhaler and spacer[2] there are no data demonstrating that these doses are appropriate and this is a consensus statement recommendation. Different doses are recommended:

- 3–6 puffs (20 μg per puff) via pMDI and spacer every 20–120 minutes combined with salbutamo[14]
- 2–4 puffs (40 μg per puff) via pMDI and spacer every 20 minutes for three doses in first hour[1,2]
- standard doses of 250–500 μg per dose for nebulised treatment seems universal.[1–5]

❸ Intravenous bronchodilators

The main problem with deciding which intravenous bronchodilator to use is that there are no good direct comparisons with the three intravenous treatments commonly used. There are certainly drug versus placebo studies but no head-to-head studies to endorse recommendations. Thus, the referenced guidelines vary with their recommendations.[1–5] The role of intravenous bronchodilators, in addition to nebulised treatment, remains unclear.[16]

Salbutamol – A study by Browne et al suggests using a bolus of 15 μg kg^{-1} (given over 10 minutes) in severe asthma[17] and this has been associated with improved outcome (reduced need for admission). This recommendation is endorsed by the BTS guidelines.[3] Continuous intravenous infusions are recommended following on, if the child does not respond, but different doses are recommended:

- 5 μg kg^{-1} over 10 minutes then an infusion of 5 μg kg^{-1} min^{-1} thereafter[1,27]
- 1-2 μg kg^{-1} min^{-1} (up to 5 μg kg^{-1} on PICU[3]
- load with 7.5 μg kg^{-1} over 2–5 minutes and then[4] use 1–10 μg kg^{-1} min^{-1}
- The USA recommendations for intravenous β_2-agonists are for terbutaline at a dose of 0.01 mg kg^{-1} every 20 minutes for three doses then every 2–6 hours as needed, but do emphasise that there is no proven advantage to systemic treatment over aerosol.[5]

Aminophylline – There is no evidence that there is a role for aminophylline in children with a mild to moderate exacerbation. However, if a child is unresponsive to maximal inhaled therapy, as above, then in the more severe and life-threatening attacks, aminophylline has been shown to have an effect on outcome (intubation).[18] Again recommended doses vary from:

- 5 mg kg^{-1} loading dose over 20 minutes if a child is not on theophyllines with an infusion[3] of 1 mg kg^{-1} h^{-1}
- 6 mg kg^{-1} loading dose followed[4] by 0.5–1 mg kg^{-1} h^{-1}
- 10 mg kg^{-1} loading dose followed by an infusion of 0.7–1.1 mg kg^{-1} h^{-1} depending on age of child[1]
- In USA, methylxanthines are not recommended because it is felt that they 'do not benefit children hospitalized with severe asthma'.[5]

This is clearly a controversial area. Aminophylline is not mentioned in other guidelines.[27] There is no doubt that vomiting is a serious side effect from the higher doses of aminophylline and this may be the reason not to use it.[18]

Magnesium – Intravenous magnesium relaxes smooth muscle and causes bronchodilation. Its exact place in the treatment of acute asthma in children has yet to be established. Doses of between 40 and 100 mg kg^{-1} as a 20-minute infusion have been used with varying effects on lung function and asthma severity scores when compared to placebo.[19] The use of intravenous magnesium sulphate is endorsed by the BTS as a possible third-line treatment after intravenous β$_2$-agonists and aminophylline[3] have failed. The USA recommendations suggest 'attempting' the use of additional treatment with magnesium sulfate if children have not responded to treatment after one hour.[5] Magnesium is not mentioned in the NAG Australia1 for use in children, nor is it mentioned in some other recommendations.[4,27]

Adrenaline (epinephrine) – This bronchodilator is not mentioned in the paediatric guidelines.[1-4] However, the GINA guidelines suggest it may be of use.[5] There is no doubt that some acute asthma may be anaphylaxis[20] and intramuscular adrenaline (epinephrine) may well have a role.[5] For acute asthma the dose suggested is 0.01 mg kg^{-1} up to 0.3–0.5 mg of 1:1000 adrenaline every 20 minutes for three doses.[5] This treatment is very rarely used in acute asthma in a paediatric population.[15]

❹ Steroids

There is no doubt that the early use of steroids for acute asthma reduces both the need for admission and morbidity.[3] If a child can take an oral dose of prednisolone there is no added benefit to administering steroid treatment intravenously.[26] There are a number of different dosing regimens suggested:

- 20 mg for children 2–5 years, 30–40 mg for children older than five years, and usually no need for more than three days[3]
- 1 mg kg^{-1} per dose daily for three days[1]
- 1–2 mg kg^{-1} d^{-1} [27]
- 1 mg kg^{-1} every six hours for 48 hours then 1–2 mg kg^{-1} in two divided doses for 3–10 days.[5]

A two-day course of dexamethasone has been shown to be as effective as a five-day course of prednisone and there are suggestions this may help adherence.[25] Currently there is inadequate evidence to suggest that high-dose inhaled steroids have any additive benefit or act as an alternative treatment to oral steroids and thus should not be initiated in preference to oral steroids.[3]

❺ Children less than two years of age

This age group can be difficult to assess and the different phenotypes of acute wheezing and indeed different labels used in different countries can cause problems when examining the literature on appropriate treatment.[3] Recent BTS recommendations for infants where asthma is considered the likely diagnosis are – oral β$_2$-agonists are not recommended in acute asthma in infants, for drug delivery in acute asthma the pMDI/spacer combination is the preferred method with a face mask, oral steroids administration early in attacks and ipratropium bromide in conjunction with an inhaled β$_2$-agonist may be beneficial for more severe symptoms.[3] NAC Australia does not make any recommendations for the younger child with asthma.[1] The main problem is differentiating bronchiolitis and asthma but this is beyond the scope of this chapter.

❻ Intensive care management

The NAC Australia recommend that once a child has severe enough asthma to require intravenous aminophylline they should be referred to a paediatric intensive care unit (PICU) even if they do not require intubation.[1] There are a number of indications for intensive care admission; deteriorating lung function, persisting or worsening hypoxia, hypercapnia, exhaustion, drowsiness, confusion, coma or respiratory arrest.[3] These features are clearly all part of the spectrum and the overall picture plus lack of response to treatment should indicate admission to high dependency or paediatric intensive care facilities. They may not necessarily require ventilation. There are no absolute criteria for ventilation but clearly this has to be done by an experienced physician/anesthetist.[3,5] Non-invasive ventilation has had some success in adults with restrictive lung conditions and it has been used in acute adult asthma.[3] None of the current paediatric guidelines recommend its use. Detailed discussion of ventilating a child with severe/life-threatening asthma is outside the scope of this chapter. Helium and oxygen mixtures have been used in adult populations but are not endorsed on current evidence.[3]

FUTURE DIRECTIONS/RESEARCH

The following are a number of themes needing further development in acute asthma research:
- Prevention of developing asthma and secondary prevention – how to best prevent asthma from causing morbidity?
- Patient education and asthma care delivery – how best to deliver asthma care and what are the best methods in education?
- Gaps in practice and delivery of care – how best to audit acute asthma care and improve implementation and use of guidelines?
- Improved assessment of acute asthma – generalised agreement on how we best assess acute asthma. What is the best predictor of need for treatment and hospital admission?
- Different phenotypes of acute asthma – are there different types of acute asthma attack that may respond differently to the different treatment modalities?
- Pharmacogenomics – are there different types of response to treatment depending on genotype?
- Intravenous bronchodilators – which one is the most effective?
- What is the best method of delivery of aerosol treatment modalities?
- Non-invasive ventilation – which modalities work in children with acute asthma?
- Antileukotriene, cytokine, Ig E antibodies – do they have a role in the management of acute asthma?

REFERENCES

1. National Asthma Council Australia 2002 Asthma Management Handbook [http://www.nationalasthma.org.au/]
2. Royal Children's Hospital, Melbourne, Clinical Guidelines 2005 [http://www.rch.unimelb.edu.au/clinicalguide/]
3. British Thoracic Society and Scottish Intercollegiate Guidelines Network 2003 British guideline on the management of asthma. Thorax 58(Suppl 1): i1–i94 [http://www.sign.ac.uk/guidelines/published/]
4. Canadian Association for Emergency Physicians 2003 Asthma management [http://www.cps.ca/]
5. Global Strategy for Asthma Management and Prevention 2002 Asthma management and prevention. A practical guide for public health officials and health care professionals 14 [http://www.ginasthma.com/]
6. Ordonez GA, Phelan PD, Olinsky A, Robertson CF 1998 Preventable factors in hospital admissions for asthma. Archives of Diseases in Childhood 78(2): 143–147
7. Robertson CF, Rubinfield AR, Bowes G 1992 Pediatric asthma deaths in Victoria: The mild are at risk. Paediatric Pulmonology 12: 95–100
8. Martin AJ, Campbell DA, Gluyas PA, Coates JR, Ruffin RE, Roder DM, Latimer KM, Luke CG, Frith PA, Yellowlee S, McLennan G 1995 Characteristics of near fatal asthma in children. Paediatric Pulmonology 20: 1–8
9. Strunk RC, Mzrazek DA, Wolfson Fuhrmann GS, LaBrecque JF 1985 Physiologic and psychological characteristics associated with deaths due to asthma in childhood. Journal of American Medical Association 254: 1193–1198
10. Gibson PG, Coughlan J, Wislon AJ et al 2001 Self-management and regular practitioner review for adults with asthma. (Cochrane Review). In: The Cochrane Library Issue 3. Update Software, Oxford
11. Madge P, McColl J, Paton J 1997 Impact of a nurse-led home management training programme in children admitted to hospital with acute asthma: A randomised controlled study. Thorax 3: 223–228
12. Wesseldine LJ, McCarthy P, Silverman M 1999 Structured discharge procedure for children admitted to hospital with acute asthma: A randomised controlled trial of nursing practice. Archives of Disease in Childhood 80: 110–114
13. Storman MO, Mellis CM, Van Asperen PP et al 1999 Outcome evaluation of early discharge of asthmatic children from hospital: A randomized control trial. Journal of Quality in Clinical Practice 19: 149–154
14. Plotnick LH, Ducharme FM 2001 Combined inhaled anticholinergic agents and β_2-agonists for initial treatment of acute asthma in children (Cochrane Review). In: The Cochrane Library, Issue 3. Update Software, Oxford
15. Kelly AM, Powell CVE, Kerr D 2003 Snapshot of acute asthma: treatment and outcome of patients with acute asthma treated in Australian emergency departments. Internal Medicine Journal 33(9–10): 406–413
16. Travers A, Jones AP, Kelly K et al 2001 Intravenous β_2-agonists for acute asthma in the emergency department (Cochrane Review). In: The Cochrane Library, Issue 3. Update Software, Oxford
17. Browne GJ, Penna AS, Phung X, Soo M 1997 Randomised trial of intravenous salbutamol in early management of acute severe asthma in children. Lancet 49(9048): 301–305
18. Yung M, South M 1998 Randomised controlled trial of aminophylline for severe asthma. Archives of Disease in Childhood 79: 405–410
19. Rowe BH, Bretzlaff JA, Bourdon C 2001 Magnesium sulphate for treating exacerbations of acute asthma in the emergency department (Cochrane Review). In: The Cochrane Library, Issue 3. Update Software, Oxford
20. Rainbow J, Browne GJ 2002 Fatal asthma or anaphylaxis? Emergency Medicine Journal 19(5): 415–417
21. Cates CJ, Rowe BH, Bara A 2001 Holding chambers versus nebulisers for β-agonists treatment of acute asthma. (Cochrane Review). In: The Cochrane Library, Issue 3. Update Software, Oxford
22. Powell CV, Maskell GR, Marks MK, South M, Robertson CF 2001 Successful implementation of spacer treatment guideline for acute asthma. Archives of Disease in Childhood 84: 142–146
23. Gazarian M, Henry RL, Wales SR, Micallef BE, Rood EM, O'Meara MW, Numa AH 2001 Evaluating the effectiveness of evidence-based guidelines for the use of spacer devices in children with acute asthma. Medical Journal of America 174(8): 394–397
24. Cheng NG, Browne GJ, Lam LT, Yeoh R, Oomens M 2002 Spacer compliance after discharge following a mild to moderate asthma attack. Archives of Disease in Childhood 87(4): 302–305
25. Qureshi F, Zaritsky A, Poirier MP 2001 Comparative efficacy of oral dexamethasone versus oral prednisone in acute pediatric asthma. Journal of Paediatrics 139(1): 20–26
26. Barnett P, Caputo GL, Baskin M et al 1997 Intravenous versus oral corticosteroids in the management of acute asthma in children. Annals of Emergency Medicine 29: 212–217
27. Sydney Children's Hospital Randwick, NSW 2001 Australia. Asthma Guidelines [http://www.sch.edu.au/h-info.asp]
28. Haby MM, Powell CV, Oberklaid F, Waters EB, Robertson CF 2002 Asthma in children: Gaps between current management and best practice. Journal of Paediatrics & Child Health 38: 284–289

6.4 PERTUSSIS

NIGEL W. CRAWFORD • COLIN V. E. POWELL

ESSENTIALS

1 Pertussis infection is most common and severe in infants less than six months of age.

2 All children less than six months with pertussis should be admitted for a period of observation.

3 Three stages of illness occur – catarrhal, paroxysmal and convalescent.

4 The mainstay of treatment is supportive. Admission allows for apnoea monitoring, oxygen and overcoming feeding difficulties.

5 Respiratory complications are the most common, with pneumonia the major cause of mortality (0.5–1%) in infants < 6 months.

6 Treatment is with macrolide antibiotics (e.g. erythromycin for two-week course), best if given early in the course of the illness.

7 Prevention is by universal immunisation with acellular pertussis vaccine in childhood, plus a booster in adolescence/adulthood.

INTRODUCTION

Pertussis or 'whooping cough' is a bacterial infection of the respiratory tract caused by the Gram-negative coccobacillus, *Bordetella pertussis*. The word pertussis itself means 'intensive cough' and was first described in 1578, when an epidemic occurred in Paris.[2] Pertussis is the preferred term because not all cases have the classical paroxysms of coughing, with an inspiratory 'whoop', which occur as a massive respiratory effort forces inhaled air against a narrow glottis.

PATHOPHYSIOLOGY

Humans are the only reservoir and the incubation period is approximately 7–10 days. Transmission is primarily by direct contact with droplets via the airborne route. The organism is highly communicable early in the illness, with attack rates of 75–100% from symptomatic individuals to susceptible contacts. Pertussis is associated with a significant morbidity and mortality, particularly in young infants.

EPIDEMIOLOGY

With the advent of universal vaccination programs in the 1940s the incidence of this disease decreased markedly. Due to concerns regarding immunisations, vaccination levels waned in the late 1970s and there was resurgence in the number of cases. Worldwide there are approximately 250 000 deaths attributed to pertussis per year. There have been epidemics every 3–4 years in Australia with epidemiological data showing an estimated incidence of 25 cases per 100 000 per year in 1996.[9]

HISTORY

The possibility of pertussis should be considered in a child presenting to the emergency department who has prominent coughing episodes. The diagnosis of pertussis is usually made on the basis of a suggestive clinical history, confirmed by isolation of the organism.

There are three characteristic stages of the illness and presentation is most commonly in the paroxysmal phase.

Stage 1: Catarrhal (1–2 weeks)
Upper respiratory tract infection symptoms, e.g. rhinorrhoea, conjunctivitis, malaise and low-grade fever.

Stage 2: Paroxysmal (2–6 weeks, can be longer)
Consists of paroxysms of coughing which may be followed by an inspiratory 'whoop'. Facial suffusion, with prominent eyes and protrusion of neck veins may be seen during these paroxysms. The paroxysms can cause fatigue, which may impair an infant's ability to take feeds. Post-tussive vomiting commonly follows the coughing episode, but between times the child may appear quite well. It is important to note that young infants may present with apnoea as the only symptom. This can result in a presentation of sudden collapse.

Stage 3: Convalescent (1–2 weeks)
The paroxysms of coughing, whooping and vomiting decrease in number and severity. The cough may persist for a number of weeks/months and future episodes of upper respiratory tract infections may restimulate the coughing paroxysms.

Pertussis is most severe in infants younger than six months of age, particularly the non-immunised. It is these high-risk infants, that particularly need to be identified and admitted for a period of observation to exclude significant apnoea events. In infants, the clinical manifestations can mimic those of bronchiolitis or other infective pneumonitis. In partially immune adults and adolescents, who have waning immunity, the presentation is less typical and can be that of a persistent cough.

EXAMINATION

The clinical findings depend on the stage of the illness when the child presents and one needs to look for potential complications (see below). Some children will kindly display a typical coughing paroxysm in the ED and reinforce the description given by parents. This may include features of facial colour changes or a whoop that will suggest pertussis as the likely cause.

Other children, may have little to find on examination, apart from mild coryza. In these, the diagnosis is based on a suggestive history and subsequent isolation of the organism. There may be visible mechanical sequelae, due to coughing and vomiting, such as petechiae or subconjunctival haemorrhages. Unless a secondary pneumonia or atelectasis due to plugging has occurred, the chest examination is generally unremarkable.

INVESTIGATIONS

The clinical diagnosis is traditionally confirmed by nasopharyngeal swab, with culture of the organism being the gold standard. The isolation rates for pertussis are best early in the course of the illness, prior to any antibiotic treatment. More recent investigations have focused on more rapid techniques, which may aid decision making in the ED. These include fluorescent antibody tests on post-nasal aspirate specimens, serology testing to anti-*B. pertussis* IgA, IgM or IgG, and polymerase chain reaction (PCR).[8]

The full blood examination, at the end of the catarrhal or early in the paroxysmal phase, can have a leucocytosis with a predominant lymphocytosis.

A chest X-ray may show perihilar infiltrates, interstitial emphysema or evidence of a secondary pneumonia.

DIFFERENTIAL DIAGNOSIS

A 'pertussis-like syndrome' may be caused by other organisms including: *Bordetella parapertussis*, adenoviral infections, *Mycoplasma pneumoniae* and *Chlamydia pneumoniae*. They often lead to a milder, shorter clinical course and can be isolated by a nasopharyngeal sample or specific serology can be performed. In young infants viral bronchiolitis may cause a very similar clinical picture.

COMPLICATIONS

Respiratory complications are frequent, with pneumonia the most common. It may be due to a secondary bacterial infection. Occasionally the pneumonia can be a severe necrotising form, which is the major cause of death. Atelectasis is common resulting from mucous plugging and air leaks (pneumothoraces, interstitial emphysema or pneumomediastinum) may occur secondary to ruptured alveoli. Bronchiectasis is a rare late sequelae.

Subconjunctival haemorrhages, rectal prolapse or inguinal hernia may occur due to increased intra-abdominal pressure. Cerebral anoxia with convulsions can occur in young children and encephalopathy is seen in approximately 1 in 10 000 cases.

TREATMENT

All infants < 6 months of age with suspected pertussis should be admitted with isolation due to the risk of apnoea and other complications. This allows for a period of observation of coughing episodes and monitoring for apnoea and desaturations. Older children will require admission should they have significant apnoea/cyanosis or feeding problems. Treatment is mainly supportive via monitoring and the provision of oxygen and fluids.

Treatment with erythromycin is most effective if given early and has little effect in the paroxysmal phase. Recent studies have looked at the equivalence of the newer macrolides and a five-day course of azithromycin or seven days of clarithromycin may be as effective at eradicating the organism.[5,6] Co-trimoxazole is the drug of choice if macrolides are contraindicated. There is minimal chance of transmission after five days of treatment. Consider broader spectrum antibiotics if there is evidence of superadded bacterial infection. The index case should be excluded from nursery/school until five days of treatment is completed.

Chemoprophylaxis of contacts

Contact tracing is difficult, but the family and close household contacts should have a course of antibiotics regardless of immunisation status.[4] There is poor placental transfer of *B. pertussis* antibodies, so pregnant women exposed around the time of delivery and their newborn infants should also receive chemoprophylaxis. The contacts should also have vaccination at the same time, particularly those under eight years who have not received their five DTPa vaccinations. There is no benefit from passive immunisation prophylaxis with human pertussis immunoglobulin.

Prevention

Immunisation first commenced in the in the late 1940s with the triple vaccine, Diphtheria Tetanus Pertussis (DTP). This was initially a whole-cell vaccine but since the 1990s an acellular vaccine has been available.[7] It has been shown to be as effective, preventing disease in 85% of cases with fewer side effects, and is now recommended.

Current immunisation schedule

DTPa: 2, 4, 6, 18 months and 4 years.

There are also multiple-combination vaccines available, e.g. DTPa-hepB. An adult-formulation pertussis-containing vaccine (dTpa) suitable for boosting adults and adolescents is recommended as a single dose at 15 to 17 years of age.[3] Complications of the vaccine may potentially present to ED and include: fever > 38 degrees (uncommonly leads to a febrile convulsion), erythema at the injection site, persistent crying, drowsiness, vomiting, anorexia, systemic allergic reaction, and hypotonic-hypo responsive episodes (rare with no long-term sequelae).

Prognosis

The severity is directly related to age with the illness normally milder in older children. Morbidity and mortality (0.5–1%) is still significant in infants under six months of age.

CONTROVERSIES AND FUTURE DIRECTIONS

❶ An encephalopathy has been controversially linked with the pertussis vaccination in the past, but the evidence is inconclusive, as the event is so rare and no causal link has been proven.[10] Pertussis vaccine does not cause infantile spasms, epilepsy or sudden infant death syndrome (SIDS).

❷ The drop in vaccination rates in the 1970s and the subsequent increase in the incidence of this preventable disease highlight the need for ongoing surveillance to monitor the uptake and efficacy of vaccinations, the frequency of adverse reactions and the incidence of epidemics. Further refinement and greater availability of the rapid diagnostic techniques will be helpful in making the diagnosis quickly and reliably. Progress in the sequencing of the genome of *B. pertussis* has also yielded a new field of research.[1] There is also a need for more studies on equivalence testing of different antibiotics for treatment of pertussis.

REFERENCES

1. Cone TR 1970 Whooping cough is first described as a disease *sui generis* by Balliou in 1640. Paediatrics 46: 522
2. Andrews R, Herceg A, Roberts C 1997 Pertussis notifications in Australia 1991 to 1997. Communicable Diseases Intelligence 21(11): 145–148
3. Heininger U, Schmidt-Schapfer G, Cherry J, Stehr K 2000 Clinical validation of a polymerase chain reaction assay for the diagnosis of pertussis by comparison with serology, culture and symptoms during a large pertussis vaccine trial. Paediatrics 104: 312
4. Aoyama T, Sunakawa K, Iwata S, Takeuchi Y, Fujii R 1996 Efficacy of short-term treatment of pertussis with clarithromycin and azithromycin. Journal of Paediatrics 129 Nov: 761–764
5. Lebel MH, Mehra S 2001 Efficacy and safety of clarithromycin versus erythromycin for the treatment of pertussis: A prospective, randomized, single blind trial. Paediatric Infectious Diseases Journal 20: 1149–1154
6. Public Health Division, Department of Human Services 1997 The blue book: Guidelines for the bontrol of infectious disease – pertussis (whooping cough). Australian Government Publishing Service, Canberra
7. Girard DZ 2002 Which strategy for pertussis vaccination today? Paediatric Drugs 4(5): 299–313
8. National Health and Medical Research Council 2003 The Australian Immunisation Handbook 8th edn – draft. Australian Government Publishing Service, Canberra
9. Miller D, Madge N, Diamond J 1993 Pertussis immunisation and serious acute neurological illnesses in children. British Medical Journal 307(6913): 1171–1175
10. Heininger U 2001 Pertussis: An old disease that is still with us. Current Opinion in Infectious Disease 14(3): 329–335

FURTHER READING

Cherry JD, Heininger U 1998 Pertussis and other *Bordetella* infections. In: Feigin RD, Cherry JD, eds. Textbook of Pediatric Infectious Diseases, 4th edn. Philadelphia, PA: WB Saunders Co, 1998; 2: 1423–1439

6.5 COMMUNITY-ACQUIRED PNEUMONIA

MIKE STARR

ESSENTIALS

1 Viruses are the most common cause of pneumonia in children, although up to 40% of cases represent mixed infection.

2 *Streptococcus pneumoniae* is the most common bacterial cause.

3 X-ray findings do not correlate with aetiology.

4 Blood tests, including full blood count, inflammatory markers and blood culture are generally unhelpful.

5 Oral amoxicillin or intravenous benzylpenicillin are appropriate for empiric therapy of most children with pneumonia.

6 The addition of a macrolide antibiotic (e.g. roxithromycin) should be considered in children over five years of age.

7 The routine use of third-generation cephalosporins provides no additional benefit over the penicillins.

INTRODUCTION

Pneumonia is a common condition with significant morbidity and mortality. It is estimated to be responsible for approximately three million childhood deaths per year, most of which occur in developing countries.[1] Even in developed countries, pneumonia remains a major cause of acute morbidity and one of the most common reasons for paediatric hospital admissions.[2] The incidence of pneumonia is approximately 40 per 1000 children per year in those under five years of age, and 15 per 1000 children per year in 5–14 year olds.[3,4]

In spite of its commonness, there is no single clinical or radiological definition that is widely accepted for pneumonia. It is investigated with a range of tests the usefulness of which is known to be incomplete, and it is then often treated without knowledge of the aetiology. Fortunately, most children recover completely with empiric treatment.

DEFINITION

There are various definitions that can be used for pneumonia. From a pathological point of view, it is defined as inflammation or infection of the lung parenchyma. In the clinical setting, the diagnosis is typically made on the basis of a constellation of clinical features, including fever, cough, tachypnoea and auscultatory findings, and confirmed by radiographic changes.

AETIOLOGY

In the majority of cases of childhood pneumonia, the causative pathogen is not identified. Blood cultures are positive in under 5% of cases of pneumonia.[5,6] Transthoracic lung aspiration yields a cause in up to 69% of cases,[7,8] but is invasive. It is difficult to obtain adequate sputum for microscopy and culture in children. Other indirect methods of identifying a cause, such as serology or immunofluorescence and culture of nasopharyngeal aspirates are neither sensitive nor specific.[9]

Although, an alveolar or lobar infiltrate on chest X-ray is considered by some to be suggestive of bacterial infection, chest X-ray changes cannot reliably predict aetiology.[10,11] Nor is any radiological pattern pathognomonic for viral or *Mycoplasma pneumoniae* infection.

Age is the best predictor of aetiology of pneumonia. In neonates, where bacterial causes predominate, Group B Streptococci and *Escherichia coli* are the most common pathogens. Viruses, particularly respiratory syncytial virus (RSV), parainfluenza, influenza and adenovirus, are the most common cause overall, particularly in young children. The occurrence of recent local outbreaks and the clinical pattern may give a clue to the likely causative virus. *Streptococcus pneumoniae* is the most common bacterial cause in childhood, although *Mycoplasma pneumoniae* infection is also prominent in children older than five years. Up to 40% of infections are mixed.[5] Staphylococcal and Group A streptococcal pneumonia are uncommon, but should be considered in children who are severely unwell with invasive disease. Gram-negative pneumonia is very uncommon in children; nontypeable *Haemophilus influenzae* is mainly seen in children with underlying lung disease, such as cystic fibrosis and bronchiectasis.

The presence of a pleural effusion does not necessarily indicate more severe disease – *S. pneumoniae* remains the most common bacterial cause, with or without effusion.

CLINICAL FINDINGS

Pneumonia should be considered in any infant or child presenting with fever, cough, difficulty breathing, tachypnoea, increased work of breathing (nasal flaring, lower chest indrawing or recession), and auscultatory findings consistent with consolidation or effusion. However, clinical signs may be unreliable in young children, particularly in those under one year. Infants may present with symptoms not obviously related to a lower respiratory tract infection, such as lethargy, vomiting, poor feeding, grunting, or poor perfusion. Children less than three months of age may present with apnoea. Tachypnoea is the most sensitive and specific sign[12] and may be the only clue in some children. Auscultatory findings, including crackles and bronchial breathing are less predictive. The presence of coryza or wheeze (particularly bilateral) suggest that bacterial pneumonia is unlikely.[6,13] Upper quadrant pain may also be a presenting feature of basal pneumonia in older children, and the infant with grunting respirations may give the initial impression of an intra-abdominal problem.

The presentation of pneumococcal pneumonia is generally abrupt, whilst *M. pneumoniae* infection more often presents with a more indolent course, less fever, and other symptoms such as malaise, headache, arthralgia and rash.

INVESTIGATIONS

Posteroanterior chest X-rays are generally used to confirm pneumonia where there is clinical suspicion. However, they need not be performed routinely in older children with mild disease. They are particularly important for confirming the diagnosis of pneumonia in children less than five years of age who present with fever and tachypnoea, unless classical features of bronchiolitis are present. Lateral X-rays do not confer much additional information in most cases.

Large effusions may be difficult to differentiate from empyema. In some cases, ultrasound may be helpful in determining whether loculations are present.

Radiological changes lag behind clinical signs, and may persist for 4–6 weeks. Follow-up chest X-rays are unnecessary in most cases of uncomplicated pneumonia, but should be considered if symptoms and signs are persistent.

Most other investigations to determine microbiological aetiology are not particularly helpful in the ED setting. Rapid viral antigen tests, such as direct immunofluorescence assay for RSV and other respiratory viruses on nasopharyngeal aspirates, do not usually alter management. However, they may inform infection control strategies for young children admitted to hospital.

MANAGEMENT

Patients should be stabilised as necessary with high-flow oxygen and fluid resuscitation. Many children will not require any specific treatment. Most children who are not too unwell and have lobar consolidation on chest X-ray can be managed as outpatients with oral amoxicillin 25 mg kg^{-1} (up to 1 g) three-times daily for seven days. Children under one year of age, and those who are more unwell or hypoxic may require inpatient management (see Table 6.5.1) and intravenous benzylpenicillin 50 mg kg^{-1} (up to 1.2 g) six-hourly. Infants less than three months of age should also be given intravenous gentamicin 7.5 mg kg^{-1} daily.

Table 6.5.1 Indications for admission

Hypoxia, apnoea
Toxic appearance, poor feeding, dehydration
Age < 1 year
Underlying lung disease or immunodeficiency
Extensive consolidation
Failed response to oral therapy

Antibiotic resistance among pneumococci is becoming more common. However, there is no difference in outcome between cases caused by susceptible and resistant strains, and amoxicillin or benzylpenicillin remains the treatment of choice.[14,15] The use of third-generation cephalosporins provides no additional benefit over these penicillins.

Children presenting with coryza, wheeze, diffuse crackles and minimal chest X-ray changes may have viral pneumonitis. Admission may be necessary, but antibiotics may be withheld. A trial of inhaled bronchodilator therapy may be useful in children who appear to have significant associated bronchospasm. A macrolide antibiotic, such as oral roxithromycin 4 mg kg^{-1} (up to 150 mg) twice daily for seven days, should be considered for those with suspected *M. pneumoniae* infection.

Only children who are severely unwell require broader spectrum antibiotics to include cover for *S. aureus*: flucloxacillin 50 mg kg^{-1} IV (up to 2 g) six-hourly *plus* cefotaxime 50 mg kg^{-1} IV six-hourly.

COMPLICATIONS

If a child remains very unwell and febrile after 48 hours of parenteral treatment, they should be reassessed for the possibility of empyema or, more rarely, lung abscess.

CONCLUSION

Pneumonia is a common illness in children. Viruses are the most common cause, and many children will not require any specific treatment. *S. pneumoniae* remains the most common bacterial cause. Conjugate pneumococcal vaccine may prevent a number of cases, and should be offered to all children under five years of age.

REFERENCES

1. Campbell H 1995 Acute respiratory infection: A global challenge. Archives of Diseases in Childhood 73(4): 281–283 [Review: 38 refs]
2. Campbell PW 1995 New developments in pediatric pneumonia and empyema. Current Opinion in Paediatrics 7(3): 278–282 [Review: 40 refs]
3. Jokinen C, Heiskanen L, Juvonen H, Kallinen S, Karkola K, Korppi M et al 1993 Incidence of community-acquired pneumonia in the population of four municipalities in eastern Finland. American Journal of Epidemiology 137(9): 977–988
4. Murphy TF, Henderson FW, Clyde WA Jr, Collier AM, Denny FW 1981 Pneumonia: An eleven-year study in a paediatric practice. American Journal of Epidemiology 113(1): 12–21
5. Juven T, Mertsola J, Waris M, Leinonen M, Meurman O, Roivainen M et al 2000 Etiology of community-acquired pneumonia in 254 hospitalized children. Paediatric Infectious Diseases Journal 19(4): 293–298
6. Starr M, Barnett P, Carlin JB, Fink AM, Harrison SK, Boldt DW et al Clinical predictors of radiological pneumonia in children (unpublished data)
7. Vuori-Holopainen E, Peltola H 2001 Reappraisal of lung tap: Review of an old method for better etiologic diagnosis of childhood pneumonia. Clinical Infectious Diseases 32(5): 715–726
8. Vuori-Holopainen E, Salo E, Saxen H, Hedman K, Hyypia T, Lahdenpera R et al 2002 Etiological diagnosis of childhood pneumonia by use of transthoracic needle aspiration and modern microbiological methods. Clinical Infectious Diseases 34(5): 583–590
9. Russell G 2001 Community acquired pneumonia. Archives of Diseases in Childhood 85(6): 445–446
10. Bettenay FA, de Campo JF, McCrossin DB 1988 Differentiating bacterial from viral pneumonias in children. Paediatric Radiology 18(6): 453–454
11. Swingler GH 2000 Radiologic differentiation between bacterial and viral lower respiratory infection in children: A systematic literature review. Clinical Paediatrics 39(11): 627–633
12. Palafox M, Guiscafre H, Reyes H, Munoz O, Martinez H 2000 Diagnostic value of tachypnoea in pneumonia defined radiologically. Archives of Diseases in Childhood 82(1): 41–45
13. British Thoracic Society Guidelines for the Management of Community Acquired Pneumonia in Childhood 2002 Thorax 57(Suppl 1): i1–i24
14. Friedland IR 1995 Comparison of the response to antimicrobial therapy of penicillin-resistant and penicillin-susceptible pneumococcal disease. Paediatric Infectious Diseases Journal 14(10): 885–890
15. Tan TQ, Mason EO Jr, Wald ER, Barson WJ, Schutze GE, Bradley JS et al 2002 Clinical characteristics of children with complicated pneumonia caused by *Streptococcus pneumoniae*. Paediatrics 110(1): 1–6

6.6 BRONCHIOLITIS

TOM BEATTIE

ESSENTIALS

1 The diagnosis of bronchiolitis is clinical, based on history and examination.

2 Bronchiolitis typically affects children under the age of 12 months, but may occur in children up to two years of age.

3 As feeding by an infant is an important index of bronchiolitis severity, a careful history of a change in feeds is paramount.

4 High-risk patients include those with underlying chronic lung disease, congenital heart disease or corrected age less than two months of age.

5 In the very young infant, apnoea may be the predominant symptom with few respiratory signs. Likewise, in neonates a non-specific sepsis-like picture with collapse may occur.

6 Oxygen saturations fall with disease severity and SaO$_2$ levels below 94% indicate a need for admission.

7 The role of chest radiography is limited and only indicated if the diagnosis is unclear or in severe cases.

8 In patients being admitted, perform a rapid NPA or PNA to analyse for RSV or other respiratory viruses for isolation control.

9 Supportive care is the mainstay of treatment of bronchiolitis.

10 The decision to admit to hospital is based mainly on considerations of the child's need for oxygen, fluids or cardiorespiratory monitoring for apnoea.

INTRODUCTION

Epidemiology

Bronchiolitis is a common presentation to emergency departments with a seasonal pattern. It typically affects children under the age of 12 months, but may occur in children up to two years of age. The peak age is between two and eight months of age, with males more commonly affected. Approximately 1% of children will require admission for bronchiolitis, which is the leading cause of admission for children with lower respiratory tract disease in the Western world.[1] Epidemics of bronchiolitis occur during each winter, with the peaking of respiratory viruses. While respiratory syncytial virus (RSV) is the commonest organism responsible for bronchiolitis, others include parainfluenza virus, adenovirus, rhinovirus and influenza. Bronchiolitis may also complicate exanthems such as measles and varicella in young children. It is estimated that by the age of two 70% of children have been exposed to RSV. Despite the frequency, mortality is low at less than 1% of hospitalised babies. High-risk patients include those with underlying chronic lung disease, congenital heart disease, neuromuscular disorders or corrected age less than two months of age.[2,3]

Pathophysiology

Infection with RSV is associated with direct invasion of epithelial cells in the respiratory tract. Primary infection in young children and infants involves the lower respiratory tract. The bronchiolar epithelium is predominantly affected and an inflammatory response follows. Lymphocytes infiltrate the affected areas and oedema develops in the submucosa. Smooth muscle spasm ensues. The net result is that small airways become narrowed by the combination of oedema and muscle spasm, giving the typical clinical picture of bronchiolitis.

The incidence of concomitant or secondary bacterial infection is low, although otitis media may occur. In the very young infant, apnoea may be the predominant symptom with few other respiratory signs. Likewise, in neonates a non-specific sepsis-like picture with collapse may occur. In reinfection with RSV or primary infection in older children, the symptoms are more limited to the upper respiratory tract, causing signs consistent with a severe common cold.

CLINICAL ASSESSMENT

History

Bronchiolitis typically presents with a prodrome of upper respiratory tract infection over 1–2 days.

When the lower respiratory tract becomes involved, the hypersecretion of mucus causes the moist cough, onset of respiratory distress and resultant feeding difficulties. As ability to feed in an infant is an important index of bronchiolitis severity, a careful history of a change in feeds is paramount.

Examination

Examination of the child will reveal a combination of signs of URTI, along with signs indicative of LRTI, which may fluctuate between examinations. The fever is usually low grade. A moist cough is common and wheeze may be audible at the bedside.

Tachypnoea and tachycardia are usually in proportion to the illness severity. Infants who are estimated to be feeding less than 50% of normal feeds usually have oxygen saturations less than 94%. Cyanosis is seen in children with severe disease.

Chest examination may reveal hyperinflation and recessions of the chest wall due to increased work of breathing. Paradoxically, as an infant fatigues, the recessions will decrease. In this situation the diminishing air entry signifies progressive disease. Auscultation reveals wheezes that are generally symmetrical. There may be inspiratory crepitations. The auscultation findings are dynamic as coughing will move secretions to more proximal airways, with resultant temporary clearing of the wheeze. A short time later, as the fluid returns to the more peripheral airways, the wheeze returns. Hence, babies referred by a local doctor with 'marked wheeze' may initially appear to be wheeze free when seen in the ED a short time later. Re-examination later will confirm the presence of wheeze.

Oxygen saturations fall with disease severity and SaO_2 levels below 94% indicate a need for admission.[4] McIntosh graded severity of bronchiolitis by simply documenting children as needing no oxygen, requiring oxygen and needing ventilation.[5] Certainly, increasing oxygen requirements will be associated with increasing severity of disease.

Assessment

In helping to assess an infant with bronchiolitis and the likely subsequent course, one needs to determine the onset of the respiratory distress or poor feeding phase of the illness. Most children have increasing work of breathing for 48–72 hours due to increasing secretions, before a plateau phase followed by resolution over 3–7 days.

The cough may persist for a further 7–10 days after resolution of the respiratory distress. In this way one can determine if a child is likely to deteriorate further, is probably stable at the peak of severity or improving at the time of the ED visit. It is the tiring consequence of the tachypnoea of bronchiolitis that impairs feeding ability, which is the important determinant of whether a child warrants interventions such as oxygen or intravenous fluids.

Assessment of the child with bronchiolitis requires several components to be considered. Several scoring systems for bronchiolitis have been developed to determine the severity of the disease. Table 6.6.1 shows the criteria used to help determine severity and management issues.

Differential diagnosis

The differential diagnosis of bronchiolitis includes cardiac failure, asthma and pneumonia (Table 6.6.2). Cardiac failure can present with many of the features of bronchiolitis – dyspnoea, tachypnoea, tachycardia, crepitations and palpable liver. Feeding may also be poor. However, infants with bronchiolitis will usually have the URTI prodrome and the onset of poor feeding is acute. The feeding difficulties in children with cardiac failure is more subacute leading to poor weight gains. Additional signs, such as a gallop rhythm or murmur, suggest an underlying cardiac abnormality. Recurrent episodes of wheeze associated with URTIs, particularly in older infants, can be difficult to differentiate from asthma. Pneumonia in infants can mimic bronchiolitis and the differentiation can be difficult. Some infants have persistent wheezing, which does not compromise activity or feeds and is unresponsive to inhaled bronchodilators.

Investigation

The diagnosis of bronchiolitis is clinical, based on history and examination. The role of chest radiography is limited and only indicated if the diagnosis is unclear or in severe cases. The typical radiological findings are hyperinflation of the lung fields, with bilateral increase in interstitial markings (particularly perihilar regions). There may be patchy atelectasis secondary to plugging or, in severe cases, collapse. Children with high fever, or a clinical impression of sepsis, may have superimposed bacterial infection, and a CXR will aid exclusion of this diagnosis.[6]

Nosocomial infection and cross-infection can occur during bronchiolitis outbreaks. In patients being admitted to hospital, a nasopharyngeal aspirate (NPA) or posterior nasal aspirate (PNA) can be done to analyse for RSV or other respiratory viruses for isolation control. The

Table 6.6.2　Differential diagnosis of bronchiolitis

- Asthma
- Cardiac failure
- Pneumonia
- Neonatal sepsis – presenting as collapse
- Happy wheezer – persistent wheezing in undistressed baby

Table 6.6.1　Bronchiolitis severity and management

Severity	Signs	Management
Mild	Alert Feeding > 50% normal Mild respiratory distress $SaO_2 \geq 94\%$ NOT high-risk patient Age > 6 weeks	Discharge home Smaller/frequent feeds Review by LMO
Moderate	Lethargic, tired Feeding < 50% normal Marked respiratory distress Dehydrated $SaO_2 < 94\%$ High-risk patient	Admit O_2 to $SaO_2 > 94\%$ Minimise handling Consider NG or IV fluids Close observations
Severe	As above but with: Increasing O_2 requirement Fatigue Signs of CO_2 retention Apnoeic episode	Cardiorespiratory monitor Consider ABG Liaise with PICU

development of near patient testing (NPT) kits for rapid diagnosis of RSV infection has aided infection control in some areas.[7] The rapid testing for RSV may be useful in cases of neonates to help with decision making where a child presents with fever, collapse or apnoea.

Other tests such as FBE are generally not useful with diagnosis. Severe cases may demonstrate CO_2 retention on ABGs or electrolyte disturbance.

TREATMENT

Supportive care is the mainstay of treatment of bronchiolitis. The decision to admit to hospital is based mainly on considerations of the child's need for oxygen, fluids or cardiorespiratory monitoring for apnoea. Treatment options depend primarily on the severity of the disease.

Mild cases require an explanation to parents and advice regarding feeding to ensure adequate hydration. Smaller volume feeds offered more frequently to the child will usually ensure adequate hydration. Hence, the child who feeds 3–4 hourly normally, should be offered feeds every 1.5–2 hours. Parents should monitor urine output, and should be advised to seek review should feeding deteriorate or urine output fall significantly. Some parents become exhausted by the constant demands of infants with bronchiolitis, and an assessment of parental coping should form part of the clinical picture. If there are concerns about parental ability to provide the increased demands of feeding, admission should be considered.

Children with moderate bronchiolitis need to be admitted. The infant will need to be monitored clinically, with regular observation of heart rate, respiratory rate, ability to feed and level of fatigue. Oxygen saturation should be monitored and supplemental oxygen should be provided to maintain Sao_2 above 95% in those with saturations below 94% or unable to feed. Oxygen may be administered by head box, nasal prong or cannula, isolette, mask or tent. The choice of method of oxygen delivery needs to be tailored to the individual case. In small infants who are obligatory nose breathers nasal prongs or cannulae may exacerbate the nasal obstruction in babies with copious secretions. Under six months of age a head box is usually the best, using an oxygen analyser to monitor the O_2 requirement. Older infants may tolerate an oxygen mask, but if distressed by this then using cot or tent oxygen may be necessary. In some infants who have self-limiting apnoeic episodes CPAP may help buy time until the disease ameliorates. However any persistence of apnoea or failure to maintain oxygenation would warrant consideration of ventilation using endotracheal intubation and admission to an Intensive Care setting. Clearly the choice of treatment will depend on available expertise and equipment. In all situations an increase in O_2 requirement to maintain saturations indicates increasing severity and the need to escalate therapy accordingly.

Feeding can be continued orally initially in those with moderate bronchiolitis, with small frequent feeds as above. If the child cannot tolerate this, naso–gastric feeds or intravenous fluids should be considered. Infants who do not have markedly increased work of breathing may come out of oxygen for feeds if tolerated.

There is no indication for antibiotic use for either mild or moderate bronchiolitis unless there is good evidence of secondary bacterial infection.

Children with severe disease need to be admitted to a facility where they can be continuously monitored by appropriate staff for ventilation should they deteriorate or have significant apnoea. Features of concern include the infant who is tiring, has escalating oxygen requirement or develops apnoeas. Early discussion with the local PICU staff will help to determine this need and organise appropriate transfer mechanism. Fluids should be given intravenously and adjusted according to volume status, urine output and electrolyte results. Children with underlying disease such as heart disease may need additional specific therapy.

Drug therapy

The role of various drug therapies in bronchiolitis is controversial and still undergoing research.

Two meta-analyses of the benefits of inhaled β-agonists in bronchiolitis have proved inconclusive.[8,9] A more recent Cochrane Review suggests some minimal benefit,[10] while Patel has recently shown no benefit with albuterol (salbutamol).[11] Isaacs suggested that if wheeze is the predominant sign then a trial of selective β-agonist may help.[1] Nebulised adrenaline (epinephrine) has similarly not been shown to provide benefit over a sustained timeframe.[11]

Systemic or inhaled glucocorticoids are widely used in some parts of the world, but the evidence for their use is variable. A recent meta-analysis has shown some marginal benefit with systemic glucocorticoid use.[12] The role of ipratropium bromide is equally unclear and there is no clear-cut benefit to use.[13]

Ribavarin and antiviral immunoglobulins are not used in the ED setting, but may have a role in high-risk groups in intensive care. Ribavirin is expensive and has only marginal benefit when given aerolysed to high-risk patients with severe disease.[14] The role of immunisation against RSV is still under investigation.

PROGNOSIS

The vast majority of children with bronchiolitis will recover over 7–10 days. The cough may persist for some weeks after the resolution of the respiratory distress. A small number may continue to wheeze and cough for several months and an indeterminate number will develop persistent wheeze and/or asthma. The exact relationship between these events is unclear. Further study is needed to elucidate the role of RSV in the development of subsequent reactive airway disease.

PREVENTION

The transmission of RSV occurs with contact with infected secretions. In the ED setting, attention to hand washing, stethoscope hygiene and cubicle use is important to prevent cross-infection between children.

CONTROVERSIES

❶ Treatment of bronchiolitis has changed little over the years, with the mainstay being supportive care. A considerable amount of research needs to be done on the classification of the severity of disease based on sound, objective data. Without this, the debate on treatment with β-agonists, glucocorticoids, anticholinergic drugs and other therapies will persist, with anecdote continuing to supplant scientific data.

REFERENCES

1. Isaacs D 1995 Bronchiolitis. British Medical Journal 310(6971): 4–5

2. Bont L, Heijnen CJ, Kavelaars A et al 1999 Peripheral blood cytokine responses and disease severity in respiratory syncytial virus bronchiolitis. European Respiratory Journal 14(1): 144–149

3. Smyth RL, Mobbs KJ, O'Hea U, Ashby D, Hart CA 2002 Respiratory syncytial virus bronchiolitis: Disease severity, interleukin-8, and virus genotype. Paediatric Pulmonology 33(5): 339–346

4. Mulholland EK, Olinsky A, Shann FA 1990 Clinical findings and severity of acute bronchiolitis. Lancet 335(8700): 1259–1261

5. McIntosh ED, De Silva LM, Oates RK 1993 Clinical severity of respiratory syncytial virus group A and B infection in Sydney, Australia. Paediatric Infectious Diseases Journal 12(10): 815–819

6. El-Radhi AS, Barry W, Patel S 1999 Association of fever and severe clinical course in bronchiolitis. Archives of Diseases in Childhood 81(3): 231–234

7. Mackenzie A, Hallam N, Mitchell E, Beattie T 1999 Near patient testing for respiratory syncytial virus in paediatric accident and emergency: Prospective pilot study. British Medical Journal 319(7205): 289–290

8. Kellner JD, Ohlsson A, Gadomski AM, Wang EE 1996 Efficacy of bronchodilator therapy in bronchiolitis. A meta-analysis. Archives of Paediatric and Adolescent Medicine 1150(11): 1166–1172

9. Flores G, Horwitz RI 1997 Efficacy of β₂-agonists in bronchiolitis: A reappraisal and meta-analysis. Paediatrics 100(2 Pt 1): 233–239

10. Kellner JD, Ohlsson A, Gadomski AM, Wang EE 2000 Bronchodilators for bronchiolitis. Cochrane Database Systems Review 2: CD001266

11. Patel H, Platt RW, Pekeles GS, Ducharme FM 2002 A randomized, controlled trial of the effectiveness of nebulized therapy with epinephrine compared with albuterol and saline in infants hospitalized for acute viral bronchiolitis. Journal of Paediatrics 141(6): 818–824

12. Garrison MM, Christakis DA, Harvey E, Cummings P, Davis RL 2000 Systemic corticosteroids in infant bronchiolitis: A meta-analysis. Pediatrics 105(4): E44

13. Everard ML, Bara A, Kurian M, Elliott TM, Ducharme F 2002 Anticholinergic drugs for wheeze in children under the age of two years. Cochrane Database Systems Review 1: CD001279

14. Everard ML, Swarbrick A, Rigby AS, Milner AD 2001 The effect of ribavirin to treat previously healthy infants admitted with acute bronchiolitis on acute and chronic respiratory morbidity. Respiratory Medicine 95(4): 275–280

6.7 CROUP

GARY GEELHOED

ESSENTIALS

1 Croup is a common childhood problem with a peak incidence of 60 per 1000 child years in those aged between 1 and 2 years.

2 The loudness of stridor is variable and is not a reliable indicator of the severity of the airway obstruction.

3 All children who present to emergency departments with croup should be treated with steroids.

4 The steroids of choice are oral dexamethasone 0.15 mg kg^{-1} or prednisolone 1 mg kg^{-1}.

5 A compromised but functioning airway should never be made worse by upsetting the child.

6 Children who require adrenaline (epinephrine) may be sent home safely if they have also received steroids and have improved over a number of hours to have no stridor at rest.

INTRODUCTION

The term *croup* describes an acute clinical syndrome of hoarse voice, barking cough, and inspiratory stridor usually seen in young children. Croup results from swelling of the upper airway, in and around the larynx, usually as a result of a viral infection. Croup occurs seasonally, peaking in winter months due to the epidemics of upper respiratory viruses. Parainfluenza virus type 1 accounts for around half the cases during winter, with parainfluenza type 2, influenza type A, adenoviruses, respiratory syncytial virus,

enteroviruses, and possibly mycoplasma pneumonia causing most of the other cases. Some of the viral exanthems, such as varicella, can cause croup by involvement of the upper airway in small children. Croup is a common childhood problem, with a peak incidence of 60 per 1000 child years in those aged between 1 and 2 years,[1] although it may be seen up to the teen years. As such, it is by far the most common cause of acute upper airways obstruction likely to present to emergency departments.

The respiratory distress caused by obstruction tends to be most marked in younger children due to the small size of their larynx, the presence of loose submucous tissues, and the tight encirclement of the subglottic area by the cricoid cartilage. In children under 8 years of age, this is the narrowest region of the airway, hence any swelling in this area due to inflammation results in a significant impingement of the airway. The younger child, who has a smaller diameter airway, mandates an increased vigilance of the degree of airway compromise.

The lower airway involvement of laryngotracheobronchitis may also cause younger children to manifest wheeze due to concurrent inflammation in the smaller peripheral airways. Likewise, older children known to have asthma may exhibit signs of asthma in the setting of croup.

PRESENTATION

History

The typical presentation of croup is in a pre–school-aged child with a history of a recent upper respiratory tract infection. The child subsequently develops a barking or seal-like cough, a hoarse voice and, if obstruction is severe enough, stridor. The stridor may initially be apparent only when a child is distressed, such as during crying. Stridor, which is inspiratory, indicates obstruction at the laryngeal level or higher. Expiratory

stridor or biphasic stridor indicates more severe laryngeal obstruction or alternatively obstruction occurring in and around the level of the trachea. The natural history of airway obstruction, when unmodified by steroids, is to increase slowly to peak over 48–72 hours. The airway compromise usually then resolves over a few days, although the laryngeal cough may persist longer.

Less common than infectious croup, older children may present with recurrent or spasmodic croup with no viral prodrome. These children may have a history of atopy and suffer from asthma more than the general population. They should, however, be treated in the same manner as in 'viral' croup. In the smaller child, particularly infants, problems with feeding, swallowing difficulties, and whether the child has been cyanosed should be ascertained.

It is important to enquire whether or not the child has had croup in the past and, specifically, whether the child has had any persistence of mild stridor in between acute attacks. This is important, as any child who has a pre-existing narrowing of the airway is more likely to proceed to severe obstruction with a superimposed acute obstruction.

An immunisation history is important to check whether the child has had Hib vaccination if there is any suggestion that the diagnosis could be epiglottitis; likewise, the very rare occurrence of diphtheria in the non-immunised.

Examination

Croup in children can generally be classified as mild, moderate, or severe (see Table 6.7.1).

Most children with mild croup are not distressed and have only a barking cough with no stridor at rest or stridor audible only with physical activity, crying, or agitation. Crying causes physiological narrowing of the airway and will increase the respiratory distress. Hence the child's obstruction will often improve by allowing

Table 6.7.1 Croup severity

Sign or symptom	Mild	Moderate or severe
Stridor	None or only if agitated	Stridor at rest
Respiratory rate	Usually normal	May be decreased
Retractions	None	+ to +++
Air entry	Normal	Normal to decreased
Colour	Normal	May be pallor
Cyanosis	None	Late sign only
Conscious state	Normal	Restless or decreased

(After Marks et al 2003.[2])

Table 6.7.2 Differential diagnoses of croup

- Epiglottitis
- Bacterial tracheitis
- Foreign body
- Congenital: laryngomalacia, subglottic stenosis, vascular ring, cord paresis
- Retropharyngeal abscess
- Allergic oedema
- Airway trauma

the child to be cuddled in the parent's arms. There may be signs due to viral illness, such as mild fever and nasal discharge. Children with mild cases can have their throats examined, but this should be deferred in more severe cases. A compromised but functioning airway should never be made worse by upsetting the child.

In more severe cases, the child may have a more pronounced stridor at rest. As airway obstruction progresses, increased work of breathing ensues and the child may exhibit increasing substernal, intercostal, and subcostal retractions. Subtle signs of hypoxia causing altered consciousness may be reflected as anxiety or restlessness in a child. An obviously fatiguing child is a worrying sign. Decreased air entry and respiratory effort, extreme pallor, and cyanosis require immediate intervention.

The child's preferred position may also give clues as to severity of obstruction or to a diagnosis other than croup. Hyperextension or other abnormal positioning of the neck may suggest epiglottitis or a retropharyngeal abscess.

The use of a croup severity score may be helpful for less-experienced staff to assess children with croup and communicate findings with a colleague when seeking advice. As previously mentioned, some children may have concomitant wheeze in addition to the upper airway stridor.

INVESTIGATIONS

Croup is usually an easy 'spot diagnosis' and requires no diagnostic tests.

Oximetry is of limited value, as children may maintain near-normal oxygen saturations even when they have significant airway obstruction.[3] Apart from monitoring in severe croup, the distress of oximeter probes will often cause increased distress by agitating the child. In stable cases, where the diagnosis is unclear, a lateral soft tissue X-ray of the neck may be helpful to distinguish croup from epiglottitis or retropharyngeal abscess. However, the possible benefits of an X-ray need to be weighed against the risks of moving or disturbing the child when the obstruction is more than mild. A nasopharyngeal aspirate in croup is not necessary for diagnosis but may be useful for infection control for patients being admitted.

DIFFERENTIAL DIAGNOSIS

It is important to establish that other, more sinister, causes of acute upper respiratory tract obstruction masquerading as croup are not present (see Table 6.7.2). Especially in the younger child, one should enquire regarding longer-term symptoms preceding the present episode, such as low-grade stridor. This might

suggest underlying congenital airway or a vascular anomaly (e.g. tracheomalacia, subglottic stenosis, bilateral cord paralysis, laryngeal web, or vascular ring compression of the trachea). One should also enquire as to possible airway trauma or toxic ingestion. Dysphagia and drooling may suggest epiglottitis, peritonsillar or retropharyngeal abscess, or foreign body in the airway or oesophagus.

Classic croup and epiglottitis are hard to confuse, as the latter usually presents as a pale, toxic, drooling child with a rapidly progressing course. Cough is generally not a prominent feature in epiglottitis. Children with epiglottitis may sit forwards, drooling saliva, and hold their neck in extension. In a child presenting with early epiglottitis, however, the distinction may be more difficult. Allergic angio-oedema may mimic croup after exposure to an allergen such as peanut. A child with 'severe croup' with a high fever, who does not respond to adrenaline (epinephrine) and steroids, may have tracheitis and will need consideration of a diagnostic laryngoscopy to provide a clear diagnosis. Likewise, the possibility of an inhaled foreign body should be kept in mind for children who don't respond to treatment or have a prolonged course. While usually parents will volunteer a history of an acute obstruction or a sudden coughing fit, the history of an inhaled object may not always be known to them. A definitive diagnosis may need to be made by directly viewing the upper airway, but this should be performed only in the hands of an experienced paediatric anaesthetist, intensivist, or emergency physician in an appropriate clinical setting (see below).

TREATMENT AND DISPOSITION

Mild or moderate croup

All children who present to an emergency department with croup should be treated with steroids.[4] The universal use of steroids for croup in emergency departments results in the relapse rate of those sent home directly dropping,[5] the average length of stay in hospital falling, and the number of children needing intensive care and intubation dramatically reducing.[6] Prior to the regular use of steroids, a general rule of thumb was to admit children with stridor at rest (moderate) to hospital for observation, while allowing those with occasional stridor and barking cough only (mild) to be managed at home. As many children will improve within a few hours of taking steroids, often they may be discharged home after a short stay in the emergency department or an observation ward. Factors such as the distance from medical care, the availability of transport, the time of day, the child's past history with regard to severe airway obstruction, and parental concern and attitude all need to be taken into account when making the decision to admit (see Table 6.7.3).

Recommended steroid doses are oral dexamethasone in a one-off dose of 0.15 mg kg^{-1},[7] or an equivalent dose of prednisolone of 0.75 mg kg^{-1}. Most children with croup will require only one dose, but if the upper airway obstruction symptoms persist (as opposed to upper respiratory tract infection manifestations), a further dose may be given 24 hours later. It is often more convenient to use prednisolone (rounded off to 1 mg kg^{-1})

Table 6.7.3 Indications for admission

- Upper airway obstruction at rest: fails to respond to steroids or adrenaline (epinephrine) and period of observation (4 hours)
- Moderate or severe croup
- Infants < 6 months
- Previous severe croup
- Underlying airway problem
- Inadequate follow-up
- Recurrent presentation

in the community, as it is more readily available. Unpublished work suggests that children treated with prednisolone may re-present more commonly than those treated with dexamethasone and would benefit from a second dose. Steroids may be administered intramuscularly or intravenously in the child with severe obstruction, when there is concern that the child may aspirate given their respiratory difficulties.

Oral dexamethasone has been found to be as effective as inhaled steroids such as budesonide,[8] and to work as fast, at a fraction of the cost. Combining dexamethasone and budesonide is no more effective than dexamethasone alone.[8] There is no place for antibiotics in a typical case of croup. The use of 'steam' or humidified air is largely unproven, despite its once common usage.[9,10]

Severe croup

Children with manifestations of severe obstruction should be given nebulised adrenaline (epinephrine). It is generally considered that adrenaline does not change the natural history of croup, such as length of stay in hospital or need to intubate, due to its short-lasting effects. It will, however, 'buy time' while waiting for the anti-inflammatory effect of steroids to work. In a worse case scenario, adrenaline can be a useful temporising measure while organising the facilities and appropriate personnel for a child who may require intubation. The recommended dose (independent of age and weight) is 5 ml of 1:1000 adrenaline, nebulised with oxygen, which can be used for all children. This may be repeated after 10 minutes if needed and may help avoid the need for intubation in children who respond to the steroids. 'Rebound' phenomenon may occur, where the upper airway obstruction may recur as the effect of the adrenaline wears off after 1–2 hours. While in the past it was recommended that any child who received adrenaline for croup should be admitted, a number of studies have now shown that children may be sent home safely if they have also received steroids and have improved to have no stridor at rest over a number of hours.[11,12]

Children receiving nebulised adrenaline require close clinical monitoring of their response, particularly the change in air entry, in order to detect any deterioration.

Intubation needs to be considered in the child who has increasing upper airway obstruction, hypoxia, decreasing conscious state, or fatigue despite nebulised adrenaline. These children should be discussed early with a paediatric intensivist in order to optimise management. The ideal setting for this to occur is in theatre or a paediatric intensive care unit environment via gaseous induction, using an endotracheal tube 1.0-mm smaller than predicted by the child's size (see *Resuscitation* section).

PROGNOSIS

Most children with croup have mild symptoms, do not need hospitalisation, and will recover within a few days. Their symptoms will be shortened even further with the use of steroids. Despite the substantial impact of steroids, the occasional child will still follow a prolonged course of cough and marked stridor for many days. While other diagnoses, such as foreign body, need to be considered, in these cases most will settle with time.

PREVENTION

For most children, croup is a one-off episode and well tolerated, especially if steroids are used. Children who suffer repeated episodes of recurrent croup, as described above, may benefit from steroid use at home at the first sign of croup symptoms. Although no trials have evaluated this approach, anecdotal evidence suggests that this practice appears to have benefit.

REFERENCES

1. Denny FW, Clyde WA Jr 1986 Acute lower respiratory tract infections in nonhospitalized children. Journal of Pediatrics 108: 635–645
2. Marks M, Wilkinson D, Munro J 2003 Paediatric Handbook, 6th edn. Blackwell Science, Victoria
3. Stoney PJ, Chakrabarti MK 1991 Experience of pulse oximetry in children presenting with croup. Journal of Laryngology and Otology 105: 295–298

CONTROVERSIES AND FUTURE RESEARCH

Although once controversial, steroids are now generally accepted for all children who present to emergency departments with croup. While it is clear that both prednisolone and dexamethasone are effective in the treatment of croup, direct comparisons have not been published as yet. Unpublished work suggests the shorter half-life of prednisolone may result in a greater number of children returning to medical care. While a once-only dose of dexamethasone is sufficient for the vast majority of children with croup, a second dose of prednisolone 24 hours later may be needed in some cases.

4. Geelhoed GC 1997 Croup. Pediatric Pulmonology 23(5): 370–374
5. Geelhoed GC, Turner J, Macdonald WB 1996 Efficacy of a small single dose of oral dexamethasone for outpatient croup: A double blind placebo controlled clinical trial. British Medical Journal 313(7050): 140–142
6. Geelhoed GC 1996 Sixteen years of croup in a Western Australian teaching hospital: The impact of routine steroid treatment. Annals of Emergency Medicine 28(6): 621–626
7. Geelhoed GC, Macdonald WGB 1995 Oral dexamethasone in the treatment of croup: 0.15 mg/kg is as effective as 0.3 mg/kg or 0.6 mg/kg. Pediatric Pulmonology 20: 362–367
8. Klassen TP, Craig WR, Moher D et al 1998 Nebulized budesonide and oral dexamethasone for treatment of croup: A randomized controlled trial.
Journal of the American Medical Association 279(20): 1629–1632
9. Neto GM, Kentab O, Klassen TP et al 2002 A randomized controlled trial of mist in the acute treatment of moderate croup. Academic Emergency Medicine 9: 873–879
10. Bouchier D, Dawson KP, Fergusson DM 1984 Humidification in viral croup: A controlled trial. Australian Paediatric Journal 20: 289–291
11. Kelley PB, Simon JE 1992 Racemic epinephrine use in croup and disposition. American Journal of Emergency Medicine 10(3): 181–183
12. Prendergast M, Jones JS, Hartman D 1994 Racemic epinephrine in the treatment of laryngotracheitis: Can we identify children for outpatient therapy? American Journal of Emergency Medicine 12(6): 613–616

GASTROENTEROLOGY AND HEPATOLOGY

7.1 ABDOMINAL PAIN

JASON HORT

ESSENTIALS

1 Only a small percentage of children presenting with abdominal pain have an underlying surgical cause.

2 The age of the child with abdominal pain influences the diagnostic possibilities.

3 The younger the child, the less reliable are the clinical signs of appendicitis.

4 The abdominal examination is the most important contributor in assessing the need for surgical consultation.

5 Providing adequate analgesia improves the reliability of physical findings and does not mask the detection of peritoneal findings.

6 Abdominal pain in children may have intra- or extra-abdominal origin.

7 Warning bells for a surgical problem include – pain that requires opiate analgesia, constant pain over a number of hours, inconsolability, a child who remains motionless despite severe pain, associated pallor or shock, reproducible localised tenderness, guarding, rebound, abdominal distension, rigidity, bilious vomiting and representation.

8 Observation with repeated examination remains very useful in indeterminate cases.

9 It is not always possible to make a definitive diagnosis in the ED. A practical, systematic approach is required to exclude serious underlying possible causes. Discharged children in whom the diagnosis is unclear need to have a clear action plan with early follow-up organised.

INTRODUCTION

Abdominal pain is a common reason for children to attend an emergency department (ED) occurring in up to 5% of all presentations in some institutions.[1] Most commonly the underlying cause is non-surgical and surgery is required in only 1–7% of children who present with abdominal pain.[1,2] It is not possible to make a definitive diagnosis in all children with abdominal pain. In one study, as many as 15% of children presenting to emergency with abdominal pain did not receive a specific diagnosis at discharge.[1] Some children arrive at the ED soon after the onset of symptoms and it may take time, ex-pectant management and review before a diagnosis becomes clear or the symptoms resolve. It is important, however, to exclude causes of abdominal pain that may require early surgical consultation, observation or investigations within the ED.

The priorities in managing children presenting with abdominal pain are:

- Triage and early appropriate analgesia
- Resuscitation with attention to ABCs as required
- Diagnosis formulation using history, examination and investigation
- Management according to the likely diagnosis.

If a clear diagnosis cannot be reached in the ED, then exclusion of serious/life-threatening diagnoses should be made. Subsequent disposition and follow-up is dependent on various factors including: likelihood of a serious diagnosis; severity of the pain; availability of review; and psychosocial factors.

PATHOPHYSIOLOGY

The sensation of abdominal pain is transmitted by either somatic or visceral afferent fibres.[3] Visceral pain from visceral peritoneum is poorly localised, whereas somatic pain arising from parietal peritoneum or the abdominal wall is well localised. Referred pain also occurs due to visceral and somatic pathways converging in the spinal column. Two examples of referred pain are diaphragmatic irritation leading to pain at the shoulder tip due to convergence of visceral and somatic pathways at C4, and somatic pain from pneumonia leading to T10–11 pain sensed in the lower abdomen.[3] Abdominal pain may occasionally be psychosomatic in origin.

AETIOLOGY

There is a broad range of causes of abdominal pain in children and one needs to initially keep an open mind regarding the diagnosis (see Table 7.1.1). The age and sex of the child need to be considered, as well as features of the abdominal pain and associated symptoms, and examination findings to determine the diagnostic possibilities.

ASSESSMENT

Each child needs initial assessment and triage with attention to securing the ABCs and providing appropriate analgesia. A detailed history and thorough examination have both to be performed.

Table 7.1.1   Causes of acute abdominal pain in children

Inflammatory Gastrointestinal Appendicitis Meckel's diverticulum Mesenteric adenitis Gastroenteritis Food poisoning Peritonitis Peptic ulcer, gastritis Hepatitis Pancreatitis Inflammatory bowel disease	**Gall bladder** Cholecystitis, cholelithiasis **Haematological** Leukemia, lymphoma Haemolytic crisis Sickle cell disease Neuroblastoma, Wilms' tumor **Endocrine** Diabetic ketoacidosis, hypoglycemia Adrenal insufficiency Hyperparathyroidism
Non-Gastrointestinal Tonsillitis, pharyngitis Pneumonia (especially basal) Pericarditis Serositis Pyelonephritis, cystitis Pelvic inflammatory disease Intra abdominal abscess Epididymitis	**Vasculitic** Henoch–Schönlein purpura Periarteritis nodosa Kawasaki disease **Renal** Renal colic Hydronephrosis Nephrotic syndrome
Generalised Infectious mononucleosis Acute rheumatic fever Herpes zoster	**Miscellaneous** Constipation Colic Toxic ingestion, e.g. lead Torsion – testicular/ovarian Ectopic pregnancy Dysmenorrhea, Mittelschmerz pain Mesenteric artery occlusion Hypokalaemia Acute intermittant porphyria Familial Mediterranean fever Abdominal migraine Psychosomatic – including abuse
Intestinal obstruction Intussusception Volvulus Adhesions Incarcerated hernia	
Abdominal trauma See trauma chapter	

Source: Adapted from reference 3.

Table 7.1.2   Serious conditions not to miss in neonates and infants

Surgical causes	*Medical causes*
Testicular torsion	Diabetic ketoacidosis
Appendicitis	Toxic, e.g. iron ingestion
Peritonitis	Sepsis
Necrotising enterocolitis	
Volvulus	Haemolytic uraemic syndrome
Intussusception	Urinary tract infection
Hirschsprung disease	
Incarcerated hernia	

HISTORY

In considering a child who has presented with abdominal pain with no history of trauma, five important questions have to be addressed:

1. The age of the child

The age of the child helps narrow the diagnostic possibilities. The most common diagnoses to consider according to age are:

Neonates and infants   Present with a change in behaviour to signify pain.[4] This may be persistent crying, irritability, inability to be consoled, fussiness, sleeplessness, and poor feeding.[4] Serious or potentially life-threatening conditions not to miss in this age group are listed in Table 7.1.2.

The diagnoses of acute gastroenteritis or 'colic' need to be made after excluding more serious causes.

Preschool   Acute gastroenteritis, urinary infection, appendicitis, viral illness (mesenteric adenitis), pneumonia, constipation and trauma-related.

School age   Acute gastroenteritis, urinary infection, trauma, appendicitis, constipation, viral-related, psychosomatic, inflammatory bowel or in older females, gynaecological causes.

In the preschool and school-aged child, the commonest cause of abdominal pain is constipation. This is a diagnosis of exclusion after carefully considering alternative causes.[6]

Adolescents   The causes of abdominal pain in adolescents expand to include various diagnoses of adulthood. In the female, pregnancy-related conditions must be considered, as well as other gynaecological conditions (see Chapter 15.1 on gynaecology).

2. Whether this is the first episode or recurrence of abdominal pain

A history of similar pain in a child may help to clarify the diagnosis. However, it is important to remember that children with chronic abdominal pain due to a myriad of causes may develop an acute abdomen and this needs to be considered at each presentation.

3. Whether there are other associated symptoms

Generally children with abdominal pain have other associated symptoms. A full symptom review is required, with particular reference to gastrointestinal symptoms. This includes vomiting, and whether it is bilious or blood stained, and the timing and quality of stool, including the presence of blood or mucus. The child with fever, voluminous diarrhoea and vomiting is likely to have gastroenteritis. However, particularly in young children one must keep an open mind to other possibilities that can mimic or complicate gastroenteritis (see Chapter 7.9 pp. 197–200 on diarrhoea and vomiting).

More general questions should assess the child's constitution – whether the child is febrile, lethargic, irritable, anorexic or has associated pallor. It is unusual for children with appendicitis to be hungry. The child with intussusception is often lethargic and pale. The presence of URTI or viral symptoms may suggest mesenteric adenitis. Dysuria or frequency may be reported in older children with a UTI. A typical rash or sore joints may indicate Henoch–Schönlein purpura as the cause of abdominal pain.

4. Whether there are any relevant pre-existing conditions

The child's past medical and surgical history should be fully explored. In older females a menstrual history may be important. Family history and racial background may be relevant, along with a psychosocial history.

5. What are the characteristics of the pain?

These include location (generalised or localised), radiation, severity, quality (constant, episodic or of a colic nature), what improves and worsens the pain, along with the timing of the pain – gradual or sudden onset and whether the pain wakes the child. Direct questioning of the verbal child often augments the description of the characteristics of the pain.

Pain that has a sudden onset may occur with perforated viscus, intussusception or torsion. The pain from appendicitis has a more insidious onset and usually increases over a period of hours. In both intussusception and mesenteric adenitis, the pain may cause episodic distress. Constant pain over a number of hours in a child usually has a significant underlying cause.

EXAMINATION

The abdominal examination of the young child with abdominal pain needs to be performed in an unhurried and gentle fashion. Toddlers may be better examined on the parent's lap. It is important to note the child's general appearance. Children with colicky pain often writhe around, whereas, the child with peritoneal irritation usually remains still as movement exacerbates the abdominal pain. Providing adequate analgesia improves the reliability of physical findings and does not mask the detection of peritoneal findings. It is best to approach the painful quadrant of the abdomen last, after the child has relaxed and become accustomed to the examination.

One of the keys to the assessment is to determine the presence of focal tenderness or true peritoneal irritation. In children this can sometimes be difficult, as many voluntarily guard the abdomen when examined, irrespective of the cause of the abdominal pain. Differentiating the presence of true peritoneal signs may be helped by distraction or by serial examination over a period of time.

Eliciting rebound should begin with gentle palpation to avoid distress and resultant voluntary guarding. Signs consistent with peritonitis include refusing or being unable to walk, slow or stooped walking, or increased pain on coughing or movement, or the child lying motionless on the bed. Likewise peritoneal irritation may be detected by asking if the child can expand or contract their abdominal wall by asking them to 'suck tummy in, then let it out'. The younger the child the less likely they are to have reliable localising signs of appendicitis and the threshold for surgical review or observation needs to be adapted accordingly.

Important features of examination include the following:

- General appearance of the child
- Temperature and vital signs
- Jaundice
- Skin markings, e.g. abdominal bruising
- Abdominal distension
- Abdominal tenderness

- Guarding or rebound and/or rigidity
- Abdominal mass
- Bowel sounds
- Palpation of testes (in the male infant)
- Presence of inguinal herniae
- Urinalysis.

Rectal examination in children, when indicated, should be performed once, and ideally by the surgeon involved. The interpretation of localised rectal tenderness is often difficult in children, as it is uncomfortable and therefore does not often add to the assessment. The inguino-scrotal regions should always be checked for an otherwise occult hernia or torsion referring pain to the abdomen. A pelvic examination may be indicated in pubertal females.

The cause of abdominal pain in children may be extra-abdominal. The child with ileus may have intra- or extra-abdominal pathology including urinary tract infection, pneumonia, or meningitis.

Important features in the examination of other systems include:

- Respiratory - signs of pneumonia
- ENT – URTI, tonsillitis or adenopathy
- Neurological – meningitis
- Endocrine – blood glucose level in diabetic ketoacidosis
- Haematological – pallor, lymphadenopathy
- Dermatological – rash, particularly purpura/petechiae of Henoch Schönlein purpura, zoster
- Renal – oliguria, haematuria, hypertension in haemolytic uraemic syndrome.

INVESTIGATIONS

Many children have the diagnosis clarified by physical examination alone. The need for investigations should be tailored to the individual case, where the diagnosis is unclear and the result of the test is likely to 'rule in or rule out' significant pathology.

Pathology

A full blood count may demonstrate leucocytosis, anaemia or film changes of haemolysis. The white cell count is not particularly useful to determine if a child has acute appendicitis. Electrolytes, urea and creatinine assess changes resulting from fluid losses and impaired renal function. This may be indicated in the child who has had significant losses from diarrhoea or vomiting. Liver function tests are indicated in children with potential hepatic and gall bladder pathology. The possibility of pancreatitis can be assessed by serum amylase and lipase levels. A blood glucose level excludes diabetic ketoacidosis in the child presenting with abdominal pain who appears acidotic or has glucose and ketones in the urine. Females of reproductive age should have a βHCG performed. Urinalysis, microscopy and culture are necessary to exclude renal pathology.

Imaging

The routine use of an abdominal X-ray is unhelpful to 'screen' children with abdominal pain. Situations where it may be helpful include: demonstrating the signs of bowel obstruction; free air, suggesting perforation; an ingested foreign body; calcification, including a faecolith in the appendix and Meckel's diverticulum; 'thumbprinting', suggesting gut ischaemia or a sentinel loop adjacent to inflammation; or a soft tissue mass. Calcification may also represent renal stones, neuroblastoma or teratoma.

An erect chest X-ray may be indicated to demonstrate gas under the diaphragm or evidence of a basal pneumonia.[3]

An ultrasound study can help evaluate liver, gall bladder and kidneys, as well as detect an intussusception, features of appendicitis (if visualised well) or evaluate a palpable mass. An abdominal CT scan may be indicated in selected cases.

MANAGEMENT

The initial management of the child with severe abdominal pain should include assessment and securing of ABCs and administration of appropriate analgesia to relieve the child's distress. Children with similar pathophysiology can have markedly varied distress levels and analgesic re-

quirements need to be individualised.[4] Concurrent anxiety may increase painful stimuli and this can be lessened by involving parents in comforting their child and using a child-friendly environment to help calm the child. Using a visual analogue scale to evaluate severity of pain may be helpful to assess response to analgesia.

There is no contraindication to providing adequate analgesia for any child presenting in pain. It is much easier to perform a reliable examination on a child who is comfortable. For severe distress, morphine titrated in increments, controls most children's pain and will not mask the abdominal signs. Oral agents such as paracetamol, codeine or ibuprofen may be used in less severe pain. Serial examination of the child's abdomen and observation of vital signs may be important to exclude significant pathology. Children with a potential surgical cause, should be given nil by mouth, until surgical review.

DISPOSITION

Children with significant abdominal findings need to have a surgical consultation. Not all children who present with abdominal pain will have a clear definitive diagnosis, after their assessment has excluded a serious cause or the need for a surgical review. Some children with severe pain, but negative physical examination findings, where the diagnosis is not clear, will warrant admission for ongoing observation. Children who are discharged home, need to have clear instructions given to parents regarding returning, should they deteriorate, and have a planned timely follow-up by the local doctor.

ACUTE APPENDICITIS

INTRODUCTION

Appendicitis is the most common non-traumatic surgical emergency in children. It occurs slightly more commonly in males at any age, although it is uncommon in those under two years, and very

rare in neonates. The peak incidence is at 9–12 years.

CLINICAL FEATURES

The clinical features of classic appendicitis are well known. Pain is felt initially in the periumbilical region due to visceral pain from obstruction of the appendix. There is often associated nausea, vomiting, anorexia and a low-grade fever. Later, there is migration of the pain to the region of the appendix. This more intense right lower quadrant pain results from irritation of the abdominal parietal lining. Up to 50% of adults have this progression of symptoms but it is less common in children.

Importantly, some children may have false localising diarrhoea or dysuria caused by irritation from an inflamed appendix. Fever is generally below 39.5°C, unless perforation has occurred. Asking the child to walk or hop to demonstrate pain with right leg movement may be useful in indeterminate cases. Likewise, manoeuvres such as the iliopsoas, obturator or Rovsing's signs may help confirm suspicion of appendicitis. In children, with clear signs of appendicitis, the rectal examination adds little value and does not alter management.[10]

Under the age of two years, vomiting (85–90%) and pain (35–77%) are the most common symptoms, with diarrhoea (18–46%) and fever (40–60%) less common. Sometimes grunting respirations (8–23%), cough or rhinitis (40%) and right hip symptoms (3–23%) may be misleading. Right lower abdominal tenderness is present in less than 50% so the diagnosis of appendicitis in this age group is often delayed, leading to perforation rates of 82–92% in this age group.

As children become older, right lower abdominal tenderness becomes more common (age 2–5 years, 58–85%), up to nearly all children in the school-age group, with some (15%) having generalised tenderness without perforation. In children 6–12 years, vomiting occurs in 68–95% of children, anorexia in 47–75%, diarrhoea in 9–16%, constipation in 5–28% and dysuria in 4–20%.

DIFFERENTIAL DIAGNOSES

These include mesenteric adenitis (less severe pain without peritoneal signs is usual and it is rare under three years of age), bacterial enterocolitis, pelvic inflammatory disease, urinary tract infection, Meckel's diverticulitis, intussusception and right lower lobe pneumonia.

INVESTIGATIONS

Children with a clear clinical diagnosis of acute appendicitis do not require investigations and delay of surgical consultation. In equivocal cases, imaging of the appendix may be helpful.

No single test is diagnostic in appendicitis, with the WBC insensitive and non-specific. On urine microscopy more than five white blood cells per high power field or the presence of red blood cells is found in 7–25% of children with appendicitis. Abdominal X-rays may show other pathology (e.g. right lower lobe pneumonia) and occasionally an appendiceal faecolith, but have questionable usefulness in diagnosing appendicitis.

Ultrasound   Has reported sensitivity of 80–92% with specificity of 86–98% and is often used when there is initial diagnostic doubt.[4] However, in one series[7] patients undergoing sonography before appendicectomy had a longer delay before operation, a higher rate of misdiagnosis, and more postoperative complications. It is not uncommon for the appendix to be difficult to visualise.

CT scan   Abdominal helical CT scan in diagnosing appendicitis shows sensitivities from 87–100% and specificities 83–97% with signs of distension of the appendix, faecolith, focal caecal wall thickening and fluid collections in ruptured appendicitis. Some institutions have used a protocol incorporating ultrasound and subsequent CT scan with patients whose diagnosis is equivocal.[5] They have shown this to be an accurate and cost-effective approach when compared with a negative appendicectomy rate of 23%.[5] Scanning with labelled ^{99m}Tc hexamethylpropylened amine oxime labelled (HMPAO) white blood cells is also described[9] with a high sensitivity (96.7%) but less specificity (80%) in a small series.

Active observation   Has also been used without investigation, with a positive predictive value of 97.9% in one series[8] and a normal appendicectomy rate of 2.6%.

MANAGEMENT

The management of acute appendicitis is appendicectomy. Some children require intravenous rehydration, ongoing analgesia and antibiotics, if perforation is suspected.

The management of the child in whom the diagnosis is not clear, but may be possible early appendicitis, is more difficult and one needs to have a clear approach.

In some children it may be useful to perform imaging of the appendix such as a CT scan or by ultrasound, particularly in older females who may have ovarian pathology as a cause of their pain. An expectant approach is appropriate in some children with a short history, with a clear plan of organised review over the next 6–12 hours. This may be achieved by actively observing the child in hospital or, if discharged, by arranging a definite early clinical review. Parents need clear instructions to return should their child's symptoms progress.

MECKEL'S DIVERTICULUM

INTRODUCTION

Meckel's diverticulum is a vestige of the omphalomesenteric duct, occurring in 2% of the population, with 2% of those with Meckel's diverticulum manifesting symptoms. The diverticulum is usually 2 ft proximal to the terminal ileum. Of symptomatic patients, 45% are under the age of two, but it can present at any age. These findings are known as Meckel's rule of twos. The majority of Meckel's diverticuli contain gastric mucosa and may secrete acid.

CLINICAL FEATURES

The presenting features of a Meckel's diverticulum vary and may include abdominal pain, gastrointestinal haemorrhage, bowel obstruction or perforation.

Meckel's diverticuli are the most common cause of significant lower gastrointestinal bleeding in children, usually from peptic ulceration within the diverticulum or adjacent ileum. It is classically painless bleeding, with stools either bright red or tarry, depending on the site and briskness of bleeding.

Diverticulitis causing crampy lower quadrant pain, can occur in older children. A Meckel's diverticulum can be a lead point in intussusception, as well as causing intestinal obstruction by the formation of intraperitoneal bands, which can lead to the possibility of a volvulus or internal herniation.

DIFFERENTIAL DIAGNOSES

These include intestinal polyps, intussusception, anal fissures, midgut volvulus and bacterial enteritis.

INVESTIGATIONS

A Meckel's scan using [99m]technetium can be used, which is 75–85% sensitive and 95% specific[11] at demonstrating the ectopic gastric tissue, when bleeding is present.

MANAGEMENT

Management is intravenous fluid support with blood transfusion for massive bleeding. A Meckel's scan can be done in stable bleeding patients, but if unstable or with peritoneal signs, urgent surgical consultation must be obtained with a view to operative intervention. Definitive treatment is surgical excision.

GASTROENTEROLOGY AND HEPATOLOGY

7

Table 7.1.3   Causes of chronic abdominal pain

Gastrointestinal causes
Chronic recurrent functional abdominal pain
Peptic ulcer disease
Irritable bowel syndrome
Inflammatory bowel disease
Chronic or recurrent pancreatitis
Biliary colic
Appendiceal colic
Constipation
Partial bowel obstruction
Parasitic infection

Endocrine disease
Hyperparathyroidism
Addison's disease
Diabetes mellitus

Cardiovascular disease
Superior mesenteric artery syndrome
Coarctation of aorta

Neurological disease
Abdominal migraine
Migraine headaches
Familial dysautonomia

Haematological disease
Sickle cell disease
Porphyrias

Gynaecological disorders
Cystic teratoma of ovary
Endometriosis
Haematocolpos
Mittelschmerz

Musculoskeletal disorders
Discitis
Linea alba hernia
Painful rib syndrome
Muscle wall sprain

Other
Uteropelvic junction obstruction
Familial Mediterranean fever
Hereditary angioneurotic oedema

Source: Adapted from reference 3.

CHRONIC ABDOMINAL PAIN

INTRODUCTION

Chronic abdominal pain is defined as the presence of at least three discrete episodes of pain occurring over a period of three months or longer.[3] The reported prevalence of abdominal pain interfering with activities is 10–15% in children between 5 and 14 years. Causes of chronic abdominal pain are diverse and are listed in Table 7.1.3.

Signs and symptoms suggesting *organic disease* causing chronic abdominal pain in school-aged children include:

- Persistent fever
- Poor weight gain or weight loss
- Child awakened from sleep
- Pain away from the umbilicus
- Radiation of pain to back, shoulder or lower extremities
- Persistent regurgitation, vomiting or dysphagia
- Bloody emesis or stools
- Associated altered bowel pattern
- Perianal disease
- Sleepiness following pain attacks
- Positive family history of peptic ulcer or inflammatory bowel disease.

ASSESSMENT

The assessment of the child with chronic abdominal pain involves a detailed history and examination. Blood pressure should be measured. The child who has no features to suggest an organic origin requires no testing, although some clinicians opt to perform a limited screen involving urinalysis, full blood count and erythrocyte sedimentation rate, and stool testing for ova and parasites and occult blood.

DIAGNOSIS

The diagnosis of recurrent functional abdominal pain is based on history and a normal physical examination. Usually the patient has no worrying features (as listed above), has periumbilical or mid-epigastric pain, and rarely wakes at night from the pain. Psychosocial stressors may be evident. There may be secondary gain from the child's abdominal pain. Reassurance is the treatment of choice, although it is important to acknowledge that the child does experience pain.

CONTROVERSIES

❶ The best approach to investigations in appendicitis has not yet been settled.

❷ There is probably little need for a rectal examination in children with abdominal pain, but more research is needed before making definitive conclusions.

MANAGEMENT

In the ED situation, the management of chronic abdominal pain depends on the possible diagnoses. Follow-up should be ensured particularly in the child with the suggestion of organic disease or the child missing a significant amount of school.

REFERENCES

1. Scholer SJ, Pituch K, Orr DP, Ditttus RS 1996 Clinical outcomes of children with acute abdominal pain. Paediatrics 98: 680–685
2. Simpson ET, Smith A 1996 The management of acute abdominal pain in children. Journal of Paediatric Children's Health 32(2): 110–112
3. Rudolph A 1996 Rudolph's Textbook of Paediatrics, 20th edn. Appleton and Lange, USA
4. D'Agostino J 2002 Common abdominal emergencies in children. Emergency Medicine Clinics of North America 20: 1
5. Garcia-Pena BM, Taylor GA, Fishman SJ et al 2000 Costs and effectiveness of ultrasonagraphy and limited computed tomography for diagnosing appendicitis in children. Paediatrics 106: 672–676
6. Browne GJ, Choong RKC, Gaudry PL, Wilkins BH 1997 Principles and practice of children's emergency care. Maclennan and Petty, Sydney
7. Emil S et al 2001 Clinical versus sonographic evaluation of acute appendicitis in children: A comparison of patient characteristics and outcomes. Journal of Paediatric Surgery 36(5): 780–783
8. Bachoo P, Mahomed AA, Ninan GK, Youngson GG 2001 Acute appendicitis: The continuing role for active observation. Paediatric Surgery International 17(2-3): 125–128
9. Yan DC, Shiau YC, Wang JJ, Ho ST, Kao CH 2002 Improving the diagnosis of acute appendicitis in children with atypical clinical findings using technetium-99m hexamethylpropylened amine oxime-labelled white-blood-cell abdomen scan. Paediatric Radiology 32(9): 663–666
10. Dunning PG, Goldman MD 1991 The incidence and value of rectal examination in children with suspected appendicitis. Annals of the Royal College of Surgeons of England 73: 233–234
11. Behrman R, Kliegman R, Jenson H 2000 Nelson's Textbook of Paediatrics,16th edn. WB Saunders, Philadelphia

7.2 GASTROINTESTINAL BLEEDING

ELIZABETH M. COTTERELL

ESSENTIALS

1 The causes of gastrointestinal (GI) bleeding in infants and children fall into age-specific diagnostic categories. They represent a different spectrum of disease, as compared to those in adults, with ulcers, varices and malignancy far less common.

2 The majority of GI bleeding ceases spontaneously, requiring no treatment or treatment on the basis of a presumptive diagnosis.

3 Eliciting a good history is important in determining the likely site of GI bleeding, the significance and acuity of the bleed and whether there are co-morbidities that will influence diagnosis and management.

4 Initial assessment is for the presence or absence of haemodynamic compromise due to the blood loss. Major GIT haemorrhage can present as a medical emergency requiring rapid assessment and stabilisation.

5 The appropriate investigation of GI bleeding is guided by history and examination findings. Specific investigations may be required to determine the likely source.

INTRODUCTION

Gastrointestinal bleeding in infants and children is an uncommon cause of presentations to an emergency department (ED) but nonetheless is an alarming symptom that concerns parents greatly. Fortunately, in the majority of infants and children, the cause is benign or relatively uncomplicated, and not associated with significant morbidity or mortality. There are, however, some less common conditions that occur in infancy and childhood that may be a cause of potentially life-threatening blood loss and require rapid assessment and resuscitation.

The epidemiology of GI bleeding in children is very limited. The reported incidence of GI bleeding of 6.4% in paediatric ICU patients[1] and the most frequent diagnoses confirmed endoscopically[2] (duodenal and gastric ulcers, oesophagitis, gastritis, and varices) represent selected populations, who most likely had more severe or protracted GI bleeding and are not representative of the ambulatory paediatric population. Overall, 20% of GI bleeding in children arises from the upper GI tract,[3] generally defined as proximal to the ligament of Treitz at the duodenojejunal flexure.

Definitions

Haematemesis Is the vomiting of blood that may be either fresh (bright red) or altered by gastric acidity and described as 'coffee ground'.

Melaena Is the passage of black, tarry stool. This is caused by bacterial degradation of haemoglobin and implies that the bleeding has occurred over a period of hours.

Haematochezia Is the passage of bright red blood per rectum. Haematemesis and melaena are usually indicative of an upper GI bleeding source. The passage of fresh blood per rectum usually indicates a source of blood from the lower GI tract. It can, however, derive from an upper GI source, especially in infants less than six months, due to rapid colonic transit times. Mild streaking of blood on the surface of stools is generally due to an anal fissure.

AETIOLOGY

The aetiology of GI bleeding is best considered within defined age groups and the likely location of the bleed, as guided by history and examination (see Tables 7.2.1 and 7.2.2). The context in which the patient presents is equally important in considering both the diagnosis and management. An infant in hypovolaemic shock from a bleeding Meckel's diverticulum clearly requires a different response than for a well child with a small amount of blood coating the stool due to an anal fissure.

The term newborn infant who is breast fed and has GI bleeding is most likely to have ingested maternal blood either at the time of delivery or from breast feeding from cracked nipples. Premature infants are at an increased risk of necrotising enterocolitis, although it can occur in term neonates with birth asphyxia or cyanotic heart disease. Any sick newborn, compromised by hypoxia, hypotension or sepsis, is at risk of GI bleeding from stress ulcers. An infant who has not received parenteral vitamin K after birth, or has interference with vitamin K absorption, is at risk of haemorrhagic disease of the newborn.

The bowel habit of the infant or child prior to onset of GI bleeding is important to note. Constipation associated with pain when straining at stool would make an anal fissure a probable diagnosis. Alternatively, an infant with diarrhoea containing blood may have developed a cows' milk protein intolerance. The older infant or child with significant neuromuscular disease, such as cerebral palsy, commonly has severe gastro-oesophageal reflux and therefore most likely has an oesophagitis-related source of upper GI bleeding.

The key factor in identifying the cause of GI bleeding in toddlers and older children is the presence of associated symptoms. Crampy abdominal pain and

Table 7.2.1 Causes of upper GI bleeding

Neonates (< 1 month)	Infants (1 month to 1 year)	Toddlers and school age
Ingested maternal blood	Ingested blood	Ingested blood
Gastritis	Reflux oesophagitis	Reflux oesophagitis
Vascular malformations	Gastritis	Gastritis
Bleeding disorders	Mallory–Weiss tear	Mallory–Weiss tear
	Peptic ulceration	Oesophageal varices
	Vascular malformation	Peptic ulceration
	Bleeding disorders	Bleeding disorders

Table 7.2.2 Causes of lower GI bleeding

Neonates	Infants	Toddlers and school age
Ingested maternal blood	Anal fissure	Anal fissure
Necrotising enterocolitis	Protein sensitive enterocolitis	Juvenile colonic polyps
Protein-sensitive enterocolitis	Hirschsprung's enterocolitis	Infectious gastroenteritis
Hirschsprung's enterocolitis	Ischaemic enterocolitis	Meckel's diverticulum
Ischaemic enterocolitis	Infectious gastroenteritis	Intussusception
Infectious gastroenteritis	Meckel's diverticulum	Ischaemic enterocolitis
Congenital bleeding disorders	Intussusception	Haemolytic uraemic syndrome
	Haemolytic uraemic syndrome	Henoch–Schönlein purpura
	Bleeding disorders	Inflammatory bowel disease
	Vascular malformation	Vascular malformation
	Inflammatory bowel disease	Bleeding disordersa

Table 7.2.3 Chart for guided history taking for GI bleeding

Is it blood?
Consider Haemoccult(r) test on stool samples and Gastroccult(r) on vomit or NG aspirates

Is it from the GI tract?
Consider other sources for the blood

Where in the GI tract is it from?
Specific symptoms reported

Is it a significant amount?
Estimate acuity of bleed by history and assess clinical signs

Are there other concerning symptoms?

Possibilities
- History of ingestion of food colouring or iron supplements
- Ingestion of maternal blood at delivery or breast feeding via cracked nipples
- History of epistaxis, post-tonsillectomy, dental work, oral injury, pharyngitis or haemoptysis
- Upper GIT – haematemasis, melaena or haematochezia for profuse or brisk bleed
- Lower GIT – haemotochezia, redcurrant jelly stools or melaena
- Haemodynamic compromise (pallor, ↑ HR, ↑ cap refill time, ↓ BP) Resuscitate immediately
- Paroxysmal abdominal pain and/or lethargy - intussusception
- Bilious vomiting – volvulus
- Abdominal pain – Henoch-Schönlein purpura
- History of chronic liver disease – oesophageal varices
- Renal or haematologic abnormalities – haemolytic uraemic syndrome
- History of prematurity – necrotising enterocolitis

diarrhoea with mucus and fresh blood may be caused by infectious gastroenteritis due to *Campylobacter*, *Shigella*, *Salmonella*, *Yersinia* and less commonly rotavirus or Norwalk virus. Intermittent colicky abdominal pain with episodes of lethargy occurring in intussusception may manifest with blood in the stools as a late sign. Henoch–Schönlein purpura will manifest with the typical palpable purpura on extremities as well as abdominal pain from a vasculitis involving the GI tract.

Certain diagnoses also have a recognised age pattern; juvenile polyps have a peak incidence of 1 to 6 years of age, intussusception peaks at 5 to 18 months, and inflammatory bowel disease more commonly presents in adolescence, although can occur at any age.

HISTORY

Eliciting a good history is important in determining the likely site of the GI bleeding, the significance and acuity of the bleed and whether there are pre-existing conditions or co-morbidities that will influence diagnosis and management. Details of the timing of the blood appearing in the vomitus or bowel motions, in relation to other events, may give a clue to alternative sources of the blood. For example, the ingestion of substances such as iron or food colourings, onset of epistaxis or recent oral or ENT surgery, will indicate a source of bleeding other than from the GI tract.

A history of recurrent retching or vomiting prior to the appearance of blood in the vomit suggests a Mallory–Weiss tear, but may occur in the absence of these symptoms. Symptoms of epigastric pain and nausea may be elicited with gastritis or peptic ulceration. Crampy abdominal pain with a passage of loose stools, with blood and mucus mixed throughout, suggest infectious or inflammatory process. Fresh blood coating the stool or wiped on the toilet paper implies a lesion in the lower rectum or anus, such as a polyp or fissure.

A positive family history may be helpful, particularly with the less common causes of GI bleeding, such as polyps, inflammatory bowel disease, coagulation disorders, haemorrhagic telangectasia and Hirschsprung's disease. A medication history, including use of non-steroidal anti-inflammatory drugs (NSAIDs), salicylates and anticoagulants may provide further clues as to the causes of the GI bleeding. Inadvertent ingestion of caustic agents and rodenticides containing warfarin-type agents should be considered in preschool-age children.

EXAMINATION

Initial assessment is for the presence or absence of any haemodynamic compromise due to the blood loss. This is uncommon in children but, if present, clinical assessment proceeds while resuscitation is commenced.

Specific findings in the physical examination of the GI tract may establish potential causes for the GI bleeding. The abdomen should be assessed for any localising tenderness or peritoneal signs. Children with minor bleeding in the setting of gastroenteritis will have a benign abdomen. The finding of hepatosplenomegaly with stigmata of chronic liver disease may suggest oesophageal varices as the cause. Palpation of a tender abdominal mass may support a suspicion of intussusception. In the neonatal nursery setting, abdominal distension in the preterm infant, in association with blood-stained nasogastric aspirates, should prompt consideration of necrotising enterocolitis.

Visualisation of an anal fissure is important to confirm the source of blood on stools when the history is suggestive. This is best done by gently spreading the perineal skin to evert the anal canal, with the defect in the rectal mucosa usually superficial and posteriorly located. In addition to the presence of fresh blood on the examining glove, a gentle rectal examination may detect palpable polyps.

Skin and mucus membrane examination may reveal signs of a bleeding tendency due to a coagulation or platelet disorder. Clinical signs of anaemia are more suggestive of a chronic, rather than acute, picture of GI bleeding. Examin-

ation of the nose and throat may show a nasopharyngeal source for ingested blood.

In addition, parents may often provide evidence of the symptoms that they have reported, such as a cloth with blood-streaked vomitus or a nappy with bloody streaks in the faeces. In the event of a fresh sample of stool or vomit being provided, testing for occult blood will verify if GI bleeding has occurred. This can be done by the guaiac and gastroccult tests respectively.

INVESTIGATIONS

The appropriate investigation of GI bleeding needs to be tailored to the most likely cause on the basis of history and examination findings.

Blood tests

Blood tests for haemoglobin level and red cell indices may indicate a hypochromic microcytic anaemia and point to a chronic, rather than acute, source of bleeding. Coagulation profile and platelet count may have to be checked if the history and examination findings suggest a bleeding diathesis or chronic liver disease.

If the GI bleeding has occurred in a breast-feeding infant, most commonly as streaks of fresh blood in the vomitus, then it may be possible to distinguish if the blood is maternal (ingested) rather than from the infant's gut. An Apt test can be performed by diluting the blood from the sample with water (1:5) and then adding 1 mL of sodium hydroxide to the centrifuged mixture. Failure to change colour is consistent with foetal haemoglobin, as it is resistant to denaturisation by alkali, as opposed to the brown-yellow colour that occurs in the presence of adult haemoglobin.

Stool testing

Stool samples for microscopy, looking for red and white cells, as well as for bacterial culture, should be sent if a bacterial enteritis is suspected.

Endoscopy

The role of endoscopy for investigating GI bleeding in the acute setting in chil-

dren is limited. It can, however, serve both a diagnostic and therapeutic role, especially in the case of oesophageal varices. A select group of patients will be defined by the severity of the GI bleed or by symptoms and signs that make the finding of pathology on endoscopy more likely. Consultation with a paediatric gastroenterologist or surgeon is helpful in determining those patients most likely to benefit from this investigation.

Imaging

Nuclear medicine studies such as technetium pertechnetate scan for ectopic gastric mucosa in a Meckel's diverticulum may have a role in investigating the cause of GI bleeding. However, the Meckel scan has a relatively low negative predictive value. This may result in the need for operative evaluation despite a negative scan, where clinical suspicion is high.[4] Other imaging techniques such as plain abdominal X-ray looking for pneumatosis intestinalis in necrotising enterocolitis, and contrast air enema for intussusception, are specific investigations that may be indicated from relevant history and examination findings.

TREATMENT

Initial assessment and stabilisation

In the event of significant GI bleeding, the child or infant will develop signs of haemodynamic compromise. Cool peripheries, delayed capillary refill and tachycardia will be the first detectable signs. Hypotension occurs as a late sign of hypovolaemia.

Resuscitation should include the administration of high-flow oxygen, insertion of two large-bore cannulae and titrated 20 mL kg fluid boluses with crystalloid. Children with significant GI bleeding require ongoing monitoring of heart rate, blood pressure, and urine output in the ED. These observations combined with frequent clinical assessment, help guide ongoing fluid therapy. Transfusion of cross-matched blood is indicated for ongoing or recurrent bleeding with haemodynamic instability unresponsive to initial fluid boluses. Correction of identified coagulopathy with fresh frozen plasma or platelet infusions may be needed to control the GI bleeding. These patients require consultation with a paediatric gastroenterologist regarding acute endoscopy.

Pharmacological treatment

Studies addressing the use of H2 antagonists for acute upper GI bleeding are restricted to the adult population. A meta-analysis of their use for bleeding gastric ulcers has shown a reduction in the incidence of rebleeding and case fatality.[5] However, the routine use of H2 antagonists in children with acute GI bleeding cannot be recommended as bleeding gastric ulcers are very uncommon. There is no evidence for the routine empirical treatment of acute GI bleeding of unspecified cause with proton pump inhibitors, such as omeprazole.

Intravenous vasopressin or somatostatin have been shown to be effective for uncontrolled bleeding oesophageal varices, however, most variceal bleeding ceases spontaneously.

Children with gastroduodenal ulceration shown to be associated with *Helicobacter pylori* infection may benefit from antibiotic eradication treatment.

Surgery

Laparoscopy or laparotomy for investigation of lower GI bleeding may be both a diagnostic and therapeutic tool in children with GI bleeding of obscure origin. A study of 17 children with GI bleeding and no identifiable source after upper endoscopy and colonoscopy found that eight patients had Meckel's diverticulum at laparoscopy, five patients had other GI pathology that accounted for symptoms

and four patients had normal findings.[6] Laparoscopic-assisted small bowel resection was successfully performed in all patients with Meckel's diverticulum.

Laparotomy may be necessary for acute abdominal emergencies such as intussusception unsuccessfully reduced at air enema, midgut volvulus or for management of continuous or recurrent active GI bleeding with haemodynamic compromise.

Endoscopic sclerotherapy

Balloon tamponade for bleeding oesophageal varices, such as Sengstaken–Blakemore tube, is not recommended due to significant complications such as aspiration and oesophageal perforation.

Injection sclerotherapy for oesophageal varices in children is well established with a reported efficacy of controlling active bleeding and eradication of varices exceeding 90%.[7] Complications including oesophageal stricture, superficial ulceration, deep ulceration and perforation are rare.

DISPOSITON

The decision to admit or discharge the infant or child with GI bleeding from the ED is very much influenced by the presumptive diagnosis. Given that the majority are self-limiting or respond readily to treatment, most patients can be managed on an out-patient basis. Those infants and children suitable for discharge will have no haemodynamic instability or significant co-morbidities at presentation to ED. Clearly, each case needs to be judged on its individual merits and high-risk patients with significant GI blood loss will need to be managed in an intensive care or high dependency unit. Children who

CONTROVERSIES

❶ The lack of evidence of benefit from the use of H2 antagonists for acute gastrointestinal bleeding has not prevented their frequent use.

❷ The role of empiric treatment with H2 antagonists or proton pump inhibitors prior to endoscopic confirmation of oesophagitis, gastritis or ulcer disease is unclear.

❸ There is debate about the use of nasogastric aspiration as a diagnostic tool to establish an upper GI tract source of bleeding as it has low specificity for active bleeding.

present with recurrent GIT bleeding of unclear cause, should be discussed with a paediatric gastroenterologist regarding the need for and timing of endoscopy.

REFERENCES

1. Lacroix J, Nadeau D, Laberge S et al 1992 Frequency of upper gastrointestinal bleeding in a paediatric intensive care unit. Critical Care Medicine 20: 35–42
2. Cox K, Ament ME 1979 Upper gastrointestinal bleeding in children and adolescents. Paediatrics 63: 408–413
3. Rodgers BM 1999 Upper gastrointestinal hemorrhage. Paediatric Review 20: 171–174
4. Swaniker F, Soldes O, Hirschl RB 1999 The utility of technetium-99m pertechnetate scintigraphy in the evaluation of patients with Meckel's diverticulum. Journal of Paediatric Surgery 34: 760–764
5. Collins R, Langman M 1985 Treatment with histamine H2 antagonists in upper gastrointestinal haemorrhage: Implications of randomized trials. New England Journal of Medicine 313: 660–666
6. Lee KH, Yeung CK, Tam YH, Ng WT, Yip KF 2000 Laparoscopy for definitive diagnosis and treatment of gastrointestinal bleeding of obscure origin in children. Journal of Paediatric Surgery 35: 1291–1293
7. Fox VL 2000 Gastrointestinal bleeding in infancy and childhood. Gastroenterology Clinics of North America 29: 37–66

7.3 GASTRO-OESOPHAGEAL REFLUX

DARYL EFRON

Essentials

1 The infant presenting with regurgitation/vomiting needs to have alternative causes considered, before concluding that the diagnosis is GOR.

2 GOR is a normal physiological phenomenon to which infants are particularly prone.

3 Infants with benign GOR appear healthy. If the child appears unwell, another cause should be considered.

4 Infants and children with uncomplicated GOR do not need any investigations.

5 Complications of GOR include failure to thrive, reflux oesophagitis, apnoea, aspiration pneumonia, and recurrent aspiration with chronic lung disease.

6 Antacids and antisecretory therapies can be helpful in reflux oesophagitis.

INTRODUCTION

Gastro-oesophageal reflux (GOR) is the regurgitation of gastric contents into the oesophagus. It is a normal physiological phenomenon at all ages. In most cases it is a benign self-limited condition. The refluxed gastric contents are generally rapidly cleared from the oesophagus without causing any problems. Complications warranting medical intervention are uncommon. When complications do occur, it is referred to as GOR disease (GORD).

PATHOPHYSIOLOGY

During periods of raised intra-abdominal pressure such as straining, there are a number of protective mechanisms which help to prevent GOR. These include contraction of the diaphragmatic crura around the lower oesophagus in the region of the lower oesophageal sphincter (LES), as well as compression of the intra-abdominal segment of the oesophagus. Many episodes of GOR are associated with transient relaxations of the LES.

In infants the LES is located above the diaphragm, rendering the above protective mechanisms ineffective. Therefore, infants are especially prone to GOR, particularly in the early months of life. However, with anatomical and physiological maturation, the natural history is of symptom resolution by late infancy in the vast majority.

Some children are particularly predisposed to develop GORD. These include premature infants, children with neurological conditions, such as cerebral palsy or neurodegenerative disorders, and children with anatomical anomalies such as tracheo-oesophageal fistula. These children have poor oesophageal motility with reduced clearance of refluxed gastric contents.

HISTORY

The cardinal symptom of GOR is visible regurgitation of milk post-feeds. This is usually called vomiting, although in GOR the expulsion of gastric contents is generally by an effortless spill, whereas true vomiting involves forceful contraction of abdominal wall musculature. In GOR, the regurgitation is not particularly forceful and the milk usually soils the child's clothing. Likewise, the physiological 'possetting' of milk, which is common after feeding, usually just spills onto the child's chin region. This is in contrast to the more projectile vomiting of pyloric stenosis, where the milk often propels to a more distant location.

The history is crucial in considering potential differential diagnoses and in identifying complications. Careful questioning regarding the relationship of vomiting to feeds, the content of regurgitated material (e.g. is there blood or bile?), apparent associated distress, and feeding behaviour, is essential. Episodic irritability related to feeds may indicate GOR. A history of associated fever suggests an infective cause. Seizures and poor feeding raise the possibility of a metabolic or neurological disorder. Infants with uncomplicated GOR thrive. Inquiry about associated symptoms such as poor weight gain and respiratory symptoms including apnoea, or wheezing is important to screen for potential complications.

EXAMINATION

Infants with benign GOR demonstrate a robust general condition. They appear well and are thriving. If the child appears unwell or lethargic another cause for the symptoms needs to be carefully considered. The presence of abdominal distension, abnormal tone, or hepatosplenomegaly suggests alternative diagnoses including anatomical anomalies, neurodevelopmental dysfunction or metabolic disorders. A pyloric tumour should be specifically palpated for in young infants. Note that occasionally, in a young infant with known GOR, a change in the character of the vomiting may indicate another diagnosis such as pyloric stenosis. Serial weight measurements should be plotted on the child's growth chart. Respiratory examination is important to identify signs of bronchospasm or recurrent aspiration, which may complicate GOR. Conjunctival pallor indicates anaemia secondary to reflux oesophagitis. The urine should be screened for an occult UTI causing vomiting.

DIFFERENTIAL DIAGNOSIS

There are many causes of vomiting in children, and it is important to consider a number of alternative causes that may mimic GOR (see Chapter 7.9 on diarrhoea and vomiting). These include: infection, e.g. urinary tract infection, gastroenteritis; surgical conditions, e.g. malrotation and volvulus, pyloric stenosis, intussusception; metabolic disorders, e.g. inborn errors, diabetes; food allergy and raised intracranial pressure, e.g. hydrocephalus, posterior fossa tumour, subdural haematoma (see Table 7.3.1).

COMPLICATIONS

GOR may result in serious complications and is then referred to as GOR disease (GORD).

Failure to thrive

Some infants with GOR have poor weight gain, which may extend to failure to thrive (crossing two major centiles on a growth chart). This may result from reduced intake – either related to dysphagia or parental reduction of feed volumes offered, in an attempt to minimise regurgitation – or from inadequate absorption of ingested food due to excessive losses.

Respiratory

A number of respiratory complications may occur with GOR. Recurrent aspiration (often silent) results in chronic wheeze or cough, and alveolar disease

Table 7.3.1	Differential diagnosis of GOR
Urinary tract infection
Gastroenteritis
Surgical: volvulus, PS, intussusception
Food allergy
Neurological
Metabolic: inborn errors
Raised intracranial pressure

may develop with signs of tachypnoea and increased work of breathing. Exposure of the oesophageal mucosa to acid can trigger reflex bronchospasm, and persistent asthma symptoms may be related to GOR in some children.[1] Intermittent (or even isolated) episodes of aspiration can cause pneumonia. Reflux of gastric contents into the upper airway can result in laryngospasm, presenting as an obstructive apnoea or apparent life-threatening event.[2]

Oesophagitis

Reflux oesophagitis has become a popular clinical diagnosis given to infants presenting with excessive crying behaviour (so-called 'silent reflux'). There are many causes for infant distress, (including temperamental factors, food allergy) and peptic oesophagitis is only responsible for a minority of cases of infant distress.[3] These infants may have episodes of blood in the vomitus or develop iron deficiency anaemia due to the red cell loss.

Sandifer syndrome is abnormal trunk and neck posturing of infants in response to oesophageal pain due to refluxed gastric acid. These uncommon episodes can be quite stereotypic, such that they may be confused with seizures.

INVESTIGATIONS

In the majority of cases, a careful history and examination will clarify the likely diagnosis of GOR. Investigations may be required to exclude differential diagnoses, when the diagnosis is unclear.

Serum biochemistry including an acid base, to exclude the evolving metabolic alkalosis of pyloric stenosis, and urine microscopy and culture to screen for a UTI, are relevant first-line tests in the vomiting infant. If the history or biochemistry is suggestive, a pyloric ultrasound should be performed to rule out pyloric stenosis.

Well and thriving infants and children with uncomplicated GOR should not be subjected to any investigations. There are a number of investigations, which may be helpful, in selected clinical situations. However, the interpretation of

studies of oesophageal function and their clinical relevance is not straightforward.

Some children may require admission under a paediatrician for observation and consideration of further tests to clarify the diagnosis.

Barium meal and follow through is used to exclude anatomical problems such as malrotation of the small bowel. The observation of GOR merely demonstrates that the infant experienced an episode of reflux at the time of the study. The frequency of GOR episodes, their correlation with clinical symptoms, or the presence of complications cannot be determined from a barium study.

Oesophageal pH monitoring over 24 hours provides representative data about the pH at the lower oesophageal mucosa. A number of indices can be calculated from the monitoring: the frequency of GOR episodes; the length of episodes; and the reflux index – the proportion of time sampled that the oesophageal pH was less than 4 (exposure to gastric acid greater than 10% is usually considered abnormal). However, the association of GOR with oesophagitis is not strong. Infants often have abnormal oesophageal pH findings in the absence of histological features of oesophagitis and, conversely, infants with oesophagitis may have no evidence of significant GOR on pH study.[3] These infants presumably have an alternative cause for their oesophagitis, such as allergy. The precise role of oesophageal pH studies is contentious. It is a good test to confirm severe GOR prior to embarking on anti-reflux surgery, and there may be other clinical scenarios where it provides useful information.

Oesophagoscopy and biopsy is required for evaluating the presence and severity of oesophagitis, as well as to characterise the changes histologically, e.g. peptic, eosinophilic (allergic), Crohn's disease, Barrett's oesophagus.

Aspiration of gastric contents into the lungs can be identified by nuclear medicine study using radiolabelled milk (can detect aspiration events up to 24 hours following a feed). A chest X-ray ± CT scan of the chest can be used to evaluate for chronic lung disease.

TREATMENT

Children diagnosed with GOR need follow-up organised with the local doctor, to ensure no alternative diagnosis is missed and to monitor for complications. Parents need an explanation of the symptoms and to be reassured that the natural history is for spontaneous resolution over months. It is unusual for GOR symptoms to persist beyond 12 to 15 months of age. If there is any doubt about the diagnosis, then a paediatric review should be arranged.

Simple measures

A number of conservative measures are commonly used to lessen the symptoms of GOR. These include posturing (elevation of cot ~ 30° head up), thickening of feeds, and changes to infant formulas. None of these have been demonstrated to modify clinical outcomes.[4] Prone sleeping position is best for reducing GOR[5] but is not generally recommended as it as associated with sudden infant death syndrome. Suggesting positioning a towel on the carer's shoulder may decrease the inconvenience of refluxed milk onto the parent during feeding.

Pharmacological

Pharmacological treatment of otherwise well, thriving infants with uncomplicated benign GOR is not indicated.

In more severe cases, the pharmacological options include antacids, antisecretory therapies, and prokinetic agents. High-dose antacids can be effective in treating oesophagitis.[6] However, prolonged use can be associated with aluminium toxicity and is not recommended. H_2-receptor antagonists such as ranitidine have been shown to improve both histological changes and symptoms.[7] Proton pump inhibitors have well-demonstrated clinical efficacy in children with reflux oesophagitis.[8,9] Prokinetic agents such as cisparide have been used extensively to treat GOR in recent years. However, a recent Cochrane Review found no clear evidence of symptom reduction,[10] and in the light of their potential for causing prolongation of the QT_c interval with risk of cardiac arrhythmias and sudden death, their use has become significantly limited.

Surgical

Antireflux surgery has a limited role in cases of severe GORD, such as neurologically abnormal infants with recurrent aspiration pneumonia. The operation of choice is usually the Nissen fundoplication. Complications of the procedure include breakdown of the wrap, dysphagia, bloating and gagging. Some surgeons are now performing fundoplications laparoscopically.

REFERENCES

1. Balson BM, Kravitz EK, McGeady SJ 1998 Diagnosis and treatment of gastroesophageal reflux in children and adolescents with severe asthma. Annals of Allergy Asthma Immunology 81: 159–164
2. Menon AP, Schefft GL, Thach BT 1985 Apnea associated with regurgitation in infants. Journal of Paediatrics 106: 625–629

CONTROVERSIES

❶ The role of oesophageal pH studies in the evaluation for reflux oesophagitis is the subject of on-going debate.

❷ Prokinetic agents have not been consistently demonstrated to reduce symptoms. Furthermore they can cause prolongation of the QTc interval, and so are not generally recommended.

3. Heine RG et al 2002 Esophagitis in distressed infants: Poor diagnostic agreement between esophageal pH monitoring and histopathologic findings. Journal of Paediatrics 140: 14–19
4. Carroll AE, Garrison MM, Christakis DA 2002 A systematic review of nonpharmacological and nonsurgical therapies for gastroesophageal reflux in infants. Archives of Paediatric Adolescent Medicine 156: 109–113
5. Meyers WF, Herbst JJ 1982 Effectiveness of positioning therapy for gastroesophageal reflux. Paediatrics 69: 768–782
6. Cucchiara S, Staniano A, Romaniello G et al 1984 Antacids and cimetidine treatment for gastroesophageal reflux and peptic oesophagitis. Archives of Diseases in Childhood 59: 842–847
7. Simeone D, Caria MC, Miele E et al 1997 Treatment of childhood peptic oesophagitis: A double-blind placebo-controlled trial of nizatidine. Journal of Paediatric Gastroenterology Nutrition 25: 51–55
8. Kato S, Ebina K, Fujii K, Chiba H, Nakagawa H 1996 Effect of omeprazole in the treatment of refractory acid-related diseases in childhood: Endoscopic healing and twenty-four hour intragastric acidity. Journal of Paediatrics 128: 415–421
9. DeGiacomo C, Bawa P, Franceschi M, Luinetti O, Fiocca R 1997 Omeprazole for severe gastroesophageal reflux in children. Journal of Paediatric Gastroenterology Nutrition 24: 528–532
10. Augood C, MacLennan S, Gilbert R, Logan S 2002 Cisapride treatment for gastro-oesophageal reflux in children (Cochrane Review). The Cochrane Library, Issue 4. John Wiley and Sons, Oxford

GASTROENTEROLOGY AND HEPATOLOGY

7.4 HYPERTROPHIC PYLORIC STENOSIS

KIM LIAN ONG

INTRODUCTION

Hypertrophic pyloric stenosis is a common gastrointestinal cause of gastric outlet obstruction in infants and presents as one of the most common surgical conditions of infancy.[1] It is caused by the idiopathic diffuse hypertrophy and hyperplasia of the circular muscle fibres of the pylorus with proximal extension into the gastric antrum resulting in construction and obstruction of the gastric outlet. In response to outflow obstruction and vigorous peristalsis, stomach musculature becomes uniformly hypertrophied and dilated. It has an incidence of 1 to 3 per 1000 live births.[2] This condition appears to be more common in infants of Caucasian decent and is rare in Asians.[3] The cause of pyloric stenosis is unknown. Genetic, familial, gender and ethnic origin can influence the incidence rates of HPS. Pyloric stenosis is more common in males than in females, up to four to five times.[4] Offspring of parents with this condition have a higher risk of developing HPS and in many series, first-born males are frequently affected.[5]

CLINICAL PRESENTATION

Pyloric stenosis is not present at birth. In the early phase, there may just be regurgitation or occasional non-projectile vomiting. The onset rarely occurs before the first week of life and it commonly present at 2–8 weeks of age. The peak usually occurs at four weeks and it is seldom delayed until the second to third month. Within one week after the onset, the vomiting becomes projectile and it generally occurs during or soon after feeding. However, at times, it may occur up to several hours later. The frequency of vomiting varies, in some infants vomiting occurs after each feed while in others it is intermittent.

Clinically, the infant is hungry and will take another feed immediately. The vomitus is non-bilious but due to the frequency and force of vomiting, it may be blood tinged. The amount of stool may be very small and infrequent depending on the amount of food that reaches the intestine. The degree of dehydration, lethargy and metabolic derangement depends on the time interval between the onset of symptoms and presentation. In some late presentations the infant may be malnourished or even moribund.

On physical examination, gastric distension or visible peristaltic waves may be seen moving from the left upper abdomen toward the epigastrium in some cases.[6] The examination may reveal the diagnostic finding of a hard, mobile and non-tender ovoid mass either to right of the epigastrium or in the midline, deep to the right rectus muscle and under the liver edge. This positive finding requires much patience as the success of such a finding is dependent on an empty stomach and a relaxed anterior abdominal wall. If the stomach is distended, aspiration using a nasogastric tube is necessary. The best position for palpation is on the infant's left side. The inability to palpate an olive-shaped mass does not rule out the diagnosis of HPS.[7]

The metabolic derangements that arise are due to the extensive and protracted vomiting, not unlike other causes of high intestinal obstruction. There are potassium and sodium deficits which may be reflected by a low serum level. The decrease in chloride concentration is most striking and the increase in pH results in the characteristic finding of hypochloremic alkalosis.

IMAGING STUDIES

Some clinicians believe that the palpation of an olive-shaped mass may obviate the need for a confirmatory imaging study as a positive examination has high specificity.[8] Plain radiographs will often have been performed, given the history of vomiting, although they are of no diagnostic value. They may show gastric distension.

Ultrasonography is the now the diagnostic test of choice. The appearance of 'doughnuts' or 'bull's-eyes' on cross-section of the pyloric channel is most characteristic. A muscle thickness of the pylorus greater than 4 mm and a pyloric channel length greater than 17 mm yield a positive predictive value of greater than 90%. For infants less than 30 days of age, these limits may be lower.[9]

In the absence of ultrasonography, barium upper gastrointestinal study is an effective means of diagnosing HPS. This study may be favoured over ultrasound as the cost-effective initial imaging study when the clinical presentation is atypical for HPS and favours other conditions more amenable to diagnosis by upper gastrointestinal study.[10] Positive findings include an elongated pylorus with antral indentation from the hypertrophied muscle. The pathognomonic finding is the appearance of a 'railroad track' sign caused by two thin parallel streams of barium traversing the pylorus. There is also a vigorously peristaltic stomach with delayed or no gastric emptying. Upper GI endoscopy is rarely used and although it would demonstrate pyloric obstruction, it would be difficult to differentiate it from pyloric spasm.

DIFFERENTIAL DIAGNOSIS

The diagnosis is made by the characteristic clinical manifestations and the finding of a pathognomic pyloric mass and inadequate bonding between mother and infant. Other causes of vomiting, especially in early life include chalasia of the oesophagus and hiatus hernia. Gastro-oesophageal reflux with or without hiatus hernia may have a similar presentation of persistent vomiting after feeding. Other non-pathological causes include poor feeding technique by inexperience caretakers.

Projectile vomiting may occur in some rare diagnosis such as pyloric membrane or pyloric duplication and a palpable mass may be felt in the case of pyloric duplication.

Metabolic causes may mimic pyloric stenosis. Adrenal insufficiency results in vomiting but it is likely to result in metabolic acidosis rather than alkalosis as is the case in pyloric stenosis. The serum potassium and urinary sodium concentration are elevated in adrenal insufficiency. Recurrent emesis with alkalosis or acidosis may be caused by some inborn errors of metabolism but usually have other associated features, such as coma or seizures.

MANAGEMENT

The definitive treatment is surgical repair by a Ramstedt pyloromyotomy, which is fairly straightforward with minimal complications. The pylorus may be accessed by various incision techniques including laparoscopic means. All methods are considered acceptable practice with minimal differences in outcomes noted.[11]

Preoperative correction of fluid and electrolyte imbalance is important. The amount of fluid resuscitation is based on the degree of dehydration. Correction of fluid and electrolyte imbalance can usually be achieved within 24–48 hours.

If resuscitation is required, the initial fluid used is normal saline or Hartmann's solution (Ringer's lactate) at 10–20 mL kg^{-1}. This is followed with N/2 + 5% dextrose solution to rehydrate over 24 hours.

Adequate amounts of both chloride and potassium are necessary to correct metabolic acidosis. The correction of potassium can be achieved by adding 10–20 mEq of KCl per 500 mL of IV fluid in patients with normal renal function. Chloride can be adequately replaced by N/2 saline + 5% dextrose. During resuscitation urine output and electrolyte determinations should be performed regularly. In general, correction of chloride level to 90 mEq L^{-1} or greater is adequate for surgery to be performed.

COMPLICATIONS

Complications are minimal when the pyloromyotomy is performed by experienced hands. The complications include incomplete pyloromyotomy, bleeding and undetected mucosal perforation.

REFERENCES

1. Schwartz MZ 1998 Hypertrophic pyloric stenosis. In: O'Neill JA, Rowe MI, Grosfeld JL et al (eds) Pediatric surgery. CV Mosby, St Louis, USA, 111–117
2. Grant GA, McAleer JJA 1984 Incidence of infantile hypertrophic pyloric stenosis (letter). Lancet 1: 1177
3. Klein A, Cremin BJ 1970 Racial significance in pyloric stenosis. South African Medical Journal 44: 1130–1134
4. Poon TS, Zhang AL, Cartmill T, Cass DT 1996 Changing patterns of diagnosis and treatment of infantile hypertrophic pyloric stenosis: A clinical audit of 303 patients. Journal of Paediatric Surgery 31: 1611–1615
5. Murtagh K, Perry P, Corlett M, Fraser I 1992 Infantile hypertrophic pyloric stenosis. Digestive Diseases 10: 190–198
6. Spicer RD 1982 Infantile hypertrophic pyloric stenosis: A review. British Journal of Surgery 69: 128–135
7. Forman HP, Leonidas JC, Kronfeld GD 1990 A rational approach to the diagnosis of hypertrophic pyloric stenosis: Do the results match the claims? Journal of Paediatric Surgery 25: 262–266
8. Godbole P, Sprigg A, Dickson A, Lin PC 1996 Ultrasound compared with clinical examination in infantile hypertrophic pyloric stenosis. Archives of Diseases in Childhood 75: 335–337
9. Lamki N, Athey PA, Round ME et al 1993 Hypertrophic pyloric stenosis in the neonate – diagnostic criteria revisited. Canadian Association of Radiology Journal 44: 21–24
10. Olson AD, Hernanadez R, Hirschl RB 1998 The role of ultrasonography in the diagnosis of pyloric stenosis: A decision analysis. Journal of Paediatric Surgery 33: 676–681
11. Hingston G 1996 Ramstedt's pyloromyotomy – what is the correct incision? New Zealand Medical Journal 109: 276–278

7 GASTROENTEROLOGY AND HEPATOLOGY

7.5 BILIOUS VOMITING

ANDREW J. A. HOLLAND

ESSENTIALS

1 Bilious vomiting generally indicates an intestinal obstruction due to surgical pathology.

2 Early referral to a paediatric surgeon is recommended.

3 Rarely bile-stained vomiting may have a non-surgical medical aetiology.

4 Malrotation with volvulus usually presents in the first few weeks of life, but can occur at any age and is always a surgical emergency.

5 Small-bowel obstruction secondary to adhesions is less common in children than in adults and rarely settles with non-operative management.

INTRODUCTION

Any child presenting to the ED with bilious vomiting has a surgical cause of intestinal obstruction until proven otherwise. Bilious vomiting occurs when the vomitus contains bile. Typically this is indicated by its bright green colour, although the discolouration may vary from a pale yellow to a dark geenish brown. Often the carer is aware of the importance of this sign and will have preserved a towel or item of clothing stained with the vomitus for inspection. For practical purposes, bilious vomiting indicates an intestinal obstruction. Some indication of the likely aetiology and level of the obstruction may be determined from the age of the child, the past medical history and length of illness prior to onset of vomiting. Rapid onset of bilious vomiting and a non-distended abdomen suggest a proximal obstruction, whereas, late onset of bilious vomiting and

abdominal distension, a distal obstruction. Immediate referral to a paediatric surgeon is indicated, as urgent surgical intervention may be required.

CAUSES

The possible causes of bilious vomiting are as shown in Table 7.5.1 and are discussed below:

Intestinal atresia

The term atresia implies maldevelopment of a lumen or opening that is normally patent. If there is just a narrowing of the lumen, this is termed a stenosis. Atresia of the intestinal tract can occur at any level, but in the context of bilious vomiting the level of obstruction is distal to the ampulla of Vater in the second part of the duodenum.

As the lesion is congenital, the child will present in the neonatal period, although increasingly, some of these infants are diagnosed on antenatal ultrasound scans.[1] Proximal lesions, such as duodenal or jejunal atresia, will usually present in the first 24 hours of life whereas more distal lesions, such as ileal or colonic atresias, can present later. Duodenal atresia may be associated with Down's syndrome and cardiac anomalies in up to 30% of cases.[2]

Table 7.5.1 Causes of bilious vomiting

- Intestinal atresia
- Anorectal anomalies
- Meconium ileus
- Hirschsprung's disease
- Malrotation with volvulus
- Irreducible inguinal hernia
- Intussusception
- Inflammatory
- Meckel's diverticulum
- Adhesions
- Non-surgical

Anorectal anomalies

Typically the anus is imperforate and the rectum communicates with the urinary tract or perineum via a fistula. It may occur as part of the VACTERL association of anomalies (Vertebral, Anorectal, Cardiac, Tracheo-oesophageal, Renal and Limb).[3] The diagnosis should normally be made as part of the routine assessment of a neonate following delivery, but is occasionally missed, leading to late onset bilious vomiting.

Meconium ileus

This condition occurs in about 10–20% of neonates with cystic fibrosis (CF), although uncommonly it may occur in the absence of CF.[4] There may be a family history of CF. The condition results from the occlusion of the bowel lumen by abnormally viscous enteric secretions in the small bowel and may be complicated by an atresia.

Hirschsprung's disease

In this condition the enteric nervous system is abnormal, leading to a distal physiological obstruction. The condition is more common in males by a ratio of 4:1.[5] In 75% of cases, so called 'classical' Hirschsprung's disease (HD), a variable extent of the rectum and sigmoid colon is involved leading to a distal colonic obstruction.[6] About 10% of children with HD will also have Down's syndrome.[7] The cardinal feature of HD is the failure to first pass meconium within 24 hours of birth, with the later development of bilious vomiting in the first few days of life.

Malrotation with volvulus

The mid-gut normally develops within a physiological hernia in utero. As this reduces towards the end of the first trimester, the mid-gut undergoes an anticlockwise rotation around the axis of the superior mesenteric vessels.[8] Failure of this process to occur results in mal-rotation. The onset of bilious vomiting usually indicates that the malrotated small bowel has obstructed as a result of twisting around its pedicle, although occasionally, this may occur as a result of associated congenital bands. There is a high risk of intestinal ischaemia, so urgent surgical intervention is required once the diagnosis has been confirmed.[9] Although malrotation most commonly presents in the first month of life, it can present later in life.[10]

Irreducible inguinal hernia

An irreducible inguinal hernia, particularly in a male, often contains bowel. The resultant obstruction of the bowel at the level of the external inguinal ring, may produce bilious vomiting. Untreated, the irreducible hernia is at risk of producing intestinal ischaemia.

Intussusception

In intussusception the proximal bowel (the 'intussusceptum') invaginates or telescopes into the distal, receiving bowel (the 'intussuscipiens'). Initially this involves the ileum invaginating into itself, but then progresses to involve the colon. Most commonly, it presents in infants or toddlers with episodic colicky abdominal pain, which may be associated with vomiting or pallor. As the disease progresses, vomiting may become bilious resulting from intestinal obstruction. The 'classical' red currant jelly stool of intussusception is a late phenomenon but occult blood can often be detected earlier.[11]

In older children above three years of age, intussusception is usually associated with a pathological lead point such as a Meckel's diverticulum (MD) or small bowel polyp.[12] It may also complicate CF and Henoch–Schönlein purpura.

Inflammatory

Complicated acute appendicitis, Meckel's diverticulitis or inflammatory bowel disease leading to the development of an inflammatory mass, may result in intestinal obstruction. This presentation usually occurs when there has been a diagnostic delay of the primary pathology, often in children under five years of age.

Meckel's diverticulum

This represents a remnant of the omphalomesenteric duct and is present in about 2% of the population.[13] For reasons that are unclear, complications of a Meckel's diverticulum (MD) are more common in males.[13] MD may lead to a bowel obstruction either as a result of acting as the lead point for an intussusception, due to an associated band adhesion with volvulus or an internal hernia, or rarely an inflammatory mass due to Meckel's diverticulitis.

Adhesions

Bowel obstruction due to adhesions are uncommon in children following abdominal surgery.[9] This is fortunate as, unlike adults, the obstruction rarely settles with non-operative intervention.

Non-surgical

A wide variety of medical conditions may occasionally present with bilious vomiting, together with a variable degree of abdominal distension. Severe gastroenteritis with prolonged vomiting, sepsis, pyloric stenosis, hypothyroidism, meconium plug syndrome and the cyclical vomiting syndrome may all lead to a clinical picture similar to intestinal obstruction.[14] However, any child presenting with bilious vomiting requires paediatric surgical consultation to exclude a surgical cause.

COMPLICATIONS

The major complication of bilious vomiting due to intestinal obstruction is the potential for intestinal ischaemia, if the diagnosis is delayed. Even short periods of ischaemia may lead to loss of the normal gut barrier function and a prolonged paralytic ileus. If there has been diagnostic delay with irreversible bowel ischaemia, perforation with peritoneal contamination can occur. In cases requiring extensive resection, short-bowel syndrome can result. In unrecognised cases, overwhelming septicaemia and even death can result.[9]

INVESTIGATIONS

A variety of investigations may be required in the child with bilious vomiting, but should not replace a focused history, clinical examination and surgical assessment.

Haematological and biochemical investigations are often normal unless the child is moderately to severely dehydrated. Acid base derangement may occur secondary to the volume and content of the vomitus. If there is intestinal ischaemia, there is usually a marked leucocytosis. The blood glucose level should always be checked and the urine screened for sepsis.

The initial radiological investigations should be directed towards demonstrating obstruction and include plain films of the abdomen and chest. Free gas from a perforation can be seen on an erect chest, erect abdomen or decubitus abdominal views. Fluid levels, consistent with intestinal obstruction, may be seen on an erect or decubitus abdominal film, but can be normal and may occasionally occur in medical causes of bilious vomiting. Dilated small bowel is identified by the presence of the valvulae conniventes of Kirkring passing across the entire lumen, as opposed to the incomplete haustral markings in the colon. In neonates, these markings are usually not visible. There may be features to suggest intussusception (see Chapter 7.1 on abdominal pain).

The use of further investigations will be directed by the likely pathology and surgical consultation. Contrast studies, either upper or lower, may be both diagnostic of the surgical cause and in the case of intussusception, therapeutic.[8,11] Ultrasound (US) has a limited role in the investigation of bilious vomiting, but may be useful as a screening tool in children with suspected intussusception and the detection of pathological lead points.[15]

TREATMENT

The treatment of intestinal obstruction in children involves analgesia, fluid and electrolyte resuscitation and definitive surgical management.

The child should be fasted. Neonates and infants require a warm environment to ensure temperature stability. Often large volumes of fluid have been lost from the intravascular space and 10–20 mL kg^{-1} fluid boluses of crystalloid solution may be required to treat shock. In addition,

CONTROVERSIES

❶ Radiological diagnosis of malrotation. False positives and negatives may occur with both contrast studies and US assessment.[16] Ultimately the clinician needs to make an assessment based on the patient's signs and symptoms in conjunction with information obtained from radiological studies.

❷ The role of laparoscopy in the assessment of small bowel obstruction in children.[17] There may be a role for laparoscopy as the first manoeuvre in the operative management of children with adhesive intestinal obstruction.

calculated maintenance and deficit fluid using half-strength normal saline with dextrose should be given. A gastric tube, at least 10 or 12F in size should be placed and regularly aspirated to decompress the stomach. Ongoing fluid losses should be charted and replaced on a mL for mL basis with intravenous normal saline.

Hypokalaemia, if present, needs to be treated appropriately (see Chapter 10.5 on fluids and electrolytes). If required, intravenous analgesia should be given in the form of morphine 100 µg kg^{-1} dose^{-1} and titrated to the response of the patient.

Most surgical causes of bilious vomiting will require operative treatment following further investigation.[9] Although adhesive obstruction may initially be treated non-operatively by a 24 to 48 hour period of gut rest, only rarely is this effective in children.

REFERENCES

1. Dalla Vecchia LK, Grosfeld JL, West KW, Rescorla FJ, Scherer LR, Engum SA 1998 Intestinal atresia and stenosis: A 25-year experience with 277 cases. Archives of Surgery 133: 490–497
2. Grosfeld JL, Rescorla FJ 1993 Duodenal atresia and stenosis: Reassessment of treatment and outcome based on antenatal diagnosis, pathologic variance and long-term follow-up. World Journal of Surgery 17: 301–309
3. Paidas CN, Pena A 1997 Rectum and anus. In: Oldham KT, Colombani PM, Foglia RP (eds) Surgery of infants and children: Scientific principles and practice. Lippincott-Raven Publishers, Philidelphia, 1323–1362
4. Fakhoury K, Durie PR, Levison H, Canny GJ 1992 Meconium ileus in the absence of cystic fibrosis. Archives of Diseases in Childhood 67: 1204–1206
5. Russell MB, Russell CA, Niebuhr E 1994 An epidemiological study of Hirschsprung's disease and additional anomalies. Acta Paediatrica 83: 68–71
6. Kleinhaus S, Boley SJ, Sheran M et al 1979 Hirschsprung's disease: A survey of members of the surgical section of the American Academy of Paediatrics. Journal of Paediatric Surgery 14: 588–597
7. Goldberg E 1984 An epidemiological study of Hirschsprung's disease. International Journal of Epidemiology 13: 479–485
8. Rowe MI, O'Neill JA, Grosfeld JL, Fonkalsrud EW, Coran AG 1995 Rotational anomalies and volvulus In: Rowe MI, O'Neill JA, Grosfeld JL, Fonkalsrud EW, Coran AG (eds) Essentials of paediatric surgery. Mosby, St Louis, 492–500
9. Madonna MB, Boswell WC, Arensman RM 1997 Outcomes. Seminars in Paediatric Surgery 6(2): 105–111
10. Powell DM, Otherson HB, Smith CD 1989 Malrotation of the intestine in children: The effect of age in presentation and therapy. Journal of Paediatric Surgery 24: 777–780
11. Losek JD, Fiete RL 1991 Intussusception and the diagnostic value of testing stool for occult blood. American Journal of Emergency Medicine 9: 1–3
12. Ong NT, Beasley SW 1990 The leadpoint in intussusception. Journal of Paediatric Surgery 25: 640–643
13. St-Vil D, Brandt ML, Panic S et al 1991 Meckel's diverticulum in children: A 20-year review. Journal of Paediatric Surgery 26: 1289–1292
14. Li BUK, Balint JP 2000 Cyclic vomiting syndrome: Evolution in our understanding of a brain-gut disorder. Advances in Paediatrics 47: 117–160
15. Bhisitkul DM, Listernick R, Shkolnik A et al 1992 Clinical application of ultrasonography in the diagnosis of intussusception. Journal of Paediatrics 121: 182–186
16. Dilley AV, Pereira J, Shi ECP et al 2000 The radiologist says malrotation: Does the surgeon operate? Paediatric Surgery International 16: 45–49
17. Holcomb GW 2002 Preface. Seminars in Paediatric Surgery 11: 195

7.6 FOOD INTOLERANCE

PATRICIA MCVEAGH

ESSENTIALS

1 A food reaction needs to be considered in any child presenting with gastrointestinal symptoms.

2 Reactions to foods may be due to a number of mechanisms. These include toxic, immune mediated, non-immune mediated intolerance, and chemical. This chapter will consider food intolerances and allergy that may present with gastrointestinal symptoms. These include:
- Infant formula protein intolerance
- Cows' milk protein-induced allergic enteropathy in toddlers
- Eosinophilic gastroenteritis
- Dysphagia due to eosinophilic inflammation of the oesophagus
- Chronic constipation due to dysmotility or allergic proctitis in children with milk allergy
- Coeliac disease
- Lactose and other carbohydrate intolerances.

3 Food protein allergies and intolerances are more common in younger children than in older children or adults. Most children who develop food reactions outgrow them by five years of age:
- Allergy to cows' milk may affect up to 5% of infants
- Treatment entails strict avoidance of the protein until the sensitisation has diminished
- The best strategy to prevent food sensitisation is to avoid the relevant allergenic proteins.

4 Care must be taken in ascribing unsettled infant behaviour (colic) to a food reaction. Crying and distressed behaviour that fits a normal developmental pattern but is in the top quartile or outside parental expectations is most commonly due to alert infant temperament and best resolved by sleep/feed/parenting/infant behavioural support.

INTRODUCTION

It is not always possible to clinically differentiate between food allergy and food intolerance. The terms are often used loosely. However, a number of symptom complexes are recognised.

Formula protein intolerance

Formula protein enterocolitis usually presents in the first eight weeks of life with spots or streaks of blood and mucus in the stool and sometimes with mild diarrhoea, vomiting, irritability or failure to thrive. Intractable diarrhoea may occur if the small bowel mucosa is involved. Cows' milk is the most common offending protein. Most affected infants are usually also allergic to other dietary proteins. About 50% also react to soy protein and some to protein hydrolysate formulas. Although this has been labelled formula protein intolerance, on rare occasions infants may react to cows' milk or other proteins present in their mother's milk. This disorder does not appear to be IgE mediated and therefore the inflammatory changes are usually confined to the gastrointestinal tract. Extra-intestinal symptoms are rare but eczema and irritability may occur.

Formula protein-induced colitis is usually not associated with positive skin tests or radioallergosorbent tests. Stool microscopy may show increased numbers of white blood cells and a peripheral blood eosinophilia may be present. Small-bowel biopsy may reveal patchy villus atrophy and a mononuclear cell inflammatory response. Rectal biopsy may demonstrate eosinophil infiltration, with clustering of eosinophils or crypt invasion by eosinophils. The finding of increased numbers of eosinophils in the colonic mucosa is highly suggestive of this condition.

Management includes instituting an amino-acid-based formula and performing food challenges once the symptoms have settled. It can take up to three weeks for symptoms to resolve or for a reaction to a food challenge to occur. Most children with this disorder lose their sensitivity by two years of age and they need to be periodically rechallenged after they reach one year of age.

For breast-fed infants, their mother should be started on a diet that eliminates common food allergens and appropriate dietary and lactation support offered. It is important to explore the mother's beliefs about feeding. Some may feel they have 'poisoned' their baby with their milk. They may be reassured that her milk is still the best option for her infant, supplying bioactive components not otherwise available to her infant, and that her milk will be more palatable to her baby than an amino-acid formula. Rarely with extreme sensitivity, an amino-acid-based formula may temporarily be needed to allow an elimination diet to be established. The mother should be supported in maintaining her lactation by expressing. The baby may tolerate small amounts of its mother's milk while the elimination diet is established.

Resolution of symptoms may take several days to three weeks. An elimination trial should continue for three weeks prior to labelling it ineffective. Once the symptoms have settled the baby can be challenged by stepwise reintroduction of foods into the mother's diet. A certain level of the offending food may be tolerated. Mothers on cow milk protein free diets will need a calcium replacement. Mothers of term babies should be counselled to follow the WHO recommendation of exclusive breast-feeding to about six months of age and be given dietary advice about the introduction of solids.[1] These infants may be very sensitive to non-human protein and breast feeding should preferably continue to at least a year.

Protein-losing enteropathy

Toddlers and preschoolers with a cows' milk products intake greater than the equivalent of 600 mL of cows' milk per day may develop anaemia due to a low iron intake. In addition, infants weaned from human milk or formula to cows' milk may present with failure to thrive associated with anaemia and pan-hypoproteinaemia, due to a chronic enteropathy with malabsorption, protein loss and iron deficiency anaemia resulting from chronic gastrointestinal bleeding. This condition is much less common than allergic colitis in infants. The stools contain occult blood, neutrophils, eosinophils and are positive for faecal α_1-antitrypsin. Jejunal biopsy demonstrates flattened villi, oedema, and inflammatory cells that may be eosinophilic. The lesion is variable and somewhat patchy. Pulmonary infiltrates are also occasionally seen (Heiner's syndrome).

Management includes a strict cows' milk protein exclusion diet. Symptoms can be expected to resolve and the histology to improve within three days of starting the diet. Symptoms usually recur within six hours of a rechallenge.

IgE-mediated food allergies

In older children and adults, food allergy is most commonly IgE-mediated and is primarily manifested by systemic symptoms, such as eczema, urticaria, respiratory symptoms, or even anaphylaxis. Peanuts, eggs, shellfish, cows' milk and soy are common causes but many foods may result in allergic reactions. IgE-mediated conditions are often associated with positive skin tests and radioallergosorbent tests. However, these tests have a low specificity and positive results need to be confirmed by food challenges. On the other hand, a negative test makes an IgE-mediated allergy to that food protein highly unlikely. Most reactions isolated to the gastrointestinal tract are caused by non-IgE-mediated mechanisms. There are two specific conditions where GI symptoms occur with IgE mediated food reaction:

1. Oral allergy syndrome

Contact of the allergen with the oropharynx results in itching or tingling and angioedema of the lips, tongue, palate, and throat. These symptoms may precede other IgE-mediated manifestations of food allergy.

2. Gastrointestinal anaphylaxis

Nausea, abdominal cramps, vomiting, and/or diarrhoea occur rapidly after ingestion of the offending allergen.

Coeliac disease

Coeliac disease is the result of intolerance to the gliadin fraction of gluten, a dietary protein present in wheat, and also oats, barley and rye. Coeliac disease needs to be considered in children presenting with diarrhoea, failure to thrive, constipation, abdominal pain, or occult nutritional deficiency states such as iron deficiency. The diagnosis is suggested by raised antiendomysial or tissue transglutaminase antibodies in a child receiving gluten in their diet and confirmed by small-bowel biopsy. Before a negative antibody result is accepted IgA deficiency must be excluded. Allergy to other food proteins does not significantly increase the risk of coeliac disease.

Eosinophilic gastroenteritis

In older children, dietary enterocolitis is usually due to cows' milk protein but it may be due to other dietary antigens such as soy, eggs, wheat, peanuts, rice, oats, chicken, and fish. Multiple food antigens are often involved. Eosinophilic gastroenteritis runs a chronic course punctuated with acute exacerbations. There is often peripheral eosinophilia and raised serum IgE levels.

Histologic findings range from mild inflammation to villous atrophy. Large numbers of eosinophils are found in biopsies of the gastric antrum or small bowel. The location of these dense eosinophilic infiltrates affects symptomatology. Mucosal infiltration is commonest and it may produce nausea, vomiting, diarrhoea, abdominal pain, gastrointestinal bleeding, protein-losing enteropathy, or malabsorption. Involvement of the muscularis may alter motility in the gastrointestinal tract leading to obstruction (especially of the pylorus). Serosal activity may produce eosinophilic ascites. The lesions respond to corticosteroids and although some children are helped by elemental diets, exclusion of dietary antigens or the use of cromolyn, most require systemic administration of corticosteroids.

Eosinophilic esophagitis

Eosinophilic esophagitis should be considered in children with ongoing reflux symptoms, anorexia, dysphagia, food impaction, and pain that are not relieved by conventional antireflux treatment. Although aggressive acid suppression may give some symptomatic relief, the eosinophilic infiltrates persist and dysphagia often continues. These children may respond to antigen elimination. Eosinophilic oesophagitis may be due to inhaled allergens. It may also occur in adults.

Eosinophilic constipation

Cows' milk protein allergy should be considered as a cause of constipation or faecal soiling in children without other cause who are not responding to laxative treatment, particularly if there is a history of cows' milk protein allergy as an infant or a family history of cows' milk protein allergy or other allergic disorders. Increased eosinophils may be found in both rectal and small-bowel biopsies. A strict cows' milk protein elimination usually results in symptomatic improvement within 2–3 weeks. This is a relatively recently described disorder and the natural history is not yet known. Periodic rechallenge with cows' milk protein would seem prudent.

A few cases of diffuse mucosal eosinophilic enterocolitis have been reported with acute abdominal pain, abdominal distension, nausea, and intractable constipation due to intestinal pseudo-obstruction. The patients improved after dietary cows' milk protein elimination and treatment with immunosuppression.

Lactose intolerance

Low disaccharidase levels in the small intestine may result in carbohydrate malabsorption due to reduced digestion and absorption of the target carbohydrate. When accompanied by clinical symptoms, such as bloating and diarrhoea, it is called carbohydrate intolerance. The main classes of disaccharidases are β-glycosidase (lactase) and α-glucosidases (sucrase–isomaltase, maltase–glucoamylase, and trehalase). The enzymes are located in the brush border of the small intestine. Each has a hydrophobic region that serves as a membrane anchor, and an active hydrophilic region that protrudes into the intestinal lumen. Lactase is found adjacent to the tips of the villi and is vulnerable in conditions that result in mucosal damage and flattening of the villi.[2] Secondary lactase deficiency following acute infectious gastroenteritis is the commonest form of disaccharidase deficiency encountered in infants and children and may also complicate conditions such as coeliac disease and inflammatory bowel syndromes.

Although symptoms of unsettled behaviour in infants are often ascribed to lactose intolerance, primary lactose malabsorption in the infant and young child is extraordinarily rare. For most of human kind, lactase levels decrease after the age of three years to about 15% of earlier values. The levels do not drop in individuals with lactase persistence. This is inherited as an autosomal dominant trait and is usual in populations where milk consumption traditionally continued into adulthood.

Human milk contains over 130 different sugars and reducing substances in the stools of breast-fed children is normal. They are not an indication of lactose intolerance. Breath hydrogen tests, oral tolerance tests, and the measurement of faecal excretion of C-enriched sugars can be used to assess carbohydrate malabsorption. Disaccharidases can be measured in intestinal juices and the histologic appearance of an intestinal mucosal biopsy may indicate whether the deficiency is primary or secondary. The histology is normal in patients with carbohydrate malabsorption due to genetically determined defects such as glucose–galactose malabsorption, sucrase–isomaltase deficiency, and adult-type hypolactasia.

In secondary lactose intolerance, a low-lactose diet may be temporarily required to hasten resolution of the symptoms. However, most children with acute gastroenteritis can be started back on their usual feed within 48 hours of the onset of diarrhoea. Breast-fed children should continue to be breast fed through the illness.

EPIDEMIOLOGY

Food hypersensitivity is more common in children than in adults. However, the manifestations of food intolerance or allergy are not specific and parents tend to over attribute incidental symptoms to foods. There is no good community data on the prevalence of food intolerance and allergy, but it appears that around 5% of young children are affected. Prospective studies of newborns have identified a prevalence of cows' milk hypersensitivity of approximately 2.5%, egg sensitivity of approximately 1.3%, and peanut sensitivity of approximately 0.5%. The prevalence of these reactions is significantly higher in children with atopic dermatitis or asthma. The incidence of allergic diseases overall has been increasing in developed countries.

Most children outgrow their food sensitivity but those who are intolerant of hydrolysed protein are more likely to have multiple food intolerances, a higher incidence of total IgE and CMP-specific IgE and are less likely to become tolerant, or become tolerant at an older age. In the first five years of life, symptoms of food reactions are mainly gastrointestinal while in older children wheezing, constipation and delayed reactions to CMP become more common. Children with persistent CMPI are more likely to have a family history of atopic disease.[3]

DEFINITION

Adverse reactions to food can be divided into toxic and non-toxic reactions and the latter into non-immune mediated and immune mediated. Food hypersensitivity or food allergy is an adverse reaction to food that is immune mediated. It may be IgE mediated or non-IgE mediated. Cows' milk, egg white and peanuts are the commonest food allergies in the under two year old. After four years of age, nuts, fruits and legumes are the commonest. Any reaction to food tends to be labelled food allergy, when in fact gastrointestinal symptoms in children are more commonly due to food intolerance rather than food allergy. These have a pharmacologic rather than immunologic basis.

PATHOPHYSIOLOGY

The GI tract has several non-immunologic and immunologic mechanisms that interact with luminal antigens with the production of IgA antibody and the induction of oral tolerance, i.e. the down regulation of immune responses at peripheral sites. Antigenic stimulation of Th1- and Th2-type cytokines activates cellular immunity and antibody production, respectively. Infants absorb more food allergen during their first year than later in life. Infants exclusively fed with human milk are exposed to human proteins. However, in some mothers, small amounts of food proteins appear in their milk and this may sensitise some infants. The precise pathways of protein intolerance and hypersensitivity are poorly understood.

In IgE-mediated reactions, food antigen binds to specific IgE antibody on mast cells and basophils releasing inflammatory mediators giving rise to a rapid onset of symptoms. On the other hand, non-IgE-mediated immune reactions are usually cell-mediated and develop over hours to days.

Combined IgE-mediated and cell-mediated reactions also occur. Genetics, host flora, and the timing, dosage, and frequency of exposure to various dietary antigens, as well as the antigenicity of food proteins, all contribute to the induction of food hypersensitivity. Children may be tolerant to novel protein, e.g. asses' milk protein. In protein-induced enterocolitis, non-IgE mechanisms predominate. Eosinophilic diseases of the GI tract may be caused by abnormal Th2 cytokine response resulting in eosinophil activation and recruitment.

HISTORY

A food reaction should be suspected in children who present with gastrointestinal symptoms without evident cause, particularly if typical symptoms occur with the introduction of specific foods or in infants who have been given formula infrequently and present after a formula feed. Non-allergic mechanisms of food intolerance, such as food poisoning or secondary lactose intolerance, should be ruled out. In children over one year, primary lactose intolerance should be considered when cows' milk allergy is suspected. The history should include:

- Gastrointestinal symptoms – vomiting, abdominal pain, diarrhoea, failure to thrive; stool character.
- Oropharyngeal symptoms – pruritus, tingling, or swelling of the lips, tongue, or palate.
- Other atopic symptoms – wheezing, flare in eczema.
- Personal and family history of atopy.
- A full feeding history:
  Timing in relation to symptoms. Immediate-type hypersensitivity responses occur within minutes up to two hours after ingestion of the offending antigen.
  Previous exposure to the suspect food.
  In breast-feeding infants – maternal diet. Cows' milk in the mother's diet is the most common identifiable cause of food-allergic reactions in breast-fed infants; reaction to peanut, soy, or egg in the mother's diet occurs less often.
  In infancy, hypersensitivity is most often associated with cows' milk or soy protein ingestion.
  Among infants and children with food allergy, 90% of reactions are to egg, milk, peanuts, soy, and wheat.

Ask also about shellfish, tree nuts and seeds. Of children with proven food allergy 75% react to only a single food. Children with allergic eosinophilic gastroenteritis are the exception, often reacting to multiple foods.

- Input-output – fluid intake; stooling, vomiting, urine output.
- Growth history.
- Genetic background, family history of coeliac disease, lactose intolerance, other bowel problems, check the basis of any diagnosis in a family member.

EXAMINATION

Examination should include growth parameters, hydration and circulatory status, markers of atopy and examination of the stool.

INVESTIGATIONS

There is no reliable single test for the diagnosis of food allergy or intolerance. Patients with IgE-mediated food hypersensitivity may be identified but unfortunately, they comprise only a small proportion of all children with food-induced reactions.

RAST testing and prick/puncture skin testing evaluate the presence of specific IgE and may be useful in patients suspected of having IgE-mediated reactions. A positive skin test result or radioallergosorbent test may be meaningful, whereas a negative test result does not rule out allergy because these tests do not detect a non-IgE mediated allergy. In older children, a positive test result for specific IgE does not mean that a specific food is the cause of symptoms as children with positive test results are often asymptomatic. Children with a negative SPT or RAST are very unlikely to have symptoms induced by IgE-mediated sensitivity to that food allergen. Total serum IgE is unreliable.

The only 'gold standard' for diagnosing food allergy or intolerance is a properly performed double-blind placebo-controlled oral food challenge. In children old enough to swallow capsules, the suspected foods are administered in capsules in progressively increasing amounts, alternating with placebo, and reactions are evaluated in a blinded fashion. These should be performed in specialised clinics. Negative results should be followed by an open challenge. When anaphylaxis has followed ingestion of a food, challenge should not be performed and the child should be referred to an allergist.

If a specialised clinic is not available the clinician usually must rely on open challenges. Open food challenges, although commonly performed, are less reliable. For food intolerance the suspected food proteins should be removed from the child's (and the breastfeeding mother's) diet. Symptoms may take up to three weeks to abate. The diet should be absolute in order to be sure of the response. This will need the support of a practising accredited dietitian or, if not available, detailed instructions to parents. On re-challenge, symptoms may take up to three weeks to recur. Because many causes can mimic food reactions, and young children should not have major food groups eliminated from their diet without just cause, 2–3 challenges is technically preferable. However, the clinician may elect not to put an infant through this.

The presence of occult blood, white cells and eosinophils on stool microscopy suggest food intolerance. A bowel biopsy is necessary to confirm eosinophilic infiltration and to exclude other causes of malabsorption. Clinicians without ready resort to a paediatric gastroenterologist may elect to observe a child's response to empiric treatment.

DIFFERENTIAL DIAGNOSIS

Depending on the presentation, other conditions to be considered include:

❶ Acute infections such as gastroenteritis and urinary tract infections.
❷ Food poisoning, e.g. by *Salmonella*.
❸ Intussusception.
❹ Causes of chronic diarrhoea, such as inflammatory bowel disease; fruit juice diarrhoea, toddlers diarrhoea.
❺ Gastro-oesophageal reflux disease.

7

❻ 'Colic' – unsettled behaviour in the very alert infant.

TREATMENT

Avoidance of the offending antigens remains the mainstay of management.[3] In a breast-feeding mother, calcium supplementation may be required. When cows' milk reactions present early, supporting the mother to relactate may be an option.

Soy-protein formulas are as allergenic as cows' milk in some infants. At least 30% of infants with cows' milk allergy also demonstrate sensitivity to soy protein. Goats' milk shares antigens with cows' milk and is not an appropriate choice for cow-milk protein sensitivity. Cows' milk casein or whey hydrolysates, in which the proteins are significantly reduced in size, may be used but some highly allergic infants have reacted to these and so amino-acid-based formulas are recommended.[5] In children and breast-feeding mothers, major food groups should not be eliminated from the diet without checking for dietary sufficiency. The help of a paediatric dietitian should be sought.

About 50% of breast-fed infants who experience proctocolitis improve with removal of cows' milk from their mothers' diet. When an infant does not respond to an elimination diet in the mother, one must decide whether the symptoms are severe enough to warrant a change in the infant's diet to include a protein hydrolysate formula. Such symptoms may include anaemia and hypoproteinaemia.

PROGNOSIS

Most gastrointestinal manifestations resolve within three days of eliminating the offending nutrient, although some may take weeks (food-induced enteropathy). Resolution of symptoms from cows' milk or soy-protein hypersensitivity is common by one year of age. Of infants with food hypersensitivity to milk proteins 85% no longer have symptoms on food challenge by three years of age. When milk is reintroduced, only a teaspoon or less should be offered at first and then increased

CONTROVERSIES AND FUTURE DIRECTIONS

❶ Because of the lack of reliable diagnostic tests for non-IgE mediated allergy and because the symptoms of food reactions may all be evoked by many mechanisms, most areas pertaining to food reactions are controversial.

❷ The future lies in the identification of infants at risk of developing food reactions and the prevention of disease expression. This can be at the level of primary prevention (inhibiting the reaction), secondary prevention (inhibiting disease expression after the reaction), or tertiary prevention (suppressing symptoms despite disease onset). Strategies aimed at primary prevention will be aided by the identification of genes or genetic markers that would identify individuals at risk.

❸ Additional studies are needed to examine the role of maternal avoidance of food allergens during lactation as a preventive measure. There are currently no studies of good methodology comparing exclusive or partial breast feeding with other infant feeds in the prevention of food allergy or intolerance. Additional studies are needed to examine the role of maternal antigen avoidance during lactation as a preventative measure. Although using hydrolysed formulas in infants not receiving human milk, and avoiding the early introduction of solid foods has been shown to reduce the development of hypersensitivity reactions in high risk infants, large-scale long term studies are needed to determine the most effective strategies in preventing the development of early and late food sensitivity. In addition, new symptom complexes and disease states due to specific food reaction are likely to be described. With time other symptom complexes and disease states are likely to be described.

progressively over a few days if tolerated. Older children and adults may lose their sensitivity to an offending food when eliminated from the diet for one to two years. Symptoms from IgE-mediated allergy to peanuts, nuts, fish, or shellfish are less likely to resolve.

PREVENTION

Controlled trials of food-allergy prevention have been performed only in high allergic risk children. Decreased dietary exposure to allergenic proteins should diminish the risk of sensitisation in atopic families and mothers should be encouraged to follow the WHO recommendation of exclusive breast-feeding to six months and continued breast-feeding thereafter with the introduction of solids.[6,7] Cow-milk protein, soy and egg introduction should be delayed until after one year and peanut until after three years. Where human milk is not given, the use of hydrolysed formulas may prevent or delay an allergic reaction.[8–10]

Current evidence suggests that avoiding highly allergenic proteins during pregnancy is not effective. Antigen avoidance during early lactation is controversial.

A new approach to preventing infant allergic reactions is the use of probiotic therapy. Kalliomaki and colleagues reported success with giving *Lactobacillus* gammaglobulin to mothers and subsequently to infants with a strong family history of cows' milk protein allergy, in reducing the incidence and severity of allergic eczema in toddlers.[10] Confirmation of this finding, and information on whether *Lactobacillus* gammaglobulin or other species of *Lactobacillus* are effective and the best means of administration, is awaited.[12]

REFERENCES

1. Heitlinger LA, Rossi TM, Lee PC, Lebenthal E 1991 Human intestinal disaccharidase activities: correlations with age, biopsy technique, and degree of villus atrophy. Journal of Paediatric Gastroenterology & Nutrition 12(2): 204–208
2. Iacono G, Cavataio F, Montalto G, Soresi M, Notarbartolo A, Carroccio A 1998 Persistent cows' milk protein intolerance in infants: the changing

faces of the same disease. Clinical & Experimental Allergy 28(7): 817–823

3. Host A, Koletzko B, Dreborg S, Muraro A, Wahn U, Aggett P, Bresson J-L, Hernell O, Lafeber H, Michaelsen KF, Micheli J-L, Rigo J, Weaver L, Heymans H, Strobel S, Vandenplas Y 1999 Dietary products used in infants for treatment and prevention of food allergy. Joint statement of the European society for paediatric allergology and clinical immunology (ESPACI) committee on hypoallergenic formulas and the European society for paediatric gastroenterology, hepatology and nutrition (ESPGHAN) committee on nutrition. Archives of Disease in Childhood 81(1): 80–84

4. Niggemann B, Binder C, Dupont C, Hadji S, Arvola T, Isolauri E 2001 Prospective, controlled, multi-center study on the effect of an amino-acid-based formula in infants with cows' milk allergy/intolerance and atopic dermatitis. Paediatric Allergy & Immunology 12(2): 78–82

5. Kramer MS, Kakuma R 2003 Optimal duration of exclusive breastfeeding. The Cochrane Database of Systematic Reviews 1 John Wiley and Sons, Chichester, UK

6. Committee on Nutrition, American Academy of Paediatrics 2000 Hypoallergenic infant formulas. Paediatrics 106: 346–349

7. Ram FSF, Ducharme FM, Scarlett J 2002 Cows' milk protein avoidance and development of childhood wheeze in children with a family history of atopy. The Cochrane Database of Systematic Reviews 4 John Wiley and Sons, Chichester, UK

8. Sinn J, Osborn D 2003 Hydrolysed formula for prevention of allergy and food intolerance in infants. The Cochrane Database of Systematic Reviews 1 John Wiley and Sons, Chichester, UK

9. Sinn J, Osborn D 2003 Soy formula for prevention of allergy and food intolerance in infants. The Cochrane Database of Systematic Reviews 1 John Wiley and Sons, Chichester, UK

10. Kalliomaki M, Salminen S, Arvilommi H, Kero P, Koskinen P, Isolauri E 2001 Probiotics in primary prevention of atopic disease: a randomised placebo-controlled trial. Lancet 357(9262): 1076–1079

11. Cross ML, Gill HS 2001 Can immunoregulatory lactic acid bacteria be used as dietary supplements to limit allergies? International Archives of Allergy & Immunology 125(2): 112–119 [Review; 75 refs]

12. The optimal duration of exclusive breastfeeding 2001 Results of a WHO systematic review. http://www.who.int/inf-pr-2001/en/note2001-07.html

FURTHER READING

Chelimsky G, Czinn SJ 2001 Techniques for the evaluation of dyspepsia in children. Journal of Clinical Gastroenterology 33(1): 11–13

Dietary Guidelines for Children and Adolescents in Australia. Endorsed 10 April 2003. http://www.health.gov.au/nhmrc/publications/pdf/n34.pdf

Hill DJ, Hosking CS, Heine RG 1999 Clinical spectrum of food allergy in children in Australia and South-East Asia: identification and targets for treatment. Annals of Medicine 31(4): 272–281

Host A, Halken S, Jacobsen HP, Christensen AE, Herskind AM, Plesner K 2002 Clinical course of cows' milk protein allergy and atopic diseases in childhood. Paediatric Allergy & Immunology 13(15 Suppl): 23–28

Iacono G, Carroccio A, Cavataio F et al 1995 Chronic constipation as a symptom of cow milk allergy. Journal of Paediatrics 126: 34–39

Olsen WA, Li BUK, Lloyd M, Korsmo H 1996 Heterogeneity of intestinal lactase activity in children: relationship to lactase-phlorizin hydrolase messenger RNA abundance. Paediatric Research 39(5): 877–881

7.7 INGESTED FOREIGN BODIES

SCOTT PEARSON

Essentials

1 Foreign bodies in the stomach or intestines are expected to pass spontaneously about 99% of the time if the child has normal anatomy.

2 Most complications occur when a foreign body is lodged in the oesophagus but a significant number of these will pass spontaneously.

3 Children who ingest a metallic foreign body and attend an ED should have X-ray localisation of the object.

4 Removal of disc batteries lodged in the oesophagus should occur urgently as mucosal injury can occur within a few hours.

INTRODUCTION

Ingestion of foreign (non-food) material is common in early childhood and often goes undetected whilst the child is playing and does not prompt a physician visit. The exact frequency of reported foreign body ingestions varies. An estimate can be obtained from Poison Centre data. There were 77 763 foreign-body ingestions reported to regional poison control centres in the United States in 2000.[1] The literature in this field can be divided into a few areas: descriptive studies of fairly large numbers of ingestion cases; studies primarily or exclusively about coin ingestion; and studies about disc batteries.[2] Common foreign bodies ingested that come to medical attention include coins, bones (fish, chicken), other metallic objects (pins, screws, keys, batteries), and plastic and rubber foreign bodies. In one large series of 1265 reported cases of foreign-body ingestions, age ranged from seven months to sixteen years with a mean of 5.2 years.[3] Most foreign bodies pass through the gastrointestinal tract without complications. The emergency physician should be aware of the few instances when emergent or semi-urgent intervention is indicated. Parents need to have clear guidelines regarding the treatment plan for children who are discharged to out-patient follow-up.

HISTORY

In most instances, a thorough history can be obtained from parents or caregivers before a requirement for intervention. The nature of the ingested item is obviously imperative, as is the time of ingestion. The ingestion may have been witnessed or may have been reported (by an older child) or implied by the child's environment at the onset of symptomatology. It can be extremely useful if a replica of the foreign body can be easily obtained, especially in determining the type and size of disc batteries. Determining the immediate environment of the child at the time of ingestion can assist in revealing any likely co-ingestants.

The symptoms experienced by the child since ingestion helps determine likely site of the foreign body but has limitations. Many children are asymptomatic at presentation, which usually (but not always) suggests that the foreign body is lying in the stomach or more distal part of the gastrointestinal tract. Symptoms of vomiting, pain or discomfort on swallowing, drooling, irritability and refusal to take food or fluids may occur and suggest oesophageal foreign body. It should be remembered that several reports note that some children will be asymptomatic with foreign bodies lodged in the oesophagus, especially the distal oesophagus.[4,5] Even in the context of sharp fishbones, a prospective study found that symptoms were a poor predictor of the presence of fishbones, except for a sharp pricking sensation on swallowing.[6] Reports of abdominal pain or blood in the bowel motions should be noted. A history of previous oesophageal or other gastrointestinal disease is significant in determining a management plan and alerting one to potential complications. Significant developmental/intellectual delay has been associated with major morbidity and mortality after foreign body ingestion.[3,7] This is often due to the vague symptomatology and delay in presentation.

EXAMINATION

For the majority of children the foreign body will have negotiated the oesophagus and general examination will be unremarkable. Vital signs should be recorded but once again are unlikely to be abnormal unless there is delayed presentation and the development of a complication.

Palpation of the abdomen will usually be normal. If the history alerts one to abdominal symptoms, the examiner may find localised tenderness or peritonism suggestive of intestinal perforation. This is rare.

Some children will have symptoms of proximal oesophageal or pharyngeal foreign body. In the older child or adolescent where this is due to bony ingestion (e.g. fish or chicken) there should be a careful examination of the oral cavity and pharynx by either indirect or direct layngoscopy. Younger children are unlikely to co-operate with these procedures.

INVESTIGATIONS

All children with a history of ingestion of coins or batteries (or other radio-opaque foreign bodies) should have an X-ray performed to localise the foreign body. There is some controversy on this issue in relation to the need for X-rays in children who have ingested coins. Some authors (mainly hospital-based) note that even previously healthy children can be asymptomatic with an oesophageal coin and advocate early removal of oesophageal coins to prevent serious sequelae.[4,5] Other authors (notably in primary care) believe that routine X-rays in children having ingested a coin are unnecessary given that asymptomatic coin ingestion is rarely if ever associated with complications in otherwise healthy children.[9] It has been recognised that those patients presenting to an ED are a selected group and would be expected to have greater severity of symptoms and higher frequency of complications.[10] Hence the recommendation that all children with a history of coin ingestion *who attend* an ED, should have X-ray localisation of the coin performed. If the ingestion is unwitnessed and the object looks like a coin on anteroposterior X-ray, be aware that a disc battery may have a similar appearance. In this situation, an additional lateral view will reveal an asymmetry, as the two sides of the disc battery are slightly different diameters. On the anteroposterior view one may also see the 'double ring' of both circumferences of the battery. Hand-held metal detectors may be an alternative where this equipment is available and emergency practitioners are experienced in its use.[8] However, the ready availability of plain X-rays, the ease of obtaining an X-ray (even in an unco-operative child) and the additional information obtained about the exact location and nature of the foreign body may explain why hand-held metal detectors are not more widely used.[2]

TREATMENT

Coins

Coins that reach the stomach almost always pass through the gastrointestinal tract without incident and further management is unnecessary unless symptoms arise. Coins that lodge in the oesophagus and have been unrecognised can cause complications such as oesophageal perforation, mediastinitis, acquired tracheo-oesophageal or aorto-oesophageal fistula formation – and death has been reported.[11] All children who are symptomatic should have a procedure to remove the coin. Asymptomatic children with proximal or middle-oesophageal coins should also have the coin removed as it is unlikely to pass spontaneously (20–30% in one series).[4] If there is a significant delay before the procedure (of more than a few hours) the X-ray should be repeated to ensure that spontaneous passage into the stomach has not occurred. Asymptomatic children with distal oesophageal coins can safely be observed as out-patients (depending on social circumstances) for 12–24 hours. The chance of spontaneous passage into the stomach has been reported to occur in 37–60% of patients.[4,5]

Glucagon has been found to be ineffective when studied prospectively in the management of oesophageal coins. Children should be referred to a specialist with expertise in paediatric endoscopy for endoscopic removal under appropriate sedation or anaesthesia. This may require transfer of the child to another institution as local resources dictate. Other techniques have been described such as oesophageal bougienage or Foley catheter extraction but most emergency physicians will not manage sufficient children with this problem to develop expertise.

Disc batteries

Disc batteries are used for hearing aids, electronic devices and children's toys and cause tissue destruction due to their alkaline nature when in contact with moist membranes. Two deaths have been reported in the literature in situations of oesophageal batteries in children with delayed presentations.[12] Children with a history of possible ingestion of a disc battery should have an urgent X-ray performed. If the battery is lodged in the oesophagus, removal should be performed on an emergent basis because mucosal injury can occur in a few hours. Litovitz and Schmitz studied 2382 cases of battery ingestion over seven years (97% were disc batteries) that were reported to a national registry.[13] There were only two major adverse outcomes, both occurring in children with oesophageal batteries.

There were no deaths. There were 16 children with oesophageal disc batteries. In 88.3% the battery passed through the gastrointestinal tract with no symptoms or minor symptoms only. In 8.4% there were unrelated or unknown symptoms. As few as 3.1% of patients suffered moderate symptoms (defined as more pronounced or multiple episodes of nausea, vomiting, fever, bloody stools or emesis or changes in vital signs). Forty-four patients had arrested transit defined as identical non-oesophageal site on successive X-rays 48 hours apart: seventeen in stomach; two in small intestine; sixteen in the colon; and in nine at unidentified sites. Although more patients had minor or moderate symptoms in this group, none had major adverse effects. Outcome was more severe when there was arrested transit in the stomach. Battery transit time was known for 1366 patients. For the great majority (86.4%) the battery passed through the gastrointestinal tract in 96 hours.

Recommendations for ingested disc batteries are:

- All oesophageal batteries to be removed urgently by endoscopy.
- Asymptomatic children with subdiaphragmatic batteries can be observed at home with appropriate instructions to return if symptoms develop. It would seem reasonable to repeat an X-ray at four days and thereafter as required to detect the small group where arrested transit has occurred.
- Symptomatic children with subdiaphragmatic batteries should have surgical consultation to consider surgical or endoscopic removal of the battery particularly if the battery case has split open or is not progressing along the gastrointestinal tract on sequential X-rays.[2]

Other metallic foreign bodies

Foreign bodies should be localised by X-ray and removed if lodged in the oesophagus. Other objects, including pins, needles and other sharp objects can be safely observed on an out-patient basis with intervention occurring only if symptoms develop. In certain situations, where the object is lodged in the stomach, it may be appropriate to repeat an X-ray to ensure passage into the intestine. In many situations repeat X-rays are unnecessary unless symptoms develop.

Non-metallic foreign bodies

Sharp foreign material such as fish or chicken bones will usually impact in the pharynx or oral cavity and are considered elsewhere. X-rays may assist in localisation but many foreign bodies are not radio-opaque. Intervention is dictated by the presence or persistence of symptoms. The vast majority of other objects pass through uneventfully. Plastic bread-bag tags have been associated with small bowel obstruction and perforation. If there are symptoms of lodgement in the oesophagus the foreign body should be removed by gastroscopy, otherwise an observant approach is adequate, with the parents or caregiver receiving clear advice on when to return to the hospital.

DISPOSITION

Most children will be managed in the ED and discharged. Some will be asked to return for further X-ray imaging but many will be advised to return only if symptoms or complications develop. Where admission is required this should be to a facility that is skilled in the endoscopic and surgical management of these children.

PREVENTION

Together with child-proofing the home to ensure that children are protected from access to potential poisons, this should extend to protection from small items that pre-school-age children can ingest. Great care should be exercised in relation to disc (button) batteries.

REFERENCES

1. Litovitz TL, Klein-Schwartz W, White S et al 2001 2000 Annual Report of the American Association of Poison Control Centers Toxic Exposure Surveillance System. American Journal of Emergency Medicine 19: 337–395
2. Brown L, Dannenberg B 2002 A literature-based approach to the identification and management of paediatric foreign bodies. Paediatric Emergency Medicine Reports 7: 19
3. Cheng W, Tam PKH 1999 Foreign body ingestion in children: experience with 1265 cases. Journal of Paediatric Surgery 34: 1472–1476
4. Soprano JV, Fleisher GR, Mandl KD 1999 The spontaneous passage of esophageal coins in children. Archives of Paediatric Adolescent Medicine 153: 1073–1076
5. Connors GP, Chamberlain JM, Ochsenschlager DW 1995 Symptoms and spontaneous passage of esophageal coins. Archives of Paediatric Adolescent Medicine 149: 36–39
6. Ngan JH, Fok PJ, Lai EC et al 1990 A prospective study on fishbone ingestion. Experience of 358 patients. Annals of Surgery 211: 459–462
7. Gilchrist BF, Valerie EP, Nguyen M et al 1977 Pearls and perils in the management of prolonged, peculiar penetrating esophageal foreign bodies in children. Journal of Paediatric Surgery 32: 1429–1431
8. Seikel K, Primm PA, Elizondo BJ et al 1999 Handheld metal detector localisation of ingested metallic foreign bodies. Archives of Paediatric Adolescent Medicine 153: 853–857
9. Connors GP, Chamberlain JM, Weiner PR 1995 Paediatric coin ingestion: a home based survey. American Journal of Emergency Medicine 13: 638–640
10. Paul RI, Christoffel KK, Binns HJ et al 1993 Foreign body ingestions in children: risk of complication varies with site of initial health care contact. Paediatrics 91: 121–127
11. Byard RW, Moore L, Bourne AJ 1990 Sudden and unexpected death: a late effect of occult intraesophageal foreign body. Paediatric Pathology 10: 837–841
12. Blatnik DS, Toohill RJ, Lehman RH 1977 Fatal complication from an alkaline battery foreign body in the esophagus. Annals of Otology Rhinology and Laryngology 86: 611–615
13. Litovitz T, Schmitz BF 1992 Ingestion of cylindrical and button batteries: an analysis of 2382 cases. Paediatrics 89: 747–757

CONTROVERSIES

❶ Methods of removal of oesophageal coins/batteries. There are some advocates of Foley catheter removal or oesophageal bougienage by emergency physicans or surgeons. Most centres utilise endoscopic removal by trained endoscopists.

❷ Hand-held metal detectors are a useful adjunct. However, more information can be obtained by X-ray examination, such as the exact location and number of foreign bodies.

7.8 HEPATIC FAILURE

DAVID KRIESER

Essentials

1 Acute liver failure implies evidence of hepatocellular failure and the presence of encephalopathy.

2 Acute liver failure is a rare but serious problem in the paediatric population.

3 Many aetiologies require consideration: infectious, toxin-mediated, congenital (structural or metabolic) or infiltrative (malignancy, storage disease).

4 Infectious hepatitis is the most common cause worldwide, paracetamol toxicity the most common in the developed world.

5 Clinical information is vital to target appropriate investigation and treatment.

6 Management is largely supportive and aims to maintain homeostasis until hepatic recovery or transplantation occurs.

7 Liason with and transport to a paediatric liver transplantation centre is usually required and should occur early.

INTRODUCTION

Acute liver failure (ALF) is a rare but devastating presentation in children. The major functions of the liver include coagulation, glucose metabolism, waste-product processing (bilirubin, nitrogenous compounds, drug elimination) and protein synthesis. ALF in children may be due to many causes (Table 7.8.1). However, the manifestations of coagulopathy, hypoglycaemia, jaundice, encephalopathy and hypoalbuminaemia, reflect common disturbances of liver function.[1] ALF may be an immediate life-threatening process or a subacute process, with a spectrum of severity between those extremes. Medical management is multifaceted and focuses on supporting vital functions while hepatic recovery occurs or liver transplantation can be performed.

Clinical and laboratory criteria lead to a diagnosis of ALF. Two criteria define ALF:

- 1. Hepatocellular dysfunction (jaundice, coagulopathy, etc.) of rapid onset, and
- 2. Encephalopathy.

Some definitions include the absence of preceding liver disease. There are, however, children with chronic liver disease who present with features of ALF. The management of such children does not differ significantly unless there are specific treatments for the underlying disease. The time interval between the onset of jaundice and the onset of encephalopathy allows classification of ALF into three groups (Table 7.8.2). This classification has aetiological and prognostic importance. O'Grady et al[2,3] and Poddar et al[4] found that, in comparison with patients suffering acute or subacute liver failure, those with hyperacute liver failure had a better prognosis.

AETIOLOGY

Table 7.8.1 demonstrates the variety of diagnoses that may cause ALF in children. The aetiology can be grouped according to onset prior or after the first year of life.

Neonates and infants

In the neonatal population, the estimated incidence of liver disease is approximately 1:2500. Biliary atresia and neonatal idiopathic hepatitis contribute 60% of all cases of cholestasis. In 80 infants under 12 months with ALF, inherited metabolic conditions were responsible for 42.5% of cases; neonatal haemochromatosis 16%, acute viral hepatitis 15%, miscellaneous causes (toxins, autoimmune, malignancy) 10% and 16% were undetermined.[5] Metabolic causes of liver failure include: disorders of the mitochondrial electron transport chain; disorders of protein, carbohydrate and lipid metabolism; and inherited causes of cholestasis.

Infectious hepatitis

Worldwide, this is the greatest cause of ALF. Five RNA viruses (hepatitis A, C, D, E and G) and one DNA virus (hepatitis B) can infect the liver. Transmission of A and E is via the faecal-oral route. The remainder are transmitted via body fluids. Acute viral hepatitis is a clinical syndrome with systemic symptoms occurring after a virus-dependent incubation period. Jaundice ensues after hepatocyte necrosis reduces the liver's capacity to metabolise bilirubin. Fulminant hepatitis occurs in less than 1% of children with hepatitis A and in 1–2% of cases of hepatitis B. Fulminant disease occurs with hepatitis D in approximately 10% of cases and is more likely with superinfection. Hepatitis C can cause acute and chronic infection and rarely fulminant hepatitis.

Toxins and medication
Paracetamol

Paracetamol toxicity is the most common cause of ALF in the developed world. Paracetamol is an analgesic and antipyretic freely available in many countries. It is metabolised by the hepatocyte and toxicity exhausts hepatic glutathione stores. Generation of toxic metabolites leads to centrilobular necrosis. Toxicity is unlikely with single doses under 150 mg kg^{-1}. Children are often given multiple doses of paracetamol and this can lead to toxicity if the cumulative daily dose is greater than 60 mg kg^{-1} day^{-1}. Treatment of toxicity is discussed in the toxicology chapter.

Table 7.8.1   Aetiology of liver failure

Neonates and infants		Older children	
Cholestasis	Biliary atresia	**Infection: viral**	Hepatitis A–D
	Choldedochal cyst		Enteroviruses
	Intra-hepatic bile duct paucity (Alagille syndrome)		EBV
	Inspissated bile syndrome		Varicella
Idiopathic neonatal hepatitis			Adenovirus
Cystic fibrosis			CMV
Endocrine	Hypopituitarism		Herpes simplex
	Hypothyroidism		Rubella
Neonatal		**Infection: bacterial**	Listeria
haemochromatosis			Tuberculosis
Infection: viral	CMV		
	Herpes simplex	**Infection: parasitic**	Toxoplasma
	virus/HHV 6/VZV		
	EBV	**Toxins and drugs**	
	Parvovirus	**Malignancy**	Leukemic infiltration
	Rubella		Lymphoma
	Reovirus type 3		Neuroblastomaa
	Adenovirus		Primary hepatic
	Enterovirus		tumours
Infection: bacterial	Bacterial sepsis	**Wilson disease**	
	Urinary tract infection	**Hepatic venous occlusion**	
	Tuberculosis	**Fatty liver**	Obesity
	Syphilis		Pregnancy
Infection: parasitic	Toxoplasma	**Hepatic hypoperfusion**	Cardiogenic shock
Metabolic disease	Peroxisome function abnormality (Zellweger's)		Hypovolemic shock
	α1-Antitrypsin deficiency		Septic shock
	Bile acid metabolism		
	Urea cycle abnormalities		
	Amino acid metabolism abnormalities		
	Lipid metabolism abnormalities (Gaucher, Wolman, Niemann Pick C)		
	Carbohydrate metabolism abnormalities (galactosaemia, fructosaemia, type IV glycogen storage disease)		
Toxins	Paracetamol		
	TPN		
	Hypervitaminosis A		
Tumour	Intra- and extra-hepatic		

Source: Modified from D'Agata ID, Balistreri WF 1999 Paediatrics in Review 20(11): 376–389.

Table 7.8.2   Classification of ALF

Interval between onset of jaundice and encephalopathy	Classification
7 days or less	Hyperacute
8 to 28 days	Acute
5 to 12 weeks	Subacute

Anticonvulsants

Sodium valproate causes intracellular fat accumulation within the hepatocyte. Impaired metabolic functions within the cell may lead to necrosis. Children under two years and those on multiple medications are at highest risk. Carbamazepine may cause hepatitis and/or cholestasis during the first months of therapy. Clinically significant hepatotoxicity is rare.

Total parenteral nutrition

The aetiology of TPN-associated liver disease is largely unknown. The associations of sepsis, surgery, and other medications, which often co-exist, cannot be ignored as possible aetiological agents. This form of liver dysfunction will present in the intensive-care setting rather than the ED.

Aspirin and Reye's syndrome

Mitochondrial dysfunction leading to acute encephalopathy, selective hepatic dysfunction and visceral fatty infiltration has been called Reye's syndrome.[6] A number of children initially diagnosed with Reye's syndrome have subsequently had metabolic disorders identified. Mitochondrial oxidative phosphorylation and fatty acid β-oxidation are the metabolic pathways affected in Reye's syndrome. Preceding viral infection (classically varicella), immune mediators and aspirin (or its metabolites) all can limit normal functioning of these pathways. The association of aspirin with this disorder remains unclear despite a study by Forsyth et al,[7] which identified a dose–response relationship, and population studies that demonstrate that the decline in Reye's syndrome mirrors a decline in aspirin usage.[6,8]

Zellweger's syndrome (cerebrohepatorenal syndrome)

Autosomal recessive inheritance of this peroxisomal abnormality leads to abnormal bile acid synthesis, and abnormal fatty-acid oxidation. Failure to thrive, due to feeding difficulties and multi-organ impairment (brain, liver and kidneys), occurs with hypotonia. Jaundice occurs in 50% of cases. Therapy has not been shown to prolong life although histological improvement may occur on liver biopsy. Biopsy demonstrates abnormal mitochondria and absent peroxisomes.

α1-Antitrypsin deficiency

Approximately 1:4000 live births are affected by this autosomal recessive disorder. Cholestasis in the neonatal period, in the context of intra-uterine growth retardation, hepatomegaly and failure to thrive is suggestive of this disease. Coagulopathy may occur in 2% of such infants and is usually responsive to vitamin K. Phenotyping of protease inhibitor (Pi) by isoelectric focus classifies children as: Pi ZZ (most commonly associated with liver disease), Pi SZ, Pi SS, Pi FZ and MZ (carrier state). Up to 50% of children with Pi ZZ will develop chronic hepatic failure leading to transplantation after development of cirrhosis. Bronchiectasis is rare in children. Liver transplantation will lead to functional restoration and phenotypic cure.

Tyrosinaemia

Deficiency of fumarylaceto acetase leads to this autosomal recessive disorder that is characterised by progressive liver parenchymal damage and renal tubulopathy with generalised aminoaciduria. Rapid progression may occur in infancy or an indolent course leading to hepatic cell carcinoma may occur.

Galactosaemia

Occurring in approximately 1 in 40 000 live births, and inherited in an autosomal recessive fashion, this deficiency of galactose-1-phosphate uridyl-transferase leads to accumulation of galactose-1-phosphate in liver, brain and renal tubules.

Clinically these infants may present with progressive jaundice, hepatic failure, hypoglycaemia or cataracts. Multifactorial encephalopathy (hypoglycaemia, liver failure) may be present. These babies have an increased susceptibility to sepsis, especially due to Gram-negative organisms. This disorder is part of the routine newborn screening programme and prenatal diagnosis is available via chorionic villus sampling.

Wilson's disease

An autosomal recessive gene defect leads to this disorder of copper metabolism that occurs in 1:30 000 live births. Symptoms include: hepatic dysfunction (ALF, chronic active liver disease, insidious progression to cirrhosis), neuropsychiatric symptoms (behavioural disturbance, tremor, dysarthria, drooling and deteriorating school performance) renal tubulopathy, haemolysis and hormonal changes. Kayser–Fleischer rings are brown bands seen at the cornea–iris border.

Alagille syndrome

This autosomal dominant condition leads to intra-hepatic biliary hypoplasia in association with cardiac, renal, ocular, facial, and skeletal abnormalities. Alagille syndrome has an incidence of 1:100 000 live births. Peripheral pulmonary arterial stenosis, with or without pulmonary valvular stenosis, is the most common cardiac defect. Vertebral anomalies described as 'butterfly vertebrae' constitute the most common skeletal defect. Retinal pigmentation and posterior embryotoxon (requiring slit lamp examination) are present in the eye. The facies are 'triangular' with a broad forehead and a pointed mandible. Failure to thrive and jaundice are common presentations. Hepatic cirrhosis can develop in up to 50% of children.

Biliary atresia

Complete absence of all extra-hepatic biliary structures is the usual malformation leading to a clinical picture of jaundice, pale (acholic) stools and dark urine due to cholestasis. A choledochal cyst may present in identical fashion and may co-exist with biliary atresia. Presentation

is usually with prolonged neonatal jaundice or delayed onset of jaundice (age 2–3 weeks). This occurs in approximately 1:10 000 live births with equal gender incidence. Following diagnostic testing (ultrasonography, nuclear medicine scan, occasionally liver biopsy), management is by surgical hepatoportoenterostomy (Kasai procedure) prior to eight weeks of age, if possible.

Mushrooms

Edible and inedible mushrooms can be difficult to distinguish. *Amanita phalloides* produces amatoxin, which is hepatotoxic. The toxin is a heat stable octapeptide. After a period of 6–48 hours the affected patient will start vomiting, complain of abdominal pain, develop diarrhoea, before neurological symptoms (coma, seizures) and hepatic failure commence. Cholinergic symptoms via muscarinic receptors may also occur and respond to atropine. Charcoal should be given to reduce absorption. Identification of the mushroom is important and may require referral to local botanists or mycologists.

PATHOPHYSIOLOGY

Exposure to hepatotoxic agents be they drugs, products of metabolism or infectious particles, initiates hepatocyte injury that may progress to necrosis. Liver failure ensues when normal regenerative processes fail. Hepatic encephalopathy occurs through the interplay of three factors:

❶ Reduction in synthesis of substances essential for normal brain function;

❷ Production of substances that are neurotoxic; and

❸ Reduced elimination of neurotoxins.

Neuronal dysfunction and altered interaction of astrocytes with neurons, in the context of hepatic failure, both contribute to the development of hepatic encephalopathy. The balance of inhibitory (e.g. GABA) versus excitatory (e.g. glutamate) neurotransmission is altered in hepatic encephalopathy.[9] Ammonia appears to augment inhibitory neurotransmission. In addition, the role of sepsis, hypoglycaemia and raised intracranial pressure may contribute to the development of encephalopathy.

PRESENTATION

History

History and examination findings are significantly influenced by the age of the child. Neonates may present with jaundice and care must be taken to differentiate physiological jaundice or 'breast milk' jaundice from pathological jaundice. The presence of acholic (pale) stools is characteristic of cholestasis. Investigation (see below) will be directed at identifying the cause of cholestasis. Jaundice in the context of dysmorphic features, cardiac murmur and ocular abnormalities suggest Alagille syndrome. The development of jaundice after a change in diet may suggest metabolic abnormalities of carbohydrate metabolism such as galactosaemia or hereditary fructose intolerance.

Infants and older children may present with a history of loss of appetite, vomiting, fevers, or abdominal pain, prior to the development of jaundice. Infectious hepatitis is the most likely cause in this situation. Hepatitis A, EBV or CMV being potential candidates. EBV infection may be suggested by a history of sore throat and lymphadenopathy. A dietary and travel history for hepatitis A may be relevant. Hepatitis B and C infection needs to be considered if a history of exposure is obtained. In adolescents the use of illicit drugs and sexual activity must be explored confidentially. In areas where strict screening is performed, children who receive blood product transfusions (e.g. malignancy, renal failure, haemophilia, haemoglobinopathy) are at very low risk for the acquisition of hepatitis B and C. An infant presenting with encephalopathy and jaundice may have a metabolic disease (fatty acid oxidation, carbohydrate metabolism) and the possibility of consanguinity needs exploration. Previous surgery for a choledochal cyst or for biliary atresia is important in the context of a child presenting with jaundice and/or hepatic failure. Exposure to hepatotoxins such as paracetamol, anticonvulsants, aspirin or mushrooms must be identified, as specific treatments can be implemented. Pruritus with jaundice, dark urine and pale stools may be the presenting features of cholestasis in an older child.

Examination

Hepatomegaly and jaundice are the most frequent findings. The character of the liver edge may offer additional information: for example a firm, nodular surface suggesting cirrhosis or fibrosis; tenderness suggesting acute hepatitis. Note that in cirrhosis liver span may be reduced. Splenomegaly suggests portal hypertension or infiltration (e.g. storage disease, extramedullary haematopoiesis, malignancy). Abdominal examination will also identify ascites if present.

As discussed above, specific diseases associated with liver failure will have other features. The phenotypes of galactosaemia, Alagille syndrome, α_1-antitrypsin deficiency and Wilson's disease may be identified by careful clinical examination. Neurological evaluation is essential and the presence of asterixis important in a child with liver failure in order to assess for hepatic encephalopathy (see Table 7.8.3). Encephalopathy may be difficult to assess in children and occurs late. Cutaneous features such as bruising, petechiae or bleeding may indicate an associated coagulopathy. In children with chronic liver disease there may be signs such as spider naevi, caput medusae or finger clubbing.

INVESTIGATIONS

Investigation of the child with hepatic failure focuses on identifying the extent of liver dysfunction and on identifying the cause. History and examination findings must guide investigation. ED screen should include FBE, LFTs including conjugated and unconjugated bilirubin, BGL, coagulation screen, renal function and ABGs. Further potentially relevant investigations such as viral serology, copper and caeruloplasmin levels, Pi typing, lactate level, drug screens, urine metabolic screen, or imaging should be determined after discussion with a paediatric hepatologist.

MANAGEMENT

The management of acute liver failure involves supportive care, complication management and specific treatment modalities

Table 7.8.3	Stages of HE					
	I	II	III	IV	
				IV a	IV b
Symptoms	Lethargy, euphoria, poor concentration	Drowsiness, erratic behaviour, disorientation	Stuporous but rousable, incoherent speech	Responsive to pain	No response
Signs	Reduced cognitive performance (drawing figures, memory)	Asterixis, incontinence, fetor hepaticus	Asterixis, hyper reflexia, rigidity	No asterixis, areflexia, flaccidity	
EEG	Normal	Generalised slowing, theta waves	Markedly abnormal, triphasic waves	Markedly abnormal bilateral slowing, delta waves, cortical silence	

Source: Modified from Suchy FJ 2000 Fulminant hepatic failure. In Behrman RE (ed) Nelson Textbook of Pediatrics, 16 edn.

where they exist. Therapy needs to be initiated in the ED prior to transfer to a paediatric intensive-care environment. The initial management issues are listed in Table 7.8.4. Intubation and ventilation may be required due to coma or respiratory failure. Respiratory failure itself is multifactorial: altered cardiac output; capillary leak; possible oliguria; and significant fluid requirements contribute. Fluid management may be complex in the face of renal failure and electrolyte imbalances. Vitamin K, fresh frozen plasma or cryoprecipitate may be required to correct symptomatic coagulopathy. Intravenous fluids containing 10% dextrose or more are usually required to correct hypoglycaemia and then maintain normoglycaemia. Lactulose is given in hepatic encephalopathy to reduce absorption of nitrogenous wastes. Neomycin and/or metronidazole, given enterally, reduce the enteric bacterial load and the production of nitrogenous wastes. Proton pump inhibitors, H_2-receptor blockers and/or sucralfate are given to limit the risk of gastric ulceration in the context of coagulopathy. Sepsis is a common and serious complication in liver failure and requires aggressive antimicrobial management.

The development of liver transplantation has allowed children with irreversible liver failure to survive. The paucity of available donors and contraindications to transplantation limit the number of children able to receive liver transplants in the acute setting. Contraindications to transplantation include: septicaemia; irreversible neurological injury; and multiorgan failure. Disease-specific treatment is available for paracetamol toxicity. Intravenous N-acetylcysteine (NAC) is given in addition to supportive measures. Herpes virus induced fulminant hepatitis may respond to aciclovir. Children with Wilson's disease may respond to chelation therapy pending transplantation. Certain metabolic diseases can be managed through dietary manipulation or metabolic pathway manipulation.

DISPOSITION

Management of the child with ALF requires a multidisciplinary team of physicians, nursing staff and allied health personnel in an intensive-care environment. The invasive nature of monitoring and maintaining such patients will necessitate transport to a paediatric intensive-care unit. Transportation will require stabilisation and continued monitoring of the above parameters, with intervention occurring en route if necessary. Liver transplantation will require the involvement of surgeons and anaesthetists in addition to those already involved within the PICU. The transplant service should be consulted early in such cases.

PROGNOSIS

The mortality of ALF is approximately 60%. Of children with Stage 4 hepatic encephalopathy, 80% will die. Sepsis is the cause of death in approximately 10% of children with ALF. The Kings' College criteria (see Table 7.8.5), based on multivariate analysis of 588 patients with fulminant hepatic failure, provide clinical and laboratory parameters predictive of mortality. A single adverse factor was associated with 80% mortality; three adverse factors were associated with 95% mortality. Paracetamol toxicity was associated with a better prognosis. If paracetamol toxicity was the reason for ALF then the presence of a single adverse risk factor places mortality risk at 55%. It is important to compare these figures with the 20–30% mortality rate of children undergoing liver transplantation.

Table 7.8.4 Initial management tasks	
Management tasks	
Observation of:	Vital signs Pulse oximetry Level of consciousness Urine output (may need indwelling catheter)
Monitoring of:	ECG Blood glucose Acid/base status (blood gases) Coagulation Liver function tests Serum electrolytes
Insertion of:	Vascular access (peripheral, central, intraosseous) Nasogastric tube (for gastric drainage and administration of neomycin and lactulose)
Supplementation of:	Glucose Potassium Albumin Coagulation factors (vitamin K, frozen plasma, cryoprecipitate, platelets) Oxygen (may require endotracheal intubation) Intravascular volume if required
Identification of:	Treatable cause if present (toxic, infectious, metabolic) Evolving encephalopathy Raised intracranial pressure

Table 7.8.5 The King's College criteria
Features associated with a poor prognosis
• Unknown aetiology • Toxin associated (other than paracetamol) • Age under 10 years • Age over 40 years • Jaundice for more than one week prior to encephalopathy • Serum bilirubin over 300 µmol L^{-1} • International normalised ratio over 3.5 • pH less than 7.3 • Serum creatinine over 300 µmol/L

Source: Data from O'Grady et al 1989 *Gastroenterology* 97: 439–445.

CONTROVERSIES AND FUTURE DIRECTIONS

❶ Lactulose, while advocated by several centres, has not shown significant improvements in outcome and may cause unwanted fluid shifts.[10]

❷ Plasmapheresis and charcoal haemoperfusion may improve hepatic encephalopathy but not long-term outcome. Cultured hepatocytes grown on hollow fibres, acting as extra-corporeal liver assist devices, require more assessment.[11]

❸ Transplantation remains the gold standard therapy and case reports of auxiliary partial orthotopic liver transplantation demonstrated that a transplanted liver lobe functioned satisfactorily until native liver recovery occured in a case of mushroom toxicity.[12]

❹ Xenotransplantation, using transplanted or extra-corporeal porcine livers, has 'bought time' in a similar fashion while waiting for human donor or hepatic recovery.[13,14]

PREVENTION

Viral hepatitis requires public health and legislative intervention to be controlled. Immunisation against hepatitis A and B, improved hygiene, reduced over-crowding and the promotion of harm-minimisation through 'safe sex' and reduction in the sharing of needles among intravenous drug users may have impacts on the incidence of viral hepatitis. Vaccines for hepatitis A and B are available but expense and distribution problems act as barriers in the developing world.

The widespread availability of paracetamol contributes to its position as the leading cause of ALF in the developed world. Limiting packet size, 'child-proofed' containers and even reducing distribution to pharmacies alone may reduce the incidence of paracetamol poisoning.

Screening of embryos or parents after the identification of a metabolic disease will assist in reducing the incidence of such diseases, if parents consider termination of pregnancy an option. Genetic counselling is mandatory in such cases. Direct gene therapy for such diseases remains elusive.

REFERENCES

1. D'Agata ID, Balistreri WF 1999 Evaluation of liver disease in the pediatric patient. Paediatrics in Review 20(11): 376–389
2. O'Grady JG, Schalm SW, Williams R 1993 Acute liver failure: redefining the syndromes. Lancet 342(8866): 273–275
3. O'Grady JG, Alexander GJM, Hayllar KM, Williams R 1989 Early indicators of prognosis in fulminant hepatic failure. Gastroenterology 97: 439–445
4. Poddar U, Thapa BR, Prasad A, Sharma AK, Singh K 2002 Natural history and risk factors in fulminant hepatic failure. Archives of Disease in Childhood 87: 54–56
5. Durand P, Debray D, Mandel R, Baujard C, Branchereau S, Gauthier F et al 2001 Acute liver failure in infancy: a 14-year experience of a pediatric liver transplantation center. Journal of Paediatrics 139(6): 871–876
6. Glasgow JFT, Middleton B 2001 Reye syndrome – insights on causation and prognosis. Archives of Disease in Childhood 85: 351–353
7. Forsyth BW, Horwitz RI, Acampora D, Shapiro E, Viscoli C, Feinstein A et al 1989 New epidemiologic evidence confirming that bias does no explain the aspirin/Reye's syndrome association. Journal of the American Medical Association 261(17): 2517–2524
8. Belay ED, Bresee JS, Holman RC, Khan AS, Shahriari A, Schonberger LB 1999 Reye's syndrome in the United States from 1981 through 1997. New England Journal of Medicine 340(18): 1377–1382
9. Jones EA 2000 Pathogenesis of hepatic encephalopathy. Clinics in Liver Disease 4(2): 467–485
10. Yee HF, Lidofsky SD 1998 Fulminant hepatic failure. In: Feldman M, Scharschmidt MH, Klein S (eds) Sleisenger and Fordtran's gastrointestinal and liver disease: Pathophysiology, diagnosis and management, 6th edn. WB Saunders, Philadelphia, 1355–1363
11. Demetriou AA, Watanabe F, Rozga J 1995 Artificial hepatic support systems. In: Boyer JL, Ockner RK (eds) Progress in liver diseases. WB Saunders, Philadelphia, 331
12. Rosenthal P, Roberts JP, Ascher NL, Emond JC 1997 Auxiliary liver transplant in fulminant failure. Paediatrics 100(2): E10
13. Makowka L, Cramer DV, Hoffman A, Breda M, Sher L, Eiras-Hreha G et al 1995 The use of a pig liver xenograft for temporary support of a patient with fulminant hepatic failure. Transplantation 59(12): 1654–1659
14. Chari RS, Collins BH, Magee JC, DiMaio JM, Kirk AD, Harland RC et al 1994 Treatment of hepatic failure with ex vivo pig liver perfusion followed by liver transplantation. New England Journal of Medicine 331(4): 234–237

7.9 DIARRHOEA AND VOMITING

CHRISTOPHER WEBBER

ESSENTIALS

1 Remember ABC, fluids in and out!

2 Not all diarrhoea and vomiting is gastroenteritis.

3 Vomiting may be a non-specific symptom of a more serious medical problem.

4 The differential diagnoses are extensive.

5 Young infants must be managed with caution.

INTRODUCTION

Common symptoms

Vomiting and diarrhoea are common symptoms that affect infants and children. These symptoms may occur separately or in combination. Clinicians must exercise caution when evaluating infants presenting with fever and vomiting, who do not have diarrhoea, as the list of differential diagnoses is extensive, including some conditions with significant morbidity and mortality.

Frequency of presentation

By far the commonest condition causing vomiting and diarrhoea in children is gastroenteritis. A urinary-tract infection (UTI) must be considered in all infants with vomiting, with or without fever. The presence of diarrhoea makes a urine infection much less likely, and in this situation the diagnosis is more likely to be gastroenteritis.

DEFINITIONS

Vomiting, reflux, diarrhoea, fever

Vomiting is an active process involving muscular contraction expelling the stomach contents orally. In comparison, gastro-oesophageal *reflux* is the passive regurgitation of gastric contents, most commonly liquid. In the newborn and young infant gastro-oesophageal reflux is common and may be considered normal if it is not associated with consequences like pain or failure to thrive.

Diarrhoea refers to the frequency and consistency of stool, being frequent, loose or liquid. The stool may also contain blood and mucous, both of which are abnormal.

Fever is present when the body's temperature is elevated above normal. Actual definitions of fever vary; but a core temperature of about 36.5–37.2°C is normal. The site used to make the measurement will also affect measured temperature. Generally aural (tympanic) temperatures are less accurate. Per-axilla temperatures are lower than rectal temperatures by about 0.5–1°C. Although rectal temperatures more closely reflect the body's core temperature, per-axilla temperatures are more convenient to measure and socially acceptable to the patient. Needless to say, an infant who is cardiovascularly compromised and peripherally 'shutdown' should have a rectal temperature checked, as a per-axilla temperature may inaccurately reflect the core temperature and falsely reassure the physician regarding the lack of fever.

CLINICAL EVALUATION

History

Presenting complaint and past history

Always listen to the parent or carer of the child! Generally, they know the infant or child best and physicians are unwise to ignore their concerns. Explore the symptoms further and in more detail, if necessary. Is there blood in the vomitus, or blood or mucous in the stool? Sometimes important associated symptoms will not be volunteered by parents, and are only alluded to when directed by a focused history. Specific information regarding the nature and content of the vomiting and diarrhoea will need clarification. In the child with a possible infectious condition, it may be important to clarify whether there have been infectious contacts or recent overseas travel. Review of the past history should include any significant medical or surgical problems and whether the child is thriving.

ABC – fluids in and out

This schema provides a simple structure for obtaining the history, and may be used to advise parents about concerning symptoms that may develop subsequently. Alertness and activity (**A**) provides information about the neurological state of the child. Lethargy and poor interactivity are concerning symptoms in a young child. The behaviour of the baby whilst feeding is also important. Parents may note poor suck and sleepiness during feeding; and the breast-feeding mother may comment more precisely about the quality of the infant's suck. Breathing (**B**), specifically rapid or laboured breathing, and poor circulation (**C**), as indicated by mottling and coolness of the peripheries, are also worrying signs.

The child's fluid intake and urine output as a percentage of usual or normal; provide a very important marker of the unwell infant or child. The number and 'wetness' of the nappies is used as the indicator of urine output. Thus, using an evaluation of 'fluids in and out', one should be concerned when these are less than 50% of normal for the child.

EXAMINATION

General observation

In the absence of a life-threatening emergency it is always worthwhile to make a careful observation of the child, either whilst talking with the carer or to the child. This general observation phase is invaluable in the paediatric assessment, particularly in young children. During this observation look and listen for the following:

❶ Airway noises (stridor, sturtor and wheeze).

❷ Tachypnoea (measure the respiratory rate!).

❸ Colour (centrally and peripherally, look for cyanosis and mottling).

❹ Alertness and activity (or inter-activity, particularly with child's carer[s]).

Note the ABCD approach (Airway, Breathing, Circulation, Disability) is utilised.

Assessment of the state of hydration is critical. It is well recognised that clinicians tend to over estimate the degree of dehydration, consequently excessive amounts of intravenous fluid may be administered. An accurate premorbid and current weight may aid this assessment. The following is a revised guide for the assessment of dehydration:

• < 3% – No clinical signs; reduced urine output.

• 3% – Mild dehydration; mild tachycardia, dry mucous membranes.

• 5% – Moderate dehydration; lethargy, tachycardia, reduced skin turgor, sunken eyes/fontanelle.

• 10% – Severe dehydration; clinical signs of shock (tachycardia, thready pulses, reduced perfusion, particularly centrally).

Always check carefully for a rash, as petechiae and purpura may be inconspicuous. Examination of the ears, nose and throat, is frequently left until the end of the examination, to avoid potential distress impairing the remainder of the examination.

Cardiovascular and respiratory status

It is important to evaluate the cardiovascular and respiratory systems in the infant with vomiting for the following reasons:

❶ Shock may be present due to either septicaemia or fluid loss from vomiting and/or diarrhoea.

❷ Septicaemia may be the cause of the symptoms.

❸ Pneumonia or other respiratory infections may cause vomiting.

❹ Effortless tachypnoea may indicate a metabolic acidosis.

The pulse rate and pulse volume may identify a rapid thready pulse indicating poor perfusion. Capillary refill is often thought to be a poor indicator of circulatory status, as the peripheral perfusion (i.e. hands and feet) may be impacted upon by environmental temperature. The comparison of central (i.e. anterior chest) and peripheral capillary refill, with other data like heart rate, pulse volume and consciousness state, will allow an assessment of the adequacy of the circulation. Remember the presence of shock indicates inadequate tissue perfusion. It is present when there is a rapid, thready pulse, delayed capillary refill, especially if central (> 2 seconds), and abnormal neurological status including agitation, lethargy, or coma. The diagnosis of shock is not reliant on the presence of hypotension, particularly in children. Delay in identifying shock until the child is hypotensive, risks severe compromise and potential progress to cardiac arrest.

Septicaemia, with or without meningitis may cause fever, vomiting and diarrhoea. Some bacterial pathogens that cause gastroenteritis may also cause septicaemia such as *Salmonella* and *Shigella*.

Respiratory examination of the infant with fever, cough and vomiting may identify tachypnoea and grunt that alerts the clinician to the possibility of pneumonia. Grunting is an expiratory noise, usually intermittent, and generates PEEP (positive end expiratory pressure) by partially closing the glottis during expiration. Percussion note for dullness may be more valuable that auscultation for crackles or bronchial breathing. Be aware of the child with abdominal pain and grunt as they may have a lower lobe pneumonia.

Abdominal examination

The abdomen is examined for distension, tenderness and guarding. Take note of the child's resting posture and how they move spontaneously or on request, both in the bed or walking. A gentle, unrushed examination will provide more information.

Presence of guarding and rebound can be elicited with gentle flexion/relaxation of the fingers of the examining hand (at the metacarpophalyngeal joint). Evaluate for organomegaly – liver, spleen and kidneys. Are there any masses? The pale, vomiting child may have intussusception. Examine for anal fissures and other perianal abnormality that may indicate inflammatory bowel disease.

Neurological examination

The child may have impaired consciousness either due to systemic illness, shock or a primary neurological problem. The unwell infant who is vomiting may have meningitis. Likewise, raised intracranial pressure (ICP) may cause vomiting. Cushing's triad includes bradycardia, hypertension and abnormal respiration, but is generally associated with a marked elevation of the ICP. On neurological examination, check for any asymmetry of movement, tone and reflexes, as a cerebral abscess may cause fever and vomiting. Focal seizures generally indicate focal pathology and should be considered the same as a focal abnormality on examination.

Temperature

Always measure the temperature of the vomiting child. If the child's circulation is compromised then consider continually monitoring the temperature with a rectal probe. The body's temperature varies over time, and in the unwell patient it is crucial to continue to monitor for fever over a period of time. Remember that some modes of measurement underestimate the core temperature or are an inaccurate reflection of the core temperature (see above). The child with overwhelming sepsis may not mount a fever and, indeed, may be hypothermic.

DIFFERENTIAL DIAGNOSES

This list is extensive and will vary depending upon the combination of symptoms, vomiting and/or fever and/or diarrhoea, as well as the examination findings:

- Gastro-oesophageal reflux
- Viral illness
  Gastritis/enteritis
  Non-specific, generalised viral illnesses
- Gastroenteritis – viral, bacterial
- Otitis media/URTI/tonsillitis/
  pharyngitis/stomatitis
- Urinary tract infection
- Septicaemia
- Meningitis/encephalitis
- Pneumonia
- Appendicitis
- Metabolic/endocrine problems
- Intestinal obstruction including
  malrotation (± volvulus)
- Cyclical vomiting
- Malabsorption including cows' milk
  protein enteropathy
- Colitis (including Crohn's disease,
  ulcerative colitis, pseudomembranous
  colitis).

The child with recurrent vomiting warrants particular attention, with consideration of diagnoses like malrotation, UTIs and cyclical vomiting. An abdominal X-ray may be helpful, but after surgical consultation an upper gastrointestinal contrast study may be required. A child thought to have cyclical vomiting should be referred to a paediatrician for follow-up. Beware of children with a pre-existing condition (or 'label') such as cyclical vomiting as they may develop other acute conditions. These children require careful reconsideration at each presentation before concluding 'just another vomiting episode'.

INVESTIGATIONS

Remember, only order tests that will aid your decision making and management of the patient. Reference ranges are frequently based on the standard deviation in a population, so a result outside the range may not necessarily indicate abnormality or pathology. This may inadvertently lead the clinician to order more unnecessary tests!

Not every child who is medically assessed requires investigations to be undertaken. The tests required will depend upon the possible differential diagnoses and the severity of illness (see Table 7.9.1).

Don't forget simple bedside tests like urine analysis (UA) and blood glucose. This information can be invaluable in assessing the child with diarrhoea and vomiting. In this context, check the specific gravity and for ketones. Glycosuria may indicate diabetic ketoacidosis. If the UA is positive for nitrites or leucocytes, then an appropriately collected urine specimen should be cultured.

The child, who is previously well and thriving, who presents with vomiting and hypoglycaemia, is likely to be hypoglycaemic from starvation if they are ketotic. In the absence of ketonuria, then metabolic and endocrine abnormalities need to be considered. It may be necessary to assay growth hormone, insulin and cortisol, as well as performing a urine metabolic screen. Consultation with a paediatrician or endocrinologist may be prudent.

Generally urine culture is unnecessary where acute gastroenteritis is likely (i.e. when there is diarrhoea) but is mandatory in the infant or baby with acute vomiting and fever. Urinary symptoms, like dysuria and frequency, can be expected in children from about four or five years of age allowing a more selective approach to those who require urine culture. 'Bag urines' (collected in an adhesive, sterile plastic bag) have a high contamination rate and are best avoided when performing a urine culture, but are satisfactory for a simple UA. Although more difficult to collect, a 'clean catch urine' provides a sample less likely to be contaminated. This is collected with an open nappy, a poised parent, with an open sterile container, waiting patiently to 'catch' the spontaneously voided urine. Those babies and infants deemed to be at higher risk of a UTI or who are more seriously unwell may require more rapid testing by either a suprapubic aspirate ('bladder tap') or an in–out catheter urine collection. Any child, who is toilet trained and requires a urine culture, should have mid-stream urine collected.

The microscopy of the diarrhoeal stool may be important. The presence of stool white cells, without a viral or bacterial pathogen, in the young infant, may indicate cows' milk protein intolerance

MANAGEMENT

Intravenous fluids

- Bolus
- Rehydration
- Glucose

The management will depend on the need for immediate resuscitation and subsequently, the provisional diagnosis. A fluid bolus is used to restore circulating volume and is therefore warranted when signs of shock are present. This must not be confused with strategies of 'rapid

Table 7.9.1 Tests that may be useful in the child with vomiting or diarrhoea

Common tests:
- Urine analysis
- Urine culture
- Stool
  Microscopy, culture
  Rotavirus antigen
  Giardia (often tested by RIA, avoiding the need for multiple samples for ova and parasites)
- Biochemistry – electrolytes, urea/creatinine, blood glucose
- Full blood count

Less common tests:
- Liver function tests
- Blood gas (venous or arterial)
- Blood culture
- Amylase
- Insulin, growth hormone, cortisol (if hypoglycaemic)
- Lactate
- Urine metabolic screen
- CXR to exclude pneumonia
- AXR to exclude intestinal obstruction

rehydration' in dehydrated children. Intravenous fluids containing dextrose must not be used as volume expanders. The choice of crystalloid fluid for a bolus is either normal saline (0.9%) or Hartmann's solution. If these crystalloids are not available, and a bolus is required, then a colloid should be used (e.g. 4% NSA, Gelofusine™, or Haemaccel®).

In dehydrated, but not cardiovascular compromised children, it is safer to commence initial intravenous rehydration with fluids that contain at least 75 mmol L^{-1} sodium, i.e. 0.45–0.9% saline solutions. Commonly available fluids include 0.45% NaCl + 2.5% glucose, 0.9% NaCl (normal saline) and Hartmann's solution. Hypoglycaemia is not infrequent, both at presentation or subsequently, thus dextrose-containing fluids are appropriate in all children, particularly in the young infant or those who have had insufficient caloric intake and are ketotic. Intravenous fluids are commonly manufactured as 'isotonic' with plasma, by varying the glucose concentration to balance the sodium chloride (e.g. 0.45% NaCl + 2.5% glucose). The addition of dextrose to many commercially available solutions (such as normal saline) will make them 'hypertonic' compared to plasma. However, due to rapid equilibration of the dextrose with extravascular space this is not clinically significant. In this context, 0.9% NaCl + 2.5% glucose is an appropriate intravenous fluid to use (made by adding 25 mL of 50% glucose to 475 mL of 0.9% saline).

Be aware of the potential of SIADH in unwell children. The rate of fluid administration may need to be altered depending upon the initial biochemistry, the diagnosis and the clinical progress of the child. Monitoring fluid balance is essential in the unwell infant or child.

Antibiotics

Any specific management, like administration of antibiotics will depend upon the provisional diagnosis, and the severity of illness. Most acute diarrhoeal illnesses are viral and self-limiting and therefore do not require antibiotics. Clearly it is preferable that appropriate cultures have been undertaken prior to the administration of antibiotics; although in the severely unwell, febrile patient, broad-spectrum antibiotics should not be delayed whilst awaiting collection of all cultures. It would be preferable, but not essential, that a blood culture be undertaken prior to such administration.

Consultation

Consultation with more experienced staff, either emergency physicians or paediatricians should be encouraged, especially for complex or severely ill infants or children. Assistance may be required for clinical evaluation and technical procedures in critically ill children.

Transfer

The child who requires transfer to a facility that provides a higher level of care, needs an experienced evaluation regarding the level of escort required to safely achieve the transfer.

CONCLUSIONS

Differential diagnostic possibilities

For each patient the differential diagnoses will vary depending upon the compilation of symptoms (fever, vomiting, diarrhoea or others). Keep an open mind and always re-evaluate clinical data. Don't be distracted by a child's previous diagnoses or labels.

General approach

Remember that 'ABC fluids in and out' is a useful tool in taking a history. Caution must be exercised in the infant who has fever and vomiting, as differential diagnoses include serious illnesses, like meningitis. The younger the infant, the more challenging the evaluation and the less reliable the clinical examination. If in doubt, seek consultation from a colleague. The telephone is a useful and powerful tool for clinicians and the value of consultation should not be underestimated.

FURTHER READING

Craig JV, Lancaster GA, Taylor S, Williamson PR, Smyth RL 2002 Infrared ear thermometry compared with rectal thermometry in children: a systematic review. Lancet 360(9333): 603–609 [Review; 48 refs]

Craver RD, Abermanis JG 1998 Dipstick only urinalysis screen for the pediatric emergency room. Paediatric Nephrology 11(3): 331–333 [1998 erratum appears in Paediatric Nephrology 12(5): 426]

Gorelick MH, Shaw KN 1999 Screening tests for urinary tract infection in children: a meta-analysis. Pediatrics 104(5): 54

Gorelick MH, Shaw KN, Baker MD 1993 Effect of ambient temperature on capillary refill in healthy children. Paediatrics 92(5): 699–702

Hewson PH, Gollan RA 1995 A simple hospital triaging system for infants with acute illness. Journal of Paediatrics & Child Health 31(1): 29–32

Shaw KN, McGowan KL, Gorelick MH, Schwartz JS 1998 Screening for urinary tract infection in infants in the ED: which test is best?. Paediatrics 101(6): E1

7.10 HEPATITIS

FRANZ E. BABL

ESSENTIALS

1 Hepatitis A, B and C are the main viral causes of acute hepatitis in children in Australia.

2 Acute hepatitides due to the various hepatotropic viruses are clinically indistinguishable.

3 The younger the child the more likely viral hepatitis will be asymptomatic or only mildly symptomatic.

4 Hepatitis B, C, D and G can cause chronic infection.

5 Hepatitis A and B are vaccine preventable and post-exposure prophylaxis is available for both.

6 In addition to toxin- and drug-related hepatitis, a variety of metabolic and systemic illnesses can present with the clinical picture of acute or chronic hepatitis in children.

INTRODUCTION[1-9]

In children the aetiology of hepatitis includes a diverse number of viral and non-viral causes. Viral hepatitis continues to be a major health problem in developing and developed countries and can present as an acute or chronic illness.

AETIOLOGY

Infection

- Hepatotropic viruses, e.g. hepatitis A, B, C, D, E, G.
- Other viruses with hepatic involvement, e.g. EBV, CMV.
- Bacterial infections with hepatic involvement, e.g. leptospirosis, brucellosis, Q fever, cat-scratch disease, gonococcal perihepatitis

(Fitz–Hugh–Curtis syndrome), syphilis, typhoid fever or associated with septicaemia.
- Amoebic.

Drug and toxin-related liver injury
- See Table 7.10.1 (page 205).

Chronic hepatitis
- Persistent viral infection (hepatitis B, C, D).
- Autoimmune hepatitis.
- Sclerosing cholangitis.
- Metabolic diseases, e.g. Wilson's disease, α-antitrypsin deficiency, cystic fibrosis.
- Systemic illnesses, e.g. inflammatory bowel disease, cardiac disease, total parenteral nutrition.

Viral hepatitis in children can present with manifestations, ranging from asymptomatic seroconversions (especially in infants), mildly symptomatic and anicteric presentations with symptoms of a flu-like illness to fulminant hepatic failure as well as chronic hepatitis leading to cirrhosis and hepatocellular carcinoma. In adults, chronic hepatitis is defined as biochemical or histologic changes that persist for more than six months. This definition in children would inappropriately delay the diagnosis of several childhood causes of non-viral chronic hepatitis, which respond to specific medical therapy. Persistence of abnormal serum aminotransferase tests beyond three months warrants aggressive evaluation to define the aetiology of the liver injury. In a child with clinical evidence of chronic liver disease or synthetic dysfunction in the absence of positive viral serology, evaluation should proceed without the three-month observation period.

HISTORY

Acute clinical viral hepatitis classically presents with a prodromal phase with non-specific symptoms of nausea, vomiting, malaise, anorexia and low-grade fever fol-

lowed by an icteric phase with jaundice and dark urine. Prodromal symptoms fade with the onset of jaundice but anorexia and malaise may persist, and localised hepatic pain or tenderness and pruritus may develop. Important historical clues indicating an infectious aetiology are attendance of childcare and possible disease among peers and childcare workers, exposure to highly endemic areas in Australia (e.g. Aboriginal communities) or overseas, attendance of schools and residential facilities for the disabled, exposure to blood products, injection drug use and high-risk sexual activity. A history of acute drug or toxin ingestion or ongoing therapeutic use of potentially hepatotoxic agents should be elicited. The history should also explore the possibility of acute or chronic presentations of metabolic and systemic illnesses associated with liver disease, e.g. neurologic complaints in Wilson's disease, respiratory difficulties in cystic fibrosis, or a history of cardiac disease.

EXAMINATION

Although jaundice is the hallmark of hepatitis many children present anicteric. Carotenaemia, which also causes a yellow–orange tinge of the skin, can be differentiated from jaundice by the lack of scleral involvement. In addition to jaundice, physical examination in acute hepatitis may show tender hepatomegaly and mild splenomegaly. Arthralgia or arthritis and macular rashes can occur with hepatitis B. Signs of chronic liver disease should be specifically looked for including clubbing, leukonychia, palmar erythema, spider naevi, bruising, scratch marks, asterixis, ascites, prominent abdominal veins, oedema and signs of fat-soluble vitamin deficiency.

INVESTIGATIONS

Laboratory tests for hepatitis can be expensive and many may not be clinically useful in the emergency setting. Initial studies should include a full blood count, total and fractionated serum bilirubins, aspartate aminotransferase (AST), alanine aminotransferase (ALT), γ-glutamyl transferase (GGT) and prothrombin time (PT). A serum alkaline phosphatase level may be difficult to interpret in growing children because levels increase with bone growth. Serum AST, ALT and GGT are indicative of hepatocellular damage rather than 'liver function tests'. Slight elevations of AST and ALT do not always predict mild disease and both can fall with end-stage liver disease. PT is the most useful indicator of synthetic function. If the aetiology of the hepatitis is unknown, anti-hepatitis A immunoglobulin M (IgM), hepatitis B surface antigen (HBsAg), IgM anti-hepatitis B core (HBc) and anti-hepatitis C virus (HCV) antibody should be obtained. If these tests are negative, other viral causes such as Epstein–Barr virus and cytomegalovirus should be considered. If no viral cause can be identified, metabolic and systemic causes of acute and chronic hepatitis should be excluded. Wilson's disease can be detected by measuring serum ceruloplasmin levels and 24-hour urinary copper excretion, cystic fibrosis by measuring sweat electrolytes, α-antitrypsin deficiency by measuring serum α_1-antitrypsin levels.

VIRAL HEPATITIS[5-10]

Over the past 35 years the knowledge about the viruses that cause hepatitis has exploded. The agents identified to cause hepatitis as their primary disease manifestation include hepatitis A virus (HAV), hepatitis B virus (HBV), hepatitis D virus (HDV) and formerly non-A, non-B designated viruses, hepatitis C (parenteral transmission) and hepatitis E (enteral transmission) and more recently hepatitis G. HBV is a DNA virus whereas the other hepatotropic agents are RNA viruses. HAV and HEV are not known to cause chronic disease whereas the others can develop chronic infection. It is virtually impossible clinically to distinguish an acute infection due to one agent from another. Diagnosis is therefore dependent on the use of serologic and nucleic-acid-based assays. Many other viruses can cause hepatitis as part of their clinical spectrum such as Ebstein–Barr virus and cytomegalovirus.

Hepatitis A[5,7,9,10]
Etiology

Hepatitis A virus (HAV) is an RNA virus classified as a member of the picorna virus group.

Epidemiology

The most common mode of transmission is person to person by the faecal–oral route. In developing countries, including Aboriginal communities in the Northern Territory, where infection is endemic, most persons are infected in the first decade of life. In developed countries, including much of Australia, infection may occur at an older age when susceptible adults travel to endemic areas. In Australia, the main patterns of hepatitis A are large, slowly evolving community outbreaks involving childcare centres, residential facilities, communities of IV drug users and male homosexuals, sporadic cases due to travel to endemic areas and point source outbreaks from contaminated food, water or an infected food handler. Faecal–oral transmission from asymptomatic infections, particularly in young children, is likely to account for many of approximately 50% of cases where the source cannot be determined.

The incubation period is 15–30 days (average 25–30 days). The highest titres of HAV in stool occur during 1 to 2 weeks before the onset of illness, when patients are most likely to transmit HAV.

Clinical course

Hepatitis A is an acute self-limited illness associated with fever, malaise, jaundice, anorexia and nausea. In children under six years of age symptomatic hepatitis occurs in only 30% and few will have jaundice. In older children and adults infection is usually symptomatic, typically lasting several weeks, and approximately 70% will have jaundice. Prolonged or relapsing disease can occur though no chronic infection occurs. Fulminant hepatitis is rare but is more frequent with underlying liver disease.

Laboratory tests

HAV specific total and IgM antibody tests are available. IgM is invariably present by the time the patient presents and indicates current or recent infection and usually disappears within four to six months. Anti-HAV IgG is detectable shortly after the appearance of IgM. The presence of total anti-HAV without IgM indicates past infection and immunity.

Management

There is no specific treatment for hepatitis A. Most patients can be managed at home. Hepatotoxic agents should be avoided. No specific dietary restrictions are required. Pruritus associated with cholestasis, which develops in 5–10% may be treated with colestyramine, an H1-receptor blocker or local therapy.

Children in childcare settings and adults with acute HAV infection who are food handlers should be excluded for one week after the onset of illness. Hospitalised patients require contact precautions for one week after the onset of illness if they are incontinent or in nappies. Patients should be admitted if signs of acute liver failure develop (repeated vomiting, deepening jaundice and increasing prothrombin time), and transfer to a liver transplant centre is indicated at the onset of acute liver failure (increased prothrombin time and clouding of consciousness).

Immunisations and post-exposure prophylaxis

Hepatitis A vaccines, which are approved for use in children older than two years of age have a protective efficacy of 94–100% in preventing clinical hepatitis A. For susceptible persons travelling to countries with high endemic rates of HAV infection or to remote indigenous communities within Australia, persons at high risk of acquiring the illness, including childcare workers, or if there is increased risk of fulminant hepatitis A, immune-prophylaxis with hepatitis A vaccine is indicated. In children under two years of age immunoglobulin (IG) is available. Hepatitis A vaccine requires 2–4 weeks to onset of protection. If immediate protection is required IG and the vaccine can be administered at the same time. Hepatitis A and B combination vaccines are available.

Post-exposure prophylaxis with IG is indicated for household and sexual contacts within two weeks of exposure and for unimmunised children and employees in outbreaks in the day-care setting and in well-defined or closed communities. IG is greater than 85% effective if given within two weeks after exposure to HAV. There are insufficient data for the use of hepatitis A vaccine alone for post-exposure prophylaxis.

Hepatitis B[5-12]
Etiology
Hepatitis B virus HBV is a DNA-containing hepadna virus. Important components include hepatitis B surface antigen (HBsAg), hepatitis B core antigen (HBcAg) and hepatitis B e antigen (HBeAg).

Epidemiology
HBV is transmitted through blood or body fluids such as semen, cervical secretions, wound exudates, and saliva of HBsAg positive persons, in particular if they are chronically infected. Modes of transmission are through blood and blood products (now rare due to screening), sharing of needles, percutaneous or mucous membrane exposure to infective body fluids and homosexual and heterosexual activity. Non-sexual transmission occurs in household settings primarily from child to child, although the exact mechanism is unknown. It is likely due to the sharing of inanimate objects as HBV can survive at ambient temperatures for one week or longer. The faecal-oral route does not transmit HBV. Prevalence of HBV infection varies markedly from country to country with low rates in Australia, the USA, Canada and Western Europe. High endemic rates occur in South East Asia, China, the Pacific Islands and other developing countries as well as some Australian Aboriginal communities. The Asian region is estimated to account for 75% of the 400 million individuals worldwide with chronic HBV infection, mostly acquired at birth or in infancy by close physical contact. The transfusion risk for HBV in Australia is currently calculated at 1 in 483 000. The incubation period is 45–160 days with an average of 90 days.

Clinical course
HBV virus infection causes a wide spectrum of diseases ranging from asymptomatic seroconversion, subacute illness with non-specific symptoms or extrahepatic symptoms and clinical hepatitis with jaundice to fulminant fatal hepatitis. Asymptomatic infection is most common in young children. Arthralgia and arthritis or macular rashes can occur early in the disease. The rate of chronic HBV infection is age dependent. It occurs in up to 90% of infants infected by perinatal infection, 30% of children one to five years of age, and 2–6% of older children and adults with HBV. Chronic HBV infection can lead to chronic liver disease and cirrhosis or primary hepatocellular carcinoma later in life, though it can occasionally occur in children. The risk of death from HBV-related cirrhosis or liver cancer is approximately 25% for persons who become chronically infected in early childhood.

Laboratory tests
Commercial antigen and antibody tests for HBV are available to detect acute infection, resolved infection, immunity after immunisation and persons at high risk of transmission. HBsAg is detectable during acute infection. If the infection is self-limited, it disappears before serum anti-HBs can be detected (the 'window phase'). IgM anti-HBc allows the detection of acute or recent infection including those in HBsAg negative patients during the 'window phase'. Persons with chronic HBV infection are positive for HBsAg as well as anti-HBc antibody. Both anti-HBs and anti-HBc antibodies are detected in persons with resolved infection, whereas anti-HBs alone is detected after hepatitis B vaccination. The presence of HBeAg and HBV viral DNA by PCR indicates ongoing viral replication, increased disease activity and infectivity.

Management
Management of acute hepatitis B is similar to hepatitis A. Interferon-α and lamivudine are the main therapeutic agents for active liver disease, though treatment indications are individualised to take into account different stages of disease activity and genetic variability of the virus and the host. Although data are scarce, children have been successfully treated with both agents. Children with chronic HBV infection should be screened periodically for disease activity and by abdominal ultrasound for hepatic complications. Liver transplantation is a possible therapy in end-stage chronic hepatitis.

Immunisations and post-exposure prophylaxis
Current hepatitis B vaccines are produced by recombinant DNA technology. They are highly efficacious, safe and provide long-term protection. The vaccines are part of universal childhood immunisations in many Western countries including Australia and should be used for other persons at high risk of exposure such as health-care personnel, haemodialysis patients, patients receiving blood products, and those with chronic liver disease. Hepatitis A and B combination vaccines are available.

The vaccine is also used for post-exposure prophylaxis in unimmunised household and sexual contacts of persons with acute HBV infection, newborns of HBsAg positive mothers, and after accidental occupational percutaneous exposure to blood that contains or might contain HBsAg. To provide immediate protection, the latter two groups should also receive hepatitis B immunoglobulin.

Hepatitis C[5-9,12,13]
Etiology
Hepatitis C virus (HCV) is a small single-stranded RNA virus with multiple genotypes, which do not elicit cross-protective antibodies. HCV is a member of the flavivirus family.

Epidemiology
Infection is spread primarily by parenteral exposure to blood and blood products. Screening of blood donors and blood

products and inactivation procedures for HCV have virtually eliminated the risk of post-transfusion hepatitis due to this agent. The transfusion risk for HCV in Australia is currently calculated at 1 in 911 000.

At increased risk are injection drug users, haemophilia patients who received untreated clotting products in the past, haemodialysis patients and persons with high-risk sexual behaviours. The risk of maternal to infant (vertical) transmission, which is the most likely source of HCV infection in developed countries, is 5–10%. In Australia there are an estimated 125–250 children infected vertically each year. Incubation time is two weeks to six months with an average of 6–7 weeks.

Clinical course

The signs and symptoms of HCV infection are usually indistinguishable from HAV and HBV infection. Acute disease tends to be mild and insidious in onset and in children most infections are asymptomatic. Jaundice occurs in 25% of patients. Persistent HCV infection occurs in 85% of patients even in the absence of biochemical evidence of liver disease. Most children with chronic HCV infection are asymptomatic. Chronic liver disease and cirrhosis can follow and primary hepatocellular carcinoma can occur in these patients in later life.

Laboratory tests

HCV infection can be detected using total anti-HCV antibody assays and HCV RNA by PCR. Antibody tests are used as screening tests and PCR testing as confirmatory tests.

Management

All patients with HCV infection should be considered infectious and refrain from donating blood products and sharing tooth brushes or razors. They should be counselled on avoiding hepatotoxic agents including medications and alcohol. Susceptible children should be immunised against hepatitis A and B. Infected children do not need to be excluded from day care. HCV is not a contraindication to breast-feeding.

In adults, interferon-α or ribavirin alone or in combination has been used for treatment of HCV infection, with combination therapy showing better outcome than single-drug therapy. Liver transplantation is indicated in end-stage liver disease. Paediatric drug data are limited, indications for therapy are unclear and HCV-infected children require ongoing care by a paediatric gastroenterologist.

Immunoglobulin (IG) has not shown efficacy for post-exposure prophylaxis and there is no hepatitis C vaccine due to the genetic diversity of the virus.

Hepatitis D[5,7,9]
Etiology

Hepatitis D virus (HDV) is a 36–43 nm particle consisting of an RNA genome and a δ-protein antigen (HDAg), both of which are coated with hepatitis B surface antigen (HBsAg).

Epidemiology

HDV causes infection only in persons with acute or chronic HBV infection. HDV requires HBV as a helper virus and cannot produce infection in the absence of HBV. It can cause infection at the same time as the initial HBV infection (co-infection) or infect a person already chronically infected (super-infection). Acquisition of HDV is similar to HBV, i.e. by parenteral, percutaneous or mucous membrane inoculation. High prevalence areas include southern Italy, parts of eastern Europe, South America and the Middle East. HDV infection is rare in Australia.

Incubation period for HDV super-infection is 2–8 weeks; in co-infection with HBV the incubation period is similar to hepatitis B (45–160 days; average 90 days).

Clinical course

The importance of HDV infection lies in its ability to convert an asymptomatic or mild chronic HBV infection into a fulminant or rapidly progressive disease. Acute co-infection with HBV and HDV usually causes an acute illness indistinguishable from acute HBV infection alone, except that the likelihood of fulminant hepatitis can be as high as 5%.

Laboratory tests

Diagnosis is made by detecting IGM-specific anti-HDV antibody and HDAg.

If markers for HDV infection exist, HBV co-infection can be differentiated from super-infection in an established HBsAg carrier by testing for IgM hepatitis B core antibody. Absence of this core antibody suggests that the person is an HBsAg carrier.

Immunisations

Because HDV cannot be transmitted in the absence of HBV infection, hepatitis B immunisation protects against HDV infection.

Hepatitis E[5,7,9]
Etiology

The hepatitis E virus (HEV) is an RNA virus and is the only known agent of enterically transmitted non-A non-B hepatitis.

Epidemiology

Transmission of HEV is by the faecal–oral route. It is more common in adults than children and has a high case-fatality rate in pregnant women. Cases have been reported in epidemics and sporadically in developing countries. HEV in Australia has been reported in returning travellers from endemic regions and in the Northern Territory. Outbreaks have been associated with contaminated water. Chronic infection does not seem to occur.

Clinical course

HEV causes a self-limited acute illness with jaundice, malaise, anorexia, fever, abdominal pain and arthralgia. Subclinical infection also occurs.

Laboratory tests

Diagnosis can be made by detecting IgM anti-HEV in serum or by detecting HEV RNA by PCR in serum or faeces.

Viral hepatitis due to other viruses[3,14]

Hepatitis G virus/GB virus (HGV/GBV-C) is a single-stranded RNA flavivirus. Although HGV can cause chronic infection, most infected persons are asymptomatic. It has been reported in patients with HBV or HBC infection, likely through co-infection. Primary route of transmission in developed countries appears to be through transfusions and injection drug use. Its prevalence in healthy Australian children is low. The incubation period is unknown.

Epstein–Barr virus, cytomegalovirus, human immunodeficiency virus (HIV), herpes virus, varicella-zoster, rubella, adenoviruses and enteroviruses as well as yellow fever and dengue fever in tropical and subtropical areas are also known agents causing acute hepatitis in children. However, hepatic involvement with these viruses is usually only one component of a multi-system disease.

Drug- and toxin-induced liver injury[4,15]

The liver is the main site of drug metabolism and is particularly susceptible to structural and functional injury from drugs and toxins. The clinical spectrum varies from asymptomatic biochemical abnormalities to fulminant liver failure. Children may be more or less susceptible than adults to hepatotoxic reactions. For example, liver injury after halothane is rare in children and paracetamol toxicity is unusual in infants compared with adolescents, whereas most cases of fatal hepatotoxicity associated with sodium valproate use have been reported in children. Excess or prolonged therapeutic administration of paracetamol combined with reduction in caloric intake may produce hepatotoxicity in children.

When considering adverse reactions to medications with liver involvement clinicians need to consider all drugs taken in the previous months including prescription medications, over-the-counter medications and complementary medicines. According to the Adverse Drug Reactions Advisory Council, in Australia the most commonly reported alternative and complementary medicines associated with hepatotoxicity are kombucha tea, echinacea, evening primrose tea and valerian.

Hepatotoxicity can be predictable or idiosyncratic. Predictable hepatotoxicity implies a high incidence in exposed persons with dose dependence. Examples are paracetamol or antimetabolites such as methotrexate. Idiosyncratic hepatotoxicity is infrequent and unpredictable.

It is not dose dependent, may occur at any time during exposure to the agent and may be immunologically mediated as a result of prior sensitisation.

The pathologic spectrum of drug-induced liver disease varies widely and is rarely specific (Table 7.10.1). The laboratory features also vary widely. After exclusion of other causes of liver disease, the cessation of a temporally related offending medication with normalisation of liver function tests is usually sufficient to establish a diagnosis. Treatment is mainly supportive. *N*-acetylcysteine (NAC) is used as a specific antidote in preventing paracetamol toxicity. The prognosis of drug- or toxin-induced liver injury depends on its type and severity. Injury is usually completely reversible with the withdrawal of the offending agent. The mortality of submassive hepatic necrosis with fulminant liver injury may, however, exceed 50%.

Chronic hepatitis[3,4,8]
Overview
Chronic hepatitis can be caused by persistent viral infection (hepatitis B, C and D), autoimmune hepatitis, sclerosing cholangitis, metabolic diseases such as

Wilson's disease, α-antitrypsin deficiency, cystic fibrosis, Indian childhood cirrhosis and other inborn errors of metabolism and systemic illnesses such as inflammatory bowel disease, cardiac disease and liver disease associated with parenteral nutrition. In addition drugs and toxins can produce chronic hepatitis.

Autoimmune hepatitis
Autoimmune hepatitis (AH) is characterized by progressive destruction of hepatocytes in association with circulating autoantibodies, but in the absence of other known causes of chronic liver disease. AH type I occurs mainly in females and presents with lethargy, jaundice and the typical findings of chronic liver disease. Antinuclear antibodies (ANA) are found in the majority. AH type II is clinically similar but ANA is negative and anti-liver-kidney microsomal antibodies are present. Liver biopsy shows piecemeal necrosis without involvement of the biliary tract. Both forms of AH can be associated with other autoimmune manifestations such as thyroiditis, glomerulonephritis, haemolytic anaemia and erythema nodosum. Of patients with AH, 70-90% respond to corticosteroid therapy.

Table 7.10.1 Patterns of hepatic drug injury

Injury	Causal agent
Centrilobar necrosis	Paracetamol Halothane
Microvesicular steatosis	Valproic acid
Acute hepatitis	Isoniacid
General hypersensitivity	Sulfonamide Phenytoin
Fibrosis	Methotrexate
Cholestasis	Chlorpromazine Erythromycin Estrogens
Veno-occlusive disease	Cyclophosphamide
Portal and hepatic vein thrombosis	Estrogens Androgens
Biliary sludge	Ceftriaxone
Hepatic adenoma or carcinoma	Oral contraceptives Anabolic steroids

Sclerosing cholangitis

Sclerosing cholangitis (SC) is characterized by chronic inflammation of the intra- or extra-hepatic biliary tree. Primary SC is associated with inflammatory bowel disease or immune deficiency, secondary SC results from an obstructive process in the biliary system such as stones or post-operative stricture. Primary SC can occasionally be associated with antibodies such as ANA. Although histology includes periductal inflammation, differentiation from other causes of chronic hepatitis often requires cholangiography demonstrating typical biliary abnormalities. Supportive therapy does not prevent disease progression and 80% develop cirrhosis in 5 to 10 years. Treatment with steroids is ineffective. Liver transplantation is required for long-term survival.

Metabolic causes of chronic hepatitis

Wilson's disease   Is an autosomal recessive disorder caused by a defect in biliary copper excretion. Excessive intra-hepatic accumulation of copper causes liver cell damage followed by fibrosis and cirrhosis. Extra-hepatic accumulation of copper in brain, cornea and kidney accounts for extra-hepatic manifestations of neurologic abnormalities and Kayser–Fleischer rings. Initial presentation of Wilson's disease may resemble acute viral, fulminant or chronic hepatitis with variable extra-hepatic findings. The importance in considering Wilson's disease, though uncommon, lies in the ability to treat patients and other family members with penicillamine, a chelating agent.

α_1-Antitrypsin deficiency   Is caused by a deficiency of the major serum protease inhibitor, α_1-antitrypisin. There are various allele combinations of α_1-antitrypsin deficiency, of which some are more prone to cause chronic liver disease than others. The course of the liver disease is highly variable. Liver transplantation is curative. There is no other effective therapy.

Cystic fibrosis   Can be associated with biliary cirrhosis and chronic liver disease. In addition, cholelithiasis may occur in the second decade of life.

Systemic disorders causing chronic liver disease   Hepatobiliary disease may complicate ulcerative colitis and Crohn's disease. Fatty liver, cholangitis, chronic hepatitis, cirrhosis, portal vein thrombosis, sclerosing cholangitis and cholelithiasis have been associated with inflammatory bowel disease. These complications are more likely to occur in patients with other extra-intestinal manifestations but there is no correlation with the severity of the inflammatory bowel disease.

Hepatic congestion and injury may occur as a complication of severe chronic or acute congestive heart failure or cyanotic heart disease. Hepatic dysfunction is due to hypoxaemia, systemic venous congestion and low cardiac output.

Liver dysfunction is the most common metabolic complication of total parenteral nutrition (TPN). Cholestasis associated with TPN is potentially fatal and is the major factor limiting long-term TPN use. The younger the child the more vulnerable they are to TPN-associated cholestasis. Pathogenesis is multifactorial. In general, with administration of oral feedings a gradual resolution of the liver disease occurs.

REFERENCES

1. Rosenthal P, Lightdale JR 2000 Laboratory evaluation of hepatitis. Paediatrics Review 21: 178
2. Harris W, Timms B, Choong R 2002 Examination paediatrics, 2nd edn. MacLennan and Petty, Sydney, 116–134
3. Jonas MM (assoc ed) 2003 The liver and bile ducts. In: Rudolph CD, Rudolph AM (eds) Rudolph's pediatrics, 21st edn. McGraw Hill, New York, NY, 1469–1518
4. Balistreri WF 2000 The liver and biliary system. In: Behrman RE, Kliegman RM, Jenson HB (eds) Nelson's textbook of pediatrics, 16th edn. WB Saunders, Philadelphia, 1194–1228
5. Ryder SD, Beckingham IJ 2001 Acute hepatitis. British Medical Journal 322: 151–153
6. Ryder SD, Beckingham IJ 2001 Chronic viral hepatitis. British Medical Journal 322: 219–221
7. Farrell GC 1998 Acute viral hepatitis. Medical Journal of Australia 168: 565–570
8. Farrell GC 1998 Chronic viral hepatitis. Medical Journal of Australia 168: 619–626
9. American Academy of Paediatrics 2000 Hepatitis A to G. In: Pickering LK (ed) 2000 Red book: report of the committee on infectious diseases, 25th edn. American Academy of Paediatrics, Elk Grove Village, IL, 280–308
10. National Health and Medical Research Council 2000 The Australian Immunisation Handbook, 7th edn. Australian Government Printing Service, Canberra, ACT
11. Leung N 2002 Treatment of chronic hepatitis B: case selection and duration of therapy. Journal of Gastrology and Hepatology 17: 409–414
12. Seed CR, Cheng A, Ismay SL et al 2002 Assessing the accuracy of three viral risk models in predicting the outcome of implementing HIV and HCV NAT donor screening in Australia and the implications for future HBV NAT. Transfusion 42: 1365–1372
13. Kesson AM 2002 Diagnosis and management of paediatric hepatitis C virus infection. Journal of Paediatric Children's Health 38: 213–218
14. Siebert DJ, Bowden DS, Tracy SL, Hardikar W 2002 Prevalence of hepatitis G/GBV-C in a healthy paediatric population. Journal of Paediatric Children's Health 38: 423
15. Ryan M, Desmond P 2001 Liver toxicity: could this be a drug reaction? Australian Family Physician 30: 427–431

CONTROVERSIES AND FUTURE DIRECTIONS

❶ Improved public health measures to minimise transmission of viral hepatitis may include universal immunisations for children and targeted immunisations for high-risk groups.

❷ The development of a vaccine against HCV infection remains a priority.

❸ The optimal monitoring, indications for therapy, and role of antiviral agents in chronic hepatitis B and C in children remain controversial.

❹ The clinical role of hepatitis G virus/GB virus and other newly discovered hepatotropic viruses is uncertain.

7.11 INTUSSUSCEPTION

KIM LIAN ONG

INTRODUCTION

Intussusception occurs when a bowel segment invaginates into the lumen of the more distal lumen. The invaginated segment is carried more distally by peristalsis while the mesentery and vessels are squeezed within the engulfing segment. The resulting venous congestion is the cause of the blood and mucous in the stool, the classic 'redcurrant jelly' stool. Intussusception occurs most commonly at the terminal ileum when the terminal ileum is carried through the ileocaecal valve into the colon (ileocolic) and in some instances it may even reach the rectum.

AETIOLOGY

Most cases are idiopathic without any mass lesion acting as a lead point or an apex of the intussusceptum. In non-idiopathic intussusception, the following may act as lead points:

❶ Meckel's diverticulum.
❷ Haemolytic uraemic syndrome.
❸ Cystic fibrosis with inspissated bowel content.
❹ Henoch–Schönlein purpura with intramural haemorrhage.
❺ Lymphoma and leukaemia involving the bowel.

EPIDEMIOLOGY

It is a common cause of abdominal pain in children and clinically, there is the classical triad of vomiting, abdominal pain and passage of blood per rectum. However, this classical triad only occurs in less than one third of patients. Most of the children are younger than one year of age, and most commonly intussusception occurs in infants between five and ten months of age. Intussusception is the most common cause of intestinal obstruction in patients between five months and three years. Patients under three years of age with intussusception usually do not have a mass lesion, that is, the cause is idiopathic and they are usually responsive to non-operative reduction. Older children often have a surgical lead point to the intussusception and require operative reduction.

The estimated incidence is 1 to 4 per 1000 live births. There is an overall male preponderance, with a male-to-female ratio of approximately 3 to 1. Mortality with treatment is rare. If untreated, this condition is fatal in two to five days. Morbidity is increased by a delay in diagnosis and is likely to be due to bowel wall necrosis and perforation. Delay will cause prolonged intestinal obstruction with persistent vomiting causing dehydration and electrolyte imbalance.

CLINICAL PRESENTATION

The patient is usually in the infant age group and is well nourished. The presentation is one of sudden onset of intermittent colicky abdominal pain. One of the descriptions sometimes given by the caregivers is the drawing up of the legs to the child's abdomen and then kicking the legs in the air. There is associated vomiting, passing of loose or watery stools, which may be followed by blood or mucous per rectum within 12–24 hours. Initially the vomiting is non-bilious but it becomes bilious when intestinal obstruction occurs. The mixture of mucus and shed blood is described as redcurrant jelly. Often there is a preceding upper respiratory tract infection. Diarrhoea can be an early sign of intussusception.

This condition is unusual in children who are malnourished. The child usually appears chubby and in good health. The child when observed has crying spells, which represent episodes of abdominal pain between periods of lethargy. In late presentation, the child may be hypotensive.

On examination, a right hypochondrium sausage-shaped mass may be palpated and this is best felt when the child is quiet between spasms of colic. The presence of fever and leukocytosis are late signs and may indicate transmural gangrene and infarction. The occurrence of intestinal gangrene and infarction can be suggested by the presence of peritonitis with the physical signs of rigidity and involuntary guarding. Often patients with intussusception do not present with classic signs and symptoms, which may lead to an unfortunate delay in diagnosis with disastrous consequences. Therefore, it is essential to maintain a high index of suspicion for intussusception when evaluating a child presenting with abdominal pain, especially those less than five years of age or those who have human serum protein (HSP) or blood dyscrasias.

INVESTIGATIONS

A plain abdominal radiograph may be performed. Early in the course of the disease it may be normal, but later in the course it may show an absence of air in the right upper quadrant and a right-sided soft tissue shadow. There may be a radiological pattern of small bowel obstruction or free air in the peritoneal cavity. The presence of stool and air fluid levels in the caecum makes the diagnosis of intussusception less likely.[1]

Traditionally, the diagnosis of intussusception is made by the use of an enema, either using air or barium. Contrast enema is a quick and reliable investigation and is often also therapeutic. Barium has traditionally been the contrast material used but perforation can result in barium and faecal peritonitis.[2–4] The availability of near-isotonic water media and the use of air as a contrast medium[5,6] have change the traditional therapeutic approach. The advantages of air reduction are its rapidity and safety compared with barium. In the case of perforation during the procedure, air enema has been shown to result in a smaller tear than hydrostatic enema with markedly less spillage of faeces.[7] In addition air has no deleterious consequences within the abdominal cavity.[8,9]

There are some recent studies to suggest that ultrasound is highly sensitive and specific for the diagnosis of intussusception. Some authors reported it to be close to 100% sensitive in identification of intussusception, even in relatively inexperienced hands.[10–12] The characteristic findings include an oval, hypoechoic mass with bright central echoes on longitudinal section (pseudokidney sign) and a hypoechoic target configuration on transverse section.

MANAGEMENT

The treatment in the ED is to provide stabilisation depending on the clinical condition. Intravenous fluids should be started for rehydration and often an initial bolus of crystalloid, e.g. normal saline, is required. The stomach should be decompressed with a nasogastric tube.

Non-operative reduction is now generally accepted as the modality of treatment for most patients. Absolute contraindications include peritonitis, perforation or profound shock.[13]

OUTCOME

Various authors have reported reduction rates of between 81% and 91% using air enema.[13–16] The perforation rate is quoted to be less than 1%.[13,14] Surgical reduction is now performed after failure to achieve reduction or when it is contraindicated to perform non-operative reduction.

The overall mortality rate of intussusception is less than 1%.[13] Mortality rates observed among children in industrialised countries is lower than those in developing countries.[17–23] Some of these deaths are preventable and may be related to reduced access to or delays in seeking health care, factors known to be associated with mortality in children with intussusception.[21–23] Therefore, early diagnosis and management play an important role in the reduction of mortality.

REFERENCES

1. Heller RM, Hernanz-Schulman M 1999 Applications of new imaging modalities to the evaluation of common pediatric conditions. Journal of Paediatrics 135(5): 632–639
2. Grobmyer A, Kerlan R, Peterson C, Dragstedt L 1984 Barium peritonitis. American Surgery 50: 116–120
3. Mahvoubi S, Sherman N, Ziegler M 1983 Barium peritonitis following attempted reduction of intussusception. Clinical Paediatrics 23: 36–38
4. Yamamura M, Nishi M, Furubayashi H, Hioki K, Yamamoto M 1985 Barium peritonitis. Report of a case and review of the literature. Diseases of the Colon and Rectum 28: 347–352
5. de Campo JF, Phelan E 1989 Gas reduction of intussusception. Paediatric Radiology 19: 297–298
6. Shiels WE II, Maves CK, Hedlund GL, Kirks DR 1991 Air enema for diagnosis and reduction of intussusception: Clinical experience and pressure correlates. Radiology 181: 169–172
7. Shiels WE II, Kirks DR, Keller GL et al 1993 John Caffey Award. Colonic perforation by air and liquid enemas: Comparison study in young pigs. American Journal of Roentgenology 160: 931–935
8. Hernanz-Schulman M, Foster C, Maxa R et al 1992 Fecal peritonitis and contrast media: Experimental protocol to assess synergistic effects and to compare relative safety of barium sulfate, water-soluble ionic media, saline and air. Presented at the 35th Annual Meeting of the Society for Pediatric Radiology, May 14–17, Orlando, Florida
9. Hernanz-Schulman M, Vanholder R, Schulman G 1994 Inhibition of neutrophil phagocytosis by barium sulfate. Presented at the 37th Annual Meeting of the Society for Pediatric Radiology, April 28-May 1, Colorado Springs, Colorado
10. Bhisitkul DM, Listernick R, Shkolnik A et al 1992 Clinical application of ultrasonography in the diagnosis of intussusception. Journal of Paediatrics 121: 182–186
11. Bowerman R, Silver T, Jaffe M 1982 Real-time ultrasound diagnosis of intussusception. Radiology 143: 527–529
12. del-Pozo G, Albillos J, Tejedor D 1996 Intussusception: US findings with pathologic correlation – the crescent-in-doughnut sign. Radiology 199: 688–792
13. DiFore JW 1999 Intussusception. Seminars in Paediatric Surgery 8: 214–220
14. Hadidi AT, El Shal N 1999 Childhood intussusception: A comparative study of nonsurgical management. Journal of Paediatric Surgery 34: 304–307
15. Gorenstein A, Raucher A, Serour F, Witzling M, Katz R 1998 Intussusception in children: Reduction with repeated delayed air enema. Radiology 206: 721–724
16. Ein SH, Alton D, Padler SB, Shandling B, Stringer D 1997 Intussusception in the 1990s: Has 25 years made a difference? Pediatric Surgery International 12: 402–305
17. Simon RA, Hugh TJ, Curtin AM 1994 Childhood intussusception in a regional hospital. Australian and New Zealand Journal of Surgery 64: 699–702
18. Ein SH, Alton D, Palder SB, Shandling B, Stringer D 1997 Intussusception in the 1990s: Has 25 years made a difference? Paediatric Surgery International 12: 374–376
19. van Heek NT, Aronson DC, Halimun EM, Soewarno R, Molenaar JC, Vos A 1999 Intussusception in a tropical country: Comparison among patient populations in Jakarta, Jogyakarta, and Amsterdam. Journal of Paediatrics Gastroenterology and Nutrition 29: 402–405
20. Meier DE, Coln CD, Rescorla FJ, OlaOlorun A, Tarpley JL 1996 Intussusception in children: International perspective. World Journal of Surgery 20: 1035–1039
21. Stringer MD, Pledger G, Drake DP 1992 Childhood deaths from intussusception in England and Wales, 1984-9. British Medical Journal. 304: 737–739
22. Adejuyigbe O, Jeje EA, Owa JA 1991 Childhood intussusception in Ile-Ife, Nigeria. Annals of Tropical Paediatrics 11: 123–127
23. Mangete ED, Allison AB 1994 Intussusception in infancy and childhood: An analysis of 69 cases. West African Journal of Medicine 13: 87–90

7.12 HERNIAE

ANDREW J. A. HOLLAND

ESSENTIALS

1 The key diagnostic steps are detailed history from the carer and careful clinical examination.

2 Radiological investigations have little, if any, role in the management of inguinal herniae in children.

3 A hernia that is not reducible may be associated with ischaemia and an urgent surgical opinion should always be sought.

4 In children, unlike in adults, it is the gonad rather than the bowel that is most at risk from an inguinal hernia.

INTRODUCTION

A hernia is defined as the protrusion of a viscus or part of a viscus into an abnormal location. The most common herniae occurring in children are inguinal and umbilical – femoral herniae are rare. A variety of descriptive terms is applied to herniae in these locations, often incorrectly. This may lead to diagnostic confusion and inappropriate delays in referral.

Herniae are usually classified based on two characteristics: anatomical location and whether or not the hernia is reducible. An irreducible hernia may result in ischaemia of either the contents of the hernia or adjacent structures. Treatment of an irreducible hernia is thus a surgical emergency. The use of the terms incarceration (irreducible) and strangulation (arrest of circulation) should be avoided, as all irreducible herniae may be associated with ischaemia.

TYPES OF HERNIAE

Inguinal

The incidence of inguinal herniae in children has been reported to be between 0.8% and 4.4%,[1] rising to between 18.9% to 30% of pre-term infants.[2,3] Inguinal herniae are six-times more common in boys and are more common in twins.[1,4] Around 1 in 10 inguinal hernias are non-reducible at presentation, although a careful history from the parents will often elucidate earlier signs and symptoms. In this group, over two-thirds are under one year of age.

In children, inguinal herniae are almost always indirect.[5] The hernia exits the peritoneal cavity via the internal inguinal ring to enter the inguinal canal, leaving the canal via the external inguinal ring. The sac is intimately related to the contents of the spermatic cord. It is compression of the testicular vessels by hernial contents that may render the testis ischaemic. In contrast, in females the risk of ischaemia to the ovary and adnexae usually occurs as a result of torsion of these structures within the hernial sac.

Inguinal herniae usually present as a swelling in the inguinal region first noticed by the carer when changing or bathing the child, especially if crying or straining.[6] The swelling may extend into the scrotum in boys or the labia majora in girls. Persistent tachycardia, overlying erythema and marked tenderness suggest an irreducible hernia complicated by ischaemia. Occasionally, an irreducible hernia may present with vomiting and abdominal distension as a result of intestinal obstruction.

A hernia can be differentiated from a hydrocoele as the later transilluminates and does not usually extend into the inguinal region. In neonates, these differences may be less obvious and a hernia may appear to transilluminate. Encysted hydrocoeles of the cord and rarely testicular torsion may also cause diagnostic confusion. Where there is any doubt regarding the diagnosis, a paediatric surgeon should be consulted.

Femoral

Femoral herniae are rare in children, accounting for between 0.4% to 1.1% of all groin herniae.[7,8] They are often not diagnosed prior to surgery and are one cause of recurrent 'inguinal' herniae in children. Typically, most present between four and ten years of age and there is an equal sex incidence. Clinically the hernia presents as a swelling that is inferior and lateral to the pubic tubercle. As in adults, femoral herniae are associated with a high incidence of complications, so early surgical intervention is required.

Umbilical and paraumbilical herniae

A true umbilical hernia occurs through the umbilical ring as opposed to a paraumbilical hernia that results from a defect *adjacent* to the umbilical ring.

Umbilical herniae are very common, occurring in up to 18.5% of infants under six month of age.[5] They are more common in Afro-Caribbean children and in premature infants, when the incidence rises to between 41.6% to 75%.[9,10] The vast majority of umbilical defects appear to close spontaneously with increasing age, largely irrespective of the size of the defect. Given the very low risk of the hernia becoming non-reducible, surgical repair is only indicated for those herniae that persist beyond three to five years of age, or in the very few that present with symptoms.[11]

Paraumbilical defects do not close with increasing age and should be referred for elective repair on diagnosis.

Epigastric herniae

These herniae occur as a result of a defect, often only a few millimetres in size, in the linea alba between the umbilicus and the xiphisternum. The child presents with a small swelling in this region that may be associated with pain, usually due to entrapment of extraperitoneal fat. Once diagnosed, elective surgical repair is required.

COMPLICATIONS

Complications of an irreducible hernia are more likely to occur if the child presents late or there is diagnostic delay. The most common adverse sequelae include gonadal ischaemia and bowel obstruction. Enteric ischaemia, perhaps leading to perforation, is rare.

TREATMENT

All inguinal hernias require surgery due to the risk of bowel ischaemia and compression of adjacent gonadal structures. If the hernia is reducible, the patient should be discussed with a paediatric surgeon regarding the timing of follow-up. Neonates and infants should be assessed within one week of presentation and scheduled for early elective surgery because of the high risk of the hernia becoming irreducible in this age group. Carers should be advised to represent

CONTROVERSIES

❶ The role of routine contralateral inguinal exploration in children with a unilateral inguinal hernia remains controversial.

❷ The use of intra-operative laparoscopy for the assessment of the presence of a contralateral inguinal hernia is increasingly being debated.

urgently if signs and symptoms of an irreducible hernia develop.

If the hernia does not spontaneously reduce, a paediatric surgeon should be contacted urgently. In the absence of signs or symptoms suggestive of ischaemia, manual reduction by an experienced clinician may be attempted. The child should be given appropriate analgesia. A two-handed technique is required: one hand from above disengages the hernia from the external ring and the other from below reduces the hernia by gentle direct pressure. If there are signs suggestive of ischaemia, emergency surgery is required.

REFERENCES

1. Bronsther B, Abrahams MW, Elboim C 1992 Inguinal hernia in children – a study of 1000 cases and review of the literature. Journal American Medical Womens Association 27: 522–525
2. Darlow BA, Dawson KP, Mogridge N 1987 Inguinal hernia and low birth weight. New Zealand Medical Journal 100: 492-494
3. Harper RG, Garcia A, Sia C 1975 Inguinal hernia: A common problem of premature infants weighing 1000 grams or less at birth. Paediatrics 56: 112–115
4. Bawkin H 1971 Indirect inguinal hernia in twins. Journal of Paediatric Surgery 6: 165–168
5. Rescorla FJ 1997 Hernias and umbilicus. In: Oldham KT, Colombani PM, Foglia RP (eds) Surgery of infants and children. Lippincott-Raven, Philadelphia, 1069–1081
6. Johnstone JMS 1994 Hernia in the neonate. In: Freeman NV, Burge DM, Griffiths M, Malone PSJ (eds) Surgery of the newborn. Churchill Livingstone, Edinburgh, 321–330
7. Kapur P, Caty MG, Glick PL 1998 Paediatric hernias and hydroceles. Paediatric Clinics of North America 45: 773–789
8. Radcliffe G, Stringer MD 1997 Reappraisal of femoral hernia in children. British Journal of Surgery 84: 58–60
9. Crump EP 1952 Umbilical hernia : Occurrence of the infantile type in Negro infants and children. Journal of Paediatrics 40: 214–223
10. Vohr BR, Rosenfeld AG, Oh W 1977 Umbilical hernia in low birth weight infants (less than 1500 grams). Journal of Paediatrics 90: 807–808
11. Meier DE, OlaOlorun DA, Omodele RA, Nkor SK, Tarpley JL 2001 Incidence of umbilical hernia in African children: Redefinition of 'normal' and re-evaluation of indications for repair. World Journal of Surgery 25: 645–648

7.13 GASTROENTERITIS

SUSAN PHIN

ESSENTIALS

1 Most children with gastroenteritis and mild-moderate dehydration can be successfully rehydrated with oral rehydration solutions either by mouth or nasogastric tube.

2 Oral rehydration solutions (ORS) should be used for oral rehydration, not fruit juices, soft drinks or sports drinks.

3 It is important to use appropriate intravenous fluids for bolus or maintenance phases of rehydration.

4 Careful instruction to parents of how to give oral fluids appropriately is vital.

5 Anti-diarrhoeal and anti-emetic medications should not be used in children.

6 Early refeeding with age-appropriate foods should be encouraged.

7 Timely reassessment is vital and, if the child does not progress as anticipated, other diagnoses and complications should be considered.

8 Other diagnoses should be considered especially in the presence of:
- An infant less than six months of age
- High-grade fever
- Bilious vomiting
- Significant abdominal pain
- No diarrhoea
- Blood in vomitus or stool
- Drowsiness/reduced level of consciousness.

❶ There is blood or mucous in the stool.
❷ There is significant abdominal pain.
❸ There is a high-grade fever.

These infective agents cause gastroenteritis by one, or more mechanisms. Some directly invade the bowel wall, e.g. *Salmonella* or *Shigella*, some produce toxins prior to ingestion, e.g. *Staphylococcus aureus*, and some multiply and produce toxins within the gastrointestinal tract, e.g. *Shigella*.

In an uncomplicated acute bout of gastroenteritis, determining the causative pathogen is usually unnecessary, as this usually does not alter the management.

HISTORY

Most children with acute gastroenteritis present with a history of diarrhoea and vomiting. Abdominal pain and fever are sometimes accompanying symptoms. It is important to ask for specific details about these symptoms, to increase the certainty of the diagnosis of gastroenteritis and also to help assess the risk of dehydration in the child.

Diarrhoea refers to loose or liquid stools. The frequency, volume (small to voluminous) and consistency (semisolid to watery) and the presence of blood or mucous are all important. Similarly, the frequency and nature (bilious or non-bilious) of the vomiting is also important. The words 'my child is vomiting everything he tries to drink' can be used by parents to describe a child who has had either two or twenty vomits in the

INTRODUCTION

Acute gastroenteritis is an inflammation of the gastrointestinal tract. It is one of the commonest reasons for children to present to an ED. Most children under five years of age have experienced an episode of gastroenteritis and most can be successfully managed without admission to hospital. Worldwide, however, gastroenteritis still remains a significant cause of morbidity and mortality.[1]

AETIOLOGY

Gastroenteritis is caused by a wide range of pathogens including viruses, bacteria and parasites (as shown in Table 7.13.1). In developed countries, the majority of episodes are due to viruses, with rotavirus

being by far the most common pathogen. The most common bacterial causes are *Salmonella* and *Campylobacter*. *Shigella*, *Yersinia* and *Escherichia coli* are less common, while *Vibrio cholerae* is seen in developing countries. Parasites such as *Giardia* and *Cryptosporidium* are sometimes the infective agent.

In general a bacterium is more likely to be the causative agent if:

Table 7.13.1	Common causes of acute gastroenteritis	
Viruses	Bacteria	Parasites
Rotavirus	Salmonella	Cryptosporidium
Norwalk virus	Campylobacter jejuni	Giardia lamblia
Enteric adenovirus	Shigella	Entamoeba histolytica
	Escherichia coli	
	Yersinia enterocolitica	
	Vibrio cholerae	

last twenty-four hours. It is important, therefore, to be specific in questioning.

The abdominal pain that can be associated with gastroenteritis is crampy in nature and more pronounced in bacterial gastroenteritis. It is not accompanied by focal or significant findings on abdominal examination. If fever is a symptom, the height of the fever can be helpful. Although children with rotaviral gastroenteritis are often febrile, it is not usually high-grade. Such fevers are more likely in bacterial gastroenteritis or in other diagnoses altogether.

Specific details about the amount of fluid tolerated by the child are vital in assessing the risk of dehydration. Parents are usually able to estimate whether, over a twenty-four hour period, the child has taken one-quarter, one-half or three-quarters of normal intake. Intake that is consistently less than half of normal is of concern.

Specific questions about urine output, i.e. heaviness and frequency of wet nappies, are also important. Less than four wet nappies in twenty-four hours is of concern when assessing dehydration.

Questions about the level of alertness and activity of the child are also important. Lethargy may simply be an indication of significant dehydration in a child. However, more severe lethargy and drowsiness (particularly if out of proportion to that expected for the dehydration) may indicate another more serious diagnosis as the cause of the child's symptoms.

EXAMINATION

The aim of the clinical examination is to exclude signs of an alternative cause of the symptoms, other than gastroenteritis (see Chapter 7.9 pp 197–200 on diarrhoea and vomiting) and to assess the degree of dehydration.

Occasionally pathogens causing gastroenteritis can cause extra-intestinal disease. This can occur particularly with *Shigella* and *Salmonella*. *Shigella* can cause central nervous system irritation, which can manifest as encephalopathy or seizures. This may occur prior to the onset of diarrhoea. *Salmonella* can cause a bacterae-

mia, which can lead to focal infections including osteomyelitis and meningitis. The infant under six months of age is particularly at risk.

Assessment of dehydration

The accurate assessment of dehydration is difficult. Studies have shown that medical personnel tend to overestimate the degree of dehydration.[2] The gold standard in assessment of dehydration is a loss of weight compared with a recent pre-illness weight. For example, a one year old weighing 10 kg a week ago who presents with gastroenteritis for three days and now weighs 9.5 kg, is approximately 5% dehydrated. However, a recent weight is rarely available in the ED. Therefore, tables such as Table 7.13.2 use a combination of clinical symptoms and signs to estimate the degree of dehydration.

It is important to remember that some of the signs and symptoms of dehydration can be affected by other factors. Mouth breathers have dry mucous membranes. Watery diarrhoea can make it difficult to assess if the child has a wet nappy. Crying can cause a sunken fontanelle to appear full. Tachycardia may be caused by a crying, anxious or febrile child, therefore it is the context and trend of the pulse that is important.

Various studies have attempted to validate combinations of these signs and symptoms with varying degrees of standardisation and scientific validity.[2–5] Difficulties arise as some of the signs are subjective and gold standards differ.

Gorelick et al[5] performed a good study in Philadelphia in 1997, which looked at the ten clinical signs shown in Table 7.13.3. Using a gold standard of serial weight gain, they found that < 3 signs correlated with < 5% dehydration, 3–6 signs correlated with 5–9% dehydration and > 7 signs correlated with > 10% dehydration.

Laboratory investigations in the assessment of dehydration

There is little data to support the usefulness of laboratory tests in the assessment of dehydration due to gastroenteritis. Dehydration is thought to typically cause a metabolic acidosis. It is true that vomiting can cause a metabolic acidosis by several mechanisms including volume depletion, lactic acidosis and starvation ketosis. However, isolated vomiting can also cause a metabolic alkalosis through loss of gastric acid. In addition, isolated diarrhoea can cause a metabolic acidosis through loss of bicarbonate in the stool, but the child who can increase oral intake to keep pace with the diarrhoeal losses

Table 7.13.2 Standard assessment scale for severity of dehydration			
Variable	Mild	Moderate	Severe
Thirst	+	++	+++
Dry mucous membranes	+	++	+++
Reduced urine output	+	++	+++
Lethargy	–	+	+++
Sunken eyes	–	+	++
Reduced skin turgor	–	+	++
Tachycardia	–	+	++
Poor perfusion	–	+	++
Tachypnoea	–	–	+
Hypotension	–	–	+

Table 7.13.3 Ten clinical signs of dehydration

1. Decreased skin elasticity
2. Capillary refill > 2 seconds
3. General appearance (ill-appearing, irritable, apathetic)
4. Absent tears
5. Abnormal respirations
6. Dry mucous membranes
7. Sunken eyes
8. Abnormal radial pulse
9. Tachycardia (HR > 150)
10. Decreased urine output

Source: Gorelick et al, ref 5

may not actually be dehydrated. Despite these confounding factors, it has been shown that serum bicarbonate is significantly lower in children with moderate or severe dehydration (mean 14.5 mEq L^{-1} and 10.3 mEq L^{-1}) than in children with mild dehydration (mean 18.9 mEq L^{-1}).[3] Raised serum urea levels have also been thought to reflect dehydration, but with even less evidence.

From a practical point of view, it is not vital to put a specific percentage on the degree of dehydration, particularly when the accuracy of such a specific percentage is questionable. What is important is to allocate the child into a broad category of dehydration, for example, mild, moderate or severe, which determines what treatment should be commenced, and then to reassess the child and the degree of dehydration within a specific timeframe.

DIFFERENTIAL DIAGNOSIS

Many other conditions can masquerade as gastroenteritis by presenting with a combination of vomiting, diarrhoea, fever, or abdominal pain. These include:

❶ Other infections, e.g. urinary tract infection, meningitis.

❷ Surgical diseases, e.g. intussusception, bowel obstruction, appendicitis.

❸ Raised intracranial pressure, e.g. blocked ventriculo-peritoneal shunt.

❹ Metabolic diseases, e.g. diabetic ketoacidosis, inborn errors of metabolism.

Features of concern to suggest the possibility of other cause include:

❶ Age less than six months.

❷ High-grade fever.

❸ Bilious vomiting.

❹ Significant abdominal pain.

❺ No diarrhoea.

❻ Blood in vomitus or stool.

❼ Drowsiness/reduced level of consciousness.

See Chapter 7.9 pp 197–200, on vomiting and diarrhoea, for more details on differential diagnosis.

INVESTIGATIONS

In uncomplicated acute gastroenteritis, it is usually not necessary to perform any investigations, as they will not alter management. Indications to consider performing investigations include:

❶ Uncertainty about diagnosis.

❷ Severe dehydration.

❸ The child's clinical course not progressing as anticipated.

❹ Commencement of intravenous rehydration.

Stool cultures do not change management in simple gastroenteritis, therefore they are not usually warranted. If bacterial gastroenteritis is suspected a stool sample may be performed, although this will not change management in the majority of cases. A stool sample may be taken for public-health reasons, or to reassure the doctor that there is not another cause for the blood and mucus in the stool.

Urine culture is usually unnecessary when the diagnosis of gastroenteritis is clear. However, if there is little diarrhoea, particularly if the child is under six months of age, it may be necessary to exclude a urinary tract infection.

Electrolytes, urea and creatinine are usually unnecessary in children with gastroenteritis who are mild to moderately dehydrated and who are to receive oral fluids, as they will not usually alter management. If, however, the child does not improve as expected, or deteriorates despite rehydration, or the child was initially severely dehydrated, these tests along with a blood glucose level and perhaps other investigations, will be required.

A full blood count and blood culture are unnecessary in acute gastroenteritis. However, if the diagnosis is uncertain it may be reasonable to perform these tests. In the younger infant, particularly the under three month age group, if bacterial gastroenteritis is likely, the possibility of systemic *Salmonella* infection should be considered and blood culture and intravenous antibiotics considered.

If significant abdominal pain is present and surgical pathology such as intussusception or bowel obstruction seems more likely than simple gastroenteritis, other investigations such as abdominal X-rays, ultrasound or air enemas may be required.

TREATMENT

1. Mildly dehydrated

Children in developed countries presenting to EDs with gastroenteritis are often only mildly dehydrated or not dehydrated at all. Most can be managed as out-patients with oral fluids alone. Educating the parents in how to give fluids, and observing them giving a trial of fluids to the child, are both important. The essential things to ensure are:

❶ The parent knows the appropriate oral fluids to give.

❷ The parent knows how, and is able, to give the oral fluids correctly to optimise success.

❸ The parent will have the child reviewed by the local doctor within 48 hours.

❹ The parent knows what worrying signs and symptoms to look for that would require representation.

If the above criteria cannot be satisfied, the child may need to be admitted. This

GASTROENTEROLOGY AND HEPATOLOGY

is particularly so in the younger infant or those with profuse gastrointestinal losses, as they have a higher risk of becoming dehydrated. See 'moderately dehydrated' for further treatment options in those patients.

Appropriate oral fluids

Oral rehydration solutions (ORSs) are the appropriate fluids to rehydrate children with gastroenteritis. These are specifically designed fluids that contain the correct amounts of sodium, glucose and other electrolytes and are of the appropriate osmolality, to maximise water absorption from the gut. They use the principle of glucose-facilitated sodium transport, whereby glucose enhances sodium and secondarily water transport across the mucosa of the upper intestine. The sodium and glucose concentrations and the osmolality are of vital importance.

The WHO ORS has a sodium concentration of 90 mmol L^{-1}. In developed countries with non-cholera diarrhoea, it is generally thought that 90 mmol L^{-1} is a little high, as non-cholera gastroenteritis does not result in the same sodium losses that are seen in cholera. Many different ORSs with varying sodium concentrations have been developed. It has been shown[6] that water absorption across the lumen of the human intestine is maximal using solutions with a sodium concentration of 60 mmol L^{-1} and this is the concentration recommended by the European Society of Paediatric Gastroenterology and Nutrition.[7] Studies have also shown that hypo-osmolar solutions are most effective at promoting water absorption.[8–10]

Studies have also examined rice-based ORSs and their effect on stool output and duration of diarrhoea when compared with glucose-based ORSs. Rice-based ORSs appear to have benefits in cholera diarrhoea but not in non-cholera diarrhoea.[11]

The composition of various ORSs and other fluids is shown in Tables 7.13.4 and 7.13.5. Fruit juices and soft drinks are inappropriate because of the minimal sodium content and the excessive glucose content and hence excessive osmolality.

Diluting these solutions will not address the grossly inadequate sodium content, nor will it result in an optimal glucose concentration or osmolality. Sports drinks are also inappropriate, with too low sodium levels and too high glucose levels and osmolalities.

Method of giving oral fluids

The important message is to give small amounts of fluid frequently, for example 0.5 mL kg^{-1} every five minutes. The fluid can be measured in a syringe and given to the child either by syringe, teaspoon or cup. The child is far more likely to tolerate these small amounts of fluid than a whole bottle at once. If the child tolerates this fluid the parent can gradually increase the volume and decrease the frequency of the fluid offered. Success can be optimised in the ED setting by giving the parents a documentation chart to fill in, which shows the fluid given and any vomits or diarrhoea or urine passed.

It is important to educate the parents that seeing a doctor will not cure the vomiting and diarrhoea. Small, frequent amounts of fluid will hopefully minimise the vomiting, but will not reduce the diarrhoea. The aim is for the input to exceed the output enough to rehydrate

and then maintain hydration. Parents will know if they are succeeding by observing their child for the following symptoms and signs.

Indications for representation

Parents should be given some indication of symptoms and signs that will prompt representation. These need to be relatively easy for a parent to detect. They will be related to two things:

❶ The child is, or is at risk of becoming, more dehydrated
  • Persistent vomiting despite small amounts of oral fluids frequently, or
  • No wet nappy for eight hours, or
  • Increasing lethargy.
❷ Gastroenteritis may not be the correct diagnosis
  • Bilious vomiting, or
  • Significant abdominal pain, or
  • Drowsiness.

Refeeding

• Breast-fed infants – breast-feeding should continue throughout the episode of gastroenteritis, including the rehydration phase.
• Formula-fed infants – full-strength normal formula should be started as

Table 7.13.4	Composition of oral rehydration solutions				
ORSs	Na		Carbohydrate		Osmolality
	(mm L^{-1})		(mm L^{-1})	(%)	(mOsm L^{-1})
WHO	90	G	111	2	331
Gastrolyte	60	G	90	2	240
Gastrolyte-R	60	RSS	6 (g L^{-1})	2.5	226
Hydralyte (solution or iceblock)	45	G	90	2.5	240

G = glucose; RSS = rice syrup solids.

Table 7.13.5	Composition of oral fluids		
Oral fluids	Na (mm L^{-1})	Carbohydrate (mm L^{-1})	Osmolality (mOsm L^{-1})
Apple juice	3	690	730
Sports drinks	20	255	330
Soft drinks	2	700	750

soon as the infant is rehydrated. This can be supplemented with an ORS for ongoing losses, for example offer 10 ml kg^{-1} after each diarrhoea. However, children with no dehydration and mild gastroenteritis are the least likely to take an ORS because of the salty taste. In this instance increased amounts of normal fluids in conjunction with age-appropriate feeding may be sufficient.

- Early refeeding – studies have shown that early refeeding does not worsen or prolong the duration of diarrhoea, nor increase vomiting or lactose-intolerance, and leads to a significantly higher weight gain after rehydration.[12] Early reintroduction of age-appropriate foods is now recommended.

2. Moderately dehydrated

Some children who present to EDs with gastroenteritis are moderately dehydrated. These children can be rehydrated in several ways. Some are successfully rehydrated with oral fluids alone, as previously described. Some fail this and require additional intervention. Increasing numbers of hospitals in developed countries are using oral rehydration therapy (ORT) via continuous nasogastric infusion.[13,14] This is where an ORS is infused continuously down a nasogastric tube with a pump such as a Kangaroo® pump. Nasogastric infusions should not be used when the child has an ileus or is comatose. Oral rehydration therapy has been the method of choice in developing countries since the 1970s. However, it has taken longer to become accepted in developed countries. This is despite numerous studies, which show that it is as effective as intravenous rehydration but less expensive[13–21] and reduces lengths of hospital stay.[13]

Different regimens are used for continuous nasogastric rehydration. The European Society of Paediatric Gastroenterology and Nutrition recommends calculating the fluid deficit and replacing that over four hours.[22] The American Academy of Pediatrics recommends that mildly dehydrated children receive 50 mL kg^{-1} over four hours and moderately

dehydrated children receive 100 mL kg^{-1} over four hours.[23] Other regimes recommend a fixed volume, for example 40 mL kg^{-1} over four hours for all mild to moderately dehydrated children followed by a reassessment and retrial of oral fluids.[24] This takes into account the tendency for medical officers to overestimate the degree of dehydration[2] and the desire to avoid subsequent over-hydration. The important thing to remember is that, whatever regimen is used to rehydrate the child, fluid status should be regularly reassessed.

Intravenous rehydration

Intravenous rehydration should be used to rehydrate children with gastroenteritis who fail nasogastric therapy or deteriorate.

The volume (mL) of replacement fluids is calculated using the formula: weight (kg) × dehydration (%) × 10. Maintenance fluids are then calculated, with one method being to give 100 mL kg^{-1} for the first 10 kg, 50 mL kg^{-1} for the second 10 kg and 20 mL kg^{-1} for each subsequent kilogram. The volumes for rehydration and maintenance are then added together and divided by twenty-four to calculate the hourly rate.

The fluid used is N/2 saline + 2.5% dextrose. This sodium concentration is halfway between the N/4 saline + 3.75% dextrose, which gives maintenance sodium requirements, and the normal saline required for the fluid deficit, which is mainly extracellular fluid with a sodium concentration of approximately 140 mm L^{-1}. As in nasogastric rehydration, it is important to regularly reassess the child's fluid status.

The type of fluid given and the rate at which it is given both need to be altered if the serum sodium level is significantly abnormal. If the child is significantly hyponatraemic (< 130 mm L^{-1}), the fluid should be changed to normal saline. If the child is significantly hypernatraemic (> 150 mm L^{-1}), N/2 saline + 2.5% dextrose can still be used, but the rate of infusion needs to be reduced to rehydrate the child over 48–72 hours. The aim is to avoid a rapid fall in the serum sodium level as this can precipitate cerebral oedema. Senior paediatric advice

should be sought if the serum sodium level is significantly abnormal.

3. Severely dehydrated

Although this is a relatively rare occurrence in developed countries, it is vital to diagnose and institute immediate treatment, as this is a medical emergency. The child is usually shocked and needs immediate intravenous access and resuscitation with a 20 mL kg^{-1} bolus of normal saline or Hartmann's solution. If the child remains shocked the bolus should be repeated. Senior advice should be sought about any child presenting in this condition. During insertion of the cannula, blood should be taken for electrolytes, urea, creatinine, glucose, full blood count and venous blood gas. Blood cultures can also be taken at the same time if indicated.

Dextrose-containing fluids such as N/2 saline + 2.5% dextrose or N/4 saline + 3.75% dextrose *should never be used for resuscitation boluses*. Although these solutions are isotonic, the dextrose is rapidly metabolised, so effectively it is as if a hypotonic solution has been given, with the resultant risk of rapid fluid shifts and cerebral oedema.

After the initial resuscitation, replacement plus maintenance fluids are given as per above. It is important to reassess the child's hydration status regularly and look for any indication that another diagnosis is the cause of the child's condition. Electrolytes, urea and creatinine need to be regularly repeated while the child remains significantly unwell.

4. Other treatments
Antibiotics
Antibiotics are rarely indicated in gastroenteritis. They are of proven benefit for treatment of only the following situations:

- *Shigella*
  Intravenous ampicillin in severe disease
  Oral ampicillin or trimethoprim-sulphamethoxazole in milder disease
  Shortens illness duration, eradicates organism.
- Invasive *Salmonella* infections – e.g. septicaemia, osteomyelitis, meningitis

215

Intravenous cefotaxime or ceftriaxone
Antibiotics prolong excretion in
gastroenteritis.

- Traveller's diarrhoea –
trimethoprim-sulphamethoxazole
- *Campylobacter* septicaemia –
erythromycin or gentamicin
Not indicated in uncomplicated
gastroenteritis.

Anti-diarrhoeal and anti-emetic medications

These medications are not indicated in
children with gastroenteritis. There is little
evidence of efficacy and a high incidence
of side effects in infants and young
children.

DISPOSITION

In the past, many children were admitted
to hospital with gastroenteritis when perhaps they did not need to be.[25] With the
emergence of 'Short Stay Wards' or
'Emergency Observation Units', where
patients can be admitted to a special area
within the ED for a finite time of less than
twenty-four hours, hospital in-patient
admission rates for children with gastroenteritis have fallen.[24] In these units
children can be rehydrated (orally or via
nasogastric infusion) over a period of a
few hours and then sent home after appropriate education and advice. This is
provided that the medical officer is confident about the diagnosis of gastroenteritis and that the criteria set out in the
'mildly dehydrated' section are fulfilled.
Care needs to be taken especially with
young infants, as they become dehydrated
more rapidly than older children and are
more likely to have another diagnosis.

Paediatric staff in non-children's hospitals can potentially be utilised to help
manage these patients in conjunction
with ED staff. An admission to, and discharge from, these 'Short Stay Wards'
causes much less disruption to the child
and family and allows hospital resources
to be used for other patients requiring
in-patient admissions. Some children,
however, still require an in-patient admission for successful management.

CONTROVERSIES AND FUTURE DIRECTIONS

❶ Interest in rapid intravenous
rehydration for children with
gastroenteritis has emerged in recent
years in developed countries. It has
long been used in developing
countries.[26,27] There have been a
number of studies in developed
countries over the last several years
that have looked at this issue.[24,28–30]
Most of the studies have used
different types of fluid over different
numbers of hours, making it difficult
to compare studies or to come to a
consensus. More research is required
to look at the safety, efficacy and
standardisation of such regimens.

❷ Interest has also arisen in the use
of probiotics such as *Lactobacillus*
GG in the treatment of acute
gastroenteritis. Early studies seem to
suggest that it may shorten the
diarrhoeal illness.[31] Further research
is necessary.

PROGNOSIS

Gastroenteritis in children is generally a
benign, self-limiting disease, with dehydration being the major potential complication. If this is recognised early and
the child is rehydrated appropriately, the
child should recover completely with no
adverse sequelae.

REFERENCES

1. World Health Organization 1995 The treatment of diarrhoea: A manual for physicians and other senior health workers. WHO, Geneva, (WHO/CDR/95.3 Rev 3 10/95)
2. Mackenzie A, Barnes G, Shann F 1989 Clinical signs of dehydration in children. Lancet 2(8663): 605–607
3. Vega RM, Avner JR 1997 A prospective study of the usefulness of clinical and laboratory parameters for predicting percentage of dehydration in children. Paediatric Emergency Care 13: 179–182
4. Duggan C, Refat M, Hashem M et al 1996 How valid are clinical signs of dehydration in infants. Journal of Paediatric Gastroenterology and Nutrition 22: 56–61
5. Gorelick MH, Shaw KN, Murphy KO 1997 Validity and reliability of clinical signs in the diagnosis of dehydration in children. Paediatrics 99(5): E6
6. Hunt JB, Elliott EJ, Fairclough PD et al 1992 Water and solute absorption from hypotonic glucose-electrolyte solutions in human jejunum. Gut 33: 479–483
7. Booth I, Ferreira R, Desjeux JF et al 1992 Recommendation for composition of oral rehydration solutions for the children of Europe. Report of an ESPGAN working group. Journal of Paediatric Gastroenterology and Nutrition 14: 113–115
8. Ferreira RMCC, Elliott EJ, Watson AJM et al 1991 Dominant role for osmolality in the efficacy of glucose and glycine-containing oral rehydration solutions: Studies in a rat model of secretory diarrhoea. Acta Paediatrica 81: 46–50
9. Hunt JB, Thillainayagam AV, Salim AFM et al 1992 Water and solute absorption from a new hypotonic oral rehydration solution: Evaluation in human and animal perfusion models. Gut 33: 1652–1659
10. International Study Group on Reduced-osmolarity ORS Solutions 1995 Multicentre evaluation of reduced-osmolarity oral rehydration salts solution. Lancet 345: 282–285
11. Gore SM, Fontaine O, Pierce NF 1992 Impact of rice based oral rehydration solution on stool output and duration of diarrhoea: Meta-analysis of 13 clinical trials. British Medical Journal 304: 287–291
12. Walker-Smith JA, Sandhu BK, Isolauri E et al 1997 Recommendations for feeding in childhood gastroenteritis. Journal of Paediatric Gastroenterology and Nutrition 24: 619–620
13. Gremse DA 1995 Effectiveness of nasogastric rehydration in hospitalised children with acute diarrhoea. Journal of Paediatric Gastroenterology and Nutrition 21: 145–148
14. Mackenzie A, Barnes G 1991 Randomised controlled trial comparing oral and intravenous rehydration therapy in children with diarrhoea. British Medical Journal 303: 393–396
15. Sharifi J, Ghavami F, Nowrouzi Z et al 1985 Oral versus intravenous rehydration therapy in severe gastroenteritis. Archives of Diseases in Childhood 60: 856–860
16. Issenman RM, Leung AK 1993 Oral and intravenous rehydration of children. Canadian Family Physician 39: 2129–2136
17. Vesikari T, Isolauri E, Baer M 1987 A comparative trial of rapid oral and intravenous rehydration in acute diarrhoea. Acta Paediatrica Scandinavia 76: 300–305
18. Santosham M, Daum RS, Dillman L et al 1982 Oral rehydration therapy of infantile diarrhoea. New England Journal of Medicine 306: 1070–1076
19. Tamer AM, Friedman LB, Maxwell SRW et al 1985 Oral rehydration of infants in a large US urban medical center. Journal of Paediatrics 107: 14–19
20. Listernick R, Zieserl E, Davis AT 1986 Out-patient oral rehydration in the United States. American Journal of Diseases in Childhood 140: 211–215
21. Nager AL, Wang VJ 2002 Comparison of nasogastric and intravenous methods of rehydration in pediatric patients with acute dehydration. Paediatrics 109(4): 566–572
22. Sandhu BK, Isolauri E, Walker-Smith JA et al 1997 Early feeding in gastroenteritis. Journal of Paediatric Gastroenterology and Nutrition 24: 522–527
23. American Academy of Pediatrics, Provisional Committee on Quality Improvement, Subcommittee on Acute Gastroenteritis 1996 Practice parameter: The management of acute gastroenteritis in young children. Paediatrics 97: 424–435
24. Phin SJ, McCaskill ME, Browne GJ, Lam LT 2003 Clinical pathway using rapid rehydration for

children with gastroenteritis. Journal of Paediatrics and Child Health 39: 343–348
25. Elliott EJ, Backhouse JA et al 1996 Pre-admission management of acute gastroenteritis. Journal of Paediatrics and Children's Health 32: 18–21
26. Slone D, Levin SE 1969 Hypertonic dehydration and summer diarrhoea. South African Medical Journal 34: 209–213
27. Rahman O, Bennish ML, Adam AN et al 1988 Rapid intravenous rehydration by means of a single

polyelectrolyte solution with or without dextrose. Journal of Paediatrics 113: 654–660
28. Reid SR, Bonadio WA 1996 Outpatient rapid intravenous rehydration to correct dehydration and resolve vomiting in children with acute gastroenteritis. Pediatrics 28(3): 318–323
29. Moineau G, Newman J 1990 Rapid intravenous rehydration in the pediatric ED. Paediatric Emergency Care 6(3): 186–188

30. Brewster DR 2002 Dehydration in acute gastroenteritis. Journal of Paediatrics and Children's Health 38: 219–222
31. Guandalini S, Pensabene L, Zikri MA et al 2000 Lactobacillus GG administered in oral rehydration solution to children with acute diarrhoea: A multicentre European trial. Journal of Paediatric Gastroenterology and Nutrition 30: 54–60

7.14 CONSTIPATION

BRUCE FASHER

ESSENTIALS

1 It is important to understand physiology and development to recognise the normal (often regarded as abnormal).

2 Constipation is a common reason for children to present to EDs with abdominal pain.

3 Management depends on the child's age and whether the problem is acute or chronic.

4 The patient's and parents' real concerns need to be acknowledged.

5 Issues to be addressed include:
- Natural history
- The aims of treatment (empty the bowel and establish pharmacological rhythm and then wean to biological rhythm)
- The likely duration of treatment
- The anticipated setbacks
- The need for a co-ordinator clinician (normally unavailable in an ED).

6 Treat from the top, once at night titrating dose according to response if possible.

7 Be able to refer to a resource who is known to be interested in managing the condition and to ensure appropriate ongoing review and support.

INTRODUCTION

Constipation in childhood engenders in clinicians unwarranted anxieties about management. Defining terms and understanding normal physiology and its variants, the frequent blurring in paediatric medicine between physical and emotional factors and their impact on normal development along with evidence-based data can provide the clinician with an algorithm for management.

Management varies according to age and whether constipation is acute or chronic. The ED is a difficult place from which to manage constipation, especially

chronic constipation, for success requires ongoing maintenance therapy and contact with a committed and interested clinician. This is best achieved through the child's local doctor, with input from a general paediatrician in difficult cases.[1,2]

Definitions
❶ *Constipation* is delay or difficulty in defecation, sufficient to cause significant distress.
❷ *Encopresis* is the passage of a normal stool in an abnormal place.
❸ *Soiling* is the frequent involuntary passage of loose or semi-loose stools in clothing. This is usually overflow

incontinence as the liquid stool escapes around an impacted rectal faecolith.

PATHOPHYSIOLOGY

The rectum and anal canal have two tasks, to store faeces temporarily and to evacuate at a socially convenient time. The distending rectum evokes a wave of contraction with inhibition of the smooth muscle tone of the internal anal sphincter, resulting in a sensation of the urge to defecate. An urgent desire to defecate occurs as the stool stretches the sensitive zone of the upper anal canal. This urge is overcome by the voluntary contraction of the external sphincter and the levator ani muscles. Eventually the rectum habituates to the stimulus of the enlarging faecal mass and the urge to defecate subsides. With time this retentive pattern can become automatic.

It is understandable, therefore, that the child who is afraid to use the non-private, wet, smelly school lavatory, will have his rectum occasionally overcome the external sphincter just as he arrives home with 'poo in the pants' – really a normal variant rather than true encopresis.

There is a wide variation of physiology and normal development as can be seen in the age range of successful potty training. To produce a stool at will is one of the child's first major achievements and most gain satisfaction from framing their success in a pot. If too much persuasion is provided, especially if full control has never been attained, the child's profound disappointments are compounded by the disapproval and hostility from the parents. Like most adults, most children seek solitude to defecate.

MANAGEMENT BASICS

❶ Be interested. The patient has often been pushed from pillar to post, with a quick fix, and reviewed in three months. Recognise that the parents and the patient have a concern, which is often the cause of major family dysfunction.

❷ Endeavour to treat from the top, orally, rather than continue to direct attention to the rectum and anus with suppositories and enemas. The exception is when a fissure needs managing with ointment or Xylocaine ointment if defecation can be anticipated.

❸ Develop a pharmacological armamentarium of stool softeners or osmotic aperients. Stimulants (e.g. senna) may cause abdominal discomfort with colic in infants.

❹ Be aware that ongoing management by a single interested clinician is necessary as the constipation will

often relapse, and gains are often small (three steps forward, two steps back).

❺ This makes constipation difficult to manage in EDs. Such departments need to have appropriate and willing referral resources. Out-patient appointments rarely work for the same reasons – difficulties with continuity of care and the ability to be seen relatively urgently (albeit that encouragement with management, behavioural modification and aperient dose titration is often all that is necessary).

❻ The significant risk of relapse dictates that a period of maintenance therapy is necessary before weaning off medications. It might be appropriate to let the patient and family know that if it has taken two years to arrive at this stage it is highly likely it will take two years or so to regain the rectum's natural motility and sensitivity.

Constipation in babies

Never again in life will the stooling pattern, and indeed the stools, be so closely examined as in the period of nappies being changed prior to toilet training. Straining at stool is often marked and then misconstrued as constipation whereas it is a simple reflection of the urge to defecate sensation. Plantar flexion of the toes is a similarly objective sign (at all ages).

Breast-fed infants may pass a stool after each feed or as infrequently as once every few weeks. As long as the stool is of normal quality (often referred to as scrambled eggs) and of great volume there is no reason for concern. For a couple of days prior to defecation the infant may be, not unreasonably, somewhat unsettled.

Just weaned, bottle-fed infants may produce dry, hard stools with difficulty and sometimes traces of fresh blood. Attention to water intake, perhaps addition of extra sugar (brown sugar is better) or sorbitol ($1–3$ mL kg^{-1} noct.) will help soften the stool. Formula switching is usually unproductive, although it is recognised that some forms of cows' milk intolerance may present with persistent constipation.

Should constipation persist and the clinician is confident that mother's description is of constipation, red flags should alert other considerations.

Fever, vomiting, bloody diarrhoea, failure to thrive, anal stenosis, abdominal distension, history of delayed passage of meconium, polydipsia or polyuria should prompt a search for physical causes.

Conditions to consider are listed in Table 7.14.1.

ACUTE CONSTIPATION

Acute constipation often occurs after febrile illnesses, change in diet or environment, especially when intake has been low (e.g. low post-operatively). A fissure in ano, usually from the passage of a hard faecolith, may cause pain, sphinc-

---

Table 7.14.1   Conditions possibly causing persistent constipation

- Anal anomalies (stenosis, stricture, malposition)
- Spinal anomalies (spinal dysraphism, sacral agenesis)
- Hirschprung's disease
- Hypothyroidism
- Metabolic – hypercalcaemia, hypokalaemia
- Coeliac disease
- Cows' milk intolerance
- Lead poisoning
- Intellectual impairment
- Child abuse
- Cystic fibrosis
- Dietary – inadequate roughage, excessive cows' milk intake
- Psychogenic – parent-child and environment issues
- Drug related – anticholinergic, sympathomimetics, codiene

ter spasm, withholding and the start of a vicious cycle leading to chronic constipation with megacolon and overflow incontinence.

Most acute constipation revolves spontaneously but given the risk of chronic constipation, especially if there has been previous tendency to constipation, it may be prudent to commence gentle oral therapy early.

CHRONIC CONSTIPATION

Chronic constipation is defined as persistent delay and difficulty in defecation often associated with soiling (overflow incontinence). Symptoms may be temporarily relieved by laxatives but relapse rapidly. This is why the ED is not the ideal place for long-term management, but may offer acute intervention for immediate relieve of unpleasant symptoms and to gain the family's confidence by explaining management and natural history.

These children usually present in the school-age group. There may be a history of fissure, pain and withholding then ongoing constipation for months or years. The colon, rectum and upper anal canal become loaded with faeces, insensitive and hypotonic. Soiling develops with loose faeces escaping around an inspissated hard faecolith. Faeces are often palpable per abdomen. Social rejection in the class, due to the malodorous state, is often the first impetus for the patient themselves to seek cure. This with loss of ability to defecate at will takes a toll on the child's emotional stability. They have often undergone multiple management regimens from dietary manipulation to manual disimpaction, delivered by a variety of health care workers.

INVESTIGATIONS

When there is doubt regarding the diagnosis, a plain abdominal X-ray is useful to demonstrate faecal loading. Demonstration of the X-ray findings to the parents may be additionally useful to aid

adherence to prolonged therapeutic strategies.

MANAGEMENT

The management of acute versus chronic constipation varies mainly in nuance and the extent and duration of treatment.

The aim of treatment is that in gaining the family's confidence the clinician recognises that there is a very real concern, and a plan can be instituted to:

❶ Exclude physical treatable causes with careful history, examination and investigations as warranted.

❷ Empty the rectum, preferably from the top.

❸ Establish a pharmacological bowel rhythm and pattern, which may need support for several years.

❹ Allow the enlarged rectum/colon to re-establish its own inherent physiological bowel pattern and tone and to regain its normal sensation.

❺ Continue maintenance for some time before considering slowly weaning off pharmaceuticals.

This will involve:

- Enthusiasm on part of managing clinicians.
- Non-punitive behaviour on part of the parents.
- Adjunctive behavioural modification interventions with achievable goals.
- Acknowledging the need for patience, determination and resolution as the most chronic cases will take years to resolve.
- Stool lubricants, paraffin oil, the taste of which has been well masked in Australia by Parachoc®, using a nocturnal dose starting at 10 mL and titrating dose according to response (not recommended less than one year old due to possible aspiration pneumonia).
- Osmotic laxative, lactulose or sorbitol, initially 3 mL kg^{-1} noct. as a 70% solution, titrating dose according to response.
- Stimulants, senna starting at 2.5 mL noct. titrating dose according to

CONTROVERSIES AND FUTURE DIRECTIONS

❶ The role of serotonin type 4 receptors in the neurochemical basis of peristalsis may provide a more logical pharmaceutical approach to the future management of constipation.

response (side effects are possible colic, and if used in combination with a lubricant it may just make the faecolith spin around).

Should oral therapy be inadequate:

- Suppositories of glycerin may be helpful, especially in acute constipation.
- Microlax enemas, also helpful in the acute situation.
- Phosphate enemas (these should be avoided in children less than two years old; persistent use may cause hyperphosphataemia, hypocalcaemia and tetany).
- Enemas, soap and water (tap water and magnesium have potential toxicity).

Disimpaction of an obstinate rectal faecolith may require:

- Polyethylene glycol – electrolyte solution lavage, 25 mL kg^{-1} h^{-1} (to 1000 mL h^{-1} by nasogastric tube); causing nausea, bloating, cramps, aspiration pneumonia. This will require the child to be admitted to hospital.
- Manual disimpaction under general anaesthesia.
- There is no evidence-based medicine to suggest the success or otherwise of anal dilatation, and some consider permanent external sphincter damage may occur.

Maintenance therapy
Focuses on the prevention of recurrence and should be instituted straight after successful disimpaction or for the child presenting without disimpaction. This involves, as above, dietary interventions, behavioural modification, laxatives, patience and enthusiasm.

Dietary changes

Those commonly advised include increased fluid intake, absorbable and non-absorbable carbohydrate, (sorbitol is found in prune, pear and apple juice). No randomised control study confirms the benefit of this. Forceful implementation would then seem undesirable.

REFERENCES

1. Clayden GS 1976 Constipation and soiling in childhood. Problems of childhood. BMA, London
2. Baker SS 1999 Constipation in infants and children: Evaluation and treatment. Journal of Paediatric Gastroenterology and Nutrition 29(5): 612–626

FURTHER READING

Liptak GS 2000 Constipation. In: Meyer et al (eds) Evidence-based paediatrics and child health. British Medical Journal Books, London

SENIOR AUTHOR RICHARD LENNON

NEUROLOGY

8.1 CSF SHUNT COMPLICATIONS

RICHARD LENNON

ESSENTIALS

1 Any child with a cerebrospinal fluid (CSF) shunt presenting to emergency with non-specific symptoms should have at least a clinical examination to exclude shunt complication.

2 The most common shunt problems involve malfunction causing an increase in ICP or are related to infection.

3 Shunt malfunction or infection can have non-specific signs and symptoms, therefore one has to have a high level of suspicion and a low threshold for investigating.

4 It is important to know as much as possible about the specific shunt hardware in each patient. This is aided by consulting old notes, parents and the child's neurosurgeons.

5 A CT scan is the preferred imaging method for detecting shunt malfunction.

6 Before performing any procedure on a shunt, it is best to consult with the treating neurosurgeon.

7 Slit ventricles on neuroimaging may be non-compliant and therefore do not exclude raised intracranial pressure.

INTRODUCTION

Many types of CSF shunt may be encountered in paediatric emergency practice. The most common form is the ventriculo-peritoneal (VP) shunt. Other systems include ventriculo-atrial, ventriculo-pleural and lumbo-peritoneal. There are also many different types of shunt hardware.

The basic structure of CSF shunts comprises a proximal tube that takes CSF, usually from the lateral ventricle, to the outer surface of the skull. At this point there is usually a subcutaneous one-way valve and possibly a pumping device. There may also be an antisiphoning device. The distal tubing is tunnelled under the skin to the drainage site, which is most commonly the peritoneal cavity. The distal catheter usually contains valves that prevent back flow.

Shunt problems that may present to an ED are listed in Table 8.1.1.

CLINICAL PRESENTATION

History

The history needs to focus on features of raised intracranial pressure and CNS infection. The presentation of shunt complications in children may be florid with acute symptoms related to increasing intracranial pressure or meningitis. Other children may have a more subacute picture with very subtle symptomatology. Parents may present very early, reporting vague and non-specific symptoms, particularly if their child has had a similar presentation of shunt malfunction previously.

The most common presentation of children with shunt obstruction is that of

Table 8.1.1	Complications of CSF shunts

- Infection
- Malfunction
  Blocked proximal catheter
  Blocked distal catheter
  Valve dysfunction
  Over shunting/slit ventricle syndrome
  Disconnection
- Abdominal pseudocyst
- Migration of distal catheter
- Invasion of abdominal organs (VP shunt)
- Peritonitis, ascites (VP shunt)
- Pulmonary emboli (VA shunt)
- Glomerulonephritis (VA shunts)
- Brain tumour metastases
- Pleural effusion (pleural shunts)

headache, vomiting and/or drowsiness. Seizures may be a presenting sign of a complication but because many children with shunts also have epilepsy, seizure alone, has a poor correlation with shunt complication. It is important to remember that distal shunt problems may present with abdominal symptomatology such as pain and distension.

Symptoms suggesting possible infection include fever, lethargy, irritability, or features of meningism. There may be concurrent symptoms of shunt obstruction.

EXAMINATION

For examination features of raised intracranial pressure see Chapter 8.2 on raised intracranial pressure. Features of infection (e.g. fever, rigors, lethargy, localised redness, swelling and peritonism (VP shunt) or pleurisy (Vpleural shunt) should be sought out.

Shunt evaluation

There may be CSF leaking around the proximal catheter and forming a fluctuant swelling around the burr hole in the skull where the shunt enters. This indicates a blocked proximal catheter or disconnection and the child will require neurosurgical consultation.

The shunt itself should be examined thoroughly. The older child is usually the best at finding the shunt hardware under his/her hair. This should be palpated and, if possible, inspected for inflammation of the skin along the shunt route. Many have a silicon-pumping bulb, which is used both for checking the patency of the shunt and for access to sample CSF.

Normally, most reservoirs can be compressed easily and rapidly refill in a few seconds. Incompressibility of the bulb is usually due to obstruction of the distal catheter. This is the less common site of obstruction. If the bulb compresses easily but does not refill, then the proximal catheter is blocked. Abnormal shunt findings should be discussed with the treating neurosurgeon.

Procedures on shunts should be deferred to neurosurgical colleagues. The exception is in the rapidly deteriorating child, where contact with the neurosurgeon is delayed. In the case of a moribund child, it may be indicated for the emergency physician to relieve the raised intracranial pressure by inserting a 25-gauge butterfly needle into the bulb at 45 degrees to the skin under aseptic technique. The pressure can be measured with a similar technique to that used in a lumbar puncture and then CSF drained off until the pressure is 10 cmH$_2$O.

In less acutely unwell children with possible obstruction the entire subcutaneous catheter should be carefully inspected and palpated for continuity and the abdomen examined for evidence of peritonitis or pseudocyst formation.

INVESTIGATIONS

In the stable child an X-ray of the entire shunt can be taken, which will demonstrate a disconnection. The CT scan is the usual preferred method of imaging, although MRI may be an option if the hardware will not be effected by the strong magnetic field. Imaging may show enlarged ventricles. However, this may be chronic and comparison with previous CT scans is usually necessary for interpretation. Obliteration of the perimesencephalic cistern is a particularly worrying sign and mandates urgent neurosurgical consultation. The scan may also show the reason for malfunction (e.g. catheter tip embedded in brain tissue) or it may show a ventriculitis when the lining of the ventricles enhances with contrast. Alternatively, neuroimaging may reveal small 'slit-like' ventricles. These are thought to be due to over shunting and may be non-compliant. This leads to sharp fluctuations in ICP with very little change in CT appearance. The management of this complication is a neurosurgical challenge. The emergency physician needs to be

Table 8.1.2 Shunt infection presenting symptoms

Symptom	Percentage of cases of infection with symptom
Shunt malfunction	33%
Fever	26%
Localised wound or shunt tract inflammation	22%
Abdominal pain or pseudocyst	19%

aware that small ventricles do not mean a normal ICP. Nuclear medicine shunt function studies are also used in some centres for diagnosing shunt blockage. An abdominal ultrasound may be useful to identify a CSF pseudocyst.

Aspects of some CSF shunt complications
Infection
The diagnosis of shunt infection is not always straightforward. In a recent retrospective case series the presenting symptoms were as listed in Table 8.1.2.

The positive predictive value of these symptoms was even greater in the first nine months following insertion of the shunt because 80% of all shunt infections occur in this time. There is also an increase in VP shunt infections after laparotomy. Case reports also mention other symptoms such as rigors whenever a ventriculo-atrial shunt is manipulated. The most useful investigation is initially the CSF white cell count, which is elevated in approximately 70% of cases. The blood white cell count is elevated in only 30% of cases. A positive CSF culture is the gold standard, although this may be negative in those children who have been on antibiotics. Bacterial antigen detection and polymerase chain reaction testing may be helpful in this situation.

Staphylococcus epidermidis is the most common bacterium isolated, followed by other coagulase negative staphylococci and *S. aureus*. Less commonly Gram-negative bacteria, such as *Propionobacter* and *Streptococcus pneumoniae*, and *Candida* infections have been reported.

Initial antibiotic therapy can be tailored to findings on Gram stain from a CSF tap and/or cultures from previous infections. Flucloxacillin or dicloxacillin should be in all empirical regimens with Gram-negative cover considered after consultation with neurosurgeons and an infectious-disease specialist. In the majority of cases the shunt will have to be removed and replaced at a later date, with some temporary measure in the mean time.

Migration and penetration of shunts

In various cases the distal end of VP shunts have migrated into the thorax, liver, bowel lumen and even out of the anus. Several liver abscesses have been reported. Spring reinforced catheters seemed to have a greater propensity to do this and these are no longer used.

Glomerulonephritis

This is a complication of ventriculo-atrial shunts, which are rarely used today. This is usually a gradually progressive illness which requires a high level of suspicion for diagnosis.

FURTHER READING

Aspner R et al 2000 The shampoo clue: Two cases of infection of ventriculoatrial shunt. Clinical Infectious Diseases 31: 1518

Roberts JR 1998 Clinical Procedures in Emergency Medicine, 3rd edn. WB Saunders Company, Philadelphia, PA

Williams DG et al 1996 Shunt infection in children: Presentation and management. Journal of Neuroscience Nursing 28(3): 155

8.2 RAISED INTRACRANIAL PRESSURE

RICHARD LENNON

ESSENTIALS

1 In the infant, prior to suture fusion, a rapidly expanding head circumference is an important sign of raised ICP.

2 The open anterior fontanelle allows direct palpation of ICP in children up to 9–18 months of age.

3 In rare circumstances an emergency procedure, such as a subdural or a ventricular tap, can be performed through the anterior fontanelle in infants.

4 A brain CT scan or MRI can rule out many causes of raised ICP, but does not exclude raised ICP itself and thus should not be the sole basis for deciding whether or not it is safe to perform a lumbar puncture.

5 Acute severe elevation of ICP is a true emergency often requiring intubation and ventilation, infusion of mannitol 1 gm kg^{-1} and early consultation with neurosurgeons.

INTRODUCTION

Normal physiology

Normal intracranial pressure (ICP) is 6–18 cmH$_2$O. It is the product of the intracranial contents mainly blood, brain and cerebrospinal fluid and the resistance of the cranial vault. Normal ICP has a diurnal cycle being higher in the early hours of the morning when one is normally supine during sleep. Therefore the symptoms of raised ICP, such as headache and vomiting are usually worse in the morning. Intracranial pressure may be raised by anything that can cause an increase in the volume of its contents or a decrease in the size of the cranial cavity (see Table 8.2.1). This section will not

cover the diagnosis and management of raised intracranial pressure associated with trauma. Those issues are covered in Chapter 3.2.

Most CSF is made by the choroid plexus in the lateral third and fourth ventricles. A normal child makes approximately 20 mL h^{-1} and the total volume is 50 mL in an infant rising to 150 mL in an adult. It flows through the foramen of Monro into the third ventricle, then down the aqueduct of Sylvius, which is usually only 2 mm wide, and 3 mm long in a child. This leads into the fourth ventricle and from there via the foramina of Luschka and Magendie to the basal cisterns. From there the CSF flows over the surface of the cerebellar and cerebral hemispheres to be reabsorbed through the arachnoid villi on the superior sagittal

Table 8.2.1   Causes of raised intracranial pressure

A. Increased CSF (hydrocephalus)
1. Decreased absorption
   - Obstructive
   - Communicating
2. Increased production

B. Swollen contents
1. Meningitis
2. Encephalitis
3. Cerebral oedema
   - Hypo/hypernatraemia
   - Post-ischaemic
   - Post-traumatic/diffuse axonal injury

C. Space-occupying lesion (SOL)
1. Tumours
   - Primary
   - Secondary
2. Haematomas
   - Extradural
   - Subdural
   - Intracerebral/intraventricular
3. Abscesses/cysts
4. Arteriovenous malformation
5. Congenital cysts

D. Decreased or fixed intracranial volume
1. Depressed skull fracture
2. Premature fusion of cranial sutures (craniosynostosis)

E. Pseudotumour cerebri (benign intracranial hypertension)

sinus. CSF can also be reabsorbed through several other channels including a small amount through the choroid plexus and via lymphatics. Intracranial pressure will be raised whenever there is obstruction to the flow or reabsorption of CSF or in the rare circumstance where CSF production is increased.

Measurement of ICP

Intracranial pressure is usually estimated from lumbar puncture manometry. When performed on a child lying in the lateral decubitus position in a relaxed posture, this is a reasonable approximation of the intracranial pressure. Measuring CSF pressure in a screaming child is likely to be inaccurate because of the temporary rise caused by high venous pressure. Similarly, the person holding the child in the foetal position for the lumbar puncture, should relax their grasp and allow the child to stretch out temporarily while the pressure is being measured. If the LP is being done under a general anaesthetic, attempts should made to normalise the Pco$_2$, so that the pressure reflects awake ICP.

PARTICULAR ISSUES IN CHILDREN

Infants

An infant's inability to communicate and smaller repertoire of behaviours makes raised intracranial pressure more difficult to diagnose.

The infant does not have a rigid cranial cavity until fusion of the sutures at approximately one to two years of age. Therefore increasing intracranial volume in the infant will cause a lesser increase in the ICP and a greater increase in the head circumference than it would in older children or adults. This is one of the reasons why acute increases in ICP in infants are often not easily detected by the infant's behaviour.

The measurement of head circumference (occipitofrontal) is a useful means of detecting intracranial pathology, particularly where imaging techniques such as CT scanning are not available or may require anaesthesia to achieve. The head circumference should be plotted on centile charts, using prior measurements, if available, to determine if there has been a trend to cross percentiles. The child's length and weight should be plotted concurrently, to evaluate if the head is disproportionately large or small. When the cranial sutures separate due to expansion, percussion of the skull makes a sound similar to that of a 'cracked pot'. This is known as Macewen's sign.

Conversely, the open anterior fontanelle allows direct palpation of intracranial pressure up to the age of nine to eighteen months. It is highly recommended that one closely observes the fontanelles of normal infants, to help one identify abnormalities in clinical practice. The normal fontanelle will bulge slightly when the infant is lying down. It will become depressed when the child is sat up. It will bulge more prominently when the infant is crying or straining. The normal fontanelle will have an arterial pulsation more apparent when the infant is upright.

The fontanelle also provides access for emergency procedures such as the draining of a traumatic subdural or a ventricular tap. Fortunately the need for these procedures in the ED rarely arises. When it does, however, it should be done by a neurosurgical specialist (or trainee if sufficiently experienced). In centres where such help is not rapidly available, over-the-phone advice from a neurosurgeon, may help with both the decision to do the procedure and the technique.

CLINICAL FEATURES OF RAISED INTRACRANIAL PRESSURE

The symptoms and signs that lead to a diagnosis of RICP will vary with the age, severity and rate of development. In slower onset conditions such as brain tumours the most common scenario in infants is the gradually progressive onset of drowsiness/lethargy, morning irritability and vomiting with an expanding head circumference. In older children there are progressive early morning headaches, but no dramatic increase in head circumference.

Brain tumours may also present with focal neurological signs before there is a significant rise in ICP due to direct invasion of neural pathways. Other symptoms may include a head tilt, which is due to unilateral 4th cranial nerve palsy causing a vertical strabismus. The child will compensate for this by tilting the head. This often occurs with posterior fossa tumours. However, there are other causes of head tilt such as sternomastoid 'tumour' in the newborn and benign torticollis. In obstructive hydrocephalus paralysis of upward gaze is common due to third nerve dysfunction. This leads to the classic picture in the infant of a big head and 'sunset' eyes. Some infants will become irritable on watching TV or looking at books because of diplopia. Parents may notice strabismus and older children will complain of diplopia.

Often there will be regression in motor milestones due to ataxia and/or weakness. Personality changes may occur.

As pressure increases the pressure itself may cause focal neurological symptoms and signs. These may be due to several mechanisms which include:

- Impingement on, or disruption of, a cranial nerve, cranial nerve nucleus or higher centre.
- Impingement on a blood vessel supplying any of the above.
- In hydrocephalus, stretching of corticospinal tract fibres around enlarging ventricles causes upper motor neuron signs in the legs.
- Focal seizures may accompany raised ICP and leave an infant with a Todd's paresis.

In the more rapid onset conditions, such as intracranial haemorrhage, rapid onset of drowsiness and vomiting with or without focal neurology is the rule. When there is a large intracerebral pressure differential across a fixed structure, such as the tentorium, the brain will herniate. There are several herniation syndromes.

The central herniation syndrome

Generalised midline or bilateral swelling above the tentorium cerebelli causes the midbrain to herniate through the tentorium. This leads to dysfunction of the midbrain and higher centres due to compression, causing:

- Drowsiness
- Initially *small* reactive pupils
- Decorticate posturing
- As the process worsens pupils become midrange
- Posture becomes decerebrate
- Bilateral 6th cranial nerve palsies may become apparent when attempting the doll's-eye reflex
- These are accompanied by Cushing's triad, i.e. hypertension, bradycardia and abnormal breathing patterns.

The lateral mass herniation syndrome

A unilateral supratentorial swelling will give rise to a pattern of events formerly known as the uncal herniation syndrome. Imaging studies now show that herniation of the uncus happens very late in the process and is not responsible for most of the signs. Features in rough sequence are as follows:

- Contralateral hemiplegia
- Drowsiness
- Ipsilateral pupillary dilatation (partial 3rd nerve palsy)
- Complete 3rd nerve palsy as pressure increases (can be bilateral)
- Ipsilateral hemiplegia (midbrain being pushed against edge of tentorium)
- Cushing's triad.

Cerebellar tonsillar herniation syndrome

A wide variety of signs and symptoms arise from posterior fossa masses. However, sometimes as the cerebellar tonsils are pushed through the foramen magnum and the medulla with its respiratory control centres are compressed the following sequence occurs:

- Patient complains of a stiff neck
- Drowsiness
- Apnoea.

OTHER EXAMINATION FINDINGS IN RAISED ICP

General observation

In the unco-operative child, general observation is a vital part of the examination. It may reveal a large and/or an asymmetric head, evidence of trauma, gait, speech or visual disturbance. Watching a playful child from a distance will yield a lot more information than the formal examination of a screaming unhappy one.

Fundi

Although often difficult to visualise in children, fundal examination is of vital importance. Using a parent as a visual distraction will often help. With patience, the disc can usually be visualised through an undilated pupil. One may be able to visualise retinal venous pulsations. The implication of these pulsations is that intracranial pressure is less than peak venous pressure. Papilloedema is less common in infants with raised ICP. Examination of the fundi is less useful in acute severe raised ICP, as papilloedema takes days to evolve. Other retinal findings associated with raised ICP include retinal haemorrhages, which have a strong association with non-accidental injury, aneurysms and arteriovenous malformation that may be associated with similar intracranial lesions and subhyaloid haemorrhages seen in patients with subarachnoid haemorrhages. In some instances it may be useful to ask an ophthalmologist to examine the child through dilated pupils.

Peripheral neurological signs

The development of 'handedness' is not apparent in normal infants under one year of age. If handedness is apparent in infancy, it is usually due to a neurological or musculoskeletal lesion, some of which are associated with raised ICP. Hydrocephalus may produce lower limb signs with gait disturbance in the ambulant child. In infants, this may be apparent when the child is held around the chest with the legs suspended in midair. Spasm of the adductors will cause scissoring of the lower limbs.

INVESTIGATIONS

Imaging the brain will often reveal the underlying pathology in children with raised intracranial pressure. However, there are several drawbacks that must be borne in mind when deciding to obtain a scan.

One must be sure that it is safe to move the child to the scanner room where facilities for resuscitation and access to the patient are less than ideal. CT or MRI scans may be falsely reassuring especially in the case of PTC or meningitis, where the appearance may be normal even when the pressure is dangerously high. To keep an unco-operative child still may require a general anaesthetic with its concomitant risks. However, as scanning technology improves, the time required for a scan is getting dramatically shorter. Many infants can often be successfully scanned with the use of a dummy (comforter) dipped in 50% dextrose and firm wrapping. Likewise, in older children, the presence of a parent in the scanner room may permit the avoidance of anaesthesia. Otherwise the decision to use general anaesthesia or procedural sedation depends on the clinical situation, local policy and skill mix, with safety always being the first consideration.

An MRI scan is more likely to require anaesthesia, as they usually take longer and patient access is more difficult. Finally, when obtaining CT scans, one must consider the risks of radiation causing cancer, which in a CT scan of the head in a child is estimated to be 1:1000–1:10000 over the lifetime of the child.[1] Head ultrasound is an option for imaging in infants. This is good at imaging the lateral ventricles and surrounding structures but dependant on operator experience. However, ultrasound is less able to image the subdural space around the vertex and the posterior fossa region.

Management of raised ICP

Acute severe increases in ICP are a true emergency and children with features of the herniation syndromes should be treated in the resuscitation area of the ED or the neurosurgical operating theatre. A neurosurgeon should be consulted as early as possible.

In this situation efforts should be directed towards maintaining ventilation circulation, by rapid sequence intubation if necessary, giving intravenous mannitol 1 gm kg^{-1} or furosemide 1 mg kg^{-1} and nursing the patient in a 30 degree head up position. There is strong evidence against prolonged hyperventilation because vasoconstriction impairs cerebral perfusion despite the reduction in intracranial pressure. $P\text{CO}_2$ should be kept between 35 and 40 mmHg unless the above measures have been unsuccessful or herniation is progressing, in which case the $P\text{CO}_2$ can be taken down to 25 mmHg for a brief period while further measures are commenced. Whilst these measures are taking effect consideration and management of the underlying cause should be undertaken. This will be aided by a concise history and some rapid bedside testing such as blood gas, which may reveal hyponatraemia. If an infant in this situation does not respond to these measures, a neurosurgeon should be urgently consulted regarding a ventricular or subdural tap. In older children who do not respond adequately the options depend on the clinical situation and the underlying cause. Therapeutic options include: consulting neurosurgeons and getting an urgent CT scan; palliating or treating an underlying cause urgently (e.g. high dose dexamethasone for vasogenic oedema or hypertonic saline for hyponatraemia); or maintaining cerebral perfusion pressure by maintaining mean arterial blood pressure at above normal levels with fluids and inotropes and reducing cerebral metabolic demand with drugs such as thiopental. Other neurosurgical interventions include: craniotomy; insertion of external ventricular drain; and insertion of a CSF reservoir or a complete CSF shunt. Where a shunt is already present this may be tapped (see Chapter 8.1 on shunt complications). Consideration should also be given to prophylactic anticonvulsants because seizure will cause a further acute rise in ICP. Once initial stabilisation is underway and neurosurgeons are involved referral to a paediatric ICU is mandatory.

Children with less severely raised ICP usually need investigation and treatment of the cause, whilst avoiding interventions that may increase ICP. One should avoid the infusion of hypotonic fluids for a vomiting child or the administration of certain drugs. Children with hydrocephalus will usually require the insertion of a shunt, although some can be treated with 3rd ventriculostomy only.

SOME PARTICULAR CAUSES OF RAISED ICP

Iatrogenic

Any child receiving intravenous fluids, especially for treatment of diabetic ketoacidosis (DKA), who develops headache and/or drowsiness and/or seizures during therapy should be considered to have raised ICP until proven otherwise. A thorough assessment should be made and electrolytes checked for disturbances that may lead to cerebral oedema. Imaging should be considered. If cerebral oedema is confirmed or not excluded then the child should be treated as above and observed in a paediatric ICU.

Pseudotumour cerebri (PTC)

This condition is characterised by sustained raised ICP causing symptoms similar to a cerebral tumour but with no

Table 8.2.2   Causes of pseudotumour cerebri

1. Idiopathic
2. Venous obstruction
3. Metabolic
   - Hypervitaminosis A
   - Hypoparathyroidism
   - Addison's disease
   - Obesity
   - Pregnancy
   - Galactosaemia
4. Drugs
   - Oral contraceptive pill
   - Glucocorticoids
   - Tetracyclines
   - Isotretinoin
   - Nalidixic acid
   - Nitrofurantoin
5. Haematologic
   - Anaemia
   - Polycythaemia
6. Infections
   - Roseola infantum
   - Chronic complicated otitis media
7. Others
   - Guillain–Barré syndrome

anatomical abnormality on neuroimaging. It is usually due to decreased CSF reabsorption. PTC has many causes (see Table 8.2.2). It often occurs in overweight pubescent girls, in which no cause is found. The presentation is usually with headaches and vomiting, which are worse in the morning. Some patients may complain of transient visual obscuration with blurring or darkening of vision that lasts less than 30 seconds. Later there may be unilateral or bilateral 6th nerve palsies causing diplopia on lateral gaze. Papilloedema is often the only positive physical finding. The most significant sequela of PTC is loss of vision. This begins with an enlargement of the blindspot associated with papilloedema, and later

progresses with erosion of the peripheral visual fields. Left untreated the patient with persistent PCT will eventually develop optic atrophy and blindness.

Investigations include CT scan or MRI, followed by lumbar puncture to measure opening pressure. Lumbar puncture may be both diagnostic and therapeutic. The cerebrospinal fluid (CSF) has a high pressure, but analysis reveals normal protein, glucose, cell count and no microorganisms.

Therapeutic CSF taps should aim to decrease the ICP by 50%. This may be curative. However, in most cases repeat lumbar punctures and/or acetazolamide are required. It is believed that acetazolamide works by reducing CSF production. In severe cases a lumboperitoneal shunt or optic nerve sheath fenestration may be required. One needs to exclude any treatable underlying cause. Anticoagulants should be given for venous thrombosis and drugs such as glucocorticoids should be ceased or weaned if possible. Referral to a paediatric neurologist is mandatory.

REFERENCES

Brenner DJ et al 2001 Estimated risks of radiation-induced fatal cancer from pediatric CT. American Journal of Roentgenology 175(2): 289–96

FURTHER READING

Behrman RE, Kliegman R, Jenson HB (eds) 2000 Nelson Textbook of Pediatrics, 16th edn. WB Saunders, Philadelphia

Roberts JR Clinical Procedures in Emergency Medicine, 3rd edn. WB Saunders, Philadelphia

8.3 SEIZURES AND NON-EPILEPTIC EVENTS

PADRAIC GRATTAN-SMITH

ESSENTIALS

1 Children commonly present to EDs with seizures.

2 The diagnosis of a seizure is based on a careful history.

3 There are many paroxysmal events or 'funny turns' in children, which can mimic seizures.

4 A bedside dextrostix should be performed on the child who is having a seizure. First-ever seizures should have blood sent for formal glucose, electrolytes, calcium, magnesium and phosphate levels.

5 The acute management of the child having a seizure involves supporting airway and breathing and the graduated use of antiepileptic drugs to terminate the seizure.

6 Parental education and reassurance is an important facet of management in the child presenting with a first convulsion.

INTRODUCTION

An epileptic seizure can be defined as a disturbance in neurological function, resulting from uncontrolled excessive neuronal activity in the central nervous system.

The subject of seizures and their differential diagnosis is large. This chapter provides essential information that may be useful in formulating diagnosis and treatment in the ED. There is insufficient space for a detailed discussion of the role of EEG and other investigations.

GENERAL COMMENTS

There are a number of conditions that must always be considered in children experiencing unusual events. Hypoglycaemia can cause both partial and generalised seizures. It may also 'illogically' produce focal neurological signs. Abnormalities of electrolytes, calcium, magnesium and phosphate can present in a similar fashion. Cardiac arrhythmias associated with prolonged QT interval may cause epileptic seizures that seem to follow the arrhythmia. Sudden loss of consciousness during, or immediately after, intense exercise or associated with strong emotion, raises the possibility of an underlying cardiac cause. A family history of premature sudden death should also raise this possibility.

Some variants of migraine may be difficult to distinguish from seizures. Acute confusional migraine often follows minor head trauma. The episodes may last for a number of hours. The child is 'concussed', confused and often vomiting. Basilar artery migraine is associated with confusion or loss of consciousness and brainstem symptoms and signs. Neither diagnosis should be made at the first presentation and without further investigation. On the other hand, occipital epilepsy can cause vomiting, visual loss and severe headache. The presence of tonic eye deviation early in the event is a strong clue that this is a seizure rather than migraine.

Pseudo-epileptic seizures and Munchausen's syndrome by proxy always need to be considered in the differential diagnosis of atypical epileptic seizures. However, the diagnosis is often difficult and the ED is usually not an appropriate setting to make a confident diagnosis of either of these conditions.

CLASSIFICATION OF SEIZURES

Seizures are conceptually divided into *generalised seizures* where the onset is from all brain regions simultaneously and *partial seizures*, where the seizure arises from one area in the brain. In *simple partial seizures* there is no alteration of consciousness. With *complex partial seizures*, alteration of consciousness occurs. Partial seizures may spread and become secondarily generalised.

Status epilepticus is said to occur where a seizure lasts more than 30 minutes or there is incomplete recovery between seizures over this time period. Status epilepticus can occur in both convulsive and non-convulsive forms.

FEBRILE SEIZURES

Febrile convulsions are not regarded as a form of epilepsy but are discussed because of their frequent presentation to EDs. Typically they occur in children between six months and six years of age. They are common, affecting around 3% of children. Most children, who have febrile convulsions have only one, but 25–30% will have a recurrence. The risk of recurrence is higher in infants less than twelve months.

Febrile convulsions most commonly occur in the setting of viral illnesses such as URTI, pharyngitis, gastroenteritis, or an exanthem such as roseola infantum. Much less commonly pneumonia or UTI may be the underlying infection. Febrile seizures typically occur relatively early in the course of an infectious illness and sometimes the convulsion is the first sign that the child is unwell.

Most febrile seizures are generalised and brief, lasting less than two minutes. The child returns to normal after a short (usually less than 30 minutes) post-ictal period. The seizures may be clonic, tonic-clonic or atonic where the child may simply seem to stop breathing. Examination should confirm the presence of a fever, identify the source of the fever, and exclude signs of CNS infection or of a focal neurological process. Most children with an uncomplicated febrile seizure who have completely recovered and have a clear source of infection, require no blood tests or other investigations.

Prolonged and complicated febrile seizures can occur. Underlying *meningitis/ encephalitis* must always be considered in the child who fails to return to normal, has multiple or prolonged seizures or has residual neurological signs. The threshold to perform a CSF examination is lower when the child is less than twelve months of age or has been on antibiotics, which may mask the usual signs of meningism. However, lumbar puncture can be dangerous in the child with focal signs such as a hemiparesis or if there has been a rapid deterioration in conscious level or an abnormality of respiratory rhythm. Consultation with senior colleagues is advised if there is doubt about the safety of a lumbar puncture.

Children with seizures are seen in the ED in two broad settings:

❶ The child who is seen after an event. Was this a seizure?
❷ The child who is still fitting.

1. THE CHILD SEEN AFTER THE EVENT

History

The diagnosis of seizures is based almost entirely on the history.

The parents or any witnesses to the event, should be taken through the episode systematically. An exact description of what took place is crucial in making a correct diagnosis. What was the child doing when it started? What was the very first sign of a problem, and what followed? If abnormal movements were present, did they principally involve one side of the body? How long did the event last? What was the child like afterwards? How long before the child was back to normal? Was there any faecal or urinary incontinence or tongue biting? Was there any apnoea or colour change?

Witnessing a sudden loss of consciousness in a child is an extremely upsetting event for any observer, particularly the parents. Many parents report that they thought their child had 'stopped breathing' and commenced various resuscitation techniques. There are obvious limitations to the history, but it remains the single piece of information most likely to provide a diagnosis. It is also worth talking to the child about what happened. Even young children can sometimes give very helpful accounts if spoken to soon after the event.

It is important to establish whether there may have been provocative factors, such as sleep deprivation, a febrile illness, head trauma or potential exposure to epileptogenic medications. A past history of similar events should be sought. It is also important to ask about a family history of seizures or unusual turns and to review the child's developmental milestones.

Examination

The physical examination is often normal, but it must be carefully performed looking for fever, evidence of intercurrent illness and abnormal neurological signs. Other important diagnostic clues include a Todd's paralysis, skin lesions of tuberous sclerosis or morphological features of a chromosomal disorder or other underlying neurological abnormality associated with seizure disorder. The finding of tongue trauma or incontinence, supports a suspicion of seizure when the diagnosis is unclear. The febrile child needs to have an underlying meningitis or encephalitis excluded.

In infants, the sudden onset of frequent seizures and failure to regain consciousness is a common presentation of child abuse and a careful retinal examination must be performed looking for haemorrhages in this setting.

Differential diagnosis

Tonic-clonic seizures, myoclonic seizures and clonic seizures, in general, can occur at any age. They are well described in standard textbooks and will not be discussed here except to discourage the tendency to loosely label any event with loss of consciousness as a 'tonic-clonic' seizure.

Although there is overlap, it is helpful to approach the problem in terms of age of presentation. For neonatal seizures refer to Chapter 2.6.

A. Infancy

Seizure types

Infantile spasms Typically take the form of 'salaam' seizures. There is characteristic sudden flexion of the arms, head and trunk in a brief spasm. Asymmetrical or extensor spasms can occur. The characteristic feature of established infantile spasms is that the episodes occur in *runs* (clusters) which can continue for ten minutes or more. In the early phases, the spasms may be mild and relatively infrequent, making diagnosis difficult.

Lennox–Gastaut syndrome In this syndrome there are multiple seizure types, including atypical absences, myoclonic seizures, drop attacks, nocturnal tonic seizures and generalised tonic-clonic seizures. In the early phases, which can be seen in late infancy, the child may present with atypical absences. These have somewhat slower onset than typical absences and there may be obscuration rather than complete loss of consciousness. Great caution should be taken with any child presenting in the first two years of life with 'absences', as this may be an early manifestation of Lennox-Gastaut syndrome.

Complex partial seizures in infancy

May present as episodes of altered consciousness, with autonomic symptoms and also with apnoea. An underlying tumour (most often in the temporal lobe) may cause this type of seizure.

Non-epileptic events of infancy

The following events can mimic seizures in young children and are usually distinguished by a careful history.

Breath-holding spells These are always provoked by an unpleasant stimulus. This is usually minor trauma, e.g. a bump on the head, but the child being scolded or frustrated may provoke them. Somewhat arbitrarily, breath-holding attacks are divided into:

❶ Pallid breath-holding attacks, where after a short cry, the infant loses consciousness, becomes pale and there may be tonic stiffening.

❷ Cyanotic breath-holding attacks, where after vigorous crying, there is breath-holding in expiration and loss of consciousness.

As in syncopal episodes there may be brief clonic jerking after an episode. The story of provocation is usually clear, but at times there can be diagnostic confusion, for example, when a child who is playing happily is found unconscious on the floor and no precipitating event was observed.

Benign neonatal sleep myoclonus Is characterised by myoclonic jerks, which can be quite violent and asymmetric, but are confined to sleep. The infant is otherwise normal.

Benign paroxysmal vertigo Sudden episodes of acute unsteadiness occur without alteration of consciousness. The child typically clutches onto whatever is nearby. The episodes are usually brief, lasting seconds to minutes. The parents may notice nystagmus during an episode. There may be multiple episodes per day.

Shuddering attacks The infant's body 'shivers' as though cold water had been poured on its back.

Self-stimulatory episodes ('infantile masturbation') These are seen in girls. The thighs are generally clenched tight, with the legs crossed at the ankles. There are pelvic undulatory movements. The infant may look extremely flushed and upset and may be sleepy afterwards.

Stereotypies There are hand-flapping or other repetitive limb movements. These are usually repeated in exactly the same way each time. Although common in children with autism, they also occur in children who are otherwise normal.

Day-dreaming Is common at all ages in childhood. The child may stare straight ahead and at times not respond to being called.

In daydreaming, stereotypic behaviours and self-stimulatory episodes, the event can usually be immediately stopped by physical interaction with the child, e.g. by tickling them.

B. Childhood
Seizure types
Absence seizures Are usually brief staring spells characterised by a sudden loss of consciousness and an abrupt end to the seizure. There is no post-ictal period. With longer absences, automatisms may occur. The events usually last less than ten seconds, and multiple episodes may occur per day.

Complex partial seizures There may be an aura (actually a partial seizure), a more prolonged episode of altered consciousness in which the child may be partially responsive and a post-ictal period characterised by drowsiness and a desire to sleep.

Benign focal epilepsy of childhood In its typical form, presents with the child awaking from sleep at around 2–4 a.m. making a 'glugging' or 'clucking' noise. This is followed by a clonic seizure involving one side of the body including the face. The child may be awake during the seizure and find it very frightening. Not uncommonly, this seizure becomes secondarily generalised.

Nocturnal frontal lobe seizures Are rare but may be mistaken for night terrors and 'pseudoseizures'. Seizures should be considered if there are multiple stereotyped events occurring in the one night, if the episodes are very brief or if they occur only in the second half of the night.

Non-epileptic events of childhood
Night terrors Usually occur within the first few hours of the child going to sleep. Typically the child screams and is found sitting up in bed with widely dilated pupils and appears to be extremely fearful. This may last for half an hour or more. The child is eventually comforted and goes off to sleep. The next morning the child has no memory of the event.

Nightmares In contrast, these usually occur in the second half of the night. The child goes into the parent's bedroom afraid because of a 'bad dream'. The child usually has a good memory of the dream, although he/she may not want to discuss it.

Paroxysmal kinesigenic dyskinesia Brief episodes of dystonic or choreoathetoid movements involving the limbs are provoked by sudden bursts of exercise. There is no alteration of consciousness.

C. Late childhood and adolescence
Seizure types
Juvenile myoclonic epilepsy This usually develops in the early teenage years. Typically there are myoclonic jerks in the morning soon after awakening. These may not be mentioned to the parents. The first presentation is often with an early morning generalised tonic-clonic seizure. A history of early morning myoclonus should always be sought in this situation.

Non-epileptic events
Syncope Is usually a vasovagal response provoked by a stressful situation, such as seeing blood or standing for a prolonged period in hot weather. There is a feeling of light-headedness, nausea and then a progressive fading out of vision. As mentioned above, there may be brief stiffening and clonic jerks in the course of syncopal episodes. Unusual forms of syncope in adolescence include 'stretch syncope' provoked by neck hyperextension and shoulder abduction while stretching and 'hair grooming syncope', which seems to be provoked by strong pulling of the hair while combing or brushing. Children with intellectual handicap may repeatedly provoke episodes of loss of consciousness by hyperventilating and then performing the Valsalva manoeuvre.

Rage attacks These consist of sudden episodes of directed anger, usually provoked by being thwarted in some way. A careful history will usually differentiate a rage attack from non-directed aggression, which can occur in the post-ictal state. This usually occurs when a patient in a confused post-ictal state is restrained or surrounded by a crowd of people.

2. THE CHILD WHO IS STILL FITTING

The child with convulsive status epilepticus

When a child is fitting on arrival to the ED, the seizure is likely to have continued for at least 15 minutes. There is a risk of brain damage or death if the seizure is not rapidly controlled and respiration appropriately supported. There needs to be a clear plan for the immediate management of the convulsing child. The child should be taken directly to the paediatric resuscitation area with ready access to anaesthetic and airway resuscitation facilities.

Airway, breathing and circulation need to be assessed and simultaneously managed. The child should receive high-flow oxygen via mask or assisted by bag and mask, if ventilation is inadequate. Basic airway manoeuvres and suctioning may be required. Oxygen saturation should be monitored continuously. Intravenous access should be gained and a dextrostix checked immediately to exclude hypoglycaemia. Blood should be taken for glucose, electrolytes, calcium, magnesium and phosphate and full blood count if the child has not previously had seizures. Children on maintenance anticonvulsants should have their drug level taken.

At the same time, a history should be rapidly obtained regarding:

- The duration of the seizure
- Previous episodes (and if there is a particular drug most likely to be effective)
- Precipitating events
- Medications the child is taking
- Whether drugs have already been given for the seizure
- The presence of underlying neurological problems.

DRUG THERAPY

If the child has received no treatment for the seizure prior to arrival, the following approach is suggested.

First line

Initial treatment is with benzodiazepines, which are rapidly acting, using intravenous (IV) diazepam 0.25 mg kg^{-1} or IV midazolam 0.15 mg kg^{-1}. If the seizure has not stopped within five minutes the dose can be repeated. The potential side effects of respiratory depression or apnoea need to be anticipated.

Second line

If after another five minutes the fit continues, IV phenytoin 20 mg kg^{-1} as an infusion over 30 minutes or IV phenobarbitone 10–15 mg kg^{-1} as an infusion over 30 minutes should be given. These 'second-line' agents need to be given *slowly* by intravenous infusion, and therefore will take time to control the seizure. If continued seizure activity is causing *respiratory compromise*, it may be necessary to use further benzodiazepines and be prepared to support respiration or to proceed to use barbiturates, which require intubation.

Third line

If there has been no response after a further five minutes, thiopental 5 mg kg^{-1} and intubation using rapid sequence induction, is the next step. The decision to intubate to control a seizure needs to involve consideration not only of the length of the seizure but also of the degree of respiratory embarrassment to the child. Mild seizure activity that is not compromising a child can be tolerated longer than a major convulsion that is impairing oxygenation. These children will need to be subsequently managed in a paediatric intensive care unit.

There are almost endless variables in this situation. If intravenous access is a problem, midazolam 0.15 mg kg^{-1} may be given intramuscularly or into the buccal space or diazepam 0.5 mg kg^{-1} may be given rectally. Intraosseous injection can be used. If the child has already received a benzodiazepine beforehand, a second dose may be given on arrival followed by phenytoin as it is less likely to cause respiratory depression, than the combination of phenobarbitone and a benzodiazepine.

In a severely handicapped child who has frequent bouts of status epilepticus where there is a desire to avoid intubation, paraldehyde 0.4 mL kg^{-1} rectally may be tried if there has been no response to benzodiazepines, phenytoin or phenobarbitone.

Absence, atypical absence and complex partial status Are much less common than convulsive status but should be considered in children who are obtunded or have bizarre behaviour without obvious cause. If there is doubt an EEG should be performed. If an EEG is unavailable and CNS infection and metabolic causes have been excluded, 'waking up' soon after an IV dose of a benzodiazepine is a useful diagnostic clue.

INVESTIGATIONS

These depend on the clinical setting but some general rules apply.

Blood tests

All children having a seizure should have a bedside dextrostix followed by a formal blood glucose to exclude hypoglycaemia. At the same time full blood count, electrolytes, calcium, magnesium and phosphate levels should be checked.

In the child who has had a first seizure but returned to normal it is worth checking the full blood count, electrolytes, calcium, magnesium and phosphate levels, although these tests have a relatively low yield. A fasting blood sugar should be considered.

Neuroimaging

As a general rule, patients with focal seizure or examination findings, features suggesting raised intracranial pressure or seizures in the setting of trauma, should have urgent neuroimaging. The CT scan of the brain has the advantage of relative ease of access but it should be remembered that the MRI scan is a better test in almost all instances except traumatic brain injury.

EEG

An urgent EEG is very useful in cases where convulsive status epilepticus has been treated but the patient remains unconscious and there is a suspicion of continuing non-convulsive status. It is also very helpful in the child presenting with an altered state of consciousness and absence or complex partial status is suspected. In the child who has recovered from a brief seizure an EEG done soon after presentation may be useful, e.g. showing focal changes that suggest a secondarily generalised seizure. There is no reason to delay getting an EEG soon after a fit but this will be limited by the resources that are available.

DISPOSITION

Children who have prolonged or multiple seizures, focal seizures, or abnormal neurological examination, or where the diagnosis is unclear, should be admitted for observation and paediatric or neurological review. Children who are having increased frequency of seizures or are known to have prolonged, or clusters of, seizures warrant admission and observation until stabilised.

Not all children presenting with an uncomplicated first seizure need to be admitted to hospital. Those who have a first generalised seizure with normal neurological examination and metabolic work up, can be followed up on an out-patient basis. This is usually best achieved by discussion with a general paediatrician or neurologist colleague to determine the timing of imaging and an EEG and formal review. Other influences on the decision to admit may include the age of the child, parental anxiety and any intercurrent illness.

If the event has clearly been a brief seizure, it is important to discuss the nature of this with the parents and provide some reassurance that it has not caused brain damage. First-aid measures should be discussed with the parents so that they have a clear plan should their child have a further seizure at home. Precautionary advice regarding the avoidance of activities that could place their

child at risk if they had another seizure should be discussed. This advice should be reviewed at the organised follow up. Children who are discharged after a febrile convulsion should be reviewed by their local doctor within 24 hours if they have not completely returned to normal. Likewise, any alteration to anti-epileptic drug doses, needs to be carefully reviewed.

FURTHER READING

Lowenstein DH, Alldredge BK 1998 Current concepts: Status epilepticus. New England Journal of Medicine 338: 970–976

Maytal J, Shinnar S, Moshe SL, Alvarez LA 1989 Low morbidity and mortality of status epilepticus in children. Paediatrics 83: 323–331

Mitchell W 1996 Status epilepticus and acute repetitive seizures in children, adolescents and young adults: Etiology, outcome, and treatment. Epilepsia 37(Suppl 1): S74–S80

The Status Epilepticus Working Party 2000 The treatment of convulsive status epilepticus in children. Archives of Diseases in Childhood 83: 415–419

Verity CM, Ross EM, Golding J 1993 Outcome of childhood status epilepticus and lengthy febrile convulsions: Findings of national cohort study. British Medical Journal 307: 225–228

8.4 ACUTE WEAKNESS

RICHARD LENNON

ESSENTIALS

1 The fact that a child has acute weakness may be obscured by an inability to communicate and a smaller repertoire of activities. The possibility of a neuromuscular problem must be consciously considered by the clinician.

2 Conversely a small child may not move a limb because of pain rather than weakness. A history and examination for evidence of trauma should be performed and appropriate diagnostic imaging considered.

3 Respiratory insufficiency due to weakness, may occur with surprising rapidity and may be compounded by aspiration. Careful assessment and close monitoring for this complication must be made.

4 Abnormal reflexes are important in localising the cause of acute weakness. If some are *absent* especially distally it suggests a lower motor neurone dysfunction. If all are *present* it suggests muscle dysfunction and if they are *increased* it suggests an upper motor neurone weakness.

5 The presence of a sensory level indicates a spinal cord lesion. One should consider investigating this with an urgent MRI to determine whether or not urgent surgery is needed.

INTRODUCTION

The acutely weak child is challenging to the emergency physician because she/he can present in many different ways with many different diagnoses. In particular, the preverbal child may present with only regression in motor milestones or bruising on the face from increased frequency of falls. The diagnosis in such children can range from a tick bite to Duchenne pseudohypertrophic muscular dystrophy.

PRESENTATION

In infants of less than three months, parents are usually quite sensitive to abnormalities of the infant's behaviour. They may bring a baby in complaining of poor feeding, decreased activity or being 'floppy'. The older infant may be noted to lose milestones such as ceasing to crawl or walk. 'Ataxia' may be the predominant feature in preschool and school-age children. Sometimes children may present with an associated feature of illness, such as the rash of dermatomyositis or an obvious engorged tick. In general, the older the child is, the more typical the presentation. However, even in this group, as in adults, there is a wide range of presentations, e.g. cranial nerve palsies in the Miller-Fisher variant of Guillain–Barré syndrome.

Trauma masquerading as weakness

Trauma is dealt with in detail in other chapters of the book. However, it should noted that non-accidental injury (NAI) can present as 'acute weakness' in the infant and young child. Shaken baby syndrome may present as a lethargic irritable child with little or no bruising. The apparent focal weakness may be due to an underlying fracture. Likewise, emotional and nutritional neglect may also lead to weakness. Hence, NAI must be considered in the differential diagnosis of the acutely weak child.

PRIMARY SURVEY APPROACH

General inspection

This is done by looking for both cause and effect of weakness. An abnormality of the primary survey severe enough to cause generalised weakness (e.g. respiratory distress) is usually the obvious presenting problem. Hypoglycaemia in a child can, in rare circumstances, present with focal weakness. It is important in the weak, floppy infant to consider the possibility of intussusception or other intra-abdominal pathology. In an infant with intussusception 'severe weakness' and lethargy may be the only presenting sign. When one comes to exposure in the primary survey of the weak child a thorough search has to take place for ticks (don't forget to look in deep skin folds) possible venomous bites and stings, and rashes, such as those caused by enteroviruses. Enteroviral rashes are usually scattered maculopapular but may be petechial. A close inspection should be made for bruises and other suggestive signs of non-accidental injury (NAI). A quick assessment of the child's nutritional state and the appropriateness of weight for age should be estimated. The size of the child's head and its proportion to the body should be noted and centiles should be plotted later in the detailed examination phase.

ABC

The effects of weakness may include airway compromise from bulbar palsy (e.g. hoarse voice, stridor, and aspiration of secretions). Severely impaired ventilation will be clinically apparent. However, mild or moderate impairment can be subtle and can rapidly progress to cause respiratory embarrassment. Therefore, if possible, respiratory function tests should be serially performed on all children presenting with neuromuscular weakness. Arterial or venous blood gases should also be considered in this assessment. (See Table 8.4.1 for predictors of needing intubation and mechanical ventilation.) Circulatory defects may arise from disturbance of the autonomic nervous system. This is characterised by labile

Table 8.4.1 Predictors of the necessity for intubation and ventilation
• Bulbar palsy
• Vital capacity < 20 mL kg^{-1}
• > 30% reduction in vital capacity from baseline
• Peak inspiratory pressure < 30 cmH$_2$O
• Peak expiratory pressure < 40 cmH$_2$O

blood pressure, heart rate and postural hypotension.

Disability

The neurological part of the primary survey can give early hints as to the site of the lesion(s) involved. The classic description of peripheral neuromuscular weakness is an alert, but anxious looking, child that has a paucity of limb movements. If respiratory failure or facial weakness have intervened this appearance will not be present. Conversely, intracranial causes of weakness are usually associated with some degree of obtundation.

The weak infant classically lies in a frog leg posture with all limbs lying on the bed, abducted at the hips and flexed at the knees. Asymmetry may be apparent in those with a focal weakness. With central causes of weakness (e.g. acute hydrocephalus) hypertonic posturing may be seen with scissoring adduction of lower limbs. Autonomic dysfunction may lead to associated fever or hypothermia. In any child with weakness one needs to consider whether the findings could be caused by a toxidrome (e.g. organophosphate poisoning).

Once the primary survey has been completed, and any abnormalities corrected then, a detailed history and examination should be performed.

HISTORY

If, on questioning, the weakness has been chronic then the list of possible diagnoses is extensive and is beyond the scope of this text. Such children should be stabilised and referred to the appropriate paediatric service for diagnosis. However, it is possible that a child with chronic weakness could undergo an acute deterioration, such as influenza in a child with a Duchenne muscular dystrophy. In infants the distinction between acute and chronic weakness is less relevant. In those children with conditions covered by this chapter, the history needs to focus initially on finding treatable causes. Detailed enquiry should be made about any possible tick bites or other venomous bites or stings. The absence of a history from a pre-verbal child, does not exclude that possibility. Enquiry should also be made about the availability of various medications and poisons around the house.

A precise time course for the illness should be obtained along with the pattern of evolution of the weakness. Whether it is *ascending* from lower limbs up, whether it is *lateralized* and whether it has *progressed* or not. A sudden onset may suggest a vascular or epileptic event. Rapid onset weakness may follow an intoxication or envenomation. Other causes are more subacute and may have progressed over weeks. The family history should be reviewed, and whether there is consanguinity. A history of recent infectious illnesses may be relevant. Immunisation history regarding polio vaccination is important and diphtheria is still a common cause of weakness in third world countries. Any overseas travel should be noted.

EXAMINATION

A detailed but focused examination is then performed, which attempts to establish the level and the nature of the lesion. The following lists the important distinguishing features of the different levels of the neuromuscular system, which may present with weakness.

❶ Muscular:
- Usually proximal more than distal weakness
- Reflexes preserved until very late
- May have tender muscles
- These children often have a positive Gower's sign.

❷ Neuromuscular junction:
- Fatigability
- Reflexes are preserved if the muscle is not fatigued or the disease is not severe.

❸ Lower motor neurone weakness:
- More peripheral than proximal weakness
- Reflexes are lost early in the illness.

❹ Upper motor neurone weakness:
- Apart from an initial flaccid phase, tone and reflexes are usually increased
- Spinal cord lesions are usually associated with a sensory level
- Intracranial problems are associated with features of encephalopathy, decreased level of consciousness, speech dysfunction, ataxia, and bulbar dysfunction.

It may be difficult to perform a formal neurological examination in an uncooperative infant or small child. Often in these situations, one can get a lot of information just by watching the child play. Another useful test is known as Gower's sign. The child is laid on their back on a firm surface and encouraged to stand. A child with proximal muscle weakness will not be able to sit up but will have to roll on to its abdomen get up on all fours and then 'climb up its legs' using its hands. Although reflexes are a good guide they are by no means fool proof. Upper motor lesions will usually have increased reflexes with increased tone. However, immediately after a spinal cord insult there may be a flaccid paralysis below the level of the lesion with absence of reflexes. Also, in transverse myelitis, there may be patchy combinations of upper and lower motor neurone signs. Early in Guillain–Barré syndrome the reflexes may be preserved and, likewise, very late in myopathic weakness, distal reflexes may be lost. Acute myositis is usually associated with tender muscles.

INVESTIGATIONS

Laboratory

Tests that may be useful in the acutely weak child include:

- A *full blood count*, which may reveal anaemia, nutritional disorders, leukaemia, or signs of infection.
- Abnormalities of *electrolytes* especially potassium, calcium, phosphate, sodium may cause weakness.
- *Urea and creatinine* – renal failure may present as generalised weakness, but more likely cause an abnormality of electrolytes.
- *Creatine kinase* is often raised in muscular causes of acute weakness.
- *Endocrine function tests* – especially thyroid and adrenal (see below).
- *Lumbar puncture* (see below).

Imaging

- *Urgent MRI* of spine.

SPECIFIC CONDITIONS CAUSING ACUTE WEAKNESS

Though not exhaustive the following sections give some detail on the more common causes of acute weakness seen in children and also the rarer ones that must be diagnosed and treated in emergency.

GUILLAIN–BARRÉ SYNDROME

Introduction

Guillain–Barré is an acute ascending polyradiculopathy. In the paediatric population it is more common in late childhood (four to nine years of age). It is uncommon, estimated at less than 1/100 000 person years in people less than 17 years of age. It is primarily a lower motor neurone disease affecting the myelin sheath with variable damage to axons. It is an immune-mediated reaction usually to a recent infection. Antibodies to various gangliosides are found in the serum of patients with GBS and matching antigens are often found in the preceding infectious agent. Infections known to be associated with GBS include *campylobacter, mycoplasma*, Epstein–Barr virus, coxsackie viruses, influenza viruses, echoviruses and cytomegalovirus. The greater the axonal damage, the longer and the less complete is the recovery.

History and examination

Children usually present with weakness, falls, regression of motor milestones or ataxia. They also complain of muscle pain in the early part of the illness. Cranial nerves are involved in 40–50% of cases, with the facial nerve most commonly involved. The Miller–Fisher variant presents with oculomotor palsies, ataxia and areflexia.

On questioning, the parents often give a history of a generalised viral, respiratory or gastroenteritis illness in the preceding two weeks. In the early part of the illness the child may have paraesthesiae. Classically the paralysis is ascending and symmetrical. The majority present with mostly distal weakness, however about 15% have extensive proximal muscular involvement.

Papilloedema is rare, but may occur in Guillain–Barré and is associated with raised intracranial pressure. Paralysis of the respiratory muscles is common and must be monitored carefully. Sympathetic nervous system involvement can produce profuse sweating, hypertension, postural hypotension and disturbances of sphincter function. Fatal cardiac arrhythmias have been reported in association with these signs. Although primarily a motor problem, sensory disturbance does occur, especially impairment of position sense. As mentioned above, reflexes are usually absent though increased reflexes and extensor plantar responses are occasionally found in the early phase of the illness.

The weakness may evolve rapidly within hours. However, it usually takes 1–2 weeks to reach the maximal weakness. Then in the 2nd to 4th week of the illness recovery is apparent and most children have recovered by two months although some take as long as eighteen months. Rarely Guillain–Barré will present in the newborn and is known as congenital GBS. They present as floppy babies that are areflexic and have elevated CSF protein.

Laboratory findings

An isolated elevation in CSF protein is the characteristic clinical finding of Guillain–Barré syndrome. The CSF cell count is usually normal, although 5% of children may have a pleocystosis of 100 or so cells.

Approximately 10% of children will have a normal CSF protein. The protein may be raised if a lumbar puncture is done later in the illness as it rises to a maximum after 4–5 weeks. Electroneurogram (ENG) characteristically shows conduction block although this may not become apparent until weeks into the illness.

Differential diagnosis

As laboratory tests may be normal in early GBS and signs may be variable, it is important to exclude other causes of acute weakness (see Table 8.4.2).

Treatment

Treatment of GBS consists of supportive therapy and either intravenous immunoglobulin or plasmapheresis. Treatment is more effective when given early. The immunoglobulin is usually given as a 2 g kg^{-1} infusion over 16 hours.

Prognosis

Prognosis is usually good in those treated and supported appropriately. Most children reach maximum weakness in the first week then remain stable for 1–3 weeks and then recover fully over a period of time that varies from six weeks to many months.

Disposition

Children with suspected GBS should be admitted and closely observed for the evolution of severe weakness that can occur. The findings outlined in Table 8.4.1 will assist in deciding who should go to an ICU/HDU and who should go to the general ward. Children with any one of these features should be monitored in a paediatric ICU and considered for elective intubation.

TICK PARALYSIS

Ticks that can cause paralysis are found throughout the world. In Australia *Ixodes holocyclus* is the main paralysing tick, it is found on the east coast. Other ticks have been known to cause paralysis, however they are rare. The toxin previously called holocyclotoxin is now thought to be

Table 8.4.2	Differential diagnosis of GBS
Diagnosis	*Features/action to exclude*
Tick paralysis	Thorough examination of hair/skin creases
Snake envenomation	History; check for bite site; coagulation screen, creatine kinase
Spinal cord lesion	Look for upper motor neurone/mixed features and a sensory level; if suspected perform MRI
Periodic paralysis	Usually a sudden or very rapid onset, reflexes are diminished but preserved; check family history; measure serum potassium; do ECG
Infant botulism	Almost exclusively in infants; ask for history of eating honey; culture stools for *Clostridium botulinum* and test for botulinum toxin
Poisoning (e.g. organophosphate, lead)	History of exposure; toxidrome; check levels where suspected
Myasthenia gravis	Often cranial nerves involved; fatigability; look for antibodies; perform Tensilon test
Vasculitis (e.g. polyarteritis nodosa)	Check urinalysis; look for autoantibodies if suspected
Myositis (e.g. dermatomyositis)	Reflexes preserved; no ophthalmoplegia; look for characteristic rash; check creatine kinase; EMG
Poliomyelitis, diphtheria, other enteroviruses	Usually has fever and sore throat in diphtheria; ask about immunisations; no sensory changes

several toxins. The toxins inhibit the release of acetylcholine from motor end plates. The paralysis usually occurs four or five days after the tick attaches. The paralysis can resemble Guillain–Barré in the form of an ascending paralysis and is an important differential diagnosis because removal of the tick is necessary for recovery. The envenomation most frequently presents with cranial nerve palsies. Although the tick is often located in the vicinity of the palsy this is not always the case and in all cases a thorough examination should be made for multiple ticks. The paralysis can be severe and require ventilation. Australian tick paralysis may get worse in the 48 hours following tick removal, and children should be monitored carefully during this time. Conversely with children presenting with paralysis one should ask if a tick was removed in the last 48 hours. Deaths have usually been due to respiratory paralysis, however there have been reports of myocarditis and autonomic effects on the heart. Treatment includes supportive therapy then careful removal of the tick(s). This can be made easier by applying a pyrethrum spray, which suffocates the creature and makes it loosen its grip. Squeezing the tick is not recommended as this may inject more toxin. If there are signs of paralysis antivenom should be administered. The antivenom is made from hyperimmunised dog serum and therefore may cause allergic and serum sickness reactions. Adrenaline (epinephrine) 1:1000 should be drawn up in the appropriate dose before the antivenom is given. The usual dose is 20 mL (200 units as a freeze-dried powder in an ampoule reconstituted with 10 mL of water for injection) of antivenom diluted to 200 mL with Hartmann's or normal saline infused slowly. The total volume can be reduced to 100 mL in small children to avoid overload.

Other envenomations

Snake and spider bites are discussed in detail elsewhere in the text. Usually the history and accompanying symptoms will give the diagnosis. Death adder envenomation is usually a purely neurological presentation so in the weak non-verbal child a thorough look for a bite site is in-

dicated. Venom detection kits should not be used to confirm the diagnosis because they can give false positives.

BOTULISM

Poisoning with botulinum toxin can present in three ways:

❶ Infant botulism
❷ Food-borne botulism, and
❸ Wound botulism.

1. Infant botulism

Although rare, several cases of infant botulism have been reported in Australia in the last few years. Infant botulism is caused by release of botulinum toxin into the bloodstream from *Clostridium botulinum* bacteria colonising the intestines. Part of the toxin enters the terminal bouton of cholinergic motor nerves and enzymatically disables the mechanism by which acetylcholine-containing vesicles attach to the cell membrane. This process is irreversible and recovery occurs by sprouting new unmyelinated motor neurones. Risk factors for babies contracting this disease include exposure to honey in the first six months (honey is not recommended for babies under one year), decreased frequency of stooling and lack of breast-feeding.

Diagnosis of this condition is characterised by:

* Age group – the infants are almost always less than six months, however there are reports in infants up to one year and older children with abnormal bowel anatomy.
* Nature of onset – the infants always start with bulbar palsies because that is where the blood supply is greatest. This is a descending paralysis.
* Fatigability, but lack of reversibility with edrophonium or neostigmine.
* Absence of fever.
* Absence of an altered mental status.
* Absence of sensory defects.
* Normal CSF.

Clostridium botulinum may be cultured from the stools and the toxin may be found in stools or serum through PCR or ELISA tests. Mouse bioassay is also available where

sterilised stools are injected into a mouse to see if it becomes paralysed. If suspicion is high, foods in the child's residence can be tested for *C. botulinum*. The electromyogram (EMG) is characteristic.

The difficulty is in early diagnosis. A weak suck is often put down to generalised illness and it is often only the mother who notices the lack of expression on the infant's face. A high index of suspicion needs to be maintained.

Treatment is by supportive care and administration of botulinum antitoxin. Antibiotics are not recommended unless there is secondary infection (e.g. pneumonia). This is because they may increase toxin release when the bacteria lyse and divulge their contents. Tube feeding is recommended as it restores peristalsis, which is essential for clearing *C. botulinum* from the gut. If antibiotics are used, aminoglycosides should be avoided because these worsen the paralysis. About half of the patients end up needing intubation and ventilation. Hospital stay is an average of one month but varies widely. Infants seem to recover completely.

There are two antitoxins available. Equine-derived antitoxin, a small amount of which is held in the Commonwealth Serum Laboratories, and botulism immune globulin (BIG), a human-derived hyper-immune globulin, which in a recent randomised controlled trial reduced hospital stay from 6.6 weeks to 2.6 weeks. It is not available outside the United States.

2. Food-borne botulism

This is due to consumption of food in which there is preformed toxin. It is associated with home-canned foods. It differs from infant botulism in that it can occur in any age group and one third of cases have gastroenteritis-like symptoms. The illness usually begins about 18 to 36 hours after ingestion, but onset can range from two hours to eight days. Presentation is similar to infant botulism but more obvious because of the patients' greater age. The treatment is similar.

3. Wound botulism

This is perhaps the rarest form. The differences from the other forms are the presence of a wound, which may be obviously infected, and the presence of fever. The incubation period is 4–14 days. This requires aggressive treatment with antibiotics and antitoxin.

SPINAL CORD LESIONS

These are usually distinguished from peripheral nerve disease by upper motor neurone signs. However, in many cases initially the reflexes and tone are diminished (e.g. 'spinal shock' after trauma). In other cases, there may be patchy upper and lower motor neurone involvement such as in transverse myelitis. Therefore spinal cord lesions need to be considered in the differential diagnosis of the weak child. The key to spinal cord lesions is the presence of a sensory level. However, in transverse myelitis and in a preverbal child this may be difficult to establish. If a spinal cord lesion is suspected the investigation of choice is an urgent MRI. This is time critical as a space-occupying lesion in the narrow canal can rapidly cause permanent damage to the surrounding cord.

Transverse myelitis (TM)

The aetiology of this acute spinal cord inflammation is still uncertain. Hypotheses include microbial antigen cross-reaction with neural elements, bacterial super-antigen inflammation and direct microbial invasion. Rarely it is associated with systemic diseases such as SLE and multiple sclerosis. It is likely that TM will be found to be several diseases and perhaps treatment will need to be tailored to the specific aetiology.

This disease usually has a rapid onset of predominantly lower limb weakness and altered sensation. Neck stiffness and fever are present early in most cases along with low back pain or abdominal pain. The sensory level is usually around the mid-thoracic region below which pain, light touch and temperature sensation are impaired. However, joint position and vibration sense are more preserved. Bladder and bowel disturbance is common, although this may be difficult to determine in a child in nappies. Tone is usually flaccid early in the illness with decreased reflexes, followed by increased tone and hyperreflexia as the disease progresses to its peak over the next 2–3 days. Sixty percent of patients recover fully over weeks to months.

Urgent MRI usually shows fusiform oedema around the site of the sensory level. CSF shows a moderate lymphocytosis and mildly raised protein.

Treatment is controversial with case-control studies indicating a benefit with glucocorticoids, whereas prospective trials show no benefit. Treatment decisions should be made in consultation with a paediatric neurologist.

Spinal cord trauma

This is discussed in the chapter on trauma.

Spinal cord space-occupying lesions

These include epidural abscess, tumours, syringomyelia and arteriovenous malformations. Since syringomyelia is almost always a chronic condition it will not be dealt with here.

Tumours

These may be intramedullary (e.g. low-grade astrocytoma), extramedullary intradural (e.g. meningioma) and extradural (e.g. lymphoma). They usually have a more gradual onset than the other diseases mentioned in this chapter but the early signs may be missed and the child may present when signs are rapidly evolving due to high intramedullary pressures. Progressive gait and bladder disturbance with back pain and absence of fever are characteristic signs. Recent onset of scoliosis may be a feature. There may be a mixture of signs with upper motor neurone signs in the lower limbs and lower motor neurone signs in the upper limbs.

Urgent MRI is the investigation of choice, followed by consultation with surgeons and/or radiation oncologists. If MRI is unavailable, CT or plain X-ray may show abnormalities. However, these should only be done if they do not delay transfer to an MRI capable centre.

Arteriovenous malformations

These are usually in the thoracic region. They may cause symptoms as a space-occupying lesion causing compression or by steal circulation from the nearby cord. The history is usually subacute, unless a haemorrhage or ischaemia has intervened. Clues to the diagnosis on examination include a cutaneous angioma over the region and a bruit on auscultation. MRI/MRA will give the diagnosis but angiography is usually required to define the lesion fully and to decide on whether to treat with surgery or embolisation.

Epidural abscess

This is a rare disease in children, who usually present with back pain and rigidity, fever, leucocytosis and a raised ESR. These symptoms, may be followed by spinal neurological signs. MRI is the investigation of choice, but there is controversy over whether treatment should be by surgery or antibiotics alone.

Tethered cord/diastematomyelia

These are two conditions that tend to fix the cord of the child, which has to 'move up' the canal as the child grows. They rarely present with acute weakness, although there may be sudden exacerbations on flexion and extension. Examination over the spine may reveal sentinel lesions such as a tuft of hair, a sacral pit, a lipoma, or a cutaneous haemangioma.

MYASTHENIA GRAVIS (MG)

This condition, which is usually due to acetylcholine receptor auto-antibodies, leads to easy and rapid fatigability of muscles. This may occur in children in three forms.

1. Transient myasthenia of newborns

This occurs where the mother has myasthenia. Maternal antibodies to the acetylcholine receptor (AChR) cross the placenta and the baby is born with fatigable muscle weakness. These babies may show very little motor activity for days after birth. Alternatively they may just have feeding difficulty that worsens during the day. This illness improves within weeks as the maternal antibody levels diminish in the child's blood. The only treatment is supportive by tube feeding and intubation and ventilation, if severe. The babies recover completely and have no increased risk of MG.

2. Congenital myasthenia

This is a lasting condition due to a genetic disorder. It is not due to antibodies to the AChR.

3. Acquired myasthenia

The incidence of this is low, though not insignificant. In an Italian study the annual incidence was 3.3 per million children < 15 years about 1% of total MG cases. The presentation is usually with ptosis, ophthalmoplegia or bulbar weakness. The clue on history is the worsening of symptoms as the day progresses due to fatigue. Peripheral muscles especially limb girdle and hand muscles are also involved. Reflexes are preserved but diminished. Clinical tests for fatigability such as getting the child to look up for 60–90 seconds and watching for ptosis, or to flap one arm 'like a bird' for a minute and then comparing its strength with the other arm are very useful.

Diagnosis can be made with three tests. First, an anticholinergic drug may be given. Edrophonium, the usual drug used in adults may cause cardiac arrhythmias in small children, so neostigmine is preferred. Atropine is given beforehand to block the muscarinic effects. These drugs should abolish the fatigability. Second, the EMG is characteristic and usually obviates the need for muscle biopsy. Third, AChR antibodies can be measured in the blood. Early diagnosis is important because, if untreated, this disease will often progress to life-threatening severity.

Associations with MG commonly found in adults, such as thymoma, are rare in children. Differential diagnosis includes botulism, chronic low-grade organophosphate toxicity and tick paralysis.

In the ED the child may present as an initial episode or because of a crisis of weakness. These crises may be myasthenic, due to exacerbation of the underlying condition or cholinergic due to excessive

anticholinesterase treatment, which leads to over stimulation and exhaustion of receptors. Classically, a cholinergic crisis has the cholinergic toxidrome features of hypersalivation, pulmonary oedema and muscle fasciculation. However, in someone with myasthenia the cholinergic crisis may only be manifest by weakness. Distinguishing between a myasthenic and cholinergic crisis may be difficult. History may give a clue if medications have been missed or an overdose of pyridostigmine has been taken. A therapeutic trial of edrophonium may help, but should not be undertaken if there is significant risk of a cholinergic crisis. In the latter case supportive treatment and measurement of blood cholinesterase activity may be the only option.

Long-term treatment of MG comprises anticholinesterases and a variety of immunosuppression IgG infusion or thymectomy.

In myasthenia gravis:

- Do not give neuromuscular blocking agents (e.g. suxamethonium, vecuronium) as these may paralyse the MG patient for days or even weeks.
- Do not give aminoglycoside antibiotics as these exacerbate the weakness.

POLIOMYELITIS AND OTHER ENTEROVIRAL INFECTIONS

Poliomyelitis is now exceedingly rare, however one should always ask about immunisation status in the acutely weak child. If the child is not immunised one should ask about contact with infants recently immunised with sabin (oral weakened live poliovirus) vaccine. Infants excrete the virus after the immunisation and this is where most recent cases of poliomyelitis have come from. The other source of infection is in developing nations, where immunisation rates are low. The illness itself usually presents with symptoms related to the virus's portal of entry through the gut and upper respiratory tract. Patients have fever, sore throat, anorexia, nausea, vomiting, generalised non-specific abdominal pain, malaise and

headache. The great majority of poliovirus infections end here or are asymptomatic. In those patients who progress there is often an asymptomatic period of 1–2 days followed by symptoms of aseptic meningitis with neck and often entire spine stiffness. There may be mild transient neurological deficits such as bladder paralysis and loss of abdominal and anal reflexes. Those who progress to paralytic polio will usually do so 8–12 hours after the superficial reflexes are lost. Poliovirus can infect and destroy neurones from the motor cortex down to the anterior horn cells. However, most commonly the paralytic form presents with patchy asymmetrical lower motor neurone weakness. Bulbar weakness is also a frequent presentation and often the picture is mixed. Rarely there are also encephalitic and ataxic presentations.

Diagnosis is based on the immunisation history, the clinical picture and a lumbar puncture showing a moderate pleocytosis, initially of neutrophils but then changing to monocytes. Serology and culture of stool, throat swab and rarely CSF will often reveal the organism. Treatment is supportive only. Infection control authorities need to be informed.

BELL'S PALSY

A sudden or rapid onset of a unilateral lower motor neurone palsy is not a rare occurrence in children. Estimated annual incidence varies from 3 to 10 per 100 000 children per year. Its aetiology is uncertain. The disease commonly begins two weeks after an infectious illness, which suggests a post-infectious autoimmune or allergic aetiology. Lyme disease has been associated and serology should be done if the patient has been in an endemic area. Epstein-Barr, mumps and herpes simplex viruses have also been associated with this disease. An association with hypertension has suggested another aetiology related to pressure necrosis of the nerve due to swelling in the narrow facial canal.

The patient often presents with pain around the ipsilateral ear and may also complain of abnormal hearing. About half have loss of taste sensation to the anterior two-thirds of the tongue.

The differential is extensive but the diagnosis can be determined by a thorough history and clinical examination. One should look for evidence of trauma (be aware of non-accidental injury), central nervous system dysfunction, aural lesions (e.g. the Ramsay Hunt syndrome), other cranial nerve dysfunctions, hypertension and Guillain–Barré syndrome. Acute lymphoblastic leukaemia and even sarcoidosis have been reported.

Treatment is controversial, as the prognosis in children is better than in adults. Complete recovery occurs in 60 to 80% of patients with near complete recovery in the remainder. In one study average time to recovery was about seven weeks with a range of nine days to seven months. Uncontrolled studies have claimed a benefit for early corticosteroid therapy. However, recent meta-analyses have disputed this. The decision to give steroids, or not, needs to take into account possible side effects and the probability of complete recovery, which may be decreased in severe cases. There is even less evidence for antiviral agents in the absence of apparent viral infection. If the eyelid does not completely close steps should be taken to protect the cornea from exposure keratopathy, i.e. artificial tears and eyeglasses during the daytime, ointment and a protective eye chamber at night.

TOXIC NEUROPATHIES

A long list of substances can cause acute weakness. Some of the more common ones are listed here.

Anticholinesterases

The organophosphates and carbamates are commonly used insecticides, which can cause poisoning through skin, oral or pulmonary exposure. They inhibit cholinesterases, allowing acetylcholine to persistently stimulate the nicotinic and muscarinic receptors, which then can become refractory and thus cause weakness. This weakness is usually accompanied by the cholinergic toxidrome (see Chapter 21.2 on toxicology) and, indeed, it is

usually the respiratory and cardiac features that predominate. However, there is an *intermediate syndrome* where 12 hours to 7 days after the initial poisoning, one finds proximal limb weakness that is unresponsive to atropine or pralidoxime. There may also be respiratory and bulbar paralysis. Recovery from this is usually complete. *Late neurotoxicity* arises 4–21 days after the acute exposure causing a mixed sensory motor deficit, which may take weeks or months to recover, or may be permanent. Diagnosis is by identification of the poison at source or in urine or serum drug screens and also by measuring serum cholinesterase activity level. Treatment is supportive and with antidotes atropine and pralidoxime. Muscle relaxants will have a prolonged effect and should be avoided if possible.

Lead and other heavy metals

Lead, mercury and arsenic are all known to cause neuropathies often taking the form of mononeuritis multiplex. It is uncommon for these to present as acute weakness. Nevertheless, a history of exposure should be sought and appropriate specimens taken if the cause of the acute weakness is unclear.

Chemotherapeutic agents

Vincristine, vinblastine and cisplatin are known to cause a peripheral neuropathy. Any child who is on, or has recently had, chemotherapy needs to have this ruled out as a possible cause.

HEREDITARY NEUROPATHY

Rarely a patient with an undiagnosed hereditary neuropathy presents with an acute exacerbation. A thorough history will reveal the chronicity of the problem. Such patients should be referred to an appropriate paediatric neurology service.

MUSCULAR DISORDERS

Juvenile dermatomyositis

Juvenile dermatomyositis is a systemic vasculitis thought to be triggered by infection. Both enteroviruses and Group

A *Streptococcus* have been implicated. This is the most common myositis of childhood. Its peak age of incidence is six years. Because of its gradual onset this uncommonly presents as acute weakness. The child may well present with the rash before weakness has become apparent.

The rash appears on sun exposed areas especially the malar region of the face and a purple discolouration of the eyelids is apparent (heliotrope rash). The rash may also be found on the extensor surfaces of the arms and legs, thorax, ankles and buttocks. The fingers develop thickening of the skin over joints called Gottron's papules. The weakness comes on about two months after the rash and is usually very slow in onset. Small children may be noted to become gradually inactive and older children have increasing difficulty with sport. Proximal muscle activities, such as climbing up stairs reveal the weakness first. The vasculopathy can effect any muscle group and children may present with aspiration dysphagia or hoarse voice due to pharyngeal muscle weakness. The affected muscles are often tender and sometimes swollen.

The vasculitis can affect any organ system. Subclinical myocarditis and conduction defects are often found at diagnosis. Less common effects include renal dysfunction, hepatosplenomegaly, retinitis, iritis, seizures, depression, bowel dysfunction and pulmonary disease.

Diagnosis is made on the clinical picture associated with a raised serum creatine kinase. There are typical changes on muscle biopsy and electromyogram. There may also be elevated autoantibodies, liver function tests and abnormalities on MRI.

Complications include calcinosis of muscles, subcutaneous fat and fascia. These are more likely if the illness is prolonged and are decreased by aggressive treatment. Calcinosis lesions may become infected and lead to septicaemia.

These children may require judicious use of pain relief and require referral to a specialist paediatric unit. Treatment options range from sunscreen for the rash through to immunosuppression with glucocorticoids and chemotherapeutic agents depending on the severity of the disease. Prognosis is generally good in children with approximately 80% making a good recovery.

Infectious myositis

Viral infections such as influenza can uncommonly cause a myositis that may in its severest form lead to rhabdomyolysis and myoglobinuria. Various bacteria including *Streptococcus* and *Mycoplasma* species have been reported to cause a focal myositis. These usually present with the other features of the infection and myalgia, rather than acute weakness. The weakness is only found on close examination, if the myalgia permits. The creatine kinase is raised. The prognosis is generally good although permanent muscle damage may ensue especially in focal bacterial myositis.

Metabolic/endocrine myopathies

Most endocrinopathies can produce weakness by several mechanisms. Often this is just myalgia and fatigue, but true myopathies can develop. This weakness usually responds to the treatment of the underlying endocrine disorder. Endocrinopathies can be associated with electrolyte disturbances that lead to weakness (e.g. hypokalaemia in Conn's syndrome) or with primary muscle diseases, such as hypokalaemic periodic paralysis with thyrotoxicosis.

The periodic paralyses are a series of genetic ion channel disorders that lead to acute episodes of weakness lasting from one hour up to more than a day. They often come on after rest, during sleep or following exercise, but never during exercise. Diagnosis is by measurement of electrolytes during an attack or response to a metabolic challenge or by gene mutation identification. Hypokalaemic periodic paralysis usually occurs in adolescence. The patient will have low potassium during attacks. Conversely, hyperkalaemic periodic paralysis usually comes on in early childhood. The attacks are more frequent occurring up to several times a day and are associated with an elevated or normal potassium. The identification of these diseases is important, as they are treatable.

SOMATISATION DISORDERS/ MALINGERING

Occasionally, children may present with a psychogenic cause of weakness. The findings of a careful neurological examination will demonstrate inconsistencies and the child will be able to perform manoeuvres that require more strength than normal walking (e.g. knees giving way but not falling). Reflexes will be normal.

Usually, no laboratory tests or imaging is necessary. However, if there is any doubt, consultation and investigation should be undertaken.

Once you have made the diagnosis it is best to take the parent or carer aside and discuss the diagnosis with them. Confrontation of the child is rarely helpful and it is often best to reassure the child that this is not serious and that they will get better. An effort should be made to find the underlying psychological reason for the presentation, which may be anything from school avoidance to sexual abuse. Consultation with social work or psychiatry may be indicated for counselling.

FURTHER READING

Behrman RE, Kliegman R, Jenson HB (eds) 2000 Nelson Textbook of Pediatrics, 16th edn. WB Saunders, Philadelphia

Emilia-Romagna Study Group on Clinical and Epidemiological Problems in Neurology 1998 Incidence of myasthenia gravis in the Emilia-Romagna region: A prospective multicenter study. Neurology 51(1): 255–258 [brief communications]

Lawn ND, Fletcher DD, Henderson, RD, Wolter TD, Wijdicks EFM 2001 Anticipating mechanical ventilation in Guillain–Barré syndrome. Archives of Neurology 58: 893–898

Odaka M, Yuki N, Hirata K 2001 Anti-GQ1b IgG antibody syndrome: Clinical and immunological range. Journal of Neurology, Neurosurgery and Psychiatry 70: 50–55

Tang T, Noble-Jamieson C 2001 A painful hip as a presentation of Guillain–Barré syndrome in children. British Medical Journal 322: 149–150

8.5 ACUTE ATAXIA

JOANNE GRINDLAY

ESSENTIALS

1 The most common causes of acute cerebellar ataxia in children are post-infectious (acute cerebellar ataxia), drug intoxication and posterior fossa tumours.

2 Clinical features suggestive of a brain tumour and hence warranting further investigation include headache, vomiting, behavioural changes and papilloedema or cranial nerve dysfunction.

3 Ataxia is not uncommonly a presenting symptom of poisoning or excessive levels of drugs, particularly anticonvulsants.

4 A number of neurological conditions may present with an unsteady gait (pseudo-ataxia) because of weakness.

5 Investigations in the child with ataxia are directed by the history and clinical features detected on examination.

6 While ataxia may be seen in post-concussion syndrome, conditions requiring acute intervention, should be sought by CT scan.

7 Most children with significant ataxia require admission for investigation and observation under a paediatrician.

INTRODUCTION

Ataxia is an uncommon, but important paediatric presentation to the ED. Ataxia is a disorder of movement manifest by the loss of co-ordination, most apparent as a disturbance of gait, with intact muscle strength. It may be associated with a disturbance of balance. Ataxia is most often caused by a loss of function of the cerebellum, which controls the co-ordination of movement. Disease of the peripheral sensory nerves or the spinal column, particularly affecting proprioception, may also lead to ataxia as a result of abnormal inputs into the cerebellum. Cortical ataxia results from cerebral cortical dysfunction, particularly of the frontal lobe, while vestibular ataxia results from disease of the inner ear. Rarely, psychiatric causes of ataxia may also be seen as a manifestation of conversion reaction. The most common diagnosis of acute ataxia in children is a post-infectious ataxia called acute ataxia of childhood (see below). This is a diagnosis of exclusion, made after consideration of other causes (Table 8.5.1). These include poisoning, metabolic disorders and organic brain lesions, such as posterior fossa tumours or neuroblastoma.

There are numerous hereditary conditions causing chronic ataxia that may present in childhood. These include Friedreich's ataxia, hereditary cerebellar

Table 8.5.1 Causes of acute ataxia in childhood

- Post-viral – acute cerebellar ataxia
- Poisoning/drug intoxication
- Tumours
  Posterior fossa, brainstem
  Paraneoplastic syndrome
- Trauma including non-accidental injury
  Haematoma
  Post-concussion
- Metabolic
  Hypoglycaemia
  Hyponatraemia
  Hyperammonaemia
  Inborn errors of metabolism
- Infections
  Meningitis – bacterial, viral
  Cerebral abscess
  Labyrinthitis
  Encephalitis
- Vascular
  Stroke
  Vasculitis
- Immune
  Multiple sclerosis
  Acute disseminated encephalomyelitis

ataxia, spinocerebellar ataxia and ataxia telangiectasia. The progressive nature of these conditions and their associated signs differentiate these from the acute ataxias.

PATHOPHYSIOLOGY

Cerebellum

The cerebellum consists of two lateral hemispheres, divided into anterior and posterior lobes by the primary fissure. The hemispheres are joined by the vermis in the midline. The cerebellum connects to the cerebral cortex and brain stem via three paired sets of peduncles, the superior, middle and inferior cerebellar peduncles.

Cerebral hemispheres and vermis

There are three functional parts of the cerebellum. These are the archaeocerebellum, the palaeocerebellum and the neocerebellum. The archaeocerebellum is formed by the flocculus, nodule and lingula of the vermis. It has only vestibular connections, which travel in the inferior cerebellar peduncle. The archaeocerebellum controls balance. Dysfunction leads to truncal ataxia characterised by a drunken gait, with swaying of the trunk and titubation when sitting, standing or walking. Typically there is no alteration in fine movements or nystagmus. Reflexes are normal and there is no tremor. The anterior lobes of the lateral hemispheres, together with uvula and pyramid of the vermis form the palaeocerebellum. The palaeocerebellum connects to the spinocerebellar tracts and is involved with postural reflexes. Dysfunction leads to postural imbalance and increased reflexes. The posterior lobes of the lateral hemispheres form the neocerebellum, which connects to the cerebral hemispheres, basal nuclei and the pontine nuclei, via the middle cerebral peduncle. It is involved in the co-ordination of fine, voluntary movements. Dysfunction leads to nystagmus, intention tremor, dysdiadochokinesis, hypotonia and decreased or pendular reflexes. The vermis and surrounding nuclei of the cerebellum form the roof of the 4th ventricle. An expanding lesion may obstruct the CSF flow with resultant hydrocephalus and truncal ataxia.

Cerebellar peduncles and connections

The cerebellum receives inputs from the vestibular and peripheral nervous systems. Outputs which co-ordinate muscle movements by modifying tone and contraction, travel in three sets of peduncles (superior, middle, and inferior) between each cerebellar hemisphere and the brainstem.

DIFFERENTIAL DIAGNOSIS

The most common causes of acute cerebellar ataxia in children are post-infectious (acute cerebellar ataxia), drug intoxication and posterior fossa tumours.

ACUTE CEREBELLAR ATAXIA

Acute cerebellar ataxia is the most common diagnosis in acute ataxia in children, particularly between two and seven years of age. It is a diagnosis of exclusion, after consideration of more sinister causes such as tumours. An autoimmune aetiology is likely with autoantibodies demonstrated in acute cerebellar ataxia following infections with Epstein–Barr virus, mycoplasma and varicella.[1] The clinical presentation is of a prodromal illness, frequently non-specific, with or without an exanthema, 5–10 days prior to the onset of acute ataxia. If a specific aetiology is present it is most commonly varicella, though a number of other viruses have been implicated (Table 8.5.2).[5–20] As more children are protected by immunisation from infections such as varicella, measles and whooping cough, the proportion of cases where there is a non-specific viral prodrome, rather than a specific diagnosis, is likely to increase. Acute cerebellar ataxia usually presents with sudden onset of severe gait ataxia, though a small number of cases have an insidious onset. Most

Table 8.5.2 Causes of post-infectious acute cerebellar ataxia

- Varicella[5]
- Coxsackie A9[6]
- Epstein–Barr virus[7]
- Mycoplasma[8]
- Mumps[9]
- Poliomyelitis[10,11]
- Typhoid[12]
- Echovirus[13]
- Pertussis[14]
- Human parvovirus[15]
- Measles[14]
- Herpes simplex virus[16]
- Enterovirus 71[17]
- Malaria[18]
- Immunization[19,20]
- Influenza
- Diphtheria

have dysarthric speech. Mild horizontal nystagmus occurs in 50% of cases. Findings of intention tremor, dysdiadochokinesis, hypotonia and decreased or pendular reflexes are seen in two-thirds of cases, but are less pronounced than the gait disturbance. Truncal ataxia is uncommon.

Investigations are aimed at excluding an alternative diagnosis, if the diagnosis is unclear. The CT scan is normal in acute cerebellar ataxia, however MRI may be abnormal. In one series, inflammatory changes were seen in the cerebellum of one of nine children.[2,3] There is a slight elevation of CSF cell count by 4–50 cells per microlitre in 32%, though occasionally (in 8%) the elevation is higher. There may also be slightly elevated protein 410–900 mg L[-1].[4]

Acute cerebellar ataxia usually begins to improve within a few days, but full recovery may take from ten days to two months. Patients who have a slower recovery are still likely to recover fully. In one series, 91% recovered fully from their ataxia, including all those with varicella, EBV or post-vaccination, but 8% had sustained learning problems. Varicella-associated ataxia recovered quicker than non-varicella.[3]

POISONING

Ataxia is not uncommonly a presenting symptom of ingestion or excessive levels of drugs, particularly anticonvulsants.

Table 8.5.3 Drugs causing acute ataxia

- Anticonvulsants
  Phenytoin
  Carbamazepine
- Benzodiazepines
- Alcohols
  Ethanol
  Isopropanol
  Ethylene glycol
- Essential oils
  Eucalyptus oil
  Tea tree oil
  Pine oil
- Cough suppressants
  Codeine
  Dextromethorphan
- Drugs of abuse
  PCP
  Solvents, petrol, glue

Accidental poisoning occurs most commonly in one- to four-year-old children. A wide variety of compounds are implicated, including alcohols, substances of abuse and essential oils, as well as medications (Table 8.5.3). In addition to ataxia, these children may have nystagmus, altered mental status and vomiting. By comparison, in acute cerebellar ataxia consciousness is unimpaired.

Anticonvulsants

Phenytoin is not an uncommon cause of toxicity in children. Serum levels of >20–30 μg mL[-1] may produce signs of ataxia, nystagmus on lateral gaze and drowsiness. Onset of symptoms following an acute ingestion is usually within one to two hours and may persist for four to five days. At >30 μg mL[-1], the ataxia and drowsiness become more marked and the nystagmus vertical.[21–23]

Carbamazepine toxicity may also lead to ataxia. There are usually associated findings of drowsiness and nystagmus. There may be progression to seizures and coma, particularly if the level is >100 μmol L[-1].[24]

Benzodiazepines

Ataxia may be the sole presenting feature of benzodiazepine ingestion in children. In one series, it was an isolated finding in one-fifth of the cases who demonstrated ataxia. Other findings included lethargy (57%), GCS <15 (35%) and respiratory depression (9%).[25]

Alcohols

Ethanol intoxication produces ataxia, disinhibited behaviour and slurred speech. A serum ethanol level will aid clarification of the diagnosis.

Ethylene glycol is the main component of antifreeze. Early symptoms of ingestion are similar to that of ethanol intoxication. Delayed features include cardiopulmonary distress and later nephrotoxicity. Ethylene glycol produces a raised anion gap metabolic acidosis with osmolal gap. Serum levels > 20 mg dL^{-1} are toxic. The ethanol level will be zero. Isopropanol, is a component of rubbing alcohol, and is also used widely as a solvent. Toxicity is evident between 0.5 and 2 hours post-ingestion and may include vomiting, ataxia, nystagmus, and altered mental state. Coma and apnoea may occur in severe poisoning.[26]

Essential oils

Eucalyptus oil is not an uncommon ingestion by children. In one series of 109 admitted children, 41% were asymptomatic. Those who were symptomatic demonstrated decreased conscious state (28%), vomiting (37%), ataxia (15%) and pulmonary disease (11%). There was a correlation between ingested dose and toxicity. An ingestion of > 5 mL 100% oil was associated with a significantly decreased conscious state, whereas < 2–3 mL was associated with minor depression of consciousness.[27] A second series of 41 presentations, however, only demonstrated effects in 20%, with no correlation with presumed dose. The clinical effects included ataxia (5%), decreased conscious state (10%) and gastrointestinal symptoms (7%).[28]

Other essential oils that may produce nystagmus include tea tree oil[29] and pine oil. In one small series of pine oil cleaner (35% pine oil, 10.9% isopropyl alcohol), symptoms developed within 90 minutes of ingestion. Lethargy was present in all symptomatic children and ataxia in four of five cases of children.[30]

Cough suppressants

Codeine is contained in a number of cough medicines as well as in analgesics. In one series of 430 children, ataxia was reported in 9% receiving codeine. Associated symptoms are somnolence 67%, rash 39%, miosis 30%, vomiting 27%, itching 10%, angioedema 9%.[31] Dextromethorphan is a common component of cough and cold medications, which acts through opiate receptors in the medulla. It may cause opisthotonus, ataxia and bidirectional nystagmus. Fatality is highly unlikely, even with one hundred-fold the therapeutic dose.[32,33]

Substances of abuse

Phencyclidine (PCP) and lysergic acid diethylamide (LSD) are rare causes of ataxia in children. More common, however, is the abuse of hydrocarbon solvents; toluene in glue, spray paints and petrol. Hydrocarbons may produce ataxia as a component of acute intoxication and also as a chronic CNS sequel.

TUMOURS

Cerebellar lesions may present with an acute, rather than insidious onset of ataxia as a result of either haemorrhage into a tumour or as a result of hydrocephalus. The ataxia may progress to chronic ataxia. Paraneoplastic syndromes including paraneoplastic cerebellar degeneration and opsoclonus-myoclonus-ataxia syndrome are uncommon causes of acute paediatric ataxia.

Clinical features suggestive of a brain tumour, and hence further investigation, include headache, vomiting, behavioural changes (particularly with frontal lobe lesions), and papilloedema or cranial nerve dysfunction.

Posterior fossa tumours include medulloblastoma, astrocytoma and ependymoma. Medulloblastoma (20–25% of posterior fossa tumours) usually presents in a child less than six years with symptoms of ataxia, which may be truncal, headache, irritability or vomiting. The tumour may be located in the 4th ventricle or vermis. Cerebellar astrocytoma (10–30% of paediatric brain tumours) is located in one of the cerebellar hemispheres. It is seen in primary-school-aged children who may display ipsilateral limb ataxia, headache and vomiting. The head may be held tilted to one side. Associated raised intracranial pressure may be life threatening. Ependymoma (8–10%), located in the 4th ventricle, causes obstruction of CSF flow and may present with headache, vomiting and ataxia, which may be truncal. Brainstem glioma (10–15% of paediatric brain tumours) develops in the pons or medulla. They typically occur in early primary-aged children. Presenting symptoms include cranial nerve palsies, ataxia and vomiting.

Hydrocephalus presents with ataxia due to stretching of frontopontocerebellar fibres. Associated features are headache, vomiting and late signs of raised intracranial pressure. Supratentorial tumours may also present with ataxia through involvement of the frontopontocerebellar fibres. An occult neuroblastoma may present with a triad of acute ataxia, opsoclonus (jerky, random, chaotic eye movements) and myoclonus (severe myoclonic jerks of the head, trunk or limbs). The most common site for the tumour is in the abdomen.[34] It is diagnosed by measuring urinary homovanillic acid and vanillylmandelic acid levels. This triad may also be seen with viral infections, including meningitis, particularly mumps. Hence a lumbar puncture should be considered. The syndrome may also occur from unknown causes.

TRAUMA

Head trauma is a frequent cause of ED presentations. While ataxia may be seen in post-concussion syndrome, conditions requiring acute intervention, should be sought by CT scan. These include haemorrhage or cerebral oedema. A base-of-skull fracture may cause ataxia by direct damage to the vestibular apparatus. Non-accidental injury should be considered in all cases of paediatric trauma.

INFECTIONS

Meningitis and encephalitis may both have ataxia as a presenting feature.[35,36] Other features to suggest an infective cause, such as headache, vomiting, fever and neck stiffness, will be evident. In labyrinthitis and vestibular neuronitis, vertigo and vomiting are prominent. There are no cranial nerve or cerebellar signs.

VASCULAR CONDITIONS

Vertebrobasilar stroke is a very uncommon cause of ataxia in children. Ataxia will not be an isolated finding. Other findings include ipsilateral cranial nerve palsies, contralateral weakness, vertigo and diplopia. Systemic lupus erythematosus vasculitis may rarely present with ataxia.[37]

OTHER NEUROLOGICAL CONDITIONS

In ataxia there is preservation of muscle strength. A number of neurological conditions may present with an unsteady gait (pseudo-ataxia) because of weakness. These include Guillain–Barré syndrome in which areflexia and ophthalmoplegia (in Miller–Fisher variant) distinguish it from acute cerebellar ataxia. Tick paralysis should also be considered in cases where the patient has been in an appropriate area. Multiple sclerosis/transverse myelitis is usually not seen until adolescent years. It may present with ataxia, optic or retinal neuritis, regional paraesthesias or weakness.[38] Acute demyelinating encephalomyelitis (ADEM), a postinfectious encephalomyelitis, where host myelin components become immunogenic, may have ataxia as one neurological sign. The diagnosis is made by abnormal CT and MRI findings.

Other neurological conditions that may present with ataxia include seizures and migraine. Because of the episodic nature of these conditions, there will be a recurrent nature to the ataxia. Basilar artery migraine may demonstrate associated headache, blurred vision, visual field defects and vertigo. It tends to have a recurrent course. Epilepsy uncommonly presents with ataxia. Ataxia may be seen post-ictally or in minor motor status or partial complex seizures. Other clues to seizure will be associated altered consciousness or motor manifestations. Benign positional vertigo is uncommon in children. Ataxia accompanies severe, repro-

ducible vertigo, nausea and vomiting. Cranial nerve examination is normal apart from nystagmus.

METABOLIC DISORDERS

A large number of metabolic disorders may have ataxia as a feature and should be kept in mind. Hypoglycaemia and hyponatraemia may present with ataxias but other signs will also be present. The inherited metabolic diseases will likely demonstrate episodes of ataxia, together with the other features of the conditions, which will point towards the diagnosis. There may be a progression to chronic ataxias. Other inborn errors are listed in Table 8.5.4.

CHRONIC ATAXIA

Chronic ataxia usually has an insidious onset but it may present as a progression of acute ataxia, or following recurrent

episodes. Causes include fixed deficits as in ataxic cerebral palsy, which makes up 10% of cerebral palsy and progressive diseases such as the hereditary ataxia, inborn errors of metabolism and tumours. Some causes are amendable to treatment. Table 8.5.4 lists some of the causes.

Hereditary ataxias/spinocerebellar degenerative

Friedreich's ataxia is an autosomal recessive condition, which manifests in a child less than ten years of age with ataxia and nystagmus. There is usually rapid progression. On examination there is impaired position and vibration sense, positive Romberg's sign and absent tendon reflexes. The plantar response is up going. Dysarthria is present. Kyphoscoliosis, distal muscle wasting and contractures and cardiomyopathy may develop. Ataxia telangiectasia is also an autosomal recessive condition with neurocutaneous manifestations. Ataxia is predominantly

---

Table 8.5.4   Causes of chronic ataxia

- Brain tumours
  Cerebellar astrocytoma
  Brainstem glioma
  Medulloblastoma
  Ependymoma
  Cerebellar haemangioblastoma (Von Hippel-Lindau)
- Hereditary ataxia
  Friedreich's ataxia
  Ataxia telangiectasia
  Dominant hereditary ataxia
  Olivopontocerebellar degeneration
  Roussy–Levy syndrome
- Hydrocephalus
- Congenital malformations
  Cerebellar aplasia/hypoplasia (autosomal recessive)
  Vermal aplasia, including Dandy–Walker malformations
  Arnold–Chiari malformations
- Inborn errors of metabolism
  Hartnup's disease
  Wilson's disease
  Refsum's disease
  Abetalipoproteinaemia
  Maple syrup urine disease
  Argininosuccinicaciduria
  Ornithine transcarbamoylase deficiency
  Multiple carboxylase deficiencies – biotinidase deficiency
  Pyruvate dehydrogenase deficiency
  Juvenile GM2 gangliosidosis
  Juvenile sulfatide lipidosis
  Leigh's syndrome
  Sphingolipidoses
  Neuronal ceroid-lipofuscinosis
  γ-Glutamyl cysteine synthetase deficiency
  Triosephosphatase isomerase deficiency
- Vitamin B_{12}, E or folate deficiency

truncal and becomes evident in early childhood. Ocular and cutaneous telangiectasia become evident between two and six years of age. Developmental delay, increased susceptibility to infection, due to thymic atrophy and IgA and IgE deficiency, and an increased incidence of neoplasia are seen.

Congenital malformations

Cerebellar aplasia/hypoplasia, Dandy–Walker malformations, Arnold–Chiari malformations or vermal aplasia may result in ataxic cerebral palsy which accounts for 10% of all cerebral palsy. Signs include, but are not limited to, ataxia, hypotonia and tremor.

EVALUATION OF THE PATIENT

The ED assessment includes history, a thorough examination to detect life-threat, such as raised intracranial pressure, and to arrive at provisional and differential diagnoses. Important aspects of the history include the timing of the ataxia. Is it acute, recurrent or chronic? What is mainly affected, is it the trunk or limbs? Are there other symptoms, such as headache, vomiting, blurred vision, altered mental status or nausea suggestive of a tumour or meningitis? The antecedent history is important, for example a recent viral illness may suggest acute cerebellar ataxia, or there may be a history of trauma or possible drug ingestion. Other symptoms, for example paraesthesia, may suggest an alternative diagnosis such as multiple sclerosis.

Examination should include a general examination to look for signs in need of urgent intervention, for example meningitis, shock, hypoglycaemia, raised ICP or head injury. A complete examination is required to detect signs that may aid in the diagnosis, such as abdominal masses, nystagmus, opsoclonus and myoclonus in neuroblastoma, or signs of infection or vasculitis.

A complete neurological examination should be performed and documented. Cerebellar signs should be carefully assessed. Dysmetria and intention tremor can be assessed in the younger child by asking him to point to the parts of a doll. Dysdiadochokinesis may, however, be difficult to perform. Gait should be assessed. If only the anterior lobe of the cerebellum or the vermis are involved, gait may be affected but the upper limb spared. With truncal ataxia the child may have difficulty keeping balance whilst seated. This imbalance increases if sitting cross-legged, standing or walking. Heel–toe walking tests are useful in detecting cerebellar problems, but unsteadiness may also be due to weakness or sensory deficits. Sensory ataxia is differentiated from cerebellar ataxia by the presence of impaired position and vibration sense and a positive Romberg's test. Lesions of the ipsilateral cerebellar hemispheres causes ataxia prominent in one direction the child will fall towards the side of the lesion. Dysmetria and hypotonia are seen on the side of the lesion. Cerebellar dysarthria (scanning speech) may be detected by repeating 'sizzling sausage'. The speech displays a slow onset and is a slurred, jerky sound with an explosive nature.

Reflexes are often decreased in cerebellar lesions and are absent in Guillain–Barré syndrome. Pendular knee jerks are seen in severe cases of cerebellar dysfunction and in those with associated pyramidal tract defects. Decreased tone is seen in cerebellar lesions with drift and static tremor on holding up the arms. Rebound may also be detected.

Nystagmus is horizontal in cerebellar lesions and maximal to the side of the lesion. It may be positional. In phenytoin intoxication, nystagmus is initially horizontal but becomes vertical at higher levels. Nystagmus in vestibular neuronitis is typically rotational. The cranial nerves should be carefully examined to look for brainstem involvement.

INVESTIGATIONS

Investigations are directed by the history and clinical features detected on examination. Acute cerebellar ataxia is a diagnosis of exclusion and investigation may be required to detect alternative conditions where urgent intervention is required.

A serum anticonvulsant level is indicated where an elevated level of a therapeutic drug is the likely cause. Other appropriate assays may include ethanol, ethylene glycol, anticonvulsants or benzodiazepines when suspected. If the drug screen is positive in an appropriate clinical setting, no other tests may be required.

Imaging by CT and/or MRI is indicated urgently where there are signs of raised intracranial pressure. It is indicated in most cases of acute ataxia unless there is a clear alternative diagnosis.

A lumbar puncture is indicated to exclude suspected meningitis or encephalitis. A CT scan should be performed to exclude space-occupying lesions and raised intracranial pressure prior to the lumbar puncture. Treatment with antibiotics and antivirals should not be delayed whilst awaiting investigation results. In Guillain–Barré the CSF protein is elevated to $0.3–1 \, g \, L^{-1}$ with no or few white cells.

Electrolytes, glucose and ammonia are indicated to assess for metabolic causes. In recurrent ataxia, or where there are features of metabolic disease, further metabolic screening should be performed in consultation with a paediatric neurologist, this may include arterial blood gas, urinalysis, liver function tests, thyroid function tests, lactate in blood and CSF, pyruvate, cholesterol and lipoproteins. Muscle biopsy may be required. If occult neuroblastoma is suspected urinary homovanillic acid and vanillylmandelic acid levels are measured. Other investigations may include an EEG if seizures are suspected.

MANAGEMENT

Treatment is aimed initially at detecting and treating emergency conditions. For example, in hydrocephalus and tumours, raised intracranial pressure is treated in consultation with the neurosurgical unit. In meningitis urgent antibiotics are given. Hypoglycaemia and other reversible metabolic causes are treated. Intoxications and poisonings are generally managed by supportive care. Acute cerebellar ataxia usually resolves over weeks to months. Occasionally there is a persistent movement disorder or behavioural and speech disorders. Supportive care is provided. Physiotherapy, occupational therapy and a wheelchair for mobility may be required.

DISPOSITION

Most children with significant ataxia require admission for investigation and observation under a paediatrician. Some children who have mild ataxia, clearly due to post-infectious cerebellitis, are appropriate to be followed as an out-patient, after discussion with a paediatrician.

REFERENCES

1. Adams C, Diadori P, Schoenroth L, Fritzler M 2000 Autoantibodies in childhood post-varicella acute cerebellar ataxia. Canadian Journal of Neurological Science 27: 316–320
2. Maggi G, Varone A, Aliberti F 1997 Acute cerebellar ataxia in children. Childs Nervous System 13(10): 542–545
3. Connolly AM, Dodson WE, Prensky AL, Rust RS 1994 Course and outcome of acute cerebellar ataxia. Annals of Neurology. 35: 673–679
4. Siemes H, Siegert M, Jaroffke B, Hanefield F 1982 The CSF protein pattern in acute cerebellar ataxia of childhood and intracranial midline tumours. European Journal of Paediatrics 137(1): 49–57
5. Dreyfus PM, Senter TP 1974 Acute cerebellar ataxia of childhood. An unusual case of varicella. Western Journal of Medicine 120(2): 161–163
6. Feldman W, Larke RP 1972 Acute cerebellar ataxia associated with the isolation of Coxsackie virus type A9. Canadian Medical Association Journal 106(10): 1104
7. Erzurum S, Kalavsky SM, Watanakunakorn C 1983 Acute cerebellar ataxia and hearing loss as initial symptoms of infectious mononucleosis. Archives of Neurology 40(12): 760–762
8. Steele JC, Gladstone RM, Thanasophon S, Fleming P 1972 Acute cerebellar ataxia and concomitant infection with *Mycoplasma pneumoniae*. Journal of Paediatrics 80(3): 467–469
9. Cohen HA, Ashkenazi A, Nussinovitch M, Amir J, Hart J, Frydman M 1992 Mumps-associated acute cerebellar ataxia. American Journal of Diseases in Childhood 146(8): 930–931
10. Gupta PC, Gathwala G, Aneja S, Arora SK 1990 Acute cerebellar ataxia: An unusual presentation of poliomyelitis. India Paediatrics 27(6): 622–623
11. Curnen EC, Chamberlin HR 1962 Acute cerebellar ataxia associated with poliovirus infection. Yale Journal of Biological Medicine 34: 219
12. Thapa BR, Sahni A 1993 Acute reversible cerebellar ataxia in typhoid fever. India Paediatrics 30(3): 427
13. Marzetti G, Midulla M 1967 Acute cerebellar ataxia associated with echo type 6 infection in two children. Acta Paediatrica Scandinavia 56: 547
14. Batton FE 1905 Ataxia in childhood. Brain 28: 487–505
15. Shimizu Y, Ueno T, Komatsu H, Takada H, Nunoue T 1999 Acute cerebellar ataxia with human parvovirus B19 infection. Archives of Diseases in Childhood 80(1): 72–73
16. Dano G 1968 Acute cerebellar ataxia associated with herpes simplex virus infection. Acta Paediatrica Scandinavia 57: 151
17. McMinn P, Stratov I, Nagarajan L, Davis S 2001 Neurological manifestations of enterovirus 71 infection in children during an outbreak of hand, foot and mouth disease in Western Australia. Clinical Infectious Diseases 32(2): 236–242
18. Senanayake N, de Silva HJ 1999 Delayed cerebellar ataxia complicating falciparum malaria: A clinical study of 74 patients. Journal of Neurology 241(7): 456–459
19. Sunaga Y, Hikima A, Ostuka T, Morikawa A 1995 Acute cerebellar ataxia with abnormal MRI lesions after varicella vaccination. Paediatric Neurology 13(4): 340–342
20. Deisenhammer F, Pohl P, Bosch S, Schmidauer C 1994 Acute cerebellar ataxia after immunization with recombinant hepatitis B vaccine. Acta Neurologica Scandinavia 89(6): 462–463
21. Murphy JM, Motiwala R, Devinsky O 1991 Phenytoin intoxication. South Medicine Journal 84: 1199–1204
22. Wilson JT, Huff JG, Kilroy AW 1979 Prolonged toxicity following acute phenytoin overdose in a child. Journal of Paediatrics 95135–95138
23. Booker HE, Darcey B 1973 Serum concentrations of free diphenylhydantoin and their relationship to intoxication. Epilepsia 14: 177
24. Tibballs J 1992 Acute toxic reaction to carbamazepine: Clinical effects and serum concentrations. Journal of Paediatrics 121(2): 295–299
25. Wiley CC, Wiley JF 1998 Pediatric benzodiazepine ingestion resulting in hospitalization. Journal of Toxicology 36(3): 227–231
26. Stremski E, Hennes H 2000 Accidental isopropanol ingestion in children. Paediatric Emergency Care 16(4): 238–240
27. Tibballs J 1995 Clinical effects and management of eucalyptus oil ingestion in infants and young children. Medical Journal of Australia 163(4): 177–180
28. Webb NJA, Pitt WR 1993 Eucalyptus oil poisoning in childhood: 41 cases in South-East Queensland. Journal of Paediatrics and Children's Health 29: 368–371
29. Del Beccaro MA 1995 Melaleuca oil poisoning in a 17-month-old. Veterinary and Human Toxicology 37(6): 557–558
30. Brook MP, McCarron MM, Mueller JA 1989 Pine oil ingestion. Annals of Emergency Medicine 18(4): 391–395
31. Von Muhlendahl KE, Kreinke EG, Scherrf-Rahne B, Baukloh G 1976 Codeine intoxication in childhood. Lancet 16: 303–305
32. Warden CR, Diekema DS, Robertson WO 1997 Dystonic reaction associated with dextromethorphan ingestion in a toddler. Paediatric Emergency Care 13(3): 214–215
33. Bem JL, Peck R 1992 Dextromethorphan: An overview of safety issues. Drug Safety 7(3): 190–199
34. Telander RL, Smithson A, Groover V 1989 Clinical outcome in children with acute cerebral encephalopathy and neuroblastoma. Journal of Paediatric Surgery 24(1): 11–14
35. Kaplan S, Goddard J, Van Kleeck M, Catlin FI, Feigin RD 1981 Ataxia and deafness in children due to bacterial meningitis. Paediatrics 68: 8–13
36. Iff T, Donati F, Vassella F, Schaad UB, Bianchetti MG 1998 Acute encephalitis in Swiss children: Aetiology and outcome. European Journal of Paediatric Neurology 2: 233–237
37. Yaginuma M, Suenaga M, Shiono Y, Sakamoto M 2000 Acute cerebellar ataxia of a patient with SLE. Clinical Neurology & Neurosurgery 102(1): 37–39
38. Rust RS 2000 Multiple sclerosis, acute disseminated encephalomyelitis, and related conditions. Seminars in Pediatric Neurology 7(2): 66–90

8.6 HEADACHE

ALISTAIR MURRAY • JOHN RYAN

ESSENTIALS

1 The primary role of the emergency physician is to exclude a significant underlying cause for the headache, most urgently that of infection, raised intracranial pressure or an intra-cerebral bleed.

2 While the majority of headaches presenting to the ED are likely to be benign, appropriate investigation and follow up of patients will ensure that serious causes are unlikely to be missed.

3 A thorough history and examination is likely to provide a diagnosis in the majority of children presenting to an ED with a headache.

4 Chronic headaches need not necessarily be investigated on an emergent basis unless they are progressive.

5 *Red flags* prompting further investigation of headache include: occipital headache; meningism; focal neurological signs; seizures; progressive nature; papilloedema; persistent vomiting; ataxia; presence of a VP shunt; age younger than three years; or early morning headaches, especially those that wake the child from sleep.

INTRODUCTION

The aim of this chapter is to give the reader a basic understanding of the aetiology of headaches in a paediatric population while offering a functional and safe approach to the management of paediatric patients with headaches in the ED. Some key points should be remembered at the outset:

- Children of different ages may require different approaches depending on factors such as age, ethnicity or socioeconomic status.
- Children under three years rarely complain of headache and this should prompt one to consider an organic cause.
- The classical history of migraine from a teenager may be more easily elicited than the history of symptoms from a shy five year old.

INCIDENCE

Approximately 1.3% of all presentations to EDs have headache as the presenting complaint.[1] Headaches in children are very common with up to 75% of children having had a headache of some form by the age of fifteen.[2] Despite the frequency, very few paediatric patients with headaches ever consult their family physician or an ED. For most EDs this equates with one to two patients presenting each day with a headache. However, this does not take account of patients who present with a different complaint such as a temperature who might also have a headache as part of a concomitant illness.

PATHOPHYSIOLOGY

The causes of headache are myriad, but the primary aim of the emergency physician should be to differentiate the patient with a headache that will run a relatively benign course from that which may be a symptom of significant underlying pathology with immediate health implications.

Multiple factors must be considered. However, the overwhelming majority of headaches will be diagnosed on history alone, with little additional information arising from either the examination or from investigations.[2-4] Furthermore, the vast majority of headaches that present to the ED are likely to be benign, but those that are not, have the potential to be life threatening.

The classification of headaches is based on the underlying aetiology.[5] The International Headache Society has developed a classification of headache, the second edition of which was published at the end of 2003.[6] This classification splits headache into two broad categories namely primary and secondary headaches, i.e. headaches that have no identifiable organic precipitant and those with a detectable underlying cause (Table 8.6.1).

The causes of some headaches are dealt with in other chapters, e.g. Chapter 8.7 on meningitis, while some of the primary headache disorders will be discussed in more detail later in this chapter. We recommend an approach whereby the emergency doctor approaches each case by initially excluding the sinister causes of the headache (Table 8.6.2).

CLINICAL ASSESSMENT

History

The first step in any medical assessment is the history and this is of vital importance in the case of headache. Depending on the age of the child, the history may be taken from the child or the parent. Important features of the headache to explore in the history include:

1. Onset of the headache

Sudden onset headaches can be considered differently in children compared to adults. The classical history of sudden onset headache being suggestive of sub-arachnoid haemorrhage in an adult is less relevant in the case of the paediatric patient. In children the most frequent underlying cause is an upper respiratory tract infection or primary headache.[1,3,4] There is a significantly higher proportion

Table 8.6.1   Summary of International Headache Society classification of headaches

Primary headaches
1. Migraine
2. Tension-type headache
3. Cluster headaches and other trigeminal-autonomic cephalgias
4. Other primary headaches

Secondary headaches
5. Headache attributed to head and/or neck trauma
6. Headache attributed to cranial and/or cervical vascular disorders
7. Headache attributed to non-vascular, non-infectious intracranial disorder
8. Headache attributed to a substance or its withdrawal
9. Headache attributed to infection
10. Headache attributed to disturbance of homeostasis
11. Headache or facial pain attributed to disorder of cranium, neck, eyes, ears, nose, sinuses, teeth or other facial or cranial structures
12. Headache attributed to psychiatric disorder
13. Cranial neuralgias and central causes of facial pain
14. Other headache, cranial neuralgia, central or primary facial pain

Table 8.6.2   Causes of headache in children

Infection
- Meningitis, encephalitis, abscess
- Influenza
- Systemic infection
- Sinusitis
- Dental infection

Vascular
- Migraine
- Intracranial haemorrhage
- Hypertensive encephalopathy

Post lumbar puncture

Raised intracranial pressure
- Brain tumour
- Hydrocephalus
- Benign intracranial hypertension
- Trauma - SDH, concussion

Toxic
- Carbon monoxide
- Lead

Functional
- Tension or cluster headache

Psychogenic

of underlying pathology in cases of acute headache, compared to chronic headache. It should also be noted that the investigation of headache of acute onset is more properly the role of the emergency physician, while chronic headaches may be best investigated by the patient's continuing care physician or paediatrician.

2. Site

Classic migraine is typically unilateral. However, childhood migraine is a little different, often being bilateral. The headache of meningeal irritation due to meningitis may involve neck pain. It should also be noted that occipital headaches are relatively uncommon in children and this has been reported to be an independent predictor of underlying pathology, particularly of the posterior fossa.

3. Pyrexia

The presence of fever will often be reported by a parent and should immediately raise the suspicion of an infectious origin. It is worth remembering that other inflammatory disorders may cause pyrexia. Equally, the absence of pyrexia does not exclude the possibility of infection. In the ED setting, febrile children with headache require consideration of the possibility of meningitis or encephalitis.

4. Progression

The temporal progression is of relevance in the patient with headache. For example, a classic migraine will last between one and seventy-two hours in a child, while a patient with a chronic headache that is becoming progressively more severe may well have an underlying organic cause. This should prompt the emergency physician who encounters a patient with such a pattern, to ensure that neuroimaging is performed.[2,7]

Nature   Headache of a throbbing nature is suggestive of migraine, while band-like headaches are often of a tension type. It has been suggested that the inability of a child to describe the nature of the headache may in itself be a predictor of underlying pathology.

Behavioural change and avoidance behaviour   This is often noted in a collateral history. While entirely non-specific, it is particularly important in raising suspicion of other causes of a headache, such as a school phobia or drug misuse in the adolescent, and may, indeed, be a pointer towards sexual assault.[8]

Sleep disturbance   Benign causes of headache rarely wake patients from their sleep and if a child is being woken by a headache this should prompt the consideration of investigation or referral.

Postural symptoms   A headache that is worse on lying flat or exacerbated by coughing may be related to raised intracranial pressure.

Neurological deficit   A history of neurological deficit, albeit temporary, should be considered highly significant and should always be enquired about. This is particularly important as some patients may have subtle objective neurological findings that could easily be overlooked in a hurried neurological examination. Most mothers will have noticed an unusual posture or limp but may not immediately mention it unless prompted. The importance of this is re-enforced by the evidence that it may take an average of seven months for a brain tumour to be diagnosed with as many as three different consultations with a physician. This is despite the results of studies showing that a significant proportion of children with tumours have abnormal neurological examinations.[9-11]

Family history (especially of migraine)   Approximately 70–90% of diagnosed cases of migraine have a positive family history. Therefore, diagnosing a migraine in the absence of a family history should be done with caution.

Analgesic use Abolition of a headache with simple analgesics or restoration of normal activities is more common in those with upper respiratory tract associated headaches. It should also be noted that chronic daily use of analgesics is in itself a cause of headaches.[12]

Examination

A number of specific points should be considered when examining the child with a headache. Headache may be a secondary symptom of a more generalised illness (see Table 8.6.2). A comprehensive physical examination is therefore mandatory. Observation of a child from a distance may be valuable. The child lying quietly unresponsive to the environment, should prompt earlier assessment than an active child who interacts normally with healthcare staff. One must also consider other causes of headache that are not readily discernible. In some cases there may be few clinical signs, such as with carbon monoxide poisoning from houses with poorly ventilated gas boilers.[13] Heavy-metal poisoning is another rare cause.

A focused examination should be directed on the basis of the history. Vital signs may provide valuable keys to the aetiology. The temperature should be recorded on more than one occasion. Likewise, it is important to measure the blood pressure as headache may be the presenting feature of co-arctation of the aorta or underlying hypertension. Checking the blood glucose may be relevant if the history suggests hypoglycaemia. It is useful to measure head circumference and plot this on centile charts, even for the older child. A disproportionately large head should prompt further investigation. The tension should be palpated in children who still have open fontanelles.

A significant proportion of children who present with headache will have a

---

Table 8.6.3 Important causes of non-benign headache

- Brain tumours and hydrocephalus
- Benign intracranial hypertension
- Intracranial haemorrhage
- Meningitis encephalitis or abscess
- Hypertensive encephalopathy

---

diagnosis of respiratory tract infection, hence the importance of a thorough ear, nose and throat examination. Occasionally a child with tonsillitis will present with headache, without any complaint of a sore throat. Dental examination may reveal percussion tenderness of an infection that may cause a referred temporal headache. The presence of nasal discharge or respiratory symptoms should prompt the clinician to seek evidence of sinus tenderness. Likewise, it should be noted that, in most children, headaches due to uncomplicated upper respiratory tract infections can be expected to settle with simple analgesics. The persistence of headache should prompt the consideration of further investigation.

A careful examination may reveal subtle evidence of trauma, which may or may not have been sustained accidentally. A mild post-concussion headache may persist for a number of days after a head injury, but may require imaging to exclude a possible subdural haematoma, particularly where the headache is severe, responds poorly to analgesia, is associated with vomiting or is prolonged. Headache has been retrospectively described as being more common in victims of sexual abuse.[8] The febrile, toxic appearing child should be examined for evidence of nuchal rigidity and other signs of meningeal irritation, which may be present in meningitis. In the child who has a ventriculoperitoneal shunt, the reservoir should be assessed by palpation (see Chapter 8.1 on shunt complications).

Ophthalmological examination, including fundoscopy, is particularly important as it may influence immediate management. The presence or absence of papilloedema should be specifically sought as this may be the only objective finding in cases of benign intracranial hypertension (BIH). In this condition the CT scan may be normal and the diagnosis based on an elevated opening pressure > 20 cmH$_2$O on lumbar puncture. This valuable test is frequently neglected in lumbar punctures performed in the ED. The CSF protein, glucose and cell counts are normal in BIH. These children may present with intermittent headache, vomiting, blurred vision or diplopia.

Retinal haemorrhages should be sought on ophthalmoscopy. Their presence is considered as evidence of significant trauma, in the absence of other causes such as hypertension or diabetes. It is difficult, if not at times impossible, to achieve successful examination of the fundi and retina of the younger child. Occasionally, one may need to use mydriatic eye drops to dilate the pupils or avail oneself of the opinion of a colleague. A deferred formal retinal assessment by an ophthalmologist may be required in cases where the possibility of non-accidental injury exists. Eye movements must be carefully examined as subtle nerve palsies may be apparent early in the child presenting with a space-occupying lesion or hydrocephalus.

The main consideration in a cardiovascular examination should be directed at the exclusion of hypertension and the palpation of femoral pulses checking for evidence of co-arctation of the aorta.

Abdominal examination is usually normal but is required as nausea, vomiting and abdominal pain are frequently associated with headache in children. It is recognised by the International Headache Society that 'cyclical vomiting' and 'abdominal migraine' are distinct entities and not infrequently progress to the typical pattern of migraine in adulthood. Hypertension of renal origin may be suggested by the presence of palpable polycystic kidneys.

A standard neurological examination should be performed. Specific features that should be sought include papilloedema, ataxia, hemiparesis, abnormal eye movements and abnormal tendon reflexes. One retrospective study in 1991 showed that in a series of 3000 children with a brain tumour, 98% of them had an abnormality of at least one of the these signs.[9] It is important to assess a child's gait and hand co-ordination to exclude any posterior fossa signs.

The patient should be fully undressed and any rash or abnormality of pigmentation specifically sought. The most urgent of these is the search for the petechial rash of meningococcal disease, but may also reveal neurofibromas and the café-au-lait spots associated with neurofibromatosis or a pigmented patch associated with tuberous sclerosis.

Investigation

The issue of how far to investigate a child with a headache in the ED is not clearly defined and remains contentious. It is clear that the cause of the majority of headaches in children presenting to the ED is a respiratory tract infection or primary headache syndrome. The key role of the emergency physician is to diagnose those headaches that may be due to significant underlying pathology. Investigation should be guided by the history and by findings on examination, as the majority of diagnoses should be suggested by these and confirmed by appropriate diagnostic tests (see Table 8.6.4).

Numerous studies have assessed the value of investigating a child with headache with most of them focusing on the relevance of neuroimaging.[14–18] Laboratory-based testing has a very low yield in paediatric patients with headaches. Occasionally they can alert the clinician to more serious underlying pathology, but their value is limited in the emergency setting. They should not delay the more specific investigations and treatment.

Lumbar puncture should be considered mandatory in any cases of suspected meningitis or encephalitis. It should be noted, however, that post-lumbar puncture headache is also a recognised complication in children, as it is in adults.[19] Such an invasive procedure may often be emotionally traumatic for a child and should not be ordinarily recommended as a routine investigation in the diagnosis of headache.

Table 8.6.4 Red flags, prompting further investigation of headache

- Occipital headache
- Meningism
- Focal neurological symptoms or signs
- Chronic progressive headaches
- Persistent vomiting
- Papilloedema
- Seizures
- Ataxia
- Presence of a VP shunt
- Age younger than three years
- Abnormal eye movements
- Early morning headaches, especially those that wake the child from sleep

Many papers have reviewed the usefulness of neuroimaging in the diagnosis of headache. The consensus is that neuroimaging has a particularly low yield in the context of a chronic, non-progressive headache with a normal neurological examination. This, however, artificially selects a cohort of patients that are unlikely to be seen in the ED. Emergency physicians are cautioned against applying such a finding to the ED population attending with a headache. The investigation of chronic headaches is not the role of the emergency physician and in the absence of an acute deterioration patients may be better served by redirection to their family physician or paediatrician.

DISPOSITION

The disposition of a patient from the ED should be considered on an individual basis though some guidelines may be helpful in minimising the risk of missing a significant diagnosis. The increasing use of observation wards can prove helpful in selected cases. Such a facility is most useful in the case where an infective cause of the headache is suspected.

All patients who present to the ED with headache should have a follow-up appointment in the short term with either their family physician or a paediatrician depending on each case. This will ensure that not only are high standards of care maintained, but unnecessary acute investigations can be avoided that would otherwise be ordered in order to exclude every possible cause of headache. Furthermore, there may be psychosocial aspects of relevance to paediatric headaches that may be more appropriately dealt with by the family physician.

MANAGEMENT

Symptomatic treatment in the ED of most headaches in children can be achieved by use of oral analgesics such as paracetamol, codeine or ibuprofen. Headaches that require stronger analgesics to control pain are an indication for admission for further evaluation.

ESSENTIALS

1 Family history of migraine is very common and a diagnosis of migraine in the absence of a family history should be carefully considered.

2 Unlike adult migraine, simple analgesics are often effective in the context of childhood migraine.

3 Childhood migraine is often bilateral.

4 Migraine is frontotemporal. Occipital headache suggests a sinister cause of headache.

MIGRAINE

INTRODUCTION

Childhood migraine is a common condition presenting to the ED. The diagnosis is often based on history. However, the diagnosis can be a little more difficult to make in the younger age group. The emergency physician should not diagnose migraine in those less than three years old or where headaches are not of a recurrent nature. Childhood migraine also has a wider spectrum of symptoms than adult migraine and should be considered in a patient who has recurrent abdominal pain, with normal investigations. It is important to remember that although the diagnosis of migraine is common, it is principally a diagnosis of exclusion.

PATHOPHYSIOLOGY

The exact mechanism of migraine is complex and incompletely understood. It has been thought to be related to alterations in the vasculature of the scalp with vasodilatation being responsible for the pulsating nature described almost universally by sufferers. Another theory has implicated the sensitivity of the trigeminal nerve as a cause while more recent approaches suggest a combination of these two theories.

It is now apparent that serotonin is integrally involved, hence the increasing popularity of the use of serotonin agonists such as sumatripan and zolmitripan in the acute treatment of adult migraine. These are increasingly being used for children although many countries have yet to license them for paediatric use.

CLINICAL FEATURES

Migraine without aura is more common than migraine with aura in children. A number of key features are listed below.[5]

❶ A history of at least five attacks, lasting 1–48 hours.

❷ Headaches pulsating or throbbing in quality.

❸ Headaches may be unilateral or bilateral (unlike adult migraine, which is typically unilateral).

❹ Headaches exacerbated by routine activities (walking or climbing stairs).

❺ Nausea and vomiting are often prominent features.

❻ Photophobia or phonophobia is frequently present.

❼ The location is frontotemporal. The presence of an occipital headache suggests a structural abnormality and not migraine.

❽ The headache is moderate or severe.

❾ Attacks may be precipitated by exercise, head trauma, foods or menstrual cycles.

In migraine with aura the headache is preceded by a period of altered visual perception that may take numerous forms. This period of altered perception can last up to sixty minutes.

Assessing the severity of headache in a young child can prove challenging. Children almost universally point to the most unhappy face on a visual analogue scale when describing a headache. More reliable answers may be achieved by asking about quality-of-life issues, such as ability to continue playing. Children who can continue playing during a headache appear to have a more benign cause to their headache.

Up to 90% of patients with migraine have a positive family history, although it is noteworthy that only one migraine gene has been identified and this is associated with only 50% of the cases of familial hemiplegic migraine, a particularly rare condition.[4]

A number of other conditions are considered to be migraine disorders in childhood, most notably cyclical vomiting and abdominal migraine. In these conditions there may be recurrent episodes of severe abdominal pain with associated vomiting but the examination and investigation of the children is often normal. These conditions are a diagnosis of exclusion, but their consideration may lead to appropriate referral and follow-up as they carry significant morbidity.

Migraine variant disorders may cause transient abnormal neurological findings such as hemiplegia, ophthalmoplegia, or confusional state. These are rare and an abnormal examination should prompt the emergency physician to investigate further.

INVESTIGATION

Migraine as a distinct entity has no specific diagnostic test. Investigations should be requested on the basis of excluding other pathology as the cause of headache. It is notable that although a significant number of migraine sufferers have abnormal EEGs, these add little diagnostic value and on current evidence should remain a research tool.[20]

TREATMENT

Most cases of childhood migraine can be adequately managed with simple analgesics such as paracetamol and ibuprofen.[21] As nausea can often be a significant feature, metoclopramide may also be of benefit. At present the tryptan group of drugs remains unlicensed for children under twelve in many countries but may prove useful in the future for more resistant cases.

DISPOSITION

All patients with a discharge diagnosis of migraine should be followed up to ensure that the headache resolves within the expected time frame and also to ensure that it does not progress. Migraine can cause significant impairment to lifestyle, if unrecognised. Follow-up should be arranged by the primary care physician with review of medication and parental understanding of the condition. Children with frequent migraine warrant referral to a paediatrician to consider preventative therapy.

CONCLUSIONS

Patients with headaches commonly present to paediatric EDs. Those children presenting with new-onset symptomatology, significant neurological symptoms/signs or evidence of abnormal physiology should be rapidly assessed with early referral for diagnostic facilities and neuroimaging being a priority. Children with chronic symptoms or recurrence of chronic symptoms should have a thorough examination and treatment. Follow-up should be arranged with the patient's paediatrician or continuing-care physician.

REFERENCES

1. Burton LJ, Quinn B, Pratt-Cheney JL, Pourani M 1997 Headache etiology in a pediatric emergency department. Pediatric Emergency Care 13: 1–4
2. Kan L, Nagelberg J, Maytal J 2000 Headaches in a pediatric emergency department: Etiology, imaging and treatment. Headache 40(1): 25–29
3. Lewis DW, Qureshi F 2000 Acute headache in children and adolescents presenting to the emergency department. Headache 40(3): 200–203
4. Lewis DW 2002 Headaches in children and adolescents. American Family Physician 65(4): 625–632
5. Headcare Classification Committee of the International Headache Society 1988 Classification and diagnostic criteria for headache disorders, cranial neuralgias and facial pain. Cephalgia 8(Suppl 7): 1–96
6. Gobel H 2001 Classification of headaches. Cephalgia 21: 770–773
7. Green SH 2002 Chronic and recurrent headache. Current Paediatrics 12: 186–190
8. Golding JM 1999 Sexual assault history and headache: Five general population studies. Journal of Nervous and Mental Disease 187(10): 624–629
9. The Childhood Brain Tumor Consortium 1991 The epidemiology of headache among children with brain tumor. Journal of Neurooncology 10: 31–46
10. Dobrovoljac M, Hengartner H, Boltshauser E, Grotzer MA 2002 Delay in the diagnosis of pediatric brain tumours. European Journal of Pediatrics 161(12): 663–667
11. Mehta V, Chapman A, McNeely PD, Walling S, Howes WJ 2002 Latency between symptom onset and diagnosis of pediatric brain tumors. Neurosurgery 51(2): 365–372
12. Vasconcellos E, Pina-Garza JE, Millan EJ, Warner JS 1998 Analgesic rebound headache in children

and adolescents. Journal of Child Neurology 13(9): 443–447

13. Hampson NB, Hampson LA 2002 Characteristics of headache associated with acute carbon monoxide poisoning. Headache 42(3): 220–223

14. Lewis DW, Dorbad D 2000 The utility of neuroimaging in the evaluation of children with migraine or chronic daily headache who have normal neurological examinations. Headache 40(8): 629–632

15. Aysun S, Yetuk M 1998 Clinical experience on headache in children: Analysis of 92 cases. Journal of Child Neurology 13(5): 202–210

16. Jordan JE, Ramirez GF, Bradley WG, Chen DY, Lightfoote JB, Song A 2000 Economic and outcomes assessment of MRI in the evolution of headache. Journal of the National Medical Association 92(12): 573–578

17. Medina LS, Kuntz KM, Pomeroy S 2001 Children with headache suspected of having a brain tumour: A cost-effectiveness analysis of diagnostic strategies. Pediatrics 108(2): 255–263

18. Alehan FK 2002 Value of neuroimaging in the evaluation of neurologically normal children with recurrent headache. Journal of Child Neurology 17(11): 807–809

19. Janssens E, Aerssens P, Alliet P, Gillis P, Raes M 2003 Post-dural puncture headaches in children. A literature review. European Journal of Paediatrics 162(3): 117–121

20. Puca F, de Tomamaso M 1999 Clinical neurophysiology in childhood headache. Cephalgia 19: 137–146

21. Hamalainen ML, Hoppu K, Valkeila E, Santavuori P 1997 Ibuprofen or acetaminophen for the acute treatment of migraine in children. Neurology 48: 1031–1037

8.7 CNS INFECTIONS: MENINGITIS AND ENCEPHALITIS

MIKE STARR

ESSENTIALS

1 Bacterial meningitis can be rapidly progressive, and result in substantial morbidity and mortality.

2 A high index of suspicion of the possibility of meningitis must be maintained in any sick infant or child.

3 Symptoms and signs are frequently non-specific, particularly with younger age.

4 Antibiotic treatment must not be delayed, although steroids can improve outcome if given before the first dose of antibiotic, and continued six-hourly for four days.

5 Careful management of fluid and electrolyte balance is critical.

6 Conjugate meningococcal and pneumococcal vaccines may reduce the incidence of bacterial meningitis.

7 HSV encephalitis must be considered in any child with features of meningitis with encephalopathy.

8 Empiric aciclovir must be given early when encephalitis is suspected.

INTRODUCTION

Meningitis and encephalitis are medical emergencies that require prompt assessment and treatment. Meningitis is inflammation of the meninges that surround the brain and spinal cord. Inflammatory cells invariably spill into the CSF from the meninges, producing an increased cell count. Encephalitis is an inflammation involving the brain parenchyma, which may occur in conjunction with inflammation of the meninges (meningoencephalitis) or spinal cord (encephalomyelitis).

MENINGITIS

CLASSIFICATION

Meningitis is usually broadly classified as bacterial or aseptic. Aseptic meningitis may be the result of a localised or systemic insult, but is most commonly caused by viruses or fungi.

AETIOLOGY

Bacteria

The bacterial causes of meningitis vary with the age of the child. In infants less than 2–3 months old, organisms acquired from the maternal genital tract predominate: Group B streptococci, *Escherichia coli* and *Listeria monocytogenes*. In older children and adults the most common causes are *Neisseria meningitidis* and *Streptococcus pneumoniae*. Other causes, including *Staphylococcus* species and Gram-negative bacilli, are occasionally seen in immunocompromised hosts or following trauma or neurosurgery. *Haemophilus influenzae* type b (Hib) is rarely seen as a cause now because of widespread immunisation. *Mycobacterium tuberculosis* is rare, other than in children who have spent prolonged periods in countries of high prevalence.

In Australia, the most common *N. meningitidis* serogroup causing invasive disease in children under 15 years is serogroup B (72%), followed by serogroup C (25%).[1] In children between 15 and 19 years, serogroup C predominates (serogroup C 51%; serogroup B 45%).[1] The most common pneumococcal serotypes causing invasive disease are those contained in the seven-valent conjugate pneumococcal vaccine currently available in Australia (14, 6B, 18C, 19F, 4, 23F, 9V).[2]

Viruses

Enteroviruses, including coxsackie and echoviruses, cause 85–95% of cases of viral meningitis. Herpes simplex viruses 1 and 2 (HSV-1 and HSV-2) and other herpes viruses (human herpes viruses 6, 7 and 8, varicella-zoster virus, cytomegalovirus and Epstein–Barr virus) tend to cause meningoencephalitis. HSV-1 and HSV-2 are perhaps the most important causes to consider, as meningoencephalitis caused by these viruses is associated with high morbidity and mortality, which may be reduced with early treatment.

Fungi

Cryptococcus neoformans is the most common fungal cause of meningitis, but occurs almost exclusively in immuno-compromised hosts.

CLINICAL FINDINGS

The unwell febrile child who presents with classical features of headache, vomiting, neck stiffness, photophobia, and altered mentation does not usually present a diagnostic dilemma. Likewise, the child who presents to emergency with florid meningococcemia is usually easy to recognise. However, it is the child who presents with early or non-specific features that one always needs to maintain a high index of suspicion about and consider the possibility of a CNS infection as the cause. Equally, the child who has recently been treated with oral antibiotics may present in a more insidious fashion, which may result in subtle clinical findings. One may have to vary the threshold for a CSF examination accordingly, particularly in the younger child or if the possibility of a partially treated meningitis exists.

The clinical manifestations of meningitis include fever, irritability, lethargy, poor feeding and vomiting. If the fontanelle is still open, it may be bulging when examined with the infant in a sitting position. Photophobia is difficult to ascertain in young children, and other signs of meningeal irritation may be absent or difficult to elicit. Kernig's sign (inability to extend the knee when the leg is flexed at the hip), Brudzinski sign (bending the head forward produces flexion movements of the legs) and nuchal rigidity may be present in older children, but have been shown to have low positive and negative predictive value in adults with meningitis.[3] Infants or young children may manifest resistance to being picked up by their parents or distress on walking due to the presence of meningeal irritation with movement.

Rashes may occur with any bacterial meningitis, although they are less common with pneumococcal infection. Petechiae or purpura are suggestive of meningococcal sepsis, but may also occur in Hib and viral meningitides.

It is impossible to reliably differentiate between bacterial and viral meningitis on clinical grounds. However, children with enteroviral meningitis are more likely to present in summer or autumn with gradual onset of non-specific constitutional symptoms including diarrhoea, cough and myalgia.

INVESTIGATIONS

Definitive diagnosis of meningitis relies on examination of the cerebrospinal fluid (CSF) with biochemical analysis, microscopy and culture. Children with suspected meningitis should have a lumbar puncture (LP) performed, unless there is a contraindication. The only absolute contraindication is raised intracranial pressure (ICP). It may be difficult to determine whether ICP is raised, but the following signs may be indicative:

- Coma (absent or non-purposeful response to painful stimulus)
- Abnormal pupillary responses
- Abnormal posturing
- Focal neurological signs or seizures
- Recent (within 30 minutes), prolonged (over 30 minutes) or tonic seizures
- Papilloedema – although this is an unreliable and late sign.

A bulging fontanelle in the absence of other signs of raised ICP, is not a contraindication to LP.

Cerebral computerised tomography (CT) should not be used to decide whether it is safe to proceed with LP in patients suspected of meningitis. In a prospective study of bacterial meningitis, CT findings obtained during the acute stages failed to reveal any clinically significant abnormalities that were not suspected on neurological examination.[4] Moreover, cerebral herniation can occur with a normal CT.[5,6]

Other relative contraindications to LP include:

- Cardiovascular compromise or shock
- Respiratory compromise
- Coagulopathy or thrombocytopenia.

Examination of the CSF

Normal CSF is clear and contains few cells (and no neutrophils). As few as 200×10^6 cells per litre will cause CSF to appear turbid. The CSF profile may help differentiate between bacterial and viral meningitis, but the findings vary. Table 8.7.1 indicates the typical profiles in normal children and those with meningitis. However, these should always be interpreted in the context of the clinical picture. In early bacterial meningitis the CSF cell count may be normal. In enteroviral meningitis there is typically a neutrophil predominance early, and this may remain so for more than 24 hours.[7]

Organisms are seen on CSF Gram stain in 60–80% of cases of meningitis, provided that prior antibiotics have not been given. The sensitivity is highest in pneumococcal meningitis. Prior antibiotics may preclude culture of the causative organism, but the biochemistry and white cell count remain abnormal for several days.

A traumatic tap occurs in 15–20% of lumbar punctures in children.[8,9] Several formulae have been devised for interpretation of CSF contaminated with blood, but the safest practice is to disregard the red cell count and treat if meningitis is suspected.

Seizures do not result in increased CSF cell count in the absence of meningitis.

Table 8.7.1   CSF findings in meningitis

	White cell count	Biochemistry		
	Neutrophils ($\times 10^6$ L^{-1})	Lymphocytes ($\times 10^6$ L^{-1})	Protein (g L(1)	Glucose (CSF:blood ratio)
Normal (> 1 month of age)	0	≤5	< 0.4	≥0.6 (or ≥2.5 mmol L^{-1})
Normal (< 1 month of age)	0	≤11 (? < 20)	< 1.0	≥0.6 (or ≥2.1 mmol L^{-1})
Bacterial meningitis	↑ (100–10 000)	↑ (Usually < 100)	↑	↓
Viral meningitis	↑ (usually < 100)	↑	0.4–1.0	Normal
Encephalitis	↑ (usually < 100)	↑	0.4–1.0	Normal

Bacterial or viral DNA can be detected in blood and/or CSF using polymerase chain reaction (PCR) analysis. Sensitivity and specificity are high, particularly for *N. meningitidis*, HSV and enterovirus. PCR for *N. meningitidis* is particularly useful in patients with a clinical picture consistent with meningococcal meningitis, but who have received prior antibiotics.

Latex agglutination allows rapid detection of bacterial antigens in CSF and urine. However, it lacks sensitivity and specificity, other than for Hib, and is therefore not clinically useful.

Other investigations

- Culture of blood, throat swab or of skin lesion may yield a causative organism.
- Gram stain on blood smear may be positive.
- Blood glucose should be measured at the same time as CSF glucose.
- A baseline sodium should be measured. Hyponatraemia occurs in about one-third of children with meningitis, and may be due to increased antidiuretic hormone secretion, increased urine sodium losses, and excessive electrolyte-free water intake or administration.
- Full blood count and acute phase reactants (e.g. C-reactive protein) may provide supportive information.

MANAGEMENT

Antibiotics

Following initial fluid resuscitation, the emphasis is on prompt commencement of parenteral antibiotics. Delay in antibiotic therapy has been associated with adverse clinical outcome in adults with bacterial meningitis.[10] The emergency physician should consider the 'door to antibiotic time' in a child with meningitis, with equal importance as the concept of time to thrombolysis in an adult patient with acute myocardial infarction.

Age < 2 months

Benzylpenicillin 60 mg kg^{-1} IV 12-hourly (week 1 of life); 6–8 hourly (weeks 2–4 of life); 4-hourly (after week 4 of life) *plus*

Cefotaxime (or ceftriaxone) 50 mg kg^{-1} IV 12-hourly (week 1 of life); 6-hourly (after 1 week of age) *plus*

Gentamicin 5 mg kg^{-1} IV daily (week 1 of life); 7.5 mg kg^{-1} IV daily (after 1 week of age).

Because of the morbidity associated with neonatal Gram-negative meningitis, and the high rates of recrudescence, many neonatologists use three drugs for empiric therapy.

Age > 2 months

Cefotaxime 50 mg kg^{-1} (maximum 2 g) IV 6-hourly (or ceftriaxone)

Vancomycin 15 mg kg^{-1} (maximum 500 mg) IV 6-hourly should be added if *S. pneumoniae* is suspected or if LP is to be deferred.

Rates of resistance to penicillin and cephalosporin amongst pneumococci are increasing in Australia.[11]

Steroids

Routine administration of steroids as adjunctive therapy has been controversial in the past. The evidence that they protect against neurological (particularly audiological) complications of childhood meningitis is strongest for Hib meningitis, when dexamethasone is given before the first dose of antibiotics, and when a third-generation cephalosporin is used. A recent large European trial in adults with meningitis showed reduction in mortality and severe morbidity with pneumococcal meningitis.[12] A recent Cochrane meta-analysis including adult and paediatric trials concluded that adjuvant steroids are beneficial for children with bacterial meningitis.[13] Evidence from animal studies shows that dexamethasone reduces penetration of vancomycin into infected cerebrospinal fluid.[14] Thus, there is concern that use of dexamethasone with vancomycin could compromise the efficacy of vancomycin in third-generation cephalosporin-resistant strains. Fortunately, the majority of cases of pneumococcal meningitis are still caused by strains that are susceptible to penicillin and third-generation cephalosporins.

Accordingly, children (> 4 weeks old) who are being treated for possible meningitis (who have not yet received parenteral antibiotics, or who have received their first dose less than one hour previously) should be given dexamethasone 0.25 mg kg^{-1} IV (maximum 10 mg) (followed by 0.25 mg kg^{-1} 6-hourly). Steroids should preferably be given 15–30 minutes before antibiotics, although antibiotic administration should not be delayed for more than 30 minutes.

Fluids

Careful management of fluid and electrolyte balance is important in the treatment of meningitis. Over or under hydration is associated with adverse outcomes. Many children have increased antidiuretic hormone secretion, and some will have dehydration due to vomiting, poor fluid intake or septic shock. Initial fluid resuscitation to treat shock should be given as required with isotonic saline. Thereafter, isotonic fluids should be given to maintain systemic blood pressure (and thereby cerebral blood flow). The optimal ongoing fluid requirement for children with meningitis is not clearly established. Previous guidelines have suggested the importance of fluid restriction. For example, in the non-shocked child with a normal serum sodium, initial maintenance fluids should be 50% of normal fluid requirements. If the serum sodium is less than 135 mmol L^{-1}, then further restriction may be required. However, more recent studies have questioned this approach.[18] Assessment of the clinical signs of hydration, including weight, measurement of the serum sodium, documentation of urine output, and clinical assessment of the neurological state should be monitored closely, and the total fluid intake adjusted accordingly.

PREVENTION

Contacts of patients with meningococcal meningitis may require chemoprophylaxis to prevent secondary spread. Those who should receive chemoprophylaxis include:

- The index case if treated only with penicillin (does not eradicate carriage)
- All intimate, household or day-care contacts who have been exposed to the index case within ten days of onset
- Any person who had mouth-to-mouth resuscitation or direct airway secretion contact with the index case.

Rifampicin 10 mg kg^{-1} (5 mg kg^{-1} less than 1 month old) PO 12-hourly (maximum 600 mg) for two days or
Ceftriaxone 125 mg ≤12 years old); 250 mg (> 12 years old) IM as a single dose or
Ciprofloxacin 500 mg PO as a single dose.

Conjugate serogroup C meningococcal vaccine is part of the routine schedule for all children from one year of age.

Conjugate seven-valent pneumococcal vaccine has the potential to prevent a considerable number of cases of childhood meningitis, and is now part of the routine schedule for vaccination in Australia.

COMPLICATIONS

Bacterial meningitis is associated with a 4.5% mortality rate, and intellectual, cognitive and auditory impairment in 10–20% of survivors.[15] The risk for sequelae is greatest in those who experience acute neurological complications at the time of their illness.[16]

Viral meningitis

Most cases are self-limiting, and treatment is symptomatic.

Brain abscess

Brain abscess classically presents with fever, headache and focal neurological deficit. Although rare, early recognition is vital as early antibiotic treatment and drainage improve outcome. Diagnosis is by cerebral CT scan or magnetic resonance imaging (MRI). Aspiration for diagnosis and neurosurgical intervention are usually required. The most common causes are oral viridans streptococci, anaerobes, Gram-negatives and *S. aureus*.

Empiric treatment is:

Flucloxacillin 50 mg kg^{-1} (maximum 2 g) IV 4-hourly *plus*
Cefotaxime 50 mg kg^{-1} (maximum 2 g) IV 6-hourly *plus*
Metronidazole 15 mg kg^{-1} (maximum 1 g) IV stat., then 7.5 mg kg^{-1} (maximum 500 mg) IV 8-hourly.

ENCEPHALITIS

AETIOLOGY

HSV is the most common cause of nonseasonal encephalitis in Australia. Other causes include enteroviruses, influenza virus, other herpes viruses and *Mycoplasma pneumoniae*. Several other viruses cause seasonal epidemics of encephalitis in specific geographic areas. Examples include Murray Valley encephalitis in the East Kimberley region, and Japanese B encephalitis in the Torres Strait Islands.

CLINICAL FINDINGS

There is considerable overlap between the features of meningitis and encephalitis, and the two frequently co-exist. Encephalitis should be considered if there is encephalopathy, that is, a change of behaviour, altered conscious state or extreme drowsiness. Convulsions (particularly focal) and focal neurological deficits are also more common in encephalitis.

INVESTIGATIONS

CSF biochemistry and microscopy findings are non-specific (see Table 8.7.1). PCR testing for HSV and enterovirus is sensitive and specific. Cerebral CT or MRI of the brain and EEG may be suggestive of HSV encephalitis, particularly if they show temporal lobe involvement.

MANAGEMENT

It is vital to consider the diagnosis of HSV encephalitis early, because treatment with aciclovir may improve the outcome. Treatment should be continued for 21 days unless HSV is excluded clinically or on subsequent investigations.

Aciclovir 20 mg kg^{-1} IV 8-hourly (age < 3 months); 500 mg m^{-2} IV 8-hourly (age 3 months to 12 years); 10 mg kg^{-1} IV 8-hourly (age > 12 years).

COMPLICATIONS

Without treatment, mortality of HSV encephalitis is up to 80%, and 50% of survivors have long-term sequelae.[17] Outcome is worse if coma is present initially.

CONCLUSION

Meningitis and encephalitis are medical emergencies that must be assessed and treated urgently to reduce the likelihood of poor outcomes.

REFERENCES

1. Australian Meningococcal Surveillance Programme 2003 Annual Report 2002. Communicable Diseases Intelligence 27: 196–208
2. Liu M, Andrews R, Stylianopoulos J, Ferreira C, Hogg G, Pyper N 2003 Invasive pneumococcal disease among children in Victoria. Communicable Diseases Intelligence 27: 362–366
3. Thomas KE, Hasbun R, Jekel J, Quagliarello VJ 2002 The diagnostic accuracy of Kernig's sign, Brudzinski's sign, and nuchal rigidity in adults with suspected meningitis. Clinical Infectious Diseases 35: 46–52
4. Cabral DA, Flodmark O, Farrell K, Speert DP 1987 Prospective study of computed tomography in acute bacterial meningitis. Journal of Paediatrics 111: 201–205
5. Rennick G, Shann F, de Campo J 1993 Cerebral herniation during bacterial meningitis in children. British Medical Journal 306: 953–955
6. Shetty AK, Desselle BC, Craver RD, Steele RW 1999 Fatal cerebral herniation after lumbar puncture in a patient with a normal computed tomography scan. Paediatrics 103: 1284–1286
7. Negrini B, Kelleher KJ, Wald ER 2000 Cerebrospinal fluid findings in aseptic versus bacterial meningitis. Paediatrics 105: 316–319
8. Mazor SS, McNulty JE, Roosevelt GE 2003 Interpretation of traumatic lumbar punctures: Who can go home? Paediatrics 111: 525–528
9. Shah KH, Richard KM, Nicholas S, Edlow JA 2003 Incidence of traumatic lumbar puncture. Academic Emergency Medicine 10: 151–154
10. Aronin SI, Peduzzi P, Quagliarello VJ 1998 Community-acquired bacterial meningitis: Risk stratification for adverse clinical outcome and effect of antibiotic timing. Annals International Medicine 129(11 Part 1): 862–869
11. McMaster P, McIntyre P, Gilmour R, Gilbert L, Kakakios A, Mellis C 2002 The emergence of resistant pneumococcal meningitis: Implications for empiric therapy. Archives of Diseases in Childhood 87(3): 207–210
12. de Gans J, van de Beek D 2002 The European Dexamethasone in Adulthood Bacterial Meningitis Study Investigators. Dexamethasone in adults with bacterial meningitis. New England Journal of Medicine 347(20): 1549–1556
13. van de BD, de Gans J, McIntyre P, Prasad K 2003 Corticosteroids in acute bacterial meningitis. Cochrane Database System Review 3: CD004305
14. Martinez-Lacasa J, Cabellos C, Martos A, Fernandez A, Tubau F, Viladrich PF et al 2002 Experimental study of the efficacy of vancomycin, rifampicin and dexamethasone in the therapy of pneumococcal meningitis. Journal of Antimicrobial Chemotherapy 49(3): 507–513
15. Baraff LJ, Lee SI, Schriger DL 1993 Outcomes of bacterial meningitis in children: A meta-analysis. Paediatric Infectious Diseases Journal 12: 389–394
16. Grimwood K, Anderson P, Anderson V, Tan L, Nolan T 2000 Twelve year outcomes following bacterial meningitis: Further evidence for persisting effects. Archives of Diseases in Childhood 83: 111–116
17. Whitley RJ, Lakeman F 1995 Herpes simplex virus infections of the central nervous system: Therapeutic and diagnostic considerations. Clinical Infectious Diseases 20: 414–420
18. Duke T, Mokela D, Frank D, Michael A, Paulo T, Mgone J, Kurubi J 2002 Management of meningitis in children with oral fluid restriction or intravenous fluid at maintenance volumes, a randomised trial. Annals of Tropical Paediatrics 22(2): 145–57

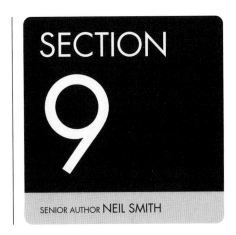

INFECTIOUS DISEASES

9.1 INFECTIOUS DISEASES

NEIL SMITH

PRACTICAL APPROACH TO THE FEBRILE CHILD

One of the most common daily problems faced by the emergency physician is the management of the febrile child. Among the diverse paediatric presentations of fever, it is important to identify which child is at risk of serious bacterial infection and know what the key markers are.

Of all children's visits to the emergency department (ED) 20–30% are with acute episodes of fever. In the first two years of life, children average four to six febrile episodes. In infants younger than three months of age, episodes of fever are less common, and an infant may present with an acute infection without mounting a fever response at all.

Measuring temperature

Temperature may be measured in a number of ways. The gold standard is rectal temperature, but parents and patients generally prefer axillary temperature assessments. The axillary temperature tends to be approximately 1°C less than rectal or central core temperature and is the measurement of choice in most paediatric departments. The use of devices such as tympanic thermometers and simple cutaneous thermometers are fraught with error and are not recommended.

A temperature of 38°C and above represents an abnormal temperature elevation or fever. The traditional teaching that normal body temperature is 37°C is too restrictive, as the upper limit of normal body temperature is currently defined as 37.7°C in adults and 37.9°C in children. Temperature also shows a diurnal variation of approx 1°C,[1] with the nadir occurring around 0600 h and peak temperature at 1800 h.

Pathophysiology of fever

Three pathophysiological mechanisms are important in managing febrile children.

First, the hypothalamic set-point in the central nervous system (CNS) is raised due to the action of endogenous cytokines released in response to various agents, most commonly viral or bacterial pathogens.[1,2] Less commonly, as in the setting of prolonged fever, the agents may be circulating immune complexes, as seen in autoimmune disease, or may be pyrogens, released by tumour cells. In such situations, antipyretics and the removal of excessive clothing may lower the fever.

Once reset, the thermoregulatory centre maintains a high body temperature through mechanisms such as cutaneous vasoconstriction, heat conservation or shivering thermogenesis.[2] Significantly, the infant's thermoregulatory response is less mature and hypothermia may occur with infection instead.

Second, fever can be due to heat production exceeding heat loss as occurs, for example, in salicylate overdose, hyperthyroidism, excessive environmental temperature and malignant hyperthermia. In such instances temperature elevations are usually above 41°C.[1]

Third, fever can be caused by defective heat-loss mechanisms, as seen in ectodermal dysplasia, heat stroke and poisoning with anticholinergic drugs. In the latter two settings, antipyretics are not effective.[3]

Vigilance is also required due to the possibility of a focal cerebral lesion affecting the function of the thermoregulatory centre, thereby causing an elevated body temperature. Lesions include CNS tumours as well as acute subdural haematomas. Therefore, look for clinical features consistent with physical abuse in the irritable infant with unexplained fever, particularly where family circumstances may raise suspicion of non-accidental injury.

Fever: to treat or not to treat?

The routine use of antipyretics in the treatment of fever has been questioned.[4] In particular, there has been concern that the use of antipyretics may prolong viral shedding and, hence, viral illness in children. In animal studies, the treatment of fever has also been shown to increase morbidity and mortality in a septic animal model.[5]

The arguments for treating fever include the following:

❶ Decreasing discomfort associated with fever often assists with settling an apprehensive child.

❷ Preventing extreme temperature elevations (>41°C) from causing permanent damage to the CNS.[2,5]

261

❸ Decreasing, in theory, the likelihood of fever-related seizures in those who have a history of seizures, even though no study to date has actually demonstrated that treatment of fever significantly decreases the incidence of recurrent febrile convulsions.

Arguments against lowering fever include:

❶ The generally recognised view that most fevers are short-lived and benign.

❷ Situations where adverse drug side effects of antipyretics outweigh the benefits of fever reduction.

❸ Situations where reducing fever may obscure diagnostic or prognostic signs, as in managing febrile neutropenic children who have recently received chemotherapy.

❹ Recent information, which suggests that fever may protect the host.[4]

It is important for the febrile child to receive adequate hydration, because the rate of fluid loss may be increased as the temperature rises. Maintenance of adequate intravascular volume also allows for better heat dissipation. Excessive clothing should be removed. Other non-pharmacological adjunctive measures, such as sponging with tepid water, are no longer recommended and may even result in an elevation of core body temperature.[3] In addition, placing a child in a cool bath adds the risk of an accidental immersion injury should the child suffer a febrile convulsion.

Aspirin, paracetamol and non-steroidal anti-inflammatory medications exert their antipyretic effects by blocking hypothalamic cyclo-oxygenase enzymes, thereby preventing the synthesis of prostaglandin E2 from arachidonic acid.[1] Because they do not suppress interleukin-2, these drugs do not diminish the proliferation of T-helper cells and, thus, do not adversely affect the body's ability to fight infection. Aspirin is not recommended for general use in children under twelve years of age due to association with Reye's syndrome, a rare form of fulminant hepatic failure, which occurs with concomitant viral infections.

General consensus amongst paediatric centres is that paracetamol is the antipyretic agent of choice. Current recommendations for the use of paracetamol include a dosage of 10–15 mg kg^{-1} per dose and an upper limit of 60 mg kg^{-1} per day, given in four- to six-hourly intervals. Serious toxicity has been reported in children with chronic daily over-dosage, mostly occurring in children who have a febrile illness and associated anorexia, vomiting and/or dehydration.[6]

The non-steroidal anti-inflammatory agent, ibuprofen can be used as an alternative to paracetamol, but only in children aged over six months, and only after four doses of paracetamol (as above) have been given. Recommendations are that it should only be used alone, not in combination with paracetamol, as this practice may lead to an increase in adverse effects, which include gastrointestinal bleeding, effects on renal function and anaphylaxis. A theoretical risk of aggravating concurrent asthma has also been described, although these adverse effects are refuted in large prospective studies.[7] The dose may vary from 5 to 10 mg kg^{-1} (up to a maximum of 500 mg per dose), given six- to eight-hourly, to a maximum of 40 mg kg^{-1} d^{-1} or 2 g d^{-1}. There is no evidence that alternating paracetamol and ibuprofen is any better at reducing fever or spares the potential hepatotoxicity related to paracetamol administration.[8]

The response to antipyretics should not be used as a clinical tool in the assessment of possible bacteraemia, which is primarily due to pneumococcal infection in children.[9] In one study, 88% of children who responded to a standard dose of paracetamol were ultimately found to have a bacteraemia.[10]

What needs to be detected in the febrile child?

The vast majority of febrile illnesses in infants and young children are due to viral infections, which are self-limiting and only require supportive therapy and expectant observation. The febrile child with no focus of infection raises the suspicion of occult bacteraemia and subsequent serious sequelae, such as bacterial meningitis or septic arthritis.

The emergency physician may take one of two approaches to the febrile child with the potential for occult bacterial infection:

❶ To minimise risk, or

❷ To minimise tests.

Risk-minimisers aim at lowering the risk of adverse sequelae from occult infections by using risk stratification to target higher-risk patient subsets for intervention in the ED. They believe that a structured, methodical and laboratory-intensive strategy minimises adverse sequelae from occult bacterial infection. Test-minimisers, on the other hand, take the greater risk of not detecting bacteraemia in such infants and children. They perform a careful clinical examination and ensure close follow-up, but do not treat with empirical antibiotics. Test-minimisers believe that the majority of children who develop serious bacterial illnesses will be identified through close follow-up and repeat ED visits.

Neither approach has been shown to be better than the other. In practice, emergency physicians often tailor their approach to suit the individual needs of the patient. Therefore, the approach chosen will depend on the patient population being treated in a particular ED and the reliability and availability of follow-up for that patient population.

A protocol that can be used for the well-appearing febrile infant is shown in Figure 9.1.1.[11]

Occult bacteraemia

Occult bacteraemia refers to a febrile illness where the infant or child does not have signs of serious illness nor a focus for fever, but has bacteria growing on blood culture. The incidence of occult bacteraemia in febrile children younger than 24 months of age is between 1.6 and 9.8%.[12,13] Occult bacteraemia is more prevalent in this group because of their difficulty in localising specific infection, due to poor opsonisation of foreign antigens by an immature immune system.[1]

Many bacteraemic children will appear well, despite being febrile. Clinical scores, such as the Rochester criteria (see Table 9.1.1), have been devised to identify children at low risk of serious bacterial

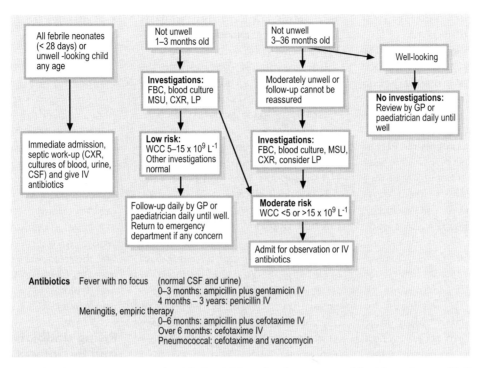

Fig. 9.1.1   Guidelines for the management of a febrile child under three years old without focus of infection. *Source*: Modified from Wentworth, South-Western & Western Area Health Services, May 2000.

Table 9.1.1   Rochester criteria
Infant appears generally well
Infant has been previously healthy
• Born at term
• Did not receive perinatal antimicrobials
• Was not treated for unexplained hyperbilirubinaemia
• Has not received antimicrobials
• Has not been previously hospitalised
• Has no chronic or underlying illness
• Was not hospitalised longer than mother
No evidence of skin, soft tissue, bone, joint, or ear infection
Laboratory values
• Peripheral WCC 5000–15 000
• Absolute band form count $\leq 1500 \ \mu L^{-1}$
• ≤ 10 WBC per high power field on microscopic urine examination
• ≤ 5 WBC per high power field on microscopic stool smear

(Modified from Jaskiewicz et al. Febrile infant Collaborative Group, as it appears in *Pediatrics* 1994)

infection.[14] However, in children younger than three months of age, the scores are unreliable, with sensitivity depending on the experience of the observer and ranging from 8 to 99%.[12,14] In children older than three months of age, the same scores only identified 30% of bacteraemic

children.[15,16] Thus, the clinician cannot rely on clinical acumen alone.

In the febrile child without an identifiable focus of infection, two additional markers can be used to identify the child at risk of bacteraemia:

❶ The height of the fever, and
❷ The total white cell count.

A peripheral white cell count (WCC) >15 000 mm^{-3} is highly indicative of bacteraemia in the highly febrile child, with sensitivities currently, in the post-*Haemophilus influenzae* type b era, reported between 79 and 86%.[13,16] Empiric antibiotic treatment of these children would result in the treatment of 19 non-bacteraemic children for each bacteraemic child treated. Lee and Harper[13] therefore suggest that empiric antibiotic treatment in children with fever > 39°C and a WCC of 18 000 mm^{-3} increases the specificity to 87%, thereby reducing the proportion of febrile children who receive antibiotics from 1 in 4 to 1 in 7. With increasing reports of antibiotic resistance, empiric antibiotic therapy for febrile children should be more restrictive.[11] A WCC of $\geq 20 000$ mm^{-3} has a higher specificity

for bacteraemia. When this higher WCC is used, fewer children will receive antibiotics with high rates of bacteraemia reported among those children treated. More importantly, significant missed bacteraemia was not identified when the higher WCC was used.

Therefore, in a child who is febrile without an identifiable cause, a full blood count and blood culture should be performed together with a screening urine examination. A prevalence rate between 4 and 7.5%,[17] makes urinary tract infection the most common serious bacterial illness among febrile infants and children (15–20% in infants < 3 months of age and 2–5% in boys 3 to 6 months and girls 3 to 12 months of age).[18] In infants, the latter requires culture of an appropriate specimen, ideally a sample obtained via urinary catheter or suprapubic aspiration. A negative urinalysis does not exclude a urinary tract infection, which may occur in the absence of pyuria.[17] A chest X-ray is often useful, even if pneumonia, in the absence of tachypnoea, is an unlikely diagnosis.

Having identified a child at risk of bacteraemia by this staged approach, the key decision is whether to treat empirically or not. The reported incidence of bacteraemia in children aged 3–36 months ranges from 2 to 12%.[11,13,14,16,18] Since the advent of *Haemophilus influenzae* vaccination, occult bacteraemia in Australia, as in the rest of the industrialised world, is essentially pneumococcal bacteraemia, which accounts for 92% of proven bacteraemia in febrile children aged 3 to 36 months.[19] Although 70–85% of these cases may resolve without treatment, between 3 and 6% risk developing pneumococcal meningitis without treatment.[12,13,16,20] The risk of developing meningitis is related to the causative organism, and is reputedly highest for *Neisseria meningitidis*, intermediate for *H. influenzae* type b, and lowest for *Streptococcus pneumoniae*.[21] Many of the bacteraemic children have persistently high fever with a long and protracted course, often taking a week for fever to resolve. In these cases, the selective use of antibiotics can be recommended, with significant improvement in the morbidity caused by fever and, concomitantly, a decrease in the risk of serious bacterial infection. It remains to be conclusively proven whether treatment with antibiotics prevents meningitis in well-looking bacteraemic children because some studies have shown no significant benefit,[13] and current estimates are that 500 children would require empiric antibiotic treatment to prevent one case of pneumococcal meningitis.[8,22]

Serious bacterial infection (SBI)

SBI includes meningitis, bacteraemia or septicaemia, urinary tract infection, pneumonia, bone and joint infection, skin and soft tissue infection and bacterial enteritis. Early consideration of which febrile infant is at risk of developing serious bacterial illness is important.

Because young children are less able to localise disease processes, they require special consideration. Factors that indicate a high risk for underlying serious disease include low birth weight or prematurity, previous frequent hospitalisation, developmental disability, poor nutrition, age < 4 weeks, rapid onset of symptoms,

social disadvantage, parental reliability problems, current antibiotic use, and prolonged febrile illness or chronic illness.[12,14]

The risk of SBI increases with the height of fever in children of all age groups, however SBI can occur when the child has low-grade fever or is afebrile. The risk of serious bacterial infection in febrile children who appear unwell, is higher the younger the child (8% age 4–8 weeks), and very high in neonates (13–25% age 0–4 weeks).[14] These infants will most likely require investigation, empirical antibiotic treatment and hospital admission.

A parental history of fever mandates careful observation, even if the infant on presentation is afebrile. Parental assessment of the wellbeing of the infant or child also deserves consideration. As in any presentation with fever, ask about a history of infectious contact and overseas travel.

Immunisation status is particularly important. The introduction of *H. influenzae* type b conjugate vaccine has been one of the greatest advances in the last decade in almost eradicating *H. influenzae* as a cause of serious bacterial infections, such as meningitis, epiglottitis, pneumonia, periorbital cellulitis and mastoiditis.[13] Emergency physicians may promote immunisation by using every consultation as an opportunity to check the infant or child's status and perform 'on-the-spot' immunisation where needed.

The 'toxic'-appearing infant is therefore at significant risk of serious bacterial illness until otherwise proven. One simple and very effective system, summarised by Hewson and Oberklaid,[23] that has proved useful in the ED, is the 'ABC, fluids-in, fluids-out' system. An infant with one or more of these symptoms or signs has a higher risk of serious illness and should be considered 'toxic' until proven otherwise:

- A – poor arousal, reduced alertness and reduced activity.
- B – breathing difficulty.
- C – poor perfusion.
- Fluids in – the frequency of feeding over the 24 h prior to presentation, < 50% of normal over 24 h prior to presentation, suggesting dehydration.

- Fluids out – significantly abnormal urine output of < 50% (fewer than four wet nappies) of usual output.

Obvious features on examination that strongly suggest a seriously ill infant include a purpuric rash, high-pitched scream, bulging fontanelle, biphasic stridor, linear burn or bruising, pallor, lethargy, decreased responsiveness, cool extremities, tachycardia, tachypnoea or irregular breathing, mottled skin and prolonged capillary return

Careful clinical examination may alternatively confirm an initial impression that the infant appears relatively well. It may also identify a focus of likely infection requiring targeted investigation and management. Clinical review is essential.

Rising antibiotic resistance and the impact of vaccination

Resistance of *Streptococcus pneumoniae* to antimicrobials has been described for decades, but changing levels of resistance (intermediate, MIC 0.12–1.0 μg mL^{-1}, and high, MIC > 1 μg mL^{-1}) to penicillin and erythromycin remains a rapidly emerging problem. With the advent of a new era of disease prevention using scientifically advanced recombinant vaccines, the prevalence of invasive disease due to common organisms is expected to be significantly altered in industrialised countries where these vaccines are easily available or form part of a national immunisation schedule. Recent laboratory surveillance data of invasive pneumococcal disease (IPD) in Australia, following the introduction of the 7-valent conjugate pneumococcal vaccine in late 2001 to high-risk paediatric groups including indigenous children, has shown a significant increase in the proportion of total isolates due to non-vaccine serotypes in vaccinated children.[24] A decrease in the number of episodes of IPD due to penicillin resistant isolates was also demonstrated. This stresses the importance of regular reviews of empiric treatment guidelines utilising continued local laboratory surveillance data.

Resistance is also increasingly reported to cephalosporins, which led to the addition of vancomycin in the treatment of suspected cases of pneumococcal bacterial meningitis. In addition, a recent meta-analysis[25] has shown that the use of corticosteroids in meningitis has the potential to decrease long-term sequelae, specifically nerve deafness due to *Pneumococcus* and *Haemophilus influenzae* type b infections. At The Children's Hospital Westmead, the recommended dose of dexamethasone is 0.4 mg kg^{-1} given twice daily for 48 hours.

Prolonged fever

Infants and children who have a fever persisting for more than 7–10 days, or a fever that appears to be occurring in a repetitive pattern, should be considered at risk of potentially serious underlying disease, but bearing in mind that viral illness still remains the most common cause of the fever. More extensive investigations are often required, such as erythrocyte sedimentation rate, C-reactive protein, repeat full blood count and film, blood cultures, specific viral and atypical mycobacterial cultures, and imaging, such as ultrasound, bone scan and, possibly, CT scan and echocardiography. Hospital admission may also be required.

Kawasaki disease is an important consideration in an infant or child presenting with prolonged fever, and is often under diagnosed. There is a degree of urgency in diagnosis because treatment, within the first ten days of fever, using high-dose intravenous γ-globulin and aspirin significantly reduces the risk of permanent coronary artery damage as occurs in up to 25% of untreated cases.[26]

EMPIRIC ANTIBIOTIC THERAPY

With the possible exception of bacterial meningitis, where Gram stain results are available to immediately guide therapy, the most appropriate antibiotic therapy in children must be based on epidemiological grounds. The most important factors determining the likely pathogens, which should be targeted by empiric therapy, are:

- Age
- Presumed focus of infection

- Presence of underlying disease or anatomical abnormality
- Whether the infection is hospital or community acquired.

In addition, the site of infection may have implications for the expected penetration of the antibiotic chosen (e.g. aminoglycosides do not penetrate into abscess cavities and are inactive in an anaerobic environment).

Resistance of bacteria to antibiotics can conveniently be divided into two categories:

❶ Intrinsic – resistance due to inherent properties of the organism or antibiotic, and

❷ Acquired – resistance gained by the organism either before or during therapy.

Important examples of intrinsic resistance (which affects 100% of organisms) include enterococci to cephalosporins, enteric Gram negatives to penicillin and flucloxacillin and anaerobes to aminoglycosides and quinolones. Important examples of increasing acquired resistance include *Staphylococcus aureus* (10–12%) and *Streptococcus pyogenes* (4–5%) to erythromycin, *Streptococcus pneumoniae* (20–30%) and *Escherichia coli* (15–20%) to cotrimoxazole and *Haemophilus influenzae* (15–20%) and *Streptococcus pneumoniae* (1–4%) to penicillin and amoxicillin.

The following are empiric intravenous antibiotic recommendations for children who have fever with no focus (including normal cerebrospinal fluid and urine microscopy) at The Children's Hospital Westmead (CHW).

At 0–3 months of age, ampicillin at 200 mg kg^{-1} d^{-1} in four divided doses and gentamicin at 7 mg kg^{-1} d^{-1} in one to three doses are recommended, specifically targeting Group B haemolytic streptococci, *E. coli* and less commonly *Listeria monocytogenes* infections. For infants aged 4 months to 4 years, benzylpenicillin at 120 mg kg^{-1} d^{-1} in four divided doses is used to cover likely streptococcal bacteraemia. In children over 4 years of age, benzylpenicillin at 120 mg kg^{-1} d^{-1} in four divided doses

and flucloxacillin at 200 mg kg^{-1} d^{-1} in four divided doses are recommended, as staphylococcal infections become more prevalent. The choice of antibiotics recommended above is according to policy guidelines at CHW and depends on local disease prevalence. Antibiotic choice should also be modified as appropriate, once relevant culture results become available.

COMMON VIRAL EXANTHEMA

Most frequently, the cause of fever in children is a viral illness. This usually occurs in a seasonal pattern – in Australia particularly the months of April through to September when there is an increase of acute infections in the community. Most of these are due to respiratory and gastrointestinal pathogens, such as respiratory syncytial virus and rotavirus, respectively. However, there is an important group of viral infections that the emergency physician needs to be familiar with that commonly present with fever and rash.

A rash or other cutaneous manifestation accompanies a large number of presentations for childhood infectious disease. An exanthema is an acute infectious disease accompanied by a rash. The most common childhood exanthemas are scarlet fever, measles, rubella, erythema infectiosum and roseola infantum. Rash and fever may be associated with other infectious agents including bacteria, e.g. meningococcal disease, a wide variety of viruses and even parasitic infection.. In addition, a rash and fever may also be associated with a wide variety of non-infectious processes.

Scarlet fever

This infection is common amongst children 3–12 years of age. The disease is transmitted by direct contact or respiratory droplets but is occasionally food-borne. It has a short incubation period of between two and four days. The illness is characterised by an abrupt onset of fever, vomiting and a sore throat, with abdominal pain, each of varying severity.

The typical rash develops within 12–48 hours after onset, and is a generalised confluent erythematous papular rash giving the skin a sandpaper-like texture. The forehead and cheeks are red, smooth and flushed, not involving the area around the mouth (circumoral pallor). Petechiae may coalesce in linear form, particularly in skin folds such as axillae and antecubital fossae, forming pathognomonic Pastia's lines. The tongue in scarlet fever is initially coated by a white fur, which after a few days is reddened by the projection of oedematous papillae through the coat. This white strawberry tongue looses its coating after four days, revealing a beefy red strawberry tongue. Resolution of the rash and other clinical manifestations usually occurs by the end of the first week, heralding a period of characteristic desquamation of skin. Desquamation progresses from face to trunk and finally to hands and feet after three to four weeks.[27]

Complications of scarlet fever may be early local upper respiratory tract disease, including cervical adenitis and otitis media, to later non-suppurative disease including acute glomerulonephritis and rheumatic fever. The causative organism, Group A-β-haemolytic *Streptococcus*, produces these clinical manifestations by an erythrogenic toxin. A ten-day course of penicillin is effective in eradication of the bacteria, but the addition of clindamycin is recommended to neutralise the effects of circulating toxin in severe infection.[28]

A throat swab for bacterial and viral culture forms the basis of investigations, but a positive result may reflect a carrier status and not necessarily invasive disease. The latter identification may be done by rapid antigen detection tests carried out on throat swabs. Elevation of anti-streptolysin O or anti-DNAse-B titres may aid diagnosis of previous streptococcal infection weeks later, but are not specific to different types of streptococcal infection.[29]

Measles

Measles is a highly infectious, acute viral illness, spread by respiratory droplets, which is characterised by fever, coryza, exudative conjunctivitis, cough and a pathognomonic buccal enanthem called Koplik's spots followed by a generalised, red maculopapular rash appearing on the fourth day of the disease. The average period from exposure to appearance of the rash, which spreads from head to feet, is 14 days, and ranges from 7 to 18 days. The infectious period is from one to two days before the onset of symptoms to four days after the appearance of the rash.

Immunisation to measles using a live attenuated measles vaccine has been well established since the early 1960s, with an uptake rate increasing steadily to over 95% with the introduction of the measles, mumps and rubella (MMR) vaccine in 1988.[30] Vaccination should be actively encouraged, given the potential complications due to measles infection of otitis media (2.5%), bronchopneumonia (4%), acute encephalitis (0.1% of cases, with a mortality rate of 10–15%) and late subacute sclerosing panencephalitis.[30] Immunisation to those with doubtful immunity to measles, given within 72 hours of exposure to measles may afford some protection, as immunity from the live attenuated vaccine appears to be more rapid than that from natural measles. Efficacy in household contacts is limited as spread can occur one to two days before symptoms and three to five days before the appearance of rash.

Normal human immunoglobulin (NIGH), given within seven days of exposure, can prevent or modify measles in non-immune persons, such as infant six to nine months of age or immunocompromised persons. The dose of NIGH is 0.25 mL kg^{-1} (0.5 mL kg^{-1} if immunosuppressed) up to a maximum of 15 mL, given intramuscularly. If there are contraindications to IM administration, immunoglobulin for IV administration can be given, in a dose of 0.4 mg kg^{-1}.[30]

Rubella (German measles)

Rubella is a mild acute infectious disease characterised by a two-to-three-day prodrome of malaise and upper respiratory tract symptoms, a three-day central, erythematous maculopapular rash and lymph node enlargement, particularly postauricular and suboccipitally. The rash, however, is not diagnostic of rubella as it can be caused by other viruses, including parvovirus and enteroviruses. It follows an incubation period of 14–21 days, and persons are infective from one week until four days after the onset of the rash. Immunity to rubella can only reliably be confirmed by serologic measurement of antibody titres.[27]

The disease itself has rare complications such as encephalitis and thrombocytopenia, but the risk to unborn foetuses of non-immune mothers exposed in the first trimester (especially 6–8 weeks gestation) of pregnancy is significant, resulting in severe developmental and structural damage in 90% of affected cases (so-called congenital rubella syndrome). The vaccine is contraindicated in pregnant women and post-exposure prophylaxis with immunoglobulin does not prevent infection in non-immune contacts.[30]

Erythema infectiosum

'Slapped cheek disease' or erythema infectiosum is caused by parvovirus B19, where a febrile illness with red, flushed cheeks and circumoral pallor, is followed by a maculopapular rash on the limbs that clears centrally, leaving a lacy pattern as it fades. The virus may precipitate a severe aplastic anaemic crisis in individuals with underlying haemolytic disease, such as hereditary spherocytosis, sickle cell anaemia and thalassaemia.

Roseola infantum (exanthem subitum, sixth disease)

Roseola infantum is caused by herpes virus type 6. It usually occurs in the first two years of life, affecting up to 30% of children. Presentation is with fever and no focus (at times a febrile convulsion), then, as the fever resolves after 3–5 days, a pink macular rash erupts, which rarely coalesces and fades within 1–2 days. Significantly, the affected infant remains alert and playful despite the significant pyrexia.

Enterovirus infection

Enterovirus infections may present in a variety of ways, including malaise and fever, often accompanied by a non-specific rash, as occurs in coxsackie B5 and echo 9. In classical hand-foot-and-mouth disease, due to coxsackie A16, vesicles occur in a typical distribution over the hands, feet and occasionally on the buttocks, with lesions in the anterior mouth often becoming painful ulcers.[27] Infections occur particularly through the summer and autumn and are usually self-limiting. The lesions may rarely become petechial, resembling that of meningococcal infection.

Varicella (chickenpox)

Varicella is typified by generalised vesicles, more predominant on the trunk than limbs, with scalp lesions a diagnostic feature. The incubation period for varicella is usually 14–16 days, but ranges from 10–21 days. Patients are most contagious for one to two days before the rash and while new lesions erupt, which can be up to five days or longer in immunocompromised patients. It is more severe in adults and can be potentially fatal in immunocompromised patients, with a mortality rate of 7–10% in the latter.[30] Cerebellitis, aseptic meningitis, transverse myelitis, thrombocytopenia and pneumonia may complicate the acute infection.

Most adults, including those with no history of chicken pox, are immune to varicella. Staff working in children's EDs who have no history of chicken pox should have serology to determine their immune status. Those that spent their childhood in tropical countries are more likely to be non-immune as adults. Non-immune staff with significant varicella exposure are candidates for consideration of varicella zoster immunoglobulin (VZIG) or early aciclovir treatment and should discuss this with an infectious disease specialist.

Children whom recently received systemic steroid therapy or who are currently immunosuppressed and with no history of chicken pox are eligible for VZIG prophylaxis following significant household or play contact of longer than one hour, or school contact with chicken pox. The parents should be warned that VZIG is only 70–80% effective, even if given within the recommended period of 96 hours. Each vial contains 1.25 mL (125 U). Give 125 U per 10 kg to a maximum of five vials.[30]

Papulovesicular acrolocated syndrome (Gianotti–Crosti syndrome)

Papulovesicular acrolocated syndrome (PALS) is an exanthem in which papular (and often vesicular) lesions are located on acral parts of limbs and occasionally the face, and may take up to ten weeks to resolve. In Australia it also commonly occurs secondary to infection by enteroviruses, particularly rotavirus, in the 2–4 year age group.[31]

COMMONLY MISSED INFECTIONS IN CHILDHOOD

Hepatitis A

Hepatitis A has an average incubation period of 28 days (15–50 days), with maximum infectivity in the two weeks prior to the onset of jaundice, and continues for up to one week after onset. This most common cause of viral hepatitis is spread by the faecal-oral route and is common in areas with poor socio-economic living conditions. ED staff should not be exposed to Hepatitis A if normal hand-washing procedures are followed. Normal human immunoglobulin, in a dose of 0.02 mL kg^{-1} is indicated for household or other close contacts of a confirmed case, and should be given within two weeks of exposure.[30]

Meningococcal disease

Neisseria meningitidis is a common cause of bacterial meningitis, but may present as a non-specific flu-like illness, which may rapidly progress to overwhelming sepsis in previously healthy young people. Suspected infection should be promptly treated with parenteral benzylpenicillin, preferably after relevant blood cultures and serum for meningococcal PCR analysis have been taken. Patients who are shocked, have raised intracranial pressure or both, should receive immediate IV ceftriaxone and fluid resuscitation,[32] which clinically may be those who are irritable, lethargic or with decreased peripheral perfusion suggesting significant bacterial sepsis.[33]

The incubation period for meningococcal disease is usually thought to be less than four days, so prophylaxis of close contacts, if indicated, should be given as rapidly as possible and will often be based on a clinical diagnosis before laboratory confirmation.

Prophylaxis is indicated for household and child-care contacts (if contact with the patient's oral secretions is likely) of a case. Medical and nursing staff do not require prophylaxis unless they have had close exposure (mouth to mouth resuscitation, intubation or suctioning). Rifampicin is most commonly used in a dose of 10 mg kg^{-1} (to a maximum of 600 mg) given twice daily for two days. Effective alternatives include a single IM dose of ceftriaxone (125 mg < 12 years of age, 250 mg if older) or an oral dose of ciprofloxacin (500 mg for adults).[30]

Pertussis

The typical incubation period for pertussis is 7–10 days, with a range of 6–20 days. Infection is highly contagious, which is maximal before the onset of characteristic whooping cough and persists for up to three weeks thereafter. Recommended chemoprophylaxis for all household and other close contacts is erythromycin (50 mg kg^{-1} d^{-1}, four doses) given orally for 14 days, regardless of immunisation status, as immunity from immunisation does not necessarily prevent infection and transmission, even though symptoms may be minimal or absent.[27] Patients are considered infectious until after five days of appropriate treatment. Immunisation appropriate for age should be ensured in child contacts less than eight years and those unvaccinated should be vaccinated with DTPa-containing vaccines.[30]

WHAT SPECIMENS AND WHEN SHOULD THEY BE ORDERED

Targeted and judicious use of laboratory investigations facilitates more rapid and accurate diagnoses of causes of infection in children presenting to the ED. In this section, general infectious disease issues, including the appropriate collection of microbiological specimens, guidelines for empiric antibiotic therapy, post-exposure prophylaxis and immunisation are addressed.

What specimens and tests are appropriate?

As alluded to earlier in this chapter, children with fever with unknown focus (FUF) are at greater risk of overwhelming systemic bacterial infection the younger they are. Generally, under 36 months children present with symptoms that localise disease less well, and this has led to the approach of the 'septic screen', which consists of a full blood count, blood urine and CSF cultures and a chest X-ray. The published protocol already mentioned may serve as a guide in selecting the appropriate tests.[11] In general, young infants < 3 months of age with FUF require a complete septic screen followed by empiric antibiotic treatment to facilitate early diagnosis, and effective and preventative treatment of potentially life-threatening bacterial infections. The age group between 3 and 36 months pose a diagnostic dilemma, but clinical acumen and objective interpretation of management guidelines should guide the choice of investigations.

Collection of microbiological specimens

It is imperative that microbiological specimens be collected appropriately, taking care not to contaminate samples during collection. Samples should also be transported to the laboratory expeditely, stored in appropriate laboratory environments and processed without undue delay.

Blood cultures
Collection

Proper hand washing technique and use of sterile gloves will avoid contamination of the sample. Peripheral blood cultures are usually collected from veins, either direct puncture or immediately aspirated from a cannula after insertion. Arterial samples may also be used, but heel prick samples are inappropriate. It is imperative to disinfect the patient site for blood collection, usually with topical aqueous chlorhexidine or large alcohol swabs and to allow the disinfecting agent to dry, which is an important part of the dis-

infection process. Swab the rubber bung on the bottle with an alcohol swab and allow drying time before introducing blood into the bottle. Blood for cultures should be collected first, before placing blood into other, non-sterile bottles for additional investigations. Avoiding needle changes to inoculate the culture bottle minimises the risk of an accidental needle stick injury.

Volume of blood and collection media

It is important to remember that the minimum amount of blood must be collected and more than the maximum amount of blood will decrease the sensitivity of the culture and thus the likelihood of identifying a microorganism. The optimum blood-to-culture broth dilution is 1:10 in most blood culture systems, and up to 5 mL of blood can be inoculated into older systems, but from 0.4 mL to 4 mL in newer collection media. Samples for anaerobic bacterial cultures are not routinely collected, with few exceptions:

- Febrile neutropenic, immunocompromised patients
- Patients with suspected intra-abdominal or pelvic sepsis
- Neonates with a high risk of anaerobic sepsis, i.e. those with prolonged rupture of membranes, offensive liquor, or maternal fever in labour.

Blood culture bottles should be correctly labelled, and optimally stored in an appropriate incubator, never in a fridge.

Interpretation

Despite appropriate collection methods, difficulties in venipuncture of young children lead to a higher rate of contamination of blood cultures with skin flora than adults, typically 5–10%. Certain organisms are always significant when isolated from blood cultures, such as *Streptococcus pneumoniae*, *Haemophilus influenzae*, *Neisseria meningitidis*, *Salmonella* spp. and *Bacteroides*. The most common contaminant organisms are Gram positive, predominantly coagulase-negative *Staphylococcus* but also *Corynebacterium* and

Bacillus spp. In immunocompetent children with community-acquired infections, these organisms can often be assumed to be non-significant. Pathogenic organisms are usually identified rapidly from blood cultures – 70% within 24 hours and 86% within 48 hours. Some potentially pathogenic organisms, such as *Haemophilus* or *Meningococcus* species, may grow more slowly.

If a child who has been discharged subsequently has a possible pathogen isolated from a blood culture, he or she should be reassessed promptly and the blood culture repeated. The pathogenic organism, which is most commonly identified in out-patients, is *Streptococcus pneumoniae* in children < 2 years of age.

Cerebrospinal fluid (CSF)

See also Chapter 23 on common procedures.

Interpretation

Typical CSF findings Characteristic features of meningitis on CSF examination may include a raised opening pressure, cloudy appearance, raised WCC with a polymorph predominance, low glucose ($<\frac{1}{3}$ of serum glucose), raised protein and the presence of organisms on Gram stain and subsequent culture. Typical CSF findings are shown in Figure 9.1.2. CSF WCC values may be low early on in bacterial infection and, conversely, polymorphs may predominate in early viral meningitis. Culture should be performed on all CSF samples. It has a high sensitivity of 70 to 85%, which falls below 50% in children treated with antibiotics prior to obtaining the sample.[27] The Gram stain remains the most important initial test on CSF and is more sensitive (up to 80%) at detecting bacterial meningitis than are bacterial antigen (capsular polysaccharides) tests.[34]

Red cells in the CSF Red blood cells (RBCs) may be present in the CSF because of a traumatic tap, certain infections (classically herpes simplex virus and *Meningococcus*), or subarachnoid bleeding. If the CSF is blood-stained, collecting small volumes in successive tubes may show clearing of blood, indicative of a

Table 9.1.2   Pattern of CSF laboratory findings suggestive of normal values, bacterial meningitis, partially-treated meningitis, viral meningitis and tuberculous (TB) meningitis

Laboratory values	Normal neonatal values	Normal values for older children	Acute bacterial meningitis	Partially treated meningitis	Acute viral meningitis (aseptic meningitis)	TB meningitis
Organisms seen on Gram stain	–	–	Usually seen	Sometimes seen	Not seen	Not seen
Cell count ($\times 10^6$ L^{-1}) • Total	0–25 (combined polymorphs & lymphocytes)	–	–	–	–	50–500
• Polymorphonuclear	0–5*		May be 1000s	10s–100s	May predominate early	May predominate early
• Lymphocyte	0–20	0–5	Occasionally seen	Lymphocytes commonly seen	100s	100s; predominant late
Protein (g L^{-1})	< 1.0 (full term) < 1.5 (premature)	0.15–0.3	Increased	Normal or increased	Normal (may be decreased in herpes simplex or mumps paramyxovirus infection)	Markedly increased
Glucose (mmol L^{-1})	> 2.5	> 2.5	Significantly decreased (< 60% of blood glucose)	Normal or decreased	Normal or increased	May be normal early Decreased late

*Proportion of polymorphs: lymphocytes should not exceed 10%.

traumatic tap. If the haematological parameters are normal, then the CSF WCC, prior to the addition of blood, can be calculated in the following way (all units in cells mm^{-3} or $\times 10^6$ L^{-1}):

Actual CSF WCC

$$= \text{Total CSF WCC} - \frac{\text{Total CSF RCC}}{700}$$

CSF antigen testing   Testing for capsular polysaccharide antigens of *Neisseria meningitidis* (Groups A and C), *Streptococcus pneumoniae*, Group B streptococci (GBS), e.g. *Streptococcus agalactiae*, *Haemophilus influenzae* type b (Hib), and *Escherichia coli*, in CSF and urine is available. It is recommended for use in facilitating the more rapid diagnosis of CSF infections and can be used to guide duration of antibiotic therapy, when:

• Negative results are present on Gram stain and CSF and blood cultures, yet CNS involvement cannot be ruled out clinically
• CSF was obtained > 24 hours after receiving IV antibiotics.[34]

As these antigen tests are most sensitive for detection of *H. influenzae* antigens while

ranging from 3 to 50% for *Neisseria meningitidis*,[35] their value in the post-*H. influenzae* era has been questioned.

Urine latex-agglutination tests for *Neisseria meningitidis/E. coli* have also been shown to have a positive predictive value too low to be clinically useful.[35] A negative test result using these tests cannot exclude the diagnosis of bacterial meningitis either.

Urine examination

A sterile urine sample enables a more accurate diagnosis of urinary tract infection (UTI) and as such the method of collection significantly influences the accuracy of the microscopic results obtained. If UTIs are over-diagnosed, other important diagnoses may be missed and the child may then be subjected to unnecessary investigations for the alleged UTI. A negative urinalysis does not exclude a UTI, and 16% are missed, if the final diagnosis is based on the urinalysis. The presence of white or red blood cells or protein does not either confirm or refute the diagnosis. All urine specimens should be sent for microscopy and culture if a UTI suspected, or if obtained via catheter/suprapubic aspirate in non-toilet-trained

children. The laboratory should always be informed of the collection method as this influences the interpretation of results.

Bag urines
A *negative* bag urinalysis may exclude a UTI, and can be used as a screen for UTIs. However, a bag urine is unlikely to be a sterile specimen, even if optimal collection by prior cleaning, and removal of bag as soon as specimen passed is performed.

Clean catch and mid-steam collection
Are both non-invasive and contamination is less likely, but they should only be used in children who are toilet trained. The 'best-catch' possible is obtained on boys with the foreskin retracted, and on girls with the labia spread continuously after cleansing with soap and water and gentle drying. The patient or parent should avoid touching skin and the specimen should be collected in mid-stream.

Catheterisation
Quick 'in-out' urinary catheterisation is a very reliable collection method and does not require the bladder to be filled. It is very unlikely that infection can be

introduced with an in-out procedure that is done with sterile technique. Only mild discomfort is usually experienced. Catheterisation should not be attempted in girls with significant labial adhesion, nor in boys with phimosis that prevents vision of the urethral meatus. We also recommend avoiding the use of feeding tubes, as they are too flexible and can become knotted, which would require subsequent laparotomy for removal.

For *female infants*, while an assistant holds the legs apart and straightened, gently clean the skin, perineum, and periurethral area. Apply a fenestrated drape for a sterile area, put finger and thumb on either side of the labia and apply gentle downward traction to visualise the urethral meatus. Insert a lubricated size 5 urinary catheter gently up to 5 cm into the urethra. Allow the first few drops to drain, then collect the sample in a sterile jar, and remove the catheter.

Clean the pubic area of *male infants* with their legs held apart, followed by gently retracting the foreskin to visualise the urethral meatus and clean it. Holding the penile shaft at 90° to the abdomen, insert a lubricated size 5 urinary catheter about 6 cm if under one year and 6–8 cm into the urethra if older than one year. Some resistance may be encountered at the prostatic area. Allow the first few drops to drain, then collect the specimen in a sterile jar and remove the catheter. A syringe is not needed to aspirate, as the urine usually drains freely.

Suprapubic aspiration

This too, allows the collection of a sterile specimen, but the infant usually needs to have full bladder. Therefore, give a drink about 20–30 minutes prior (or after a 'dry' tap) and try to percuss a full bladder before commencing the procedure. Ultrasound assistance is very useful if available. Clean the skin with an alcohol swab or aqueous chlorhexidine and allow it to dry. Then insert a 23-gauge needle and syringe about 1 cm above the pubic symphysis at 90° (roughly at the level of the skin creases, aspirating gently while the needle advances. Urine will fill the syringe easily if the bladder is successfully located. Remove the needle and cover the

site with a Band-Aid™. Any growth on a culture of suprapubic aspirate is significant. Bladder tap is contraindicated in children thought to be anuric, or those with abdominal distension due to gastrointestinal disease.

Interpretation

Reagent-impregnated dipstick A dipstick urinalysis can be used to detect the presence of nitrite-forming bacteria or estimate the presence of pyuria using a leucocyte esterase test strip, thereby allowing a quick presumptive diagnosis of a UTI and early treatment in an unwell child. Blood, protein and ketones can also be detected. The poor sensitivity for nitrites (40%) and pyuria (70%), however, means that a high false negative rate (of 50% and 20% respectively) for detection of true infection by this method exists.[36] Non-nitrite-forming bacteria such as *Enterococcus* spp. may also cause UTIs, and pyuria is not always present in UTIs, which makes a negative urinalysis less likely to exclude a UTI.

Microscopy A urinary white cell count $> 10 \times 10^6$ L^{-1} together with a positive leucocyte esterase is a very sensitive screening test for UTIs, but still has a false negative rate of 15%.[36] The presence of > 10 leucocytes mm^{-3} on direct microscopy has been shown to have a low positive predictive value (56%) for UTI but, combined with the presence of bacteria, this constitutes the most accurate screening test in detecting positive urinary cultures.[17]

Culture UTI is ultimately diagnosed on demonstration of significant bacteriuria, which implies counts of $> 10^8$ L^{-1} of a single pathogen in a fresh, uncentrifuged clean catch or mid-stream urine sample. Any growth on a sample obtained by urinary catheter or suprapubic aspirate is also diagnostic. The interpretation of urine culture results varies between laboratories and the method of collection used. *E. coli* remains the most common pathogen isolated in children under five years (84% in a recent Australian study), followed by *Proteus* spp. (6.6%), *Klebsiella* spp. (4.7%) and *Enterococcus faecalis* (3.4%).[36]

Stool specimens

Viral gastroenteritis is the most common cause of paediatric hospital attendance during the spring and early summer months. The organism involved is usually rotavirus, which is usually self-limiting and is readily detected by enzyme-linked immunoassay or latex agglutination. Laboratory analysis is usually not warranted during seasonal endemic periods as most causes of diarrhoea are usually self-limiting and identification will not alter management in most cases. Indications for stool analysis are:

- Chronic diarrhoea > 5 days
- Blood in stool
- Recent overseas travel to typhoid endemic areas
- Immunocompromised children.

Collection

Diarrhoeal stool (5–10 g) should be collected in a sterile container with a secure fitting lid. Testing the stool pH using a reagent strip may be a useful indicator for rotavirus gastroenteritis as it causes an acidic stool (pH < 5). Similarly, testing stool for reducing substances would be positive in cases of secondary lactose intolerance.

Interpretation

Children who are admitted for dehydration treatment are nursed applying universal infection precautions. Some causes of bacterial gastroenteritis, e.g. *Salmonella* spp. are notifiable to Public Health Authorities.

Throat swab

Throat swabs may be performed both for bacterial and viral culture, although for the latter a nasopharyngeal aspirate or nasal wash is usually more helpful.

Collection

Use a bright light to illuminate the oropharynx and depress the tongue with a spatula. Rub the tonsillar areas, posterior pharynx and any purulent exudate firmly with a sterile swab. Viral throat swabs are performed separately using a cotton swab, which is placed in viral culture medium.

Interpretation

Group A *Streptococcus* (GAS) is the commonest cause of bacterial tonsillitis, although Groups C and G streptococci may rarely be implicated. The problem clinically is to distinguish colonisation with GAS, which may be long-term, from infection. Repeated isolation of GAS from the throat swab may indicate colonisation rather than treatment failure. Age (over five years) and the presence of tender cervical adenopathy are the most helpful clinical indicators of GAS infection, but are insensitive. The great majority of children younger than three years will have viral pharyngitis unless they are household contacts of an older GAS infected child.

Nasopharyngeal aspirate (NPA)

NPA is the preferred method for recovering viruses from the upper respiratory tract. This is helpful in children with the clinical syndrome of bronchiolitis, both for a specific diagnosis and to facilitate infection control procedures. Nasal lavage is an alternative to NPA, but swabs of the nose and throat have a lower yield.

Collection

An 8FG suction catheter, with a mucus extractor built into the circuit, is passed into posterior nasopharynx and secretions are aspirated. The suction catheter and sputum trap are sent together to the laboratory. Nasal lavage is performed by gently instilling 2 mL of phosphate buffered saline at room temperature into each nostril. This is simultaneously suctioned from the anterior nares into a standard mucus extractor. Specimens sent for virology or pertussis culture should not be placed on ice and transported to the laboratory immediately.

Interpretation

Most respiratory viruses can be detected by direct immunofluorescence of exfoliated respiratory epithelium, as viral antigens are expressed on the cell surface. If available, this allows rapid diagnosis of infection. Viruses can also be cultured. The positive and negative predictive values of both NPA and nasal lavage in diagnosing RSV infection are over 90%.

Bordetella pertussis may be identified by serum PCR if a definitive diagnosis is required before culture results of NPA are available.

Pernasal swab

A pernasal swab is the classic method for collection of diagnostic specimens for diagnosis of pertussis. However, a nasopharyngeal aspirate is also satisfactory. The crucial need is for prompt transport to the laboratory.

Collection

A small-tipped nasopharyngeal swab is passed into the posterior nasopharynx. Do not use a swab with a cotton tip as this may be inhibitory to the organism. The swab is left in place for at least 30 seconds, if possible.

INFECTION CONTROL IN THE ED

Adhering to strict universal precautions (i.e. treating all blood and body fluids as potentially infectious) is an integral part of containing the spread of infections in any healthcare setting. Nowhere more so than in paediatric EDs, where communicable viral respiratory and enteric infections are the most common causes of presentations. Cross-infection can be eliminated by strict hand-washing measures by both staff and parents, as well as avoiding toy sharing by patients in ward situations. Prophylaxis with human immunoglobulin following significant exposure to communicable diseases, such as hepatitis A and B, measles and varicella, is easily available, as well as rifampicin prophylaxis for significant exposure to meningococcal and Hib disease.

NEEDLE STICK INJURY (NSI)

The child presenting with a needle stick injury

Intravenous drug abuse in major metropolitan areas will always pose a risk of accidental needle stick injuries, to the general population and children in par-

ticular, from needles recklessly discarded in parks or on beaches. A child presenting to the ED after an NSI is therefore not too infrequent an occurrence. The main concern arises about the risk of transmission of parenteral infections like hepatitis B and C and HIV. As the prevalence of all three infections is very low in Australia, and highest for hepatitis C, for which no prophylaxis exists, treatment of accidental NSI in children remains unclear. Hepatitis C is most common in IV drug abusers, among whom the incidence in Australia is estimated at 80%, with a 65 to 80% chance of infectivity should blood be positive for anti-Hep C antibodies.[37] However, like HIV, hepatitis C very rapidly loses its potency in environmental conditions, whereas hepatitis B virus may remain potentially viable for an undefined period. Prophylaxis after accidental NSIs in children and adults is therefore targeted towards hepatitis B, for which effective active and passive immunoprophylaxis exists. Due to the usually small amount of potentially infective inoculate in discarded syringes, hepatitis B immunoglobulin is rarely offered to the child following an NSI. Instead the best option may be accelerated hepatitis B immunisation, given at 0.1 and 2 months. This would be expected to be effective, as hepatitis B viral replication does not occur for 4–6 weeks, in the unlikely event that the offending needle had contained sufficient infectious material to cause infection.

After obtaining informed parental consent, serologic testing of the recipient for hepatitis B and C and HIV is recommended immediately following the NSI, and at six weeks, three and six months after the exposure for HIV and hepatitis C in particular.

Hospital staff exposure to hepatitis B

In general, NSIs occur more often in the hospital environment, where a lack of universal precautions in handling or discarding contaminated needles or sharps have occurred. It is advisable that all staff working in the hospital environment should be adequately immunised against hepatitis B and that serological confirmation of immunity is performed. If significant exposure (percutaneous, ocular, or mucous membrane) to blood or potentially blood-contaminated secretions has occurred in persons who are unimmunised, testing of the source should be done as well as the recipient. A single dose of hepatitis B immunoglobulin (HBIG 400 IU for adults and 100 IU for children) is then offered to the recipient who is HBs-negative, or the source is HBsAg positive or cannot be identified.[30] This should be given within 72 hours after exposure.

IMMUNISATION

Immunisation of staff

It is in the best interests of all healthcare workers, and their patients, that staff in paediatric centres have a serologically proven immunisation record against communicable illnesses such as measles, mumps and rubella and hepatitis B, and receive the relevant immunisation as appropriate.

Opportunistic immunisation

The ED visit also presents an invaluable opportunity to monitor the immunisation status of children and offer 'catch-up' immunisation to those who have missed vaccinations or commence the appropriate vaccination schedule. The current NH&MRC immunisation schedule is available in the Australian Immunisation Handbook.[30] (See also Table 1.1.8).

REFERENCES

1. Powell KR 2000 Infectious diseases. In: Behrman RE, Kliegman RM, Jenson HB (eds), Nelson textbook of pediatrics. WB Saunders, Philadelphia
2. Saper CB, Breder CD 1994 The neurologic basis of fever. New England Journal of Medicine 330(26): 1880–1886 [comment; review; 61 refs]
3. Meremikwu M, Oyo-Ita A 2003 Cochrane Database of Systematic Reviews 3
4. Kramer MS, Naimark LE, Roberts-Brauer R, McDougall A, Leduc DG 1991 Risks and benefits of paracetamol antipyresis in young children with fever of presumed viral origin. Lancet 337(8741): 591–594 [comment]
5. Mackowiak PA, Boulant JA 1996 Fever's glass ceiling. Clinical Infectious Diseases 22(3): 525–536 [review; 147 refs]
6. Riordan M, Rylance G, Berry K 2002 Poisoning in children 2: painkillers. Archives of Diseases in Childhood 87(5): 397–399
7. Lesko SM 2003 The safety of ibuprofen suspension in children. International Journal of Clinical Practice 135(Suppl): 50–53 [review; 3 refs]
8. Fleisher GR, Rosenberg N, Vinci R, Steinberg J, Powell K, Christy C et al 1994 Intramuscular versus oral antibiotic therapy for the prevention of meningitis and other bacterial sequelae in young, febrile children at risk for occult bacteremia. Journal of Pediatrics 124(4): 504–512 [comment]
9. Alpern ER, Henretig FM 2000 Fever. In: Fleisher GR, Ludwig S (eds), Textbook of paediatric emergency medicine. Lippincott Williams & Wilkins, Philadelphia
10. Yamamoto LT, Wigder HN, Fligner DJ, Rauen M, Dershewitz RA 1997 Relationship of bacteremia to antipyretic therapy in febrile children. Pediatric Emergency Care 3(4): 223–227
11. Browne GJ, Ryan JM, McIntyre P 1997 Evaluation of a protocol for selective empiric treatment of fever without localising signs. Archives of Disease in Childhood 76(2): 129–133
12. Baraff LJ, Bass JW, Fleisher GR, Klein JO, McCracken GH Jr, Powell KR et al 1993 Practice guideline for the management of infants and children 0 to 36 months of age with fever without source. Pediatrics 92(1): 1–12
13. Lee GM, Harper MB 1998 Risk of bacteremia for febrile young children in the post-*Haemophilus influenzae* type b era. Archives of Pediatrics & Adolescent Medicine 152(7): 624–628 [comment]
14. Jaskiewicz JA, McCarthy CA, Richardson AC, White KC, Fisher DJ, Dagan R et al 1994 Febrile infants at low risk for serious bacterial infection—an appraisal of the Rochester criteria and implications for management. Febrile Infant Collaborative Study Group. Pediatrics 94(3): 390–396
15. Teach SJ, Fleisher GR 1995 Efficacy of an observation scale in detecting bacteremia in febrile children three to thirty-six months of age, treated as outpatients. Occult Bacteremia Study Group. Journal of Pediatrics 126(6): 877–881 [comment]
16. Kuppermann N, Fleisher GR, Jaffe DM 1998 Predictors of occult pneumococcal bacteremia in young febrile children. Annals of Emergency Medicine 31(6): 679–687
17. Hoberman A, Wald ER, Reynolds EA, Penchansky L, Charron M 1994 Pyuria and bacteriuria in urine specimens obtained by catheter from young children with fever. Journal of Pediatrics 124(4): 513–519 [comment]
18. Baraff LJ, Schriger DL, Bass JW, Fleisher GR, Klein JO, McCracken GH Jr et al 1997 Management of the young febrile child. Commentary on practice guidelines. Pediatrics 100(1): 134–136
19. McIntyre PB, Chey T, Smith WT 1995 The impact of vaccination against invasive *Haemophilus influenzae* type b disease in the Sydney region. Medical Journal of Australia 162(5): 245–248
20. Dershewitz RA, Wigder HN, Wigder CM, Nadelman DH 1983 A comparative study of the prevalence, outcome, and prediction of bacteremia in children. Journal of Pediatrics 103(3): 352–358
21. Shapiro ED, Aaron NH, Wald ER, Chiponis D 1986 Risk factors for development of bacterial meningitis among children with occult bacteremia. Journal of Pediatrics 109(1): 15–19
22. Kramer MS, Shapiro ED 1997 Management of the young febrile child: A commentary on recent practice guidelines. Pediatrics 100(1): 128–134
23. Hewson P, Oberklaid F 1994 Recognition of serious illness in infants. Modern Medicine of Australia July: 89
24. Watson M, Bayley K, Bell JM, Gilbert G, Hogg G, Keil AD et al 2003 Laboratory surveillance of invasive pneumococcal disease in Australia in 2001 to 2002 – implications for vaccine serotype coverage. Communicable Diseases Intelligence 27: 478–487
25. van de Beek D, de Gans J, McIntyre P, Prasad K 2003 Corticosteroids in acute bacterial meningitis. Cochrane Database of Systematic Reviews 3: CD004305
26. Burns JC 2001 Kawasaki disease. Advances in pediatrics 48: 157–177
27. Gershon AA, Hotez PJ, Katz S 2004 Krugman's infectious diseases of children, 11th edn. Mosby, Philadelphia
28. Zimbelman J, Palmer A, Todd J 1999 Improved outcome of clindamycin compared with β-lactam antibiotic treatment for invasive *Streptococcus pyogenes* infection. Pediatric Infectious Diseases Journal 18(12): 1096–1100
29. Bell F, Finn A 1996 Exanthemata. In: Isaacs D, Moxon E (eds), A practical approach to pediatric infections. Churchill Livingstone, Edinburgh, 371
30. Australian Technical Advisory Group on Immunisation 2003 The Australian immunisation handbook, 7th edn. Canberra, Australia
31. Rogers M 1996 Non-specific patterns of viral exanthem. In: Isaacs D, Moxon E (eds), A practical approach to pediatric infections. Churchill Livingstone, Edinburgh
32. Welch SB, Nadel S 2003 Treatment of meningococcal infection. Archives of Diseases in Childhood 88(7): 608–614
33. Brogan PA, Raffles A 2000 Short report. The management of fever and petechiae: Making sense of rash decisions. Archives of Diseases in Childhood 83(6): 506–507
34. Maxson S, Lewno MJ, Schutze GE 1994 Clinical usefulness of cerebrospinal fluid bacterial antigen studies. Journal of Pediatrics 125(2): 235–238 [comment]
35. Boyer D, Gordon RC, Baker T 1993 Lack of clinical usefulness of a positive latex agglutination test for *Neisseria meningitidis/Escherichia coli* antigens in the urine. Pediatric Infectious Disease Journal 12(9): 779–780
36. Craig JC, Irwig LM, Knight JF, Sureshkumar P, Roy LP 1998 Symptomatic urinary tract infection in preschool Australian children. Journal of Paediatrics & Child Health 34(2): 154–159
37. New South Wales Health Department 1997 Blood-borne infections – management of healthcare workers potentially exposed to HIV, hepatitis B and hepatitis C. Circular 97/12. New South Wales Healthnet, Australia [electronic citation]

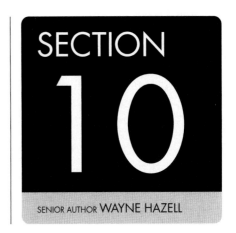

SECTION

10

SENIOR AUTHOR WAYNE HAZELL

ENDOCRINE AND METABOLIC

10.1 METABOLIC EMERGENCIES

PETER FRANCIS

Essentials

1 Inborn errors of metabolism are individually rare but as a group are not uncommon.

2 The possibility of an inborn error of metabolism needs to be considered in any child with unexplained hypoglycaemia, acidosis, altered conscious state, neurological presentation or vomiting.

3 Prompt recognition is important to allow appropriate therapy and to avoid decompensation.

4 Precise identification of the defect in the ED is not generally important as long as appropriate initial therapy is commenced and this usually consists of dextrose.

INTRODUCTION

Inborn errors of metabolism are a group of diverse disorders that result from a defect or absence of a enzyme or transport system. The resulting symptoms and signs may be due to the deficiency of an important precursor, accumulation of a precursor, alternative pathway utilisation, product deficit or product excess (Table 10.1.1).

These conditions commonly present to the emergency department (ED) in children who have not been known to have the disease or may be known to have the disease but have experienced an acute decompensation.

EPIDEMIOLOGY

The conditions tend to be inherited as a simple Mendelian trait. Most are inherited as autosomal recessive diseases but X-linked and autosomal dominant inheritance does occur. The incidence of each individual defect is uncommon to rare varying from 1 in 2000 to 1 in >1 000 000. Some demonstrate significant racial clustering with others being evenly spread. The number of these diseases continues to escalate as new ones are recognised. The large number of individual conditions now numbering many hundreds, means that the cumulative incidence is relatively high.

Some produce clinical syndromes before birth and some only in adult life.

PHYSIOLOGY

The process by which living matter is built up (anabolism) or broken down (catabolism) is termed metabolism. The interaction of the environment and an individual's genes in combination controls the metabolic process. The effect of any individual géne defect is dependant upon the individual protein coded for and the role that this protein plays within the cellular metabolism.

The types of role that may be involved include:

❶ Transport of substrate into a cell. If the transport protein is defective then the intracellular levels of precursor may be deficient, thereby leading to product deficit.

❷ Reduced intracellular enzyme activity. This may lead to accumulation of immediate and remote precursors of the reaction.

❸ Alternative pathway utilisation. The products of alternative pathways of metabolism may interfere with other cellular processes.

❹ Product deficit. An enzymatic lack may lead to inadequate product.

❺ Product excess. Excessive production due to enzyme over activity or lack of feedback mechanisms may cause dysfunction.

The urea cycle defects, organic acidaemias and aminoacidopathies are three large groups of inborn errors of metabolism that may confront the emergency physician.

ORGANIC ACIDAEMIAS

All cells utilise the oxidation of carbohydrates, fats and amino acids to produce ATP, carbon dioxide, water and (from amino acids) ammonia. This occurs via a series of enzymatic steps with intermediate products that are predominantly organic acids. The excessive accumulation of these acids leads to acidosis, neurological dysfunction, impaired hepatic function and gluconeogenesis and may cause

Table 10.1.1	Some clinical finding associated with inborn errors of metabolism	
Symptoms or signs	*Disease example*
Neurological abnormalities	Almost any
Metabolic acidosis	Organic acidaemias
Poor feeding, persistent vomiting, failure to thrive	Organic acidaemias, urea cycle defects
Liver disease	Galactosaemia, tyrosinaemia, hereditary fructose intolerance
Hypoglycaemia	Glycogen storage diseases Fatty acidation defects
Jaundice	Tyrosinaemia galactosaemia

bone marrow failure with thrombocytopenia and neutropenia.

UREA CYCLE DEFECTS

All cells metabolise nitrogen with ammonia as an end product. Ammonia is then converted to urea via the urea cycle.

Elevated ammonia levels leads to neurological dysfunction.

AMINOACIDOPATHIES

These result from the inability of the patient to utilise certain amino acid pathways. Any of the above mentioned mechanisms of pathology may come into play and a wide variety of clinical manifestations may result.

CLINICAL FEATURES

These are many and varied due to the wide ranging nature of these inherited metabolic problems. Despite this there are still cardinal features that should alert the clinician to the possibility of metabolic disease.

Some of the more common serious presentations to the ED include neonatal collapse, where the child is well at birth and within a few days to weeks disease becomes manifest. The baby may become drowsy, listless with accompanying vomiting and loss of muscle tone.

This description is typical of the non-specific nature of many neonatal presentations and the differential diagnosis should include sepsis, cardiac, respiratory and neurological disorders. Very few infants should be considered to have a metabolic disorder when unwell without having had a septic workup and treatment for sepsis.

Recurrent coma in infants and children

This may occur because of hypoglycaemia or accumulation of a toxic product or metabolite. Episodes may be precipitated by minor illnesses, particular foods or prolonged fasts.

The episodic nature of these illnesses make it vital for the emergency physician to consider the diagnosis both for the initial management but also for the diagnostic workup. Because the clinical manifestations are the product of the genetics and the environment the biochemical and metabolic markers of many of the diseases are present only at the time of stress and may disappear with treatment. This means that if a disease picture such as hypoglycaemia is treated initially with dextrose and the patient's signs and symptoms are lost then the biochemistry that would allow the diagnosis of a particular defect is lost. The patient is then left with the options of provocation testing, with its inherent risks, or no formal diagnosis leaving them at potential risk in the community.

MANAGEMENT

The treatment of a child suspected of having an organic acidaemia, urea cycle defect or aminoacidopathy has three primary goals:

❶ Correction of abnormalities
❷ Reduction of toxic compound production
❸ Enhancement of excretion of toxic compound.

Correction of abnormalities In an organic acidopathy the major abnormalities tend to be severe acidosis and hypoglycaemia. Hypoglycaemia needs to be corrected as a matter of urgency.

The infusion of glucose at 10 mg/kg/min is enough to correct hypoglycaemia and also is a sufficient source of calories to turn off endogenous protein catabolism to minimise further production of organic acids.

Other therapies that may be useful, usually with in-patients, include bicarbonate therapy (contraindicated in accompanying renal tubular acidosis and in urea cycle defects unless severely acidaemic), l-carnitine therapy and specific antidotes for some of the organic acidaemias. It may take days or even weeks, with no further significant production of organic acids for the detoxification of some children due to the sequestration of acids within adipose tissue.

The urea cycle defects are managed on similar grounds with an infusion of 10% dextrose to minimise protein catabolism by providing calories and stimulating insulin secretion that promotes protein synthesis. The maintenance of adequate circulating blood volume and adequate renal blood flow is vital to promote renal ammonia excretion and may require the use of saline infusion. Unless the patient has severe acidaemia then bicarbonate therapy should not be given as this alkalises the urine, which makes it less favourable for NH_4^+ excretion and encourages conversion of NH_4^+ to NH_3, which more readily crosses the blood-brain barrier.

In severe cases dialysis may be required and is effective.

All cases of aminoacidopathies, organic acidurias or urea cycle defects should be admitted for specialist care, diagnosis of the specific problem and have a long-term management plan. This plan should consist of: details on what diet to commence the patient on when they are unwell, notes on any specific therapies that are available for the condition, and genetic counselling.

HYPOGLYCAEMIA

Hypoglycaemia is defined as blood glucose less than 2.5 mmol L^{-1}. A blood glucose should be performed in all children who are unwell as they are more prone to hypoglycaemia from metabolic stress than adults are. Any child who has an altered conscious state, convulsions, unexplained irritability or signs of increased adrenergic activity should have a Dextrostix blood sugar level performed immediately with laboratory confirmation of any hypoglycaemic reading.

The infant who is less than one year old is most likely to have hyperinsulinism. Between two and ten years of age ketotic hypoglycaemia is the most common condition.

PHYSIOLOGY

Glucose is an essential energy substrate for the continued normal functioning of human cells. It provides a vital source of ATP production with 38 molecules of ATP produced for every glucose molecule oxidised via the aerobic pathway. It can be stored as fat, protein or glycogen. It is the preferred substrate for cerebral energy metabolism and accounts for almost all of the brain's oxygen consumption.

Normoglycaemia is maintained by a system of interaction between the autonomic nervous system and hormones that act to defend against hypoglycaemia by enhancing glucose production through enzymatic control of glycogenolysis and gluconeogenesis whilst limiting peripheral glucose utilisation.

A lack of substrate, enzyme defect or counter regulatory hormone may cause hypoglycaemia in the young. An oversupply of insulin driving sugar levels down may also occur. Permanent neurological sequelae are common in patients who present with severe hypoglycaemia, particularly those under six months of age or those with recurrent hypoglycaemia. These changes may include atrophic gyri and cortex and reduced white matter myelination.

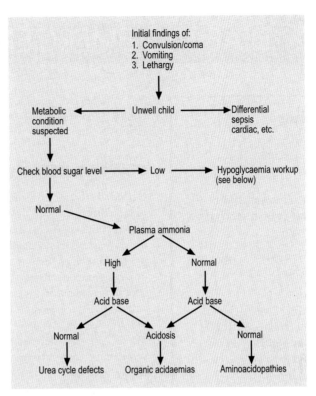

Fig. 10.1.1   Clinical approach to the child with a suspected metabolic disorder.

CLINICAL FEATURES

Historical features of recurrent episodes of altered mentation with illness, failure to thrive, poor weight gain, medications, intolerance of fasting or viral illness should be sought (Fig. 10.1.1).

Physical features on examination should include height and weight. Midline defects and micropenis may suggest hypopituitarism, cataracts and hepatomegaly may suggest a storage disorder and hyperpigmentation points to adrenal insufficiency.

INVESTIGATIONS

Investigations should be quickly obtained before treatment but treatment must not be unduly delayed if there is difficulty obtaining blood.

The tests include those looking at the hormonal regulation of the blood sugar

level and the metabolic consequences of the pathways of gluconeogenesis.

Blood:

- Glucose
- Lactate
- Ammonia
- Ketones and free fatty acids
- Amino acids
- Electrolytes
- Acid base – pH, bicarbonate
- Acyl-carnitine profile.

Urine:

- Ketones, glucose, reducing substances
- Metabolic screen – amino acids and organic acid profile.

MANAGEMENT

Symptomatic hypoglycaemia requires urgent treatment with intravenous glucose (0.25–0.5 g kg^{-1}) or dextrose (2–5 mL kg^{-1} 10% dextrose, 1–2 mL kg^{-1} 25% dex-

trose). Glucagon should not be used in the initial treatment when diagnosis is not known as it does not work to increase glucose concentrations in some of the metabolic conditions.

All children who present with hypoglycaemia that is not related to diabetic control require admission for ongoing blood sugar monitoring and potential dextrose replacement. An ongoing glucose requirement of greater than 10 mg kg^{-1} min^{-1} is consistent with hyperinsulinism.

CONCLUSION

The child with a metabolic condition may present in a variety of ways to an ED and the diagnosis should be considered in all children with unexplained serious illness. There should be a low threshold for performing a blood glucose in the young and initial investigations and management should be instituted expeditiously.

10.2 DIABETIC EMERGENCIES IN CHILDREN

KAM SINN

Essentials

1 Diabetes mellitus is one of the most common chronic diseases in childhood.

2 The incidence of childhood diabetes has been increasing over the last decade.

3 Both Type I (IDDM) and Type II (NIDDM) have increased in incidence.

4 As obesity becomes more prevalent in childhood, Type II diabetes has started to present in younger and younger adolescents.

5 Type I Diabetes remains the major (> 90%) cause of childhood diabetes.

DIAGNOSIS

The classic symptoms of polyuria, polydipsia and weight loss may be present for a few weeks before parental concern is raised.

The diagnosis should be confirmed by a random blood glucose level (> 11.1 mmol L^{-1}) in addition to urine analysis for glucose and ketone.

Once the diagnosis is confirmed, initial management is dictated by the severity of dehydration, presence of shock, degree of acidosis, hyperglycaemia and osmolality.

In a child with no past history of diabetes the initial diagnosis may be misled by non-specific symptoms such as abdominal pain, weight loss, drowsiness, fever, secondary enuresis and dyspnoea. Beware of tachypnoea due to metabolic acidosis, intercurrent infection in a new diabetic, abdominal pain related to diabetic ketoacidosis (DKA) and drowsiness in a child. In such children, diabetes should be excluded as a possible cause with a random blood glucose.

DIABETIC KETOACIDOSIS

Diabetic ketoacidosis is the major cause of mortality in diabetic children. It often presents in newly diagnosed Type I diabetic children. In established diabetics, it occasionally presents in the midst of intercurrent febrile illness or poor adherence to management.

Diabetic ketoacidosis is caused by insulin deficiency, leading to hyperglycaemia, osmotic diuresis, hyperosmolar dehydration, lipolysis, ketosis and acidosis. It may be defined by the combination of:

- Hyperglycaemia
- Ketosis and ketonuria
- Acidosis (pH < 7.3, bicarbonate < 15)
- Dehydration or shock.

Management starts with rapid assessment, resuscitation and meticulous replacement of fluid, electrolyte and insulin infusion.

Like all medical emergencies, assessment of airway, breathing and circulation (ABC) is vital. Ketotic breath, degree of tachypnoea and respiratory distress should be noted. Degree of shock or dehydration should be assessed. Initial level of consciousness should be noted, and hourly neurological observation commenced. It is also important to look for a focus of infection and sepsis.

Initial investigations should include venous blood glucose, electrolytes, urea, creatinine, venous or arterial blood gases, full blood count, blood culture, urine culture and chest X-ray.

RESUSCITATION

Intravenous access should be established; ideally with two IV cannulae so that further venous sampling of blood glucose levels (BGL) and electrolyte may be undertaken easily.

In children with shock, noted to be hypotensive and poorly perfused, resuscitation should start immediately with facial mask oxygen and intravenous fluid bolus. Normal saline 0.9% 10 mL kg^{-1} should be given over ten minutes. The normal saline bolus (10 mL kg^{-1}) should be repeated if the child remains shocked upon reassessment in 10–30 minutes.

Careful and frequent monitoring should continue for the next 24–48 hours. Monitoring should include all vital signs, including neurological assessment, urine output and ECG monitoring.

FLUID

After the initial resuscitation, IV fluid consisting of maintenance fluid and deficit replacement should be calculated and replaced over 48 hours. The child's degree of dehydration should be assessed clinically, including an accurate weight.

The calculation of maintenance fluid is based on the child's weight or surface area.

Dehydration in the form of deficit in percentage of body weight would allow calculation of an estimated volume to be replaced over the next 48 hours. Maintenance and deficit replacement should be given as normal saline 0.9% until the BGL falls to 12–15 mmol L^{-1}. Once the BGL falls to 12–15 mmol L^{-1}, the IV fluid should be changed to half normal saline with glucose 2.5–5% (0.45% saline with 2.5–5% glucose).

Beware of giving deficit replacement too rapidly, which decreases intravascular osmolality and may contribute towards cerebral oedema.

INSULIN

Insulin infusion should only be started after shock has been resuscitated with normal saline intravenously as above. The BGL would fall rapidly during the resuscitation phase with fluid replacement alone.

Insulin infusion with rapid acting insulin (soluble or regular) should be started with maintenance IV fluid. An initial bolus of insulin is not recommended, as it may reduce the BGL and osmolality too rapidly. The infusion is made up by diluting soluble or regular insulin in normal saline to a concentration of 1 U mL^{-1}, to be given in an electronic IV syringe pump. The infusion is started at a rate of 0.05 U to 0.1 U insulin kg^{-1} h^{-1}. The insulin infusion rate can be titrated to achieve a fall in BGL of 4–5 mmol h^{-1}.

Once the BGL falls to the normal range, the insulin infusion should continue until the child is ready to change over to subcutaneous insulin. As DKA is caused by Type I diabetes, the insulin infusion should not be stopped or decreased in rate of infusion below 0.03 U kg^{-1} h^{-1}; until subcutaneous insulin can be started, despite a normal BGL. Insulin is required to suppress lipolysis and clear ketosis. If there is a concern about hypoglycaemia, the glucose concentration in the maintenance IV fluid can be increased.

The change over from IV insulin to subcutaneous insulin is often most conveniently performed at mealtime; when the child is no longer acidotic, but is alert and able to tolerate an oral meal.

POTASSIUM

The initial serum potassium may be high, normal or low, despite a low total body potassium. Potassium replacement should be given intravenously once resuscitation is completed and there are no ECG changes of hyperkalaemia or severe renal impairment.

The measured serum potassium goes up by 0.6 mmol L^{-1} for every 0.1 drop in pH. As the acidosis gets corrected with fluid resuscitation and insulin, serum potassium will drop rapidly in exchange for H+ ions.

The potassium requirement may be as high as 4–5 mmol kg^{-1} d^{-1} in the first 24 hours. Initially, potassium chloride 40 mmol is usually added to each litre of normal saline for rehydration. It is important that serum electrolyte is checked frequently in the first 12 to 24 hours of DKA management.

SODIUM

Serum sodium is a major determinant of osmolality. Rapid change and fall in serum sodium should be avoided to minimise the risk of cerebral oedema. The measured sodium is initially affected by hyperglycaemia.

The corrected sodium can be calculated by:

Corrected Na = Measured Na + (BGL /3)

If there is hypernatraemia with a corrected serum sodium > 150, rate of rehydration should be slowed down further to 72 hours, to minimise rapid changes in osmolality and fluid shift.

BICARBONATE

Bicarbonate is not indicated despite metabolic acidosis. Bicarbonate may increase CNS acidosis and worsen hypokalaemia and hypernatraemia. Blood gas should be repeated at frequent intervals if the initial pH is below 7.1.

PHOSPHATE

Serum phosphate is often low initially. It is controversial whether replacement of phosphate makes any difference to outcome.

COMPLICATIONS

Approximately 0.5% children develop cerebral oedema as a complication of DKA. The warning signs are changes in level of consciousness, irritability, headache, cranial nerve palsies and seizures. Treatment includes slowing the rehydration infusion, IV mannitol, intubation and assisted ventilation.

Careful and close observation of vital signs, frequent review of clinical status and laboratory values of BGL, electrolytes, and acid-base status are vital in the first 24–48 hours of DKA to minimise complications.

Hypoglycaemia and hypokalaemia can be minimised by frequent monitoring of BGL and electrolytes, followed by the adjustment of rehydration fluid and insulin infusions.

HYPOGLYCAEMIA

Hypoglycaemia is a common complication in all diabetics. Education and ongoing support for the diabetic child and his/her family is the key to preventing and managing hypoglycaemia when it does occur.

Hypoglycaemia can be caused by insulin excess (e.g. 'honeymoon period'), overdose of oral hypoglycaemic (in Type II diabetes), intercurrent illness (e.g. gastroenteritis), vigorous exercise and other metabolic/endocrine disorders (e.g. Addison's disease).

Hypoglycaemia is often defined as a BGL < 2.5 mmol L^{-1}. However, symptoms of hypoglycaemia may appear with a BGL < 4.0 mmol L^{-1} in a diabetic. Therefore, the level of BGL in a child with diabetes should be maintained above 4 mmol L^{-1}.

Hypoglycaemia may cause symptoms related to neuroglycopenia and autonomic activation.

In mild to moderate cases, where the patient remains conscious, treatments include ingestion of rapidly absorbed simple carbohydrate such as sugar, followed by more complex carbohydrate and medical review of the cause of the hypoglycaemia.

In severe hypoglycaemia, the patient may present with seizure or coma. Treatment includes stabilisation of airway, breathing and circulation.

- If IV access is available, glucose 25% 1–2 mL kg^{-1} can be given as an IV bolus.
- If IV access is not available, IM or deep SCI glucagon should be given.

The dose of glucagons is 0.5 U (0.5 mg) for children and 1 U (1 mg) for adolescents.

In the recovery phase of severe hypoglycaemia, close monitoring of BGL, medical review of insulin dosage, diabetic control, IV infusion of glucose containing crystalloid solution and/or additional oral complex carbohydrate would be required.

In all children with diabetes, education for the parents, patient, teachers and other carers on symptoms and management of hypoglycaemia, sick-day management, and the availability and use of glucagons are vital.

Some form of wearable identification (e.g. Medic-Alert bracelet) for the child would also help in the management of hypoglycaemic coma.

LONG-TERM MANAGEMENT

The key to good long-term management of children with diabetes is a team and holistic approach to education for the affected child and his/her parents.

Regular medical review of insulin dosage, diet, exercise, medium-term control and complications should be undertaken with a paediatrician, diabetic educator and dietician. It is beyond the scope of this chapter to deal with the details of long-term management of childhood diabetes.

10.3 THYROID EMERGENCIES

MALCOLM HIGGINS

Essentials

1 Life-threatening paediatric thyroid emergencies are rare.

2 Children with undiagnosed thyrotoxicosis or hypothyroidism may present to the ED with a range of acute symptoms and signs.

3 The identification, appropriate management and referral of children with congenital hypothyroidism is important as this condition may cause severe neurological impairment if untreated.

4 The onset of clinical hypothyroidism in Hashimoto's thyroiditis may occur in adolescents.

THYROTOXICOSIS

Hyperthyroidism is generally a disease of adult women but occasionally may present in adolescents. Although there are a number of causes the most common is Graves' disease, which is thought to have an autoimmune basis. In approximately 1–2% of cases the presentation of hyperthyroidism is acute and severe. This has been called the 'thyroid storm' and is potentially life threatening. Other causes of hyperthyroidism in children include thyroiditis, iodine-induced hyperthyroidism, thyroid stimulating hormone (TSH) hypersecretion, excessive ingestion of thyroid hormone and thyroid neoplasms. Hyperthyroidism is one of several endocrinopathies associated with McCune-Albright syndrome.

Clinical features

Raised levels of circulating thyroid hormone have predictable clinical effects depending on the organ system and are similar to the symptoms and signs of catecholamine excess (see Table 10.3.1). The onset of symptoms in Graves' disease is usually insidious and variable in severity between patients. Severe ophthalmopathy or dermopathy is rare in children.

The clinical presentation of thyroid storm is of abrupt onset of high fever and marked tachycardia and hypertension with exaggerated features of hyperthyroidism (Table 10.3.1). Altered mental state is invariably present and may progress to seizures and coma.

Diagnosis

In most cases, low thyroid stimulating hormone (TSH) with raised free T_4 and T_3 will be diagnostic of hyperthyroidism. Other investigations such as thyroid autoantibodies and radionuclear scans are not usually part of the ED assessment.

Thyroid storm is a clinical diagnosis and treatment should not be withheld while waiting for laboratory results.

Treatment

Further investigation and management of hyperthyroidism in children and adolescents will optimally occur following referral to a paediatric endocrinologist or general paediatrician. Therapy will depend on the cause but may include antithyroid drugs. β-Blockers are useful for

Table 10.3.1 Signs and symptoms of thyrotoxicosis
Symptoms
• Nervousness/irritability
• Heat intolerance and increased sweating
• Weight loss
• Behaviour problems and poor school performance
• Fatigue
• Restless sleep/insomnia
• Palpitations
• Diarrhoea
• Menstrual irregularities
Signs
• Tachycardia, hypertension
• Thyroid enlargement with bruit or thrill
• Tremor
• Warm, moist skin
• Muscle weakness
• Eyelid lag and retraction
• Brisk tendon reflexes
• Growth acceleration

initial control of symptoms, particularly in thyroid storm.

Thyroid storm is a medical emergency. Attention to airway, breathing and circulation are the initial priorities

NEONATAL THYROTOXICOSIS

This rare condition is usually due to the transplacental transfer of thyroid-stimulating antibodies from a mother with autoimmune hyperthyroidism. Importantly, antibody levels sufficient to cause neonatal thyrotoxicosis may not cause clinical hyperthyroidism in the mother.

The infant may develop clinical features of hyperthyroidism. Poor weight gain, cardiac dysfunction and hepatosplenomegaly may also be present. Although symptoms usually resolve spontaneously this condition is associated with significant morbidity and mortality.

HYPOTHYROIDISM

Insufficient thyroid hormone leads to slowing of bodily functions and can impair the function of many organ systems. The most important causes in the paediatric patient are congenital hypothyroidism and autoimmune (Hashimoto's) thyroiditis.

Table 10.3.2 Symptoms and signs of congenital hypothyroidism

- Poor feeding, growth and development
- Constipation
- Umbilical hernia, enlarged fontanelle
- Enlarged, protruding tongue
- Prolonged neonatal jaundice
- Hypotonia
- Hoarse cry
- Bradycardia, cool extremities

CONGENITAL HYPOTHYROIDISM

Inadequate thyroid hormone production in newborn infants can occur from anatomic defects of the thyroid, an inborn error of thyroid metabolism, or from maternal iodine deficiency. Thyroid hormone is vitally important to brain growth and development. Profound mental retardation is the most serious effect of untreated congenital hypothyroidism.

Fortunately the majority of infants with congenital hypothyroidism are diagnosed soon after birth via the newborn screening program. A small number of cases will be missed and present for medical attention because of symptoms of hypothyroidism. Suggestive symptoms and signs are listed in Table 10.3.2.

Diagnosis of congenital hypothyroidism is confirmed by demonstrating de-

---

Table 10.3.3 Symptoms and signs of Hashimoto's thyroiditis

- Weakness and lethargy
- Weight gain
- Cold intolerance
- Constipation
- Depression, emotional lability and personality changes
- Forgetfulness and poor concentration
- Hoarse/husky voice
- Goitre
- Menorrhagia and menstrual irregularity
- Bradycardia
- Hypothermia
- Delayed relaxation of deep tendon reflexes

creased levels of serum thyroid hormone (total or free T_4) and elevated levels of TSH. Urgent referral for further investigation and initiation of therapy is important.

HASHIMOTO'S THYROIDITIS

Autoimmune thyroiditis is generally a condition of adult women. Adolescents may be affected. The clinical features are of insidious onset (Table 10.3.3). Diagnosis is confirmed with a TSH assay supplemented by thyroid hormone levels, thyroid autoantibodies and a thyroid scan. Referral to an appropriate specialist is highly recommended.

10.4 ADRENAL CRISIS

YURESH NAIDOO

Essentials

1 The prompt recognition of the possibility of adrenal crisis or the risk of adrenal insufficiency is paramount to early and appropriate management.

2 Adrenal crisis should be considered as a possible contributor in any child with acute severe cardiovascular collapse.

3 In children, the majority of cases are due to primary adrenal failure, with congenital adrenal hyperplasia the most common.

4 A crisis can be precipitated in a child with known adrenal insufficiency, who develops an intercurrent illness or other physiological stress.

5 Signs of glucocorticoid deficiency include hypoglycaemia, hypotension (absolute and postural), and refractory shock.

6 Signs of mineralocorticoid deficiency include dehydration (often out of proportion to estimated fluid losses), hyperkalaemia, hyponatraemia, acidosis, and pre-renal failure.

7 Patients are at risk of hypoglycaemia.

8 The management of adrenal crisis involves immediate fluid resuscitation, replacement of corticosteroid and treating hypoglycaemia.

9 The differential diagnosis of a collapsed neonate (particularly male) in the first 14 days includes adrenal insufficiency.

10 Prevention of adrenal crisis in susceptible children may be possible by following a predetermined action plan during intercurrent illnesses.

INTRODUCTION

Adrenal crisis is a life-threatening emergency caused by acute insufficiency of the adrenal hormones, cortisol and aldosterone. This can occur in situations of stress where the adrenal gland would normally respond by an increase in glucocorticoid secretion. A crisis can be precipitated in a child with known adrenal insufficiency, who develops an intercurrent illness or other physiological stress (e.g. burns, surgery, trauma, and sepsis). In this situation, the increased cortisol requirements of the stress or the altered oral intake of normal replacement therapy results in a relative insufficiency and rapid clinical deterioration. Likewise, the ED visit may be a new presentation of adrenal insufficiency in a child previously unrecognised to have the subtle, often non-specific symptoms of lack of adrenal hormones or a child who is at risk due to suppression by prolonged steroid therapy. The prompt recognition of the possibility of adrenal crisis or the risk of adrenal insufficiency is paramount to early and appropriate management. These children are at risk of hypoglycaemia and this needs to be anticipated and managed accordingly.

Adrenal insufficiency can be primary, due to a failure of secretion of the adrenal cortex, or secondary to hypothalamic or pituitary dysfunction. In children, the majority of cases are due to primary adrenal failure, with congenital adrenal hyperplasia the most common. The incidence of neonatal congenital adrenal hyperplasia in Australia is estimated at 5.9 cases per 100 000 births.

❶ *Primary* causes include:
- Congenital adrenal hyperplasia
- Addison's disease (autoimmune)
- Adrenal aplasia/hypoplasia
- Adrenal infarction secondary to haemorrhage/sepsis
- Other – trauma, tumour, post-surgical.

❷ *Secondary* causes include:
- CNS tumour or trauma
- Idiopathic
- Exogenous steroid therapy.

CLINICAL PRESENTATION

History
- Prior steroid use, including inhaled steroids for asthma or other condition.
- Known congenital adrenal hyperplasia or other adrenal insufficiency on replacement therapy.
- Severe physiological stress (sepsis, trauma, burns, surgery).
- On anticoagulants, haemorrhagic diathesis.
- Neonate with collapse and/or hypoglycaemic event or ambiguous genitalia.
- Symptoms of glucocorticoid deficiency – weakness, fatigue, lethargy, anorexia, vomiting, diarrhoea, weight loss.

Examination
- Signs of glucocorticoid deficiency – hypoglycaemia, hypotension (absolute and postural), refractory shock.
- Signs of mineralocorticoid deficiency – dehydration (often out of proportion to estimated fluid losses), hyperkalaemia, hyponatraemia, acidosis, pre-renal failure.
- Signs of excess ACTH secretion – pigmentation of skin, lips, nipples, skin creases.
- Signs of glucocorticoid therapy – Cushing's syndrome.

- Signs of associated hypothalamic/pituitary abnormality – growth abnormality, midline defects, hypogonadism, diabetes insipidus, hypothermia.

Investigations

- Bedside: Dextrostix (hypoglycaemia), ECG (hyperkalaemia).
- Biochemical: glucose, urea and electrolytes, arterial blood gas, save clotted blood for cortisol level and 17 hydroxyprogesterone, if no underlying diagnosis is known.

Differential diagnosis

- Other causes of hyponatraemia – SIADH, nephrogenic or cerebral salt wasting, gastrointestinal or urinary losses.
- Other causes of shock – septicaemia, profound dehydration, duct-dependant cardiac lesion.

Treatment

The management of adrenal crisis involves immediate fluid resuscitation, replacement of corticosteroid and treating hypoglycaemia. Treatment of the underlying illness causing the stress needs to be treated on merits and potential complications, such as hyperkalaemia, may require intervention. In children not previously known to be adrenal deficient, blood (prior to administration of glucocorticoid) should be held for analysis to determine if an underlying condition exists.

Fluid management

Patients known to have adrenal deficiency who are not dehydrated or shocked can have a trial of enteral fluids in the ED. They should be considered to have vomited or potentially not absorbed their normal replacement adrenal medication, and should be administered IM hydrocortisone 2 mg kg^{-1} to ensure delivery.

Children who are dehydrated or shocked require intravenous resuscitation with crystalloid. Initial boluses of 20 mL kg^{-1} normal saline should be titrated to restore peripheral circulation in those children who have shock. Remaining estimated deficit plus maintenance volumes should then be replaced with 5% dextrose and normal saline over a 24-hour period. The maintenance fluid requirements are 1.5 times normal in this setting and clinical and biochemical (electrolytes and glucose) reassessment is required to tailor fluid therapy to the individual.

Replacement of corticosteroid

Hydrocortisone should be given intravenously, unless access is significantly delayed, where it should be administered IM as an interim alternative. The appropriate dose can be determined by age:

- Neonate: 25 mg stat., then 10–25 mg 6-hourly
- 1 month–1 year: 25 mg stat., then 25 mg 6-hourly
- 1–3 years: 50 mg stat., then 50 mg 6-hourly
- 4–10 years: 75 mg stat., then 75 mg 6-hourly
- > 10 years: 100 mg stat., then 100 mg 6-hourly.

Maintenance doses of glucocorticoid and mineralocorticoid are introduced after the child has been stabilised as an inpatient. Generally, glucocorticoid replacement dose is 10–15 mg m^{-2} d^{-1} PO and mineralocorticoid dose is 0.1–0.2 mg d^{-1} for salt-wasting children.

Hypoglycaemia

The management of hypoglycaemia is treated in the routine fashion using a lower concentration of intravenous dextrose in smaller children. Maintenance fluid will generally require 5–10% dextrose solution added to normal saline.

- Neonate/infant: 5 mL kg^{-1} of 10% dextrose stat.
- Older child: 2 mL kg^{-1} of 25% dextrose stat.
- Maintenance fluid: 5–10% dextrose-containing solution.

Hyperkalaemia

Treat if > 7 mmol L^{-1} with ECG changes.

- 0.5 mL kg^{-1} of 10% calcium gluconate over 3-5 minutes
- 0.1 U kg^{-1} h^{-1} of insulin + 2 mL kg^{-1} h^{-1} of 50% dextrose infusion.

DISPOSITION

All children with an established adrenal crisis require in-patient admission.

Discharge may be considered in milder cases, after a period of six hours observation for those susceptible patients who respond well to treatment with oral fluids and increased dose of intramuscular hydrocortisone.

PROGNOSIS

In the absence of bilateral adrenal haemorrhage, the survival rate of patients with adrenal crisis (that is diagnosed and treated appropriately) approaches that of patients without acute adrenal crisis with similar severity of illness. Because the true incidence of adrenal crisis and bilateral adrenal haemorrhage is unknown, the actual mortality rate is also unknown.

CONTROVERSIES AND FUTURE DIRECTIONS

❶ The role of screening for congenital adrenal hyperplasia (CAH). In Australia there is currently no programme in place.

❷ Research indicates that early screening may reduce the morbidity or mortality associated with adrenal crisis.

❸ National newborn screening awaits the development of a more cost-efficient test.

❹ New research suggests that critically ill children with adrenal crisis may be best managed with a single intravenous bolus dose of hydrocortisone followed by a constant rate infusion. This in preference to the six-hourly boluses used currently.

❺ A further recent research development is that CAH can be diagnosed and treated prenatally if a mother has previously had a child with CAH.

PREVENTION

At risk children with an intercurrent illness may prevent an adrenal crisis by having an action plan for parents to follow:

- If moderately unwell and/or temperature is 38–39°C give 3× oral dose of oral hydrocortisone.
- If more unwell and/or temperature > 39°C give 4× dose of oral hydrocortisone.
- If vomiting give IM 2 mg kg^{-1}.

- If gastroenteritis or diarrhoea give 4× dose of oral hydrocortisone.

NB. Increase only dose of hydrocortisone (not fludrocortisone). When stress is over revert to previous dose without tapering.

FURTHER READING

Charmandari E, Lichtarowicz-Krynska EJ, Hindmarsh PC, Johnston A, Aynsley-Green A, Brook CG 2001 Congenital adrenal hyperplasia: Management during critical illness. Archives of Diseases in Childhood 85(1): 26–28

Fischer JE, Stalmach T, Fanconi S 2000 Adrenal crisis presenting as hypoglycaemic coma. Intensive Care Medicine 26: 105–108

Kirkland L 2003 Adrenal crisis. eMedicine. www.emedicine.com

Macdessi JS, Randell TR, Donaghue KC, Ambler GR, van Asperen PP, Mellis C 2003 Adrenal crisis in children treated with high-dose inhaled corticosteroids for asthma. Medical Journal of Australia 178(5): 214–216

Royal Children's Hospital 2005 Clinical Practice Guidelines. Adrenal Crisis. www.rch.org.au

The Children's Hospital at Westmead 2005 The New Children's Hospital Handbook. Acute adrenal insufficiency. www.chw.edu.au

Van der Kemp HJ, Noordham K, Elvers B, Van Baarle M, Otten BJ 2001 Newborn screening for congenital adrenal hyperplasia in the Netherlands. Paediatrics 108(6): 1320–1324

10.5 DISORDERS OF FLUIDS, ELECTROLYTES AND ACID-BASE

WAYNE HAZELL • BARRY WILKINS

ESSENTIALS

1 The three most common causes of hypovolaemic shock in paediatric patients are sepsis, dehydration and trauma.

2 Aggressive restoration of the circulating volume reduces mortality in hypovolaemic shock.

3 Isotonic or near-isotonic fluids such as 0.9% saline, 4% albumin in 0.9% saline, blood products, Hartmann's or Ringer's solutions are appropriate for volume resuscitation. Hypotonic solutions including 5% glucose, 0.18%, 0.225% or 0.45% saline are inappropriate.

4 After resuscitation of circulating volume, residual dehydration should be corrected slowly with physiological solutions, such as Hartmann's solution or 0.9% saline, or 0.45% saline in the presence of hypernatraemia.

5 The degree of dehydration is easily overestimated.

6 The concept of maintenance fluids applies only after resuscitation of circulating volume and repair of dehydration or water overload, and even then fluids must be individualised to the patient's particular needs.

7 Hyponatraemia generally reflects water excess, and creates a risk for cerebral oedema. Hypotonic fluids are contraindicated until the plasma sodium is corrected.

8 Cerebral oedema may develop rapidly in hyponatraemic children, especially after administration of hypotonic fluids, which are therefore contraindicated.

9 Rapid correction of hyper- or hyponatraemia is contraindicated.

10 Hyperkalaemia with ECG changes requires urgent potassium-lowering treatment.

11 Metabolic acidosis is common in sick children.

12 The anion gap remains useful in determining the cause of metabolic acidosis.

13 Treatment of acidosis is aimed at correcting the underlying cause. Alkali therapy is rarely indicated.

14 Metabolic alkalosis is caused by vomiting, especially pyloric stenosis, or as a compensation for chronic respiratory failure.

INTRODUCTION

Disorders of blood volume, body fluids, sodium, potassium and acid-base are common in acutely ill children. The 'ABC' principle of resuscitation is overriding, even in acute illness where shock and dehydration are dominant – always manage the airway and ventilation first. In resuscitation of the circulation aggressive replacement of blood volume deficit is urgent, but correction of residual dehydration is not. Maintenance fluids are the last consideration.

PHYSIOLOGY

Although there are many physiological differences between adults and infants, there are a few specific features that must be taken into account in managing fluid therapy. Infants have greater total body water, up to 80% instead of 60% of body weight, the extra being mostly extracellular, 30–40% instead of 20% of body weight[1,2] (Fig. 10.5.1). The ionic composition of intracellular and extracellular fluid is shown in Table 10.5.1. Small children drink more to accommodate a higher

metabolic rate and excrete a higher solute load, and thus urine volume is greater.

The following physiological differences apply to paediatric patients:[1,2,3]

- The infant is more dependent on heart rate for cardiac output.
- There are fewer myocardial actomyosin elements and fewer mitochondria per unit cross-sectional area and smaller noradrenalin (norepinephrine) stores than adults. Therefore, there is less ability to increase contractility.

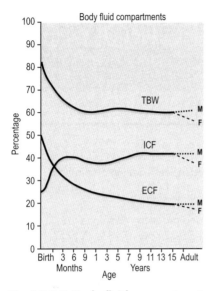

Fig. 10.5.1 Body fluid compartments in children
Source: Adapted from Henning, 1995.

Cations and anions	Intracellular fluid (mEq L^{-1})	Interstitial fluid (mEq L^{-1})	Plasma (mEq L^{-1})
Sodium (Na$^+$)	10	145	140
Potassium (K$^+$)	150	4	4
Magnesium (Mg^{2+})	30	2	2
Calcium (Ca^{2+})	0	5	5
Chloride (Cl$^-$)	5	114	104
Bicarbonate (HCO$_3^-$)	10	24	24
Protein (Pr$^-$)	65	6	15
Phosphate (PO$_4^-$)	95 (organic)	4 (inorganic)	4 (inorganic)
Sulphate (SO$_4^-$)	20	1	1

Table 10.5.1 Ionic distribution of body fluid compartments

- The infant's ventricle is less compliant than the adult. Higher atrial pressures are required for the same degree of ventricular filling.
- The child is more dependent on the extracellular concentration of calcium.
- Storage and release of calcium from the sarcoplasmic reticulum in the infant's myocardium is less efficient.
- The infant tolerates more tachycardia and hypotension than an adult.
- The lack of degenerative diseases in children.
- The capacity of the infant's brain and heart for anaerobic metabolism is greater than the adult.
- The infant's kidney is less able to concentrate urine and to handle a sodium load in the first two years of life. Thus they are less able to compensate for fluid loss.
- The renal blood flow and glomerular filtration rate is less per unit body surface area.
- The infant has less capability to acidify the urine. This renders the infant less able to deal with a hyperchloraemic acidosis caused by too much chloride administration.
- Total body water and extracellular fluid are proportionally higher in the first six months of life.

- In later childhood extracellular fluid declines and intracellular fluid increases due to cell multiplication.
- Limited glycogen stores exist. Hypoglycaemia occurs in periods of stress in infants and young children.

CLINICAL ASSESSMENT

In assessing the degree of dehydration, sequential body weight measurement is the most accurate way of determining the percent loss in body weight due to dehydration. However, previous normal body weight is seldom available in the ED.

Capillary refill times were studied in 32 children, aged 1–26 weeks, admitted to hospital with dehydration.[4] Based on their findings, the authors recommended a cut-off value of two seconds, below which minimal or no dehydration exists. A capillary refill time of 2–3 seconds suggests a 50–100 mL kg^{-1} water deficit; 3–4 seconds 100–120 mL kg^{-1} and over 4 seconds > 150 mL kg^{-1}. Further studies have, however, demonstrated that ambient temperature could affect capillary return.[5]

It has been found that in children less than four years old clinicians overestimated the degree of dehydration by 3.2%.[6] Other studies have suggested that the sensitivity of clinical examination for diagnosing dehydration is 74%, 33% and 70% for mild, moderate and severe dehy-

dration respectively.[7] See Tables 10.5.2 and 10.5.3 for clinical signs associated with dehydration and electrolyte imbalance.[8]

The addition of a plasma bicarbonate concentration may be the single most useful laboratory test. Plasma bicarbonate less than 17 mmol L^{-1} indicates moderate or severe dehydration. Addition of this to the clinical scale improves the sensitivity of diagnosing moderate and severe dehydration to 90 and 100% respectively. Plasma bicarbonate was a better predictor than plasma urea and creatinine.[7]

Shock is a disorder characterised by a decrease in end organ oxygenation and/or perfusion. This is not solely reliant on blood pressure or pulse rate. Blood pressure can be maintained in the infant with shock being present. Hypotension is a preterminal sign.

Estimation of end organ perfusion can best be ascertained by assessing the conscious state, capillary return, urine output and degree of metabolic acidosis.

Haemorrhagic shock

Clinical signs are of value in assessing degree of haemorrhage.[9] See Table 10.5.4. Note that hypotension is a preterminal sign.

Fluid deficit

In the case of dehydration once the percentage loss of body weight (PLBW) is estimated from clinical and laboratory tests the fluid deficit can be estimated.

Table 10.5.2   Degree of dehydration based on percentage of body weight lost*

Variable[a]	Mild (3–5%)	Moderate (6–9%)	Severe (10% or more)
Blood pressure	Normal	Normal	Normal to reduced
Quality of pulses	Normal	Normal or slightly decreased	Moderately decreased
Heart rate	Normal	Increased	Increased[b]
Skin turgor	Normal	Decreased	Decreased
Fontanelle	Normal	Sunken	Sunken
Mucous membranes	Slightly dry	Dry	Dry
Eyes	Normal	Sunken orbits	Deeply sunken orbits
Extremities	Warm, normal capillary refill	Delayed capillary refill	Cool, mottled
Mental status	Normal	Normal to listless	Normal to lethargic or comatose
Urine output	Slightly decreased	$< 1\ mL\ kg^{-1}\ h^{-1}$	$<< 1\ mL\ kg^{-1}\ h^{-1}$
Thirst	Slightly increased	Moderately increased	Very thirsty or too lethargic to indicate thirst

*For each dehydration category, the percentages of body weight lost varied among authors.
[a]See Table 10.5.3 for the physical signs of hypernatraemia and hypokalaemia in dehydration.
[b]Bradycardia may occur in children with severe dehydration.
Source: Based on Burkhart, 1999.

Table 10.5.3   Signs of hypernatraemia and hypokalaemia in dehydration

Hypernatraemia

Cutaneous signs
Warm, 'doughy' texture
Possibly decreased skin-fold tenting in severe dehydration, thereby giving appearance of lower level of dehydration

Neurological signs
Hypertonia
Hyperreflexia
Lethargy common, but marked irritability when touched

Hypokalaemia

Weakness
Ileus with abdominal distension
Cardiac arrhythmias

Source: Based on Burkhart, 1999.

Fluid deficit (litres)
= PLBW% ×
Estimated body weight (kg)

Thus a 10 kg, one year old who is 10% dehydrated has a fluid deficit of:

10% of 10 kg = 1 kg = 1000 g
= 1 litre or 1000 mL

As this is an estimate, ongoing clinical parameters must be assessed including aiming for a urine output of >1.0 mL $kg^{-1}\ h^{-1}$.

Oedema

Oedema suggests that considerable water and salt retention has occurred. Mild sodium and water retention do not cause clinical oedema, nor does water retention without sodium retention, e.g. the syndrome of inappropriate antidiuretic hormone secretion rarely causes oedema. Oedema is most obvious in dependent and distensible subcutaneous tissue such as the genitalia, eyelids, lower legs and lower back. Firm pressure for at least one minute is needed to detect some cases. Causes include:

- Heart failure
  Structural cardiac disease
  Myocarditis
  Cardiomyopathy

  Arrhythmias, especially supraventricular tachycardia
  Effusion
- Liver disease
  Acute hepatic failure
  Chronic hepatic failure
- Renal disease
  Nephrotic syndrome
- Protein-losing enteropathy
- Hereditary angio-oedema
- Excessive water and sodium intake
- Other causes of hypoalbuminaemia.

INVESTIGATIONS

Most children with gastroenteritis do not warrant an IV or investigations. However, the following biochemical tests should be performed in children presenting with shock or significant problems of water and electrolyte imbalance that require intravenous treatment or where such disorders are expected, e.g. respiratory disease, renal disease, liver disease and encephalopathy:

- Plasma sodium, potassium, urea, creatinine, osmolality, glucose, bicarbonate, lactate.
- Plasma calcium, magnesium, phosphate, liver function tests, albumin.
- Arterial pH and gases if shocked.

Venous or intraosseous blood samples give a satisfactory measurement of electrolytes, and of respiratory and metabolic acid-base status.

- Urine sodium, potassium, urea, creatinine, osmolality, glucose, and dip-stick test for protein, red cells and casts (random spot sample).

A urine sample aspirated from a cotton-wool ball placed at the perineum is satisfactory for all measurements except urine calcium.

Plasma osmolality can be calculated as well as measured in order to detect an osmolar gap.

$$\text{Osmolality (mosmol kg}^{-1})$$
$$= 2 \times (Na + K) + Glucose +$$
$$Urea \text{ (all in mmol L}^{-1})$$

If measured osmolality is greater than this figure by 5 mosmol kg^{-1} or more, then an unmeasured solute is present such as an alcohol, e.g. ethanol or ethylene glycol. Ingestion of alcohols may cause a high anion gap ketoacidosis and hypoglycaemia.

Accurate timed urine collections are rarely possible in the emergency department. A useful indication of urine flow rate can be obtained from a spot urine sample, based on the relatively constant creatinine excretion between individuals. For example, a urine creatinine of 2000 μmol L^{-1} represents urine flow of 2–4 mL kg^{-1} h^{-1}, and 8000 (μmol L^{-1}) represents 0.5–1 mL kg^{-1} h^{-1}.

Fractional sodium excretion (FE_{Na}) is a useful diagnostic tool. It represents the proportion of filtered sodium that is not reabsorbed and is < 1% in health. It is given by the formula:

$$FE_{Na} = \frac{Urine\ Na}{Urine\ creatinine} \times \frac{Plasma\ creatinine}{Plasma\ Na}$$

A high FE_{Na} suggests any cause of natriuresis, including acute renal failure, a renal salt-wasting disorder or diuretics. Hyperosmolar urine with high urine creatinine and low FE_{Na} suggests dehydration of non-renal cause. Diabetes insipidus causes hypo-osmolar urine, low urine creatinine (often < 1000 (μmol L^{-1}) and plasma hyperosmolality. Plasma urea is high in most cases of dehydration because of reduced urea clearance.

TREATMENT

Replacement of circulating volume

Also called volume resuscitation, this is an urgent priority in any cause of hypovolaemic shock, e.g. haemorrhage, sepsis, burns, anaphylaxis and dehydration. It requires isotonic fluids (Table 10.5.5). Hypotonic fluids are inappropriate. Crystalloids are inexpensive and readily available. Colloids have a theoretical advantage of increasing the colloid oncotic pressure of plasma, thus helping to maintain fluid in the vascular space. However, in a capillary leak syndrome such as septic shock, the colloid may pass into the interstitial space. Albumin in saline solution has recently been tested against 0.9% saline in adult intensive care patients.[10] There was no diference in mortality or ICU stay between the two therapies. More saline was administered than albumin (ratio 1.38:1), suggesting that albumin may be superior in patients where excessive water administration may be harmful, e.g. pulmonary oedema, pul-

Table 10.5.4 Classes of haemorrhagic shock[9]

Class of haemorrhage	Blood volume lost (%)	Signs
I	< 15	Minimal, slight tachycardia
II	15–30	Tachycardia, tachypnoea, diminished pulse pressure, systolic BP unchanged, prolonged capillary refill, minimal decrease in urine output, anxiety
III	30–40	Tachycardia, tachypnoea, decreased BP, decreased urine output, mental status changes
IV	> 40	Hypotension, anuria, loss of consciousness

Source: Based on Morgan, O'Neill, 1998.

Table 10.5.5 Common crystalloid and colloid IV fluids

Content per litre	0.9% NaCl (normal saline)	0.45% NaCl (half-normal saline)	3% NaCl	4% glucose/ 0.18% NaCl (fifth-normal saline)	5% glucose	Hartmann's solution	Albumin	Haemaccel®
Na+ (mmol L^{-1})	154	77	500	30		130	140	145
K+ (mmol L^{-1})						4–5	5	
Cl− (mmol L^{-1})	154	77	500	30		109	134	145
Ca2+ (mmol L^{-1})						3		6
Lactate (mmol L^{-1})						28		
Glucose (g L^{-1})				40	50			
Osmolarity (mosmol L^{-1})	285	145	900	282	278	274	280	293
Other							Octanoate 6	
Number average molecular weight (M_n)							69 000	24 500
Weight average Molecular weight (M_w)							69 000	35 000
Duration of action							6 hours	3–4 hours
Survival in the body							21 days	7 days

monary hypertension and encephalopathy. There was a suggestion that albumin may be superior in sepsis but inferior in traumatic brain injury.[10] A problem with saline is that it has no bicarbonate and relatively high chloride, so it can lead to hyperchloraemic acidosis. Hartmann's and Ringer's solutions are more physiological, containing buffer (as lactate which is converted to bicarbonate) and calcium.[10-12]

In dehydration the loss of fluid and electrolytes is similar to the composition of extracellular fluid; as this is predominantly where the loss comes from. Thus the deficit is best replaced with a solution that approximates extracellular fluid, i.e. 0.9% saline (normal saline).

However, as fluid replacement is not an exact science, and due to the fact that maintenance fluids also need to be given, a solution somewhere between 0.9% saline and 4% dextrose plus 0.18% saline is given. Saline (0.45%) with added glucose (2.5%) and sometimes potassium would be appropriate. Clinical parameters and serum biochemistry are sequentially measured and the fluid is adjusted accordingly.

Overall 24-hour fluid requirement =
Fluid deficit + Maintenance +
Ongoing losses

Remember, an initial bolus or boluses of 20 mL kg^{-1} to treat shock may be part of this initial fluid deficit.

Most crystalloids are acidic, pH 5-6, albumin and Haemaccel® are buffered to a pH of approximately 7.

The crystalloids (except Hartmann's) tend to cause a metabolic acidosis because they cause a dilution of bicarbonate, the principal buffer in extracellular fluid. A relative hyperchloraemia will develop with the sodium chloride preparations.

Hartmann's is a more physiological solution. The lactate is rapidly metabolised to bicarbonate.

Glucose may be added to the sodium chloride preparations.

How much fluid?

Fluid should be given in shock to cause the signs of shock to improve and disappear.

The blood volume of an infant is approximately 70–80 mL kg^{-1}. Decompensation in haemorrhagic shock starts to occur in class 3 haemorrhagic shock. At this stage it can be presumed that at least 30% or approximately 20 mL kg^{-1} of blood has been lost.[9]

Thus a bolus dose of 20 mL kg^{-1} is a logical bolus dose of fluid with which to begin resuscitation.

However, it must be remembered that in dehydration and sepsis much larger fluid losses and shifts have occurred and the total body water and extracellular fluid are likely to be depleted far more than 20 mL kg^{-1}. If crystalloid is given not all of the fluid will stay in the intravascular space. Capillary leakiness and third space losses in sepsis will contribute to the ongoing loss of fluid from the vascular space.

Thus in dehydration repeated boluses may be necessary. Give a bolus, wait ten minutes and reassess the patient again. Do not wait ten minutes if it is clear that more than 20 mL kg^{-1} will be required.[13-15]

In severe sepsis such as meningococcaemia 80–100 mL kg^{-1} may be required. Good evidence exists that early and aggressive resuscitation improves morbidity and mortality in paediatric sepsis and meningococcaemia.[16] The volume and the rapidity of resuscitation seems to be more important than the type of fluid used.[17-19]

In haemorrhagic shock boluses of 10 mL kg^{-1} of whole blood or packed cells may be given. If FFP is required this can also be given in 10 mL kg^{-1} aliquots.

How to administer fluid in shock

Intravenous access is often difficult in a shocked young infant. However, it is essential that this is achieved as soon as possible. If intravenous access has not been achieved within 90 seconds and/or three failed attempts have occurred intraosseous access should be gained.

Poiseuille's law states that the flow through a hollow tube is proportional to the radius to the power of four and inversely related to the viscosity of the fluid and length of the tube. The small radius can be overcome by applying a larger pressure differential across the tubing. Fluid can be drawn up in a 20 or

50 mL syringe and injected rapidly. It is harder to push fluid through a small cannula with a 50 mL syringe.

A three-way tap can be connected to a normal giving set attached to your IV fluid of choice. The tap can be turned off to the patient allowing fluid to be drawn into the syringe. The tap can then be turned off to the giving set and fluid can rapidly be injected into the patient.

Ideally, blood should be given through the largest cannula that can be inserted. As well as the usual complications of blood transfusion that an adult might get the paediatric patient is at risk of hyperkalaemia from cell lysis as the cells are pushed through the small cannula.

Remember that infants have a higher surface area to body weight ratio and lose heat more quickly. Overhead radiant warmers or fluid warmers are recommended for large rapid volume replacement when it is felt that hypothermia is a risk.

Investigation and management of fluids in different conditions

Gastroenteritis and dehydration

Dehydration is a common presenting feature in children. Causes are outlined in Table 10.5.6.

Table 10.5.6 Causes of dehydration
Gastrointestinal loss
• Diarrhoea
• Non-obstructive vomiting
• Obstructive vomiting
• Third space loss into bowel wall and peritoneum
Renal loss
• Renal tubular disease
• Acquired tubulopathies
• Chronic renal failure including obstructive uropathy
• Adrenal failure
• Congenital adrenal hyperplasia (salt-losing)
• Diabetes insipidus (central and renal)
• Osmotic diuresis (e.g. DKA)
• Diuretics
Insensible loss
• Burns
• Sweating
• Hyperthyroidism
• Hyperventilation with reduced intake
Reduced intake (rarely causes dehydration)

Table 10.5.7   American Academy of Pediatrics (AAP) recommendations for oral rehydration therapy (ORT) in children based on estimated degree of dehydration*

No dehydration
- Oral rehydration therapy: not generally needed unless the child is feeding poorly or is not taking other fluids well; then give 10 mL kg^{-1} of an oral rehydration solution for each diarrhoeal stool
- Feeding: continue age-appropriate diet[a]

Mild dehydration (3–5% body weight loss)
- Oral rehydration therapy: give 50 mL kg^{-1} of an oral rehydration solution *plus* replace ongoing fluid losses[b] over a four-hour period; re-evaluate hydration and estimate ongoing fluid losses every two hours
- Feeding: resume age-appropriate diet[a] as soon as dehydration is corrected and emesis resolves

Moderate dehydration (6–9% body weight loss)
- Oral rehydration therapy: in a supervised setting, give 100 mL kg^{-1} of an oral rehydration solution *plus* replace ongoing fluid losses[b] over a four-hour period; re-evaluate hydration and estimate ongoing fluid losses every hour
- Feeding: resume age-appropriate diet[a] when dehydration is fully corrected

Severe dehydration (10% or greater body weight loss; implies shock or near-shock)
- Intravenous therapy: give a rapid intravenous bolus of 20 mL kg^{-1} of normal saline solution or Ringer's lactate; repeat as needed until the child is haemodynamically stable and shock resolves; if the child does not respond to one or more boluses, consider causes or shock other than fluid loss from diarrhoea and emesis
- Oral rehydration therapy: when the child is stable and alert, begin administration of an oral rehydration solution; keep intravenous line in place until the child is drinking well
- Feeding: resume age-appropriate diet[a] when dehydration is corrected

*These recommendations cover children from one month to five years of age with no pre-existing comorbid conditions who live in developed countries. Specifically excluded are children who have diarrhoea lasting more than ten days, diarrhoea associated with failure to thrive and/or vomiting in the absence of diarrhoea. If the physician is unsure of the dehydration category for a specific patient, the therapy for the more severe category should be used.
[a]The diet should emphasise complex carbohydrates, lean meats, yogurt, fruits and vegetables. Fatty foods, and foods and fluids that are high in simple sugars should be avoided.
[b]Replacement of ongoing fluid losses should include an amount for the estimated volume of emesis and 10 mL kg^{-1} for each diarrhoeal stool.
Source: Based on Burkhart, 1999.

It has been shown that gastroenteritis patients can be successfully resuscitated, even in shock situations, with oral rehydration.

Oral rehydration either by mouth or nasogastric tube is the method of choice for rehydration unless shock exists. It is safe, cheap and effective. It can be effective even in the case of vomiting.[21,23–26]

Recommendations for oral and intravenous hydration in gastroenteritis as given by the American Academy of Paediatrics are contained in Table 10.5.7. Oral rehydration should occur with one of the recommended oral rehydration solutions (Table 10.5.8). No evidence exists to show that one formula is more effective than another[22]. These fluids resemble 0.45% saline and 2.5% glucose with added potassium, which was mentioned earlier as being a useful intravenous solution in this condition.[8]

Note that clear liquids or soft drinks are not to be encouraged. These may be high in carbohydrate and osmolality and lead to osmotic diarrhoea. Hyponatraemia may occur due to their low sodium content. Chicken broth is inappropriate as it may lead to hypernatraemia[8] (see Table 10.5.9).

Some trials suggest frozen oral rehydration solution is better tolerated than the liquid form.[27] A study in the *Annals of Emergency Medicine*[28] suggested that children with a serum bicarbonate greater than 13 mmol L^{-1}, and whom were vomiting, could be treated with rapid intravenous rehydration (20–30 mL kg^{-1} of isotonic crystalloid over 1–2 hours) in the ED. They could then go on and tolerate oral rehydration and be discharged home. Shorter stays in the ED were also enabled compared to times reported with oral rehydration solution. This was a small study of 58 children and the admission rate was used as an end point.

Hypernatraemia and hypernatraemic dehydration

Hypernatraemia is usually caused by water depletion, or water plus sodium depletion in dehydration states where there is relatively more water depletion. Most causes of dehydration (see Table 10.5.5) can cause hypernatraemia. Rarely hyperaldosteronism or salt poisoning cause sodium excess.

The clinical features are usually those of dehydration. Coma and seizures may occur, especially if plasma sodium is >160 mmol L^{-1} at any time, especially if there are rapid changes in circulating volume or plasma chemistry. Thrombocytopenia suggests a CNS vascular insult. Some neurological deficit may result from the encephalopathy of severe hypernatraemia.

Fractional sodium excretion is low because of a normal physiological response to dehydration, but may be high if the cause is an osmotic diuresis, excessive diuretic use or in salt poisoning. The urine will be concentrated (osmolality >600 mosmol kg^{-1}) except in diabetes insipidus.

Shock should be treated with isotonic fluids until haemodynamically stable, then 0.225–0.45% saline, with potassium as needed (40 mmol L^{-1} if not hyperkalaemic). The estimated dehydration should be corrected over 48 hours with slow correction of plasma sodium at no more than 0.6 mmol L^{-1} h^{-1} (15 mmol L^{-1} d^{-1}).

Table 10.5.8　Oral rehydration solutions commercially available in the United States

Product	Electrolyte content (mEq L^{-1})					Calories (per fl oz)	Osmolality (mOsm kg^{-1})	How supplied
	Na$^+$	K$^+$	Cl$^-$	Citrate	Carbohydrate			
Rehydralyte solution	75	20	65	30	25 g L^{-1} of dextrose	3	310	240 mL, ready to use
Infalyte oral solution	50	25	45	32	30 g L^{-1} or rice syrup solids	4.2	200	1 L, flavoured, ready to use
Resol solution	50	20	50	32	20 g L^{-1} of glucose	2.5	Not reported	240 ml, ready to use
Pedialyte solution	45	20	35	30	25 g L^{-1} of dextrose	3	250	240 ml and 960 ml, unflavoured or flavoured, ready to use
Pediatric electrolyte	45	20	35	48	25 g L^{-1} of dextrose	3	250	1 L, flavoured
Pedialyte freezer pops	45	20	35	30	25 g L^{-1} of dextrose*	3	250	2.1 fl oz flavoured freezer pops, 16 per pack
WHO oral rehydration solution salts, mixed	90	20	80	30	20 g L^{-1} of glucose	2.5	310	Dry packets, mixed with 1 L water
Home mix (recipe developed by WHO)	90	20	80	30	20 g L^{-1} of glucose or 40 g L^{-1} of sucrose	2.5	310	Mix 3.5 g (one half teaspoon) or table salt, 1.5 g (one half teaspoon) of potassium chloride or potassium salt, 2.5 g (one half teaspoon) of baking soda and either 20 g (two tablespoons) of glucose or 40 g (four tablespoons) of sucrose in 1 L of water)

Na$^+$, sodium; K$^+$, potassium; Cl$^-$, chloride; WHO, World Health Organization.
*Pedialyte freezer pops also contain phenylalanine and aspartame.
Source: Based on Burkhart, 1999.

Table 10.5.9　Electrolyte and carbohydrate content of common 'clear liquids'

Liquid	Electrolyte content (mEq L^{-1})				Osmolality (mOsm kg^{-1})
	Na$^+$	K$^+$	HCO$_3^-$	Carbohydrate (g L^{-1})	
Cola	2	0.1	13	50 to 150, glucose and fructose	550
Ginger ale	3	1	4	50 to 150, glucose and fructose	540
Apple juice	3	20	0	100 to 150, glucose and fructose	700
Chicken broth	250	5	0	0	450
Tea	0	0	0	0	5
Gatorade	20	3	3	45, glucose and other sugars	330

Na$^+$, sodium; K$^+$, potassium; HCO$_3^-$, bicarbonate.
Source: Based on Gremse, 1995.

If there is salt excess without dehydration, then give less than maintenance water with no sodium, aiming for a very slow correction of plasma sodium, < 0.6 mmol L^{-1} h^{-1}. A diuretic may be considered and, in extreme cases, dialysis.[29–31]

Diabetes insipidus
Diabetes insipidus should be treated with glucose/water, replacing the previous hour's urine volume plus 10–20 mL kg^{-1} d^{-1} for insensible losses. Hyperglycaemia may result. An intravenous vaso-

pressin infusion may be needed, but only if the urine output is stable, which means usually after admission to a ward or ICU, and always after consulting an endocrinologist.

Hyponatraemia and hyponatraemic dehydration
Hyponatraemia may be caused by water excess (e.g. water intoxication, inappropriate antidiuretic hormone), water and salt retention where the water excess is greater than the sodium excess (e.g. nephrotic syndrome, heart failure, renal failure or liver failure), dehydration where sodium depletion is greater than the water depletion (e.g. renal loss, gastrointestinal loss, third-space loss, congenital adrenal hyperplasia, acute adrenal failure), abnormal solute in extracellular fluid (e.g. glucose in uncontrolled diabetes), causing water shift from intra- to extracellular space.

Hyponatraemia may cause nausea, lethargy, depressed consciousness, raised

ICP and seizures, especially if of rapid onset.

Urine osmolality and plasma urea are high in dehydration, but low in water intoxication. FE_{Na} is high in salt-losing states, inappropriate ADH and often in acute renal failure.

Treatment of shock remains the same and can be instigated safely with normal saline. Severely symptomatic patients with plasma sodium less than 120 mmol L^{-1}, such as those with seizures or coma (which is likely to be associated with cerebral oedema), should have their sodium corrected rapidly to 125 mmol L^{-1} (but no higher), using 3% saline (0.5 mmol mL^{-1}).

The following formula may be useful for this:

$$\text{Sodium required (mmol)} = (125 - \text{Plasma sodium (mmoL/L)}) \times 0.6 \times \text{Weight (kg)}$$

Excessive rapid correction of hyponatraemia can lead to central pontine myelinolysis, but it is not clear whether this relates to the severe hyponatraemia itself or the rapid correction. Convulsions and decreasing level of consciousness may occur at any time in treatment, especially if there are rapid changes in circulating volume or plasma chemistry. Some neurological deficit may result from the encephalopathy of severe hyponatraemia.

After treatment of shock, residual dehydration should be managed by replenishing extracellular space with 0.9% sodium chloride, slowly over 48 hours. Residual hyponatraemia should correct itself slowly.

Water intoxication needs water restriction to half maintenance and sodium supplementation if there is evidence of natriuresis.

Syndrome of inappropriate antidiuretic hormone secretion (SIADH)

This condition is over diagnosed. Plasma concentration of antidiuretic hormone, vasopressin, is elevated, despite physiological conditions which should suppress it, namely hypo-osmolality and water overload. Hyponatraemia and hypo-osmolality are accompanied by marked oliguria, but with high fractional sodium excretion and very high urine osmolality

and sodium (often > 200 mmol L^{-1}). The child is sodium depleted but water overloaded, so the management of choice is water restriction, the IV fluid being given as 0.9% saline. Furosemide causes a diuresis in SIADH and may contribute to management.

Pyloric stenosis

Shock is treated with 20 mL kg^{-1} boluses of 0.9% saline. Saline (0.9%) with 40 mmol L^{-1} of KCl is the appropriate rehydration solution. Glucose will need to be added. This remedies the loss of chloride and potassium, and slowly corrects the alkalosis.

Sepsis and meningococcal disease

There is no compelling argument for crystalloid or colloid in the paediatric literature.[18-20] A study of septic shock[14] found that fluid resuscitation in excess of 40 mL kg^{-1} in the first hour was associated with improved survival, decreased occurrence of persistent hypovolaemia and no increase in the risk of ARDS or pulmonary oedema. No restriction was placed on the type of resuscitation fluid used.

A study of severe meningococcaemia[17] looked at 336 patients retrospectively and found a decreased mortality, both in the general population and in high-risk groups, when FFP was not used.

Thus, early aggressive fluid management is the key.

Haemorrhagic shock

Initial resuscitation can take place with crystalloid or colloid. Whole blood at 10 mL kg^{-1} can be given and repeated as necessary until blood pressure is restored.

FFP should be thawed if a large transfusion is expected, and platelets requested. FFP only comes in adult-sized bags and doses of 10 mL kg^{-1} are appropriate with repeating of coagulation times.[9]

Head injury

Aggressive treatment of shock should be undertaken to maintain cerebral perfusion pressure.[32]

Interest has been generated over the use of 7.5% saline in head-injured patients. A recent article in *Paediatric Critical Care*[33] studied 35 patients with head injury

in a prospective randomised fashion comparing Ringer's lactate with 7.5% saline. They found that children treated with hypertonic saline had a statistically significant decrease in complications, intracranial pressure and ICU stay. There was no difference, however, in survival or duration of hospital stay. Neurological outcome was not well documented. More evidence is required.[33-35]

Burns

The original Parkland formula of 3–4 mL kg^{-1} per percentage burn is still applicable to burns patients. Remember that this is over the first 24 hours and starts at the time of the burn not their admission to ED.

Originally 50% of this was to be given in the first eight hours and the rest over the remaining sixteen hours. However, recent evidence suggests that restoration of urinary output and vital signs occur earlier if 50% is given in the first four hours. Many burns patients require more fluid than is provided by the Parkland formula. Aim for urine output greater than 1 mL kg^{-1} h^{-1}.[35]

Some evidence also exists that paediatric burns patients tolerate hypoalbuminaemia well and may not require albumin.[36]

Diabetic ketoacidosis

Treatment of shock should include boluses of 20 mL kg^{-1} of colloid or normal saline. Remember Haemaccel® has potassium in it and should ideally not be used in hyperkalaemic renal failure.

Rehydration over 48 hours is desirable so as to minimise the risk of cerebral oedema.

Cerebral oedema is almost exclusively a condition of the newly diagnosed young diabetic with 95% of cases occurring under 20 years of age in one series.

The fluid of choice is controversial. One article suggests that normal saline be used till restoration of glucose and then a change should be made to 0.45% saline. Potassium replacement should be started when the urinary output is adequate.[37]

Hyperkalaemia

Hyperkalaemia is often discovered incidentally on routine chemistry, but may be suggested by ECG changes. It may be associated with renal failure, hypoxia–ischaemia or acidosis (there may not be potassium excess but rather potassium shift from intra- to extracellular fluid), β-blockers, rhabdomyolysis, haemolysis, potassium sparing diuretics, acute adrenal failure and potassium poisoning.

Mild hyperkalaemia may be asymptomatic but potassium levels > 6 mmol L^{-1}, especially when acute, may cause weakness, peaked T-waves and wide PR interval on ECG, and then loss of P wave, heart block and asystole.

Investigations should include a blood gas, creatine kinase (CK) and glucose.

Any plasma potassium > 6 mmol L^{-1}, or < 6 but rising fast, demands urgent treatment. If K > 7 or there are ECG changes consider giving calcium 0.1–0.15 mmol kg^{-1}, which does not change plasma potassium but protects cell membranes. Beware of subcutaneous infiltration of the infusion. Sodium bicarbonate may also be given, especially if acidotic, 1–3 mmol kg^{-1} over 30–60 minutes, but its value is not certain. If plasma potassium > 6.5 mmol L^{-1}, consider arranging early dialysis. Discuss with the nephrology and intensive-care services.

Milder degrees of hyperkalaemia respond to 5–10 μg/IV salbutamol over a few minutes (or 2.5–5 mg of inhaled nebulised salbutamol if there is no IV cannula), to promote potassium entry into cells. This is more effective and longer lasting than glucose/insulin (0.1 U kg^{-1} insulin plus 0.5 g kg^{-1} glucose over 30–60 minutes).

Resonium, 1 g kg^{-1} every 4–6 hours oral or rectal, may eliminate 1–2 mmol kg^{-1} of potassium.

All cases of hyperkalaemia should be admitted with ECG monitoring.

Hypokalaemia

Hypokalaemia is often an incidental finding on blood chemistry and usually represents potassium depletion. Causes of potassium depletion include vomiting, diuretics, secretory diarrhoea, ureterosigmoidostomy, renal tubular acidosis, hyperaldosteronism, anorexia nervosa and diabetic ketoacidosis. Causes of hypokalaemia without depletion include salbutamol use, alkalosis and familial periodic paralysis.

Mild hypokalaemia is often asymptomatic but tachyarrhythmias, ileus, weakness and rhabdomyolysis may occur. Hypokalaemia associated with alkalosis usually corrects itself as the pH corrects.

Treat potassium depletion by slow potassium supplementation at 2 mmol kg^{-1} d^{-1} or greater. Never give 0.5 mmol kg^{-1} in one hour without ECG monitoring and frequent repeat measurement. Concentration > 40 mmol L^{-1} of infusion fluid should be given into a central venous catheter.

Maintenance fluids

The concept of maintenance fluids refers to healthy children, where the kidneys are able to conserve or excrete water and salt over a wide range in each case according to intake and non-renal losses. 'Maintenance' is a volume of water intake, which maintains urine output in the middle of the normal range with an osmolality about that of extracellular fluid. However, changes in total body water and sodium and other electrolytes are common in many diseases. Insensible skin loss of water may be high because of fever and the higher surface area:weight ratio in infants. Maintenance is only relevant after restoration of circulating volume and total body water, and is therefore relevant to ongoing rather than ED care. A maintenance amount should be a starting amount in your thinking. It may be excessive for any sick child where there may be diminished ability to excrete water.

Maintenance rates of 0.18% sodium chloride with 20 mmol L^{-1} added potassium provides 40–100 mL kg^{-1} d^{-1} of water, 1.5–3 mmol kg^{-1} d^{-1} of sodium and 0.7–1.5 mmol kg^{-1} d^{-1} of potassium, which are normal quantities in healthy children.

A common formula for calculating 'maintenance' water requirements in healthy a child is as follows:

- For the first 10 kg of body weight: 100 mL kg^{-1} d^{-1} or 4 mL kg^{-1} h^{-1}
- For the second 10 kg of body weight: 50 mL kg^{-1} d^{-1} or 2 mL kg^{-1} h^{-1}
- For every subsequent kg of body weight: 25 mL kg^{-1} d^{-1} or 1 mL kg^{-1} h^{-1}.

Reduce this by one-third initially, or even one-half if there is risk of cerebral oedema, e.g. in meningitis or brain injury, especially if hyponatraemia already exists. Less than 'maintenance' water should be given when water retention is likely, such as in sepsis and severe respiratory disease (0.7×'maintenance'), cardiac failure (0.5×'maintenance'), renal failure or other oliguric states without hypovolaemia (0.3×'maintenance' plus urine output) (see Table 10.5.10). Greater than 'maintenance' is often advocated when water losses are expected, e.g. spontaneous hyperventilation or fever, but it is probably more appropriate to increase fluids only if urine output falls to 0.5 mL kg^{-1} h^{-1}. The most appropriate maintenance IV fluid in the acutely ill child is 0.45% saline because at half-'maintenance' rates this provides 1–3 mmol kg^{-1} d^{-1} of sodium, but separate consideration should always be given to sodium and other electrolyte requirements. Do not include dehydration deficit in maintenance; consider this separately and use 0.9% saline or Hartmann's solution.

ACID-BASE DISORDERS

Disorders of physiological control of acidity of body fluids are common in acutely ill children. The system of defining acid-base state by changes in P_{CO_2} (respiratory) and standardised base excess (metabolic) according to the Copenhagen school remains the most familiar way of analysing acid-base disorders. Base excess is mostly bicarbonate deficit, but includes a small amount of buffering by albumin, and a larger amount by haemoglobin. Standardised base excess is provided by blood gas machines derived by microprocessor rather than the original nomograms. The philosophy of base excess has been challenged because it does not take into account the actual plasma albumin concentration and assumes a notional haemoglobin concentration of 50 g L^{-1} across blood and extracellular fluid in all patients. It can be argued that the bicarbonate concentration alone is a sufficient measure of the degree of metabolic acidosis or alkalosis.

Table 10.5.10   Guide to ongoing water therapy

Weight (kg)	0.7× 'maintenance' – the commonest starting point		Full 'maintenance'	
	($mL\ h^{-1}$)	($mL\ kg^{-1}\ d^{-1}$)	($mL\ h^{-1}$)	($mL\ kg^{-1}\ d^{-1}$)
4	11	70	16	100
6	17	70	24	100
8	22	70	32	100
10	28	70	40	100
12	31	62	44	88
14	34	57	48	82
16	36	55	52	78
18	39	53	56	75
20	42	50	60	72
30	49	39	70	56
40	56	34	80	48
50	63	30	90	43
60	70	28	100	40
70	77	27	110	38

The anion gap remains a useful tool in determining whether any bicarbonate deficit is caused by organic acid (high anion gap) or by chloride excess (normal anion gap). It is obtained from the formula:

$$\text{Anion gap} = Na^+ + K^+ - Cl^- - HCO_3^- \text{ (all in mEq } L^{-1})$$

The normal is 16 mEq L^{-1} and is essentially the negative charge on albumin and phosphate. Any excess is accounted for by abnormal unmeasured acid and/or lactate. Most modern laboratories, including blood gas machines, measure lactate. A more accurate way of determining the unmeasured component is from the formula:

$$\text{Unmeasured anion} = Na^+ + K^+ + Mg^{2+} + Ca^{2+} - Cl^- - HCO_3^- - \text{Albumin} \times (0.123 \times pH - 0.631) - \text{Phosphate} \times (0.309 \times pH - 0.469) - \text{Lactate}^- \text{ (all in mEq } L^{-1})$$

Note that Mg^{2+} and Ca^{2+} are divalent and so are 2 × mmol L^{-1}.

Albumin × (0.123 × pH – 0.631) is the negative charge on albumin, derived from its known buffer curve.

Phosphate × (0.309 × pH – 0.469) is the negative charge on phosphate, derived from its known buffer curve.

Plasma albumin at 40–45 g L^{-1} is 0.6 mmol L^{-1} but contributes 12 mEq L^{-1} to the anion at pH 7.4. Phosphate at 1.5 mmol L^{-1} contributes 2.7 mEq L^{-1}.

The normal value for unmeasured anion is 5–6 mEq L^{-1}, including 1 mEq L^{-1} of lactate. Any excess is abnormal. This may be lactate in hypoxia–ischaemia, acetoacetate or β-hydroxybutyrate in DKA, ketones in starvation, organic acids in inborn errors of metabolism or alcohol poisoning or toluene inhalation.

Most metabolic acid-base disturbances do not need treatment. Compensating mechanisms should generally not be treated; otherwise the primary disturb-ance is exacerbated. It is not necessary to restore pH to normal.

Metabolic acidosis

Normal physiology maintains extracellular pH close to 7.4 in health, but permits metabolic acidosis at times of anaerobic metabolism without danger. Metabolic acidosis may be advantageous because it is thought to protect cells against the effects of hypoxia, and assists oxygen unloading from haemoglobin by shifting the oxygen/haemoglobin dissociation curve to the right.

Acidosis is alleged to cause negative inotropy or failure of inotropes to work at pH < 7.2, but this has little experimental support. Acidosis causes pulmonary vasoconstriction and may predispose to arrhythmias caused by other electrolyte abnormalities.

In metabolic acidosis, bicarbonate deficit (mmol kg^{-1}) is given by:

$$\text{Weight (kg)} \times (24 - \text{Plasma bicarbonate [mmol } L^{-1}]) \times 0.5$$

A plasma lactate estimation should be performed if there is significant base deficit or high anion gap. Urine for drug screen may be indicated. For suspected inborn error of metabolism if the anion gap is greater then 20, send a urine for metabolic screen.

First treat the underlying disease (see Table 10.5.11), including general management of renal, hepatic failure, cardiac failure, hypoxia, shock and hypovolaemia. Alkali is not usually needed for mild acidosis (pH > 7.2) because the acidosis itself does not cause any compromise. Even extreme acidaemia (pH < 6.8) can be followed by full recovery, and bicarbonate therapy is only indicated if there is severe hyperkalaemia or tricyclic poisoning. Sudden changes in acid–base status should be avoided. Sodium bicarbonate has many alleged adverse effects, especially when given rapidly, such as hypokalaemia, decreased plasma ionised calcium, sodium load, osmolar load, increased haemoglobin/oxygen affinity, exacerbation of effects of hypophosphataemia, and late metabolic alkalosis. There is no evidence for increased intracellular acidosis. Sodium bicarbonate is especially

Table 10.5.11 Causes of acidosis

High anion gap	Normal anion gap
• Diarrhoea (starvation/ketosis) • Sepsis • Diabetic ketoacidosis • Renal failure • Hepatic failure • Drugs and poisons (e.g. salicylates, ethanol, methanol, ethylene glycol) • Inborn errors of metabolism (especially in babies) • Hypoxia • Circulatory failure	• Renal tubular acidosis • Other renal tubulopathies which include bicarbonate loss • Gastroenteritis • Intestinal fistulae or enterostomies • Excessive sodium chloride administration • Hypoaldosteronism

unlikely to be helpful in lactic acidosis because the patient will end up sodium overloaded with a metabolic alkalosis as the lactic acid is metabolised to bicarbonate during recovery.

Slow sodium bicarbonate treatment may have a role in the management of normal anion gap acidosis where excessive chloride therapy would exacerbate hyperchloraemia. A suitable recipe is 2 mmol kg^{-1} d^{-1}. In diabetic ketoacidosis bicarbonate is not recommended acutely, even in severe acidaemia with pH < 7.0. However, ketoacids are excreted by osmotic diuresis in preference to chloride, so it may be helpful to include about a fifth of the sodium replacement as bicarbonate given just as slowly as the rest of the repair. This may avoid the patient ending up hyperchloraemic and tachypnoeic after the metabolic disorder is corrected. There is, however, no intravenous fluid preparation available that contains bicarbonate.

Correct hypoglycaemia. If an inborn error of metabolism is suspected give glucose at > 8 mg kg^{-1} min^{-1}, correct electrolyte imbalance, and partially correct acidosis with bicarbonate, giving this over at least one hour (see above).

Metabolic alkalosis

Metabolic alkalosis may be caused by chronic potassium and/or chloride depletion, e.g. vomiting, especially pyloric stenosis (accompanied by volume depletion) or renal (including diuretic use). It may be compensatory (chronic renal bicarbonate retention) in chronic respiratory failure, in which case it should not be treated. Acute alkalosis can cause tetany by lowering plasma ionised calcium in which case it should be treated.

After correction of dehydration, chloride deficit is approximately 6 mmol kg^{-1} for every 10 mmol L^{-1} fall in plasma chloride. A suitable fluid for treating alkalaemic patients is 0.9% or 0.45% sodium chloride plus 40 mmol L^{-1} potassium chloride with added glucose. Hypotonic solutions, which may exacerbate hyponatraemia, should not be used. Intravenous hydrochloric acid (or arginine hydrochloride) is indicated in rare severe cases when alkalosis may be depressing respiratory drive, and when the chloride deficit is not accompanied by sodium deficit. Give hydrochloric acid (150 mmol L^{-1} solution) by central intravenous catheter. Give half-correction over at least one hour.

$$\text{Dose of HCl for full correction (mmol) =}$$
$$\text{Weight (kg)} \times (\text{Plasma bicarbonate [mmol L}^{-1}] - 24) \times 0.5$$

Acidifying diuretics such as acetazolamide may be indicated in metabolic alkalosis where there is sodium and water retention.

CONTROVERSIES

❶ Use of albumin in sepsis and meningococcal disease.

❷ Crystalloid vs. colloid argument in paediatrics.

❸ Which colloid if any colloid?

❹ Evidence for aggressive early fluid resuscitation.

❺ Hypertonic saline in hypovolaemic shock.

❻ Hypertonic saline in traumatic brain injury.

❼ Oral vs. IV rapid rehydration therapy in the ED for patients with gastroenteritis.

❽ Frozen rehydrating solution.

❾ Which fluid and how quickly in DKA?

❿ Hypertonic saline for head injury and haemorrhagic shock.

REFERENCES

1. Henning R 1995 Fluid resuscitation in children. Emergency Medicine. Second Australian Symposium on Fluid Replacement 57–62
2. Cullen P 1996 Fluid resuscitation in infants and children. Current Anaesthesia and Critical Care 7: 197–205
3. Tobias JD 1996 Shock in children: The first 60 minutes. Pediatric Annals 25: 330–338
4. Saavedra JM, Harris GD, Li S, Finberg L 1991 Capillary refilling (skin turgor) in the assessment of dehydration. Am J Dis Child 145: 296–298
5. Gorelick MH, Shaw KN, Baker N 1993 Effect of ambient temperature on capillary refill in healthy children. Pediatrics 92: 699–702
6. Mackenzie A, Barnes G, Shann F 1989 Clinical signs of dehydration in children. Lancet ii: 605–607
7. Vega RM, Avner JR 1997 A prospective study of the usefulness of clinical and laboratory parameters for predicting percentage of dehydration in children. Paediatric Emergency Care 13: 179–182
8. Burkhart DM 1999 Management of acute gastroenteritis in children. American Family Physician 60: 2555–2563
9. Morgan WM, O'Neill JA 1998 Hemorrhagic and obstructive shock in pediatric patients. New Horizons 6: 150–154
10. The SAFE Study Investigators 2004 A comparison of albumin and saline for fluid resuscitation in the Intensive Care Unit. New England Journal of Medicine 350: 2247–2256
11. Schierhout G, Roberts I 1998 Fluid resuscitation with colloid or crystalloid solutions in critically ill patients: A systematic review of randomised trials. British Medical Journal 316: 961–964
12. Emery EF, Greenhough A, Gamsu HR 1992 Randomised controlled trial of colloid infusions in hypotensive preterm infants. Archives of Diseases in Childhood 67: 1185–1188
13. Schexnayder SP 1999 Pediatric septic shock. Paediatrics in Review 20: 303–307
14. Carcillo JA, Davis AL, Zaritsky A 1991 Role of early fluid resuscitation in pediatric septic shock. Journal of American Medical Association 266: 1242–1245
15. Goh AYT, Chan PWK, Lum LCS 1999 Sepsis, severe sepsis and septic shock in paediatric multiple organ dysfunction syndrome. Journal of Paediatric Child Health 35: 488–92
16. Pollard AJ, Britto J, Nadel S, DeMunter C, Habibi P, Levin M 1999 Emergency management of meningococcal disease. Archives of Diseases in Childhood 80: 290–296
17. Busund R, Straume B, Revhaug A 1993 Fatal course in severe meningococcemia: Clinical predictors and effect of transfusion therapy. Critical Care Medicine 21: 1699–1705

18. McClelland B 1998 Human albumin administration in critically ill patients. British Medical Journal 317: 882 [letter]

19. Cochrane Injuries Group Albumin Reviewers 1998 Human albumin administration in critically ill patients: Systematic review of randomised controlled trials. British Medical Journal 317: 235–240

20. Nadel S, De Munter C, Britto J, Levin M, Habib P 1998 Albumin: Saint or sinner? Archives of Diseases in Childhood 79: 384–385

21. Moyer VA, Elliott EJ 2000 Evidence-based pediatrics: The future is now. The Journal of Pediatrics 136: 282–284

22. Mackenzie A, Barnes G 1991 Randomised controlled trial comparing oral and intravenous rehydration therapy in children with diarrhoea. British Medical Journal 303: 393–396

23. Gremse DA 1995 Effectiveness of nasogastric rehydration in hospitalised children with acute diarrhea. Journal of Pediatric Gastroenterology and Nutrition 21: 145–148

24. Barnes GL 1996 Oral rehydration solutions in gastroenteritis before and after admission to hospital. Journal of Paediatric Child Health 32: 16–17

25. Eliason BC, Lewan RB 1998 Gastroenteritis in children: Principles of diagnosis and treatment. American Family Physician 58: 1769–1776

26. Wittenberg DF, Ramji S 1995 Paediatric diarrhoea – rehydration therapy revisited. South African Medical Journal 85: 655–658

27. Santucci KA, Anderson AC, Lewander WJ, Linakis JG 1998 Frozen oral hydration as an alternative to conventional enteral fluids. Archives of Paediatric Adolescent Medicine 152: 142–146

28. Reid SR, Bonadio WA 1996 Outpatient rapid intravenous rehydration to correct dehydration and resolve vomiting in children with acute gastroenteritis. Annals of Emergency Medicine 28: 318–323

29. Ng PC, Chan HB, Fok TF, Lee CH, Chan KM, Wong W, Cheung KL 1999 Early onset of hypernatraemic dehydration and fever in exclusively breast fed infants. Journal of Paediatric Child Health 35: 585–587

30. Moritz ML, Ayus JC 1999 The changing pattern of hypernatremia in hospitalised children. Paediatrics 104: 435–439

31. Dunn K, Butt W 1997 Extreme sodium derangement in a paediatric inpatient population. Journal of Paediatric Child Health 33: 26–30

32. Scalea TM, Maltz S, Yelon J, Trooskin SZ, Duncan AO, Sclafani JA 1994 Resuscitation of multiple trauma and head injury: Role of crystalloid fluids and inotropes. Critical Care Medicine 22: 1610–1615

33. Simma B, Burger R, Falk M, Sacher P, Fanconi S 1998 A prospective, randomised, and controlled study of fluid management in children with severe head injury: Lactated Ringer's solution versus hypertonic saline. Pediatric Critical Care 26: 1265–1270

34. Sheikh AA, Matsuoka T, Wisner DH 1996 Cerebral effects of resuscitation with hypertonic saline and a new low sodium hypertonic fluid in hemorrhagic shock and head injury. Critical Care Medicine 24: 1226–1232

35. Cocks AJ, O'Connell A, Martin H 1998 Crystalloids, colloids and kids: A review of paediatric burns in intensive care. Burns 24: 717–724

36. Sheridan RD, Prelack MS, Cunningham JJ 1997 Physiological hypoalbuminemia is well tolerated by severely burned children. The Journal of Trauma: Injury, Infection and Critical Care 43: 448–452

37. Edge JA 1996 Management of diabetic ketoacidosis in childhood. British Journal of Hospital Medicine 55: 508–512

FURTHER READING

Arieff AI 1998 Postoperative hyponatraemic encephalopathy following elective surgery in children. Paediatric Anaesthesia 8: 1–4 [editorial]

Arieff AI, Ayus JC 1991 Treatment of symptomatic hyponatremia: Neither haste nor waste. Critical Care Medicine 19: 748–751 [editorial]

Arieff AI, Ayus JC, Fraser CL 1992 Hyponatremia and death or permanent brain damage in healthy children. British Medical Journal 304: 1218–1222

Bickell WH, Wall MJ, Pepe PE et al 1994 Immediate versus delayed fluid resuscitation for hypotensive patients with penetrating torso injuries. New England Journal of Medicine 331: 1105–1109

Bohn D 2000 Problems associated with intravenous fluid administration in children: Do we have the right solution? Current Opinion Paediatrics 12: 217–221

Chan JCM, Gill JR (eds) 1990 Kidney electrolyte disorders. Churchill Livingstone, New York

Coulthard MG, Haycock GB 2003 Distinguishing between salt poisoning and hypernatraemic dehydration in children. British Medical Journal 326: 157–160

Doyle JA, Davis DP, Hoyt DB 2001 The use of hypertonic saline in the treatment of traumatic brain injury. Journal of Trauma 50: 367–383

Duke T, Molyneux EM 2003 Intravenous fluids for seriously ill children: Time to reconsider. Lancet 362: 1320–1323

Feld LG 1996 Hyponatraemia in infants and children: A practical approach. Journal of Nephrology 9: 5–9

Finberg L, Kravath RE, Hellerstein S (eds) 1993 Water and electrolytes in pediatrics. Physiology, pathology and treatment, 2nd edn. WB Saunders, Philadelphia

Fraser CL, Arieff AI 1997 Epidemiology, pathophysiology and management of hyponatremic encephalopathy. American Journal of Medicine 102: 67–77 [review]

Gerigk M, Gnehm HPE, Rascher W 1996 Arginine vasopressin and renin in acutely ill children: Implication for fluid therapy. Acta Paediatrica 85: 550–553

Halberthal M, Halperin ML, Bohn D 2001 Acute hyponatremia in children admitted to hospital: Retrospective analysis of factors contributing to its development and resolution. British Medical Journal 322: 780–782

Holliday MA, Segar WE 2003 Reducing errors in fluid therapy management. Pediatrics 111: 424–425 [Commentary]

Ichikawa I, Yoshioka T (eds)1990 Paediatric textbook of fluids and electrolytes. Williams and Wilkins, Baltimore

Kamel KS, Wei C 2003 Controversial issues in the treatment of hyperkalaemia. Nephrology, Dialysis and Transplantation 18: 2215–2218

Kellum JA 2002 Saline-induced hyperchloremic metabolic acidosis. Critical Care Medicine 30: 259–261

Laureno R, Karp BI 1997 Myelinolysis after correction of hyponatremia. Annals of Internal Medicine 126: 57–62

McClure RJ, Prasad VK, Brocklebank JT 1994 Treatment of hyperkalaemia using intravenous and nebulised salbutamol. Archives of Diseases in Childhood 70: 126–128

Meyers A 1994 Fluid and electrolyte therapy for children. Current Opinion in Paediatrics 6: 303–309

Myers CT 1995 Minimal volume, hypotense resuscitation. Emergency Medicine. Second Australian Symposium on Fluid Replacement 51–56

Phin SJ, McCaskill ME, Browne GJ, Lam LT 2003 Clinical pathway using rapid rehydration for children with gastroenteritis. Journal of Paediatric Child Health 39: 343–348

Rodriguez-Soriano J 1995 Potassium homeostasis and its disturbances in children. Paediatric Nephrology 9: 364–374

Ronco C, Bellomo R (eds) 1998 Critical care nephrology. Kluwer Academic Publishers, Dordrecht

Tuthill DP, Hewson M, Wilson R 1998 Paediatric resuscitation – by phone. Journal of Paediatric Child Health 34: 524–527

Wilkins B 1999 Fluid therapy in acute paediatrics: A physiological approach. Current Paediatrics 9: 51–56

SECTION

11

SENIOR AUTHOR ROBERT PITT

HAEMATOLOGY AND ONCOLOGY

11.1 THE USE OF BLOOD PRODUCTS IN CHILDREN

JOSEPH TING

Essentials

1 Blood components are appropriately used when clinical benefits of administration outweigh potential hazards and are generally safe.

2 Use specific component(s) appropriate to a clinical problem whenever possible.

3 Trauma with associated haemodynamic derangement requires rapid packed red blood cell (PRBC) transfusion while a decision is made regarding the need for surgical haemostasis.

4 Anaemia that does not pose a hypoxic risk to the asymptomatic child may not require transfusion.

5 Platelets are used in massive transfusion associated with platelet count $< 50 \times 10^9$ L^{-1}, in non-trauma situations when platelet count $< 10 \times 10^9$ L^{-1} and may be given prophylactically in children undergoing invasive procedures or surgery to maintain platelet count $> 50 \times 10^9$ L^{-1}.

6 FFP is used to treat significant coagulopathy associated with massive transfusion, excessive anti-coagulation with warfarin and liver disease.

7 Albumin is used for volume expansion or to replenish serum protein.

INTRODUCTION

Blood components should only be given when the expected benefits to the child outweigh the potential hazards. A range of clinical signs and symptoms viewed within the context of a clinical need is essential for the decision to transfuse. In the setting of massive transfusion or acute blood loss, whole blood should be used. Otherwise, there is no indication for the use of whole blood when specific component(s) appropriate to a clinical problem are available. Emphasis on blood component safety, standardisation of appropriate guidelines for use of blood components and informed consent for blood component administration have led to a substantial reduction in the potential risks and complications of their use as well as increasing their appropriate usage. Informed consent with regards to the risks and benefits of blood component therapy needs to be obtained in the light of community concerns about transfusion safety, particularly the potential for infection transmission. The indication, risks, benefits, alternatives to transfusion, parental consent, response to treatment and any adverse event should be clearly documented.

Whole blood

Whole blood is rarely used, being specifically used for exchange transfusion and haemorrhage with uncontrolled coagulopathy.

Packed red blood cells (PRBC)

Indications

Each PRBC unit contains 200–250 mL of red cells with a haemoglobin concentration of 100–150 g L^{-1}. PRBC is indicated if the oxygen-carrying capacity of blood is so reduced that the degree of anaemia poses a risk to the child or there is ongoing blood loss. Transfusion of PRBC in an asymptomatic child is not appropriate in most situations. PRBC transfusion is likely to be appropriate when haemoglobin is less than 70 g L^{-1}, especially when the child is compromised from anaemia with tachycardia and tachypnoea. Use of PRBC with haemoglobin in the range 70–100 g L^{-1} is appropriate if the child is at risk of hypoxia (cardiac, respiratory disease) and should be supported by the need to relieve clinical symptoms and signs. Criteria for PRBC in patients aged less than four months are different from those for older children. Infants in the former group have smaller blood volumes, decreased erythropoietin production (especially if premature) and there may be physiologic anaemia of infancy.

Additional indications for PRBC include:

- Emergency surgery in a child with significant preoperative anaemia
- Anaemia related to chemotherapy or radiotherapy
- Sickle cell disease with ischaemic organ events
- Chronic congenital or acquired anaemia such as B-thalassaemia.

Administration

In haemorrhagic shock, RBC infusion at an initial volume of 20 mL kg^{-1} should be considered when loss of blood volume approaches 30% and shock is refractory to non-blood fluid resuscitation. If haemorrhage or haemolysis is accompanied by life-threatening hypoxia then uncross-matched group O rhesus negative packed cells may be required. In less-urgent cases, type-specific or cross-matched RBC is preferred. Rh type specific blood takes 15 minutes to cross match. If the child has no immediate need for RBC replacement and there is no ongoing bleeding or haemodynamic instability, cross-matched RBC may be administered over four hours.

The volume required for elective top-up transfusion in mL is:

$$\text{Weight (kg)} \times \text{Haemoglobin rise required (g L}^{-1}) \times 3$$

Alternatives

Autologous blood (patient's own blood is collected before surgery) is suitable for elective surgery but has no role in urgent situations. Peri-operative blood scavenging may be useful in reducing exposure to donor blood. Red cell substitutes such as cell-free haemoglobins and perfluorocarbon emulsions require 100% oxygen to be effective and are still being trialled.

Adverse reactions

Fatal acute haemolytic reactions occur in 1:250 000–1:1 000 000 transfusions, with half caused by ABO incompatibility as a result of mismatching the blood with the patient or other administrative errors. Another 1:260 000 patients have a haemolytic reaction due to minor red-cell antigen incompatibility and 1:1000 patients experiences delayed haemolytic reaction.

Platelets

Indications

In haemorrhagic shock, platelet infusion should be considered in massive transfusion associated with platelet count less than 50×10^9 L^{-1}. Platelet transfusion may be appropriate in children with failure of platelet production and platelet count less than 10×10^9 L^{-1}, as there is a risk of intracerebral bleeding. Routine use of platelets is not indicated in children with autoimmune thrombocytopenia and idiopathic thrombocytopenic purpura because autoantibodies rapidly destroy transfused platelets. In thrombotic thrombocytopenic purpura platelet transfusion predisposes to thrombosis. Platelets should not be used in haemolytic-uraemic syndrome. Platelets may be given prophylactically in children undergoing invasive procedures or surgery to maintain platelet count $> 50 \times 10^9$ L^{-1}. In children with platelet dysfunction (inherited or acquired), platelets are administered to treat active bleeding. Platelets are indicated in thrombocytopenic premature infants with active bleeding or prior to an invasive procedure.

Administration

Each unit is 40–70 mL in volume and contains at least 5.5×10^{10} platelets.

Infusion of 5–10 mL kg^{-1} of platelets will lead to a rise in platelet count of $50–100 \times 10^9$ L^{-1}.

Adverse reactions and other problems

Platelets are stored at room temperature to maintain their ability to aggregate, and this promotes bacterial growth. Compared with other blood components, the risk of bacterial contamination of platelets is relatively high at 1:2000 units and sepsis is the most frequent fatal complication of platelet use. Platelets older than five days lose their ability to aggregate and are therefore less effective. Alloimmunisation due to the development of platelet alloantibodies from repeated transfusions may lead to refractory thrombocytopenia.

Fresh frozen plasma (FFP)

FFP contains all coagulation factors, except VII, including approximately 150 units of factor VIII. FFP is used to treat coagulopathy associated with massive transfusion for haemorrhagic shock when 50% or more of circulating blood volume has been replaced. FFP may be considered for treatment of acute disseminated intravascular coagulation (DIC) and thrombotic thrombocytopenic purpura (TTP). Less urgent indications include children with coagulopathy undergoing invasive procedures/surgery, liver disease-related coagulopathy, replacement of single coagulation factor deficiency, where a specific factor concentrate is not available, and reversal of life-threatening bleeding due to warfarin. FFP should not be used for volume expansion or plasma-exchange procedures.

Administration

In life-threatening exsanguination requiring massive transfusion, FFP may be required to minimise the dilutional coagulopathy. As a guide, one unit of FFP is required for every four units of packed cells but titrate FFP use against the coagulation profile if possible. FFP contains all coagulation factors including approximately one unit of factors VIII and V for each millilitre of FFP. FFP is administered at an initial dose of 10–15 mL kg^{-1} with a paediatric bag containing 50 mL. After thawing, FFP needs to be used within 24 hours.

Cryoprecipitate

Cryoprecipitate contains factors VIII, XIII, fibrinogen, von Willebrand's factor and fibronectin. Approximately 200 units each of these factors are contained in a 15 mL bag. This allows more rapid administration than FFP, whilst reducing the risk of fluid overload. In infants, a dose of 10–15 mL is sufficient to achieve haemostasis.

Clotting factor concentrates

Bleeding or thrombosis in children with proven coagulation or antithrombotic factor deficiency may require specific factor replacement. These factors have become safer with the advent of synthesis using recombinant genetic technology. Recombinant factor VIII concentrate is used to treat haemophilia A whereas recombinant factor IX is the treatment of choice for haemophilia B. Antithrombin III, protein S and protein C concentrates are used to treat patients with these specific factor deficiencies.

Albumin

Indications

Albumin is derived from human plasma pools and is indicated for rapid volume expansion in children with evidence of shock or poor perfusion. In paediatric emergency practice, albumin may be used in the initial fluid resuscitation for hypovolaemic shock, although it is no better than crystalloids or other colloids in this setting in adults. Other indications include the treatment of hypoproteinaemia, severe burns after the first 24 hours and plasma exchange. There is no evidence for albumin use as a nutritional supplement or for the treatment of ascites or oedema related to portal hypertension.

Administration

Albumin 4% (40 g L^{-1}) at 10–20 mL kg^{-1} is used for volume expansion. Albumin 20% (200 g L^{-1}) is used for plasma albumin repletion on a gram-for-gram basis.

Adverse effects and risks

There is evidence that albumin may increase mortality and morbidity in critically-ill adults, aside from those with severe burns, but no such evidence in young children. Albumin may worsen capillary leak in acute respiratory distress syndrome, thereby impeding oxygenation. The relative risk of viral disease transmission is less compared with cellular blood components.

Normal human immunoglobulin (NIGH)

Human immunoglobulin affords passive immunity against many infectious agents for several weeks. NIGH is derived by Cohn fractionation from pooled plasma and contains antibodies to viruses that are prevalent in the general population. Subclasses are present in the approximate proportions G1 60%, G2 30%, G3 6% and G4 4% but there is no such thing as generic IgG. The 'new' purified commercial products are all a little different with different minor reaction rates. NIGH is administered IM for pre- or post-exposure prophylaxis against measles, varicella zoster and hepatitis A. IV NIGH (either Intragam® or Sandoglobulin®) is used to treat idiopathic thrombocytopenic purpura (ITP), Kawasaki's disease, perinatal AIDS, GBS, demyelinating disease, immunological disorders associated with antibody deficiency (such as primary hypogammaglobulinaemia) and sepsis with secondary immunodeficiency. Allergic reactions and rarely anaphylaxis may occur. NIGH is contraindicated in children with selective IgA deficiency and evidence for its role in the treatment and prevention of neonatal sepsis is conflicting. Immune response to live virus vaccines (with the exception of yellow fever vaccine) may be inhibited by NIGH given three weeks before or three months after immunisation.

Hyperimmune immunoglobulins (Ig)

Maternal administration of Rhesus (Rh) Ig prevents the development of Rh antibodies in an Rh-negative mother who gives birth to an Rh-positive baby. This reduces the risk of maternal Rh sensitisation and maternal-neonatal Rh-incompatibility in subsequent pregnancies. CMV Ig is used in the prevention and treatment of CMV in children at risk of adverse sequelae from CMV infection, such as with immunodeficiency and following renal and bone-marrow transplantation. Zoster Ig (ZIG) is advisable within 72 hours after varicella exposure in children with cellular immune deficiency, immunosuppression, neonates whose mothers are susceptible to primary varicella infection and infants who are less than 28 weeks gestation at birth. Infants born to HbsAg-positive mothers should receive hepatitis B Ig and commence primary hepatitis B vaccination within 12 hours of birth. Respiratory syncytial virus (RSV) Ig is used prophylactically in infants at high risk of severe RSV infection, including those with bronchopulmonary dysplasia. Tetanus Ig passively protects non-tetanus immune children who sustain a tetanus-prone wound and a tetanus Ig infusion is used to treat clinical disease.

RISKS OF BLOOD COMPONENT USE

These are categorised as acute or delayed, haemolytic or non-haemolytic, allergy-based or not. Other complications include those associated with massive transfusion (fluid overload, hypothermia, coagulopathy, dilutional thrombocytopenia) and with gaining venous access. Mild non-haemolytic febrile reactions can occur with any blood component and need to be distinguished from major reactions. If a major reaction occurs, the transfusion is discontinued and threats to the airway, breathing and circulation are attended to. Specific treatment for anaphylaxis, sepsis and blood group incompatibility may be required, in consultation with a haematologist. Recipient and donor blood samples are sent for immunological and microbiological testing. Critical adverse incidents should be notified to the blood bank and followed up as a quality assurance activity with appropriate adjustments made to hospital transfusion protocols to reduce risk of recurrence.

Infections

Even though blood components are the safest they have ever been, infection transmission risk remains emotive and highly publicised. Infection acquired from a blood component is a rare occurrence by itself, and when compared with non-infectious complications. The estimated risks per actual blood unit transfused are 1:200 000–1:2 000 000 for HIV, 1:30 000–1:250 000 for hepatitis B and 1:30 000–1:150 000 for hepatitis C. Disease transmission occurs primarily during the window period when a blood donor is infectious and the infection is immunologically silent and therefore undetectable on screening tests. Other infectious agents encountered include hepatitis A and G, HTLV I and II, parvovirus B19, syphilis, malaria, babesiosis, *Salmonella* and *Trypanosoma cruzi*. There is no current evidence to suggest that variant Creutzfeldt–Jakob disease can be transmitted by blood transfusion. Donor selection and exclusion, donated blood screening, post-collection leucodepletion and viral inactivation help to minimise risk of infection transmission. Using pooled blood components allows contamination of the entire pool from one infectious donor and is therefore less safe than components derived from a single donor. Bacterial contamination of blood components, either from prolonged/faulty storage or acquired from the donor, is most frequently due to occult donor bacteraemia and donor skin organisms. *Yersinia enterocolitica* and other Gram negatives are most frequently implicated.

Transfusion-related acute lung injury

Acute respiratory distress syndrome with non-cardiogenic pulmonary oedema occurs within four hours in 1:5000 transfusions, with 90% of patients recovering. This reaction may be difficult to distinguish from fluid overload and is related to immune-mediated increased pulmonary capillary permeability.

Transfusion-mediated immunomodulation

Allosensitisation, disturbed immunomodulation (both due to contamination by donor leucocytes) as well as infection transmission may be reduced by leucocyte-depletion, psoralens and UV irradiation of blood components and using non-pooled blood components from a single donor. Whether exposure to donor blood significantly predisposes to increased postoperative infection and cancer recurrence is unclear.

Transfusion-associated graft-versus-host disease (TA-GVHD)

This occurs as a result of transfused lymphocytes engrafting and proliferating in the transfusion recipient. TA-GVHD is fatal in 90% of cases because of induction of marrow hypoplasia. Irradiation of cellular blood components is effective prevention.

CONTROVERSIES AND FUTURE DIRECTIONS

❶ The threshold for red cell transfusion at which benefits outweigh risk in children and non-critically ill adults remains unclear.

❷ The role and potential harm of albumin in adult resuscitation has not been identified in paediatric resuscitation and the role of immunoglobulins in severe sepsis remains uncertain.

❸ Oxygen-carrying red cell substitutes such as cell-free haemoglobins and perfluorocarbon emulsions may offer the same benefits as red blood cells without the infection-transmission risk.

❹ The role of non-blood alternatives such as autologous blood donation, perioperative blood salvage and directed parental transfusion are not clearly defined in children.

FURTHER READING

American Association of Blood Banks 2003 Facts about blood and blood banking. http://www. aabb.org [accessed 29 January 2003]

Christensen RD 2000 Hematologic problems of the neonate. WB Saunders Company, Philadelphia

Goodnough LT, Brecher ME, Kanter MH, AuBuchon JP 1999 Transfusion medicine. Blood transfusion. New England Journal of Medicine 340: 438–447

Goodnough LT, Shander A, Brecher RE 2003 Transfusion medicine: Looking to the future. Lancet 361: 161–169

Behrman RE, Kleigman RM 2002 Intercontinental childhood ITP registry. In: Nelson essentials of pediatrics, 4th edn. WB Saunders, Philadelphia

Kruskall MS 1997 The perils of platelet transfusions. New England Journal of Medicine 337: 1914–1915

Miller DR, Bachner RL 1995 Blood diseases of infancy and childhood. In the tradition of Carl H Smith. Mosby-Year Book, 7th edn. Mosby, St Louis, MO

National Health and Medical Research Council 2002 Clinical practice guidelines on the use of blood components (red blood cells, platelets, fresh frozen plasma, cryoprecipitate). Australian Society of Blood Transfusion, Canberra

National Health and Medical Research Council 2002 Blood components: A guide for patients. Australian Society of Blood Transfusion, Canberra

Regan F, Taylor C 2002 Recent developments. Blood transfusion medicine. British Medical Journal 325: 143–147

Sadowitz PD, Ammanullah S, Souid AK et al 2002 Hematologic emergencies in the pediatric ER. Emergency Medicine Clinics of North America 20: 177–88, vii

Smith H 1996 Diagnosis in paediatric haematology. Churchill Livingstone, New York

11.2 ANAEMIA

MARIAN LEE

Essentials

1 The normal haemoglobin concentration and type is age and sex dependent.

2 Clinical effects of anaemia depend on the tempo of development, the magnitude of the anaemia and the underlying cause.

Iron-deficiency anaemia is the commonest cause of microcytic and hypochromic anaemia.

4 Intravascular haemolysis is Coombs' test positive and free haemoglobin is present in the plasma.

5 Extravascular haemolysis is Coombs' test negative and haemoglobin is released in the reticuloendothelial system.

6 Autoimmune haemolytic anaemia (AIHA) is caused by a variety of infective agents. Additionally, autoantibodies can be triggered by a number of systemic illnesses.

7 Non-immune haemolytic anaemia can be due to infective agents, medications and chemical exposures.

8 Erythrocyte fragmentation syndromes are due to direct mechanical damage to the erythrocytes, resulting in haemolysis.

9 Haemolytic uraemic syndrome (HUS) is the commonest cause of acute renal failure in children and the most commonest cause is *E. coli*.

10 Thrombotic thrombocytopenic purpura affects children over the age of 10 years. The clinical features are similar to HUS with the addition of neurological deficit. The renal failure is less severe.

11 G6PD deficiency is an X-linked enzymatic inborn error in which haemolysis is triggered by exposure to an oxidant.

12 Thalassaemia is a relatively common inherited defect in the synthesis of the globin chain.

13 Sickle cell disease is an inherited condition with a globin chain that is unstable in the deoxygenated state and undergoes haemolysis.

14 Hyposplenism can be congenital or functional and potential bacterial infections must be treated aggressively.

15 Hypersplenism refers to splenomegaly and resulting increased sequestration and destruction of red blood cells, neutrophils and platelets. The most common cause is splenic congestion due to portal hypertension.

16 Treatment options for hypersplenism include total or partial splenectomy, and partial splenic embolisation.

17 Splenic sequestration in SCD is defined clinically as an enlarging spleen with an associated fall of the haemoglobin greater or equal to 20 g L^{-1} from the patient's baseline value.

INTRODUCTION

Anaemia is a reduction in the haemoglobin concentration due to a reduction in the total erythrocyte (RBC) mass. Haemoglobin is the major functional constituent of the RBC responsible for the task of carrying oxygen to the tissues with the RBC acting as the carrier through the cardiovascular system. The normal haemoglobin level is age and sex dependent.

After a trough level of 114 g L$^{-1} \times 90$ g L^{-1} between 8 and 12 weeks of age, the haemoglobin rises again to reach the lower threshold of the adult range with a further increase in adolescence.

Erythropoietin, the hormone that regulates the production of erythrocytes, is produced in the foetal liver and, after birth, in the renal peritubular cells. In normal erythropoiesis there is a condensation of the nuclear material with con-

tinual production of the haemoglobin until it is 90% of the mass of the RBC. The nucleus is then extruded so the RBC has no synthetic or replication ability. The implication is a limited lifespan of 120 days in a normal RBC and much less if there are any intrinsic abnormalities. Haemoglobin is composed of an iron-containing molecule known as haeme coupled with two globin chains of polypeptides. There are six types of

303

Table 11.2.1 Causes of anaemia

Haemorrhage
1. Traumatic
2. Non-traumatic
   - Acute or chronic

Production defect
1. Primary bone marrow failure
   - Aplastic anaemia (congenital or acquired)
   - Diamond-Blackfan syndrome
   - Transient erythroblastopenia of childhood
2. Erythropoietin production problem
   - Chronic renal disease
   - Hypothyroidism
3. Abnormal cytoplasmic maturation (microcytic anaemias)
   - Iron deficiency
   - Sideroblastic anaemia (congenital or acquired)
   - Lead toxicity
   - Thalassaemia syndrome
4. Megaloblastic anaemia
   - Vitamin B_{12} deficiency
   - Folate deficiency
   - Thiamine-responsive megaloblastic anaemia
   - Orotic aciduria (rare, associated with megaloblastic anaemia)
5. Others
   - Primary dyserythropoietic anaemias
   - Erythropoietic protoporphyria
   - Marrow infiltration, e.g. malignancy or myelofibrosis

Decreased RBC survival (haemolytic anaemia)
1. Hereditary haemolytic anaemias
   a. Haemoglobin variants
      - Thalassaemias
      - Sickle cell disease
   b. Abnormal RBC membranes
      - Hereditary spherocytosis
      - Hereditary elliptocytosis
      - Hereditary stomatocytosis
   c. Abnormal enzymes
      - Glucose-6-phosphotase dehydrogenase deficiency (G6PD)
      - Pyruvate kinase deficiency
2. Acquired haemolytic anaemias
   a. Autoimmune haemolytic anaemia (AIHA)
   b. Non-immune haemolytic anaemia
   c. Fragmentation haemolysis
      - Haemolytic uraemic syndrome (HUS)
      - Thrombocytopenic thrombotic purpura (TTP)

Table 11.2.2 Anaemia in the neonate

1. Physiological anaemia
2. Abnormal RBC production
   a. Nutritional deficiency
   b. Secondary to infection
3. Blood loss
   a Overt blood loss
      - Iatrogenic during delivery
      - Obstetric accidents
   b. Occult blood loss
      - Twin-to-twin transfusion
      - Fetoplacental haemorrhage
      - Fetomaternal haemorrhage
4. Decreased RBC survival (haemolysis)
   a. Immune-related: isoimmunisation
   b. Infection-related
5. Hereditary haemoglobin variants, enzyme abnormalities, membrane abnormalities

haemoglobin present at different stage of life from the embryo to the adult but HbF (foetal Hb) and HbA (adult Hb) comprise nearly 100% of the haemoglobin at birth. Minor amounts of HbA_2 are present at all ages and HbF disappears by about three months of age.

OVERVIEW

The principles of management of anaemia in the ED are:

❶ Resuscitate the patient with circulatory collapse.

❷ Remove or treat the precipitant if known.

❸ Treat the cause if it can be initiated in the ED (see Tables 11.2.1 and 11.2.2).

Causes of life-threatening anaemia include uncontrolled haemorrhage, acute intravascular haemolysis in glucose-6-phosphatase deficiency (G6PD) or autoimmune haemolytic anaemia (AIHA), sequestration crisis in sickle cell disease (SCD) and acute decompensation in chronic anaemia (see Table 11.2.1). Initial assessment is directed at circulation and

respiration. The anaemic patient may be tachypnoeic with tissue hypoxia. The adequacy of ventilation should be ascertained and supplemental oxygen provided. Circulatory compromise in acute haemorrhage and acute haemolysis requires cardiorespiratory monitoring and intravenous access for fluid resuscitation (see Chapter 2.5 on shock). Packed red blood cells are used if haemorrhage or haemolysis is life-threatening. If tissue oxygenation is not critically affected, the circulatory volume should be sustained with colloid or crystalloid until group-specific or cross-matched RBCs are available. If the bleeding is controlled with further bleeding unlikely, the signs mentioned above are stable and the haemoglobin concentration is greater than 70 g L^{-1}, a cross-match should be performed and the packed RBCs should be held in reserve for 24 hours. Early consultation with a haematologist is important in acute haemolytic anaemia especially if the underlying cause has not been diagnosed.

Anaemia is a clinical finding rather than a disease in its own right and symptoms depend on the tempo of development, the severity and the underlying cause. The presentation is frequently not specific to anaemia. Common presenting features consistent with insidious onset anaemia include:

- Lethargy, irritability, sleep or settling difficulty

- Pallor or yellow skin hue
- Loss of appetite ± weight loss ± pica
- Bruising, bleeding or infection.

Patient factors to note are age, ethnicity and the presence of other significant disease. Iron-deficiency anaemia is uncommon in the first six months in term infants and SCD is unlikely to present as anaemia under the age of four months. Haemolytic uraemic syndrome (HUS) mainly affects those under four years of age, whereas thrombotic thrombocytopenic purpura (TTP) affects children from ten years of age. Iron deficiency is common in adolescent females whereas G6PD deficiency occurs mainly in males. The association between ethnicity and various types of hereditary anaemia is shown in Table 11.2.3. Family history of anaemia will also suggest hereditary anaemia.

Dietary history can provide important clues. Iron-deficiency anaemia is likely in prolonged breast-feeding beyond six months of age in term infants and sooner in preterm infants if no iron supplementation is provided, if there is excessive dependence on cows' milk as a food source or if food sources are restricted, e.g. food fads. Ingestion of clay and dirt is found in lead toxicity and iron defi-ciency. Ingestion of fresh uncooked broad beans is a potent precipitant of haemolysis in G6PD along with medications.

Recent infections may precipitate AIHA, non-immune haemolytic anaemia, HUS and TTP. Hyperbilirubinaemia caused by haemolysis leads to jaundice, cholelithiasis, cholecystitis and dark urine. Mechanical destruction of RBCs is caused by vascular malformations, shunts, abnormal native or prosthetic cardiac valves. Septic shock, bleeding disorders, chronic renal disease, severe burns and hypothyroidism may all cause anaemia.

The salient physical findings in the context of anaemia relate to general appearance, cardiovascular status and abdominal examination. Frontal bone expansion and frontal bossing seen in thalassaemias is due to expansion of the medullary spaces and Diamond-Blackfan anaemia is also associated with physical abnormalities. Hepatosplenomegaly is a feature of some the hereditary haemolytic anaemias. Purpuric or petechial rashes are due to coagulation disorders or vasculitis. Dark urine from bilirubinuria is consistent with haemolysis and haematuria must be confirmed by microscopy to distinguish haemoglobinuria from haematuria.

The anaemia is confirmed by the lowered haemoglobin concentration and decreased RBC count. An age-related reference range must be used. Abnormalities in the other cell lines should be noted. The mean cell volume (MCV) may suggest an underlying cause. The upper limit of normal in adults is 96 fl but MCV in children is less than in adults and average values may be estimated by adding 0.6 fl per year of age to 84 fl. The reticulocyte count is expressed as a percentage of the circulating RBC mass with a normal range of 0.5–1.5%. A low reticulocyte count is found in abnormalities of RBC production and a high reticulocyte count is found in increased destruction or from RBC loss, provided there is no concurrent bone-marrow pathology. Morphological features of RBC may be diagnostic of the underlying cause as shown in Table 11.2.4.

There are many additional investigations apart from full blood count (FBC) to assist in identification of the underlying cause. Some that are undertaken in the ED include:

❶ Hyperbilirubinaemia because elevated unconjugated component suggests haemolysis.
❷ Elevated urea and creatinine to detect renal failure in HUS and TTP.
❸ Iron studies (serum iron , total iron binding capacity, transferrin saturation).
❹ Coombs' tests to identify immune-related haemolysis.
❺ Haemoglobin electrophoresis.

Identification and treatment of the underlying precipitant, where appropriate and possible, is a crucial part of the management of anaemia in the ED. Packed RBCs are indicated in the treatment of severe anaemia with cardiovascular compromise. A dose of 4 mL kg^{-1} of packed RBCs will raise the haemoglobin concentration by 10 g L^{-1}. This dose can be given hourly or slower in the presence cardiac failure. Furosemide 1 mg kg^{-1} may be given if there is evidence of volume overload. Involvement of a paediatric haematologist is recommended for all but the simple nutritional anaemias.

Table 11.2.3   Ethnicity and anaemia

1. Thalassaemia syndromes
   - α-Thalassaemia – descendents from China, Malaysia, Indonesia and Africa
   - β-Thalassaemia – descendents from Africa, Middle East, Mediterranean, India, Pakistan, China
2. Sickle cell disease
   - Descendents of population from Africa, Southern Arabia, Turkey, Greece, central India
3. Hereditary spherocytosis
   - Descendants of population from northern Europe
4. G6PD deficiency
   - Descendants from Africa, China, south east Asia and the Mediterranean

---

Table 11.2.4   Morphological features of RBCs to assist the diagnosis of anaemia

Schistocytes	Erythrocyte fragmentation syndromes
Sickle cells	Sickle cell disease
Spherocytes	Immune-mediated haemolytic anaemia Hereditary spherocytosis
Blister or bite cells with poikilocytosis	G6P deficiency

NEONATAL ANEMIA

In the term neonate, the haemoglobin at birth is in the range of 159–191 g L^{-1} and rises in the first 24 hours. Subsequently it falls to a trough level of 114 g $L^{-1} \times 90$ g L^{-1} between eight and twelve weeks of age. This initial anaemia is due to a combination of haemodilution at birth, a comparatively lesser life span of the neonatal RBC and a sharp decline in haemopoiesis a few days after birth.

Physiologic

Immune-related haemolysis is the commonest cause of anaemia in the neonate. Maternal antibodies pass through the placenta leading to foetal cell lysis. Haemolysis occurs when the target foetal cells are the RBCs. The commonest antigen responsible is the Rhesus antigen on the RBC surface followed by ABO incompatibility. The sensitisation of the mother occurs when Rhesus incompatible foetal cells gain access to the maternal circulation. Foetal RBCs can be found from eight weeks' gestation onwards.As little as 0.05–0.10 mL is enough to cause primary immunisation but the volume and the risk increases with obstetric procedures, miscarriages and toxaemia. Foetal harm occurs during a subsequent pregnancy with a Rhesus positive fetus in a Rhesus negative mother. The resultant intravascular haemolysis of the fetus can be devastating. The clinical significance is due both to the severity of the anaemia and kernicterus from the hyperbilirubinaemia. ABO incompatability produces less severe jaundice and anaemia during the second week of life.

Prevention relies on identification of the Rhesus status of all pregnant women. This is an essential task for any doctor involved in antenatal care. Prophylaxis therapy using anti-D immunoglobulin (Ig) is given to all Rhesus negative women with per vaginal bleeding or requiring any obstetric procedures that may lead to foetomaternal haemorrhage. The recommended dose is 250 IU if the sensitizing event occurs in the first trimester and 625 IU beyond this gestation period. This passive immunisation is given intra- muscularly. If required in the postpartum period the immunoglobulin is administered intravenously.

Infection and haemolysis

Infections cause anaemia by producing bone-marrow suppression of erythropoiesis or by haemolysis. The infections of relevance in the neonate are cytomegalovirus (CMV), rubella, toxoplasmosis and congenital syphilis. The human parvovirus may lead to spontaneous miscarriage in early pregnancy and, in late pregnancy, can selectively depress erythropoiesis producing severe foetal anaemia. In the older child, parvovirus is the cause for fifth disease, which can be complicated by aplastic crisis or chronic haemolysis. Vertical transmission of malaria to the foetus is a major cause of anaemia in the neonate in endemic regions. HIV infection in the neonate is predominantly acquired via perinatal transmission from the mother. The transmission rate is in the range of 20–40%. The mechanism is bone-marrow suppression and associated pancytopenia as well as chronic multi-system disease.

Haemoglobinopathies and enzymopathies

G6PD deficiency is an important global cause of neonatal jaundice. Haemolysis from other enzymopathies and haemoglobin variants, such as thalassaemias and SCD, is usually unmasked beyond the neonatal period when the proportion of foetal haemoglobin falls. It is important to consider congenital causes of anaemia in children with a family history of hereditary anaemia or persisting neonatal jaundice.

Blood loss

Blood loss may arise from twin-to-twin transfusion, or obstetric procedures, or as part of the delivery of the neonate in the perinatal period. Haemorrhage from an underlying haematological disorder must be considered. Vitamin K deficiency is normally present at birth but only a minority of neonates will develop generalised bleeding. Breast milk has a small amount of vitamin K and, in the breast-fed baby, maternal medications may compound the deficiency. The likely ones are warfarin, phenytoin, rifampicin and isoniazid. Nutritional vitamin K deficiency has been associated with prolonged breast-feeding without supplementation, malabsorption, chronic diarrhoea, and prolonged use of oral antibiotics. Vitamin K prophylaxis is normally given at birth. Haemophilia can rarely lead to spontaneous haemorrhage in the newborn.

ANAEMIAS OF CHILDHOOD

Iron-deficiency

Iron deficiency is uncommon in the first six months in the term infant due to the efficient recycling of the iron from the haeme component of the haemoglobin when it is metabolised. In the preterm and low-birth-weight neonate, iron deficiency occurs earlier, often at the time of doubling of the birth weight. In the second six months of life, iron deficiency is found in 20% of Australian children with associated anaemia in 3%. The respective figures in the second year are 35% and 9%. It is even more common in indigenous children and children from non-English-speaking backgrounds. In school-age children, iron deficiency is present in 1–2% but is found in up to 9% of adolescent girls.

Stages

The first stage of iron deficiency is a low serum ferritin level. Iron-dependent body functions, including erythropoiesis, are affected in stage two. Microcytes and an elevated erythrocyte protoporphyrin level are detectable and the serum iron falls. The third stage is the presence of a microcytic hypochromic anaemia.

Causes

The commonest cause globally is insufficient intake of dietary iron. In developing countries, the two most significant factors are the failure to obtain iron-rich nutrients and malabsorption from intestinal pathology. The aetiology is different in developed countries, such as Australia, where prolonged breast-feeding beyond six months of age without supplementation with iron-rich foods is a common finding. Breast milk has easily absorpable iron in modest amounts. The quantity is inadequate for the rapid growth in the second six months. Cows' milk has minimal iron content, which exists in a poorly absorbable form and is not recommended under the age of twelve months. Cows' milk can cause gastrointestinal bleeding in the immature gut and children who have an excess intake of cows' milk will have a lower appetite for other foods. More than two serves of milk per day is not advisable. Iron-fortified cereals should be introduced from five months of age.

Adverse effects

Iron deficiency before 24 months can lead to impaired development of cognitive and psychomotor skills, which may be only partially reversible when the deficiency and the associated anaemia is corrected. Many parents report loss of appetite, irritability and inability to concentrate. Pica may be present. Iron deficiency affects neutrophil and lymphocyte function in vitro and is indicated as one of the investigations of recurrent infections.

Diagnosis

Iron deficiency is the commonest cause of microcytic hypochromic anaemia and is characterised by a low serum iron, a high total iron binding capacity and a low transferrin saturation. The reticulocyte count is less than 2% unless iron had been reintroduced into the diet. The diagnosis is not confirmed until iron supplementation is followed by a reticulocytosis within 1–2 weeks and a rise in the haemoglobin over 2–4 weeks. Other conditions producing microcytic anaemia must be considered if there is poor response to iron supplementation.

Treatment

Dietary advice and education are the basis of prevention and treatment in developed countries. If iron supplementation is required, the ferrous form is more effectively absorbed either as syrup or tablets at 2–3 mg kg^{-1} d^{-1}. The treatment dose for severe anaemia is up to 6 mg kg^{-1} d^{-1}, but side effects of nausea, vomiting, and constipation are dose-related. Transfusion is only ever required if there is cardiovascular compromise. Parents should be informed regarding the toxicity of iron in overdose so that they store the medication safely.

HAEMOLYTIC ANAEMIAS

Haemolysis is normal and 1% of the RBC population is removed and replaced per day. In the older age group, the bone marrow's capacity to accommodate an increase in erythropoiesis can compensate for mild pathological haemolysis. In the infant and young child the bone marrow is maximally active with minimal ability to increase erythropoiesis and anaemia accompanies pathological haemolysis.

Intravascular vs. extravascular haemolysis

Intravascular haemolysis is a Coombs'-test-positive process where free haemoglobin is liberated in plasma and combines with haptoglobin resulting in decreased serum haptoglobin. RBC fragmentation, spherocytes and sometimes tear-shaped cells are found on the peripheral blood film. Spherocytosis and other characteristic red-cell changes are due to membrane loss as splenic macrophages attack antibody-coated red blood cells. LDH, an RBC enzyme, is raised and free haemoglobin and haeme-albumin may be found in the plasma. Extravascular haemolysis is a Coombs'-test-negative process where haemoglobin is liberated in the reticuloendothelial system. It is associated with haemoglobinaemia, haemoglobinuria and haemosiderinuria.

ACQUIRED HAEMOLYTIC ANAEMIAS

Autoimmune haemolytic anaemia (AIHA)

A variety of infectious agents (EBV, CMV, mumps, mycoplasma and tuberculosis) can cause severe anaemia in the younger child. The antibody involved is mainly cold haemagglutinins—IgM, but can be IgG. Other diseases that trigger autoantibodies include systemic lupus erythematosus, rheumatoid arthritis, thyrotoxicosis, ulcerative colitis, malignancy and immunodeficiency syndromes. Idiopathic autoimmune anaemia can be rapidly progressive over days in the young infant and chronic and relapsing in the older child.

In children the pattern is most frequently an acute episode of severe anaemia with resolution within three months. Haemoglobin drops to less than 60 g L^{-1} in over 50%. A slower onset is more likely to follow a chronic and relapsing course with guarded prognosis.

A reticulocytosis may not be present initially due to rapid onset. Associated immune thrombocytopenia is present in a third. Direct Coombs' antiglobulin test is positive. IgG causes warm AIHA while IgM and complement are responsible for cold AIHA. The former has maximum activity at 37°C and the latter are active between 0 and 30°C. Serology may be useful in identifying the infective agent. Hyperbilirubinaemia is present.

IgG-induced AIHA responds to prednisone 2–10 mg kg^{-1}. This is not effective in cold agglutinin disease, which may require plasmapheresis. Both may respond to immunoglobulin, 1 g kg^{-1} IV, and require exchange transfusion if disease is severe. Splenectomy is a last resort in IgG-induced AIHA. A haematologist should be consulted regarding specific treatment.

Non-immune haemolytic anaemia

Non-immune haemolytic anaemia can also be caused by a variety of infectious agents (malaria, Gram-positive and Gram-negative organisms), medications (salicylates, sulfasalazine, nitrofurantoin) and chemicals (naphthalene). Clinical features are similar to AIHA but Coombs' test is negative. Treatment is supportive focusing on the identification and treatment of the underlying cause.

Erythrocyte fragmentation syndrome

These are haemolytic anaemias due to direct physical or mechanical damage to the erythrocytes. They are characterised by red cell fragmentation with schistocytes and spherocytes in the peripheral blood film and the features of intravascular haemolysis mentioned previously. There are two groups.

MACROANGIOPATHIC HAEMOLYTIC ANAEMIA

Macroangiopathic haemolytic anaemia results from RBC damage upon passage through large vessels and the heart and is associated with structural cardiac abnormality or large vessel disease (coarctation of the aorta). It can follow cardiac surgery but infection or failure of the prostheses must be considered if it occurs distinct from the surgical period. It is less likely with xenografts and also when prostheses are covered by endothelium. The damage is from a combination of shearing forces from turbulent flow and interaction between the cells and the abnormal surfaces. The anaemia is usually mild and severe haemolysis is uncommon. Treatment of the underlying cause is important.

MICROANGIOPATHIC HAEMOLYTIC ANAEMIA

Microangiopathic haemolytic anaemia is due to RBC damage as they pass through diseased or partially occluded arterioles and capillaries and is often acute and severe with associated thrombocytopenia. The commonest causes are HUS under four years of age and TTP in the child ten years and older but connective tissue disease, haemangiomas and severe burns can all be causes.

Haemolytic uraemic syndrome (HUS)

HUS is the commonest cause of acute renal failure in children. In warmer climates it may be endemic but in cooler climates it occurs sporadically. More than 90% of affected children are under the age of four years with peak incidence in children between the age of four months to two years. Numerous infections can trigger HUS including *Shigella*, *Salmonella*, *Yersinia*, *Campylobacter*, *Streptococcus pneumoniae*, echovirus, coxsackievirus A and B, and varicella. The commonest

organism is *E. coli* and verocytotoxin is the toxic agent.

HUS is usually preceded by an infection with vomiting and bloody diarrhoea. Fever is present and oliguria occurs within days. Hypertension may be present. The thrombocytopenia is mild and severe bleeding is uncommon. Rarely, cardiomyopathy, cerebral infarcts or haemorrhage, bowel perforations and diabetes may complicate HUS.

The peripheral blood film will show the typical schistocytes. A leucocytosis with left shift often accompanies the anaemia and thrombocytopenia. Stool samples should be tested for verocytotoxin. Raised urea and creatinine indicate renal failure.

This is directed at the acute renal failure with early dialysis indicated in some cases. Transfusion of packed RBCs may be required. Platelet transfusion is not indicated unless there is active bleeding. Careful monitoring is essential.

The long-term outcome for the acute renal failure is good. Atypical HUS following an upper respiratory tract infection may manifest severe hypertension and renal failure. The prognosis for the latter is poor. Recurrence of the disease occurs in 50%.

Thrombotic thrombocytopenic purpura (TTP)

This clinical syndrome is similar to the above with the addition of neurological deficit. The latter may take the form of an altered level of consciousness ranging from confusion, to seizure or coma. Cranial nerve palsies may also be present. The renal failure is not as severe compared to HUS but the thrombocytopenia is more severe. TTP usually affects children older than ten years. Possible triggers include mycoplasma and viral infections, HIV and subacute bacterial endocarditis but none is evident in the majority of patients. Underlying immunological disease may be relevant as is pregnancy and genetic predisposition. Treatment is supportive mainly via exchange transfusion using FFP. If there is no improvement in 24 hours then plasmapheresis is considered. Transfusion of packed RBCs is rarely needed for severe anaemia. Involvement of a paediatric haematologist is mandatory.

HEREDITARY HAEMOLYTIC ANAEMIA

Glucose-6-phosphatase (G6PD) deficiency

G6PD deficiency renders the RBC vulnerable to haemolysis when exposed to an oxidant. G6PD is the enzyme in the pathway leading to generation of NADPH which maintains glutathione in its reduced form. Reduced glutathione is an essential factor in the degradation of cellular peroxides that may otherwise damage cellular proteins including haemoglobin. The enzyme activity is higher in the younger RBCs but deteriorates as the cell ages so older RBCs are more prone to haemolysis.

G6PD is an X-linked recessive condition with wide variability of expression depending on the biochemical type, the oxidant stress and the sex of the patient. Homozygous females are rare and the disease is predominantly found in males. The severity of the disease varies and levels of enzyme at or above 40% of normal will rarely result in clinically significant haemolysis. A number of different variants are found in patients of African, Chinese and Mediterranean descent.

Viral and bacterial infections can both cause acute haemolysis especially in children less than 2 to 3 years of age. Oxidant drugs and chemicals that commonly cause haemolysis include naphthalene, sulphonamides, antimalarials, nitrofurantoin, diazoxide and dapsone. Favism refers to the acute haemolysis resulting from the ingestion of broad bean (*Vicia faba*) or inhalation of the pollen in those with the Mediterranean variant but not those with the African variant. The haemolytic agent in the broad bean can be passed to the infant by breast milk. The anaemia is present within 3–36 hours and usually lasts for 2–6 days. Death can occur within 24 hours of the haemolysis. Definitive diagnosis of G6PD deficiency is via a quantitative assay of the enzyme. Treatment is non-specific. Prevention is crucial with avoidance of oxidating medications and prompt treatment of infections.

THALASSAEMIAS

Thalassaemia is one of the commonest inherited haemoglobin variants. Defective synthesis of globin chains leads to abnormal pairing of the globin chains in the haemoglobin molecule. Excess chains tend to aggregate, precipitate and cause damage to the RBCs. The nomenclature depicts the missing chain, e.g. β-thalassaemia refers to a deficiency of the β-chain. In general, the homozygote state is incompatible with life and haemolysis occurs in the heterozygous patient. Haemoglobin electrophoresis defines the haemoglobin variants.

β-Thalassaemia major

Each carrier parent must donate one abnormal gene to the offspring and there is a 25% chance of a homozygote progeny with β-thalassaemia major. No β-chains are produced so presentation is in the first month of life when the foetal haemoglobin is falling with an increasing reliance on adult haemoglobin. Excess unpaired α-chains aggregate to form an unstable tetramer, which is functionally useless. Haemolysis and severe anaemia occur unless there are sufficient RBCs with HbF to sustain life. Extramedullary haemopoiesis with hepatosplenomegaly accompanies expansion of the marrow, which results in skeletal changes (e.g. bossing of the frontal bone). The peripheral blood film shows a microcytic hypochromic anaemia with marked poikilocytosis, target cells and reticulocytosis. Basophilic stippling may be seen in the RBCs. Iron and folate deficiency may be demonstrated. The prognosis is bleak. Transfusion dependency occurs to prevent marrow expansion but this results in iron overload.

β-Thalassaemia minor

There is enough β-chain production and normal haemoglobin to avoid symptomatic anaemia. The life span of the RBCs is only slightly decreased. The anaemia is microcytic and hypochromic with target cells and elliptocytes. HbA_2 level in the range of 3.5–7.0% is almost diagnostic of the β-thalassaemia trait. The bone marrow is hyperplastic. Attention to potential iron and folate deficiency is important. The absence of an age-related rise in the MCV and MHC in a patient of the relevant ethnicity should prompt further investigations.

α-Thalassaemia

Two genes on chromosome 16 code for the α-chain, producing four possible phenotypes. Deletion of one α-gene is asymptomatic with a minority having a microcytic hypochromic anaemia. Deletion of two α-genes produces mild anaemia. Deletion of three α-genes results in HbH disease due to aggregation of β-chains, which leads to an unstable haemoglobin. There is a chronic haemolysis with anaemia in the range of 70–110 g L^{-1}, jaundice, cholelithiasis, hepatomegaly and leg ulcers. Deletion of four α-genes results in intrauterine death and stillbirths usually after 25 weeks' gestation. Live births have a severe anaemia, which may lead to congestive cardiac failure. The fetus is grossly oedematous. The haemoglobins present are HbH, Hb Barat (four γ-chains) and small amounts of Hb Portland (two ζ and two γ). None of these are functional.

SICKLE CELL DISEASE

Sickle cell disease (SCD) is an inherited condition in which glutamine in the sixth position of the globin chain is replaced by valine. In the homozygote with HbSS the haemoglobin is unstable in the deoxygenated state. It precipitates in the RBC and leads to a change in the biconcave shape to a configuration resembling a sickle. This change is initially reversible. The consequences are multiple. It is detrimental to the RBC and the end-organs. Sickle cells have a reduced life-span of 10–20 days and occlude the microvasculature leading to end-organ ischaemia. The precipitants for the sickling are:

- Tissue hypoxia
- Tissue acidosis
- Dehydration
- Vascular stasis
- Increased 2,3-diphosphoglycerate (2,3-DPG) levels in the RBC.

Clinical features

The baseline haemoglobin in SCD is in the range of 60–90 g L^{-1} with a reticulocytosis of 5–15%. Vaso-occlusive crises are acute episodes of severe pain from tissue infarction resulting from vessel occlusion by the sickled cells. The major organs involved are bones, lungs, liver, spleen, brain and the penis. Painful bone crisis is the commonest with minimal signs on examination. In aplastic crisis, the reticulocytosis falls to less than 1%. The haematocrit may fall as rapidly as 10–15% per day. The precipitant is usually an infection. Spontaneous recovery is usually the case. Supportive therapy may involve transfusion of RBCs. Acute splenic sequestration can occur suddenly with acute pallor, weakness, abdominal pain and distension with features of hypovolaemic shock. The precipitant is usually an intercurrent infection. The key finding is circulatory shock in a child with atraumatic abdominal pain and distension. A massive tender spleen is unmistakable. The haematocrit is usually less than 50% of baseline. Reticulocytosis and moderately severe thrombocytopenia are present. Splenic sequestration of RBCs affects those SCD sufferers who are young enough to still have a spleen as autosplenectomy from infarction commonly occurs. Hepatic sequestration may also occur but the volume of trapped RBCs is unlikely to lead to devastating hypovolaemia due to the tight hepatic capsule. Treatment is resuscitation of the intravascular volume. Prevention of sickling of those RBCs remaining in the circulation is important as is the prompt treatment of the infective precipitant.

Diagnosis

Diagnosis is made on the family history and presentation. It is confirmed by haemoglobin electrophoresis and the 'sickle prep' test outside the neonatal age group. The 'sickle prep' uses sodium metabisulfite, which extracts oxygen from the RBC and causes sickling. Parents can be tested for further confirmation.

CONTROVERSIES

❶ The evidence for the detrimental effects of iron deficiency on psychomotor development in children under the age of three years is unclear. There is also a lack of clear evidence for the beneficial effects of iron therapy on psychomotor development in this group. There is a need for a large randomised controlled trial of iron-replacement therapy in children with iron-deficiency anaemia.

❷ Acute splenic sequestration (ASS) is a life-threatening complication of sickle cell disease (SCD) occurring in 7–30% of patients under the age of two years with homozygous SCD. It has also been reported in heterozygous cases. ASS recurs with the interval between episodes being less each time. Splenectomy, partial or total, is one of the methods used to prevent ASS and also to reduce the mortality from SCD.

❸ Following splenectomy, the younger the child the greater the risk of septicaemia. The alternative is a regime of periodic blood transfusion but, in developing countries, a schedule of repeated red-cell transfusion is unlikely to be reliably and safely obtained.

❹ Patients with splenectomy in developing countries may not have access to vaccines, such as those against pneumococcus and meningococcus infections, and splenectomy in this context also places the patient at an increased risk of falciparum malaria infection. Hence, treatment is on an individual basis and varies according to region.

Sickle cell trait

Sickle cell trait is a carrier state with a ratio of HbS to HbA of 40:60. The RBCs have a normal lifespan. Other heterozygote variants have milder forms of the disease.

FURTHER READING

Browne GJ 1997 Blood disorders and malignancies. In: Browne GJ, Choong RKC, Gaudry PL, Wilkins BH (eds), Principles and practice of children's emergency care. Maclennan and Petty, Sydney, 277–293

Buchanan GR 1987 Hemorrhagic disease. In: Nathan DG, Oski FA (eds), Hematology of infancy and childhood. WB Saunders, Philadelphia, 104–127

Cohen AR 1988 Hematological emergencies. In: Fleisher G, Ludwig S (eds), Textbook of pediatric emergency medicine, 2nd edn. Williams & Wilkins, Baltimore, 521–547

Dosage guidelines for prevention of RhD haemolytic disease of the newborn. 2002 CSL RhD Immunoglobulin Product Information

Eberst ME 2000 Acquired hemolytic anemia. In: Tintinalli JE, Kelen GD, Stapczynski JS (eds), Emergency medicine—a comprehensive study guide, 5th edn. McGraw-Hill, 1387–1391

Fitzpatrick M 1999 Haemolytic uraemic syndrome and E coli 0157. British Medical Journal 318: 684–685

Haemolytic uraemic syndrome. 2003 www.chw.edu.au/prof/handbook/section 18

Hegenbarth MA 1996 Acute childhood exanthems and classic childhood diseases. In: Harwood-Nuss AL, Linden CH, Luten RC, Shepherd SM, Wolfson AB (eds), The clinical practice of emergency medicine, 2nd edn. Lippincott-Raven, Philadelphia, 1125–1131

Hinchcliffe RF 1987 The haemolytic anaemias. In: Hinchcliffe RF, Lilleyman JS (eds), Practical paediatric haematology: A laboratory worker's guide to blood disorders in children. Wiley, Chichester, 315–358

Hinchcliffe RF, Clark SJ 1987 The haemoglobin disorders. In: Hinchcliffe RF, Lilleyman JS (eds), Practical paediatric haematology: A laboratory worker's guide to blood disorders in children. Wiley, Chichester, 231–280

Iron deficiency in children. 2003 www.ironpanel.org.au/AIS/AIS docs/index/html

Joseph J, Irwin MD, Jeffrey T, Kirchner DO 2001 Anemia in children. American Family Physician 64: 1379–1386

Kelton JG, Brain MC 1987 The destruction of red cells by the vasculature and reticuloendothelial system. In: Nathan DG, Oski FA (eds), Hematology of infancy and childhood. WB Saunders, Philadelphia, 427–442

Newland AC, Evans TGJR 1997 Clinical review. ABC of clinical haematology: Haematological disorders at the extremes of life. British Medical Journal 314: 1262–1265

Oski FA 1987 The erythrocyte and its disorders. In: Nathan DG, Oski FA (eds), Hematology of infancy and childhood. WB Saunders, Philadelphia, 16–43

Platt OS, Nathan DG 1987 Sickle cell disease. In: Nathan DG, Oski FA (eds), Hematology of infancy and childhood. WB Saunders, Philadelphia, 655–698

Pomelli SG 1987 Pd deficiency and related disorders of the pentose pathway. In: Nathan DG, Oski FA (eds), Hematology of infancy and childhood. WB Saunders, Philadelphia, 583–612

Shreiber AD, Gill FM 1987 Autoimmune haemolytic anemia. In: Nathan DG, Oski FA (eds), Hematology of infancy and childhood. WB Saunders, Philadelphia, 413–426

Stevens RF 1987 Congenital and acquired coagulation defects. In: Hinchcliffe RF, Lilleyman JS (eds), Practical paediatric haematology: A laboratory worker's guide to blood disorders in children. Wiley, Chichester, 281–314

Stevens RF 1987 Leukaemia and myeloproliferative disorders. In: Hinchcliffe RF, Lilleyman JS (eds), Practical paediatric haematology: A laboratory worker's guide to blood disorders in children. Wiley, Chichester, 195–230

Walters MC, Abelson HC 1996 Interpretation of complete blood count. Paediatric Clinics of North America 43(3): 599–602

Weatherall DJ 1997 ABC of clinical haematology: The hereditary anaemias. British Medical Journal 314: 492–496

Zipursky A 1987 Isoimmune hemolytic diseases. In: In: Nathan DG, Oski FA (eds), Hematology of infancy and childhood. WB Saunders, Philadelphia, 44–73

11.3 DISORDERS OF COAGULATION

FIONA REILLY

HAEMOPHILIA

INTRODUCTION

Haemophilia A (classical haemophilia) is a coagulation disorder caused by a deficiency of factor VIII occurring in 1 per 7500 male births. Haemophilia B (Christmas disease) is caused by factor IX deficiency occurring in 1 per 30 000 male births. Both are due to defects in a single gene at the tip of the X chromosome, which are usually X-linked recessive in transmission (70% of cases) but can occur as spontaneous gene mutations (30% of cases). Acquired haemophilia is rare and occurs when autoantibodies develop against factor VIII. Median time to diagnosis is seven months in those with a family history of haemophilia but up to 30 months in those without a family history. Antenatal diagnosis is becoming available and has greater than 90% sensitivity. Female carriers of haemophilia have clotting factor activity of 50% or greater and do not express the disease clinically. In the absence of a family history, mild haemophilia with activity in the range 5 to 30% may not be diagnosed until late childhood.

CLINICAL PRESENTATION

Haemophilia A and B are clinically indistinguishable. Patients with mild haemophilia bleed only after major trauma or surgery but those with less than 5% activity bleed after minor injury and those with under 1% activity bleed into muscle either spontaneously or following trivial trauma. The early manifestations include easy bruising and mucous membrane bleeding. The first haemarthrosis usually occurs between two and four years of age when mobility is developing. The joints most frequently involved are the large joints of the knee, ankle, hip, elbow, wrist

and shoulder. Symptoms in the young child include inability to weight bear, limp, swelling, warmth and redness of a joint, or non-specific symptoms such as paraesthesias. Soft tissue bleeds are generally apparent as a painful swollen area on the involved limb but more extensive bleeds and fractures may result in limb-threatening compartment syndrome. Greenstick and buckle fractures are less prone to significant bleeding.

Intracranial haemorrhage occurs with increased frequency after head trauma in haemophiliac patients. Retroperitoneal haematoma may occur spontaneously or following trauma and may mimic appendicitis. Gastrointestinal haemorrhage is a less-common manifestation of haemophilia in children. Haematuria may be macroscopic or microscopic. Soft tissue haemorrhage in the head or neck is potentially life-threatening due to the risk of airway obstruction. Haemophiliac patients may also present with transfusion-borne viruses including hepatitis B and C and HIV. These are rare in the current paediatric haemophiliac population as most cases of transmission occurred prior to 1985.

INVESTIGATIONS

Haemophilia A and B both cause a prolonged activated partial thromboplastin time (aPTT) with a normal prothrombin time. Individual factor assays can then be performed to confirm the diagnosis. Haemophiliacs presenting with suspected intracranial or retroperitoneal bleeds need CT scanning. Plain radiographs will exclude fractures associated with traumatic haemarthroses.

TREATMENT

Analgesia should be provided as required but aspirin should be avoided. Other NSAIDs may be used on the advice of the treating haematologist. Narcotic

analgesia has limitations associated with use in treating a chronic condition. Cryoprecipitate revolutionised treatment of haemophilia in 1965 and patients could anticipate a normal lifespan for the first time. Factor concentrates were introduced in 1978 but the realisation in the 1980s that they could transmit hepatitis and HIV viruses has led to today's use of more expensive recombinant factors and virus-inactivated plasma-derived factors. In Australia, the latter are produced by CSL and come in vials of 250 and 500 units. The half-life of factor VIII is 12 hours so repeated doses may be required. The main goals of treatment are to control bleeding by clotting factor replacement, control of pain and elimination of inhibitors.

Factor replacement may be given following a confirmed bleed or as prophylaxis against potential bleeding, for example prior to dental extraction. Early and appropriate treatment reduces the risk of deterioration to disabling arthropathy and chronic pain. Many patients now initiate treatment for minor bleeds at home. The amount of clotting factor required depends on the patient's weight and on the type and severity of the bleed. Prophylactic factor replacement , usually two- to three-times a week at home with increased doses given for any breakthrough bleeds, has led to a marked reduction in the number and severity of bleeding episodes. Lacerations generally require factor replacement to prevent excessive bleeding. Head injury requires a high index of suspicion and a very low threshold for factor treatment. A negative cranial CT scan does not preclude the need for factor replacement.

Desmopressin (DDAVP) is a synthetic analogue of vasopressin that elevates factor VIII levels for several hours after administration by stimulating release from endothelial stores. It is usually used to treat von Willebrand disease but can also be used to treat mild haemophilia A. In an emergency situation where no

CONTROVERSIES AND FUTURE DIRECTIONS

❶ Haemophilia is particularly suited to gene therapy intervention because the disease is due to deficiency of a single gene product. Gene therapy is still at the stage of small human trials.

clotting factor is available, FFP or cryoprecipitate can be administered. Inhibitors are alloantibodies that develop against clotting factors. They are present in 10–20% of those with haemophilia A and 3–5% of those with haemophilia B. Inhibitors may mean that large amounts of clotting factor are required, or that clotting factors will not work at all. Treatment options include a prothrombin complex concentrate (prothrombinex) or recombinant activated factor VIIa. Elimination of inhibitors is possible in a proportion of patients using immune tolerance therapy, where daily low-dose factor infusions will lead to the development of neutralising anti-inhibitor antibodies.

FURTHER READING

Fischer K et al 2001 Changes in treatment strategies for severe haemophilia over the last 3 decades: Effects on clotting factor consumption and arthropathy. Hemophilia 7: 446–452

Knobel K et al 2002 Inhibitors in the Swedish population with severe haemophilia A and B: A 20-year survey. Acta Paediatrica 91(8): 910–914

Liras A 2001 Gene therapy for haemophilia: The end of a 'royal pathology' in the third millennium? Hemophilia 7: 441–445

Minhas H, Giangrande P 2001 Presentation of severe haemophilia – a role for accident and emergency doctors? Emergency Medicine Journal 18(4): 246–249

Petrini P 2002 Treatment strategies in children with hemophilia. Paediatric Drugs 4(7): 427–437

VON WILLEBRAND DISEASE

INTRODUCTION

Von Willebrand disease (vWD) is the most common inherited disorder of coagulation and is present in 1% of the population. It demonstrates autosomal dominant inheritance with variable penetrance and expressivity. Males and females are affected equally. Rarely, vWD may be acquired in the context of SLE or nephroblastoma. Von Willebrand factor (vWF) is a large multimeric, multifunctional protein that facilitates the adherence of platelets to the vascular endothelium enabling a platelet plug to be formed. In addition, vWF is necessary as a carrier protein for factor VIII. Quantitative or qualitative abnormality of vWF is the primary defect in vWD. The coagulation defects can be due to abnormal platelet adhesion expressed by a prolonged bleeding time and abnormal blood coagulation expressed by low factor VIII levels or activity.

Three types of vWD exist, with four subtypes:

- Type 1 – 80% of cases with partial quantitative deficiency of vWF.
- Type 2 – 17% of cases with qualitative deficiency of vWF.
  Type 2A, B and M with abnormal interaction between vWF and platelets. Type 2N with reduced interaction between vWF and factor VIII.
- Type 3 – 3% of cases with total quantitative deficiency of vWF and decreased factor VIII activity.

CLINICAL PRESENTATION

The clinical features of vWD are milder than those seen in haemophilia. Mucosal bleeding is more common and prolonged bleeding is seen after surgical procedures. In small children, the classic presentation of vWD is bruising and bleeding out of proportion to the severity of the injury. Many will report a family history of a bleeding disorder. Haemarthroses and intracranial and intra-abdominal bleeds are much less common and tend to occur only with the severe type 3 vWD. Von Willebrand disease is eventually identified in 10 to 20% of women and adolescents with menorrhagia and in 15% of children with recurrent epistaxis.

INVESTIGATIONS

The initial abnormality detected is often a prolonged bleeding time. In most patients the activated partial thromboplastin time (aPTT) and platelet count are normal and a prolonged aPTT should prompt a measurement of factor VIII levels to exclude haemophilia A. The diagnosis and typing of vWD is difficult and usually requires a specialist laboratory. The panel of investigations required to determine the type and severity of vWD includes:

- vWF assay
- Ristocetin co-factor assay
- Factor VIII activity
- Platelet activity.

An acute phase reactant, vWF levels are low in children and those with Type O blood group and are elevated by exercise or stress. Ristocetin is normally able to induce platelet aggregation in vitro but is unable to in patients with vWD.

TREATMENT

The aim of treatment in vWD is to correct the haemostatic defects by increasing plasma levels of vWF and factor VIII. Treatment is given in response to bleeding or prophylactically prior to surgical or dental procedures. Plasma-derived factor VIII concentrates contain both vWF and factor VIII. Recombinant factor VIII does not contain vWF and is no use. These plasma-derived products are the treatment of choice for type 2A, 2B (in which DDAVP is contraindicated) and type 3 vWD. They are pasteurised to prevent transmission of blood-borne viruses including HIV and hepatitis B and C. FFP contains both vWF and factor VIII but very large volumes would be required to raise vWF to satisfactory levels.

Desmopressin (DDAVP) is a synthetic analogue of vasopressin that releases factor VIII and vWF from endothelial storage sites causing a transient rise in levels. DDAVP is effective in type 1 vWD and will increase plasma levels of vWF by up to 200%. It is usually ineffective in types 2A, M and N, and type 3 vWD and is contraindicated in type 2B vWD because it may cause thrombocytopenia and thus worsen bleeding. Overall, 85% of those with vWD will respond and a trial of intravenous DDAVP should be given at the time of diagnosis because DDAVP is the treatment of choice. The dose is 0.3 µg kg^{-1} given intravenously in 30–50 mL normal saline over 30 minutes. The most common adverse effects are facial flushing, headache and tachycardia, which usually respond to slowing the infusion. Repeat doses may need to be given each 6–12 hours but tachyphylaxis occurs after approximately 48 hours. DDAVP should be used with caution in children under three years of age in whom there have been case reports of water intoxication and hyponatraemia. An intranasal DDAVP preparation is available but may be less reliable in children if part of the dose is swallowed. The dose is 2–4 µg kg^{-1}.

Adjunctive treatments include tranexamic acid for bleeding involving the oral or nasal mucosa, either alone or in conjunction with DDAVP. Synthetic oestrogens cause an unpredictable rise in vWF but may be useful in controlling menorrhagia.

FURTHER READING

Battle J, Noya M, Giangrande P, Lopez-Fenandez M 2002 Advances in the therapy of von Willebrand disease. Haemophilia 8: 301–307

CONTROVERSIES AND FUTURE DIRECTIONS

❶ Recombinant vWF has undergone animal trials with promising early results. No human trials have yet been completed.

Montgomery R, Kroner P 2001 Von Willebrand disease: A common pediatric disorder. Pediatric Annals 30(9): 534–540
Rodeghiero F 2002 Von Willebrand disease: Still an intriguing disorder in the era of molecular medicine. Haemophilia 8: 292–300
Sandoval C et al 2002 Clinical and laboratory features of 178 children with recurrent epistaxis. Journal of Pediatric Hematology and Oncology 24(1): 47–49

11.4 PLATELET DISORDERS

KIERAN CUNNINGHAM

Essentials

1 Abnormal bleeding can occur from disorders of total numbers of platelets or platelet function.

2 The normal platelet count is between 150 and 400 × 10^9 L^{-1}.

3 Idiopathic thrombocytopenic purpura (ITP) is the commonest platelet disorder in childhood.

INTRODUCTION

In normal haemostasis, blood loss is initially limited by the formation of a platelet plug and cross-linked fibrin at the site of injury. In platelet disorders this platelet plug is not formed or is ineffective and abnormal bleeding occurs. Small petechial skin haemorrhages less than 3 mm in diameter are characteristic of platelet defects. Platelet abnormalities can be either quantitative or qualitative.

The normal platelet count is between 150 and 400 × 10^9 L^{-1} and the commonest platelet disorder is thrombocytopenia (low platelet count). Thrombocytosis (elevated platelet count) is seen in inflammatory reactions including Kawasaki disease, patients with malignancy and polycythaemia rubra vera. Thrombocytosis of itself is rarely of clinical importance but platelet levels greater than 1000 × 10^9 L^{-1} can be associated with acute thrombosis or haemorrhage. Significant thrombocytopenia has a characteristic bleeding profile of spontaneous bruising, petechiae, epistaxis and mucosal bleeding. Bleeding complications usually only occur at levels of less than 50 × 10^9 L^{-1} with spontaneous bleeding possible at levels below 10 × 10^9 L^{-1}. As most platelet counts are performed by electronic particle counters, an inappropriately low platelet count can result from the spontaneous platelet clumping that can occur in EDTA collection tubes. This is confirmed by direct inspection of the peripheral blood smear for platelet clumping.

In qualitative disorders of platelet function the abnormal bleeding occurs despite a normal platelet count. Platelet dysfunction occurs in hepatic failure, renal failure, some myeloproliferative disorders, with some drugs (e.g. aspirin) and in rare inherited disorders of platelet function (Glanzmann, Portsmouth, Hermansky–Pudlak, May–Hegglin and Bernard–Soulier syndromes).

IDIOPATHIC THROMBOCYTOPENIA PURPURA (ITP)

Introduction

Idiopathic thrombocytopenic purpura or immune-mediated thrombocytopenic purpura (ITP) is the commonest platelet disorder in children. It is an autoimmune disorder characterised by the development of antibodies to the body's own platelets. ITP in children is usually a benign self-limiting disorder that is most common between the ages of two and ten years, when children experience the greatest frequency of viral infections.

Clinical presentation

Typically there is a short history of bruising or mucosal bleeding in an otherwise well child. Apart from a purpuric rash, bruising and any mucosal haemorrhages, the physical examination is normal.

Differential diagnosis

The presence of a limp, hepatospleno-megaly or lymphadenopathy suggest the possibility of an underlying lymphopro-liferative disorder. In infants with bruising, intentional injury must be excluded. In Wiskott–Aldrich syndrome eczema is present in the first year and the platelets are smaller than normal. The presence of other congenital abnormalities might be a clue to Fanconi's anaemia. Thrombocy-topenia in Down's syndrome may be the precursor of megakaryoblastic leukaemia. In older children, particularly those with a chronic course, a systemic autoimmune disorder such as lupus or antiphospholipid syndrome should be considered.

Investigation

The blood count and film is normal apart from the thrombocytopenia. Large platelets may be seen on the film. In Wiskott–Aldrich syndrome the platelets are smaller than normal. Anaemia or lymphopenia suggest some other under-lying disorder. Other causes of throm-bocytopenia should be considered and clinically excluded if the child is other-wise healthy. If they cannot be clinically excluded then further work up is re-quired. In infants, exclude CMV and consider immunoglobulins and T/B lymphocyte subsets to exclude immune disorders. In school-age children an autoimmune screen including ANA, dsDNA, anticardiolipin antibodies and lupus anticoagulant should be considered. Refer to a paediatric haematologist and consider bone marrow examination if the diagnosis is uncertain or if any specific therapy for ITP is considered. Bone mar-row aspiration is usually performed after four weeks if there is no evidence of remission or if the bleeding symptoms are out of proportion to the platelet count.

Management

Most children recover spontaneously within six to eight weeks and have only cutaneous or mild bleeding. They re-quire no specialist treatment and can be managed as ambulatory patients. Parents should be supported with good written advice on the condition and given a tele-phone contact name and number. Written

advice should include information about avoiding contact sports, bangs to the head, aspirin and other drugs that inter-fere with platelet function. They should watch for bleeding and report to hospital if new episodes occur. In the initial stages the platelet count can be reviewed weekly but this can be extended to every two to four weeks once it is improving. School can be recommenced when platelets are greater than 20×10^9 L^{-1}. By six months around 85% will have a normal platelet count. Patients with platelet counts greater than 150×10^9 L^{-1} can be discharged but warned that occasional relapses are seen and to represent if symptoms recur.

Consider admission of patients with initial platelet counts below 20×10^9 L^{-1}. Serious bleeding is rare in ITP and appears to be restricted to those with platelet counts less than 10×10^9 L^{-1} but deaths have occurred. All children with counts less than 10×10^9 L^{-1} during the course of the illness should be admitted. The decision to admit may be influenced by the social circumstances and parents' coping ability. Consider treatment if bleeding is severe enough to drop the haemoglobin, e.g. troublesome epistaxis, GI bleeding or menorrhagia. If treat-ment is required, there are a number of established options. Most of these treat the low platelet count and not the under-lying disorder. Hence, relapse is com-mon. All these treatments can have significant side effects, so it is important to weigh up the risks and benefits. This has lead to different practice guidelines around the world. To address this an Intercontinental Childhood ITP Registry was established in 1997 to pro-spectively investigate the clinical course, management and outcome of children with ITP. In the future, this should bring consensus to the optimum treatment strategy for individual children with ITP.

Current treatments

Treatment of choice for the rare serious haemorrhage is intravenous immuno-globulin (IVIG) infusion. Rapid platelet count rise occurs usually within 48 hours and lasts two to four weeks. As a pooled blood product IVIG carries the risk of viral transmission and is expensive. A

range of side effects have been reported. IVIG had been thought more effective than a short course of prednisolone at a dose of 1–2 mg kg^{-1} for up to two weeks but recent work has shown shorter courses at higher doses (4 mg kg^{-1} d^{-1} for four days) may raise the count as quickly as IVIG. Short-term steroid therapy is rela-tively harmless but long-term steroids in childhood ITP should be avoided if possible. Anti-D is effective in Rh-posi-tive children only, but has the advantage of being a rapid single injection and re-sults are comparable to IVIG. Splenec-tomy has been overused in the past and is now reserved for life-threatening hae-morrhage (see below) or children who have failed to respond to medical treat-ment with significant bleeding and who are at least six months from diagnosis (see chronic ITP). Post-splenectomy patients have an increased risk of sepsis despite pneumococcal vaccination and antibiotic prophylaxis

Medical emergencies

The risk of intracranial haemorrhage is less than 1% but persists as long as the platelet count is very low. This is the main reason why prophylactic treatment has been and still is recommended by some physicians. Children with ITP get the same sort of headaches as any other child and in a well child they can be managed in the same way. Severe headache with neurological signs requires urgent inves-tigation with cranial CT and immediate

CONTROVERSIES

❶ The Intercontinental Childhood ITP Registry was established in 1997 to prospectively investigate the clinical course, management and outcome of children with ITP. Since then a Splenectomy Register and a prospective database on both paediatric and adult patients with chronic ITP have also been set up. Information from these databases should provide the evidence base for the optimum treatment strategy for individual children with ITP in the future.

treatment if indicated with IVIG and steroids. Life-threatening haemorrhage is the only instance where platelet transfusions should be used as the antibodies in ITP target all platelets including donor transfusions. As a result the benefit of any transfusion is very short-lived and may be ineffective or even detrimental if the diagnosis is wrong (DIC, TTP). Emergency splenectomy is a last resort but the bleeding ceases when the spleen is removed.

CHRONIC ITP

Around 10–20% of children fail to remit within six months but spontaneous remission will occur in up to two-thirds of these patients in subsequent years. A chronic course is most often seen in older children, particularly adolescent girls. Some may have underlying conditions such as lupus. Most do not have significant bleeding problems or a need for regular treatment.

FURTHER READING

Bolton-Maggs PH 2000 Idiopathic thrombocytopenic purpura. Archives of Diseases in Childhood 83(3): 220–222

Buchanan GR 2001 Idiopathic thrombocytopenic purpura in childhood. Paediatric Annals 30: 527–533

Intercontinental Childhood ITP Registry 2005 http://www.unibas.ch/itpbasel/

Kuhne T, Imbach P, Bolton-Maggs PH, Berchtold W, Blanchette V, Buchanan GR 2001 Newly diagnosed idiopathic thrombocytopenic purpura in childhood: An observational study. Lancet 358: 2122–2125

11.5 VASCULITIS

RUTH BARKER

Essentials

1 Childhood vasculidities are a heterogeneous group of disorders that are poorly understood.

2 The most common childhood vasculidities are Henoch–Schönlein purpura (HSP) and Kawasaki disease.

3 HSP is largely a clinical diagnosis. Presentation is characterised by palpable purpura, polyarthritis, nephritis and colicky abdominal pain. Rash is present in 100% of cases but rash development may lag behind the other symptoms.

4 Kawasaki disease is a clinical diagnosis, supported by evidence of raised inflammatory markers. The clinical manifestations involve persisting unexplained high fever lasting more than five days, together with mucositis, cervical lymphadenopathy, conjunctivitis, rash and peripheral cutaneous manifestations.

INTRODUCTION

Primary vasculitis is an inflammatory disease process affecting arteries and veins. It is the common end point of several different disease processes and no one mechanism can explain the pathogenesis in this heterogeneous group of conditions. Although abnormalities in polymorph, lymphocyte, platelet and endothelial function and humoral and T-cell immune function have been described, it is difficult to differentiate primary from secondary pathological findings. In serum sickness, circulating immune complexes are trapped in vessel walls at sites of increased vascular permeability with resultant complement activation, attraction of polymorphonuclear leucocytes and vessel wall damage due to local release of enzymes and free radicals. Immune complexes have not been identified in all forms of vasculitis and immune complex deposition does not always correlate with sites of vessel inflammation. Endothelial and leucocyte factors have been identified that facilitate leucocyte binding to and migration through the endothelial surface. Up-regulation of these factors (predominantly cell-surface immunoglobulins and other proteins) has been demonstrated in some vasculitic processes. Antibody-mediated vascular damage has also been demonstrated in Goodpasture syndrome (antiglomerular basement membrane antibodies). Antineutrophil cytoplasmic antibodies (ANCA) and anti-endothelial antibodies (AEA) have been demonstrated in other vasculitic processes. However, the presence of these autoantibodies is inconstant and generally not diagnostic alone.

CLINICAL PRESENTATION

The clinical presentations of the different vasculitic disorders vary according to the extent and nature of organ involvement. Skin manifestations are frequent and often give a clue to the size of the vessel involved. Lesions are commonly purpuric but may be urticarial, ulcerative, vesicular or resemble erythema multiforme. Vasculitis in subacute bacterial endocarditis is a secondary to septic emboli, but the clinical appearance and constellation of symptoms resembles a primary vasculitic process. Any process that causes occlusion to a vessel can clinically resemble vasculitis. When the vasculitic process is severe, vessel destruction leads to tissue infarction. This can result in ischaemia of extremities and gangrene.

CLASSIFICATION

The primary vasculitic disorders can be divided according to the size of the vessel involved. Classification relies on a combination of clinical, laboratory, histologic and radiographic features.

LARGE VESSEL VASCULITIS

Takayasu disease is the third commonest form of vasculitis in childhood after Henoch–Schönlein purpura (HSP) and Kawasaki disease. The cause is unknown, but genetic factors and tuberculosis may play a role. A panarteritis primarily involving large arteries results in stenosis, occlusion and aneurysmal dilatation of affected vessels. Systemic symptoms of fever, night sweats, anorexia and weight loss are followed by hypertension, heart failure and pulse deficits. Arterial insufficiency may result in limb length discrepancies. ESR may be normal and the diagnosis may hinge on angiographic findings. Treatment involves immunosuppression and possibly antitubercular therapy.

MEDIUM VESSEL VASCULITIS

This group includes Kawasaki disease (see below) and polyarteritis nodosa (PAN). PAN is a necrotising vasculitis involving medium-sized muscular arteries. It is rare in childhood and the aetiology is unknown. Antineutrophil cytoplasmic antibodies (ANCA) are present in some forms of PAN. PAN is a systemic illness with a wide spectrum of clinical presentations depending on the organs involved. Symptoms of fever, malaise abdominal pain and arthropathy are common. Skin manifestations may resemble those of HSP or erythema multiforme or may be necrotic with peripheral gangrene. Other features include myalgia, ischaemic heart

pain, nephritis and cerebral manifestations of stroke, visual loss and psychosis. Diagnosis relies on elevation of inflammatory markers (ESR and CRP) and biopsy showing characteristic histopathologic changes in affected vessels.

SMALL VESSEL VASCULITIS

Vasculitides involving predominantly small vessels include HSP (see below), hypersensitivity angiitis, Wegener granulomatosis and Churg–Strauss syndrome. The latter two conditions are extremely rare in childhood. Hypersensitivity angiitis is a serum-sickness-like reaction in infants that includes an erythema-multiforme-type rash, arthropathy and fever. Like acute urticaria in infancy, it most frequently follows the use of penicillin or cephalosporins (particularly Ceclor). The skin manifestations in both conditions include oedema of the dorsum of the hands and feet, nodular, purpuric, urticarial or erythema-multiforme-like lesions. Arthralgia and arthritis are common and respond to non-steroidal anti-inflammatory agents with short-term oral steroids reserved for the more severe cases. The condition is self-limiting but recurs on re-exposure to the same agent.

SECONDARY VASCULITIS

Vasculitis may occur in association with a variety of connective tissue disorders such as systemic lupus erythematosus, dermatomyositis and scleroderma. Occlusive endarteropathy correlates with cutaneous ulcerative lesions in dermatomyositis. Many infectious diseases are associated with vasculitis, predominantly with cutaneous manifestations. Papulovesicular acrolocated syndrome (PALS or Gianotti-Crosti syndrome) is a vasculitis associated with multiple viral and other triggers, including hepatitis B antigenaemia, EBV, CMV, parvovirus B19, HIV, rickettsial diseases and streptococcal infections. Multiple skin-coloured or red, flat-topped papules occur in an acral distribution with sparing of the trunk. Subacute bacterial endocarditis with bacterial or

fungal agents results in a vasculitic process secondary to the spread of septic emboli. There is an increased association with vasculitis in patients with familial Mediterranean fever with several patients described with PAN and HSP features.

HENOCH SCHÖNLEIN PURPURA (HSP)

Introduction

HSP is the most common acute vasculitis in childhood with an overall incidence about 10 per 100 000. The aetiology is undefined, but several infective agents and drugs have been implicated. Boys are more commonly affected more than girls and most are between two and eight years of age.

Clinical presentation

HSP is characterised by palpable purpura, polyarthritis, nephritis and colicky abdominal pain. Skin lesions occur in 100% of cases and rash is the usual reason for presentation. They begin as maculopapules that initially blanch and develop to palpable purpura, which may include macules, papules, vesicles, bullae, nodules and urticaria. These appear in crops lasting 3–10 days and are maximal on lower limbs and buttocks. They may be painful with associated fever and angioedema. Local angioedema of scalp, eyelids, lips, hands, feet, back, scrotum and perineum is common in younger children and the oedema may precede the skin lesions.

Arthritis is present in the majority of patients. It is mainly large joint especially knees and ankles with serous effusions, which may recur but eventually resolve leaving no residual joint deformity. Two-thirds have gastrointestinal symptoms including colicky abdominal pain, vomiting and bloody diarrhoea. Over half of all patients have occult blood in stools. Some children present with isolated abdominal symptoms or arthritis and the diagnosis may only become apparent when the rash develops days to weeks later. Nephritis occurs in under half and may be delayed for up to four or more weeks. Other less-common features include intussusception (usually ileo-ileal), orchitis and cerebral involvement, including seizures.

Investigations

The diagnosis is largely clinical but may be difficult in the absence of rash. Screening for the variety of agents that have been implicated (hepatitis B, HIV, adenovirus, mycoplasma, human parvovirus B19, HSV) is unnecessary in uncomplicated cases. There is no clear link between group A streptococcal infection and HSP. However, the collection of a throat swab, C3/C4 and ASOT may be useful in distinguishing post-streptococcal arthralgia from HSP where the clinical picture is not full-blown. All patients should have BP recording, urinalysis and renal function assessment at presentation. In the absence of nephritis, urinalysis should be repeated each month for three months until other symptoms have resolved. Women with a history of HSP as children should have BP and urinary protein excretion monitored closely during pregnancy. Renal biopsy is reserved for patients with nephritis complicated by nephrotic syndrome, hypertension or renal failure.

Prognosis

The condition is self-resolving over a period of six to eight weeks. However, the disease recurs in up to one-third of patients and a small percentage of children develop persistent renal disease. Estimates vary but recent population-based studies have suggested that the frequency is approximately 1% with less than 0.1% developing serious renal disease. Those with isolated haematuria and proteinuria without renal insufficiency completely recover.

Management

Steroids are thought to reduce the severity and speed the resolution of the abdominal pain, but neither seem to ameliorate other symptoms nor prevent recurrence. Children can usually be managed as outpatients but may require admission for blood-pressure management and analgesia. Follow-up should involve blood-pressure surveillance and urinalysis for three months after the acute attack.

KAWASAKI DISEASE

Introduction

Kawasaki disease is an acute multi-system illness associated with a systemic vasculitic process affecting medium and small muscular arteries with a predilection for coronary arteries. It is the second most common vasculitic disease of childhood after HSP. The disease frequency varies globally with a preponderance in Asians. In Japan, the incidence is between 50 and 200 per 100 000 children under five years. This contrasts with rates in the USA of between 6 and 15 per 100 000, again with a preponderance in Asian-American children. It predominantly affects children under the age of five. Aetiology is unknown but genetic and infective factors seem to be involved. No specific pathogen has been defined.

Clinical presentation

Diagnosis requires persisting, unexplained high fever lasting more than five days and four out of the following five clinical features:

❶ Cervical adenopathy with one lymph node 1.5 cm or greater.
❷ Bilateral conjunctival injection with perilimbal sparing.
❸ Polymorphous rash (maculopapular, multiforme or scarlatiniform).
❹ Peripheral cutaneous changes to palms and soles including erythema, swelling and induration.
❺ Mucous membrane changes to lips and/or oral cavity (fissuring of the lips, pharyngitis, and strawberry tongue).

Extreme irritability in a toddler with persisting fever of unknown origin should always prompt consideration of Kawasaki disease. As the disease evolves there is desquamation beginning with periungual desquamation 10–18 days after onset of fever. Other associated findings are carditis (pericarditis, myocarditis, valvular involvement), aseptic meningitis, arthritis, sterile pyuria, uveitis, hepatitis and hydrops of the gall bladder.

Investigations

Early in the disease there is a leucocytosis with left shift, raised ESR, and a pro-gressive rise in the platelet count up to 1000×10^9 L^{-1}. Mild hepatitis may be evident with a rise in the transaminases and elevation of the conjugated bilirubin may reflect functional biliary tract obstruction. CSF analysis is not necessary for diagnosis but, if undertaken, shows a mononuclear pleocytosis with normal glucose and protein and sterile culture. An ECG is routinely performed looking for conduction delay with PR or QT prolongation. All cases should have an echocardiogram looking for coronary aneurysms.

PROGNOSIS

The high, spiking fever with minimal response to antipyretics usually persists for one to two weeks if untreated. Aneurysmal dilatation of coronary arteries is the main concern and develops within one to four weeks of the onset of fever. These may be small (< 4 mm), medium (4–8 mm) or large (> 8 mm). Small to medium aneurysms usually regress within five years although the vessels are likely to remain abnormal with poor response to dilating agents. Large aneurysms carry a poor prognosis with frequent thrombosis and resultant myocardial ischaemia. Kawasaki disease is thought to play some aetiological role in adult coronary artery disease as there are case reports of young adults suffering myocardial infarctions where coronary aneurysms have been found.

Management

The mainstay of treatment is intravenous immunoglobulin (IVIG) together with high dose aspirin 100 mg kg^{-1} per day until the fever subsides then at 5 mg kg^{-1} d^{-1} for seven to eight weeks or until coronary abnormalities settle. Both high dose (1000 to 2000 mg kg^{-1} over four to six hours) and low dose (400 mg kg^{-1} d^{-1} for four days) IVIG regimens have been used. Since the introduction of IVIG, the case fatality rate has dropped from 2% to 0.3% and the rate of aneurysm development has been reduced from up to 25% to less than 10%. Prognosis is better if the IVIG is given before day ten of the illness. Children who do not respond

CONTROVERSIES AND FUTURE DIRECTIONS

❶ Childhood vasculitidies are a heterogeneous group of disorders with overlapping clinical manifestations. Most progress in the epidemiological and pathological understanding of these diseases has been made with the more common diseases, HSP and Kawasaki disease. It is hoped that a better classification of these diseases may follow a better pathological understanding of clinical vasculitic manifestations. This understanding will likely be extrapolated from adult data, where disease presentation is more common. Whether this extrapolation is valid remains uncertain.

after the first dose of IVIG may respond to a second dose (1000 mg kg^{-1}) although it is not know whether this prevents development of aneurysms. A group of patients remain resistant to IVIG therapy. The use of steroids is contraindicated because of an increased rate of coronary artery aneurysm. Follow-up includes regular echocardiography, the duration of which will be determined by the degree of coronary artery involvement. Stress testing in adolescence is required if there has been cardiac involvement and angiography may be indicated. Long-term anti-platelet or anticoagulation therapy may be indicated.

FURTHER READING

Athreya BH 1995 Vasculitis in children. Paediatric Clinics of North America 42(5): 1239–1261
Barron KS 1998 Kawasaki disease in children. Current Opinion in Rheumatology 10(1): 29–37
Dillon MJ, Ansell BM 1995 Vasculitis in children and adolescents. Rheumatic Diseases Clinics of North America 21(4): 1115–1136
Rowley AH, Shulman ST 1999 Kawasaki syndrome. Paediatric Clinics of North America 46(2): 313–329
Saulsbury FT 1999 Henoch-Schönlein purpura in children. Report of 100 patients and review of the literature. Medicine 78(6): 395–409
Yalcindag A, Sundel R 2001 Vasculitis in childhood. Current Opinion in Rheumatology 13(5): 422–427

11.6 ACUTE LEUKAEMIA

JOSEPH TING

INTRODUCTION

The leukaemias are a group of diseases characterised by the clonal proliferation of malignant immature white blood cell precursors. They differ in the lineage and degree of differentiation of cells involved, being broadly divided into two groups: lymphoid and myeloid. These two categories are further subdivided into an acute form that progresses more rapidly than the chronic disease, which is relatively indolent. Causal factors are unclear and the majority of children affected have no identifiable predisposing factors. However, certain congenital conditions such as Down's and Fanconi syndromes pose a definite risk. Preconceptional germ cell and post-natal environmental exposure to radiation and carcinogens may play a role. Previous chemotherapy and radiotherapy are associated with increased risk of a secondary malignancy. The triggering event most likely occurs during faulty B- or T-cell germ-line rearrangement, leading to failure of cell-proliferation control and the creation of a leukaemic clone. Acute lymphoblastic leukaemia (ALL) constitutes the majority (up to 82%) of childhood leukaemia with acute myeloid leukaemia (AML) and chronic myeloid leukaemia (CML) accounting for 16% and 2%, respectively. Together they account for one-third of the malignancies in children under 15 years old. Although children of all ages are affected, the peak incidence is between two and six years.

CLASSIFICATION

Leukaemogenesis represents clonal proliferation of white blood cells arrested at various stages of differentiation, lending itself to diagnostic and prognostic classification based on the cell line affected, degree of differentiation, immunophenotyping, cell receptor, cell antigen and chromosomal studies. Classification of leukaemia is complex, with the French–American–British (FAB) categories being useful for AML and immunotyping better suiting ALL. For instance, the most frequent immunophenotype encountered in ALL is common ALL (c-ALL), which expresses CD 19, CD 24 and CD 10 antigens. More detailed classification systems can be found elsewhere.

CLINICAL PRESENTATION

Signs and symptoms in ALL and AML are similar and depend on the degree of marrow infiltration and extent of extramedullary spread. Classic findings in acute leukaemia include fever/infection, pallor/lethargy/easy fatigability and bruising/mucosal bleeding due to febrile neutropenia, anaemia and thrombocytopenia respectively. Marrow infiltration leads to bone pain and extramedullary spread leads to painless adenopathy (including mediastinal), hepatomegaly, splenomegaly, skin or periorbital infiltrates and rash. Difficulty with diagnosis arises in differentiating early acute from chronic disease, when symptoms (night sweats, arthralgia, bone pain, constitutional symptoms) and signs (enlarged liver and spleen, lymphadenopathy) are variable and non-specific. CNS involvement occurs in 4% of children (cranial nerve palsy, headache) and testicular leukaemia in 10% of boys (painless enlarged testes). Hyperviscosity results in tissue infarction (CNS, pulmonary) and rarely priapism results from leucocyte sludging and cavernosal obstruction.

DIFFERENTIAL DIAGNOSIS

Children with pancytopenia may have acute leukaemia, aplastic anaemia or marrow failure from infiltration by non-haematological malignancy. However, hepatosplenomegaly and adenopathy is unusual with the alternative diagnoses. Viral infections may lead to lymphadenopathy and hepatosplenomegaly accompanied by atypical lymphocytes rather than blast cells. Leukaemoid reactions with leucocyte counts greater than $50 \times 10^9 \, L^{-1}$ may rarely occur with acute infections and inflammatory disease such as rheumatoid arthritis. Marked lymphocytosis without leukaemic cells occurs in pertussis. Isolated thrombocytopenia in childhood may follow a viral infection or be associated with idiopathic or thrombotic thrombocytopenic purpura rather than leukaemia.

INVESTIGATIONS

Full blood count reveals anaemia and thrombocytopenia in 80% of cases. The majority of children have leucocyte counts below $20 \times 10^9 \, L^{-1}$. Those with leucocyte counts up to $900 \times 10^9 \, L^{-1}$ usually have extramedullary involvement as evidenced by hepatosplenomegaly and lymphadenopathy. The neutrophil count is often depressed to below $1.0 \times 10^9 \, L^{-1}$. Circulating blast cells are a frequent finding on blood film examination. Blood typing is necessary if red-cell transfusion is anticipated. A screen for atypical antibodies is warranted if there have previously been multiple occasions of blood product use. Cultures of blood and other potential infection sites are done prior to antimicrobial administration. Blood cultures may be positive in up to 25% of cases of newly diagnosed leukaemia. Tumour lysis syndrome due to massive cell death during

treatment causes hyperkalaemia, hyperuricaemia, hyperphosphataemia, hypocalcaemia and acute renal failure. Mediastinal masses are visible on chest X-ray in 5–10% of cases and pneumonia may require exclusion. Osseous abnormality occur in half the skeletal surveys performed. Bone-marrow aspiration and trephine (BMAT) is essential for specific diagnosis and prognostication, including complex tests such as immunophenotyping, cytogenetics, molecular studies and cell-cycle kinetics. AML is rarely complicated by a coagulopathy that progresses to DIC, so that a coagulation profile and fibrinogen level may be helpful.

PROGNOSIS

The cure rate for ALL is 50–80% compared with only 30–50% for AML, depending on whether adverse prognostic factors are present. Poor-risk AML has a dismal outlook, with less than 20% achieving long-term remission. Adverse prognostic factors include certain chromosomal translocations (such as t(4;11) in infant ALL), a very high-presenting leucocyte count, poor response to first-course treatment, recurrent disease, below one year or above ten years at age of onset and transition of non-Hodgkin's lymphoma to acute leukaemia. Low-grade CNS disease is no longer considered a disadvantage.

MANAGEMENT

Management requires close collaboration with a paediatric haematologist/oncologist. ED supportive treatment focuses on the sequelae of acute leukaemia: febrile neutropenia and sepsis (broad-spectrum antimicrobial agents), bleeding from thrombocytopenia (platelet transfusion) and correction of acute or symptomatic anaemia, which are described elsewhere. Combination chemotherapy used during the induction, intensification and maintenance phases may give rise to manifestations of bone-marrow suppression, which are similar to the sequelae of acute leukaemia. Definitive treatment includes surgery, chemotherapy and radiotherapy.

CONTROVERSIES AND FUTURE DIRECTIONS

❶ The future management of leukaemia will be influenced by new and improved risk stratification of the disease based on gene profiling studies with better understanding of biology, i.e. the tempering of therapy according to risk group.

❷ In future, high-risk patients may receive more therapy than standard-risk patients. Increased treatment success in the former group outweighs higher incidence of treatment related side-effects and complications.

❸ Late effects of therapy are becoming an increasing problem, e.g. second malignancies; endocrine deficiencies; osteoporosis; etc. New management agents are likely to be 'biologic' agents rather than cytotoxic agents, e.g. retinoic acid in the treatment of acute promyelocytic leukaemia and imatinib in Philadelphia chromosome (Ph') positive chronic myeloid leukaemia and Ph' positive ALL.

AREAS OF CONCERN

Although offering improved treatment success, greater intensity of chemotherapy increases the risk of a second treatment-related malignancy, reduced fertility and late anthracycline cardiotoxicity. CNS irradiation, now infrequently performed, damages the hypothalamic-pituitary structures and may lead to impaired growth. Many patients will undergo bone-marrow transplant, which entails profound immunological dysfunction and increases septic complications.

FURTHER READING

Saha V, Lilleyman JS 1998 Leukaemia. Current Paediatrics 8: 73–77

HAEMATOLOGY AND ONCOLOGY

11.7 FEBRILE NEUTROPENIA

JOSEPH TING

INTRODUCTION

Infection is a major cause of death in children with haematological malignancies following bone marrow or solid organ transplantation, iatrogenic immunosuppression, and chemotherapy. The major factor predisposing to infection in these patients is neutropenia, which is defined as decreased circulating neutrophils in the peripheral blood. The normal reference range for neutrophil counts varies with age of the child, being highest in the neonatal period. Neutropenia in childhood results from reduced production (marrow underactivity or infiltration); increased destruction, consumption, or sequestration with reduced survival (immune-mediated or overwhelming sepsis); or is associated with congenital or familial syndromes. It may be intrinsic, such as in cyclical neutropenia, or occur in relation to extrinsic factors such as immune-mediated destruction of neutrophils by drugs, infection, connective tissue disorders, and neonatal–maternal blood incompatibility. Neutropenia may be isolated or be part of a pancytopenia. Regardless of cause, the incidence of infection increases as the neutrophil count falls below $0.5 \times 10^9/l$ and is highest below $0.1 \times 10^9/l$.

Implicated organisms are usually bacterial, infrequently fungal or viral, and may be recognised pathogens or commensals that become opportunistic because of reduced host immunity. Neutropenic children receiving chemotherapy for leukaemia are at significant risk from Gram-negative sepsis, including *Pseudomonas aeruginosa* and *Escherichia coli*, and from systemic fungaemia, including aspergillosis and candidiasis. In bone marrow transplant (BMT) patients, half the infections are bacterial, evenly split between Grampositives (such as *Staphylococcus aureus*) and Gram-negative organisms; 40% are due to viruses like cytomegalovirus; and about 10% are due to fungi. Vascular catheter–related infections are usually related to Gram-positive skin organisms. Anaerobic infections rarely occur with neutropenia. Other important considerations in febrile neutropenia include the presence of central vascular access devices; alteration of microbial environments favoring resistant organisms, due to prophylactic or inappropriate antimicrobial use; and abnormal neutrophil function, with the last occurring despite normal neutrophil count.

The principles of management of febrile neutropenia in the emergency department are:

- resuscitation of the patient with overt septic shock
- careful physical examination to detect the source of infection
- detection of the patient with compensated septic shock
- definitive treatment with appropriate broad-spectrum antimicrobial therapy.

PRESENTATION

Young children compensate for impending shock and remain normotensive in the early stages of systemic sepsis. The earliest reliable sign of vascular redistribution is delayed capillary return, because tachycardia and tachypnoea can be secondary to the fever. Neutropenic or immunosuppressed children may have attenuated or altered signs of infection. The absence of neutrophils to localise an infection makes it difficult to determine the source of infection by physical examination alone. Pay special attention to body regions vulnerable to bacterial infection, such as oropharynx, ears, skin, and perianal area. Digital rectal examination or rectal thermometers may cause Gram-negative bacteraemia in neutropenia and should be avoided. Evidence of respiratory, circulatory, renal, and metabolic derangement indicates severe sepsis.

INVESTIGATIONS

Microbiological samples from potential infection sources such as blood, urine, cerebrospinal fluid, throat, skin, and central access devices should be obtained prior to, but not delay, treatment. Full blood count with white cell differential confirms and quantifies neutropenia. Thrombocytopenia and coagulopathy are early markers of disseminated intravenous coagulation. Chest X-ray may indicate lower respiratory involvement or cardiac decompensation.

TREATMENT

Fluid resuscitation and inotropic support may be required in septic shock. Urgent empiric intravenous therapy with combination broad-spectrum antimicrobials that have excellent Gram-negative cover is essential in febrile neutropenia. The pattern and severity of infection varies according to location, clinical context, and level of immune suppression. Regularly reviewed institution- and scenario-specific treatment protocols developed in conjunction with infectious diseases physicians and microbiologists that take into account local patterns of infection and their susceptibilities help to deliver and standardise optimal treatment. The Victorian Drug Committee's Therapeutic Guidelines for Antibiotics is an excellent resource for centres that do not have their own febrile neutropenia protocols but should be adapted to local requirements.[1]

Prior to a causative organism(s) and susceptibility being available, intravenous gentamicin 4–6 mg kg^{-1} daily plus either intravenous ceftazidime 50 mg kg^{-1} up to 1 g t.d.s. or intravenous ticarcillin or clavulanate 50 mg kg^{-1} up to 3.1 g q.i.d. is recommended to cover multiple possibilities, including frequently encountered Gram-negative rods like *P. aeruginosa* and *E. coli*. Vascular catheter–related Gram-positive sepsis requires the addition of intravenous vancomycin 40 mg kg^{-1} per day in two or four divided doses to cover coagulase-negative staphylococci and *S. aureus*. The central device may require removal if it becomes a persistent nidus of infection. If a specific organism is isolated, antimicrobials are adjusted according to in vitro sensitivities. Antibiotic levels, such as trough gentamicin levels, are monitored for therapeutic effect and to avert toxicity. An empiric antifungal agent such as liposomal amphotericin may be added if fever and neutropenia persist after 72 to 96 hours despite broad-spectrum antibiotics. Antibiotics can be discontinued if there is no proven infection, cultures remain negative, and neutrophil count improves to above 0.5×10^9/l.

Bone marrow stimulation with colony-stimulating factors reduces the severity and duration of neutropenia, the duration of fever, and antibiotic requirements in children undergoing BMT, and may be effective in premature infants at high risk of infection as well as children with severe neutropenia and Gram-negative sepsis. Corticosteroids are effective in *Pneumocystis carinii* pneumonia (PCP) and have been used in conjunction with immunoglobulin to treat immune-mediated neutropenia.

PROGNOSIS

The short-term outcome for febrile neutropenic children is better than that in adults, with 66% successfully responding to initial empiric antibiotics and a mortality of 1%. Mortality and morbidity increase if febrile neutropenia remains unrecognised. Long-term prognosis is determined by the underlying cause of the neutropenia. Persistent fever, prolonged neutropenia prior to fever, and shock are poor prognostic indicators, as are increased duration and degree of neutropenia, and low monocyte count.

PREVENTION

Neutropenic children require meticulous asepsis during invasive line placement, and BMT patients require barrier and isolation nursing. Good orodental hygiene and routine immunisation prevent infections. Prophylaxis against PCP with co-trimoxazole and inhaled pentamidine is important in neutropenia due to chemotherapy for leukaemia. Acyclovir is given prophylactically to BMT recipients and is required in clinical viral disease. Zoster immunoglobulin reduces serious infection after contact with varicella zoster virus.

CONTROVERSIES AND CHALLENGES

Granulocyte infusions are no longer used because of questionable efficacy but may have a role in refractory neonatal sepsis. The emergence of highly resistant and virulent organisms is increasingly recognised as a barrier to improved outcomes, especially in the context of immunosuppression.

REFERENCES

Victorian Drug Committee 2000 Therapeutic Guidelines for Antibiotics, 11th edn. Victorian Drug Committee, Victoria

FURTHER READING

Hann IM 2000 Management of infection in children with bone marrow failure. Bailliere's Clinical Haematology 13: 441–456

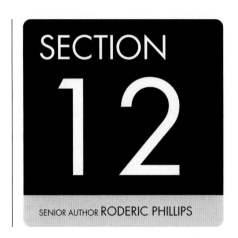

SECTION

12

SENIOR AUTHOR RODERIC PHILLIPS

DERMATOLOGY

12.1 DERMATOLOGY

RODERIC PHILLIPS • DAVID ORCHARD • MIKE STARR

Essentials

1 Look at the rash.
- Are there any blisters? Finding fluid-filled lesions greatly narrows the range of possible diagnoses.
- Is the rash red? Redness is from haemoglobin. Most red rashes blanch, i.e. the redness disappears with pressure. If not, the haemoglobin is outside the blood vessels giving purpura.
- Is the rash scaly? If so, the epidermis is involved in the disease process. The epidermis may be broken to give weeping, crusting or fissures ('eczematous rash'), or it may be intact ('red scaly rash').

2 Examine all the skin including the anogenital region.

3 Do not ignore a skin condition even if unrelated to the emergency visit. You may not deal with it yourself but you can organise appropriate follow-up for it.

INTRODUCTION

Approximately 65 000 children a year attend the emergency department (ED) at the Royal Children's Hospital in Melbourne and about 15 000 of these have some skin findings relevant to their visit. For 4000 children (6%), skin findings are a primary reason for their visit. These figures are likely to be representative of other tertiary teaching hospital EDs in Australasia. Diagnosing and managing these children requires a careful history and astute observation, particularly focusing on the appearance, site and development of their rashes.

For children who present to the ED with the primary symptom in another organ, the physician has an opportunity to observe cutaneous signs of disease, which may be relevant or may be coincidental to the child's presentation, for example, a five-year-old boy (Fig. 12.1.1) who presents with gastroenteritis. You notice the mild comedonal rash on his forehead and recognise that this is unusual at this age. Examination shows that he is tall for his age and has inappropriate penile (but not testicular) growth. His hyperadrenergic state can be investigated and treated years before it might otherwise have been recognised.

The discussion of diseases in this chapter is based on the features of the presenting rash and follows the algorithm given in Essentials. Diseases are grouped under their main morphology, e.g. vesicular, papular, eczematous, or purpuric. Mouth, anogenital, hair and nail problem are considered separately.

ERYTHRODERMA AND SKIN FAILURE

Erythroderma is one form of skin failure and refers to any condition that causes most of the skin surface to become red, often with some degree of scaling. Skin failure is rarely taught as a concept but is analogous to failure of any other organ system. Skin failure refers to the inability of the skin to adequately perform its functions, such as fluid and electrolyte balance, temperature control and protection from infection. Any child presenting with extensive areas of skin pathology or skin loss has some degree of skin failure. This may be well tolerated in otherwise healthy children but may be life threatening, especially in infants and those children with associated disorders.

Children presenting with erythroderma will usually be found to have one of the

Fig. 12.1.1   Mild prepubertal acne on the forehead of a five-year-old boy who presented with the unrelated problem of gastroenteritis. Examination and investigation confirmed that he had a variant of congenital adrenal hyperplasia requiring treatment.

following: atopic eczema (with or without secondary staphylococcal infection); an allergic reaction; or sepsis with toxin mediated skin involvement. Less common causes include: psoriasis; pityriasis rubra pilaris; several forms of inherited ichthyosis; some other genodermatoses; and internal lymphoid malignancies. In 10–20% of children with erythroderma, no cause can be found.

Management

- The aim is to restore and maintain the core functions of skin. Many sensible management decisions can be made before the diagnosis is clear.
- Have a low threshold for admission to hospital.
- Restore skin-barrier function by using an ointment emollient frequently.
- Monitor temperature, as the child may readily become hypothermic or, less commonly, hyperthermic.
- Monitor fluids and electrolytes.
- Monitor cardiac output, particularly if the child has known cardiac pathology.
- Skin and/or systemic sepsis may have caused the skin failure or may be secondary to it. Temperature control may be affected, so fever may not be present. Have a low threshold for giving systemic antibiotics, particularly to cover *Staphylococcus aureus* and streptococcal species.
- Local or systemic pain relief may be required.
- Cease all non-essential drugs.
- Identify and treat the underlying cause.
- Manage any associated conditions (e.g. diabetes, renal failure, congenital heart problems, metabolic disorders).

VESICULOBULLOUS RASHES

Vesicles are usually caused by infections (herpes simplex virus, varicella zoster virus, enterovirus, tinea, scabies or impetigo) or contact dermatitis. Also, consider drug reactions, erythema multiforme and photosensitivity. Dermatitis herpetiformis is a rare cause of itchy vesicles and papules. Larger blisters occur with staphylococcal infections, tinea, erythema multiforme, Stevens-Johnson syndrome, immune-mediated blistering disorders, arthropod bites, contact dermatitis, fixed and bullous drug reactions, mastocytosis, burns or trauma.

Many vesicles and blisters are fragile and rupture easily. A vesicular disease may present with a number of shallow monomorphic erosions but no vesicles. A bullous disease may present with several larger shallow erosions with surrounding loose epithelium but no bullae. Vesicles present for more than a couple of days become cloudy and vesiculopustular.

VARICELLA (CHICKENPOX)

Varicella is caused by infection with varicella-zoster virus. It usually occurs in children less than 15 years of age, and is highly contagious. The incubation period is 2–3 weeks. The contagious period begins two days before the rash and continues until the lesions are crusted. Clinical disease begins with a fever and malaise but these are usually mild. Lesions on the skin appear initially as erythematous macules, rapidly becoming small vesicles and then crusting. Over the next few days, anything from a few to hundreds of lesions may develop, initially on the face and trunk and gradually spreading onto the extremities. Superficial ulcers may be seen on all mucosal surfaces. Itch is not always present but may be marked. Diagnosis is clinical but can be confirmed by serology or immunofluorescence of vesicular scrapings for varicella-zoster virus antigen. Complete resolution occurs in most children but some scarring is common.

Children with varicella usually remain systemically well and afebrile after the first few days. If persistent fever and malaise is present, search for complications. In previously well children, the most common complications are:

- Bacterial skin infection with group A Streptococci or *Staphylococcus aureus*. Look for bullous, indurated, spreading or cellulitic lesions. Treat with oral antibiotics.
- CNS dysfunction. Encephalitis, meningitis, transverse myelitis, Guillain–Barré syndrome or Reye's syndrome (sudden onset of vomiting, coma and liver abnormalities) may occur. Cerebrospinal fluid analysis, including polymerase chain reaction (PCR) assay for varicella-zoster virus DNA may be useful in suspected encephalitis.
- Pneumonia. Cough and respiratory distress begin a couple of days after onset of the rash.
- Cerebellar ataxia may appear as the rash is clearing and resolve within weeks.

In neonates, immunocompromised children and adolescents, varicella can be more severe and occasionally fatal.

Management

- Treatment of otherwise well children with varicella is supportive with bland emollients and oral antihistamine if necessary. If the child is unwell, look for secondary complications.
- Avoid aspirin or other salicylates because of the association with Reye's syndrome.
- Treat secondary skin infection with flucloxacillin.
- Immunocompromised children should be treated with intravenous aciclovir 20 mg kg^{-1} per dose (2–12 weeks), 500 mg m^{-2} per dose (12 weeks–12 years), 10 mg kg^{-1} per dose (adult) 8-hourly given over 1 h.
- Premature neonates (less than one month old) with varicella should be treated with intravenous aciclovir.
- Term neonates should be admitted, and treated with aciclovir if they have severe disease.
- Give zoster immune globulin to at-risk contacts (immunocompromised children, those on prednisolone 2 mg kg^{-1} d^{-1} or more, newborns of mothers who have varicella any time from five days before until two days after delivery, any infant under 28 days of age). Give within four days of exposure (6 mL for adults, 4 mL for children 6–12 years of age, 2 mL for children up to five years of age).
- Exclude from school until all lesions are crusted.

- Offer varicella-zoster vaccine to non-immune contacts – the vaccine has been shown to prevent or attenuate infection if given within five days of exposure.

ZOSTER

Zoster is uncommon in childhood but can occur at any age, even in the neonatal period. It occurs in children who have previously had primary varicella infection. Zoster in a young child is usually associated with primary varicella having occurred in infancy. Zoster occurring in a young child with no previous history of varicella infection may be attributable to reactivation of varicella-zoster virus after an unrecognised intra-uterine infection.

Radicular pain may be the first symptom of zoster but pain is less common than in adults and may not be present. Vesicles on an erythematous background appear in one or more groups aligned in a dermatomal distribution, frequently with a striking midline cut-off. The affected area can be an isolated group of a few vesicles suggestive of herpes simplex virus infection. Alternatively, there may be extensive involvement of one or more dermatomes. Lesions continue to appear for a few days and then resolve over two weeks, generally without sequelae. Post-herpetic neuralgia is very uncommon after childhood zoster.

Complications include generalised dissemination during the first week of the rash, sometimes with pulmonary or brain involvement. This can be seen in both normal and immunocompromised children. Zoster on the head is occasionally accompanied by an aseptic meningitis, which resolves fully without treatment. Zoster lesions on the tip of the nose imply involvement of the nasociliary branch of the ophthalmic nerve and may accompany ocular involvement including keratitis and conjunctivitis. Facial nerve palsy and ear involvement can occur (Ramsay Hunt syndrome).

Immunocompromised children are much more likely to develop zoster. In such cases, zoster may be severe, extensive and prolonged. Significant dermatomal scarring can result.

Management

- If the diagnosis is unclear, collect epithelial cells from the base and roof of the vesicles for immunofluorescence and viral culture. This is not 'just a swab' and it requires some persistence to collect enough cells.
- In an otherwise well child, the occurrence of typical zoster does not require investigation for underlying immunodeficiency states. However, unusually severe or extensive zoster should raise this possibility.
- Oral antiviral agents are not indicated in an otherwise well child as the risk of significant symptoms or post-herpetic neuralgia is very small. If a child has underlying chronic illness or immunodeficiency, give intravenous or oral aciclovir.

HAND, FOOT AND MOUTH DISEASE

Hand, foot and mouth disease is one presentation of enteroviral infection, usually coxsackie A16 virus. There may be a mild prodrome of fever, malaise and sore throat. Discrete vesicles about 6 mm in diameter on an erythematous base appear first in the mouth, sparing the lips and usually sparing the gingiva. One to two days later, 3–7 mm vesiculopustules on an erythematous base appear on the palms, soles and around the fingers and toes. Lesions are also often found on the buttocks. They are often greyish and oval rather than circular in shape. In some cases, the mouth, hands or feet may not be involved. Resolution occurs within a week. The incubation period is about five days and epidemics are common. Virus is excreted in the faeces for weeks and exclusion is not recommended. Supportive care leads to complete recovery.

HERPES SIMPLEX INFECTION

Herpes simplex infection in childhood is common. Intrauterine, intrapartum and neonatal infection are considered elsewhere. Primary herpes infection after the neonatal period may be either primary herpetic gingivostomatitis or primary cutaneous herpes simplex. In children with impaired immune function, herpes simplex infection can present as indolent, slowly growing, irregular ulcers.

Primary cutaneous herpes simplex can present at any age. There may be a history of a family member with a recently activated herpes simplex lesion on the lip ('cold sore'). However, the virus is ubiquitous and transmission more often occurs from an unknown source. Painful grouped vesicles on an erythematous base can appear at any site. Multiple lesions rupture, crust and coalesce into larger erosions with scalloped edges. There may be associated fever, malaise and lymphadenopathy.

Management

- Supportive care.
- Bathing of crusts.
- Analgesia.
- Aciclovir is not routinely indicated unless risk factors for complications exist (e.g. underlying disease, immunosuppression).

Recurrent cutaneous herpes simplex can occur weeks or months after the primary episode. Recurrences usually get milder and less common with time but exacerbations can occur throughout childhood and later life (Fig. 12.1.2). Recurrences can lead to significant time off school. Prophylactic antiviral drugs will stop recurrences of HSV infection and should be used if the morbidity of the recurrences justifies this.

Herpes simplex can involve the fingers, especially the thumbs and index fingers (herpetic whitlow). At these sites, the thick skin does not readily rupture and children present with painful, coalesced pustular collections, often misinterpreted as bacterial abscesses. Any history of 'abscesses' occurring at the same site on a finger on more than one occasion is suggestive of herpes simplex. Management includes taking a swab for immunofluorescence and viral culture to confirm the diagnosis, analgesia and supportive care.

Fig 12.1.2 **(A)** This erythematous, slightly vesicular rash around the eye of a four-year-old boy had appeared over twelve hours. Because his other eye was blind, he was treated with oral aciclovir. Immunofluorescence confirmed herpes simplex virus. **(B)** One day later.

ECZEMA HERPETICUM

Herpes simplex infection in children with eczema is quite common. It occurs in children with any severity of eczema including children with mild eczema under excellent control. Many cases are misdiag-nosed either as an exacerbation of the eczema or as bacterial infection (Fig. 12.1.3). Grouped vesicles may be prominent, but more often vesicles are rudimentary or absent and the infection may present as a group of shallow 2–4 mm monomorphic erosions on an inflamed base. In more-severe cases, evolution is rapid and large crops of vesicles can arise daily. Ulcers may coalesce into larger erosions with scalloped edges. The infected area may not be painful or itchy.

In an atopic child, a high index of suspicion is needed about any patch of skin where small erosions or crusts are present and not responding to standard eczema therapy with moisturisers and topical cortisone derivatives. One reason for the under diagnosis of this condition is that even without treatment, resolution usually occurs in 1–4 weeks. However, dissemination may occur leading to multifocal and extensive erosions, malaise and secondary bacterial infection. In the past, disseminated eczema herpeticum had a significant mortality but this has declined with the recognition and aggressive treatment of secondary bacterial infections.

After complete resolution, recurrences may occur at the same or different sites, sometimes as often as every few weeks. Recurrences can be widespread and severe but usually decrease in severity over one to two years.

Management

- Clinical differentiation between herpetic and bacterial infection may be difficult; investigation and empiric treatment for both may be necessary.
- Collect epithelial cells from the base and roof of the vesicles for herpes simplex virus immunofluorescence and viral culture. This requires some persistence to collect enough cells.
- Local stable disease in an otherwise well child requires regular observation but does not need antiviral therapy.
- Milder cases demonstrating progression or facial involvement can be managed with oral aciclovir.
- Admission to hospital and treatment with intravenous aciclovir (20 mg kg^{-1} per dose (2–12 weeks), 500 mg m^{-2} per dose (12 weeks–12 years), 10 mg kg^{-1} per dose (adult) 8-hourly should be considered for children with any of fever, multiple sites of cutaneous herpes infection, widespread eczema, eye involvement, immunosuppression or age less than six months.

Fig. 12.1.3   Eczema herpeticum. Typical monomorphic vesicles can be seen away from the central weeping area.

Fig. 12.1.4   Bullous impetigo in a seven-year-old girl.

- Secondary bacterial infection is common. Swab for microscopy and culture. Soak to remove excessive crusts. Consider addition of intravenous or oral flucloxacillin.
- Monitor for eye involvement, particularly scleral redness. If present, this should be managed with topical or systemic aciclovir, or both, and urgent review by an ophthalmologist.
- The underlying eczema can be treated with moisturiser or wet dressings until the herpetic lesions are under control and then, if necessary, restart topical cortisone treatment.
- Prophylactic antiviral drugs will stop recurrences and are often warranted in older children with recurrent eczema herpeticum.

IMPETIGO (SCHOOL SORES)

This is caused by *Staphylococcus aureus* or group A Streptococcus or both.

Non-bullous impetigo presents initially as small erythematous vesicles that rapidly rupture to form yellow-crusted lesions, commonly on the face.

Bullous impetigo is due to *Staphylococcus aureus* and presents as flaccid blisters on normal skin. Lesions are rounded and well demarcated and may be single, grouped or widespread. Their onset and spread may be rapid or occur over days. New blisters appear and existing blisters rupture to give shallow moist erosions that can be many centimetres in size. There is often loose epithelium and/or brown crusting peripherally and some degree of central healing (Fig. 12.1.4). In more chronic cases, lesions may appear annular.

Impetigo is often secondary to itchy conditions such as scabies infection (especially hand impetigo), atopic eczema and head lice.

Impetigo can be followed by glomerulonephritis in the ensuing two months. This may cause oedema, hypertension and haematuria and is usually self-limiting. Contrary to long held beliefs, it now seems likely that chronic impetigo may also be a precursor of rheumatic heart disease in communities where medical conditions are poor and skin hygiene is suboptimal (McDonald et al).

Management

- Swab for microscopy and culture if the diagnosis is unclear or in widespread or complicated disease.
- Bathe off crusts.
- Apply topical mupirocin 2% ointment 8-hourly if very localised, or oral flucloxacillin 15 mg kg^{-1} (maximum 500 mg) orally, 6-hourly if extensive.
- Isolate the child from other children or from sick adults unless all lesions are covered or antibiotic treatment has commenced.
- Treat any underlying condition such as scabies or eczema.
- Blisters or erosions often continue to occur for a couple of days after antibiotic therapy. If new blisters continue to form after this time, the incorrect antibiotic may have been chosen, or the child may have an immune-mediated blistering disorder rather than impetigo.
- Children with chronic impetigo should be examined for any signs of heart disease. Families should be aware that rheumatic heart disease may be delayed by some years in this setting. Older siblings are likely to have had chronic impetigo in the past and therefore to also be at risk of heart disease and should be examined.
- In any child with chronic impetigo where ongoing care may be suboptimal, review with urinalysis to monitor for glomerulonephritis is warranted. In other cases, families should be aware of the possibility of renal involvement.

STAPHYLOCOCCAL SCALED SKIN SYNDROME

This is usually seen in younger children or children with renal impairment. It is mediated by an epidermolytic toxin released from an often insignificant staphylococcal focus (e.g. eyes, nose or skin). Fever and tender erythematous skin are early features. Exudation and crusting develop, especially around the mouth. Wrinkling, flaccid bullae and exfoliation of the skin are seen and can be extensive. Nikolsky sign is present ('normal' skin separates if rubbed). Blisters are very superficial and heal without scarring.

Management

- Admit to hospital. Monitor temperature, fluids and electrolytes if large areas are involved. Increase oral (or intravenous) fluids to increase toxin excretion. Give analgesia.
- Consider alternative diagnoses including Stevens-Johnson syndrome and toxic epidermal necrolysis. If the diagnosis is unclear, a skin biopsy will confirm the diagnosis by showing the split is in the granular layer in the upper epidermis.
- Flucloxacillin 50 mg kg^{-1} (maximum 2 g) IV 6-hourly if there is evidence of sepsis or systemic involvement.
- Look for a focus of infection. Drain any foci of pus if present.
- Handle skin carefully and use an emollient ointment.

ERYTHEMA MULTIFORME

This is a specific hypersensitivity syndrome that occurs at any age, often preceded by facial herpes simplex virus infection. It is over diagnosed in EDs. Most children diagnosed with erythema multiforme have urticaria, often with large lesions with annular or polycyclic borders. In erythema multiforme, the primary lesions are red papules, usually symmetrical and involving the forearms, palms, feet, face, neck and trunk. They can be found anywhere. There may be few or many lesions. At least some of the papules will form classical target lesions – these have an inner zone of epidermal injury (purpura, necrosis or vesicle), an outer zone of erythema and sometimes a middle zone of pale oedema. These papules and target lesions are not migratory. The involvement of mucous membranes is common

but unlike Stevens–Johnson syndrome, is limited to isolated patches. Most cases are caused by herpes simplex virus, including most of the cases that occur without prior symptoms. Drugs are an uncommon cause. Erythema multiforme does not evolve into Stevens-Johnson syndrome. They are different conditions.

Management

- Fluid maintenance.
- Analgesia if required.
- Apply emollient ointment to the lips, if needed.
- If the condition is recurrent, it is highly likely to be related to herpes simplex virus. Prophylactic aciclovir prevents recurrences and should be considered if recurrences are frequent, severe and affecting the quality of life.
- Prednisolone alleviates symptoms but probably prolongs the duration of the condition and may cause recurrence of herpes simplex virus infection.

STEVENS–JOHNSON SYNDROME/TOXIC EPIDERMAL NECROLYSIS

Stevens–Johnson syndrome and toxic epidermal necrolysis are believed by many to be variants of the one condition. Most cases are thought to be triggered by medications, especially antibiotics (sulfonamides, penicillins), anticonvulsants (lamotrigine) and non-steroidal anti-inflammatory drugs. Mycoplasmal and other infections may be the cause in some children. Fever, myalgia, arthralgia, headache and other organ involvement are usually present as a prodromal illness for several days. The rash evolves suddenly, characterised by widespread blisters on an erythematous or purpuric macular background, often with extensive mucous membrane haemorrhagic crusting. Lesions are usually on the face and trunk or generalised rather than acral, and typical target lesions are not seen. There may be tender erythematous areas with a positive Nikolsky sign ('normal' skin separates if rubbed). Mucous membrane involvement can be extensive, severe and painful. Conjunctivitis, corneal ulceration and

blindness can occur. Anogenital lesions can lead to urinary retention.

Management

- See general advice under 'skin failure'.
- Admit to hospital. A multidisciplinary approach including dermatology, paediatrics, ophthalmology, surgery and paediatric intensive care is required. Good nursing care is paramount. In severe cases, nurse in a specialised burns unit.
- Apply emollient ointment to the skin, lips and anogenital areas – this may be required many times a day.
- Regular eye examination with specialist review is required. Topical steroid eye drops may be needed.
- Give intravenous γ-globulin 2 g kg^{-1}. Commence ciclosporin (5–6 mg kg^{-1} d^{-1} orally for a few days, then taper to 3-5 mg kg^{-1} d^{-1} for 2–3 weeks). Data about the efficacy of any treatment regimes is limited but is sufficent to justify treatment. Stevens–Johnson syndrome has a significant mortality and has a high rate of permanent visual scarring including blindness as well as other problems.
- Maintain good nutrition, with nasogastric feeding if needed.
- Intubation may be needed if the child is unable to protect the airway because of severe oropharyngeal involvement.

Note: Stevens–Johnson syndrome is not severe erythema multiforme. They are distinct conditions. Permanent sequelae are rarely seen in severe erythema multiforme and concurrent drug use is unlikely to be the cause. Skin lesion distribution and morphology are the best discriminating factors. Mucous-membrane involvement can be seen in both conditions but is more widespread in Stevens–Johnson syndrome.

DERMATITIS HERPETIFORMIS

Dermatitis herpetiformis is an uncommon autoimmune blistering disease that may present at any age as itchy papules or vesicles. Rapid excoriation means that intact vesicles are rarely seen. Lesions occur on extensor surfaces of the limbs, buttocks, trunk and scalp. Most patients have gluten enteropathy (coeliac disease) and may have abdominal discomfort, diarrhoea or anaemia. Some degree of villous atrophy will be seen on small bowel biopsy in most cases, but coeliac disease is often asymptomatic at the time of presentation of dermatitis herpetiformis. Growth retardation has been reported with dermatitis herpetiformis, probably secondary to intestinal involvement.

Recurrence some years after successful treatment has been reported.

Management

- Perilesional skin should be biopsied for immunofluorescence to demonstrate the diagnostic granular IgA deposition.
- Investigate for coeliac disease with total IgA, antigliadin IgA and IgG, antitransglutaminase and endomysial IgA. Antitransglutaminase antibodies are the most specific for dermatitis herpetiformis. A small bowel biopsy is required but may be equivocal early in the disease course.
- Anaemia, usually megaloblastic secondary to malabsorption, may be found.

Skin lesions (but not intestinal symptoms) respond well to dapsone, but haemolysis and other side effects can limit its use. A gluten-free diet normalises gut function and, in most children, leads to eventual clearing of skin lesions.

OTHER IMMUNE-MEDIATED BLISTERING DISORDERS

As with dermatitis herpetiformis, the many diseases in this group are characterised by circulating autoantibodies directed against one or other of the structural proteins that give the epidermis its integrity. All are uncommon in childhood, linear IgA dermatosis (chronic bullous disease of childhood) being the most common. An immune-mediated blistering disorder should be considered in an otherwise well child if vesicles, blisters,

or crusted erosions continue to appear for more than a couple of weeks.

If there is a split below the basement membrane, lesions may be tense, long-lasting bullae, as seen in dermatitis herpetiformis, linear IgA dermatosis, systemic lupus erythematosus and pemphigoid. If the split is higher in the epidermis, lesions are flaccid, short-lived blisters that rapidly give crusted erosions with loose epithelium around the edges. These are seen in pemphigus variants. Lesions can mimic local or generalised impetigo. Mucous membranes may be involved. Despite the widespread and often dramatic appearance of the rash, the child is usually well. Accurate diagnosis always requires histology and immunofluorescence in addition to clinical findings. Management requires immunosuppressive therapy and long-term follow-up.

SUNBURN AND PHOTOSENSITIVITY

Excessive solar radiation to the skin causes erythema and tenderness commencing at least half an hour after the beginning of the exposure. Tenderness worsens for a day and resolves in four days. In more severe cases, oedema and blistering may be widespread. Healing is accompanied by desquamation and intense itch. Sunburn occurs more rapidly when the sun is overhead (summer, closer to the equator, 11 a.m. to 3 p.m.), and when the skin is less pigmented, but can occur with any skin type. Children with sensitive skin can burn significantly within 15 minutes of midday exposure in summer.

Any child presenting to the ED with sunburn or with a rash in sun-exposed areas may have an underlying photosensitivity disorder. These can be considered in four groups.

❶ Primary photosensitivity disorders.
❷ Inherited disorders including porphyrias.
❸ Diseases with a photosensitive component (systemic lupus erythematosus, dermatomyositis).
❹ Exogenous photosensitivity from drugs or plants.

A high index of suspicion is needed to diagnose photosensitivity. There have been examples of sunburn in children that were attributed to parental neglect but were actually due to a photosensitivity disorder. These diseases are common but diagnostic traps abound. For example, sun-induced rashes may develop in spring with the first sun exposure of untanned skin after winter, but not later in summer. The rash may develop on areas usually covered in winter such as the neck and arms and not on the face. Sun-induced rashes may require a few minutes or several days of sun exposure and may commence days after the exposure. In erythropoietic protoporphyria, sun exposure induces pain without skin changes initially. Viral exanthems may occur exclusively or mainly in areas of sun-exposed skin. Children with solar urticaria develop urticaria on sun-exposed areas.

Management

- Assess for associated causes (below) of increased sun sensitivity. Many children presenting to the ED with 'sunburn' have an associated photosensitive trigger. Any child who experiences symptoms within half an hour of sun exposure should be assumed to have an underlying condition.
- Assess the family situation, especially with younger children. Significant sunburn in a young child can occur in the setting of sub-optimal child care, although usually it is due to an oversight by otherwise caring parents.
- Within the first few hours of exposure, before blistering has developed, application of topical potent steroid creams can considerably reduce the severity and duration of symptoms.
- Cool compresses and wet dressings will alleviate symptoms. Topical anaesthetics should not be used. Admission and oral analgesia may be required in severe cases. Maintain adequate fluid intake.
- Educate about prevention.

Prevention

Prevention of sunburn is important. Episodes of sunburn are linked to later development of naevi and melanoma.

Parents need to balance the psychological and physical benefits of activities associated with sun exposure (including increased fitness, increased independence, healthier bones and decreased obesity) with the increased risk of skin cancers of all types. In summer, children should minimise sun exposure during the middle four hours of the day, wear broad-brimmed hats and long-sleeved shirts in the sun, and use a sunscreen with SPF 30 or greater on exposed parts.

Sunburnt infants regularly present to the ED, partly because of widespread advice that sunscreens are not recommended below the age of six months. This recommendation is not based on any evidence of problems in infants. It is based on the premise that it is usually easy to protect young babies who can't crawl by keeping them out of the sun and appropriately dressed. However, if a young baby is going to be in the sun, sunscreen should be used.

PRIMARY PHOTOSENSITIVITY DISORDERS

Polymorphous light eruption (PMLE) Presents in spring or early summer as skin-coloured or erythematous itchy papules or vesicles on the face, ears, neck or arms. It is recurrent. Recurrences usually occur at the same sites in that child.

Juvenile spring eruption Is a specific variant of PMLE and is common in 4–12-year-old boys as a recurrent blistering of the ears each spring.

Hydroa vacciniforme Is rare and can begin at any age in childhood as a sun-induced vesicular eruption on the cheeks during spring and summer. The cheeks, ears, nose, dorsum of the hands and rarely the eyes can be involved. Recurrences occur for many years.

Diagnosis can be difficult and may require formal evaluation in a photobiology unit including assessment of the response to different wavelengths of light. Management requires sun avoidance and often both UVA and UVB sun protection.

Solar urticaria Presents as urticaria within minutes or hours of exposure and settles within one day. Sharp margins are seen at the edges of clothing. Skin chronically exposed to the sun, such as face and hands, is often spared.

PORPHYRIAS AND OTHER INHERITED DISORDERS WITH PHOTOSENSITIVITY

The porphyrias are a group of inherited enzymatic defects in haem synthesis leading to increased levels of porphyrins, some of which cause photosensitivity.

Erythropoietic protoporphyria Is the most common childhood porphyria. Infants and young children present after brief sun exposure with acute discomfort, burning sensations, itching, erythema, oedema, urticaria and occasionally vesicles, particularly on the face and dorsum of the hands. Episodes are recurrent and with time affected skin appears prematurely aged. Erythrocyte protoporphyrin levels are elevated.

Congenital erythropoietic porphyria Is rare and presents in early childhood with extreme photosensitivity leading to painful blisters filled with red fluid on the face and dorsum of the hands. Progressive scarring can be severe.

Familial porphyria cutanea tarda Presents in childhood with chronic blistering on hands, arms and face leading to poorly healing ulcers, atrophic scarring and mottled hypo- and hyper-pigmentation.

If a porphyria is suspected, measure blood, urine and faecal levels of porphyrins. Management requires intensive avoidance of solar radiation including UVA and UVB. β-Carotene is useful in erythropoietic protoporphyria.

Many genodermatoses including xeroderma pigmentosum, Cockayne syndrome, Rothmund-Thomson syndrome and trichothiodystrophies are associated with photosensitivity and increased photodamage to skin, but do not usually present with blistering.

PHOTOSENSITIVITY AND BULLOUS REACTIONS TO DRUGS

Blisters may be the presenting feature of a number of different types of drug reactions. A high index of suspicion is required to diagnose these conditions. Families must be asked about all ingested and topical products including herbal, recreational and prescription drugs and unusual food patterns (e.g. daily cups of celery juice). Families will occasionally not remember the causative drug and deny taking anything, only to recall the vital information days later.

Many medicines can cause increased sun sensitivity leading to erythema, oedema and blistering on sun-exposed areas. Doxycycline (particularly at doses higher than 100 mg d^{-1}), tetracyclines, griseofulvin, isotretinoin, non-steroidal anti-inflammatory drugs, sulfonamides, fluoroquinolones and diuretics are typical causes in children. In one series of children receiving naproxen, 12% developed photosensitivity reactions on the face. Other causes include tars, perfumes, cosmetics, sunscreens, artificial sweeteners and many dyes. As with other photosensitivity syndromes, the rash can occur rapidly or days after the sun exposure and is most prominent on sun exposed areas. The photosensitivity can persist for up to three months after withdrawal of the medication. Prominent hyperpigmentation may persist for months after resolution.

Fixed drug eruptions in children are usually caused by paracetamol, non-steroidal anti-inflammatories or sulfonamides. They are quite common and present as single or multiple, usually circular red patches that may blister. With subsequent exposures, eruptions recur at the same site and sometimes at other sites. Post-inflammatory hyperpigmentation is prominent and may be the only sign of the drug reaction.

Many plants and herbal products contain chemicals that can induce drug reactions including fixed drug reactions, bullous drug reactions and photosensitivity reactions.

Management

- Recognise and stop the causative drug.
- Institute strict sun protection measures. Photosensitivity can persist for three months after cessation of the drug.
- If the patient is taking multiple drugs, the timing of the eruption and the frequency of reactions with each of the medications may suggest the causative drug.
- If continued drug ingestion is necessary, reducing the dosage may prevent the reaction.

PHOTOSENSITIVITY REACTIONS TO PLANTS

Many plants contain furocoumarins, which are naturally occurring psoralens. UVA light induces covalent bonding of psoralen into DNA leading to cell death. Typically, a child is playing outside in spring or summer and comes into close contact with a psoralen-containing species (e.g. species of celery, parsley, parsnip, fig, hogweed, limes and other citrus fruits). Several hours later, erythema, oedema and occasionally blistering develop. While contact dermatitis from plants can also present with streaky, often linear vesicular eruptions on areas of contact after exposure, photosensitivity reactions are more often painful, are usually sharply limited to sun exposed areas, and typically heal to leave striking patterns of hyperpigmentation that can persist for months or years.

Management

- Sun protection measures including a UVA sunscreen will prevent phytophotodermatitis.
- Offending plants can be removed.
- Treat as for sunburn.

CONTACT DERMATITIS – PLANTS

In children, contact dermatitis reactions from agents other than plants usually do not blister and these conditions are discussed under eczematous rashes (p. 347).

Many plants, including *Rhus* and *Grevillea* species, can cause an allergic contact dermatitis. Some species only cause reactions at specific times of the year and contact with the plant at other times does not cause a rash. One to three days after exposure, erythema, oedema and vesiculation develop at sites of contact, often in linear distribution. Lesions may persist for three weeks. Periorbital erythema and vesiculation is often misdiagnosed in the ED as cellulitis needing antibiotics. Clues to the correct diagnosis are that pruritus is the main symptom, the degree of pain and tenderness is much less than would be expected for cellulitis, systemic features, such as fever, are absent, the outline of the rash often has irregular patterns corresponding to the contact areas and a careful examination will often reveal other lesions on sensitive parts of the body. In particular, genital skin may develop lesions from secondary spread of the allergen via the fingers. Patients with allergic contact dermatitis may be extremely uncomfortable. Treatment often requires a few days of oral prednisolone, topical potent steroid ointments, cool compresses and supportive care. Unlike plant-induced photosensitivity, contact dermatitis from plants does not induce long-term hyperpigmentation.

Irritant contact dermatitis to components of stinging nettles, chilli peppers, mustard, horseradish and other plant products can lead to irritation, stinging, and occasionally blisters. Burning, oedema and blistering in the oral cavity can occur in small children after chewing irritant plants.

CONTACT DERMATITIS – ID REACTIONS

Repeated exposure to an allergen can result in a papulovesicular eruption at sites distant from the area of contact. This is thought to be a result of systematised contact sensitisation. The id reaction may be local or generalised. Examples include non-infective blisters erupting on the hands of a child with chronic tinea infection of the feet, and a severe generalised itchy vesicular rash on an adolescent using topical neomycin ointment.

ISOLATED BLISTERS

For a child who presents with a single blister or a few blisters as an isolated finding, consider:

- Mastocytoma. Usually in an infant with a history of recurrent blistering or crusting at the site of a brownish macule, often misdiagnosed as recurrent localised impetigo. There may be one brownish lesion or as many as hundreds.
- Insect bite. There may be a few lesions in one area. Non-blistered papules may have a tiny central red bite punctum.
- Irritant contact dermatitis.
- Spider bite. These can grow over days to become a non-tender blister with a diameter of many centimetres. They are uncommon. Regular dressings may be required. Debridement is rarely necessary. White-tailed spiders and huntsman spiders do not cause chronic necrotic ulcers.
- Scalds or burns from cigarettes or other hot objects. Look for characteristic patterns in the burn, as well as other factors on the history or examination suggestive of non-accidental injury or suboptimal caring practices.
- Fixed drug eruptions, e.g. from tetracyclines, sulfonamides, non-steroidal anti-inflammatory drugs or paracetamol.
- Friction. If minor friction appears to cause more blistering than expected on hands and/or feet in children, consider the possibility of a mild inherited blistering disorder (e.g. mild epidermolysis bullosa simplex). There may be a positive family history of childhood blistering that settled in later life.
- Artefactual lesions caused by either the child or a carer.
- Bullous Sweet syndrome or pyoderma gangrenosum.

CHRONIC EROSIONS OR ULCERS

Several primary skin conditions can cause chronic erosions or ulcers in children including itchy conditions such as scabies and papular urticaria. Also consider:

- Immunodeficiencies. Recurrent boils can be seen in chronic granulomatous disease and hyper IgE syndrome. Poor wound healing is a feature of leukocyte adhesion defects.
- Skin fragility syndromes. In junctional and dystrophic forms of epidermolysis bullosa, chronic ulcers related to minimal skin trauma may be seen in association with failure to thrive, anaemia and gastrointestinal tract involvement.
- Porphyria. Several enzyme defects in haem metabolism are associated with chronic erosive lesions, photosensitivity and hyperpigmentation. Episodes of acute pain or neurological dysfunction are rarely seen in childhood porphyrias.
- Artefactual lesions caused by either the child or a carer.
- Pyoderma gangrenosum.
- *Mycobacterium ulcerans* infection.

NEONATAL VESICLES

A neonate with vesicles or blisters requires urgent assessment, as potential causes include infection with herpes simplex virus, varicella-zoster virus and *Staphylococcus aureus*, including bullous impetigo. Neonates who acquire herpes simplex virus at birth usually present at a few days of age with grouped vesicles, often on the scalp. Lesions may rapidly spread and coalesce. Collect epithelial cells from the base and roof of a vesicle for immunofluorescence and viral culture. This is not 'just a swab' and it requires some persistence to collect enough cells. CSF must be examined for herpes simplex virus DNA, as 30% of neonates with apparently localised skin disease also have CNS involvement. Empiric intravenous aciclovir is essential until herpes infection has been excluded.

Non-infective causes of neonatal vesicles include:

- Epidermolysis bullosa. Over forty inherited diseases are associated with skin fragility. Presentation ranges from a few isolated blisters in otherwise well children to extensive blistering at any site of handling with associated systemic problems.

- Miliaria. Very superficial blistering in hot or occluded areas.
- Ichthyosis. Bullous subtypes present as blisters or erosions on red skin, which gradually becomes more scaly.
- Langerhans cell histiocytosis – vesicles and/or purpuric crusted lesions (see p. 340).
- Incontinentia pigmenti. This disease is X-linked and fatal in male foetuses. Girls present with lesions distributed in linear patterns. Lesions evolve through vesicular and warty phases to eventually leave permanent hyperpigmented streaks. Seizures and developmental, ocular and dental problems may occur.
- Mastocytosis. Urtication and blistering occur spontaneously or on top of oval brown macules.

PUSTULAR RASHES

Consider acne, folliculitis, drug reactions, pustular psoriasis, scabies, perioral dermatitis, tinea and localised bacterial infection. All vesicular rashes can become pustular if the vesicles persist for more than a couple of days. Vesicles on areas of thick skin can be white and look like pustules, e.g. on the toes in hand, foot and mouth disease. If in doubt, prick one lesion to reveal the clear fluid within.

ACNE

Acne mainly affects the forehead and face but can involve other sebaceous gland areas (neck, shoulders and upper trunk). Early lesions include blackheads, whiteheads and papules. In more severe cases there may be pustules or inflammatory cysts that can lead to permanent scarring. Acne is common in adolescence. It is treatable and no person with acne should be told it is an inevitable part of adolescence. Several topical and oral acne therapies are available and should be used to treat the disease. Under-treated acne is a major medical cause of significant morbidity in adolescents and has a recognised mortality as a factor in teenage suicide. It can also lead to permanent

scarring in 10% of untreated cases. Significant acne in an adolescent attending the ED for another reason should not be ignored any more than other findings such as proteinuria. The adolescent should be offered information, initial treatment and referral for ongoing management.

Management

- Most cases are mild and either require no intervention or can be managed with topical treatments. A first-line topical treatment is benzoyl peroxide 2.5% applied once or twice a day. Warn the adolescent that improvement with topical therapy occurs steadily over 1–4 months (not in a few days). Other topical agents include topical antibiotics for inflammatory lesions (clindamycin, erythromycin or tetracycline), topical retinoids (isotretinoin, adapalene) or azelaic acid. These can be used singly or in combination. All of these topical agents have potential side-effects with which practitioners must be familiar.
- If there are prominent red papules or pustules, a course of oral antibiotics for 3-6 months in combination with a topical treatment is warranted (e.g. tetracycline 500 mg twice daily, erythromycin 500 mg twice daily, doxycycline 50-200 mg d^{-1}). Oral hormone therapy can help female patients.
- If the acne is severe, or if antibiotics and topical treatment have not resulted in considerable improvement in three months, oral isotretinoin (Roaccutane®) is indicated. Prescription of isotretinoin is tightly controlled because it is expensive and because it is teratogenic, requiring absolute avoidance of any pregnancy risk in girls. In boys, and in girls who do not become pregnant, it is safe and highly effective. Most adolescents with troublesome acne can be cured with oral isotretinoin.
- Some acne sufferers develop scarring. This can be quite subtle and can occur with otherwise fairly mild disease. Any scarring is an indication for oral antibiotics and early consideration of oral isotretinoin. Similarly, the presence of any cysts should alert you

to the likelihood of scarring and the need for oral therapy.

ACNE AND DEPRESSION

Both adolescence and acne can be associated with depression. Significant depression is an indication to consider oral isotretinoin therapy. For several years, the issue of whether isotretinoin can trigger depression and suicide has been investigated. Current medical evidence suggests that treatment of severe acne with oral isotretinoin may decrease the risk of suicide. Assessment and treatment of any depression is required.

ACNE FULMINANS

Acne fulminans typically occurs in young males being treated for acne. There is sudden onset of fever, malaise, arthralgia, myalgia, lymphadenopathy and/or hepatosplenomegaly in association with a rapid worsening of acne over the trunk and shoulders. Many painful cystic lesions develop and become haemorrhagic and ulcerated. Many laboratory abnormalities have been noted, including elevations of white cell count, erythrocyte sedimentation rate, C-reactive protein and liver enzymes. The cause is unknown but may be an abnormal immunological response rather than a primary bacterial infection. The response to oral antibiotics is slow and indeed these adolescents are often taking oral antibiotics at the time of onset.

Management
- Oral prednisolone 0.5–1 mg kg^{-1} daily for 4–6 weeks (thereafter slowly reduced to zero).
- Oral isotretinoin being added to the regimen at the fourth week, initially at 0.5 mg kg^{-1} daily and gradually increased to achieve complete clearance.

ACNE WITH GRAM-NEGATIVE FOLLICULITIS

This can develop in patients treated for acne with long-term antibiotics. It is more common in adolescents with an oily complexion. It presents as rapidly worsening acne with pustular lesions on the face. Several common Gram-negative pathogens may be involved. Treat with oral trimethoprim and oral isotretinoin.

EARLY ONSET ACNE

Acne normally appears after the onset of pubertal changes such as testicular enlargement, pubic hair and breast development, and increases in severity for several years. However, comedonal and occasionally papular lesions may be the first manifestations of puberty in a child. These changes can begin up to two years before other signs of puberty. Early onset of comedonal lesions, even if mild, is associated with more severe acne several years later.

If comedones or acneiform papules are noted before puberty (see Fig. 12.1.1), you should consider the possibility of pathological androgen secretion (see below). Look for increased growth, genital development and advanced radiological bone age.

ATYPICAL ACNEIFORM RASHES

Acne that is atypical in age of onset, distribution, morphology or severity may be associated with systemic disease. Consider:

- Glucocorticoid excess, either exogenous or endogenous. This can give a monomorphic acneiform rash on the face and trunk. Other cushingoid stigmata may be present. In children on corticosteroid treatment, the rash may appear as the dose of corticosteroid is being weaned. Glucocorticoid acne may be due to *Malassezia* folliculitis. If there is no response to tetracycline, treatment of *Malassezia* folliculitis with topical or oral antifungals may be required (see Folliculitis below).
- Androgen excess. Other features depend on the age and sex of the child. In younger children accelerated growth, body odour, pubic hair, clitoromegaly (but not breast development) and penile (but not testicular) enlargement may be present. In teenage females, polycystic ovary syndrome is commonly the cause. Other causes include late-onset congenital adrenal hyperplasia, and virilising tumours. Investigations may include X-rays for bone age, pelvic ultrasound, plasma androgens, fasting glucose and insulin, and response to dexamethasone suppression.
- Precocious puberty.
- Several drugs can induce an acneiform rash with monomorphic papules and pustules in post-pubertal children. The distribution is different from acne vulgaris, often involving arms, legs or trunk, and comedones are not present. Affected individuals often have a history of troublesome acne vulgaris. Possible causative agents include anti-epileptic medications, especially phenytoin and phenobarbital, glucocorticoids, testosterone, isoniazid, lithium and iodides.
- Apert syndrome and related craniofacial syndromes can present with more severe widespread acne.

FOLLICULITIS

Infection of the hair follicles is usually due to *Staphylococcus aureus*. Predisposing factors include a moist environment, a heavy bacterial load (e.g. adjacent to wounds or anal region) and excessive occlusive ointment, particularly on the trunk. Treatment involves avoidance of the predisposing factors, use of topical cleansers such as chlorhexidine and, rarely, oral antibiotics. Folliculitis often occurs repeatedly over a period of months and may require continued topical measures for 3–6 months. In resistant cases, daily use of topical benzoyl peroxide lotion may be helpful.

Folliculitis can occur in a child with moderate or severe eczema. Oral antibiotics are usually beneficial in this setting.

In adolescents, *Malassezia* folliculitis is common and presents as a persistent itchy rash with many tiny monomorphic erythematous papules and pustules on the back, shoulders and upper trunk. It is often associated with occlusion or sweating. Daily application of keto-conazole 2% shampoo is effective in gaining control. For resistant cases, use oral ketoconazole 400 mg weekly for six weeks taken with a glass of grapefruit juice followed by indefinite weekly shampooing with selenium sulfide 2% shampoo.

Occasionally, pruritic papules and pustules can develop many hours after soaking in a hot spa. Lesions usually occur under the bathing costume and are caused by *Pseudomonas aeruginosa*. Oral antibiotics are not usually needed.

ACUTE GENERALISED EXANTHEMATOUS PUSTULOSIS (AGEP)

Acute generalised exanthematous pustulosis appears as a rapidly developing facial or truncal erythema with hundreds of tiny sterile pustules. Oedema is often seen in the affected areas. Fever and malaise may be present. Healing is associated with extensive superficial peeling. In some cases, children presenting with acute generalised exanthematous pustulosis have an underlying psoriatic tendency.

Many common medications, including amoxicillin, erythromycin, azithromycin, sulfonamides, anticonvulsants (especially carbamazepine) and non-steroidal anti-inflammatory drugs, can cause this. Acute generalised exanthematous pustulosis drug reactions often begin within hours of commencing the drug. Other causes include Group A streptococcal infection.

Treat by stopping any offending medication. Give oral antibiotics for underlying streptococcal infection if required.

PUSTULAR PSORIASIS

Psoriasis can present with pustules on an erythematous background. The pustules are sterile. The affected area may be limited to fingers, palms and soles, or local areas of skin, often with an annular arrangement of pustules. Alternatively, there may be erythroderma, high fever, malaise and arthralgias with widespread pustules coalescing into sheets of pus. Local pustular psoriasis can be treated topically (see psoriasis, p. 341). Generalised pustular psoriasis requires admission to hospital, rest, skin emollients and/or wet dressings, monitoring of fluid balance, electrolytes, renal and cardiac function and oral therapy (see erythroderma p. 325 and psoriasis p. 341).

NEONATAL PUSTULES

In the neonatal period, pustules may be part of several transient benign conditions. Pustules or vesicles may also be a marker of serious underlying illness, even in the absence of fever and lethargy. Consider:

- Infection, either congenital or acquired, e.g. *Staphylococcus* species, Group B streptococci, *Haemophilus influenzae*, *Candida* species.
- Neutropenia from any cause. Superficial bacterial pustules may be the only sign of congenital neutropenia.
- Toxic erythema of the newborn. In this benign condition, well term babies develop many tiny papules or pustules on an erythematous macular background in the first few days of life. Lesions clear within several days.
- Transient neonatal pustular dermatosis. Loose pustules are present from birth, and disappear within two days. This condition is more common in dark-skinned babies.
- Acropustulosis of infancy. Itchy vesicles and pustules appear on the hands and feet, usually commencing in the first couple of months of life and continuing for some months. New crops appear each two to four weeks. Sleep disturbance is common. In some infants, it appears to follow previously treated scabies infection. Pustules contain neutrophils and are sterile. Multiple scrapings may be necessary to exclude active scabies infection. Potent topical steroids assist control of flares, and the condition remits over 1–2 years.
- Eosinophilic pustular folliculitis (scalp). Yellowish pustules appear on the scalp and face within the first days of life. Lesions crust over and new lesions develop for some weeks. Pustules contain eosinophils and are sterile but secondary infection can occur. Mid-potency topical corticosteroids are helpful to control itch.
- Milia (white papules on the face) and sebaceous hyperplasia (yellowish papules, particularly around the nose) can be misinterpreted as pustules. Both resolve within a few weeks of birth.

NEONATAL PITYROSPORUM FOLLICULITIS

This extremely common eruption is referred to as 'milk spots', the 'six-week eruption' or 'infantile acne'. This is not true acne and comedones are not present. It is due to an inflammatory reaction to *Pityrosporum* yeast as the newborn sebaceous glands, activated during pregnancy, are returning to their quiescent childhood state. It is self-limiting and often needs no treatment. In more severe cases, application of ketoconazole 0.2% solution (dilute the 2% shampoo) by cotton bud to affected areas twice daily leads to rapid clearing.

PAPULAR (RAISED) RASHES

If a child has itchy papules, consider scabies, urticaria, serum sickness, papular urticaria, molluscum, *Malassezia* folliculitis, dermatitis herpetiformis or Langerhans cell histiocytosis. If papules are not itchy, consider urticaria, molluscum, warts, acne, skin appendageal tumours, melanocytic naevi, Spitz naevi, pilomatricomas, keratosis pilaris, vasculitis and papular acrodermatitis. For raised red circles or rings, consider urticaria. For softer red, purple or blue swellings, consider haemangiomas or vascular malformations. For haemorrhagic papules, consider Henoch–Schönlein purpura and other causes of vasculitis. If papules are yellowish when blanched, consider juvenile xanthogranulomas or xanthomas.

Papules or nodules may also occur in a number of disorders including acute rheumatic fever, juvenile chronic arthritis, systemic lupus erythematosus and neuro-fibromatosis, but are rarely the presenting feature.

SCABIES

Scabies infection occurs as a result of close, usually repeated, contact with an infected individual. Scabies mites eat into the upper skin forming burrows a few millimetres in length around the fingers, palms, wrists, elbows, axillae, nipples, penis, and soles. Early burrows may be vesicular. Usually only a few mites are present.

An intensely itchy secondary papular eruption develops 2–6 weeks after first exposure to the *Sarcoptes scabiei* mite or 1–4 days after subsequent reinfestation. This secondary eruption represents an immune response to the scabies antigen and does not mean that mites are spreading all over the body. Papules can occur anywhere including the palms, soles, axillae and genitalia, but are most prominent on the abdomen, buttocks and thighs. The scalp and head may be involved in infants and young toddlers. Inflammatory nodules may also develop, especially on covered areas. Excoriations and secondary impetigo may be present. Scabies is pandemic and affects both adults and children.

Not all itchy parasitic rashes are scabies. Many species of parasite can cause small itchy papules on the skin, in some cases hundreds of lesions. Bird mites, fleas, body lice, mosquitoes, sand flies, horse flies, bed bugs, ticks, chiggers, midges and harvest mites can all masquerade as scabies. Parasites can be collected from the skin on transparent adhesive tape. The CSIRO Australian National Insect Collection provides an identification service on 02 6246 4263.

MANAGEMENT

- Treatment of scabies is expensive and upsetting. If there is any doubt about the diagnosis, confirm by scraping to find a scabies mite, or refer before treating.
- Permethrin 5% cream.
- An alternative, recommended for pregnant or neonatal cases, is sulfur 6% in yellow soft paraffin. This is unpleasant and has no proven safety advantages over permethrin in these groups. The following are not recommended: lindane 1% (contraindicated in infants or women who are pregnant or breast-feeding) or benzyl benzoate 25% (too irritant for children and ineffective if diluted).
- Apply to dry skin (not after a bath) from the neck down to all skin surfaces. For infants, apply to the scalp as well (not face). Use mittens if necessary to prevent finger-sucking.
- Leave the cream on for at least eight hours.
- Wash the cream off. Wash clothing, pyjamas and bed linen at this time.
- Remove soft toys from the bed. The scabies mite cannot live for long periods away from the body, and insecticide sprays and cleaning of furniture and carpets are not warranted.
- Exclude from school until after treatment has commenced.
- Treat all family members and any other people who have regular close skin contact with the affected individuals.
- The itch takes a week or two to settle and can be treated with topical or oral corticosteroid. Nodules may take months to resolve despite successful treatment of the scabies infestation.
- Reinfestation is common. To minimise the risk of reinfestation, the family should notify all social contacts (e.g. crèche, school or close friends) to ensure that all those infected receive treatment.
- Treat secondary impetigo with oral flucloxacillin.
- Post-streptococcal glomerulonephritis may be seen after chronic impetigo secondary to scabies in the indigenous population. Oedema, hypertension and haematuria may occur over the next two months. In a child with long-standing infected scabies where ongoing care may be suboptimal, review and urinalysis to monitor for renal involvement is warranted. Examination of the child and siblings for signs of rheumatic heart disease is also warranted in this patient population.

PAPULAR ACRODERMATITIS OF CHILDHOOD

Papular acrodermatitis of childhood usually occurs in children aged one to three years but can occur outside this range. It is a reaction pattern to many infectious agents, including coxsackie viruses, echoviruses, *Mycoplasma* species, Epstein–Barr virus, adenovirus, respiratory syncytial virus, rotavirus, cytomegalovirus, hepatitis B virus and others. It has also been reported after all standard childhood vaccines. It is common and a regular source of confusion in EDs.

Papular acrodermatitis of childhood is characterised by the acute onset of monomorphic, red or skin-coloured papules mainly on the limbs, buttocks and face, with striking sparing of the trunk (Fig. 12.1.5). In any given patient, the papules tend to all look the same, typically firm and dome shaped, measuring 2–4 mm in diameter. However, in different patients, the papules can vary from tiny, skin-coloured papules to larger urticarial plaques. Lesions may coalesce into patches on the extensor surfaces of the elbows and knees. Lesions may be papulovesicular (particularly on the limbs) or purpuric (particularly on the face). Hundreds of lesions may appear over several days. It is usually asymptomatic but may be itchy. Complete resolution occurs in 4–8 weeks.

Affected children may be otherwise well or may have features of the underlying infection, such as mild fever, malaise, coryza, sore throat, lymphadenopathy and splenomegaly. Lymphopenia or lymphocytosis may be present. In some cases, no history of a preceding or intercurrent illness can be found.

Fig. 12.1.5 Papular acrodermatitis of childhood showing almost complete sparing of the trunk.

Papular acrodermatitis of childhood was formerly known as Gianotti–Crosti syndrome and was initially described as a manifestation of hepatitis B infection in Italy. This association has not been shown to be of general relevance, and papular acrodermatitis of childhood has been recognised as benign and much more common than previously thought.

Management

- Reassure and advise that clearing can take a few weeks.
- Children with papular acrodermatitis of childhood do not routinely require investigation to determine the underlying cause.
- Itch may require topical mid-potency corticosteroids and/or oral antihistamine.
- No exclusion from school or crèche is needed.

PAPULAR URTICARIA

This is a clinical hypersensitivity to insect bites. New bites appear as crops of asymmetrical, small, red papules, usually in warmer weather. Older bites appear as 1–5 mm papules, sometimes with surface scale or crust, or with surrounding urticaria. Vesicles or pustules may form in the centre of lesions. Individual lesions may resolve in a week or, if scratched, may last for months and may repeatedly flare up after fresh bites elsewhere. Itch is often intense and secondary ulceration or infection can occur. Full resolution usually occurs within nine months. However, scratching can lead to secondary changes, with non-healing erosions, ulceration, scarring and nodule formation. These lesions remain itchy and a cycle of scratching and skin destruction can persist for years or decades if not treated. Improve-

ments occur with new treatments but relapses are common without considerable medical support.

Management

- If the diagnosis is unclear, skin biopsy is useful as the typical histological findings are specific for insect-bite reactions.
- Prevent bites , e.g. by adequate clothing, modifying behaviour that leads to exposure, occasional use of repellent, and the treatment of pets and house for fleas and mites if necessary. The commonest source of bites is from mites in roof-dwelling animals such as birds, rats and possums. Surface spray of ceiling vents can be very useful.
- Treat the itch with an agent such as aluminium sulfate 20% (Stingose®), liquor picis carbonis 2% in calamine

lotion, potent steroid ointment or antihistamines.

- Protective dressings (e.g. Duoderm®) can speed the healing of lesions. In older children, intralesional injection of corticosteroid is effective.
- Treat secondary infection with topical mupirocin ointment 2% or oral flucloxacillin.
- For more persistent and severe lesions, an intensive regimen may be necessary, including in-patient admission for moisturiser, potent topical steroid ointment and wet dressings, combined with continued intensive care of any relapse for weeks or months. Treatment needs to be modified according to response.

MOLLUSCUM

Molluscum is caused by a pox virus and is very common. Most children get at least a few molluscum at some stage between the ages of one and twelve years. Uncomplicated molluscum lesions are easily recognised as firm, pearly, 1–4 mm dome-shaped papules with central umbilication. They are sometimes misdiagnosed as vesicles on initial examination. A child may develop a few or a great many lesions and individual lesions may last for months. Lesions can come and go for up to three years without causing any problems in most children. Complete resolution will not happen until an immune response develops, which may take from three months to three years.

Rarely, individual lesions can grow to over 1 cm in diameter. Individual lesions can become inflamed and, uncommonly, can develop secondary abscesses. More commonly, presentation to the ED is triggered by the development of widespread itchy and excoriated eczematous lesions in surrounding skin, usually on the lateral chest and axillary region or between the thighs. In such cases, recognition can be difficult, as the secondary changes can obliterate the primary lesions. A carefully taken history of the initial lesions is usually diagnostic.

Molluscum is common in the anogenital area and occurrence at this site does not suggest child sexual abuse. Molluscum is common on the face and occurrence at this site does not suggest underlying undiagnosed immunodeficiency.

Molluscum may occur on the eyelid margin or adjacent area. This can cause a persistent unilateral conjunctivitis. The molluscum may be isolated and subtle and go unnoticed for months during which the child may receive multiple courses of antibiotic treatment for conjunctivitis (Fig. 12.1.6).

Management

- Most children with molluscum require no treatment.
- Children with molluscum should not share towels but should not be restricted in their activities. Swimming should not generally be restricted. It is possible that spread to other parts of the body and to other children may be reduced by advising the child not to soak in warm water (baths, spas, heated pools). This is a significant restriction for many children with long-term sequelae if they miss their school swimming lessons. If restrictions are imposed on the child, lesions must be actively treated to ensure rapid clearing.

- Any child having problems with molluscum should be treated.
- The treatment depends on the age of the child, the location of the lesions and any secondary changes. Uncomplicated lesions not causing problems and not spreading can be left alone.
- If the presenting problem is the itch from secondary eczema, treatment of the eczema with mild or mid-potency topical steroid ointment may be all that is required. Try not to overuse as it is possible that this may encourage spreading of molluscum lesions.
- It is not difficult to destroy molluscum lesions. Simply deroofing the central umbilication is almost painless and leads to the papule becoming inflamed and resolving. In older children, this can be achieved with superficial needle pricking or light cryotherapy. Benzoyl peroxide 5%, a variety of chemical irritants and tape stripping can all be used but these can tend to flare any surrounding eczema.
- Topical cantharidin (e.g. Cantharone®) is the most rapid and effective way of dealing with molluscum in many situations. This is painless on application and causes small blisters at the site over the next several hours.

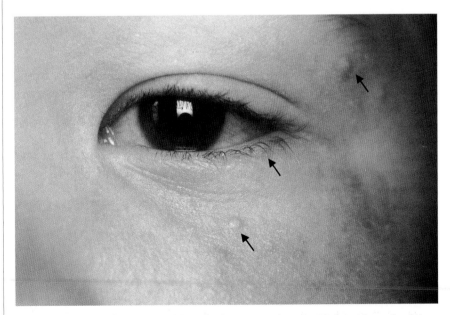

Fig. 12.1.6 **This six-year-old boy had presented to the ED four times in six months with recurrent unilateral conjunctivitis.**
Molluscum can be seen on the surrounding skin and a small papule towards the lateral end of his lower lid margin is also a molluscum. Treatment of the molluscum cured the conjunctivitis.

Importation of cantharidin requires a personal TGA permit and is not warranted unless you see many children with troublesome molluscum.

- Imiquimod 5% cream, noct. for several days, is expensive and unproven but may be useful for small numbers of lesions at difficult-to-treat sites.
- Several treatment options exist for molluscum around the eye and causing conjunctivitis. One or two lesions in older non-anxious children can be treated physically as for elsewhere on the face. Imiquimod 5% cream can be tried. If there are many lesions elsewhere, treating all the other lesions away from the eyes often induces rapid resolution of the eye lesions as well. In anxious children with significant problems with conjunctivitis, sedation or a brief general anaesthetic may be warranted.
- Inflamed lesions rarely warrant antibiotic treatment or drainage.

ADNEXAL TUMORS – PILOMATRICOMA

Many different benign tumours of the various cell types in hair follicles, sebaceous glands and sweat glands can present as papules during childhood. The most common by far are pilomatricomas. These present at any age in childhood as a slow-growing papule on the head, face or neck (or occasionally elsewhere) that can be 4–40 mm in size. They may be skin-coloured, white or bluish and are usually firm or hard, often due to calcification within the lesion. They may be lobulated. The main differential is an epidermal cyst. An ultrasound may confirm the diagnosis by demonstrating calcium shadows, which are not present in epidermal cysts. Pilomatricomas do not usually regress. Surgical removal is usually recommended but is not urgent.

KERATOSIS PILARIS

This is a rough, somewhat spiky papular rash, mainly on the upper outer arms, thighs and/or cheeks with variable erythema. It affects 50–80% of all adolescents and approximately 40% of adults. About 30–50% of patients have a positive family history. Autosomal dominant inheritance with variable penetrance has been described. It appears in infancy and persists throughout life. However, it tends to improve towards adulthood. Rarely, the erythema and papules are florid and distressing and treatment is warranted.

Management

- Reassure the patient that this is rarely a problem. Soap avoidance and moisturisers can improve the spiky feeling. Most children need no further treatment. Steroids do not help.

GRANULOMA ANNULARE

Granuloma annulare is not common in children. It begins as a small skin-coloured or red papule that spreads outward over many weeks or months to give an annular, asymptomatic ring, usually on the hands or feet. Although often misdiagnosed as tinea, the epidermis is not scaly and discrete subcutaneous papules can be felt all around the ring. It is slow growing and takes months to reach a size of 2 cm. Resolution usually occurs within a year or two. No investigation is necessary. Most children should be reassured and don't need treatment.

LANGERHANS CELL HISTIOCYTOSIS

Langerhans cell histiocytosis may present in several ways and should be considered as a possible diagnosis in any unusual, non-healing rash in infancy.

In neonates, Langerhans cell histiocytosis may present as a congenital self-healing form. One or a few papules are present at birth or shortly thereafter. They can be many millimetres in diameter and classically have a raised border and central necrosis. The papules usually show complete regression within months. Recurrence years later with visceral involvement or disseminated disease has been reported, and long-term monitoring is warranted.

In infants, Langerhans cell histiocytosis can present as recalcitrant 'cradle cap' with scaly, papular and petechial scalp lesions, often mistaken initially for severe seborrhoeic dermatitis. Flexural areas, especially the groin and anogenital area, can be involved, presenting as a chronic weeping 'nappy rash'. The presence of papules and/or petechiae, sometimes with ulceration, and the lack of response to treatment for napkin dermatitis should raise suspicion.

In infants and older children, there may be widespread, often itchy, small haemorrhagic papules mimicking a vasculitis. Erythematous and purpuric scaling and papules may be present on the hands and feet and nails may become dystrophic. Mucosal involvement can lead to ulceration on the gums or palate.

Extracutaneous disease can involve the liver, lymph nodes, marrow, bone and CNS. Diabetes insipidus can occur.

Management

- Confirm the diagnosis with a skin biopsy.
- Investigate for other organ involvement with skull, chest and skeletal X-rays, dental examination, full blood examination and liver function tests.
- Skin lesions can be treated with topical corticosteroid application or may require topical nitrogen mustard. Systemic treatment is usually reserved for children in whom progressive organ involvement is leading to problems.

JUVENILE XANTHOGRANULOMAS

Juvenile xanthogranulomas are the commonest cause of yellow papules in children. Occurring in early childhood, lesions appear as low, dome-shaped papules 2–5 mm in diameter. They may be yellow or red-brown lesions that become yellow when blanched. They are often on the scalp but can occur elsewhere. There may be one or multiple papules appearing over weeks or months. Biopsy may be required to confirm the diagnosis. Resolution without treatment usually occurs within a few years. Juvenile xanthogranulomas

DERMATOLOGY

are not associated with lipid disorders.

Children with neurofibromatosis who develop juvenile xanthogranulomas have an increased risk of developing myeloid leukaemia and should be monitored more closely for this complication.

Children less than two years old with multiple juvenile xanthogranulomas should have an ophthalmology assessment. Ocular juvenile xanthogranulomas leading to glaucoma have been reported in this subgroup of patients.

XANTHOMAS

True xanthomatous papules associated with elevated cholesterol levels are rare in childhood. They may present as multiple eruptive xanthomas, tuberous xanthomas (usually distributed over the elbows, knuckles, buttocks, knees and heels) and tendinous xanthomas (usually on tendons around the elbow, wrist, hand, or ankle). Investigation to exclude hyperlipidaemias is mandatory. Consider:

- Primary hyperlipoproteinaemias. Skin lesions may present between five and fifteen years of age, sometimes as tendinitis or tenosynovitis. Look for signs of atherosclerotic disease, and a family history of high cholesterol, early myocardial infarcts or strokes.
- Secondary hypercholesterolaemia. This can occur in hypothyroidism, biliary cirrhosis, diabetes mellitus, glycogen storage disease and nephrotic syndrome.

ANGIOFIBROMAS IN TUBEROSCLEROSIS

Facial angiofibromas may be the first sign of tuberosclerosis. They appear as small, red-brown papules (not pustules) on the cheeks from about 5–6 years of age and can be misinterpreted as flat warts or early-onset acne.

RED SCALY RASHES

Redness and scale indicate a combination of vasodilatation and epidermal involve-

ment. Atopic eczema is the commonest cause of red scaly rashes in children (see p. 343). Other red scaly eruptions include seborrhoeic dermatitis (infants), psoriasis, tinea corporis, pityriasis rosea and pityriasis versicolor. If itch is present, consider any of the causes of eczematous rashes (p. 343).

PSORIASIS

Psoriasis can occur at any age. Every year in a city of two million people, 400 children will present with psoriasis for the first time. Lesions typically begin as small, red papules that develop into circular, sometimes itchy, sharply demarcated, erythematous plaques with prominent silvery scale. However, psoriasis can present in many ways, including isolated thick scaly scalp lesions, scaly plaques on the hairline and behind the ears, annular lesions, pustular lesions, palmoplantar psoriasis, guttate psoriasis and flexural psoriasis. Therefore, psoriasis must be considered in the differential diagnosis of any red, scaly rash, particularly if well-demarcated and not particularly itchy.

Guttate psoriasis describes the eruption of hundreds of small, scaly papules on the trunk and limbs, often following a streptococcal throat infection.

Flexural psoriasis can involve any of the skin folds, particularly the anogenital area, and is more common in children than in adults. Psoriasis at flexural sites presents as moist, non-scaly erythema, often painless but sometimes with secondary fissuring or streptococcal infection.

Minor nail pitting is often seen in childhood psoriasis.

Management

- Presentation to the ED is often precipitated by the onset of guttate psoriasis or by secondary problems with long-standing anogenital psoriasis. The treatment depends on the site and extent of disease and the age of the child. Guttate psoriasis is often most easily managed with an extemporaneous tar cream, e.g. liquor picis carbonis (LPC) 3%/salicylic acid 2% in sorbolene cream, 500 gm.

Adolescents are less tolerant of tar creams.
- Minimise skin trauma. Use regular moisturiser.
- Treat isolated skin plaques with either topical steroids (e.g. mometasone) or topical calcipotriol, or both, for four weeks, with clinical monitoring. Topical steroids are not used for large areas in childhood psoriasis because of the possible development of rebound pustular disease. Thick scalp plaques can be softened overnight with a tar cream and removed with a tar shampoo. Generally avoid tar cream on the face, flexures and genitalia as it can be irritating.
- Use hydrocortisone 1% or pimecrolimus 1% cream on the face, flexures and anogenital region.
- Palmoplantar psoriasis can be resistant to treatment. Initially treat with topical potent corticosteroid and calcipotriol ointment.
- Secondary infection including perianal streptococcal infection may require treatment with oral penicillin. Recurrent or persistent streptococcal infection or carriage should be considered but is uncommon.
- A mild normocytic (occasionally microcytic) anaemia of chronic disease can occur in more severe cases.
- Appropriate medical follow-up is essential. Psoriasis will recur. Widespread or resistant psoriasis may need treatment with one or more of dithranol, ultraviolet therapy, acitretin, methotrexate or ciclosporin, all of which are effective.
- Widespread involvement may lead to erythroderma with metabolic and other complications (see erythroderma, p. 325).

TINEA CORPORIS

Tinea corporis (often called ringworm) is a common skin disorder, especially among children, but it may occur in people of all ages. It is caused by mould-like fungi (dermatophytes). Tinea infections can be transmitted by direct contact with affected individuals or by contact with contaminated items such as combs, clothing, shower, or pool surfaces. They can also be transmitted by contact with pets that carry the fungus (cats are common carriers). The typical lesion is a slow-growing erythematous ring with a clear or scaly centre. Scale is usually most prominent on the outside of the annular ring. However, tinea corporis can present in a wide variety of ways. It can be pustular or vesicular, particularly on the soles (Fig. 12.1.7), or it can spread to many sites within days. Between the toes, it presents as an itchy, white, scaly and macerated rash. Previous treatment with steroid ointments often leads to partial improvement in symptoms but causes spreading of the rash, the development of papules and the masking of diagnostic features. Tinea should be considered in any red, scaly rash where the diagnosis is unclear, particularly if there

Fig. 12.1.7 Inflammatory bullous fungal infection. (A) The foot with **(B)** secondary id reaction involving the hands.

is a gradually spreading eruption with inflammatory edges.

Management

- Confirm the diagnosis by scraping the scale for microscopy and culture.
- The family should identify and treat the source animal if any.
- Treat focal lesions with terbinafine cream (twice daily for 1 week) or an imidazole cream (e.g. clotrimazole, miconazole or econazole 2–4 times daily for four weeks).
- Rapidly spreading or widespread lesions, or involvement of hair-bearing areas usually requires oral griseofulvin (20 mg kg^{-1} d^{-1} in divided doses).
- Combined steroid and antifungal ointments (e.g. Kenacomb®) are often ineffective for clearing tinea corporis.
- Exclude from school until one day after treatment has commenced.

PITYRIASIS ROSEA

Pityriasis rosea is common from one to ten years. The cause is uncertain, but is thought to be viral. Human herpes virus, HHV-6 and HHV-7, has been implicated. A similar eruption may occur in response to a number of drugs. A pink scaly patch 2–4 cm in diameter near the shoulders or hips (herald patch) is the first sign in about 50% of children and is often misdiagnosed as tinea corporis because of its central clearing. However, unlike tinea, the scale is usually most prominent on the inside edge of the inflammatory ring. A few days or weeks later (or as the first feature if no herald patch is present), many pink/red, scaly, oval macules appear, mainly on the trunk, arms and thighs. The face, palms, lower legs and soles are largely spared. There may be thin scale within the lesions and oval lesions may align with skin lines to give a 'Christmas tree' pattern on the back and trunk. Pityriasis rosea usually persists for 1–2 months. It may be mildly itchy but is often asymptomatic.

Pityriasis rosea may be atypical. Lesions may be papular, crusted, vesicular or purpuric. The distribution may involve neck and extremities.

Secondary syphilis can appear in a similar fashion, but mucosal and acral lesions are usually present. Secondary syphilis should be excluded in any adolescent at risk of sexually transmitted disease who presents with pityriasis rosea, particularly if palms and soles are involved.

Management

- Reassure the patient.
- Sunlight (or ultraviolet light in troublesome cases) will hasten clearing. Topical corticosteroids do not help. Emollients, or occasionally oral antihistamine, are useful for itch.
- In an adolescent at risk for sexually transmitted diseases, arrange VDRL test.

SECONDARY SYPHILIS

Secondary syphilis presents 1–2 months after the primary chancre (which may be unreported). Erythematous, slightly scaly, macules or papules appear mainly on the trunk. There may be darker red macules on the palms and soles, as well as smooth or eroded papules on the tongue and oral mucosa, moist perineal papules (condylomata lata), annular lesions and pustules. Lymphadenopathy is usually present. Secondary syphilis can mimic pityriasis rosea and other red scaly disorders.

SEBORRHEIC DERMATITIS

The term 'seborrhoeic dermatitis' has been used to describe a number of different clinical entities. It is most widely used for a particular dermatitis that occurs in areas of skin that have a high density of sebaceous glands, namely the scalp, the central 'T-zone' of the face, and the upper chest and back (not the anogenital area, see p. 366). It is due to a reaction to a *Pityrosporum* yeast, which is part of the normal flora at these sites.

As true seborrhoeic dermatitis can only occur in the setting of active sebaceous glands, the diagnosis should only be made in the first three months of life or after puberty has begun. The sites of predilection are the scalp, inner eyebrows and paranasal folds. The quality of the scale is more greasy than that of an eczema at other sites and the degree of pruritus and discomfort is usually minimal. The degree of erythema varies and mild cases present as neonatal cradle cap or adolescent dandruff.

Atopic eczema is common on the scalp of infants and is differentiated from seborrhoeic dermatitis by increased pruritus and discomfort, a harsher drier scale and occurrence after the age of two months. It is important not to diagnose scalp eczema as seborrhoeic dermatitis as eczema will be further irritated by shampoos and 'cradle cap' creams.

Management

- Gently debride any built up crust with a non-irritating product such as olive oil, bath oil or a soap substitute. Only if very thick scale is present should salicylic acid creams be used.
- Settle erythema with 1% hydrocortisone cream.
- The use of an anti-yeast shampoo (e.g.. 2% ketoconazole) may be helpful in more recalcitrant cases.
- Adolescents with seborrhoeic dermatitis may have to wash their hair more frequently.

LICHEN STRIATUS

Lichen striatus usually presents on a limb as a unilateral linear eczematous rash following the developmental lines of the skin. On close inspection, there are often collections of tiny flat-topped papules, coalescing into scaly lines that may stretch the full length of the limb. It may remain static for a period of months or a couple of years, before spontaneously resolving. It may be pruritic but usually not significantly so.

The cause of the eruption is an inflammatory reaction in a streak of skin that has a genetic abnormality (mosaicism). The genetic difference of the streak is so subtle that the skin is phenotypically and functionally normal until a trigger, mostly a viral infection, induces an inflammatory reaction against the abnormal skin. As the condition is self-limiting,

no treatment is necessary if the condition is asymptomatic. Moderate-strength to potent topical steroid creams can help with any pruritus.

ECZEMATOUS RASHES

The term 'eczematous rashes' covers several common conditions that are characterised by erythema, itching and disruption to the epidermis with oozing, crusting, fissures or excoriations. The degree of epidermal disruption may be minimal so that the presentation of atopic eczema may be with just red dry patches. Alternatively, the degree of epidermal disruption may be severe with oedema and widespread vesiculation (e.g. plant contact dermatitis which is discussed under vesiculobullous rashes, p. 333).

ATOPIC ECZEMA – GENERAL ISSUES

The term 'atopic eczema' covers a range of presentations that depend on the age of the child and on the child's individual sensitivities. Several of these presentations are best seen as separate diseases. Clinical features and specific management suggestions are discussed under the individual headings below. However, some generalisations apply to most children with atopic eczema subtypes.

Atopic eczema usually begins in infancy. It commonly involves the face, and often the trunk and limbs as well. In older children, the rash may be widespread but is often localised to flexures. Erythema, weeping, excoriation and rarely vesicles may be seen in acute lesions. Chronic lesions may show scale and lichenification. In some children, the lesions are more clearly defined, thickened discoid areas that may intermittently be itchy. There is usually a cyclical pattern of improvement and exacerbation.

Families who present to the ED with atopic eczema often have children with chronic and severe disease requiring frequent, time-consuming applications of topical medicines and wet dressings. These children may have recurrent infections,

particularly with *Staphylococcus aureus* or herpes simplex. Failure to thrive may be present. A mild, normocytic (occasionally microcytic) anaemia of chronic disease can occur. Severe psychosocial and behavioural problems are common in these children although often hidden from medical staff. Parents may be under enormous stress with financial, marital and other problems secondary to the child's eczema. These problems need to be identified and addressed.

ATOPIC ECZEMA – GENERAL MANAGEMENT PRINCIPLES

- *Education.* Parents need to know that treatments are effective in controlling the disease. They should be aware of the principles of avoiding relevant triggers and settling the inflammation. Environmental and food allergens may contribute to the exacerbation of symptoms in some patients. Allergen avoidance in these children may be of benefit.
- *Avoid irritants.* The following may worsen atopic eczema: soaps, bubble baths, prickly clothing, including clothing worn by adults carrying babies, seams and labels on clothing, car seat covers, sand, carpets, overheating or contact with pets. Smooth cotton clothing is preferred.
- *Avoid heat.* Overheating increases itch. Most parents overdress young children. Outer clothing should be removed when entering warm environments. Bedding and baths should be kept comfortably cool.
- *Keep the skin moist.* Use a moisturiser such as sorbolene with 10% glycerine, aqueous cream or paraffin ointment (50:50 white soft paraffin/liquid paraffin) as often as a few times a day if necessary.
- *Treat inflammation.* In mild or moderate cases, steroid creams can be used intermittently with good effect. Hydrocortisone 1% is usually adequate. If not, moderate potency (e.g. betamethasone valerate 0.02%) or potent (e.g. mometasone 0.1% or

methylprednisolone 0.1%) ointment can be used for exacerbations. Widespread regular use of moderate potency steroids to the skin can cause atrophy or striae, especially on the face, the nappy area of infants, and sites of rapid growth such as the thighs of pubertal girls. Although expensive, pimecrolimus 1% is a useful alternative in some situations. Oral steroids are rarely indicated in atopic eczema. For chronic atopic eczema on the limbs, zinc and tar combinations are alternatives to steroids. Topical calcineurin inhibitors (tacrolimus and pimecrolimus) are increasingly used as an adjunct to topical steroid therapy but are expensive.

- *Control itch.* Advise parents to avoid saying 'stop itching' all the time and to distract the child instead. Wet bandaging is very helpful if warranted. Antihistamines are often unhelpful but if the itch is not controlled by other measures, they may be tried. Terfenadine (Teldane®) and astemizole (Hismanal®) should not be used because of occasional fatal interactions if erythromycin is also taken.

- *Wet dressings.* Wet dressings are bandages applied over topical moisturiser or corticosteroid ointments two to four times a day. They cool the skin and are effective in controlling flares of eczema, settling troublesome focal patches of eczema and reducing the need for corticosteroid. They are well tolerated by children although cumbersome to apply. However, if the initial application is done by a parent at home, acceptance of the treatment may be prejudiced by pre-existing conflict between the child and parent over treatment regimens. If possible, wet dressings should ideally be commenced by trained staff in hospital.

- *Treat infection.* Weeping and yellow crusted areas that do not respond to therapy may indicate secondary bacterial or herpetic (see p. 328) infection. Take cultures and treat with simple wet dressings and oral antibiotics (e.g. cefalexin or flucloxacillin). For recurrent bacterial infection, use antiseptic wash/bath oil.

- *Severe cases.* Do not accept that nothing more can be done. Children with chronic severe eczema need to be referred for psychosocial support and for assessment as to whether they warrant admission to hospital, oral prednisolone, narrow-band ultraviolet B therapy or oral ciclosporin therapy.

ATOPIC ECZEMA – DIETARY PRINCIPLES

A normal diet is indicated in most children with eczema. If a child has immediate urticarial reactions to a particular food, that food should be avoided. No alteration should otherwise be made to an infant's or child's diet unless appropriate conventional therapy, as above, has not worked. In difficult cases, particularly in infants, consider a formal allergy assessment. Restrictive diets without professional supervision should be avoided.

Babies with a first-degree relative with eczema have a 50% chance of developing eczema. For these babies, no modifications to the mother's diet are recommended during pregnancy and breast feeding. Exclusive breast feeding for the baby is recommended for a minimum of four months for a number of reasons. If exclusive breast feeding is not possible, supplementation with partially hydrolysed formula may reduce the risk of eczema. The use of soy formula has no role in the prevention of allergy. Peanuts and other nuts should be avoided until one year of age.

ATOPIC ECZEMA – ADMISSION TO HOSPITAL

Children with eczema who attend EDs often do so because the parents have become increasingly desperate to get their child's skin under control. Admission to hospital can be very helpful. You should consider admitting the child if any of the following circumstances apply:

- A child is missing school because of atopic eczema. If so, they should generally be admitted to hospital for intensive treatment.

- A child has severe impetiginisation or you have concerns about sepsis.

- A child has widespread eczema herpeticum.

- The family has social, financial or mental-health issues that make home treatment difficult.

- Education of the parents in an emergency setting is difficult because they speak a language other than English.

- The parents exhibit significant stress or impending breakdown.

- Outpatient management has not given a satisfactory response.

- An adolescent has widespread chronic eczema that affects their lifestyle (wears long clothing in summer, won't swim, etc.).

ATOPIC ECZEMA – USE OF TOPICAL STEROID PREPARATIONS

The use of topical steroids remains a pivotal component of eczema management. It is important to settle the eczema and restore the natural integrity of the skin. If eczema is left untreated, the natural barrier of the skin remains disrupted and the skin is more prone to react to other eczema triggers. Any scratching will further flare the skin and a worsening cycle is created. Topical cortisone preparations are used to break this cycle and heal the skin. They should not be used as prophylaxis on normal skin. The preparations are best prescribed in ointment formulation as these are more moisturizing. Creams may be used if ointments are poorly tolerated. As a general rule, topical corticosteroids are extremely safe. Side effects are very uncommon if used appropriately.

Always ask parents if they are treating their children with herbal creams. Any herbal cream that gives dramatic clearing should be assumed to contain corticosteroid products until proven otherwise. A British study in 2003 looked at a number of herbal creams given to children for eczema.[1] Over 80% of those tested had illegal potent or very potent corticosteroid additives. Similar results have been found in previous studies.

Systemic effects of topical steroid use
Suppression of the pituitary–adrenal axis can occur if potent topical corticosteroids are used over most of the skin surface continuously for many weeks, but this is an uncommon clinical scenario. If a child is using large amounts of topical corticosteroids in combination with inhaled corticosteroids and/or occasional oral cortisone therapy, you should consider adrenal suppression. Steroid therapy should not be abruptly stopped in this situation.

Local effects of topical steroid use
Irritation or allergy to one of the constituents of the topical steroid occurs in a few children. Apart from this, local side effects should not occur. Inappropriate use can lead to atrophy, striae, telangiectasia, purpura, cataracts and juvenile rosacea. Care is required when treating the face, anogenital areas, flexures and any areas of rapid growth where the skin is already under tension (e.g. breasts in adolescent females). In these situations, permanent striae can occur within weeks (Fig. 12.1.8). Precipitants of eczema should continue to be sought if the need for topical corticosteroids is ongoing. It should be explained to patients that once

the eczema has cleared, the topical corticosteroids should be ceased. This is more important in darker-skinned individuals where post-inflammatory hyperpigmentation may be mistaken by the patient for active disease.

The topical calcineurin inhibitors, tacrolimus and pimecrolimus, are now available as steroid-sparing agents. However, their expense currently limits their use and long-term safety data in children is not yet available.

ATOPIC ECZEMA – GENERALISED INFANTILE

Some infants present in the first six months of life with red, scaly and excoriated lesions covering much of the trunk and often the limbs, scalp and face as well. These infants are typically sleeping poorly. They are irritable and feeding poorly. The parents are often highly stressed by the difficulties with managing the child. Appropriate treatment usually leads to a dramatic change in the baby's behaviour and the family dynamics.

A detailed history should be taken to identify any exacerbating factors in the

child's environment. Examination will often reveal considerable dermographism and urticarial change. Allergy to foods is common in this setting and allergy testing is useful. Consider whether admission for wet dressings is required. Consider whether secondary bacterial or herpes infection is present. Treat with a bland emollient such as paraffin ointment once or twice daily. Use hydrocortisone 1% ointment on the face and methylprednisolone 0.1% to the body daily to gain rapid control of the skin. Arrange follow-up within a week or two if using significant amounts of potent topical steroid preparations. Skin prick testing and appropriate allergen avoidance may be useful in the longer term.

ATOPIC ECZEMA – FACIAL

Some infants will present with facial lesions. There may or may not be eczema elsewhere. Facial eczema may be secondarily infected with *Staphylococcus aureus*, resulting in weeping and crusting (Fig. 12.1.9). Saliva is a significant exacerbating factor. It is less common after one year of age. Herpes simplex virus infection needs to be considered (look for the typical monomorphic erosions, see p. 328). Treat with ointment moisturiser several times daily and, if indicated, oral flucloxacillin for one week. If appropriate follow-up can be assured, use methylprednisolone 0.1% ointment for a few days to gain rapid control of the skin. Arrange follow-up within a week to avoid problems from prolonged steroid use. Avoidance of irritating factors and general management measures are required to prevent relapse.

ATOPIC ECZEMA – PERIORAL ECZEMA VS. JUVENILE ROSACEA

Perioral eczema Refers to eczema round the mouth. This is common in infancy and early childhood. Irritation from saliva is the main cause. Occasionally, intolerance or allergy to foods

Fig. 12.1.8   Striae in the cubital fossa of a pubertal twelve-year-old girl after four weeks of potent corticosteroid cream. The underlying rash is acanthosis nigricans but was misinterpreted as eczema. (Courtesy of Dr Novick)

Fig. 12.1.9   Facial eczema with secondary impetiginisation in a ten-month-old boy.

can play a role in the older child. Confluent patches of erythema with weeping and superficial erosion occur in acute eczema. Management involves settling the active patches with a brief period of topical corticosteroid ointment and then trying to minimise irritation from saliva. This is difficult in the dribbling infant. Thicker moisturisers such as 50% white soft/liquid paraffin (Dermeze®) may be used both as a moisturiser and as a barrier on the skin. In persistent cases, use pimecrolimus 1% cream or tacrolimus 0.03% ointment.

Juvenile rosacea   Is often called 'perioral dermatitis' and confused with perioral eczema but it is not a true dermatitis. It is better thought of as a subset of rosacea. The most common clinical setting is following the use of topical steroids in a young child who is genetically predisposed to develop this condition. The morphology is quite different from perioral eczema. Erythematous papules occur around the mouth but spare the skin immediately adjacent to the lips. Other facial areas may be involved. The papules are essentially distinct from each other but may coalesce at times. Topical steroids tend to temporarily settle the

inflammation and then cause a rebound flare, and patients are often under the false impression that the topical steroids are the only effective therapy. Treatment involves the cessation of all topical steroids on the skin in this area and the introduction of an appropriate antibiotic. Use erythromycin in children or tetracyclines in adolescents. Pimecrolimus 1% cream may give added benefit. Resolution usually takes 3–4 weeks of therapy. It is important to warn patients who have been actively using topical steroids that there will be a rebound flare before they begin to see improvement.

ATOPIC ECZEMA – PERIORBITAL

Periorbital eczema is usually associated with sensitivity to airborne allergens, especially house dust mites, cat dander and pollens. Consideration of the occasions when the itch is worst will often indicate the causative agent. Formal skin prick testing, allergen avoidance measures, moisturiser, pimecrolimus 1% cream and follow-up are required. In atypical cases, consider allergic contact dermatitis, irritant contact dermatitis and molluscum.

ATOPIC ECZEMA – SUDDEN WORSENING OR URTICARIAL FLARE

Children with eczema occasionally present to the ED with an acute worsening of previously stable eczema. This should prompt a search for an underlying cause. Look for any evidence of scabies, which can easily be overlooked amongst the background eczema – other family members may be itchy. Look for secondary bacterial infection. Consider if herpes simplex virus infection (p. 328) may be present. Small papules in widespread patches of eczema may be from subtle molluscum lesions. The child may have developed an irritant or allergic contact sensitivity to their topical treatments or other agents. Search for and treat any exacerbating factors. Arrange early follow-up for management of the underlying eczema.

Often a sudden worsening with a dramatic increase in itch in a child with previously mild eczema is caused by viruses or allergy to drugs, food or environmental agents. They are often dermographic (i.e. they urticate in response to pressure on the skin) and it is likely that the cause of the flare is a subtle urticaria. When they itch, the scratching causes more urticaria, thereby causing more itch and escalating problems. These flares will often abate over a few days or weeks and the addition of a regular antihistamine will considerably help to control the symptoms.

ATOPIC ECZEMA – MOLLUSCUM

Molluscum infection can trigger a marked local or generalised reaction in children. Presentation to the ED follows the development of widespread itchy and excoriated eczematous lesions in surrounding skin, usually on the lateral chest and axillary region or between the thighs. If the child has a previous history of atopic eczema, the molluscum lesions may be overlooked or hidden in the eczema. A careful history may reveal that clear, firm papules were present at some stage. A careful examination may reveal some typical molluscum or some residual papules in the centre of eczematous patches. Treat as previously described (under molluscum, p. 339).

ATOPIC ECZEMA – FLEXURAL

While flexural eczema is the most common form of atopic eczema in children, it is rarely a cause for attendance at the ED unless sudden worsening has been triggered by secondary bacterial infection, secondary herpetic infection, acute irritant or allergic contact sensitivity or molluscum infection. Search for and treat any exacerbating factors. General principles of moisturisation, reducing overheating and avoiding irritants are usually adequate to regain control.

ATOPIC ECZEMA – DISCOID

Discoid eczema is characterised by chronic focal circular crusted lesions 1–5 cm in diameter. These children may have an associated psoriatic tendency. The discoid lesions are thickened, oozing and itchy. They are relatively resistant to therapy. Secondary staphylococcal infection is present in most cases. Intensive therapy is needed to break the cycle of itch, lichenification and infection. Oral flucloxacillin, ointment moisturiser, potent topical steroid ointment and regular wet dressings for two weeks may be adequate, but therapy may need to be prolonged. Follow-up is mandatory. Hospital admission, intralesional steroid injections, ultraviolet light therapy or oral ciclosporin may all be considered.

ATOPIC ECZEMA – JUVENILE PLANTAR DERMATOSIS

Juvenile plantar dermatosis is characterised by erythema, dryness and cracking of the anterior sole and the under surface of the toes. It is usually seen in mid-childhood. The child may or may not have atopic eczema elsewhere. Both feet are usually symmetrically involved. Juvenile plantar

dermatosis may persist for years and exacerbations may be associated with painful fissures. The differential includes tinea (which should be excluded by culture), psoriasis and contact dermatitis, which can all present with red scaly lesions on the soles. Cotton socks, leather shoes and regular ointment moisturiser three-times daily should be used. Cotton socks can be worn over the moisturiser. Minimise exposure of cracked skin to carpets and other irritants. Topical potent corticosteroid ointments may be necessary. Follow-up is needed.

ATOPIC ECZEMA WITH SYSTEMIC ASSOCIATIONS

Eczematous skin lesions can also be associated with:

- Immunodeficiency syndromes. Thrombocytopenia, immunodeficiency and eczema are seen in Wiskott–Aldrich syndrome. Petechiae, failure to thrive, recurrent infections, diarrhoea or haematological abnormalities may suggest this or other immunodeficiencies that are variably associated with eczema. Netherton syndrome should be considered if neonatal-onset eczema is associated with failure to thrive and sparse hair.
- Multiple food allergies with consequent dietary restrictions and secondary nutritional and psychosocial problems.
- Metabolic or nutritional disorders. Phenylketonuria often presents with eczema. Less typical eczematous lesions, more prominent in periorificial areas, are seen in biotin, essential fatty acid and zinc deficiency syndromes. Malnutrition and organoacidaemias, e.g. methylmalonicacidaemia, can result in similar lesions.

IRRITANT CONTACT DERMATITIS

The most common forms of irritant contact dermatitis in children are irritant napkin dermatitis (p. 366), juvenile plantar dermatosis (see above) and lip licking.

Lip licking refers to a dermatitis caused by chronic exposure to saliva. Usually the application of saliva by the child is presumed by the carers to be secondary to the dermatitis rather than causative, and may not be mentioned. Lip licking often presents with a clearly defined ring of dermatitis around the mouth but the pattern of involvement may vary considerably depending on the behaviour of the child. Any habit that spreads saliva in a particular direction will affect the pattern of the dermatitis. Acidic foods, artificial colours, preservatives and toothpaste may contribute to the irritation. Treatment requires education, frequent topical ointment barrier applications (initially many times daily) and immediate treatment of any relapse. A short period of topical pimecrolimus 1% cream may be needed. Secondary bacterial or candidal infection is rarely present.

ALLERGIC CONTACT DERMATITIS

Acute allergic contact reactions (e.g. to plants) often cause vesiculation and are considered under vesiculobullous rashes (p. 333). Chronic exposure to a contact allergen presents with erythema, itch and lichenification. The site of reaction usually suggests the cause; axillary rashes from deodorants, ears from earrings, lips and eyes from make-up, lower abdomen from nickel buttons on pants, wrist from watch, perioral from toothpaste and so on. However, the trigger may be overlooked. For example, an itchy eczematous patch on the scalp may be due to a metal stud in a cap that is not being worn at the time of presentation to the ED. Consider allergic contact dermatitis if a child has persistent eczema in an unusual distribution.

ALLERGIC CONTACT DERMATITIS – 'BLACK HENNA' REACTIONS

In recent years, several children have presented to EDs with an allergic reaction to 'black henna'. Henna is widely used in Asian countries as a traditional skin colouring agent. It is dark brown. Many street vendors use cheap black hair dye instead, calling it 'black henna'. These tattoos last for some weeks. These tattoos contain para-phenylenediamine, a strong contact sensitiser that should not be applied to the skin.

Three to ten days after the application of the tattoo, the child may notice discomfort, itch, erythema and swelling. This may progress over the next two weeks to blistering and scabbing of the tattoo site, sometimes with ulceration. Generalised itch and urticaria may be present and it may take months for complete resolution to occur. These children may develop a long lasting cross-sensitivity to sun screens, hair dyes, black clothing and cosmetics.

Treat with ointment moisturiser and potent topical corticosteroid. Review in one week.

GENERALISED DRY SKIN – ICHTHYOSIS

Ichthyosis refers to generalised scaly skin. There are several forms. Some ichthyoses only affect the skin but several have associated abnormalities in other organs.

Ichthyosis vulgaris is the commonest of the ichthyoses. It has autosomal dominant inheritance, and occurs as an isolated finding in 1 in 200 children.

X-linked ichthyosis is less common and may be undiagnosed for years or decades. About one-third of affected boys are diagnosed for the first time by an observant clinician during an emergency attendance for an unrelated problem. A fine scaling at birth is later replaced by larger brown scales. Diagnosis is confirmed by enzyme analysis for the affected steroid sulfatase gene. Boys with X-linked ichthyosis are usually otherwise normal but need to be monitored for hypogonadism, cryptorchidism, anosmia, short stature and mental retardation. Female carriers may have obstetric difficulties leading to prolonged labour.

In Sjögren–Larsson syndrome, a yellow-brown lichenified appearance is present in infancy. This evolves into a more florid scaling with a symmetric spastic paralysis and mental retardation. In some trichothiodystrophies, ichthyosis is associated with brittle hair and mental and growth retardation. Several ichthyoses are linked with deafness, cataracts or other eye problems. Mild, generalised scaling may be the first feature in later-onset Refsum disease, before development of multiple visual problems, deafness and neuropathy.

Eczema does not usually present as generalised dryness in babies. Unless there is a clear history of familial ichthyosis vulgaris, an infant with significant dryness should be referred for assessment by a skin specialist.

Ectodermal dysplasias are a heterogeneous group of conditions characterised by congenital, non-progressive abnormalities of hair, teeth, nails and sweat glands. The skin is dry and may be hyperpigmented. Deficient sweating may cause overheating in infants at any time and in older children in summer. Children may present with undiagnosed recurrent fevers or with heat prostration, collapse or death. Teeth are often poorly developed or absent. Cleft lip and palate, limb abnormalities and mucous retention in the upper airway and ear may be present. Accurate diagnosis, genetic counselling, dental and audiological review, appropriate moisturiser and topical cortisone use if needed, education about avoiding overheating and regular follow-up are all required.

RED BLANCHING RASHES (ERYTHEMATOUS)

Erythematous rashes are common in children. They are most commonly caused by viral infections (e.g. Coxsackie virus, echovirus, Epstein-Barr virus, adenovirus, parainfluenza, influenza, parvovirus B19, human herpes virus 6, rubella and measles) or by a drug reaction. Consider also septicaemia, scarlet fever, Kawasaki disease and *Mycoplasma* infection.

FEVER AND EXANTHEM

Fever and rash is a common presentation to the ED. The most common cause is a viral illness. Some infections have specific clinical features that aid diagnosis, e.g. measles and erythema infectiosum. However, in most instances, a specific viral diagnosis cannot be made with certainty. To manage such a child, consider:

- Is the child sick? Is the child lethargic, or peripherally cold? Are they young? Consider meningococcal disease, other bacterial sepsis, Kawasaki disease. These children require resuscitation if needed, urgent investigation and appropriate treatment guided by the findings.
- Is the child taking medications? Consider ceasing any medication.
- Are there other people at risk? If relatives are immunosuppressed or pregnant, consider serology, stool viral culture, and advising the at-risk person to consult their doctor.
- Is the rash papular? Consider papular acrodermatitis (p. 337).
- Is the rash itchy? If so, it may be primarily urticaria or a dermatitis.
- If the answer to all the above is 'no', reassurance and review is probably appropriate.

SCARLET FEVER

Group A streptococci cause a variety of diseases including scarlet fever, pharyngotonsillitis, impetigo, cellulitis, otitis media, streptococcal toxic shock syndrome, necrotising fasciitis, glomerulonephritis and rheumatic fever. Group A streptococcal infection usually occurs in school-age children.

Scarlet fever begins with a prodrome consisting of sudden onset of high fever, vomiting, malaise, headache, and abdominal pain. This is followed within a few hours by rash. The typical rash is a diffuse, pink-red generalised 'flush' with pinhead spots, that feels like sandpaper. The rash blanches. It is first noted on the upper chest, before spreading to the trunk, skin folds, neck, and extremities. The face is often flushed with circumoral sparing. It does not usually involve the palms or soles. Other features include strawberry tongue (initially white, then red day 4–5), pharyngotonsillitis and tender cervical and submaxillary nodes.

Confirm diagnosis by throat swab and serology. Notification is not required. Transmission occurs by direct contact. Isolate the child from school or crèche for three days after the start of treatment. Treat with phenoxymethylpenicillin (penicillin V) 250 mg orally (under 10 years), 500 mg orally (over 10 years) twice daily for 10 days. For penicillin-sensitive patients, use roxithromycin.

TOXIC SHOCK SYNDROME

Toxic shock syndrome is an acute, febrile illness with a characteristic rash and multiple system involvement. It has potential complications that include shock, renal and myocardial failure, coagulopathy and respiratory distress syndrome. Toxic shock syndrome has been associated with *Staphylococcus aureus* and group A streptococcal infection.

Presentation is initially similar to that of scarlet fever, but other features include myalgia, profuse diarrhoea, conjunctival injection and hypotension. Desquamation of digits, palms, soles and perianal region occurs 7–21 days later.

Initial management should focus on resuscitation. Antibiotic treatment should include flucloxacillin 50 mg kg^{-1} 4–6-hourly. Clindamycin should be added as it has been shown to inhibit the release of toxin in vitro.

KAWASAKI DISEASE

Kawasaki disease (see Chapter 5.7) is mainly seen in children between the ages of six months and five years. It is an acute, self-limiting vasculitic illness and a major cause of acquired coronary artery disease in Australian children. An understanding of the timing of clinical features aids diagnosis. The cardinal feature is a high fever persisting for 1–4 weeks with unusually severe irritability unresponsive to antipyretics. Dilatation of conjunctival vessels is seen within a few days of the onset of fever in 90% of children but may be subtle and there is no conjunctivitis or purulent discharge. In 60% of children, cervical lymph nodes are enlarged as a firm mass at the onset of fever. In older children, there may be striking, unilateral tender lymphadenopathy thought to be cervical adenitis but unresponsive to antibiotics.

Within a few days of onset of fever, 90% of children develop a widespread erythematous rash. This may include urticarial and maculopapular lesions that increase to several centimetres in diameter. There is usually involvement of the anogenital area. There are no vesicles or crusting but there may be a few pustules on elbows or knees. The rash lasts for 1–7 days.

Within a day or two of the rash, 90% of children develop changes of the lips and mouth. The lips become red, dry, fissured and occasionally crusted and bleeding. The oral mucosa is red without ulceration. These changes can persist for 2–3 weeks.

Within a day or two of the development of a rash, about 95% of children develop erythema of the palms and soles, often with associated oedema to give a shiny swollen appearance to the hands. The swelling can persist until the fever resolves. About two weeks after the onset of fever, desquamation begins at the finger tips and spreads to involve the palms, followed a few days later by desquamation of the toes then soles. Fingertip desquamation will usually be seen even if no palm or sole involvement was noted earlier. This is an important feature as palm and sole involvement in a widespread eruption is otherwise uncommon.

Less common features include arthritis, diarrhoea, vomiting, coryza, cough, and hydrops of the gall bladder.

In babies under six months of age, and sometimes in older children, Kawasaki disease may present as prolonged fever with only one or two of the above features. Untreated, about 25% of children with Kawasaki disease develop coronary artery changes. These can occur up to 6–8 weeks after the onset of fever and may ultimately be fatal. Any child with persistent fever of unknown cause should be carefully screened for any manifestations of Kawasaki disease. Investigations should include full blood count, ESR, liver function tests and serology to exclude possible differential diagnoses. If Kawasaki disease is suspected, echocardiography should be performed at least twice: at presentation and again at 6–8 weeks. Treatment with intravenous γ-globulin (2 gm kg^{-1}, repeated if fever persists) and aspirin (10 mg kg^{-1} 8 hrly while febrile, then 3–5 mg kg^{-1} orally daily for at least 6–8 weeks) may be life-saving. Regardless of the initial echocardiogram result, treatment should be given as early in the course of the illness as possible, to minimise the risk and severity of cardiac problems.

ERYTHEMA INFECTIOSUM

Erythema infectiosum, also known as slapped cheek disease or fifth disease, is caused by parvovirus B19. It begins with a non-specific prodrome of fever (15–30% of cases), malaise, myalgia and headache. The distinctive rash has three stages:

❶ Slapped cheek appearance (1–3 days).
❷ Maculopapular blanching rash on the proximal extensor surfaces, flexor surfaces and trunk. This fades over several days with central clearing and then forms a reticular pattern (after 7 days).
❸ Reticular rash reappears with heat, cold and friction (weeks/months).

Arthralgia and arthritis occur infrequently in infected children, but are common in adults. Other potential complications include aplastic crises in children with haemoglobin abnormalities and chronic anaemia in children with HIV infection.

Treatment is supportive. Children with erythema infectiosum are highly infective before the onset of illness and are probably not infective once the rash appears. They do not need to be excluded from school or childcare. Seek specialist advice if the child is known to have a blood disorder or to be immunosuppressed.

Pregnant women who contract parvovirus B19 have a small risk of foetal anaemia and death but do not have an increased risk of foetal abnormalities. It is not practicable to prevent exposure at home, and exclusion of pregnant women from work is not recommended.[2] Pregnant women in contact with a child with parvovirus B19 infection should be advised to consult the doctor supervising their pregnancy.

ROSEOLA INFANTUM

This common viral exanthem is caused by human herpes virus 6 (HHV-6), and in some cases by HHV-7. Ninety-five percent of children have been exposed to HHV-6 by the age of two years. Up to 30% of all infants will present with the clinical features of roseola. Typically, an infant has a high fever for 2–4 days and is often prescribed oral antibiotics. Despite the high fever, the child remains well and active. Occipital and cervical lymphadenopathy is frequently present. The fever then disappears, but at the same time a widespread erythematous rash appears on the face and trunk. This commonly leads to presentation to the ED. Recognition of this condition is important so that both doctor and family realise that the rash is not a reaction to the antibiotics. After the appearance of the rash, the child remains well and no isolation is necessary.

ENTEROVIRUSES

Coxsackie A, B and echoviruses are all enteroviruses that cause a range of childhood illnesses, particularly in the summer months. They can cause several types of exanthem, including maculopapular, erythematous, vesicular and petechial rashes. Hand, foot and mouth disease represents one particular syndrome, usually caused by coxsackie A16 virus, and less commonly by other group A and group B coxsackie viruses and enterovirus 71 (EV71) (see p. 327). Pharyngitis is a frequent feature of enteroviral infection. Encephalitis is a less-common accompanying presentation.

INFECTIOUS MONONUCLEOSIS

This syndrome is most commonly caused by Epstein–Barr virus, but may also be associated with cytomegalovirus and other viruses. Clinical features include fever, generalised lymphadenopathy, exudative tonsillopharyngitis, palatal petechiae, and hepatosplenomegaly. Children usually have milder disease than adults.

Rash occurs in up to 20% of children in the first few days of the illness. The rash may be erythematous, maculopapular or morbilliform. There is an increased incidence of rash in children with infectious mononucleosis if treated with amoxicillin or other penicillins. This rash is typically maculopapular and pruritic, and occurs mainly over the trunk.

Epstein–Barr virus has a number of other less-common dermatological manifestations, including papular acrodermatitis, oral hairy leukoplakia and cutaneous lymphoproliferative disorders.

Diagnosis can be confirmed by full blood examination, liver function tests and serology. Isolation is not required. Children with significant throat symptoms may need admission for supportive care. Oral prednisolone for five days may assist resolution of symptoms. Children with splenomegaly should be advised to avoid contact sports until approved by their doctor.

MEASLES

As a result of widespread measles immunisation, this disease is now seen infrequently. However, outbreaks continue to occur in most parts of the world. The hallmarks of measles are cough, conjunctivitis and rash. The rash appears 3–4 days after the prodrome of fever, conjunctivitis, coryza, cough and Koplik spots (white spots on a bright red buccal mucosa). The rash is initially red, blanching and maculopapular. It begins around the ears and hairline; and spreads to the trunk and the proximal arms and legs. It becomes confluent by the third day. High fever often persists after onset of the rash. Uncommonly, a child will develop otitis media, pneumonia or encephalitis. Subacute sclerosing panencephalitis is a rare, fatal, late complication.

Measles vaccination gives a transient mild exanthem in about 5% of cases. If a child has been previously immunised with killed measles vaccine and later contracts measles, the presentation may be unusual. This 'atypical measles' often has high fever and malaise, no cough, no eye signs, no Koplik spots, and a rash that is more distal and often purpuric. Australian children are routinely immunised with attenuated live virus and atypical measles is rarely seen here.

Measles is highly contagious and spread by airborne droplets or direct contact with infected nasal or throat secretions. Suspected cases presenting to the ED should be managed in a separate area to other patients in the department, preferably in a negative pressure room. Diagnosis should be confirmed by immunofluorescence (rapid) and culture of a nasopharyngeal aspirate or throat swab and serology with paired sera. Laboratory confirmation and notification to the health department is essential to prevent epidemics. The child should be excluded from school or crèche for five days.

If an unimmunised child over nine months of age has contact with measles, measles infection can be prevented by MMR vaccination within 72 hours. This is because the incubation period of the vaccine strain is shorter (4–6 days) than the incubation period of wild measles virus (10–14 days). Older contacts who do not have documentation of immunisation with measles vaccine, should be tested for measles IgG if this can be performed within 72 hours. If seronegative, or if serology cannot be performed, contacts should be immunised within 72 hours. Infants under nine months old who have contact with measles should be given normal human immunoglobulin within seven days.

RUBELLA

Rubella infection is asymptomatic in 25–50% of children. Affected children are usually only mildly unwell. The prodrome lasts up to five days and consists of low-grade fever, malaise, headache, coryza, and post-auricular, occipital and posterior triangle lymphadenopathy. The rash is characterised by small, fine, discrete, pink maculopapules. It starts on the face and spreads to the chest and upper arms, abdomen and thighs, all within 24 hours.

If a child is over one year of age and known to have received rubella vaccination, a subsequent exanthem is highly unlikely to be rubella and investigation is not required. If rubella is suspected in younger children or you cannot confirm that the child has been previously vaccinated, immunofluorescence (rapid) and culture of a nasal or throat swab should be performed. This can be taken out of hours and kept cold until morning for testing. If diagnosis is confirmed, notification to state health departments is required in most states. The child should be excluded from school or crèche for five days. Pregnant women in contact with a child with rubella infection must consult the doctor supervising their pregnancy without delay.

UNILATERAL LATEROTHORACIC EXANTHEM

Unilateral laterothoracic exanthem has only been well recognised in the past decade but is another common presentation to the ED. It usually occurs between one and four years. There is often a mild fever with gastrointestinal or upper respiratory symptoms one to three weeks before the onset of rash. The rash begins on one side of the chest as erythematous, urticarial, eczematous or papular lesions. Uncommonly, the rash may start in the inguinal region or on the thigh. Over a period of a week, the rash spreads to give a strikingly unilateral involvement of the lateral chest, axilla and arm. Over the next two weeks, there may be some spread to the other side and other areas. Itch may be present but is not marked. Coryza, pharyngitis, and regional lymphadenopathy may occur. Complete resolution occurs without sequelae within a total of four to six weeks.

Although the epidemiology of unilateral laterothoracic exanthem suggests an infective cause, no causative agent has been identified despite exhaustive searching. No isolation or restriction of activi-

ties is needed. Moderate potency topical corticosteroids may give some relief but often no treatment is needed.

URTICARIA

Urticaria is common. It is characterised by the rapid appearance and disappearance of multiple raised red wheals on any part of the body. Circular erythematous macules or swellings, sometimes with central pallor, appear, migrate and disappear over minutes or hours. Individual lesions are often itchy and resolve within one day. There may be central clearing to give ring lesions. (These are not the target lesions of erythema multiforme, which always persist for several days.)

In some children the urticarial wheals do not fully blanch with pressure. As the lesions migrate or grow circumferentially, they leave a purplish non-blanching tinge on the skin, indicating some degree of leakage of red cells from capillaries. Frank purpura is not usually present. Typically, these children are otherwise well and are reacting to the same group of possible triggers as children with normal urticaria. Occasionally, this may be a presentation of serum sickness or cutaneous or systemic vasculitis. Features that raise suspicion about an underlying vasculitis include weals lasting more than 24 hours, bruising within weals, painful lesions or associated fever, arthralgia, abdominal pain or haematuria.

Urticaria usually occurs in otherwise well children as an isolated finding. The most common trigger for acute urticaria is a viral infection, but it may be triggered by any environmental or food allergen, or by prescription and non-prescription drugs. In most cases of short duration the urticaria resolves rapidly and the cause cannot be determined. Occasionally, the parents will strongly suspect some food or environmental agent that the child contacted before the onset of the urticaria.

Urticarial drug reactions in children are often associated with penicillin group antibiotics, cefaclor, other antibiotics, aspirin, other non-steroidal anti-inflammatory drugs and latex. Latex allergy is most common in children with recurrent ex-

posure to latex such as repeated catheterisations or surgery, and may present as local urticaria, oedema or anaphylaxis. Banana, avocado and kiwifruit can cross-react with latex and after ingestion, children may present with itch, oedema, urticaria and wheezing.

Urticaria can be precipitated by sunlight, pressure, water, cold, heat and other physical factors.

Urticarial episodes usually resolve over days or weeks and rarely last longer than three months. Chronic urticaria refers to lesions being present virtually every day for more than three months. Rarely, this can last for many years. Urticaria may be recurrent with individual episodes resolving quickly but occurring many times over weeks, months or years. Recurrent or chronic urticaria is usually of unknown aetiology but may be related to underlying inflammatory conditions such as systemic lupus erythematosus, juvenile chronic arthritis, other vasculitic diseases, and parasitic infection. Painful urticaria may be a presenting feature of erythropoietic protoporphyria.

In a child who is very unwell with urticaria, consider anaphylaxis or Kawasaki disease. If individual lesions last longer than two days or are tender or purpuric, consider investigation for cutaneous vasculitis including Henoch–Schönlein purpura and urticarial vasculitis.

Management

- Urticaria may be the first sign of anaphylaxis. If there is associated angio-oedema (prominent subcutaneous swelling) or wheeze, continued observation and appropriate treatment is required (see Chapter 22.5 on anaphylaxis).
- Investigation is usually not required.
- Identify the cause if possible. Ask about illnesses, medications, recent unusual foods and environmental contacts. Document these clearly.
- Treat the itch with oral antihistamine. Oral prednisolone, 1 mg kg^{-1} per day (maximum 50 mg), for a few days may be warranted by the severity of the itch but is usually not needed.
- If any purpura is present or the child is significantly lethargic or less

responsive than usual, assess and investigate to exclude meningococcal sepsis and other causes of purpura. Check urine for blood.

- For recurrent or chronic urticaria, look for trigger factors. Consider mast-cell-degranulating drugs (including opiates, aspirin, and other non-steroidal anti-inflammatory drugs), foods, alcohol, animals, parasitic infections, heat, cold, sunlight and physical pressure. Consider investigating with a throat swab (for streptococcal carriage), full blood examination (for eosinophilia and anaemia), IgE, antinuclear antibodies, urine culture for bacteraemia, nocturnal check for threadworms and a possible challenge with any suspected agent. Assessment of erythrocyte protoporphyrin is warranted in young infants with sun-induced, painful urticaria.
- For recurrent or chronic urticaria that is unresponsive to conventional H1 antihistamine antagonists, adding cimetidine, 10–15 mg kg^{-1} (maximum 200 mg) orally 6-hourly, to the antihistamine may help.
- For recurrent urticaria, or for chronic urticaria where there is a clear history of regular exacerbations in the severity of the lesions, a diary recording all happenings in the 24 hours before each relapse may be rewarding in identifying the cause.

SERUM SICKNESS

Serum sickness (sometimes called 'serum-sickness-like-reactions') consists of the triad of fever, urticaria and arthralgias. It can occur at any age. Historically, about 50% of serum sickness reactions in Australian children are idiopathic and 50% have been associated with a recent course of cefaclor. Other medications may also be implicated.

Symptoms begin 5–21 days after commencement of the cefaclor and persist for five to ten days. Previous courses of cefaclor may have been taken uneventfully, but more rapid onset can be seen in those children previously exposed. The child presents with an urticarial rash,

which can be dramatic in appearance and cause considerable alarm to parents. The lesions may be more fixed than typical urticaria and may bruise or be tender Arthralgia and joint swelling, possibly with effusion, is observed. Polyarthralgia occurs in up to 80%. Fever, lymphadenopathy, malaise, nausea, vomiting and abdominal pain are less common. Symptoms resolve fully in a few days. Laboratory investigations are unrewarding and infectious studies negative.

Management (see also urticaria)

- If associated with cefaclor, or another medication, cease the medication and give written information about this to the family and treating doctor.
- Joint symptoms may require analgesia and bed rest.
- Oral antihistamines may provide symptomatic relief. A few days of oral prednisolone, 1 mg kg^{-1} d^{-1} (maximum 50 mg), may be warranted by the severity of the symptoms.
- Hospitalisation and supportive care may occasionally be needed.
- Rechallenge with cefaclor may result in a recurrence of serum sickness although the risk of recurrence is unknown. A serum sickness reaction to cefaclor is not a contraindication to having another cephalosporin.

LUPUS ERYTHEMATOSUS

Systemic lupus erythematosus may present as erythematous, well-demarcated facial lesions, occasionally urticarial or slightly scaly. These lesions occur most commonly in a characteristic butterfly distribution over both cheeks and the base of the nose. In children, the facial rash may be the only manifestation (cutaneous lupus) or there may be systemic involvement. There is usually an epidermal and a dermal component. Therefore the lesion is usually more indurated than a dermatitis and more scaly than an urticaria.

In more widespread disease, patchy lesions may be present over the ears, neck and less commonly the limbs. Erythematous macules, petechiae and small infarcts

can also be seen around the nail beds and on the tips of the fingers and toes. Erythematous macules may appear on the palms of the hands and soles of the feet. Florid urticaria, blistering and erythema nodosum are uncommonly seen.

Fever, arthralgias and arthritis affecting many joints imply systemic involvement. Lymphadenopathy, anorexia, weight loss, muscle weakness, pulmonary disease (especially pleuritis), cardiac disease (myocarditis and coronary artery disease), nephritis and a wide range of neuropsychiatric symptoms can be seen in childhood systemic lupus erythematosus.

If lupus is suspected, a detailed history and examination should look for systemic organ involvement, and investigations should include antinuclear and anti-double-stranded DNA antibodies, erythrocyte sedimentation rate, full blood count, renal assessment and/or brain imaging as indicated. Localised cutaneous lesions generally respond well to moisturiser, sun protection and potent topical corticosteroid preparations. Systemic disease requires oral corticosteroid therapy initially. Regular follow-up and monitoring for renal and other organ involvement is essential in all cases.

NEONATAL LUPUS ERYTHEMATOSUS

Neonatal lupus erythematosus occurs in infants whose mothers are positive for anti-Ro(SSA) and/or anti-La(SSB) antibodies. Most of these mothers are asymptomatic and unaware of their antibody status. About 5% of infants of antibody-positive mothers develop neonatal lupus.

Skin lesions in neonatal lupus can first appear from a few days to a few months after birth. Widespread, erythematous, often annular and growing lesions develop on the face, scalp, trunk, extremities and neck. These can be misdiagnosed as tinea or eczema. They persist for months before clearing as the maternal antibodies clear. Moderate potency topical steroid assists clearing. Sunlight and ultraviolet light can precipitate or worsen the rash.

The other major manifestation of neonatal lupus is complete heart block (from the third trimester). This is permanent and often fatal and requires a pacemaker. Interestingly, about half of all babies with neonatal lupus have complete heart block and about half have the characteristic skin lesions but only a few have both.

All infants with neonatal lupus presenting with skin lesions require ongoing follow-up as they appear to have an increased risk of developing autoimmune thyroid or rheumatological disorders during childhood. Subsequent siblings may be normal but 25% develop neonatal lupus in either the skin or cardiac form. Subsequent pregnancies should therefore have serial echocardiogram monitoring. Most mothers eventually develop rheumatological disease and they also require referral for follow-up.

DERMATOMYOSITIS

Childhood dermatomyositis affects skin and muscle. Children may present with skin changes years before any muscle involvement or may present with acute or subacute development of fever, rash, pain and weakness. The earliest features in many children are an erythematous, sometimes violaceous, rash on the eyelids, periorbital oedema, a malar erythematous rash, and erythematous papules over the extensor surfaces of the joints of the hands. In more severe cases, there may be widespread desquamation and ulceration around the eyes, fingers and skin folds.

Muscle weakness may not have been noticed at presentation but may be present on testing. Investigations should include erythrocyte sedimentation rate, full blood count, and creatine kinase. Magnetic resonance imaging has replaced muscle biopsy as a means of assessing muscle inflammation. Therapy involves high-dose oral corticosteroid therapy initially, maintenance immunosuppression for a couple of years, and regular follow-up.

JUVENILE CHRONIC ARTHRITIS

An erythematous maculopapular rash is often seen in the systemic form of juvenile chronic arthritis. This rash usually has a salmon pink colour, and tends to come and go, being particularly evident at the time when the fever is at its height. It may be urticarial.

ERYTHEMA NODOSUM

Erythema nodosum can occur at any age and presents with the fairly abrupt onset of painful and tender subcutaneous erythematous lesions up to 5 cm in diameter, mainly on the anterior lower legs. The arms, soles and trunk may be affected. Malaise, fever, and arthralgia may be present. Histologically there is a septal panniculitis.

In about 50% of children, erythema nodosum occurs in association with another condition, either as the presenting feature or as part of the evolution of an already diagnosed disease. Causes include chronic streptococcal disease, tuberculosis at any site, inflammatory bowel disease, chronic gastrointestinal infections, sarcoidosis, *Mycoplasma* infection, lymphoma, secondary syphilis, deep fungal infections and the oral contraceptive pill.

Lesions pass through colour changes similar to aging bruises. Resolution occurs in three to six weeks in most cases. Chronic or recurrent erythema nodosum can persist for months or years, particularly if an underlying cause has not been removed.

Management
- Search for any underlying cause.
- Investigations may include throat swab, full blood examination, erythrocyte sedimentation rate, serology for *Streptococcus*, *Mycoplasma* and Epstein–Barr virus, stool culture, Mantoux testing and chest X-ray.
- Depending on the severity of symptoms, bed rest or limitation of activities for a few days may be required.
- Non-steroidal anti-inflammatory treatment will help settle inflammation and pain. The use of oral prednisolone is controversial.
- In troublesome, prolonged or recurrent cases, potassium iodide

(10% solution, 2.5 mL = 250 mg three-times daily for older children, taken with milk or juice for two weeks) is effective.[3]

NECROBIOSIS LIPOIDICA

This presents as large, irregularly shaped, red-yellow patches on the lower legs, usually in adolescents. With time, the central area may become atrophic or sclerosed. Necrobiosis lipoidica may be the first sign of diabetes in childhood and a fasting serum glucose should be arranged with follow-up.

PALMOPLANTAR HIDRADENITIS

Palmoplantar hidradenitis, (previously known as childhood neutrophilic eccrine hidradenitis or plantar erythema nodosum), occurs in otherwise well children, typically aged 2–14 years, during spring or autumn. There may be a history of considerable physical exertion in the days before the lesions appear, often with exposure to cold or water. Erythematous, dusky tender lesions appear on the soles (Fig. 12.1.10), and sometimes on the hands. *Pseudomonas* infection within the sweat glands may be the cause in some or most cases. Antibiotics are not needed and spontaneous resolution occurs within three weeks. If you are confident of the diagnosis, no investigation is necessary. Recurrences are common.

PERNIO (CHILBLAINS)

Pernio usually presents after exposure to cold such as playing outdoor sport in winter. Tender red/purple swellings occur on the fingers and or toes. Initially there is no epidermal change but lesions can persist for weeks and dusky scaling can develop. Symptoms are usually mild. Most children presenting with pernio are otherwise well and do not routinely need investigation. In persistent and troublesome cases, baseline investigations may include anti-Ro, antinuclear and anti-

Fig. 12.1.10 Palmoplantar hidradenitis. (Photo courtesy of Dr Cremer)

phospholipid antibodies, rheumatoid factor and cryofibrinogens. Recurrences are common. Manage by avoiding cold.

SPIDER TELANGIECTASIA

A spider naevus presents as a tiny red macule or papule with a surrounding network of fine telangiectasias, best appreciated by compressing the lesion to make it disappear then watching it reappear in the characteristic centripetal pattern, filling from the centre. These appear during mid-childhood in about 50% of children, typically on the face, hands or arms. Most resolve within a few years. Investigation is not needed. If the cosmetic concern is severe, removal by electrodessication or laser can be arranged.

Multiple spider naevi are of no medical significance in healthy children. Multiple telangiectatic vessels of non-spider type may raise suspicion of hereditary haemorrhagic telangiectasia or a photosensitivity syndrome.

OTHER ERYTHEMATOUS RASHES

Many conditions that present with red, scaly or purpuric rashes may appear erythematous initially, including guttate psoriasis, pityriasis rosea and Henoch–Schönlein purpura. Sometimes, most of the lesions may be erythematous but a few may reveal the more typical features of the underlying condition, such as scale or purpura.

Many haemangiomas (vascular tumours) will initially present as erythematous macules. This possibility should be borne in mind in any infant presenting with an erythematous macule on the face. Early review may show some progression of the lesion. If so, urgent referral for treatment may minimise potentially severe long-term problems from florid facial haemangiomas (p. 358).

PURPURIC RASHES

Purpuric rashes in childhood may be due to vascular dysfunction, coagulation disorder or a low platelet count. Fever may or may not be present. Purpuric rashes are associated with several life-threatening diseases and require urgent assessment.

FEVER AND PETECHIA

Petechiae are pinpoint, non-blanching spots, less than 2 mm diameter. There are many causes of fever and petechiae. These include:

- Viral infections including enteroviruses and influenza.
- *Neisseria meningitidis* (meningococcal) disease.
- Other causes of bacteraemia including *Streptococcus pneumoniae* and *Haemophilus influenzae*.

- Other diseases including Henoch–Schönlein purpura, idiopathic thrombocytopenic purpura and leukaemia.
- Illness associated with vomiting or coughing causing petechiae around the head and neck.

The majority of children with fever and petechiae do not have a cause identified – they are presumably due to viral infections. Few children with fever and petechiae (< 5%) will have meningococcal disease. Recognition and early treatment of these children with meningococcal disease is paramount. Clinical signs and laboratory investigations will help determine those who should be treated for suspected meningococcal disease. All children with fever and petechiae should be reviewed by a senior doctor.

FEVER AND PETECHIA IN AN UNWELL CHILD (INCLUDING MENINGOCOCCAL SEPSIS)

If a child with fever and petechiae meets any of the following criteria, they should be presumed to have meningococcal sepsis until proven otherwise and treated accordingly (see meningococcal and other septicaemia below, p. 355).

- Impaired conscious state (lack of alertness, lethargy, irritability).
- Abnormal signs (tachycardia, tachypnoea, desaturation in air, widened pulse pressure).
- Poor perfusion (cold extremities).
- Any purpuric lesions greater than 2 mm (unless the clinical picture is suggestive of Henoch–Schönlein purpura, see below).
- Abnormal blood indices (including WCC $> 15 \times 10^9$ L^{-1} and $< 5 \times 10^9$ L^{-1} or raised CRP > 8).

FEVER AND PETECHIA IN A WELL CHILD

If a child with fever and petechiae is well and does not meet any of the criteria for meningococcal sepsis in the preceding paragraph, the petechiae may be due to an obvious mechanical cause. These children do not require investigation and may be discharged with review planned within 12–24 hours. Mechanical causes of petechiae include:

- Coughing or vomiting leading to petechiae around the head and neck.
- Local physical pressure such as a tight tourniquet or being held tightly for procedures.
- The practice seen in some ethnic groups of treating a febrile child by rubbing or suctioning the skin with a variety of implements, producing bizarre circular and linear patterns of petechiae.

If no mechanical cause is identified in a well child with fever and petechiae, the child is likely to have a viral infection (Fig. 12.1.11), and should be managed as follows:

- Investigate with a full blood count, C-reactive protein and blood cultures.

- Observe for four hours.
- If the initial test results are normal and there is no clinical deterioration or progression of the rash over the four hours, discharge with review the next day.

Children who have received antibiotics prior to presentation can be managed the same way, but the possibility of partially treated meningitis or sepsis may lead to a lower threshold for admission or early review.

MENINGOCOCCAL AND OTHER SEPTICAEMIA

Septicaemia with purpura is usually due to meningococcal disease. There may be an upper respiratory prodrome followed within hours by high fever, malaise and headache. Skin lesions may begin as tender erythematous macules or as petechiae on the skin and mucous membranes.

Lesions develop purpuric centres and large haemorrhagic areas may form. Purpuria may also be due to sepsis with *Haemophilus influenzae*, group A streptococci, *Staphylococcus aureus* and some Gram-negative organisms. Infective endocarditis, typhus, typhoid fever and certain viral haemorrhagic fevers may cause purpuric lesions.

Early management (a detailed updated protocol for meningococcal management can be accessed online[4]):

- Give oxygen.
- Gain intravenous or intraosseous access.
- Immediate investigations (if blood can be obtained without delay) including blood culture, blood smear, blood PCR, full blood count/ differential, glucose, urea and electrolytes, clotting, if appropriate.
- Administer cefotaxime (50 mg kg^{-1} per dose – maximum 3 g, 6-hourly). Chloramphenicol may be used in children with a type 1 hypersensitivity

Fig. 12.1.11 Fever and rash in a six-year-old boy. (A) The rash appears erythematous. **(B)** Close inspection reveals many petechiae.

to cephalosporins. Do not allow investigations to delay this.

- Meningococcaemia is often associated with hypovolaemia, give 20 mL kg^{-1} of normal saline. More fluid will often be needed to improve blood pressure and peripheral perfusion (40 mL kg^{-1} in the first hour is common).
- Isolate cases (if possible) until they have had > 12 hours antibiotic treatment.
- Contact paediatric intensive care unit.
- Subsequent investigations include throat swab, lumbar puncture (unless contraindicated). Urinary or CSF 'rapid antigen' testing is not recommended because of poor sensitivity and specificity.

VASCULITIS AND HENOCH–SCHÖNLEIN PURPURA

Vasculitis is a reaction pattern that presents as non-itchy, painless macules, papules or urticarial lesions with purpuric centres. There are many causes of vasculitis including infections (streptococcal, hepatitis viruses and others), autoimmune diseases (systemic lupus erythematosus, Behçet disease), allergy (drugs) or idiopathic.

Henoch–Schönlein purpura is an IgA-mediated condition and is the commonest cause of vasculitis in children. It can occur at any age but is most common between the ages of two and ten years. There is sometimes a preceding streptococcal or non-specific viral illness. Over a couple of days, lesions occur in a symmetrical distribution, mainly on the buttocks and lower legs, and occasionally on the genitalia, arms and elsewhere (Fig. 12.1.12). In many children, most lesions are purpuric, ranging from pinpoint petechiae to 2 cm in diameter. In other children, only a few purpuric areas may be noted amongst many erythematous or urticarial lesions. There may be associated abdominal pain, arthralgia, arthritis or haematuria. Renal involvement leading to chronic renal failure is rare, but can occur irrespective of the severity of the rash and other symptoms, and may be delayed until weeks or months after the onset of the illness.

A child with Henoch–Schönlein purpura may warrant a full blood examination to exclude thrombocytopenia. Check blood pressure and urine for blood or protein. Bed rest and analgesia may be needed if discomfort is considerable. Oral prednisolone may reduce the duration of abdominal pain and may reduce the likelihood of renal problems. Severe renal involvement may require immunosuppression, plasmapheresis or hypertensive therapy but this is rare. In children with no renal involvement at presentation, blood pressure and urinalysis should be done weekly for one month, then monthly for three months, then yearly for life.

THROMBOCYTOPENIC PURPURA

Purpura in association with a low platelet count is often associated with bruising and signs of bleeding elsewhere. Children need to be examined and investigated for splenomegaly, leukaemia and pancytopenia. Drug-induced thrombocytopenia or aplastic anaemia may be present (chloramphenicol, antithyroid medications).

Idiopathic thrombocytopenic purpura is the most common cause. Bruises, petechiae or purpuric lesions appear over a period of days or weeks, mainly in sites of frequent mild trauma. The child is otherwise well. Full blood examination will be normal apart from a low platelet count.

LEUKAEMIA

Leukaemia should be suspected in a child with generalised petechiae or purpura in the absence of trauma. Features may include tiredness, pallor, limp, malaise and gum hypertrophy. Thrombocytopenia is usually present. An urgent full blood examination should be obtained (see Chapter 11.6 on acute leukaemia).

Fig. 12.1.12   Vasculitis. Henoch–Schönlein purpura.

Two subtypes of acute myeloid leukaemia typically present with skin lesions. Acute monocytic leukaemia may present with skin infiltrates and gum hypertrophy. Acute promyelocytic leukaemia often presents with a purpuric rash anywhere on the body in association with disseminated intravascular coagulation. The long-term prognosis is good provided treating staff recognise this presentation as a medical emergency needing urgent treatment and coagulation support.

COAGULATION DISORDERS

Extensive purpuric lesions in a well child without a history of significant trauma may be due to an underlying coagulation disorder. This may be inherited or acquired. There may be a history of joint pain or swelling, or bleeding from other sites.

CHILD ABUSE

Twisting, compression, pinching and hitting can all cause petechial or purpuric lesions. Look for bruises of bizarre shapes and different ages or evidence of fractures or other injuries. Assess the child's affect and relationship with carers. A complete examination is mandatory. If child abuse is suspected, admission or immediate referral to a paediatrician may be needed for complete assessment and further investigations (see Chapter 18.2 on child abuse).

ARTEFACTUAL PURPURA

Older children sometimes present with self-induced purpuric lesions. These are often in bizarre, non-physiological shapes, sometimes with obvious marks of finger trauma. They occur in exposed areas. Lesions may have recurred for months or longer in an otherwise well and generally unconcerned child or adolescent. The history typically has inappropriate or contradictory details and a lack of concern about the lesions. The diagnosis and management of artefactual disease in children may be difficult and requires confidence in interpretation of the skin findings and ongoing paediatric and psychological follow-up of the child and family. Occasionally, admission to hospital may be required.

PAPULAR-PURPURIC GLOVES AND SOCKS SYNDROME

Papular-purpuric gloves and socks syndrome is caused by parvovirus B19 and probably by several other common viruses. Adolescents develop vague symptoms of fever, fatigue and pains. Redness and swelling of the palms and soles progresses rapidly to petechial and purpuric lesions that do not extend onto other body parts. There may be oral vesicles or erosions. The adolescent remains generally well and the eruption clears in two weeks. Interestingly, unlike erythema infectiosum, adolescents with papular-purpuric gloves and socks syndrome are thought to be infective during the period of rash.

DUSKY PURPLE NODULES ON HANDS AND FEET

For tender red/purple areas (not usually purpuric) on hands and feet in otherwise well children, consider pernio (p. 353) and palmoplantar hidradenitis (p. 353).

CHRONIC PIGMENTED PURPURA

Chronic petechiae in childhood are usually due to chronic pigmented purpura. This typically presents as several 2–3 cm patches of petechiae. In each patch, both new and old petechiae can be seen giving red, purple and brown dots (like cayenne pepper). Patches may be subtle, the child is otherwise well, the condition is benign, but lesions recur for months or years.

OTHER CAUSES OF CHILDHOOD PURPURA

Unusual patterns or presentations of purpura in childhood may be associated with vasculitic diseases, glucocorticoid excess, any cause of abnormal skin elasticity and scurvy. In children with scurvy, irritability, bone pain, gum sponginess and bleeding may be present. Wrist X-rays are diagnostic.

Langerhans cell histiocytosis may present with persistent anogenital or scalp petechiae in infants, or with widespread, itchy, haemorrhagic papules, including on the hands and feet (see p. 340).

NEONATAL PURPURA

Purpuric rashes in the neonatal period may be an early presentation of any cause of childhood purpura (see above). In addition, consider:

- Congenital infection including rubella, cytomegalovirus, toxoplasmosis, and herpes simplex.
- Haemolytic disease of the newborn.
- Malignancy, including neuroblastoma, Langerhans cell histiocytosis and leukaemia.
- Iatrogenic injury, including birth trauma, extravasation of drugs and arterial injury during catheterisation.
- Protein C or S deficiency.

VASCULAR TUMOURS – HAEMANGIOMAS AND HAEMANGIOMA VARIANTS

HAEMANGIOMAS OF INFANCY

Haemangiomas are tumours of vascular endothelial cells. While haemangiomas may be present at birth, most appear in the first days or weeks of life. The appearance depends on whether the haemangioma involves the skin. If the skin is involved, the first sign is often a patch of pallor, followed by the development of an erythematous macule. Over a few weeks, this may grow and thicken into a soft, partly compressible, well defined, crimson or purple nodule (the so-called 'strawberry haemangioma'). There may be a substantial subcutaneous mass. Haemangiomas that do not involve the skin are often first noticed as firm, blue or skin-coloured swellings. Haemangiomas can occur anywhere on the body and may involve internal organs such as the liver or trachea.

Haemangiomas may remain as tiny one millimetre lesions or involve extensive areas of the body. Growth may be slow but can be rapid and frightening, even with intensive treatment.

Haemangiomas usually grow for 3–9 months and then slowly involute over the next 2–10 years. Involution is first noticed as a decrease in the intensity of the surface crimson colour with development of small islands of greyish skin. The haemangioma becomes softer and gradually shrinks in size. Half resolve by age five, and 90% by age nine. Resolution may not be complete. Particularly with larger lesions, there may be residual telangiectatic vessels, fibro-fatty tissue or redundant skin. Some haemangiomas show little resolution.

Most haemangiomas never cause problems and are best left alone and allowed to involute spontaneously. However, haemangiomas can rapidly lead to problems such as extreme disfigurement, ulceration, blindness, destruction of cartilage, respiratory obstruction, coagulation failure or death. Urgent assessment by a clinician experienced in this field is needed in the following circumstances:

Association with stridor   Stridor, especially increasing stridor of recent onset in a child of a few months of age, may be due to a laryngeal or tracheal haemangioma. This risk is greatest in children with a superficial haemangioma involving the beard area. About half of all children with an airway haemangioma will have a visible superficial haemangioma.

Eye involvement   Even quite small haemangiomas on the eyelid or adjacent to the globe of the eye can cause impaired vision on that side, either by directly obstructing the visual axis or more commonly by pressing on the globe to cause astigmatism. In both cases, amblyopia may result and may lead to permanent blindness if not treated.

Involvement of facial structures   Haemangiomas may deform structures such as the lip, ear cartilage, nasal cartilage, dentition or jaw growth. This deformity will remain after resolution of the haemangioma. Deforming lesions require aggressive treatment.

Ulceration   Ulceration is more common in haemangiomas at sites exposed to trauma, including areas of friction, anogenital lesions and lesions involving the lips. Ulcers may be very painful and can spread within days to give necrotic lesions several centimetres in size. There may be full tissue loss of lips, nose and eyelids with permanent disfigurement and loss of function. Early treatment with topical metronidazole and paraffin ointment several times daily usually leads to healing. Laser to the ulcer base or surgical excision may be warranted.

Macular facial lesions   A macular (flat) capillary lesion on the face of a neonate is likely to be a capillary malformation, not a haemangioma, and does not require urgent treatment. However, it may be the first sign of an extensive facial haemangioma. This can commence as a large macular capillary lesion that is indistinguishable from a capillary malformation until thickening and rapid growth occurs (Fig. 12.1.13). These haemangiomas cause extreme disfigurement and after thickening has commenced, treatment is difficult. Treatment with vascular laser can dramatically help if given during the brief macular phase, but is of little value after thickening has commenced. If you are suspicious about a large macular capillary lesion in a neonate (e.g. onset after birth, changing colour, any sign of thickening), monitoring and/or referral should be done with an awareness of the possible urgency of treatment.

Sudden onset of swelling and bruising in a large haemangioma   This may presage the development of a consumptive coagulopathy – see Kaposiform haemangioendothelioma/tufted angioma (p. 359).

Multiple haemangiomas (diffuse neonatal haemangiomatosis)   Infants with five or more cutaneous haemangiomas have a considerably higher risk of haemangiomas at other sites, including liver, gut and lungs. Investigations should include a hepatic ultrasound, full blood examination, platelet count, fibrinogen level, clotting profile, urinalysis, liver function tests, and stool analysis for blood. An electrocardiogram and chest X-ray may be needed. Liver haemangiomas in particular are associated with high flow cardiac failure and a significant mortality. If small hepatic lesions are found on imaging, follow up is required to ensure that undetected rapid growth does not occur.

Management

- Most parents just need education and reassurance about the inherently benign nature of these lesions.
- If complications, as described above, are considered likely, the initial treatment option is often oral prednisolone for six weeks, 3–5 mg kg^{-1} d^{-1} for two weeks before weaning. Intralesional corticosteroids, intravenous vincristine, subcutaneous α-interferon, vascular laser, surgery and embolisation may all be warranted, either at presentation or if the response to oral prednisolone is insufficient. Early treatment will prevent or minimise complications in most cases.
- Any infant with a midline lumbosacral or anogenital haemangioma or other vascular malformation should be checked for genitourinary abnormalities and have imaging to exclude a tethered cord. To image the spine prior to three months of age, an ultrasound examination is generally satisfactory. In older children, a magnetic resonance imaging (MRI) examination is warranted.

RAPIDLY INVOLUTING CONGENITAL HAEMANGIOMA

Rapidly involuting congenital haemangiomas have recently been recognised as a distinct type of haemangioma. They are present at birth as raised violaceous vas-

A

B

C

Fig. 12.1.13   Untreated segmental facial haemangioma.
(**A**) At one week; (**B**) at two weeks (easily misinterpreted as a capillary malformation); and (**C**) at six weeks, by which time thickening has occurred. Urgent referral for laser and oral prednisolone treatment prior to thickening is required.

cular tumours, often many centimetres across. They can be associated with high-flow cardiac failure, and can be mistaken both on clinical and radiological assessment for arteriovenous malformations or vascular sarcomas. The distinction is important because they resolve within 12–18 months without treatment.

KAPOSIFORM HAEM-ANGIOENDOTHELIOMA TUFTED ANGIOMA

These may be present at birth. Growth can be rapid and extend over much of a leg or buttock. The texture is often firmer than felt with typical infantile haemangiomas.

Kaposiform haemangioendothelioma and tufted angioma are associated with platelet trapping and a consumptive coagulopathy (Kasabach–Merritt syndrome). This has a significant mortality if untreated. Crises usually manifest clinically as rapid swelling of the lesion with the lesion appearing bruised and becoming hard and tender. Assess platelet count, clotting profile and fibrinogen level. High-dose oral corticosteroids and vincristine are used to treat crises. α-Interferon may be needed.

PYOGENIC GRANULOMA

Pyogenic granulomas are benign acquired vascular tumours that often present to EDs with a history of bleeding. They usually occur after infancy, on the face and neck, hands, or elsewhere on the body. There may be a history of preceding trivial trauma to that site. Over several days, a dark red/bluish papule appears and grows to 10 mm in height. The surface may be moist, scaly or warty. Bleeding is common and may be recurrent.

Management

• Bleeding will stop with the application of pressure. Pedunculated lesions can be ligated at the base without anaesthetic. Alternatively, or if recurrence occurs, surgical curettage is curative. Usually, local anaesthesia is adequate. Any solitary feeding arteriole beneath the papule may need cautery. A protective dressing will minimise the risk of rebleeding before surgery.

VASCULAR MALFORMATIONS

Vascular malformations are developmental lesions composed of dilated blood vessels and/or lymphatic channels. They are present at birth but may not become evident until infancy or occasionally later in childhood. Malformations include common capillary malformations on the face (port-wine stain), more extensive capillary lesions, localised venous malformations, venous malformations involving large areas with associated overgrowth and other changes, arteriovenous malformations, lymphatic malformations (e.g. cystic hygroma) or any combination of these.

They are not tumours and do not have a growth phase or resolution phase as haemangiomas do. They are generally static lesions. However, changes can occur over time leading to increasing problems. Particularly at puberty, there may be growth of the malformation leading to its appearance for the first time, or leading to problems such as pain in a previously asymptomatic lesion.

The appearance depends on the nature and site of the malformation. Purely capillary malformations appear as red macules on the skin. They blanch partially or fully. Venous involvement manifests as dilated veins or soft compressible bluish lumps that empty when elevated. Phleboliths are common and may be palpable. Significant arterial involvement may allow a thrill to be felt on examination. Lymphatic lesions give diffuse swelling of a limb or soft subcutaneous masses. Lymphatic involvement on the skin surface results in a mass of firm warty 2 mm papules that may be clear but often are dark blue or black because of haemorrhage into the lesions.

Vascular malformations can be associated with many chronic and acute problems that can precipitate attendance at an ED. Chronic problems include concerns about the appearance, psychological problems, social isolation, pain, deformity, dental problems, overgrowth, leg length discrepancy, arthritis and bone erosion. Acute problems may be related to any of these and also include pain, haemorrhage, infection, thrombosis and pulmonary emboli.

NEONATAL VASCULAR MALFORMATIONS

A neonate with a substantial vascular malformation should be examined thoroughly for associated malformations, for high-flow cardiac compromise and for other abnormalities in any system. Investigation includes ultrasound and radiological imaging.

FACIAL CAPILLARY MALFORMATIONS ('PORT WINE STAIN')

Facial capillary malformations are usually present at birth and persist throughout childhood, becoming a bit darker and thicker during adolescence. Treatment with vascular laser in early childhood leads to clearing of most of the lesion in most children.

Children with vascular malformations around the eye should be screened for glaucoma and other eye abnormalities. Children with capillary malformations involving the forehead and upper eyelid have a 10% risk of intracranial involvement and a smaller risk of developing epilepsy, strokes, hemiplegia or mental retardation (Sturge–Weber syndrome).

Beware of any facial 'capillary malformation' that appears after birth or becomes darker or thicker in the first weeks of life. This may actually be a haemangioma requiring urgent treatment. (see 'macular facial lesions', p. 358)

PAIN, SWELLING

Chronic discomfort and pain is common with large venous malformations, particularly those involving the legs. Pain is worse after standing for prolonged periods. Sudden onset or worsening of pain is also common. In venous malformations, it may arise from localised microthrombi and microinfarction. In venous and lymphatic malformations, it may be due to secondary infection. Sudden pain may be accompanied by a sudden increase in swelling and may lead to a rapid compromise of a body function, depending on the site. Sudden, severe pain in an adolescent, with or without fever, may be the presenting feature of Fabry disease (see below).

HIGH-FLOW LESIONS

Arteriovenous malformations are dangerous. Any vascular lesion with a thrill should be presumed to be an arteriovenous malformation. They can present in many ways to the ED – as a new swelling, an area of skin necrosis, skin ulceration, bleeding, or with the sequelae of internal bleeding, including intracranial bleeding. They can expand and erode surrounding structures. If a high-flow lesion is suspected, Doppler ultrasound should be arranged to confirm this. Follow-up is essential.

BLEEDING, COAGULOPATHY

Large venous malformations are associated with chronic consumption of clotting factors, low fibrinogen, somewhat reduced platelet count and bleeding. (This is not Kasabach–Merritt syndrome, which is associated with vascular tumours.)

INTESTINAL BLEEDING

Multiple cutaneous and visceral vascular malformations occur in blue rubber bleb syndrome and may cause intestinal bleeding. In hereditary haemorrhagic telangiectasia, telangiectasias usually appear on the face, mouth and nose. Nose bleeds become frequent in late childhood and gastrointestinal bleeding occurs in adult life.

BLADDER OR BOWEL DYSFUNCTION IN OLDER CHILDREN

Congenital lesions over the lumbosacral area may be associated with occult spinal abnormalities such as a tethered cord. These spinal anomalies may not cause problems until later in childhood when they can present insidiously with irreversible bladder, bowel or limb dysfunction. These problems can be prevented by early screening with magnetic resonance imaging (MRI) and surgical correction. Congenital lesions that have been associated with underlying spinal problems include haemangiomas, capillary malformations, lipomas, dimples, sinuses and hairy patches.

LEG-LENGTH DISCREPANCY

Children with a significant vascular malformation involving a leg need to be monitored for unequal leg growth. This can present as a limp or as a secondary problem including scoliosis, back pain, joint pain and headache.

MULTIPLE TELANGIECTATIC VESSELS

Multiple telangiectatic vessels of nonspider type may raise suspicion of hereditary haemorrhagic telangiectasia or a photosensitivity syndrome. Multiple spider naevi do not require investigation.

FABRY DISEASE

Fabry disease is X-linked and primarily affects males. Females can be variably affected. Angiokeratomas (flat or raised, slightly warty, red/purple lesions) appear in mid-childhood on the lower trunk, pelvis and thighs. Tiny vascular lesions may be seen on the lips or in the mouth. Corneal opacities are invariably present. Children or adolescents may present to the ED with paresthesia of the hands and feet, or with sudden severe pain involving the limbs. Renal, cardiac and central nervous system problems occur later.

Management of vascular malformations

- Management of vascular malformations can be demanding and complex. For example, interventional embolisation of a large venous malformation of a limb may achieve an excellent result but only after perhaps twenty or more general anaesthetics each of a few hours duration.
- Management requires a multidisciplinary approach using expertise from surgical, paediatric, dermatological, radiological and psychological fields.
- Children with lumbosacral vascular malformations should have magnetic resonance imaging to exclude a tethered spinal cord.
- Compression stockings may reduce chronic pain in venous malformations. Low-dose aspirin may reduce episodes of pain in venous malformations. Heparin will minimise the coagulopathy from large venous malformations (but does not help the coagulopathy associated with Kasabach–Merritt syndrome seen with some vascular tumours).

- Partial or complete surgical resection may be needed for venous, lymphatic or arteriovenous malformations.
- Orthotic or surgical correction may assist with a leg length discrepancy.

HYPERPIGMENTATION

DIFFUSE HYPERPIGMENTATION

Diffuse hyperpigmentation is rare in children and investigation to identify the cause is required. Generalised darkening of the skin is often most obvious on the palmar creases, linea alba and areola, on the buccal mucosa and on the sun-exposed areas of the face, neck and extremities. Consider:

- Endocrine disease. Addison disease (also thickening of the skin and signs of increased androgen production), Cushing syndrome of pituitary origin (also acne, hirsutism, striae, purpura), exogenous ACTH administration, acromegaly (thickened, greasy, more hairy and often with many skin tags) and hyperthyroidism can all cause hyperpigmentation.
- Renal failure may cause greying of the skin.
- Haemochromatosis. In children, this is usually secondary to transfusions.
- Lipoidoses. A yellow-brown darkening of skin, most prominent in sun-exposed areas, can occur in the Niemann–Pick diseases. Look for waxy indurated skin, purpura, hepatosplenomegaly and neurological deterioration. Although a similar colour can be seen in adult-onset Gaucher disease, it is not a feature of the earlier onset forms.

LOCALISED MACULAR HYPERPIGMENTATION – INCLUDING CAFÉ-AU-LAIT MACULES

Many normal children have one or two well-defined pigmented macules, generally not present at birth but appearing in the early years. In a child with pigmented macular lesions of normal texture, consider:

Neurofibromatosis Six or more café-au-lait spots greater than 0.5 cm in diameter are strong evidence for neurofibromatosis. Examine for other features including axillary 'freckling' (usually not seen until mid-childhood), pigmented or thickened skin over plexiform neurofibromas (present in early childhood), iris pigmentation, optic tumours, skeletal abnormalities, short stature, skin neurofibromas, hypertension, macrocephaly and learning difficulties. The diagnosis may be uncertain early in life but full penetrance of neurofibromatosis is usually seen by eight years of age. Regular follow-up is needed, including assessment of intellectual progress and audiological and ophthalmological review. In children under five years old, magnetic resonance imaging of optic tracts to exclude optic glioma is warranted. Other investigations are not required unless suggested by clinical findings. Most children with neurofibromatosis never develop any of the significant medical associated features.

McCune–Albright syndrome A child with one or more large unilateral brown macules may have McCune–Albright syndrome. Endocrine or bony abnormalities should be looked for on examination. A bone scan should be performed at three years of age, and the child should be monitored for any signs of increased hormonal secretion. Routine endocrine investigations are not warranted in the absence of abnormal clinical signs.

Incontinentia pigmenti If the earlier phases have occurred in utero, hyperpigmented linear streaks may be present at birth.

Peutz–Jegher syndrome Small, pigmented macules present on the lips and mucosa from birth are associated with intestinal polyposis. Care must be taken when assessing any episodes of abdominal pain as these children are at higher risk of intussusception and collapse. Intestinal bleeding may be the presenting feature.

Linear and whorled hyperpigmentation and hypopigmentation Streaks, lines and whorls of hyperpigmentation and/ or hypopigmentation may be present from birth. These patterns reflect mosaicism. Usually these children are otherwise normal but a wide range of associated malformations in other systems have been reported, particularly eye, teeth, brain and skeletal malformations. Apart from audiological and ophthalmological examination, investigations are not required unless suggested by clinical findings, but these children should be reviewed until settled in school.

Post-inflammatory hyperpigmentation This occurs particularly in dark-skinned people. Many inflammatory skin disorders may heal leaving diffuse, hypo- or hyperpigmented macules that can persist for months or years. They usually resolve.

Pellagra Hyperpigmentation and erythema on sun-exposed areas, cheilitis, perineal inflammation and diarrhoea may be seen in niacin deficiency.

Naevus of Ota This presents at birth or during childhood as a bluish brown patch around the eye, sometimes involving the sclera. Glaucoma has been reported with naevus of Ota.

LOCALISED RAISED HYPERPIGMENTATION

If local areas of hyperpigmentation are roughened, raised or warty, consider:

- Congenital and acquired pigmented naevi (see below).
- Genodermatoses such as dyskeratosis congenita. Congenital nail dystrophy, pancytopenia, skeletal and eye anomalies may be present.
- Acanthosis nigricans. Rough 'dirty' skin on the neck or axillary folds is associated with obesity, polycystic ovary syndrome, other insulin resistance syndromes and hypothyroidism. Early acanthosis nigricans can be seen in many overweight children. If weight continues to increase, the acanthosis nigricans will progress to become cosmetically obvious and widespread. Early intervention and follow-up is required.

CONGENITAL PIGMENTED NAEVI

Congenital melanocytic naevi are thickened, sharply defined, tan, dark brown or black birthmarks. They range in size from common small lesions less than 2 cm in diameter to rare giant lesions that may cover entire parts of the body, such as the trunk. Larger lesions may have irregular colour, texture and hairiness with areas of thick redundant skin. Large congenital melanocytic naevi often are associated with many smaller lesions elsewhere on the body, some of which appear in the first two years of life.

Management

- The risk of malignancy in isolated small congenital melanocytic naevi is very small and does not require surgical excision. Decisions about removal are based on the site and potential effects of the child's psychosocial development. Excision, if desired, can be done early in life, or later if undecided.
- Giant congenital melanocytic naevi are associated with major psychosocial problems. Early dermabrasion can markedly decrease the colour of the naevus and is usually warranted. Results may be better if surgery is performed within the first two weeks of life. Urgent contact with a plastic surgeon experienced in this area is necessary. Pigment lasers have also recently been used and may be a treatment option in the near future.
- A second concern is malignancy. The lifetime risk of melanoma in a giant congenital melanocytic naevus is small (less than 5%). Parental instruction about reporting changes in the naevus will allow early biopsy of changing areas.
- Congenital melanocytic naevi of the scalp or spine can be associated with neurocutaneous melanosis and other CNS abnormalities. Most of these abnormalities remain asymptomatic, and screening with magnetic resonance imaging (MRI) is controversial. A reasonable approach is to screen if there is any suggestion of obstructive hydrocephalus, if there

are large lesions involving the axial spine and posterior scalp or multiple cannonball-shaped lesions (look for Dandy–Walker malformations), or if there are lesions over the lower spine (look for tethered cord). Early imaging in the first weeks of life allows the use of ultrasound where possible and the use of MRI without the need for a general anaesthetic.

- Regular follow-up is needed throughout childhood to monitor the naevi and psychosocial development.

ACQUIRED PIGMENTED NAEVI

During childhood, most children develop multiple acquired melanocytic naevi. Sun exposure in white children is associated with the development of an increased number of naevi. Acquired melanocytic naevi begin as small, flat, well demarcated pigmented lesions (junctional melanocytic naevi). A small percentage of junctional melanocytic naevi become raised and dome shaped (compound melanocytic naevi) often with a darker centre. Enlargement and darkening of naevi just before and during puberty is common.

Melanoma is very rare in childhood and uncommon in adolescence. Children and adolescents continue to acquire new melanocytic naevi until age twenty. Therefore, the presence of a new naevus is not in itself suspicious. You do need to be concerned if atypical features are present, particularly in adolescents. Any rapid change over a few weeks leading to an increase in asymmetry, an irregular border, multiple colours especially with non-brown areas within brown areas, and growth beyond 10 mm may suggest malignancy.

Immune-suppressed children and those who have had chemotherapy are at greater risk of skin malignancy and should have regular skin review.

Children with a great many lentigines (small, dark brown 1–2 mm macules) may have associated findings (e.g. LEOPARD syndrome) and require screening for hearing and cardiac problems and regular follow-up.

DYSPLASTIC NAEVI

These are a subtype of acquired pigmented naevi. Dysplastic naevi are usually macular, greater than 5 mm in diameter, with a less-regular border, some erythema, and some variability in colour. They may develop during childhood or after puberty. The presence of multiple dysplastic naevi is associated with a significant increased risk of melanoma. However, the great majority of melanomas that occur in this population are found in unaffected skin or normal moles rather than in pre-existing dysplastic naevi. Removal of a dysplastic naevus is only indicated if there is concern that a naevus may represent a melanoma. Regular photography and follow-up are indicated to aid in the detection of melanoma at an early stage.

Children with a family history of malignant melanoma and/or multiple dysplastic naevi are at a higher risk of developing melanoma and require regular skin review.

HALO NAEVI

Halo naevi appear as a sharply defined area of depigmentation 5–15 mm in diameter, centred on a regressing mole. They are common in childhood and benign.

SPITZ NAEVI

Spitz naevi are fairly common, benign melanocytic lesions. They usually present prior to puberty as single, red or red/brown papules that can grow to 1 cm in diameter. They are vascular and blanch to reveal the underlying pigmentation.

- Management is controversial. Spitz naevi are benign but usually do not resolve. Removal may be indicated because of uncertainty about the clinical diagnosis or for cosmetic reasons. Lesions on the central face that are only a few millimetres in diameter at presentation are likely to grow considerably and early surgical excision may be desirable. Histological interpretation is sometimes difficult with findings that overlap with malignant melanoma. Assessment by an experienced dermatopathologist is required.

NAEVUS OF OTA

Naevus of Ota is present at birth in 50% of cases and appears at puberty in most others. It can occur in any racial group and is one manifestation of dermal melanocytosis. It presents as a unilateral, well-demarcated, blue-black patch of skin on the cheek, forehead and periorbital area. The sclera of the associated eye may also be pigmented. It is benign but in white children may have an increased lifetime risk of melanoma. Cover-up cosmetics or laser depigmentation have been used to treat the discolouration.

MONGOLIAN SPOTS

Mongolian spots are another manifestation of dermal melanocytosis. They are extremely common and can be found on most Asian and dark-skinned babies as poorly-circumscribed, blue-black patches. The most common site is on the lower back, but they can occur elsewhere, and may be multiple and widespread. They are benign and usually fade over many years. No treatment is required. When at unusual sites, they can be mistaken for bruises.

HYPOPIGMENTION

Localised patches of depigmentation (total loss of pigment of skin or hair) can be seen in vitiligo, halo naevi, naevus depigmentosis and piebaldism. Localised patches of hypopigmented skin or hair may be due to pityriasis versicolor (usually in adolescence), pityriasis alba (usually in mid-childhood) and post-inflammatory loss of pigment. Focal pale patches may be the only marker of leprosy in an individual from an endemic area.

PITYRIASIS VERSICOLOR

This is common in adolescents, and caused by an increased activity of commensal yeasts. Multiple oval macules, 3–10 mm in diameter and usually covered with fine scale, appear on the trunk or upper arms. In young children, lesions may present on the face or neck. The lesions coalesce and may appear paler or darker than the surrounding skin. If depigmentation is present, it is distinguished from vitiligo by the presence of scale and residual pigment. Scrapings can be sent for microscopy to confirm the diagnosis. Treat with topical imidazole creams or with anti-yeast shampoos. For example, apply selenium sulfide 2% shampoo or ketoconazole 2% shampoo. Leave on for 30 minutes, if tolerated, rinse, and treat daily for one week and then monthly. If there are cosmetic concerns, a short course of oral ketoconazole followed by the above measures may be warranted. The yeast is readily treated, but the post-inflammatory hypopigmentation takes months to resolve. Relapses are common unless ongoing monthly treatments are used for a year or so.

PITYRIASIS ALBA

This condition is common in pre-pubertal children and simply represents post-inflammatory hypopigmentation secondary to mild eczema. Single or multiple, poorly demarcated hypopigmented (but never completely depigmented) 1–2 cm macules are seen on the face or upper body. Lesions are not itchy but often have a fine scale. Usually no treatment is needed. If desired, treat with emollients. Treat any erythema with hydrocortisone 1%. Resolution takes weeks and requires sun exposure for full repigmentation.

VITILIGO

This condition is characterised by sharply demarcated, often symmetrical areas of complete pigment loss. Eventual repigmentation in childhood vitiligo is common and is helped by topical steroids. In troublesome cases refer to a specialist for advice regarding treatment (e.g. corrective cosmetics or ultraviolet therapy). Vitiligo in children is weakly associated with other organ specific autoimmune conditions. Children with vitiligo should

be reviewed for features of diabetes and thyroid dysfunction.

POST-INFLAMMATORY HYPOPIGMENTATION

This condition occurs particularly in dark-skinned people. Many inflammatory skin disorders may heal leaving diffuse, hypo- or hyperpigmented macules that can persist for months or years. Repigmentation eventually occurs.

LINEAR AND WHORLED HYPOPIGMENTION ('HYPOMELANOSIS OF ITO')

See linear and whorled hyperpigmentation and hypopigmentation, p. 362.

TUBEROSCLEROSIS

Hypopigmented patches may be the first sign of tuberosclerosis. These patches can be regular or irregular in shape. A couple of isolated hypopigmented patches in a young child are far more likely to be simple achromic naevi than to be the first sign of tuberosclerosis. Tuberosclerosis becomes much more likely if the child has a history of epilepsy. Look also for forehead plaques (pink, initially flat but later slightly raised) and shagreen patches (rough, slightly thickened skin usually over the back). Other skin findings such as periungual fibromas and facial angiofibromas usually appear in older children. The diagnosis of tuberosclerosis may require imaging of eyes, brain, heart and kidneys and investigation of relatives. Regular paediatric follow-up is required.

GENERALISED HYPOPIGMENTATION

Generalised hypopigmentation, blonde hair and grey-blue eyes are seen in several genodermatoses involving chromosomes 11 or 15. The clinical presentations vary from mild to complete loss of pigmentation and individuals may go undiag-

nosed unless compared to their siblings and parents. Early diagnosis and investigation is important to ensure early ophthalmological intervention and rigorous sun protection. Look for:

- Poor vision, photophobia and nystagmus. Type 1 oculocutaneous albinism usually results in more severe disease than type 2.
- Bleeding diathesis, due to a platelet defect in Hermansky-Pudlak syndrome.
- Recurrent infections in Chédiak-Higashi syndrome.
- Mental retardation and obesity. Both Angelman and Prader-Willi syndromes can present with albinism.

SKIN TEXTURE

LAX SKIN

Lax, hyperextensible skin is seen in the several Ehlers-Danlos syndromes. There may be bruising, scarring at sites of minor trauma, joint hyperextensibility and arthritis, and recurrent urinary infections.

FIRM OR THICKENED SKIN

Scleredema (do not confuse with scleroderma) is a rare condition in childhood, which presents over some weeks with gradual thickening of the skin of the head, neck and upper trunk. It may be related to preceding streptococcal infection. Diagnosis can be confirmed by skin biopsy showing mucopolysaccharide intradermal staining. Resolution usually occurs over months.

Unusually firm skin is an early feature of systemic sclerosis. In children, there is usually widespread skin involvement. Raynaud phenomenon may be present and involvement of lungs, heart, kidneys and gastrointestinal tract usually occurs within a few years.

Waxy indurated skin may accompany neurological degeneration and hepatosplenomegaly in type A Niemann-Pick disease. Thickened skin may be seen in acromegaly and Addison's disease.

MOUTH DISORDERS

Most of the conditions covered in the section on vesicular disease can involve the oral mucosa. Oral vesicles break rapidly so that usually only erosions or small ulcers are seen. Oral involvement is often the first feature of hand, foot and mouth disease, manifesting as a few lesions involving the tongue and palate followed a day or two later by vesicles on the extremities. Oral erosions may be seen occasionally in varicella and rarely in zoster.

PRIMARY HERPETIC GINGIVOSTOMATITIS

Primary herpetic gingivostomatitis presents in infants and young children with malaise, high fever, soft-tissue swelling, lymphadenopathy and vesicles and erosions on the buccal mucosa, gingivae, lips and adjacent face. Drinking and eating is painful. Management includes supportive care, bathing of crusts and analgesia. Aciclovir is not routinely indicated unless risk factors for complications exist (e.g. underlying disease, immunosuppression).

HERPANGINA

Several echoviruses and Coxsackie viruses can cause the sudden onset of malaise, high fever, sore throat and vomiting, sometimes with abdominal pain. Examination of the pharynx and posterior mouth reveals a large number of small, 2 mm vesicles or erosions coalescing on an erythematous background to form painful ulcerations. Diagnosis can be confirmed by throat or faecal swab. Complete resolution occurs with supportive care over five days.

TRANSIENT LINGUAL PAPILLITIS

Transient lingual papillitis is probably the same condition as eruptive familial lingual papillitis. It was first described in 1996 and is not mentioned in major paediatric or dermatology texts but is much more common than generally realised. Most reported cases have been in the families of hospital staff. In one survey of 200 hospital staff, 50% of families appeared to have experienced this condition.[5] In most cases, an infant appears to be the index case and many other family members are then affected. Older children present with a burning sensation on the tip or sides of the tongue. Younger children present with irritability and poor feeding of unknown cause. The tongue is normal apart from small papules or 'scalloping' along the anterior and lateral tongue margins without ulceration. Affected individuals are otherwise well without any fever, lethargy, respiratory or gastrointestinal problems. Symptoms and signs last from 2–20 days. Recurrent episodes may occur for many weeks and again years later. Manage with symptomatic treatment and education.

ANGULAR CHEILITIS

Angular cheilitis can occur during childhood and is common in older children. It presents as persistent erythema, scaling and fissuring at the corners of the mouth and surrounding skin, sparing the buccal mucosa. Discomfort and pain may be worsened by stretching, during yawning for example, and by salty or tart foods. Most cases are primarily attributable to atopic eczema but are multifactorial. Contributing factors include saliva, licking, drooling at night, significant dental malocclusions, irritant and allergic dermatitis (e.g. cosmetics, medicated lip balms, sunscreen lip creams, toothpaste, fluoride and sucked or chewed lollies). *Staphylococcus aureus*, *Candida albicans* or streptococcal species may all be cultured from affected skin.

Rarely, angular cheilitis may be the presenting feature of nutritional deficiencies including riboflavin, iron, zinc, pyridoxine, biotin and protein metabolic disorders. Malabsorption, malnutrition, oral corticosteroids and oral antibiotics may contribute.

- Management requires avoidance as much as possible of any factors that may be contributing.
- Minimise acidic foods such as tomatoes and citrus fruit.
- A trial of non-fluoride toothpaste and supervised rinsing after teeth cleaning helps in some children.
- Topical unmedicated ointment or paste up to several times a day will assist recovery. Topical 1% hydrocortisone ointment is useful. If microscopy reveals evidence of *Candida* or bacterial pathogens, topical miconazole or mupirocin, respectively, can be added.
- Allergy to a component of the treatment schedule should be suspected if the condition persists despite treatment, and patch testing may be warranted.
- In difficult cases, consider an uncommon underlying cause as above, and a trial of iron, vitamin and mineral supplementation.

GEOGRAPHIC TONGUE

Geographic tongue is typically seen under four years of age but can occur in older children. Most children are asymptomatic but some complain of tenderness or pain with salty foods. Irregular smooth patches are seen on the tongue in a pattern that changes from day to day. The cause is unknown. Geographic tongue is more common in psoriasis but most children (> 90%) who have geographic tongue never develop psoriasis. No treatment is needed unless some foods cause discomfort in which case avoidance of those foods for a while is usually sufficient. If needed, topical corticosteroid can alleviate symptoms.

RECURRENT MOUTH ULCERS

These are most often due to aphthous stomatitis. Aphthous ulceration usually presents as a few, painful, 4–8 mm ulcers on an erythematous base on the non-keratinised mucosa (the 'softer' areas) rather than the gums or hard palate. They resolve in a few days. Less commonly, ulcers can be larger and persist for weeks. Any atypical features should lead to a consideration of less-common causes of recurrent mouth ulcers including:

- Iron, folate or vitamin B_{12} deficiency.
- Recurrent erythema multiforme.
- Pemphigus, pemphigoid and other immune-mediated blistering conditions.
- Gastrointestinal disorders. Coeliac disease, Crohn's disease and ulcerative colitis are all associated with mouth ulceration. Recurrent abdominal pain, intermittent diarrhoea and failure to thrive may be present.
- Connective tissue disorders. Patients with Behçet disease usually present in late childhood with ulcers at one site (mouth or genitals) and it may be many years before a second site is involved. Systemic lupus erythematosus and juvenile rheumatoid arthritis may cause recurrent mouth ulcers.
- Immunodeficiency states, human immunodeficiency virus (HIV) infection, cyclic neutropenia and periodic fevers.
- Malignancy and chemotherapy. Lymphoma and Langerhans cell histiocytosis can present with non-healing mouth ulcers.
- FAPA syndrome of fever, aphthous ulcers, pharyngitis, adenitis.

Troublesome episodes of aphthous ulceration can be managed by:

- Investigating for an underlying cause as above.
- Topical anaesthetic gels.
- Topical steroid paste (e.g. triamcinolone acetonide).
- Oral colchicine.

ANOGENITAL RASHES

Anogenital rashes are common in infancy. Most anogenital rashes seen in infants that wear nappies are primarily caused by reaction with urine or faeces (irritant napkin dermatitis). Soaps, detergents and secondary yeast infection may contribute. In atypical or persistent anogenital rashes in infancy, consider psoriasis, Langerhans cell histiocytosis, zinc deficiency and malabsorption syndromes. In older children, consider perianal streptococcal infection (if painful), psoriasis, lichen sclerosis, and atopic eczema. Kawasaki disease may be associated with a tender anogenital rash in an unwell child.

Treatment of rashes in the anogenital area requires caution. The moistness and occlusion of these areas increases the penetration and effectiveness of topical agents. For example, the absorption of topical hydrocortisone per square centimetre of anogenital skin can be several times greater than trunk skin. Adrenal suppression may occur after use of excessive topical hydrocortisone under the nappy area in small infants. Anogenital skin is also more likely to develop local steroid side effects, such as atrophy and striae. Any child using cortisone products in this area should have written instructions and appropriate medical follow-up.

IRRITANT NAPKIN DERMATITIS

Irritant napkin dermatitis is the most common cause of napkin dermatitis in infants and typically presents as confluent erythema that spares the groin folds. Variant presentations include multiple erosions in the natal cleft secondary to diarrhoea, scaly or glazed erythema, and satellite lesions at the periphery. Satellite pustules are suggestive of secondary *Candida* infection. *Candida* infection is much less common with breathable disposable nappies.

Gluteal granulomas are purple/brown papules or nodules, often oval shaped, which can develop around the skin folds in infants with troublesome napkin dermatitis. Most cases are associated with the inappropriate use of potent topical steroid in this area. These lesions slowly resolve over several months provided the underlying irritant napkin dermatitis is treated.

Irritant or traumatic anogenital rashes may be seen in circumstances of suboptimal care, emotional abuse or physical abuse.

Management

- Keep the area clean and dry. Leave the nappy off whenever possible.
- Clean the anogenital area by hand under warm water or with diluted bath oil on cotton wipes. Avoid commercial 'wipes', which can be irritating.
- Gel-based disposable nappies or a non-wettable under-napkin can be helpful. Cloth nappies should be thoroughly washed and rinsed.
- Use topical zinc cream or paste for mild eruptions. This functions as a barrier and should be applied thickly so that some is still present at the next nappy change. The cream or paste does not need to be completely removed at each change.
- Add hydrocortisone 1% cream if inflamed. Do not use stronger steroids.
- Consider mupirocin 2% cream if not settling. Antifungal therapy is usually not needed even if *Candida* is present.

CANDIDA NAPKIN DERMATITIS

This occurs secondary to irritant napkin dermatitis and antibiotic use, leading to erythema and white material in the folds and satellite pustules. Treat the underlying cause as above and add topical imidazole cream if necessary.

ANOGENITAL SEBORRHEIC DERMATITIS

The term 'seborrhoeic dermatitis' has been used to describe an anogenital eruption in infants, with or without scalp or flexural involvement. Traditionally, it is differentiated from irritant napkin dermatitis by accentuation in the skin folds. However, this distinction is far from clear. The napkin area is not a seborrhoeic site. Many presentations with anogenital 'seborrhoeic dermatitis' represent either atopic eczema with irritant napkin dermatitis or psoriasis with anogenital involvement, or a combination of the two. Treat as for irritant napkin dermatitis, or anogenital psoriasis if suspected.

ANOGENITAL PSORIASIS

Anogenital psoriasis can present at any age from infancy to adolescence. Sharply demarcated, non-scaly, brightly erythematous plaques can be seen and may involve any or all of the perianal and intragluteal region, inguinal folds and the genital area in both boys and girls (Fig. 12.1.14). Symptoms are often surprisingly minimal. If pain and/or fissuring are present, swab for secondary streptococcal infection. This leads to a marked increase in discomfort and pain and is often the cause for presentation in an older child who may have had months or years of asymptomatic redness. Anogenital psoriasis may be an isolated finding or there may be similar lesions in other intertriginous areas, such as the axillae, or more typical signs of psoriasis elsewhere. Occasionally, in infants, anogenital psoriasis will lead to a few lesions on the lower trunk and then a rapid eruption of lesions elsewhere including scalp, face and trunk. This settles within weeks.

Manage by treating streptococcal infection, if present, and then treat as for irritant napkin dermatitis (p. 366). Medical follow-up is essential to ensure clearing, as children and adolescents are often unaware of quite significant asymptomatic anogenital psoriasis or fail to report it because of embarrassment.

PERIANAL STREPTOCOCCAL DERMATITIS

A painful, red, perianal rash in a child between the ages of one and ten is likely to be due to perianal streptococcal dermatitis. The usual presentation is a child who has had a sore anal region for weeks or months. Defecation is painful and constipation is present, but treatments aimed at relieving the constipation have not helped. Bright red blood may be present on the stool or toilet paper. On examination, a localised, well-demarcated erythema that covers a circular area of 1–2 cm radius around the anus can be seen. Fissures or macerated skin may be seen.

Perianal streptococcal dermatitis is caused by group A streptococci, although occasionally *Staphylococcus aureus* is present. It may be secondary to any cause of perianal itching. Constipation usually follows painful defecation, rather than being the cause of it. It takes a long while for the child to recover confidence in defecation after successful treatment.

Management

- Take perianal and throat cultures to confirm the presence of group A *Streptococcus*.
- Apply paraffin ointment three-times daily to the perianal area for symptomatic relief. Topical mupirocin three-times daily has a role. Treat with phenoxymethylpenicillin (penicillin V) orally BD 250 mg (under 10 years), 500 mg (over 10 years) for a minimum of two weeks. Several weeks of therapy may be required. Intramuscular benzathine penicillin can be used if there are concerns about compliance.
- Keep stools soft with oral liquid paraffin.
- Perianal emollient ointment and stool softeners should be continued for a further two months after resolution of symptoms to prevent relapse, which is otherwise common.

STAPHYLOCOCCAL-MEDIATED ANOGENITAL RASHES

Bullous impetigo may present in the anogenital area as small vesicles or pustules that coalesce to give areas of peeling skin with peripheral margins of loose epidermis. These may be asymptomatic and the infant is otherwise well. Oral antibiotics (e.g. flucloxacillin) can be given. Provided the baby is well, the disease is localised and the parents will follow instructions regarding follow-up, an alternative is to treat with topical mupirocin 2% and general measures for napkin care.

HERPES SIMPLEX VIRUS

Primary herpes simplex virus infection and eczema herpeticum can both occur in the anogenital area. Initially, small vesicles on an erythematous base may be seen but these rapidly become small monomorphic erosions, crusting and coalescing, sometimes into an extensive, painful, erosive rash. Herpes simplex virus infection in the anogenital area of young children is usually innocent, contracted from a cold sore on a carer but the possibility of child sexual abuse should be considered. The possibility

Fig. 12.1.14   Anogenital psoriasis in a one-year-old boy.

of child sexual abuse is higher in older children. For management see p. 327.

VARICELLA

Varicella lesions may initially be localised to the anogenital area in young children. Immunofluorescence and culture may be required to avoid an incorrect diagnosis of herpes simplex.

THREADWORMS

In older children, threadworms (*Enterobius vermicularis*) are a common cause of an itchy anogenital rash. Look for the worms at night and treat with oral mebendazole 50 mg (< 10 kg), 100 mg (> 10 kg) (not in pregnancy or less than six months) or oral pyrantel 10 mg kg^{-1} (maximum 500 mg) as a single dose. A repeat dose two weeks later helps reduce the high rate of reinfestation. Emphasise the importance of wearing clean underwear at night, preventing perianal scratching at night, hand washing immediately on awakening, avoidance of thumb sucking and good toileting hygiene.

LICHEN SCLEROSIS

Lichen sclerosis presents with chronic itch, discomfort or pain in the vulval area of girls aged three years or older. On examination, there may be an area of atrophy with white shiny skin, purpura or telangiectasia in the perivulval region. Cases have been misdiagnosed as sexual abuse. Management is with moisturisers and brief courses of moderately potent or potent steroid ointment. About 50% of cases resolve spontaneously. Relapses after successful treatment are common and children with this condition may have ongoing troublesome symptoms and vulval abnormalities into adulthood. Long-term follow-up is required.

VULVAL ITCH/VULVITIS IN PREPUBERTAL GIRLS

Prepubertal girls with vulval itch usually have an identifiable dermatological con-

dition. (Do not call this 'vulvovaginitis' as the vagina is not involved.) Girls between the age of two and ten present with months or years of vulval itch, occasionally with stinging or pain on micturition. On examination, the labia majora may appear normal or may show erythema, scale, lichenification and excoriation. The introitus is normal. The great majority of these girls have atopic eczema. There may be signs of this elsewhere or signs may be limited to the vulval area. Management is as for atopic eczema at other sensitive sites and involves avoidance of chemicals, soaps, bubble baths and other irritants, and use of cotton underwear and ointment moisturiser. Use of corticosteroid or pimecrolimus creams needs to be monitored by a doctor familiar with their use at this site. Measures to 'oestrogenise the vagina' are either irrelevant or counterproductive and oestrogen creams should not be used.

Less common causes of vulval itch include psoriasis, lichen sclerosis, staphylococcal folliculitis or infection with group A streptococci. In all these cases, clinical signs suggestive of the associated condition are likely to be present.

ZINC AND OTHER NUTRITIONAL DEFICIENCIES

Zinc deficiency may be due to an inherited defect in zinc handling or may be an acquired deficiency as a result of prematurity, malabsorption syndromes or abnormally low maternal breast-milk zinc levels. Breast milk normally provides some protection from the inherited form, so presentation of inherited zinc deficiency is usually after breast-feeding has ceased. By contrast, acquired zinc deficiency can present earlier, in the neonatal period.

Zinc deficiency causes acrodermatitis enteropathica. A sharply defined, red, often extensive, anogenital rash is an early and prominent manifestation. Look for perioral, perinasal and acral (hand and foot) dermatitis, alopecia, diarrhoea, and failure to thrive. Serum zinc levels do not correlate well with body zinc status. Oral zinc leads to a rapid improvement of the rash within days. Long-term follow-up

to monitor the child's zinc and copper status is essential.

Biotin and essential fatty-acid deficiency syndromes can give a similar picture.

MALABSORPTION

Malabsorption from any cause (e.g. cystic fibrosis) can present with diarrhoea, erosive dermatitis and failure to thrive. There may be a progressive intractable napkin rash contributed to both by the diarrhoea and by secondary nutritional deficiencies. If malabsorption continues, the rash may become glazed and generalised in association with oedema and malaise. Identify and treat the cause of the malabsorption. Manage the anogenital area as for irritant napkin dermatitis. Topical pastes are thicker than ointments and may be required.

LANGERHANS CELL HISTIOCYTOSIS

Langerhans cell histiocytosis may present in infancy as a chronic inguinal or anogenital rash, with brownish/red scale and petechiae, which is often erosive and unresponsive to treatment. A scaly, papular, eruption on the scalp or trunk may appear. Purpura, fever, diarrhoea or hepatosplenomegaly may be present, see p. 340.

CONSTIPATION

Constipation by itself does not cause perianal erythema and pain. Look for another cause, e.g. eczema, psoriasis or streptococcal infection.

ANOGENITAL PAPULES AND LUMPS

Anogenital warts   Are soft fleshy warts that occur at the mucocutaneous junctions, especially around the anus. They may be isolated, flesh-coloured nodules or may coalesce into large cauliflower-like masses. Management options include awaiting resolution, topical podophyllotoxin, imiquimod, curettage and diathermy and carbon dioxide laser.

The presence of genital warts in a young child is not an indication for mandatory reporting to government protective services. Genital warts in young children should prompt consideration of the possibility of sexual abuse, but transmission is usually by normal intimate parent-child contact, including at birth. Unless there are other risk factors for sexual abuse on history or examination, referral for sexual abuse investigation is inappropriate. If in doubt, seek paediatric advice. In children older than five years, the association between anogenital warts and sexual abuse increases and assessment by a paediatrician is warranted.

Molluscum In the anogenital area are often misdiagnosed as warts. Close examination of all lesions usually reveals a few to have the classical umbilicated pearly appearance. Molluscum in the anogenital region are common and are not a marker of child sexual abuse.

Congenital syphilis Erosions and moist warty lesions in the perianal area may be seen in infants with congenital syphilis. There may be erythema on the palms and soles, fever, failure to thrive and hepatosplenomegaly.

IMMUNODEFICIENCY STATES

Immunodeficiency from any cause may present in infancy as diarrhoea with a chronic erosive napkin dermatitis or widespread seborrhoeic dermatitis. Secondary infection with bacteria and/or viruses can complicate the clinical appearance. Look for other features of immunodeficiency including failure to thrive, erythroderma, lymphadenopathy, unusual infections and petechiae with eczema.

HAIR PROBLEMS

For an itchy scalp, consider tinea capitis, atopic eczema and head lice. For patches of hair loss, consider alopecia areata, traumatic alopecia, tinea capitis and kerion. For diffuse hair loss, consider telogen effluvium and nutritional causes. Long-standing sparse hair can be associated with ectodermal dysplasias and with many primary genetic abnormalities of hair and hair anchoring.

HEAD LICE

Head-lice infestation is common. Epidemics of head lice regularly sweep through primary schools in all areas. Nits (eggs) can be seen as small white specks firmly attached (unlike dandruff flecks) to hairs. Adult lice may occasionally be seen as small brown insects, about 4 mm long, walking across the scalp. Itching and excoriation are common. Presentation to an ED usually follows secondary eczematisation and infection causing extending weeping and crusted scalp lesions and neck lesions.

Suitable treatments include pyrethrin 0.165% (e.g. Pyrifoam®), maldison 0.5% and permethrin 1% (e.g. Nix® and Lyclear® cream rinse). Wash the hair with soap and water. Thoroughly moisten the hair with the treatment and leave for ten minutes. Rinse well and comb out with a fine-toothed lice comb. Reapply one week later to kill any eggs that have subsequently hatched. Reinfestation is common. A regular physical inspection, use of conditioner and combing of the hair are as important as chemical treatment. Resistance to chemical preparations is increasingly common and combination chemical and physical therapies may be required. A shorter hair cut can make this more manageable.

TINEA CAPITIS

In Australia, tinea capitis is usually caused by *Microsporum canis* contracted from cats or dogs or by *Trichophytum* species contracted from other infected children or animals. The incidence of tinea capitis is much higher in children with racially determined tightly curled black hair. Any child of African background with an itchy scalp should be assumed to have tinea until proven otherwise. Apart from itch, tinea capitis is characterised by patches of hair loss with some short, lustreless, broken hairs a few millimetres in length. Redness and scaling are present in the patch. Occasionally, inflammatory pustular swellings may be present (see kerion below). Hair loss without any epidermal changes is not likely to be fungal.

Confirm the diagnosis by greenish fluorescence of the hair shafts (not present with some fungi) with Wood's light and with microscopy and culture of hair and scale. Treatment usually comprises griseofulvin orally 20 mg kg^{-1} in divided doses (maximum 0.5–1 g, after meals with milk) daily for 8–12 weeks or until non-fluorescent. Terbinafine and itraconazole are also effective. Ketoconazole 2% shampoo twice-weekly can be used by all family members for six weeks to reduce cross-infection. Exclude from school until two days after treatment has commenced.

KERION (INFLAMMATORY RINGWORM)

This represents an inflammatory scarring immune response to tinea capitis. It is an erythematous, tender, boggy swelling, often several centimetres in diameter, that discharges pus from multiple points. The swellings appear fluctuant and are often misinterpreted in EDs as pyogenic abscesses. Skin incision and drainage should be avoided as it leads to delayed healing and increased scarring. Scrapings and/or some extracted hairs should be sent for microscopy and culture. Treatment is as for tinea capitis combined with a brief course of oral steroids to suppress the immune response. Antibiotics for secondary infection may occasionally be useful. Other inflammatory granulomas can mimic kerions. Exclude from school until two days after treatment has commenced.

ALOPECIA AREATA

Typically one or more oval patches of hair loss develop over a few days or weeks. These patches are usually completely bald but some hairs may remain within the patches. Rarely, the hair loss is diffuse. The scalp appears normal and does not show scaling, erythema or scarring. Most cases in childhood resolve spontaneously but progression to total scalp or body-hair loss or recurrent alopecia can occur. Regrowth can occur decades later.

Management

- For isolated small patches present for weeks without further progression, no treatment is needed.
- In older children who are bothered cosmetically, intralesional corticosteroid injections are the treatment of choice.
- For recent or progressive hair loss, treatment with potent topical steroids for a few weeks may help. In difficult cases, other therapies, including contact sensitisation, irritant agents and pulsed corticosteroids, need to be considered.

TRAUMATIC ALOPECIA

This condition is usually caused by rubbing (as on the occiput of many babies), cosmetic practices (e.g. tight braiding) or hair pulling as a habit (trichotillomania). Trichotillomania may be largely nocturnal and parents are often unaware of it. The affected areas are usually angular and on the anterior or lateral scalp. The areas contain hairs of different lengths and are never completely bald, unlike alopecia areata. Presentation to EDs may be triggered by the hair loss or by the sequelae of eating the hair, including acute intestinal obstruction (trichobezoar) in severe cases.

MANAGEMENT

- Recognition of the problem and a careful explanation to the family is often sufficient. Alert the family to the risk of trichobezoar.
- Trichotillomania in younger children does not usually indicate that significant psychological problems are present. It is a habit similar to thumb-sucking or nail-biting and a low-key approach similar to that used in those conditions is appropriate. In

older children, it may be part of an obsessive trait or other psychological problems that require professional and pharmacological support.

DIFFUSE HAIR LOSS

Diffuse hair loss in children is usually from telogen effluvium. This is characterised by an increased number of hairs going synchronously into the resting (telogen) phase and subsequently being shed several weeks later. Shed hairs have a small club-like appearance at the proximal end. Telogen effluvium presents as diffuse, often quite dramatic hair loss 4–16 weeks after the causative event. In children, this is commonly a high fever for a few days. Other causes include car accidents and acutely stressful events. Complete regrowth always occurs.

Dramatic widespread diffuse hair loss may be from alopecia areata.

Diffuse hair loss occurs after cancer chemotherapy. Diffuse hair loss without an obvious cause may require investigation to exclude treatable causes, such as zinc or iron deficiency, malnutrition, excess vitamin A, oral retinoids for acne, hypothyroidism or antithyroid medications, hypopituitarism, hypoparathyroidism, diabetes, and thallium poisoning.

Long-standing sparse or irregular hair is a feature of many genetic diseases. In some, such as monolethrix, the child is otherwise normal. In others, such as ectodermal dysplasias, many associated features may be present. These include decreased or absent sweating, pointy or missing teeth, dysplastic nails and dry skin. Clinical findings may be subtle. In any young child with unusual nails, skin or teeth who presents with fever and collapse, ectodermal dysplasia with inability to sweat and dysfunctional temperature control should be considered. Treatment includes cooling to restore normal body temperature, ongoing parental education and support to avoid similar overheating crises.

HYPERTRICHOSIS

Generalised hypertrichosis (increased hair in all areas) may be an isolated finding or

may be related to inherited syndromes (including Hurler and De Lange syndromes), medications (especially minoxidil, phenytoin and ciclosporin), gastrointestinal disease (including coeliac disease), anorexia nervosa, hypothyroidism, and porphyria (look for photosensitivity and blisters).

Local patches of hypertrichosis can be seen as an isolated finding or in association with lichenified eczema and topical corticosteroid use (temporary), pigmented lesions (congenital pigmented naevi, acquired naevi, Becker's naevi), plexiform neurofibromas, other naevoid lesions, chronic rubbing or over the sacral area in association with underlying spinal anomalies ('Faun's tail'). A small degree of increased hair growth over the sacral area is common in many racial groups and this is not a marker of spinal anomalies.

HIRSUTISM

Hirsutism refers to an increase in male pattern terminal hair. Increased pubic or axillary hair in young children may be due to adrenal, gonadal or CNS disease and requires investigation. Hirsutism in adolescent females may be an isolated finding or may be seen with obesity and amenorrhea in polycystic ovary syndrome. Cushing syndrome, mild congenital adrenal hyperplasia, virilising adrenal and ovarian tumours, exogenous androgens and thyroid dysfunction may cause hirsutism.

NAIL PROBLEMS

Infants' nails are often thin and exhibit a degree of koilonychia (spoon shape) that requires no investigation. Congenitally abnormal nails are usually atrophic and can be the presenting feature of rare inherited conditions, such as ectodermal dysplasias (these children may present with fever and heat prostration), dyskeratosis congenita, pachyonychia congenita (thickened nails), congenital malalignment of the great toenails and the nail-patella syndrome. Nails may have appeared normal at birth and become dystrophic over the first year of life.

Acquired nail disease is usually a result of paronychia, fungal infection, psoriasis, ingrown toenails or 20-nail dystrophy. It may also be seen in association with diseases, such as alopecia areata and lichen planus. Nail-biting and picking can lead to marked deformity of involved nails.

PARONYCHIA

Acute paronychia (inflammation of the nail fold) Is usually caused by *Staphylococcus aureus* or group A *Streptococcus*. It can be seen during therapy with oral isotretinoin for acne. One or more nail folds become red painful and swollen. Pus may be present at the nail margin. Any cause of prolonged wetness or minor trauma (e.g. finger sucking, nail picking, finger eczema, preceding chronic paronychia) predisposes to acute infection by breaching the seal between nail and skin. Treatment requires identification and avoidance of the trigger factors, warm compresses, drainage if needed, oral antibiotics (e.g. flucloxacillin, or if oral anaerobes from nail biting suspected, penicillin V), topical paraffin ointment and ongoing nail care. If due to oral isotretinoin, dose reduction and treatment as above usually resolves the problem.

Chronic paronychia Is traditionally associated with *Candida albicans*, which can be found in specimens from most cases. However, *Candida* is now seen by many authorities as a secondary feature that may not be particularly relevant to the onset and maintenance of the condition. The primary event is disruption of the nail cuticle resulting in inflammation of the proximal nail fold. Chronic paronychia may be a primarily eczematous condition caused by many factors including finger sucking, nail picking, finger eczema and any increased exposure to moisture. Affected nail folds are often dusky red or purple with loss of the cuticle and without significant pain. The nail often has several horizontal ridges corresponding to episodes of inflammation of the proximal nail fold. The nails may become increasingly dystrophic with time but do not tend to thicken.

Chronic paronychia may be present for months or years with occasionally acute exacerbations that respond to oral antibiotics without clearing the underlying problem.

- Management requires topical potent corticosteroid application daily for several weeks.
- Avoid all factors that predispose to continuing irritation or allergen exposure. Nails should be kept dry. Repeated applications of Vaseline or even a hydrocolloid dressing over the cuticle can assist in this. At times when wetting is unavoidable, such as when the child washes the dishes after dinner, cotton gloves under rubber gloves should be used.
- In difficult or unresponsive cases, consider an unusual infection or rare underlying cause such as mucocutaneous candidiasis (especially if oral *Candida* infection is present), hypoparathyroidism and malignancy.

NAIL PSORIASIS

Psoriasis can present as isolated nail disease and can mimic acute or chronic paronychia and onychomycosis. Features of nail psoriasis include pitting, thickening and brownish subungual discoloration. There may be repeated episodes of pain associated with the collection of pus under the nail. Drainage leads to relief but antibiotics don't help. Cultures are sterile. Detailed history and examination of the rest of the child may reveal other features of psoriasis. Initially treat with potent topical steroid ointments.

INGROWN TOENAIL

The nail of the large toes can grow into the lateral nail fold and cause pain, redness, swelling and occasionally pus secondary to *Staphylococcus aureus*. The chronic inflammatory process leads to progressive granulation tissue formation. Management involves avoidance of shoes where possible, avoidance of tight-fitting shoes, careful cutting of the nails and use of pledgets between the nail and lateral nail fold. Oral antibiotics are not usually required. Surgical removal of granulation material is helpful. Trimming of the lateral nail alone usually results in recurrence of the problem. In troublesome cases, surgical ablation of the lateral nail plate may be warranted.

TINEA UNGUIUM (ONYCHOMYCOSIS)

Dermatophyte infection may affect one or more nails. White or yellow patches develop at the distal and lateral nail edges. The rest of the nail may become discoloured, friable and deformed with accumulation of subungual debris. Multiple nails may become involved over years. Tinea may also present on the adjacent skin. It can be difficult to clinically distinguish between psoriasis and fungal infection in nails. Always confirm the diagnosis by microscopy and culture of nail clippings before commencing treatment. If cultures are negative, repeat the cultures but do not start oral treatment. In very mild cases only, treatment with physical debridement and anti-fungal nail lacquer (e.g. amiolfarone) may be effective. Most cases require oral therapy with terbinafine or griseofulvin for months. School exclusion, although specified in some states, is not medically warranted or appropriate.

ITCH WITHOUT RASH

Some children present with an itch without an obvious rash. Other children may have multiple excoriations without obvious cause, or they may have much more severe pruritus than would be expected for the eruption present. All such children need to be evaluated for:

- Atopy.
- Scabies.
- Symptomatic dermographism.
- Dermatitis herpetiformis.
- Iron deficiency.
- Food allergy.
- Drug use. Most pharmaceutical, recreational and herbal drugs can cause itch.

- Systemic disease, including hepatitis C infection, diabetes, uraemia, conjugated hyperbilirubinaemia, paraproteinaemia, polycythaemia and thyroid disease.

REFERENCES

1. Ramsay HM, Goddard W, Gill S, Moss C 2003 Herbal creams used for atopic eczema in Birmingham, UK, illegally contain potent corticosteroids. Archives of Disease in Childhood 88(12): 1056–1057
2. Gilbert G, Starr M 2002 Parvovirus. In: Palasanthiran P, Starr M, Jones C (eds), Management of perinatal infections. Australasian Society for Infectious Diseases, Sydney, 30–32
3. Sterling JB, Heymann WR 2000 Potassium iodide in dermatology: A 19th century drug for the 21st century uses, pharmacology, adverse effects, and contraindications. Journal of the American Academy of Dermatology 43(4): 691–697
4. http://www.rch.org.au/clinicalguide
5. Whitaker SB, Krupa JJ, Singh BB 1996 Transient lingual papillitis. Oral Surgery, Oral Medicine, Oral Pathology, Oral Radiology and Endodontics 82: 441–445
6. McDonald M, Currie BJ, Carapetis JR 2004 Acute rheumatic fever: a chink in the chain that links the heart to the throat? Lancet Infectious Diseases 4: 240–245

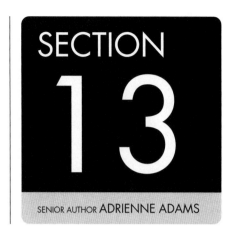

SECTION

13

SENIOR AUTHOR ADRIENNE ADAMS

EYES

13.1 OPHTHALMOLOGICAL EMERGENCIES

ADRIENNE ADAMS

ESSENTIALS

1 Conjunctivitis in the new-born needs gonococcus excluded.

2 Eye examination in young children is often opportunistic.

3 A history should always be taken regarding contact lens use in the red eye.

4 An absent or abnormal red reflex necessitates ophthalmology referral.

5 Visual acuity should be assessed as practical and if decreased in the acute setting requires ophthalmology referral.

6 Eye patching in corneal injury has no place.

7 In eye trauma thorough examination is required to exclude a penetrating injury or ruptured globe. However, the eye should not be forced open.

8 Treatment should be instituted immediately with chemical burns.

INTRODUCTION

There are very few ophthalmologic emergencies that relate exclusively to children.

Although the pathology may be the same, the general approach, examination, compliance with treatment is very different depending on the age and development of the child. Also, the long-term sequelae of serious eye injury or disease are much greater.

HISTORY

An accurate history is vital. In some instances, particularly caustic burns and the child in pain, treatment should coincide with history taking.

It is important to elicit a historical assessment of visual acuity:

- What is their vision like usually?
- Do they usually wear glasses?
- Do they wear contact lenses? This is especially important in the patient who presents with a red eye as bacterial keratitis is much more likely.

EXAMINATION TECHNIQUES (GENERAL)

Emergencies affecting the eye are often associated with a high degree of anxiety for the parent and the child. There is always a concern that sight may be affected.

As in all encounters with children, gaining the child's trust will greatly assist in eliciting the physical signs. This particularly applies to the examination of the eye. If examination is suboptimal and there is concern regarding serious injury or disease, examination under sedation or general anaesthetic is often necessary. Eyes can be alternatively patched/covered if it is suspected that an eye is not seeing.

Verbal children

Gaining trust is important and finding interesting things to look at in general conversation can ascertain the child's gross visual acuity. It may be difficult to ascertain if failure to answer appropriately is due to development, lack of co-operation or visual disturbance.

In testing each eye, children will try to 'cheat', so ensure the eye is well occluded and no peeping is occurring. The easiest way to occlude the eye is with patched glasses, which can make the examination 'fun'.

There are a number of eye charts. The best known is the Snellen Chart, which requires recognition of letters. If there is doubt about reliability, the child should show that they can perform the task close

up first. Other charts are the illiterate E chart, and the Landolt C chart but you must ensure that the child understands what you want them to do. Other child-appropriate charts are probably not available in most EDs, but include letter matching to a card a child is holding and the picture Snellen Chart.

Another factor in testing with the Snellen chart is 'boredom'. So, starting at normal visual acuity is important, rather than 6/60.

Pre-verbal children

Babies may be more easily examined if they are well wrapped. Babies also find faces very interesting and should fix on faces from 6–10 weeks of age. Nystagmus beyond this age may signify pathology. Examining the baby while feeding may be useful.

Pre-verbal children cannot co-operate and follow commands, but you can still elicit many signs, with the greatest chance being in the presence of a trusted care-giver. Often time is required to establish trust, which is helped by establishing rapport with parents.

If the eye is not swollen shut, assessment should be possible without touching the child:

- Eye movements.
- Pupil size, shape, reaction, including afferent pupil defect (see later).
- Conjunctivae.
- Limbal blush.
- Swelling.
- Red reflex.
- Corneal clarity and light reflex.

Depending on the child's interest, the simple light of an ophthalmoscope may be adequate to gain attention, but often bright, attractive toys or sweets, such as 'hundreds and thousands', may be more successful.

If visual acuity is reduced vision should be checked with the pinhole test, as this will reveal a refraction rather than an eye problem.

THE RED REFLEX

The red reflex is used to screen for abnormalities of the back of the eye, and for opacities in the visual media, such as cataract and corneal opacity.

The technique is as follows:

- The ophthalmoscope is held close to the examiners eye and focuses on the pupil 30–45 cm from the patient.
- A + 3–5 lens should be dialled up on the ophthalmoscope.
- The examination should be performed in a darkened room to promote dilatation of the pupil.

A normal reflex is red and symmetrical. The following are all abnormal:

- Dark spots in the reflex.
- Blunted red reflex on one side.
- Lack of red reflex.
- White reflex.

All children with an abnormal red reflex must be referred to an ophthalmologist.

'THE SWINGING LIGHT TEST'

This test is for afferent pupillary defect. A light is shone into one pupil for three seconds, then swung to the other side. The second pupil should remain constricted when the light is shone on it, i.e. each pupil should have the same degree of constriction. If it dilates, this is abnormal and reflects that there is damage to the optic nerve or retina slowing impulses from the afferent limb of the consensual light reflex. This is repeated for the other eye.

OTHER GENERAL TIPS

❶ If local anaesthetic is required proxymetacaine should be used as it stings less than tetracaine.
❷ If pupils are to be dilated 0.5% cyclopentolate should be used in the child < 1 month. In the older child use 1%. These can induce drowsiness.
❸ Eye drops are less painful if warmed to body temperature before instillation.

INFECTION

CONJUNCTIVITIS

Conjunctivitis is an inflammation of the mucous membranes of the eye, and can be caused by bacteria, *Chlamydia*, viruses, allergy or toxins.

Ophthalmia neonatorum

This is conjunctivitis in infants <1 month of age and is the most common infection in the first month of life. The most serious cause is gonococcal infection. It is essential to treat immediately. Ocular perforation can occur within 24 hours without treatment.

Differential diagnosis

- Bacterial conjunctivitis[1]
  Haemophilus influenzae – 17%
  Streptococcus pneumoniae – 17%
  Staphylococcus aureus – 11%
  Enterococcus – 8%.[4]
- Gonococcal conjunctivitis.
- Chlamydial conjunctivitis.
- Herpes conjunctivitis – nearly all viral conjunctivitis in the new born is herpetic.
- Chemical conjunctivitis.
- Nasolacrimal duct obstruction (occurs in up to 6% of neonates).

History

Important points to establish are:

❶ Delivery history – most cases are acquired during vaginal delivery. Rates are much lower in caesarean section deliveries, unless the membranes have been ruptured for >3 hours. However, in-utero infections have been reported in babies born by elective caesarean section.
❷ Antenatal history – antenatal swabs and if mother and partners have been adequately treated.
❸ Maternal sexual-health history
  - Have there been multiple partners?
  - History of herpes infection past and present.
  - No genital signs in the mother can be present in 30% of babies delivered with herpes

conjunctivitis.[2] If the mother has active genital herpes 40–60% of newborns are infected if they are delivered vaginally. If it is a primary infection, transmission is much higher than a secondary infection.
❹ Type of discharge – although this is often unhelpful. Gonorrhoea is usually associated with thick green/yellow discharge.

Prophylactic silver nitrate eye drops are used routinely in some countries to prevent gonococcal conjunctivitis. These are not used in NZ or Australia.

Conjunctivitis presenting at > 24 hours is unlikely to be chemical in nature.

Examination

Both eyes are examined taking care not to cause cross-contamination by means of physician contamination. Note is made of the discharge colour and type, although relying on this will lead to frequent misdiagnosis (up to 50%).

The conjunctivae are examined. In all cases of conjunctivitis they are inflamed, compared to nasolacrimal duct obstruction where the eye is not red and the conjunctivae are not inflamed.

Bacterial conjunctivitis is usually bilateral. Chlamydial conjunctivitis may be unilateral.

If herpes is suspected, the eye should be examined with fluorescein, looking for a dendritic ulcer (branching ulcer on cornea). If this is present, herpes is very likely but its absence does not rule out herpes infection. A general examination should also be carried out as herpes is always systemic, and the eye is the least of the child's problems.

Chlamydia infection can cause an associated cough and pneumonia. *Neisseria* can cause meningitis.

Pre-auricular lymphadenopathy rarely occurs in neonates due to their immature immune system.

Investigations

Swabs are mandatory in neonatal conjunctivitis. These need to be done firmly as conjunctival scrapings increase yield.

These need to be transported quickly to the laboratory as isolation of *Neisseria gonorrhoeae* is most successful if plated immediately onto chocolate agar.

A Gram stain may be diagnostic and should be acted on. If it is negative, conjunctival scrapings should be done for *Chlamydia*. PCR or LCR antigen testing is available, although sometimes chlamydial culture is also done.

Treatment

Treatment is aimed at the causative agent. Bacterial conjunctivitis (excluding gonorrhoea) is treated with antibiotic eye drops.

- Gram-positive organisms on Gram stain:
  Erythromycin eye drops, or Chloramphenicol eye drops.
- Gram-negative organisms on Gram stain:
  Gentamicin eye drops.

Pseudomonas conjunctivitis is rare in the healthy neonate, but is seen in the sick NICU patient and requires intensive hourly fortified topical antibiotics (gentamicin and cefuroxime), and systemic antibiotics. Ophthalmology consultation is paramount as there is a great risk of perforation and endophthalmitis.

GONORRHOEA

The baby with gonorrhoea conjunctivitis needs to be hospitalised and treated immediately. Treatment is started on seeing Gram-negative diplococci. Systemic treatment with IV antibiotics is mandatory. Depending on local resistance patterns, treatment is either third-generation cephalosporin (cefotaxime 50 mg kg^{-1} IV 8-hourly for one week), *or* penicillin 30 mg kg^{-1} d^{-1} IV 12-hourly during the first week of life or 6-hourly in the child over 1 week old for a total of one week.[3]

Eye toilet and irrigation decreases bacterial load – endo- and exotoxins can be extremely toxic and in some cases cause corneal stromal melt and perforation. The use of topical eye drops is debated, as is the length of treatment. Erythromycin 50 mg kg^{-1} orally in divided dose in 24 hours for three weeks is also necessary to treat presumed co-infection with *Chlamydia*. The mother and her sexual partners should also be treated.

CHLAMYDIA

Untreated chlamydial ophthalmia neonatorum can cause conjunctival scarring and corneal infiltrates.

Chlamydia also causes systemic disease, particularly pneumonitis, so systemic treatment is mandatory. Treatment is oral erythromycin 50 mg kg^{-1} d^{-1} for three weeks. There is no evidence that topical antibiotics provide any benefit.[3]

VIRAL CONJUNCTIVITIS

As mentioned previously, herpetic infection confined to the eye in the neonate is rare (only 1%). Most cases are disseminated and therefore require intensive treatment for systemic disease.

Intravenous aciclovir 10 mg kg^{-1} 8-hourly for ten days, plus topical ivifluridine five times a day. Ophthalmologic consultation and follow-up is necessary.

CONJUNCTIVITIS IN THE CHILD > 1 MONTH

The pathogenesis is the same, although causative agents change. In particular, viruses are much more common.

History

Important points to elicit in the history are:

- Usual visual acuity.
- History of trauma.
- Use of contact lenses.
- Nature of discharge.
- Sexual history in the adolescent.

Examination

The eye will be red – may be unilateral or bilateral. Visual acuity should be normal, as should the red reflex and the swinging light test.

Infection caused by adenovirus is often associated with pre-auricular lymphadenopathy (65%). This can sometimes be so haemorrhagic that the eye actually bleeds.

Visual acuity should be checked in an age-appropriate manner and the cornea should be fluorescein stained to exclude herpetic dendritic ulcers, foreign body or corneal abrasion.

Allergic conjunctivitis is associated with itching, excess lacrimation and eyelid oedema.

INVESTIGATIONS

Except when *H. influenzae*, *Neisseria* or *Chlamydia* is suspected, a trial of broad-spectrum topical antibiotics without culture may be practical, but if in doubt a swab done prior may aid treatment. See investigations in neonatal conjunctivitis.

Treatment

Treatment is aimed at the cause (see Table 13.1.1). Antibiotics shorten the duration of bacterial conjunctivitis.[4] Antibiotic ointments have higher penetration, but cause blurring of vision, so are often used at night, with drops during the day.

KERATITIS

BACTERIAL KERATITIS

This is a bacterial infection of the cornea and presents with a red eye, decreased visual acuity and a 'white spot on the cornea' in severe cases.

Aetiology

Most cases only occur where there is a defect in the corneal epithelium. However, *Neisseria gonorrhoeae*, *Corynebacterium diptheriae*, *Listeria* and *Haemophilus* can produce corneal infection in the presence of an intact epithelium.

Patients most at risk of bacterial keratitis are:

❶ Contact-lens wearers, especially 'extended-wear soft lenses'
❷ Those with ocular surface disease
❸ Those on immunosuppressants.

Investigations

Microbiological examination of corneal scrapings is mandatory.

Local anaesthetic is instilled and then under slit lamp the margins of the ulcer

Table 13.1.1   Treatment of conjunctivitis in children >1 month of age

Bacterial	Topical eye drops: Chloramphenicol, or polymyxin B, neomycin, or gramicidin 1–2-hourly in severe cases to 6-hourly as the infection improves[3]
Viral	Symptomatic: Cold compresses Artificial tears Analgesics
Herpetic	Aciclovir drops five times a day Oral aciclovir Ophthalmology referral
Contact-lens wearers	May need anti-*Pseudomonas* cover Gentamicin 1.5% Ophthalmology referral Abstain from wearing contact lenses
Allergic	Remove from allergen if possible Topical mast cell stabiliser or topical antihistamine Cold compresses
Gonorrhoeal	IV ceftriaxone 50 mg kg^{-1} daily for 3 days Concurrent chlamydial treatment Treat sexual partners Consider sexual abuse
Chlamydial	Oral erythromycin or azithromycin 20 mg/kg (max 1g) single dose in child >1 year[3] Treat sexual partners Consider sexual abuse

are scraped with a sterile 21 G hypodermic needle. Yield is increased if plated at the bedside. This is best done in the ophthalmology department. However, if an ophthalmologist is not readily available and treatment needs to be started, plating may be done in the ED. Scrapings should be plated onto glass slides and horse blood (HB) and chocolate agar for culture. Most cases (80%) are bacterial, with the remainder usually due to herpes simplex virus or a fungus.

Treatment (bacterial)

Broad-spectrum topical antibiotics, which need to start immediately post-investigation to reduce the risk of perforation.

Combined therapy gentamicin drops 1.5% and cefuroxime 5%, *or* monotherapy ciprofloxacin 0.3%[3] instilled hourly when awake for first 5 days. Ciprofloxacin drops can be used in children >1 year.

All cases need referral and admission under ophthalmology.

There is controversy regarding the use of steroids, however they are never prescribed acutely.

HERPES SIMPLEX DISEASE

Primary herpes infection typically occurs in children from six months to five years and is usually self-limiting.

Herpes simples blepharoconjunctivitis is infection of the eyelids and peri-orbital region and associated conjunctivitis. It is usually unilateral.

Treatment is symptomatic and antiviral ointment (aciclovir) is used five-times per day for 27 days.

Even without treatment keratitis is rare. It should, however, be actively sought.

HERPES SIMPLEX KERATITIS

This is infiltration of the cornea by the virus. In early stages there may be fine defects in the cornea on staining with fluorescein, but these can progress to the classic findings of a 'dendritic ulcer'.

Treatment is with topical antiviral ointment (aciclovir) 5-times per day and urgent ophthalmology referral.

There is no benefit from adding oral aciclovir as in herpes zoster ophthalmicus (shingles), where oral aciclovir, if started early, reduces the incidence and severity of eye disease.

Prognosis

With appropriate treatment 95% heal well with minimal adverse effects. Steroids are catastrophic in herpes simplex disease.

EYLID INFECTIONS

The major eyelid infections and treatments are shown in Table 13.1.2.

PERIORBITAL AND ORBITAL CELLULITIS

It is very important to differentiate between periorbital and orbital cellulitis. Both can present with fever, swollen lids and pain.

Orbital cellulitis however involves the eye with infection deep to the orbital fascia. Eye movements are limited and painful, visual acuity is reduced and proptosis can occur.

Differential diagnosis

- Insect bite. Clinically the child is afebrile and close examination will usually reveal a bite.
- Allergic reactions, which are typically bilateral and itchy.
- Trauma. (Trauma can predispose to secondary infection.)

Aetiology

Pre-*Haemophilus influenzae* vaccination this was a common cause in the child less than five years old. Now *Staphylococcus aureus* and *Streptococcus pneumoniae* are the most common causative agents.

Investigations

In cases of orbital cellulitis investigations are:

- Blood culture.
- Full blood count.
- CT scan – with contrast to identify possible subperiosteal abscess.

Table 13.1.2   Eyelid infections

	Definition	Treatment
Stye (hordeolum)	Infection of an eyelid follicle *Staphylococcus aureus* 90–95%	Hot soaks 5–10 minutes QID and lid hygiene
Chalazion	Meibomian cyst – chronic inflammation	Hot soaks 5–10 minutes QID for 1 month and lid hygiene Surgical excision if does not settle
Blepharitis	Inflammation of eyelid margin secondary to *Staphylococcus aureus*	Lid hygiene with baby shampoo Antibiotic ointment
Dacryocystitis	Infection of the lacrimal sac Peak < 2 years	Broad spectrum antibiotics and warm compresses May need admission for IV antibiotics if systemically unwell

- Visual acuity and optic-nerve function tests – colour vision/APD.

In the very unwell child, lumbar puncture may be considered, though this should be delayed until the child is stable and the CT has been performed.

Investigations in all but very minor periorbital cellulitis would be FBC and blood culture.

Treatment and disposition
Orbital cellulitis
- All need admission under ophthalmology as surgical decompression may be necessary.

- IV antibiotics – flucloxacillin 50 mg kg^{-1} 6-hourly, plus cefotaxime 50 mg kg^{-1} 8-hourly or ceftriaxone 50 mg kg^{-1} daily.
- General resuscitation for sepsis.

Peri-orbital cellulitis
- Controversy exists as to whether all cases of peri-orbital cellulitis need admission.
- Some authors advocate admission for all children < 5 years. In the older child who is clinically well, has a suitable home environment and ability for good follow-up, oral antibiotics amoxicillin/clavulanic

acid 12.5 mg kg^{-1}, up to 500 mg, 6-hourly.
- < 5 years – 3rd generation cephalosporin and flucloxacillin if staph suspected. > 5 years – flucloxacillin.

COMPLICATIONS

These include meningitis and septicaemia, abscess formation, cavernous sinus thrombosis and visual loss.

REFERENCES

1. Sandstrom K, Bell T, Chandler J, Kuo C, Wang S, Grayston J, Foy H, Stam W, Cooney M 1984 Microbiological causes of neonatal conjunctivitis. Journal of Pediatrics 105(5): 706–711
2. Whitley RJ, Chien LT, Alford CA 1975 Neonatal herpes simplex virus infection. In: Pavan-Langston DC (ed), Ocular viral disease. Little Brown, Boston, 141
3. Therapeutic Guidelines 2000 Antibiotic Guidelines Version 11. Therapeutic Guidelines Limited, Level 2, 55 Flemington Road, North Melbourne, Victoria 3051 Australia
4. Sheikh A, Hurwitz B, Cave J 2004 Antibiotics versus placebo for acute bacterial conjunctivitis (Cochrane Review). The Cochrane Library, Issue 4. Wiley, Chichester, UK

FURTHER READING

Cuculino G, Di Marco C 2002 Common ophthalmological emergencies: A systematic Approach to evaluation and management. Emergency Medicine Reports 23(13): 163–178
Nelson LB 1993 Pediatric ophthalmology. The Pediatric Clinics of North America 40(4): 693–890
Seak DV, Bron AJ, Hay J 1998 Ocular infection – investigation & treatment in practice. Martin Dunitz, London

13.2 CONGENITAL, DEVELOPMENTAL AND NEOPLASTIC CONDITIONS

GREG STEVENS

Congenital, developmental, and neoplastic disorders of the eye in children require an appropriate index of suspicion when confronted with abnormal clinical findings, and generally require referral to a paediatric ophthalmologist.

STRABISMUS

Abnormalities of the binocular alignment of the eyes, strabismus, may present with a concern from a parent that their child has a squint, and this may be confirmed by careful examination of the corneal reflex and use of the cover-uncover test.

Strabismus may be convergent (esotropia), divergent (exotropia), upwards (hypertropia) or downwards (hypotropia).

The angle of strabismus may be large, especially in congenital esotropia, however small-angle strabismus is important to detect.

Strabismus may also be a dynamic process, occurring in relation to alterations in the accommodative reflex with refractive errors.

The importance of strabismus lies in the development of amblyopia, which is the decrease in visual acuity occurring in visually immature children due to the lack of a clear image provided to the retina. It is usually unilateral. Strabismus may also be an early sign of significant visual pathology, e.g. retinoblastoma, retinitis of prematurity and Coats' disease.

If the diagnosis is suspected, a paediatric ophthalmology opinion should be requested.

PAEDIATRIC CATARACTS

These can be detected as an abnormality of the red reflex. There is an association with several chromosomal, metabolic and intrauterine infective causes.

All require referral to a paediatric ophthalmologist.

CONGENITAL NASOLACRIMAL DUCT OBSTRUCTION

This is a common disorder, occurring in up to 6% of children. It presents with excessive overflow of tears. It has a good outcome with 96% resolving by the age of one year.

A paediatric ophthalmologist should be consulted.

INFANTILE GLAUCOMA

Glaucoma in children is rare, but if undetected may cause blindness.

Because of the elasticity of the paediatric eye, significant enlargement of the cornea may occur, with subsequent clouding of the cornea. Excessive lacrimation and photophobia may be present. It is a cause of irritability in the infant.

A paediatric ophthalmology consultation is required and the treatment is usually surgical.

OCULAR TUMOURS

Tumours may present with an evident deformity, with proptosis, or with an alteration in the visual axis. Any of the tissues in the orbit and eyelids may give rise to tumours.

RETINOBLASTOMA

This is the most common primary intra-ocular tumour in childhood.

Hereditary and non-hereditary forms exist. The heredity forms are usually bilateral and multifocal. There is a defect of a tumour suppressor gene located on chromosome 13.

Leukocoria, a white pupillary reflex, may be present.

A paediatric ophthalmology opinion is required. When the tumour is confined to the eye there is a good cure rate (>90%).

RHABDOMYOSARCOMA

This is the most common primary intra-orbital tumour in childhood and usually occurs in the first decade.

It presents with proptosis, which may be rapid, and requires an urgent paediatric ophthalmology opinion.

13.3 OCULAR TRAUMA

JENNIE MARTIN

Ocular trauma is a preventable cause of visual impairment, and is the commonest cause of unilateral blindness in children. The peak incidence is seen around 11–15 years and boys are more usually affected (4:1). The usual cause of injury is sports activities and projectiles (from air guns, stones, darts, sticks, toys).

The management parallels that of the adult. However, thorough examination may be hampered by a lack of co-operation in the child and thus a lower threshold for referral may result. Unlike the adult patient, sedation (oral midazolam) or procedural sedation may be required for adequate examination and in some cases referral for general anaesthesia. About 16% of ocular trauma in children involves a penetrating globe injury.

EYELID

An ecchymosis of the eyelid or periorbital haematoma (black eye) are common traumatic injuries. Careful examination is required to exclude associated injury to the globe or orbit ('blow out fracture'), an anterior fossa fracture (suggested by a subconjunctival haemorrhage without a posterior limit) or a base-of-skull fracture ('raccoon' or 'panda eye').

Care must be exercised when opening the lids that pressure is not exerted on the globe until a ruptured globe is excluded. If the eyelids are markedly swollen, examination of the eye is often difficult. Placing one's thumb on the infraorbital and supraorbital rims, the swollen eyelids can be separated without placing pressure on the eyeball.

After other injury is excluded, the eyelid haematoma requires no specific management. Cold compresses may provide analgesia. The eye should be re-examined in 24 hours to ensure that an injury has not been missed. A laceration to the eyelid may be partial or full thickness. The laceration may involve the lid margins, canthal tendons, levator complex or canalicular system.

It is important to perform a thorough and complete eye examination to exclude an injury to the globe. Pressure exerted by attempts at cleaning and repair may apply pressure to a potentially ruptured globe. Incomplete examination can lead to an inaccurate assessment of the depth of the wound. Thus, children who are unable to be co-operative, should be referred for examination under anaesthesia. If the child is co-operative, toothed forceps can be used to assist separation of the wound edges to allow assessment of the depth of penetration of a laceration.

The mechanism of injury should be determined to assess the risk of a foreign body (e.g. windscreen shattering), whether a bite (human or animal) has taken place, and whether significant contamination may have occurred. Children are more likely than adults to conceal the mechanism of injury due to fear of discipline or implicating a friend.

Lacerations which require referral include:

- Bites and those with significant contamination, which may require debridement of necrotic tissue.
- Lacerations involving the eyelid margin should be referred for formal repair to prevent notching of the margin.
- Lacerations nasal to the upper or lower eyelid punctum, as there is a risk of injury to the canalicular system
- Deep lacerations with involvement of the levator aponeurosis of the upper eyelid (which produces ptosis) or the superior rectus muscle. Exposure of orbital fat is suggestive that the orbital septum has been lacerated as there is no subcutaneous fat in the lids themselves. Deep lacerations not fulfilling the above criteria require careful closure in layers, specialist referral is best.
- Those with significant tissue loss.

Wounds requiring referral should be cleaned with normal saline and have foreign material removed. Following cleansing the wound should be covered with a moist dressing and prophylactic antibiotics commenced for bites or significantly contaminated wounds. Tetanus prophylaxis is necessary.

If injury to the globe is suspected, or there is suspicion of a retained foreign body, a CT scan of the orbit with axial and coronal views should be performed.

If the laceration is suitable for repair in the ED, the eyebrow should not be shaved as long-term cosmetic alterations may result and the hair direction assists in correct alignment of the wound. Tissue should not be removed, as the good blood supply of the eyelid generally ensures viability. Partial-thickness lacerations should be repaired with 6/0 silk or synthetic suture and full-thickness lacerations should be repaired in layers. In general, non-absorbable sutures used in the repair of eyelid lacerations should be removed in 4–7 days.

CONJUNCTIVAL TRAUMA

Subconjunctival haemorrhage presents as a red eye with a painless collection of bright, smooth blood confined to a sector of the bulbar conjunctiva, which is sharply demarcated at the limbus and does not pass beyond the limbus. The visual acuity is normal.

Causes include: trauma (isolated or associated with a retrobulbar haemorrhage or ruptured globe), idiopathic, hypertension, bleeding diathesis, valsalva (cough, heaving, lifting, straining). If due to blunt or penetrating trauma, a ruptured globe, penetrating injury and retrobulbar haemorrhage should be excluded with caution. Pain with extra-ocular movement, reduced vision, hyphaema, pupil abnormality and/or bloody chemosis raise suspicion of a globe injury.

Subconjunctival haemorrhages without a posterior border suggest a skull fracture. No specific treatment is required for an isolated subconjunctival haemorrhage. The haemorrhage will clear spontaneously within 1–2 weeks.

Conjunctival lacerations present as a red eye with a foreign-body sensation and usually a history of trauma. Conjunctival and subconjunctival haemorrhages may be present. Thorough examination is required to exclude a scleral perforation or a subconjunctival foreign body. If necessary, the conjunctival edges can be separated gently with a moist cotton-tipped applicator following topical anaesthesia. If the diagnosis is uncertain – refer. If the conjunctival laceration is isolated, treatment with antibiotic ointment or drops is required for 4–7 days. Such lacerations rarely require repair, with only very large lacerations needing referral.

CORNEAL INJURY

Corneal lacerations may be partial or full thickness (ruptured globe). Partial-thickness lacerations have not entered the anterior chamber and the cornea has not been perforated. Complete examination (which may necessitate ophthalmologic referral) is required to exclude a penetrating injury of the cornea or sclera. Ensure the anterior chamber is not deep and there is no hyphaema.

Superficial partial-thickness lacerations will heal spontaneously with antibiotic cover. However, daily review is necessary to exclude the development of infection until healing is complete and this may necessitate referral. Deep partial-thickness lacerations should be referred for consideration of repair.

Seidel's test can be used (see ruptured globe). For management of full-thickness lacerations refer to ruptured globe.

Corneal abrasions are very painful and present with tearing, a foreign-body sensation and photophobia. Visual acuity may be reduced, depending on the size of the abrasion and the position over the visual axis. Conjunctival injection, iritis and eyelid swelling may be associated. The non-verbal child may manifest this as a refusal to open the eyes associated with intense distress. The application of a topical local anaesthetic provides temporary pain relief and will assist in allowing the eye to be opened for examination. Place a drop at the medial canthus and when the eye is opened the drops flow in. This technique is also diagnostic as symptoms that are relieved by topical anaesthesia must be due to a disruption of the corneal or conjunctival surface.

Topical anaesthesia should never be provided to the patient for continued installation and home use as this can impair healing, inhibit protective reflexes and permit further injury.

The diagnosis is made by demonstrating an epithelial-staining defect with fluorescein using either an ophthalmoscope or a slit lamp. The ophthalmoscope should be used at + 12 or greater to allow magnification of the abrasion. The red reflex will be intact.

The lids should be everted to exclude a subtarsal foreign body (an upper lid foreign body is suggested by a linear vertical abrasion – the ice-rink sign). Conjunctival foreign bodies (palpebral or bulbar) should be removed after topical anaesthesia with irrigation or a cotton-tipped applicator. A simple manoeuvre, which is often successful, for the removal of a conjunctival foreign body located on the under surface of the upper lid is to pull the upper lid by its eyelashes, out and down over the lower lid and let go, thus removing the foreign body from the small groove running parallel and close to the lid margin where it is most commonly found.

Corneal foreign bodies should be removed at the slit lamp with a foreign-body spud or 25-gauge needle, bevel down. Ophthalmologic referral for removal of the foreign body should be made if the foreign body is central, if difficulty is anticipated or the child is not fully co-operative.

Topical antibiotic treatment should be commenced and a cycloplegic (to relieve ciliary spasm) may be required for comfort if associated traumatic iritis is present (suspect with photophobia, limbic blush in addition to conjunctival injection and miosis). Eye patching does not reduce pain nor aid healing and has been shown to contribute to difficulty in walking in children. It should thus be avoided.

Contact-lens wearers require coverage for *Pseudomonas* (tobramycin or ciprofloxacin) and the lens should not be worn in the affected eye. Patients who wear contact lenses and those with central or large abrasions should be referred for examination daily until healing has occurred.

TRAUMATIC IRITIS

Traumatic iritis presents with the onset of a dull throbbing and aching pain, photophobia, and tearing within three days of trauma. The pupil may be small, perilimbal injection of the conjunctiva and pain in the affected eye when a light is shone into either the affected or non-affected eye are clues to the diagnosis if a slit lamp is not available for use.

There may be a reduction in visual acuity. White blood cells and a flare is seen within the anterior chamber when examined under the slit lamp. This is best seen by placing the slit lamp beam at 45 degrees with full intensity and a short, narrow slit. The appearance is like dust in a room illuminated with a torch. Referral for a cycloplegic and consideration of steroid use is required.

RUPTURED GLOBE AND PENETRATING EYE INJURY

A ruptured globe occurs when the integrity of the sclera or cornea is disrupted. This may be due to blunt trauma or direct perforation. A tear-shaped pupil is suggestive of occult rupture. Bloody chemosis may overlie the laceration. Severe subconjunctival haemorrhage (may involve the entire bulbar conjunctiva), chemosis, reduced visual acuity, loss of the red reflex, nausea, distortion of the anterior chamber (deep or shallow), extrusion of the intra-ocular contents, hyphaema, scleral laceration or loss of ocular motility may be indicative. Leakage of vitreous appears as clear jelly.

A Seidel test can be used if the diagnosis is unclear. Seidel's test is performed by applying a moistened fluorescein strip (and thus concentrated fluorescein dye) over the potential site of perforation. Using the blue light of the slit lamp and the leak from a perforation will manifest as a green dilute aqueous stream within the darker dye.

Always consider a penetrating injury if the history is suggestive (struck by a projectile, sharp trauma, metal against metal).

Do not apply pressure to the globe if penetration or rupture is suspected. Do not attempt to remove a protruding foreign body from the globe. Do not force the lids open as pressure on the globe may cause extrusion of the ocular contents.

Once perforation or penetration of the eye is suspected, further ED examination is unnecessary. Protect the eye with an eye shield. If a formal eye shield is unavailable, one can be created from the base of a Styrofoam cup. The shield should rest on the bony prominences. Keep the patient fasted and record the fasting time. Commence an antiemetic and analgesia as necessary. Bed rest the patient. Further eye drops should not be used and *never* use eye ointment on an open globe. Ensure tetanus prophylaxis. Commence systemic antibiotic prophylaxis such as cephazolin. Contact the ophthalmologist.

If an intra-ocular foreign body or globe rupture is suspected orbital imaging with axial and coronal CT will be necessary following discussion with an ophthalmologist. In those patients with a very high-risk history, immediate referral to an ophthalmologist may be indicated if the child is particularly unco-operative or the lids are so swollen that it is too difficult to obtain a good view of the eyeball.

HYPHAEMA

Hyphaema occurs when blood arises from the iris or ciliary body and is seen in the anterior chamber layered inferiorly if the patient is sitting or standing. Hyphaemas may result from blunt or penetrating trauma. Pain, photophobia, mydriasis or miosis and blurred vision may result. In traumatic mydriasis the pupil is large and less reactive (caused by damage to the pupillary sphincter muscle). Somnolence and restlessness is particularly common in children. The red reflex will be intact (use the ophthalmoscope at +10). The size may vary from microscopic (suspended red blood cells seen as rust-coloured specks under magnification in the slit lamp – microhyphaema) to blood involving the whole anterior chamber.

The eye should be examined for other anterior-segment injuries and ophthalmologic referral is required for all patients.

If the pupil is dilated, it is important to differentiate between traumatic mydriasis (present only in the affected eye) and an afferent pupillary defect (swinging light test – paradoxical initial dilatation of the affected pupil when light is shone quickly from the unaffected to the affected eye). A positive test may suggest an optic nerve or severe retinal injury.

Black and Mediterranean patients require screening for sickle cell trait or disease as spontaneous hyphaema may occur.

Hospitalisation is generally required.

Treatment includes bed rest with head elevation, eye shield, antiemetics, simple analgesics (not NSAIDs or salicylates), cycloplegics and steroids. Rebleeding occurs in up to one-third of patients, usually after a few days.

Amblyopia may be a risk if vision remains reduced in the eye for more than a few days in children at the critical age for vision development.

FRACTURES

In adolescents, blow-out fractures result from blunt trauma and refer to fractures of the orbital floor. There is often a haematoma of the eyelid. Look for diplopia usually on upward gaze (due to haemorrhage and oedema of the orbital fat, entrapment of the inferior rectus or inferior oblique muscle or direct injury to the extra-ocular muscle), enophthalmos and infra-orbital nerve anaesthesia. Facial X-rays (+/− facial CT) and referral are required.

RETROBULBAR HAEMATOMA

Retrobulbar haematoma is seen in both blunt and penetrating trauma. Presents with pain, nausea and vomiting, proptosis, tense globe, diffuse subconjunctival injection extending posteriorly, chemosis, reduced acuity and sometimes restricted ocular motility. All patients require ophthalmological referral. If an afferent pupillary defect or elevated intra-ocular pressure is present emergency decompression by an ophthalmologist will be required.

CHEMICAL BURNS

Chemical burns are unusual in childhood but potentially very serious. Treatment should be instituted immediately, even before visual acuity is documented. Anaesthetise the eye (procedural sedation may be required in young children) and then copiously rinse the eye with at least 1–2 litres of normal saline or Hartmann's for at least 30 minutes. Use IV tubing connected to the litre bag, this assists the process. Ensure the eye is irrigated with the upper lid everted and the lower lid pulled down to ensure irrigation of the fornices. About five minutes after irrigation has been completed, check the pH with litmus paper and continue irrigation until a neutral pH of 7 is achieved. Many litres may be required for some chemical burns. Particulate matter requires removal and this may require general anaesthesia.

Alkali burns produce liquefactive necrosis and are often more severe than acid burns. Many domestic cleaning products are alkaline.

Once irrigation has been completed, the severity of the injury can be assessed with a slit lamp and fluorescein stain. Moderate or severe burns (suggested by significant epithelial loss, chemosis, corneal oedema, blanching of the conjunctival vessels or opacification) should be referred immediately. Ophthalmologic assessment can be delayed to the next day for mild burns. Treatment with antibiotic drops/ointment, analgesia and cycloplegics is required.

NON-ACCIDENTAL INJURY

Any eye injury can be the result of abuse and a high index of suspicion is required if the injury is inconsistent with the given history or the history is inadequate. Retinal haemorrhages are found in 80% of cases of shaken baby syndrome. The presence of retinal haemorrhage in a child < 1 year is most commonly due to a NAI. Other conditions seen include any of the above traumatic injuries, traumatic mydriasis, detached retina, cataract, subluxed lens and optic atrophy.

THE RED EYE

The differential diagnosis is similar to adults, and includes conjunctivitis, corneal ulceration, keratitis, episcleritis and scleritis, iritis and glaucoma.

The commonest cause of red eye in children is conjunctivitis (see above) and other diagnoses are uncommon. Systemic illness should be excluded, e.g. Stevens–Johnson syndrome (erythema multiforme major), Kawasaki disease, or measles. Thorough examination is vital to accurately establish the eye signs. Unilateral redness, reduced vision, severe pain, intense grittiness or photophobia are suggestive that conjunctivitis is not the diagnosis.

Use a light to inspect the pupil shape, size and reaction to light. Is the red reflex present? Is the redness unilateral or bilateral? Examine the pattern of bulbar injection.

An intact red reflex and normal reaction of the pupil to light suggests conjunctivitis. If the pupil is irregular, unreactive to light or the red reflex is not present, consider iritis, or uveitis.

Conjunctivitis is almost always bilateral. The unilateral red eye should prompt consideration of a corneal ulcer, foreign body, trauma, and iritis or herpes infection.

CORNEAL ULCER

Corneal ulcer presents with a red eye, pain, photophobia, and watering, there may be decreased visual acuity or a discharge. Corneal sensation should be assessed prior to the application of topical anaesthetic.

The causes include traumatic, bacterial, HSV, uncommonly fungal (from plant injury), and *Acanthamoeba* (contact lens wearers). Always exclude a subtarsal foreign body when a corneal ulcer is found. A dendritic (herpes simplex virus) ulcer may present painlessly as corneal sensation is diminished. Consider HSV in children with a unilateral red eye, recent fever, cold or flu-like illness and in particular those with labial herpes or herpetic vesicles around the eye. Preauricular adenopathy is frequently present. If the diagnosis is suspected, referral for review and follow up is required.

UV KERATITIS

Due to excess sunlight exposure, UV keratitis presents with pain, burning and watering. Examination reveals a punctate keratopathy (fine spots on the cornea with fluorescein staining) with a macroscopic diffuse corneal haziness. Treatment involves cycloplegics and topical antibiotics.

IRITIS (ANTERIOR UVEITIS)

Signs of iritis include a ciliary flush (red injected sclera at limbus), reduced visual acuity, pain, photophobia, tearing and blepharospasm. There is usually a pupil irregularity or miosis. Relief of pain when the eye is topically anaesthetised is a relatively sensitive and simple method of excluding the diagnosis of iritis. On slit-lamp examination a flare and cells in the anterior chamber are seen, a hypopyon in severe cases.

Causes include idiopathic, juvenile rheumatoid arthritis (girls with oligo-articular juvenile chronic arthritis who are ANA positive are more at risk), sarcoidosis and post-trauma. Contact ophthalmology

if the diagnosis is suspected. In children iritis is more often related to infectious or neoplastic causes than it is in adults.

SCLERITIS AND EPISCLERITIS

Scleritis and episcleritis are strongly associated with systemic disease and presents with epiphora, with localised areas of tenderness and inflammation. Ophthalmologic referral is necessary.

ACUTE GLAUCOMA

Acute glaucoma is very rare in children unless it is due to a subluxed lens (Marfan syndrome, homocystinuria) or a hyphaema. An enlarged, clouded cornea is seen associated with tearing (epiphora) and photophobia. Ophthalmologic referral should be made immediately. Congenital glaucoma presents at or soon after birth with an enlarged, hazy cornea and tearing in an infant. Red eye may be present and the condition is commonly bilateral. Prompt diagnosis is essential to prevent visual loss.

UNCOMMON EYE CONDITIONS IN CHILDREN

- Sun-gazers' retinopathy; eclipse burn.
- Migraine, including common migraine with aura; ophthalmoplegic migraine (produces paralysis of one or more of the extra-ocular muscles, which resolves with resolution of the headache); visual migraine without headache; hemiplegic migraine; retinal migraine; basilar artery migraine. Ophthalmoplegic migraine is most common in children less than ten years. The third nerve is most commonly affected, followed by the sixth nerve. A personal or family history of migraine is seen. Migraine is a diagnosis of exclusion and neurology referral is necessary.
- Sudden visual loss with optic neuritis.
- Functional visual loss. Usually teenage girls who are unconcerned about their

visual loss. Functional blindness is a diagnosis of exclusion and ophthalmologic review is necessary.

- Gradual onset of decreased visual acuity is seen with optic glioma and craniopharyngioma.

FURTHER READING

Datner EM, Tilman Jolly B 1995 Paediatric ophthalmology. Emergency Medicine Clinics of North America 13(3): 669–679

Flynn CA, D'Amico F, Smith G 1998 Should we patch corneal abrasions? A meta-analysis. Journal of Family Practice 47: 262–270

Hamid RKA, Newfield P 2001 Paediatric eye emergencies. Anesthesiology Clinics of North America 19(2): 257

Kanski JJ 1999 Clinical Ophthalmology. A Systematic Approach, 5th edn. Butterworth Heinemann, Oxford

Levin AV 1991 Eye emergencies: Acute management in the paediatric ambulatory care setting. Paediatric Emergency Care 7(6): 367–377

Linden JA, Renner GS 1995 Trauma to the globe. Emergency Medicine Clinics of North America 13(3): 581–605

Michael JG, Hug D, Dowd MD 2002 Management of corneal abrasion in children: A randomised clinical trial. Annals of Emergency Medicine 40(1): 67–72

Opthalmology 2004 Emedicine www.emedicine.com

Repka MX 1993 Common pediatric neuro-opthalmologic conditions. Pediatric Clinics of North America 40(4): 777–788

Rychwalski et al 1999 Evaluation and classification of pediatric ocular trauma. Paediatric Emergency Care 15(4): 277–279

Kunimoto DY, Kanitkar KD, Matar MS (eds) 2004 Office and emergency room diagnosis and treatment of eye disease. The Wills eye manual, 4th edn. Lippincott Williams & Wilkins, Philadelphia, USA

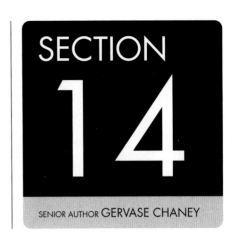

SECTION
14

SENIOR AUTHOR GERVASE CHANEY

ENT AND DENTAL

14.1 THE EAR

GERVASE CHANEY

ESSENTIALS

1 Otitis externa usually results from excessive exposure to heat and moisture and is usually very painful. Treatment involves cleaning, keeping dry and topical antibiotics.

2 Acute otitis media is a very common emergency presentation, but not all red ear drums are due to otitis media. Management with adequate analgesia is essential. However, antibiotic use is hotly debated.

3 Discharging otitis media due to chronic suppurative otitis media usually presents with painless and offensive discharge. Treatment is with ear toilet and topical antibiotics. Oral antibiotics have little or no role.

4 Otitis media with effusion is very common in children, but treatment is unnecessary in the majority with resolution over three months.

5 Mastoiditis continues to be a problem in the antibiotic era and in many cases is the first presentation of ear disease. Admission, myringotomy and IV antibiotics constitute the mainstays of medical management.

6 Complication rates are significant. Ear trauma is uncommon. Accidental ear injuries are usually unilateral and isolated. Ear trauma is rare in the first year of life and may indicate non-accidental injury. Haematomas should be removed by aspiration or excision.

OTITIS EXTERNA

INTRODUCTION

Otitis externa includes various conditions from the most common acute diffuse otitis externa (swimmer's or tropical ear) to otomycosis, localised (furunculosis) or chronic otitis externa. It occurs commonly in hot, humid climates or in the summer of temperate climates. Risk factors also include swimming and other water exposure, local trauma, loss of the protective coating of the ear canal, including cerumen and obstruction of the ear canal. Allergy may also play a role.

HISTORY

It may initially present with aural fullness or itch, but usually progresses to pain with or without discharge. The pain is often severe and is worse with chewing.

Otomycosis or fungal otitis externa makes up 10% of cases and has a more insidious onset

EXAMINATION

Oedema and erythema of the canal with serous or purulent discharge is usual. The tragus is very tender to manipulation. With increased severity the canal becomes occluded with periauricular oedema and lymphadenopathy. Differentiation from acute otitis media with perforation or chronic suppurative otitis media is important. Usually in these conditions, the tragus and canal are not tender and there is no erythema and oedema of the canal.

Acute localised otitis externa (furunculosis) occurs in the posterosuperior aspect on the ear canal. Otomycosis has only mild canal wall inflammation and thick otorrhoea.

INVESTIGATIONS

Investigations are largely unnecessary. The organisms found in diffuse otitis externa are most commonly *Pseudomonas aeruginosa* and *Staphylococcus aureus*. Furunculosis is usually *S. aureus* and otomycosis – *Aspergillus* or *Candida* species. Consideration of cultures – aerobic, anaerobic and fungal is worthwhile in cases resistant to routine therapy or if there is more extensive disease – such as associated cellulitis.

TREATMENT

Acute diffuse otitis externa is managed with gentle cleaning of the canal, along with avoidance of water (swimming prohibited). Ototopical medications are the mainstay of treatment, usually topical antibiotics such as framycetin/gramicidin/dexamethasone combinations. Ciprofloxacin is also effective. Insertion of a wick or ribbon gauze is also helpful.

Furunculosis treatment is by local heat application and oral antibiotics (flucloxacillin or cefalexin) or incision and drainage. Otomycosis will require canal cleaning and antifungal drops or gentian violet.

PREVENTION

Keeping the ear canal dry and avoidance of trauma to the canal are the mainstays of prevention.

COMPLICATIONS

Progression to cellulitis of the nearby skin/soft tissue and/or lymphadenitis may occur. Oral antibiotics are usually then indicated, with cefalexin a reasonable first choice, but anti-pseudomonal antibiotics may be necessary. Less commonly, involvement of the parotid gland, temporomandibular joint or base of skull may occur.

Chronic otitis externa may occur, but may be a sign of an underlying dermatological disease such as seborrhoeic or atopic dermatitis.

ACUTE OTITIS MEDIA

INTRODUCTION

Acute otitis media is one of the most common primary care paediatric presentations, including to EDs. Its diagnosis is not always clear, particularly in the young child with a non-specific presentation. Diagnosis is not straightforward and it is frequently over diagnosed. It can be caused by both viral and bacterial organisms and its management, particularly in relation to use of antibiotics, continues to be debated. There are significant variations in the rates of antibiotic use between different countries, but it remains the most frequent reason for antibiotic use in countries like the United States. This is a significant contributor to the development of antibiotic-resistant bacteria.

HISTORY

Classic symptoms include fever, malaise and ear pain. The pain can be severe and during the night may wake the child. Other systemic features such as nausea and vomiting can occur. In younger children, presentation is often non-specific, with crying and irritability. Eardrum perforation and otorrhoea may occur (see complications).

Middle-ear effusions occur in 100% and spontaneously resolve gradually within three months in 90% of cases.

EXAMINATION

Redness of the eardrum is a non-specific finding and may be seen with a high fever or following crying. Alone, therefore, it is not predictive of otitis media. More reliable signs to predict otitis media are clouding and bulging of the eardrum. The presence of an effusion (a visualised fluid level or reduced mobility on pneumotoscopy) may assist in differentiation.

INVESTIGATIONS

If available, tympanometry is a reasonably reliable way to demonstrate an effusion (reduced compliance or a 'flat or type-B tympanogram' with an intact ear drum). It will not be able to indicate whether an effusion is infected. Other investigations are usually not indicated.

When it has been performed, tympanostomy reveals that two-thirds of patients are bacterial-culture positive, with a predominance of *Streptococcus pneumoniae*, *Moraxella catarrhalis* and *Haemophilus influenzae*.

TREATMENT

The administration of adequate analgesia is paramount to the management of acute otitis media. Paracetamol alone may not be adequate and the combination with codeine may be required. Topical anaesthetics, such as benzocaine in glycerol are also a useful adjunct. Decongestants and antihistamines have not been shown to be effective and are not recommended.

The majority of cases of otitis media will resolve spontaneously. However, antibiotics have been used routinely ever since their introduction. A recent Cochrane review concluded that antibiotics confer a small benefit for acute otitis media in children. There is a small, but significant reduction in pain, with no difference in complications. The authors conceded that antibiotics might play an important role in prevention of mastoiditis in populations where it is more common. Unfortunately, despite it being such a common presentation, there are very few well designed studies of an adequate size to demonstrate the most appropriate antibiotic regimen and one review concluded that routine antibiotic use for otitis media is unproven.

Amoxicillin is a reasonable first-line antibiotic choice. The usual recommended dose is 40 mg kg^{-1} d^{-1}, but high doses are recommended (80–90 mg kg^{-1} d^{-1}) when penicillin-resistant pneumococci are more likely. Amoxicillin + clavulanate is the next choice for poor responders. Cefaclor has a significant rate of serum sickness reactions in children and should be used with caution. A number of studies have suggested that children can be observed for 48 hours and antibiotics used if required.

The recommended length of antibiotic course varies, but generally has shifted from ten days to five days. The reasons for this include, reduced cost, improved adherence, reduced development of antibiotic-resistant organisms and only minor differences in outcome. The longer course is still recommended for severe or complicated otitis media and for children less than two years of age.

COMPLICATIONS

The most common complication is perforation of the drum and otorrhoea. Other complications are very unusual but potentially severe. Most are due to bacterial spread and include extracranial complications such as mastoiditis, cholesteatoma and facial nerve paralysis and intracranial complications such as epidural abscess, meningitis and lateral sinus thrombosis. Mastoiditis is now very uncommon even when antibiotics are withheld, and there is no evidence that antibiotic use for otitis media will prevent meningitis.

PREVENTION

Prophylactic antibiotics confer a small decrease in recurrence at best, and are likely to contribute to increasing antibiotic resistance and generally are not recommended. Other means of reducing recurrence are more worth pursuing, such as cutting passive smoke exposure, reducing day-care attendance and immunisation (conjugate pneumococcal and influenza).

DISCHARGING OTITIS MEDIA – CHRONIC SUPPURATIVE OTITIS MEDIA

INTRODUCTION

Discharging otitis media is most common in developing countries and certain high-risk populations in developed nations, such as Aboriginal Australians. It generally occurs following perforation of the eardrum from acute otitis media. It also occurs as a complication of tympanostomy tube (grommet) placement. Otorrhoea has been reported to be as high as 83% of cases within 18 months of tube placement, with a mean duration of 16 days.

HISTORY

There is usually an absence of pain and a variable history (often weeks) of discharge that is purulent and offensive. It is often recurrent.

EXAMINATION

The canal is usually non-tender and there is usually no inflammation or some chronic inflammation. If the tympanic membrane can be visualised, usually only after ear toilet, there will be a perforation or tympanostomy tube in situ.

INVESTIGATIONS

Investigations are largely unnecessary. If performed, the organisms found on ear swabs are most commonly *Pseudomonas aeruginosa* and *Staphylococcus aureus*.

TREATMENT

Ear toilet (using a dry tissue spear) and topical antibiotics particularly quinolones (such as ciprofloxacin with hydrocortisone) or framycetin/gramicidin/dexamethasone combinations, have been demonstrated to be effective in acute resolution of otor-

rhoea. Long-term outcomes are still to be determined. Systemic antibiotics alone are not as effective and addition to topical treatment does not improve outcome.

COMPLICATIONS

Chronic perforation and discharge are the main issues, although hearing impairment may be a problem. Cholesteatoma occurs in a small proportion of affected children.

OTITIS MEDIA WITH EFFUSION

INTRODUCTION

Otitis media with effusion (OME) is the presence of a middle-ear effusion in the absence of acute inflammation. It is unlikely to be a presenting complaint in an ED setting. It is more likely to be found as an incidental finding. It is extremely common, particularly in pre-school children. Its significance is in relation to its effect on conductive hearing.

HISTORY

Older children may present with aural fullness or reduced hearing. OME is usually asymptomatic in young children.

EXAMINATION

The eardrum may appear dull and non-erythematous and the effusion is most easily recognised by the presence of bubbles or a fluid level. If these are not present pneumatic otoscopy will demonstrate impaired mobility.

INVESTIGATIONS

Middle-ear effusion can be confirmed by tympanometry. A 'type B' or flat tympanogram in the presence of an intact tympanic membrane indicates the presence of a middle-ear effusion. More im-

portantly, in persistent cases audiology is recommended to determine any significant hearing loss.

TREATMENT

As the majority of OME cases will resolve spontaneously (90% by three months) a period of observation is recommended. Persistent OME is more likely to follow acute otitis media in the first year of life.

Many different treatments have been tried and recommended over the years. Antibiotics, nasal decongestants, nasal insufflation, and corticosteroids have all failed to be proven treatments. Persistent OME with significant hearing loss would warrant referral to an ENT surgeon. If ventilation tubes (grommets) are sited, hearing should be reassessed to establish that any loss has improved and that there is not an underlying sensorineural hearing loss.

COMPLICATIONS

The principle concern for persistent OME is conductive hearing loss and potential impact on language and cognitive development. There are potential long-term changes to the tympanic membrane and middle ear that may cause hearing loss (e.g. tympanosclerosis). Less clear is whether other problems such as clumsiness and behavioural disorders are related to OME.

MASTOIDITIS

INTRODUCTION

Mastoiditis is the infection of the mastoid air cells. It is an infrequent presentation with a rate of between 1.2 and 4.2 per 100 000 person years in developed nations. Incidence rates are reported variously as unchanged and decreasing. Ages at presentation range from two months up, with a median of 12–48 months.

HISTORY

Presentation with mastoiditis is almost always accompanied by acute otitis media. However, acute mastoiditis is the first presentation of pathology in the ear in 38.5–82% of patients in many series. Mean time from onset of illness to signs of acute mastoiditis has been reported as just over four days. Presentation is with ear or retroauricular pain, irritability, fever (28–79% of cases) and otorrhoea (16–36%). Frequently the patient is already on antibiotics.

EXAMINATION

Examination findings include protrusion/displacement of the auricle, post-auricular redness, oedema and tenderness and ear-canal narrowing. The tympanic membrane is usually abnormal and may be perforated.

INVESTIGATIONS

Routine use of CT scanning is recommended due to the low rate of diagnosis of subperiosteal abscess by clinical examination. MRI scanning may also be valuable. Bacteriological diagnosis is made either by myringotomy (54% of cultures positive) or mastoidectomy. Cultures show *Streptococcus pneumoniae* to be the most common organism followed by *Streptococcus pyogenes*, but many organisms are possible.

TREATMENT

Management has frequently been cortical mastoidectomy. However, a number of series report successful treatment of the majority of cases with myringotomy and IV antibiotics. Broad-spectrum antibiotics such as third-generation cephalosporins are generally recommended, although antipseudomonal antibiotics may be required.

COMPLICATIONS

Complication rates are significant (13–35%) and include subperiosteal abscess, facial nerve paralysis, sigmoid sinus thrombosis, epidural abscess and meningitis.

TRAUMA

INTRODUCTION

Paediatric ear trauma is an uncommon presentation to an ED. Accidental ear trauma is almost always unilateral. There is the usual male predominance, with a majority between one and seven years of age. Accidental ear trauma is rare in the first year of life and such presentations should be assessed for possible non-accidental (inflicted) injury. Other suggestive findings are bilateral ear injuries and associated injuries, particularly retinal haemorrhages and subdural haematoma.

HISTORY AND EXAMINATION

The most common mechanism is falls, followed by blows from an object and self-inflicted penetrating injuries. The most common object inserted are cotton buds. Dog bites of the ear also occur. Lacerations are the most common injury, followed by bruising, abrasions and haematomas. Blood in the canal is a common finding in the penetrating injuries, making assessment of the eardrum difficult at the time of initial presentation. Burns are rare and are likely to be associated with more extensive burns. Pressure injuries from explosions, loud noises and airflights are uncommon, but occur.

Assessment should include assessment of the facial nerve and hearing.

INVESTIGATION

Acute investigations are rarely required. However, follow-up audiology is indicated in penetrating and pressure-type injuries. This would usually be in conjunction with ear, nose and throat surgeon follow-up.

TREATMENT

Minor lacerations may be managed with steristrips, glue or suturing under local anaesthesia. Complex or larger lacerations will often require a general anaesthetic and surgical repair. Haematomas can lead to cartilage necrosis, infection and chondritis or fibrous organisation. All of these have potential to cause significant deformity. Therefore removal of the haematoma is indicated. Smaller haematomas can be aspirated and larger or recurrent collections should be evacuated. Appropriate contoured dressings are then required to avoid reaccumulation. Penetrative injuries will often require ENT surgeon referral. Unless minor, burns will require evaluation by a burns specialist.

COMPLICATIONS

The main concerns are cosmetic deformity from haematomas, lacerations and burns, and hearing loss from penetrative injuries.

FURTHER READING

Acuin J 2002 Extracts from 'concise clinical evidence': Chronic suppurative otitis media. British Medical Journal 325(7373): 16

Acuin J, Smith A, Mackenzie I 2000 Interventions for chronic suppurative otitis media. Cochrane Database of Systematic Reviews 2 John Wiley and Sons, Chichester

Ah-Tye C, Paradise JL, Colborn DK 2001 Otorrhea in young children after tympanostomy-tube placement for persistent middle-ear effusion: Prevalence, incidence, duration. Paediatrics 107(6): 1251–1258 [comment]

Bitar CN, Kluka EA, Steele RW 1996 Mastoiditis in children. Clinical Paediatrics 35(8): 391–395

Brook I 1999 Treatment of otitis externa in children. Paediatric Drugs 1(4): 283–289

Butler CC, Van Der Voort JH 2000 Oral or topical nasal steroids for hearing loss associated with otitis media with effusion in children. Cochrane Database of Systematic Reviews 2002 4 [update of Cochrane Database of Systematic Reviews 4 CD001935, PMID: 11034736]

Byington CL 1998 The diagnosis and management of otitis media with effusion. Paediatric Annals 27(2): 96–100

Cantor RM 1995 Otitis externa and otitis media. A new look at old problems. Emergency Medicine Clinics of North America 13(2): 445–455

Cohen-Kerem R et al 1999 Acute mastoiditis in children: Is surgical treatment necessary? Journal of Laryngology & Otology 113(12): 1081–1085

Combs JT 2003 Diagnostic accuracy of otitis media. Paediatrics 112(1): 205–206

Dagan R, McCracken GH Jr 2002 Flaws in design and conduct of clinical trials in acute otitis media. Paediatric Infectious Disease Journal 21(10): 894–902 [comment]

Del Mar CB, Glasziou PP 1999 Should we now hold back from initially prescribing antibiotics for acute otitis media? Journal of Paediatrics & Child Health 35(1): 9–10

Dowell SF et al 1998 Principles of judicious use of antimicrobial agents for pediatric upper respiratory tract infections. Paediatrics 101(1): 163–165.

CONTROVERSIES AND FUTURE DIRECTIONS

❶ Acute otitis media:
- Antibiotic usage for acute otitis media in Australia, the UK and USA has been about 97–98%. Due to concerns over the emergence of antibiotic resistance, the Netherlands has limited antibiotic use (31%) with good results leading to a review of use in high-prescribing countries. The concern about lower rates of antibiotic use is the potential for increased complications (see mastoiditis).

❷ Discharging otitis media – chronic suppurative otitis media:
- Concern has arisen with the use of potentially ototoxic antibiotic ear drops in the presence of a tympanic-membrane perforation, despite routine use by ENT specialists with few reported cases of ototoxicity.
- A series of nine cases of iatrogenic topical vestibulotoxicity, all secondary to gentamicin-containing eardrops, has been reported. As a result agents such as ciprofloxacin are being increasingly used.

❸ Otitis media with effusion
- Ventilation-tube (grommet) insertion remains one of the most common surgical procedures performed in children.
- It is effective at improving hearing in the short term. There has been conflicting evidence for its long-term benefit on language and cognitive development.

❹ Mastoiditis
- There is a higher incidence of mastoiditis in the Netherlands where there is a low antibiotic prescription rate for acute otitis media (31%), compared to some countries, such as Australia, Canada, UK and USA, where there are very high prescription rates (>90%).
- However Norway and Denmark have high prescription rates (67 and 76%) and have similar incidence rates to the Netherlands. If the effect is real there would be two extra cases of acute mastoiditis per 100 000 children per year. The Netherlands has so far achieved its aim of a low rate of pneumococcal resistance (1.1% in 1995) to penicillin compared to countries with high prescription rates. These two factors have to be weighed up in the choice of management of acute otitis media.

Dowell SF et al 1998 Otitis media – Principles of judicious use of antimicrobial agents. Paediatrics 101(1): 165–171

Flynn CA, Griffin G, Tudiver F 2001 Decongestants and antihistamines for acute otitis media in children. Cochrane Database of Systematic Reviews 2002 1 [update of Cochrane Database Systematic Review 2. CD001727, PMID: 11406002]

Froom J et al 1997 Antimicrobials for acute otitis media? A review from the international primary care network. British Medical Journal 315(7100): 98–102

Garbutt J, Jeffe DB, Shackelford P 2003 Diagnosis and treatment of acute otitis media: An assessment. Paediatrics 112(1): 143–149

Glasziou PP et al 2000 Antibiotics for acute otitis media in children. Cochrane Database of Systematic Reviews 2000 4.[update of Cochrane Database Systematic Review 2. CD000219, PMID: 10796513]

Holmes RE 1999 Management of traumatic auricular injuries in children. Paediatric Annals 28(6): 391–395

Hughes E, Lee JH 2001 Otitis externa. Paediatrics in Review 6: 191–197

Kozyrskyj AL et al 2000 Short course antibiotics for acute otitis media. Cochrane Database of Systematic Reviews 2.

Little P et al 2001 Pragmatic randomised controlled trial of two prescribing strategies for childhood acute otitis media. British Medical Journal 322(7282): 336–342

Little P et al 2002 Predictors of poor outcome and benefits from antibiotics in children with acute otitis media: Pragmatic randomised trial. British Medical Journal 325(7354): 22 [commentary: research directions for treatment for acute otitis media]

Pond F, McCarty D, O'Leary S 2002 Randomized trial on the treatment of oedematous acute otitis externa using ear wicks or ribbon gauze: Clinical outcome and cost. Journal of Laryngology & Otology 116(6): 415–419

Rovers MM et al 2000 The effect of ventilation tubes on language development in infants with otitis media with effusion: A randomized trial. Paediatrics 106(3): e42

Rovers MM et al 2001 Randomised controlled trial of the effect of ventilation tubes (grommets) on quality of life at age 1–2 years. Archives of Disease in Childhood 84(1): 45–49 [comment]

Ruohola A et al 2003 Antibiotic treatment of acute otorrhea through tympanostomy tube: Randomized double-blind placebo-controlled study with daily follow-up. Paediatrics 111(5-1): 1061–1067

Segal S et al 2003 Inner ear damage in children due to noise exposure from toy cap pistols and firecrackers: A retrospective review of 53 cases. Noise & Health 5(18): 13–18

Spratley J et al 2000 Acute mastoiditis in children: Review of the current status. International Journal of Pediatric Otorhinolaryngology 56(1): 33–40

Steele BD, Brennan PO 2002 A prospective survey of patients with presumed accidental ear injury presenting to a paediatric accident and emergency department. Emergency Medicine Journal 19(3): 226–228

Straetemans M et al 2002 Pneumococcal vaccines for preventing otitis media. Cochrane Database of Systematic Reviews 2

Van Zuijlen DA et al 2001 National differences in incidence of acute mastoiditis: Relationship to prescribing patterns of antibiotics for acute otitis media? Paediatric Infectious Disease Journal 20(2): 140–144 [comment]

Vassbotn FS et al 2002 Acute mastoiditis in a Norwegian population: A 20 year retrospective study. International Journal of Paediatric Otorhinolaryngology 62(3): 237–242

14.2 THE NOSE

GERVASE CHANEY

ESSENTIALS

Rhinitis and sinusitis

1 Acute rhinitis is common and largely due to viral infections.

2 Mucopurulent discharge does not mean bacterial infection.

3 Antibiotics are only indicated in prolonged cases of nasal discharge (> 10–14 days duration), indicating likely sinusitis.

4 Constant nasal discharge may be due to perennial allergic rhinitis.

Epistaxis

1 Epistaxis is common and largely responds to simple first aid – compression of the nose.

2 Those cases failing to respond to first aid can be managed with nasal antiseptic cream or silver nitrate cautery.

3 Severe cases are uncommon, but are a medical emergency, requiring nasal packing and urgent ENT referral.

4 Underlying bleeding tendency should be excluded in cases with a family history of bleeding tendency or those with severe recurrent epistaxis.

Nasal trauma

1 Nasal trauma is common.

2 Most injuries will require little or no intervention. However, a careful examination to exclude septal haematoma is essential.

3 Septal haematoma requires urgent ENT referral.

4 Acute assessment can be difficult and a review, once the swelling has settled, is required to manage any deformity.

RHINITIS AND SINUSITIS

INTRODUCTION

Most children with nasal discharge have a viral infection, such as the common cold. Children will commonly experience three to eight colds per year, even more if attending day care. Despite recommendations against such practice, antibiotics have been frequently prescribed for the common cold, often due to the finding of green or mucopurulent discharge. Bacterial sinusitis has been estimated as complicating 0.5–5% of upper respiratory tract infections.

HISTORY

The common cold usually commences with a throat irritation and clear, thin nasal discharge and progresses to a thick, mucopurulent discharge after a few days. This does not indicate bacterial infection. Sneezing, nasal obstruction, systemic features such as malaise and low-grade fever, and cough are common. Generally the duration is about seven days.

Persistence of mucopurulent nasal discharge without improvement for longer than 10–14 days or more severe acute symptoms, such as high fever, headache, facial pain and/or swelling are more indicative of bacterial sinusitis.

Persistent clear nasal discharge is more likely due to perennial allergic rhinitis. This may be associated with sneeze, and itchy eyes and/or nose. Unilateral nasal discharge, particularly offensive, is suggestive of a nasal foreign body.

EXAMINATION

In rhinosinusitis, nasal discharge is the usual finding. This may be clear or mucopurulent and, as already discussed, is not indicative of cause. A red throat is a common association. In allergic rhinitis, the nasal mucosa will be pale and swollen. Facial swelling, such as orbital/peri-orbital and/or facial tenderness may occur in sinusitis.

INVESTIGATIONS

Investigations are not indicated for the common cold. Rhinoviruses and coronaviruses make up about 60% of infections and are difficult to identify.

Sinusitis is also a clinical diagnosis. Radiological investigations for acute sinusitis are difficult to interpret, as similar findings may be found in the common cold or even asymptomatic children. Also, the sinuses of young children are poorly developed, with frontal and sphenoid sinuses not appearing till 5–6 years of age. Radiological investigations should be reserved for those cases with complications, such as intraorbital or intracranial, or possibly in recurrent cases.

If aspirated under general anaesthesia, sinusitis fluid most commonly cultures *Pneumococcus*, followed by *Haemophilus influenzae*, *Moraxella catarrhalis* and then viruses. Nasopharyngeal cultures are not predictive and therefore not useful.

TREATMENT

Antibiotics are not indicated for the common cold and have been shown neither to alter the course of the illness nor prevent the development of complications. Symptomatic treatment with antihistamines has been shown to reduce nasal secretions and sneezing. Perennial allergic rhinitis responds best to intranasal corticosteroids, but these are often not tolerated well by children.

Even in bacterial sinusitis, the majority of cases will resolve spontaneously. Nasal decongestants may provide some short-term relief. If antibiotics are used, amoxicillin is recommended as first-line treatment for 10–14 days duration. Amoxicillin + clavulinate can be kept for those cases failing to respond in 48–72 hours.

COMPLICATIONS

Bacterial complications of the common cold do occur, such as otitis media, but cannot be prevented by antibiotic use.

Asthma is frequently precipitated by upper respiratory tract infections.

Ethmoid sinusitis can spread to cause orbital cellulitis or intracranially, causing an abscess or cavernous sinus thrombosis.

PREVENTION

Breast-feeding has a protective effect on the number of upper respiratory tract infections experienced by young children. Day care attendance and environmental tobacco exposure increase the number of episodes.

EPISTAXIS

INTRODUCTION

Although epistaxis is common in childhood (affecting about 6–9%), it is usually mild and usually does not require any medical intervention, let alone presentation to an ED.

HISTORY

If epistaxis presents for medical assessment, is usually recurrent and occasionally severe. When recurrent, it can be very frequent. It occurs at any age, during both day and night.

EXAMINATION

Bleeding can be unilateral or bilateral. Crusting and vessels in Little's area are commonly seen.

INVESTIGATIONS

Investigation for bleeding disorders is frequently performed. However, the vast majority of these will be normal unless there is other indications of bleeding tendency or family history. A more severe history of epistaxis, with frequent bleeds of greater volume and duration, is more suggestive of a bleeding disorder such as Von Willebrand disease and warrants appropriate testing.

TREATMENT

First aid treatment of epistaxis is firm compression of the alar nasae, thereby applying pressure over Little's area. This will result in cessation of bleeding in the majority of cases. For both primary and recurrent epistaxis, nasal antiseptic cream is equally effective as nasal cautery and easier to use. Nasal packing or other more major intervention is rarely required in children, but may be indicated along with urgent ENT referral for severe acute epistaxis.

COMPLICATIONS

Rarely, recurrent epistaxis is sufficient to cause anaemia.

NASAL TRAUMA

INTRODUCTION

Nasal trauma is common in children and the nasal bone is the most commonly fractured bone in the human body. It can occur at any age, but is most frequent in early primary-age groups. Like most injuries there is a male predominance.

HISTORY AND EXAMINATION

The most common mechanism of injury is falls, usually at home, followed by sports injuries. Fights are a not infrequent cause of nasal injury. Child abuse (inflicted injury) should be considered, particularly in the younger (non-mobile) child. A careful history is therefore required.

The types of injury are varied, from abrasions and lacerations of the soft tissues to skeletal injuries – fractures, dislocations and cartilage damage. More than minor epistaxis is unusual. Due to swelling it is often difficult to make a thorough assessment of the extent of injury in the acute setting – particularly for deformity. Examination must include an examination of the nasal cavities. Deviation, swelling and/or discolouration of the nasal septum may indicate a septal haematoma and urgent ENT consultation for evacuation is indicated.

Unco-operative children may require an anaesthetic for adequate assessment.

INVESTIGATIONS

Radiological evaluation is rarely of assistance and is generally only proposed for medicolegal reasons.

TREATMENT

Most nasal injuries require no intervention beyond analgesia. However, follow-up is essential, to determine the extent of deformity. The timing of this is recommended to be about 3–4 days post-injury, as the swelling has usually resolved by then, and, if required, earlier treatment instituted.

COMPLICATIONS

Septal haematoma, ± abscess formation, is the main complication that causes long-term damage and therefore concern. It

CONTROVERSIES

EPISTAXIS

❶ The choice of which children to test and extent of investigation for bleeding disorders is still uncertain. Although for the severe recurrent cases, thorough coagulation testing, including for Von Willebrand disease, would appear appropriate.

NASAL TRAUMA

❶ Open rhinoplasty for nasal deformities may affect nasal growth in itself and should be used as conservatively as possible.

may present later down the track and may have been missed on earlier assessment. Haematomas can be very painful and frequently causes nasal obstruction. On its own, a septal haematoma can cause nasal cartilage damage, including aseptic necrosis. However, the development of an abscess is almost always associated with cartilage damage and potentially severe nasal deformity. *Staphylococcus aureus*, *Streptococcus pneumoniae* and *S. pyogenes* have all been cultured. Meningitis or cavernous sinus thrombosis may also complicate a septal abscess.

FURTHER READING

Canty PA, Berkowitz RG 1996 Hematoma and abscess of the nasal septum in children. Archives of Otolaryngology Head & Neck Surgery 122(12): 1373–1376

Crockett DM, Mungo RP, Thompson RE 1989 Maxillofacial trauma. Paediatric Clinics of North America 36(6): 1471–1494

East CA, O'Donaghue G 1987 Acute nasal trauma in children. Journal of Paediatric Surgery 22(4): 308–310

Ghosh A, Jackson R 2001 Towards evidence based emergency medicine: Best BETs from the Manchester Royal Infirmary. Cautery or cream for epistaxis in children. Emergency Medicine Journal 18(3): 210

Ginsburg CM 1998 Nasal septal hematoma. Paediatrics in Review 19(4): 142–143

Katsanis E et al 1988 Prevalence and significance of mild bleeding disorders in children with recurrent epistaxis. Journal of Paediatrics 113(11): 73–76

Makura ZG, Porter GC, McCormick MS 2002 Paediatric epistaxis: Alder Hey experience. Journal of Laryngology & Otology 116(11): 903–906

Nyquist A-C et al 1998 Antibiotic prescribing for children with colds, upper respiratory tract infections, and bronchitis. Journal American Medical Association 279(11): 875–877

O'Brien KL et al 1998 Acute sinusitis—Principles of judicious use of antimicrobial agents. Paediatrics 101(1): 174–177

Rosenstein N et al 1998 The common cold—Principles of judicious use of antimicrobial agents. Paediatrics 101(1): 181–184

Ruddy J et al 1991 Management of epistaxis in children. International Journal of Paediatric Otorhinolaryngology 21(2): 139–142

14.3 THE MOUTH AND THROAT

GERVASE CHANEY • RICHARD WIDMER

ESSENTIALS

Stomatitis

1 Acute herpetic gingivostomatitis is the most common cause of stomatitis in young children.

2 Early treatment with aciclovir is effective if commenced in the first 72 hours.

3 Aphthous stomatitis or ulcers are more common in young adults, but do occur in children.

Pharyngitis/tonsillitis

1 Most sore throats in children are due to viral infections.

2 Throat-swab culture ± antigen detection can be used to confirm Group A streptococcal infection and the need for antibiotics.

3 Ten days of penicillin is the recommended course of treatment for bacterial infection.

Peritonsillar abscess

1 Peritonsillar abscess is the most common abscess of the head and neck.

2 Diagnosis is not always straightforward.

3 Management is analgesia, antibiotics, fluids and draining the abscess.

Post-tonsillectomy haemorrhage

1 Tonsillectomy remains a relatively common procedure.

2 Post-tonsillectomy bleeding occurs in about 1.5% and although most may be managed conservatively, for some, transfusion and/or surgery are necessary.

Oral/dental trauma

1 Oral/dental trauma is common in children.

2 A careful examination of the orofacial structures is required.

3 Dental consultation is indicated for all but the minor cases.

Oral/dental infection

1 Dental infections are the most common cause of facial cellulitis.

2 There are usually underlying dental caries and tooth extraction is often required.

STOMATITIS

INTRODUCTION

Acute herpetic gingivostomatitis is the most common cause of stomatitis in young children (1–3 years). It is also the most common clinical presentation of primary herpes simplex infection in young chil-dren. It can also occur in older children and adults. Untreated, the course of the illness is 10–14 days. Aphthous ulcers usually occur as single ulcers and are often recurrent.

HISTORY

Acute herpetic gingivostomatitis may pre-sent suddenly or insidiously – initially with fever and irritability. Mouth pain, often severe, plus drooling and refusal to eat will usually follow. Dehydration can occur if the child refuses to drink. Gingival bleeding can occur

Aphthous ulcers present as recurrent painful lesions of the oral mucosa, usually single and less than 1 cm diameter.

397

EXAMINATION

Early herpetic lesions are vesicles, but usually not seen, due to early rupture. Multiple ulcers up to 1 cm then occur on any part of the oral mucosa and initially are covered with a yellow-grey membrane. Associated gingivitis is usual.

INVESTIGATIONS

Viral swabs and immunofluorescence or viral culture for herpes simplex can confirm the diagnosis if required. However, if this is not readily available, clinical diagnosis is reasonably accurate.

For recurrent aphthous ulcers, checking a neutrophil count to exclude cyclical neutropenia is appropriate.

DIFFERENTIAL DIAGNOSIS

Initially presentation is non-specific and can be confused with a general viral infection. If the tonsils are involved early, acute tonsillitis or herpangina may be diagnosed. Oral candidiasis is often suspected.

Aphthous ulcers are easily distinguished, as these are usually single. Recurrent aphthous ulcers can be seen in cyclical or congenital neutropenia and PFAPA syndrome (fever, malaise, aphthous stomatitis, tonsillitis, pharyngitis and cervical adenopathy).

TREATMENT

Traditional treatment has been symptomatic, in the form of analgesia and hydration. Analgesia usually requires a combination of topical anaesthetic agents and oral analgesics, such as paracetamol or ibuprofen. Topical lidocaine gel can be very effective. Rehydration may require the use of nasogastric or intravenous fluids.

Recent studies, including a placebo-controlled study, have demonstrated the efficacy of oral aciclovir, if commenced in the first 72 hours of the illness. They have shown a significant reduction in duration of fever, feeding and drinking

difficulties and viral shedding. A dose of 15 mg kg^{-1} per dose (up to 200 mg) five times a day for five to seven days is recommended.

Aphthous ulcers with an adherent/dental base can be treated with topical corticosteroids (e.g. triamcinolone).

COMPLICATIONS

Acute dehydration has been mentioned. Secondary bacterial infection is uncommon. Primary herpetic infection may progress to generalised vesicular eruption. Also, autoinoculation can occur, particularly to the eye.

Recurrent labial herpes is common and more of an inconvenience. It occurs following exposure to sunlight, stress, trauma or cold. Topical aciclovir may be of use, when applied with the first evidence of symptoms.

PHARYNGITIS/TONSILLITIS

INTRODUCTION

Sore throat is an extremely common presentation and Group A streptococcal infection, makes up about 10–20% of cases. This is age dependent, increasing with age (infants < 1 year < 5%). The rest are largely viral infections. The concern over potential complications from streptococcal infection, such as rheumatic fever and glomerulonephritis, has led to many children being prescribed unnecessary antibiotics. Most people do not seek medical care for sore throats and the problem resolves spontaneously.

HISTORY

Older children will present with a complaint of sore throat, while younger children may be non-specifically unwell. A reluctance to take food or drinks may indicate a sore throat. Associated symptoms include fever, headache, vomiting and abdominal pain, but are not predictive whether bacterial or viral.

EXAMINATION

Ulcerative pharyngitis (herpangina) is a helpful finding indicating viral infection, such as coxsackie. Otherwise, it is difficult to differentiate between bacterial and viral causes. Features that suggest bacterial infection are tender cervical lymphadenopathy and absence of other symptoms such as coryza, cough, conjunctivitis and diarrhoea. Tonsillar exudate or pus is not an accurate predictor of bacterial infection and is frequently seen in viral causes such as infectious mononucleosis EBV and adenovirus. EBV infection may be suggested by the presence of more widespread lymphadenopathy, particularly if there is associated splenomegaly.

Scarlet fever is suggested by a widespread, fine, maculopapular rash with a sandpaper-like feel, with associated pharyngitis and possibly a 'strawberry-tongue'. Although the scarletiniform rash is highly specific for streptococcal infection, it only occurs in a minority of cases.

INVESTIGATIONS

In those being considered for antibiotics, accurate diagnosis does require laboratory confirmation. Culture of a throat swab is the recommended standard and in one study throat culture with treatment of only those positive for group-A β-haemolytic streptococcus (GABHS) was the most effective and least costly treatment option. Rapid antigen detection is available, but is not as sensitive and is more expensive. Most recommend doing culture as well.

Blood tests are usually done for investigation of infectious mononucleosis, although in children, the monospot/monotest has a high false negative rate and serology is more reliable.

TREATMENT

For the majority of sore throats, due to viral pharyngitis/tonsillitis, no antibiotics are necessary. Analgesia in the form of paracetamol or ibuprofen will provide symptomatic relief. For confirmed streptococcal pharyngitis, phenoxymethyl-penicillin (250 mg or 500 mg) twice daily for ten days is the recommended treatment with a cure rate of approximately 90%.

Antibiotics should be routine in groups at high risk of rheumatic fever, those with existing rheumatic heart disease and those with scarlet fever.

COMPLICATIONS

Complications from sore throats are uncommon. Suppurative complications of streptococcal infection include peritonsillar abscess, sinusitis and otitis media. The principle concerns, however, are with the non-suppurative complications: rheumatic fever and glomerulonephritis. Acute tonsillitis can cause airway obstruction, particularly with pre-existing tonsillar hypertrophy and may even warrant admission for monitoring.

PERITONSILLAR ABSCESS

INTRODUCTION

Peritonsillar abscess is the most common deep space head and neck infection in children. It is likely to be an extension of acute tonsillitis. However, it has been suggested that some cases may arise from obstruction and infection of Weber's glands (mucous glands located in the superior tonsillar pole). It can occur at any age.

HISTORY AND EXAMINATION

Presentation is usually with sore throat or neck pain, which is often severe. Odynophagia, dysphagia, and fever are also common. A muffled (or hot potato) voice and trismus occurs in about one-third of cases. Only a minority will have a prior history of tonsillitis (20–30%).

Examination findings include cervical lymphadenopathy, unilateral tonsillar erythema, bulging of the superior aspect of the tonsil and uvular deviation. The differential is peritonsillar cellulitis, where there is no abscess. Clinical differentiation between the two is difficult.

INVESTIGATIONS

The definitive investigation is needle aspiration, but not all children will be co-operative. CT scan or ultrasound may assist diagnosis. Microbiological identification of abscess contents probably does not alter management. If performed, the predominant organism found is *Streptococcus pyogenes*.

TREATMENT

Initial treatment is rehydration, analgesia and antibiotics (penicillin). Acute drainage is generally recommended, with either intra-oral drainage, abscess tonsillectomy or needle aspiration. Needle aspiration alone would appear to be effective in a majority of cases (>90%). Sedation or general anaesthesia may be required.

Abscess tonsillectomy should be reserved for recurrent tonsillitis abscess, but many of these can still be managed with aspiration and delayed tonsillectomy.

COMPLICATIONS

Dehydration is common and will require medical intervention. Uncommon, but dangerous, complications include infection spread, such as to the parapharyngeal space, airway obstruction and aspiration of pus causing pneumonia.

POST-TONSILLECTOMY HAEMORRHAGE

INTRODUCTION

Tonsillectomy remains a very commonly performed procedure. The most common complication of tonsillectomy is bleeding. Secondary (delayed) haemorrhage, which occurs after the first 24 hours following surgery, is the predominate group with rates of about 1.5% (up to 10%). The mean time of presentation is about seven days, with a range up to fifteen days. Rarely haemorrhage is catastrophic and life threatening.

HISTORY

Bleeding is usually obvious, although occasionally will be swallowed and not immediately apparent. Evidence of infection, such as a temperature, should be sought. A history of bleeding or bruising tendency should have been picked up prior to such surgery, but still should be inquired about. Also, whether coagulation testing has previously occurred.

EXAMINATION

Initial assessment is of a primary resuscitation type with pulse, capillary refill and blood pressure, to assess volume status. Examination of the tonsillar fauces for evidence of active bleeding is then important.

INVESTIGATIONS

Checking the patient's haemoglobin is routine, along with cross-matching blood. Coagulation profile testing rarely demonstrates abnormality, but is warranted in major haemorrhage.

TREATMENT

Immediate, preferably large-bore, intravenous access is indicated with cross-matching of blood and commencement of antibiotics (usually intravenous amoxicillin). Early involvement with of an ENT surgeon for children with active bleeding is indicated. Silver nitrate cautery can be attempted in the co-operative patient. Transfusions have been reported as being required in 10–12% of secondary haemorrhage. However, a more conservative approach is probably possible with use of other intravenous fluids and close monitoring. Surgical intervention under general anaesthesia is less frequently required according to a retrospective Australian study (4.3%).

COMPLICATIONS

Post-tonsillectomy bleeding is potentially life threatening, largely from hypovolaemic shock. Massive bleeding may also cause airway obstruction.

ORAL/DENTAL TRAUMA

INTRODUCTION

As with all emergencies, management of oral facial emergencies can be upsetting for both child and parent/carer. The prompt attention to orofacial injuries is valuable as it can significantly lessen the sequelae associated with, for example, altered jaw growth, extensive tooth loss and, damaged unaesthetic soft tissues.

The most common reasons why infants and children will present to the ED are orofacial injuries as a result of accidents (MVA, sports, animal bites, falls) or child abuse. However, other potentially serious, but uncommon, presentations can involve spontaneous oral bleeding and trauma from dental appliances, fixed or removable.

HISTORY

A thorough history is naturally valuable in treatment planning with particular emphasis on past or current dental treatment, where and how the accident occurred, and comments on any hard or soft tissues that have been damaged. In particular, any specific damage to teeth (fractured or avulsed) is essential. It would be prudent to investigate all hard and soft tissue injuries of the mouth with a dental consultation, unless obviously of a minor nature.

EXAMINATION

The physical examination should review all orofacial structures with careful scrutiny, digital palpation and observation of normal function. Externally and internally the orofacial region should exhibit consistent symmetry and any departure from this, be it an area of altered facial soft tissue architecture associated with a swelling or altered bony architecture associated with a fracture, will be important. For example chin point trauma is a common

injury associated with mandibular condylar fracture. Assessment of mandibular opening and closing is also vital. Beware of the likelihood of full-thickness soft tissue injuries, especially of the lips. Or, if a child has fallen while playing with an object held in their mouth (often a toothbrush!), it is essential to check the posterior palate for laceration.

The key points in recognition of a facial fracture are pain, facial swelling, stepping (of the bony border), limited jaw opening, palatal or sublingual haematoma, altered occlusion and paraesthesia. Tetanus prophylaxis needs to be considered and antibiotics prescribed. Usually (penicillin and metronidazole) should be given for a compound fracture in the mouth.

Often initial swelling of the lower lip, in particular, can hide the true nature of the through and through injury by everting the lower lip thus hiding the dermal injury and emphasising mucosal damage.

Intra-orally, the assessment includes checking of the occlusion and health of the teeth (fracture/avulsion) and gingivae/mucosa (contusions, lacerations, tears). Areas of haematosis, especially in the submental region and sublingual areas are strongly indicative of mandibular fracture, likewise conjunctival haemorrhage is very suggestive of maxillary fracture. As well, paraesthesia of the upper or lower lip can also be suggestive of similar fractures.

A common error when assessing a child's occlusion is to fail to recognise that an anterior open bite (associated with a prior digit or object sucking habits) is a normal anterior relationship for that child and not necessarily evidence of a fracture in the maxilla/mandible. Check the posterior teeth for appropriate occlusion in this situation. The child will usually be able to tell you if the teeth 'feel right' when they bite.

INVESTIGATIONS

The most relevant extra-oral radiograph is the orthopantomography (OPG). This radiograph will give an excellent view not only of the body of the mandible, the dento-alveolar area, but also of the temporomandibular joints. If a temporomandibular joint (TMJ) view is

specifically required it will be important to notify the radiographer. Other plain films that may be useful include lateral head films, PA skull films and occlusal films. Also, CT scans may be very useful.

TREATMENT

Management will obviously depend upon the exact diagnosis, which may include the following five factors:

1. Luxation

This is defined as a slight movement of the teeth as a result of trauma with or without associated gingival bleeding (luxation, subluxation). These injuries can occur in either the primary or permanent teeth and can be in any direction, i.e. intrusively, extrusively or laterally. Active intervention may or may not be needed depending on the extent of movement and interference with the occlusion. These sorts of injuries can be quite subtle and require a long-term follow-up as they can have consequences that manifest several years post injury, especially for the permanent teeth.

The appropriate treatment in luxation cases may include extraction of the damage tooth/teeth or repositioning of displaced teeth and placement of a dental splint with associated suturing of damaged soft tissues.

2. Avulsion

This is defined as the complete loss of a tooth, primary or permanent. In all situations, if there is any doubt about the nature of the tooth (that is whether it is primary or not) and given that permanent teeth are always reimplanted, it is prudent, as first-line advice to suggest that all avulsed teeth are placed in milk or an appropriate tissue-culture medium, if available. The appropriate tissue-culture medium is Hanks balanced salt solution. This can be kept frozen in the ED in a small vial. It will provide up to twelve hours' working time before replanting the avulsed tooth is necessary. It is important not to store the tooth in water. If milk or tissue-culture medium is not available it is crucial to keep to the tooth moist by wrapping it in a clingfilm or a gauze that is kept moist with saline or the patient's saliva. As a general rule the primary teeth are not reimplanted. Reasons include the potential damage to the developing permanent teeth, difficulties in securing the tooth/teeth in place and the level of co-operation that is required.

Ideally, avulsed permanent teeth should be repositioned/reimplanted in the tooth socket as soon as possible. It is crucial not to handle the root of the tooth. Manipulate using the crown only. This avoids damage to the periodontal ligament cells, which line the root surface and are critical in re-establishing the tooth back in the mouth as a functioning unit. Once reimplanted, avulsed teeth need to be splinted in place. Temporary splints can include moulded aluminium foil around the teeth or a fishing line and super glue. It will be crucial to stress dental follow up to try and avoid the sequelae that lead to tooth loss.

3. Root factures

The root of the tooth, which is buried in the alveolar bone can also be fractured, often with minimal damage to the crown of the teeth. This may present at review, if not initially obvious. A particularly mobile or loose tooth/teeth, that is/are slightly extruded are classic signs of associated root fractures.

4. Hard tissue injuries

This involves a chip off the tooth, whether it is just enamel or involves the deeper layers – such as the dentine. It may involve all three layers of the tooth and 'expose' the dental pulp. If a tooth is exposed then it is important that the exposure is treated immediately so as to preserve the vitality of the dental pulp and thus enable the root to grow to its full length and thickness. This is very important for the tooth's long-term maintenance as a useful member of the dentition. It is important to locate any missing tooth fragments as these may have been ingested/inhaled or lodged in soft tissues. Usually the fragments are ingested or lost externally rather than inhaled but it is important to locate all missing tooth fragments or teeth. It would also be important to check tetanus status and place the child on antibiotics if the wounds are significant.

5. Soft-tissue injuries

The soft tissues of the mouth involve the gingival tissues, mucosa and muscle. The soft tissue lacerations, especially of the gingival tissues need to be carefully assessed for degloving and may need to be repositioned and sutured. Where teeth are significantly displaced there will be associated displacement and laceration of soft tissue and it is very important for the long-term periodontal of the traumatised teeth that displaced soft tissues are adequately repositioned and sutured. Alveolar bone should not be left exposed to granulate over.

Other causes of soft tissue injuries include aphthous ulcers and traumatic ulcers associated with post-dental anaesthesia and children falling over with objects in their mouths. Aphthous ulcers are usually sited around the mouth in such places as the depth of the buccal sulcus at the reflection of the mucosa or on the palate. They can be described as major or minor depending on presentation. Treatment is symptomatic.

PREVENTION

Advice on prevention is never misplaced and recommendation of well-made and fitted mouth guards is encouraged.

ORAL/DENTAL INFECTION

INTRODUCTION

Dental infections are the most frequent cause of acute facial cellulitis, accounting for about 50% of all cases. Therefore, for children presenting with a facial swelling associated with raised temperature and general malaise, a dental cause must be high on the list of differentials.

HISTORY

Facial cellulitis will present as above, with facial redness and tenderness. The upper face is affected more frequently, particularly in younger children. The lower face is affected relatively more often in older children, probably related to caries patterns.

A history of previous dental contact is relevant in deciding on a dental cause for such swelling but is not exclusive for determining an odontogenic origin to the swelling.

EXAMINATION

A thorough examination, particularly intraorally is required and early dental involvement is very helpful in determining a dental source.

INVESTIGATIONS

Appropriate radiographs are frequently indicated to determine a dental aetiology. These may be extra-oral, e.g. an OPG, and/or intra-oral. If cultured, the most common organism is α-*Streptococcus*.

TREATMENT

The usual treatment involves the use of antibiotics (usually penicillin will be adequate) and repair or removal of the offending tooth/teeth. Metronidazole maybe added in cases of significant infection requiring hospitalisation.

PREVENTION

A significant cause of tooth decay in infants and young children is inappropriate feeding habits centring on the use of a night-time feeding bottle containing sweetened liquids, which end up causing extensive dental damage. Advice should be given to parents to go from breast to cup with their babies or to wean from the bottle by twelve months. Also, infants should not be put to bed with a bottle.

OTHER DENTAL ISSUES

SPONTANEOUS ORAL HAEMORRHAGE

Oral bleeding is still a very important sign for the diagnosis of underlying generalised bleeding disorders. It is important to determine the actual site of the bleeding and consequently a through oral examination will be required. Try to rinse the child's mouth with water or saline and use gauze to remove any blood clots and identify the source of the oral bleeding. In many instances this may be a tooth socket associated with a recent extraction. However, life-threatening disorders such as haemangiomas and arterio venous malformations will present with a history of oral bleeding.

If a tooth-extraction socket is identified as the cause of bleeding, local measures to control the bleeding would be as follows: first, firmly compress the alveolar bone between finger and thumb and then, second, apply pressure over the tooth socket with a tightly folded gauze pad (or tampon if nothing else is available) for at least fifteen minutes. Also topical thrombin may be placed on the pack to aid in haemostasis. In some situations, where a child is unco-operative, sedation/analgesia may be required. Other measures include placing resorbable gels into the socket and suturing/resuturing as appropriate with local anaesthetic containing adrenaline (epinephrine).

INTERMITTENT FACIAL/DENTAL PAIN

Dental pain is a relatively common presentation to the ED. Children who present suffering from spontaneous dental pain, especially at night, will usually require dental care. Such a presentation is indicative of untreated dental caries. Such pain can be very severe and consequently those who suffer it can be very difficult to manage without some form of sedation/anaesthesia. Tooth extraction is often required and is more frequent in younger children.

DENTAL APPLIANCES

Occasionally dental appliances can be a source of an acute presentation to EDs. A child may have damaged their appliance(s) such that wires or fractured edges of a denture base are traumatising the soft

CONTROVERSIES

PHARYNGITIS/TONSILLITIS

❶ Although antibiotics have a protective effect in the prevention of rheumatic fever, the evidence does not support a similar effect on prevention of glomerulonephritis.

TONSILLECTOMY

❶ Antibiotics post-tonsillectomy do lessen morbidity, in particular pain, analgesic use and delay in resumption of oral diet. Amoxicillin and amoxicillin + clavulinate have been shown to be effective. The studies have not had the numbers to demonstrate whether this is also true for post-tonsillectomy haemorrhage.

ORAL/DENTAL TRAUMA

❶ The management of avulsed permanent teeth centres on the prescription of routine antibiotics post-reimplantation in an effort to limit the unwanted side effects associated with reimplantation, such as an ankylosis of the teeth and inflammatory root resumption. This prescription of antibiotics is not universally accepted.

❷ The immediate deimpaction of the traumatically intruded permanent tooth/teeth using orthodontic appliances is proposed as the most appropriate care, especially when trying to limit the unwanted sequelae of poor alveolar bone height and gingival attachment. However, there is a school of thought that proposes to partially deimpact surgically, and then complete the job of realignment orthodontically.

ORAL/DENTAL INFECTION

❶ Antibiotic choice is not universally agreed in either delivery (oral vs. intravenous) or type (penicillin vs. cephalosporins).

tissues. Treatment will involve removal of the non-fixed appliances or cutting off the offending wire/s and initiating a dental follow-up.

FURTHER READING

Amir J et al 1997 Treatment of herpes simplex gingivostomatitis with aciclovir in children: A randomised double blind placebo controlled study. British Medical Journal 314(7097): 1800–1803 [comment]

Cmejrek RC, Coticchia JM, Arnold JE 2002 Presentation, diagnosis, and management of deep-neck abscesses in infants. Archives of Otolaryngology Head & Neck Surgery 128(12): 1361–1364

Dawes LC, Bova R, Carter P 2002 Retropharyngeal abscess in children. Australian and New Zealand Journal of Surgery 72(6): 417–420

Del Mar CB, Glasziou PP, Spinks AB 2000 Antibiotics for sore throat. Cochrane Database of Systematic Reviews 4 [update of Cochrane Database of Systematic Reviews 2: CD000023; PMID 10796471]

Delaney JE, Keels MA 2000 Paediatric oral pathology. Soft tissue and periodontal conditions. Paediatric Clinics of North America 47(5): 1125–1147

Edmond KM et al 1996 Streptococcal pharyngitis in a paediatric emergency department. Medical Journal of Australia 165(8): 420–423

Febres C, Echeverri EA, Keene HJ 1997 Parental awareness, habits, and social factors and their relationship to baby bottle tooth decay. Paediatric Dentistry 19(1): 22–27

Gianoli GJ et al 1991 Retropharyngeal space infection: Changing trends. Otolaryngology Head & Neck Surgery 105(1): 92–100

Goldenberg D, Golz A, Joachims HZ 1997 Retropharyngeal abscess: A clinical review. Journal of Laryngology & Otology 111(6): 546–550

Graham DB, Webb MD, Seale NS 2000 Paediatric emergency room visits for nontraumatic dental disease. Paediatric Dentistry 22(2): 134–140

Herzon FS, Nicklaus P 1996 Paediatric peritonsillar abscess: Management guidelines. Current Problems in Paediatrics 26(8): 270–278

Irani DB, Berkowitz RG 1997 Management of secondary hemorrhage following paediatric adenotonsillectomy. International Journal of Paediatric Otorhinolaryngology 40(2–3): 115–124

Myssiorek D, Alvi A 1996 Post-tonsillectomy hemorrhage: An assessment of risk factors. International Journal of Paediatric Otorhinolaryngology 37(1): 35–43

Nussinovitch M et al 1999 Group A beta-hemolytic streptococcal pharyngitis in preschool children aged 3 months to 5 years. Clinical Paediatrics 38(6): 357–360

Ripa LW 1988 Nursing caries: A comprehensive review. Paediatric Dentistry 10(4): 268–282

Schraff S, McGinn JD, Derkay CS 2001 Peritonsillar abscess in children: A 10-year review of diagnosis and management. International Journal of Paediatric Otorhinolaryngology 57(3): 213–218

Schwartz B et al 1998 Pharyngitis: Principles of judicious use of antimicrobial agents. Paediatrics 101(1): 171–174

Schwartz SS, Rosivack RG, Michelotti P 1993 A child's sleeping habit as a cause of nursing caries. Journal of Dentistry for Children 60(1): 22–25

Sharma HS, Kurl DN, Hamzah M 1998 Retropharyngeal abscess: Recent trends. Auris, Nasus, Larynx 25(4): 403–406

Spruance SL et al 2002 Acyclovir cream for treatment of herpes simplex labialis: Results of two randomized, double-blind, vehicle-controlled, multicenter clinical trials. Antimicrobial Agents & Chemotherapy 46(7): 2238–2243

Tsevat J, Kotagal UR 1999 Management of sore throats in children: A cost-effectiveness analysis. Archives of Paediatrics & Adolescent Medicine 153(7): 681–688 [comment]

Unkel JH et al 1997 Comparison of odontogenic and nonodontogenic facial cellulitis in a paediatric hospital population. Paediatric Dentistry 19(8): 476–479

van Everdingen T, Eijkman MA, Hoogstraten J 1996 Parents and nursing-bottle caries. Journal of Dentistry for Children 63(4): 271–274

Wilson S et al 1997 Nontraumatic dental emergencies in a paediatric emergency department. Clinical Paediatrics 36(6): 333–337

Windfuhr JP, Chen YS 2001 Hemorrhage following paediatric tonsillectomy before puberty. International Journal of Paediatric Otorhinolaryngology 58(3): 197–204

14.4 RETROPHARYNGEAL ABSCESS

JAMES TILLEARD

ESSENTIALS

1 The potential for airway compromise and other complications necessitates early diagnosis and treatment.

2 Retropharyngeal abscess should be suspected in children with neck pain, fever, dysphagia, neck swelling or torticollis.

3 The differential diagnosis of meningitis should be considered in the unwell febrile child with neck pain.

4 Antibiotics must be initiated early.

5 Patients should be managed in an institution with appropriate paediatric medical surgical anaesthetic and intensive-care facilities.

INTRODUCTION

Retropharyngeal abscess is an uncommon condition with the potential for significant complications including airway compromise. A retrospective analysis at the Sydney Children's Hospital over a twelve-year period treated only 21 cases. The median age in this study was three years and three months with 86% of patients less than six years old.

Incidence in the developed world may be reduced by early use of antibiotics. The aetiology of retropharyngeal abscess in the paediatric population is usually secondary to upper respiratory tract infection and suppuration in retropharyngeal lymph nodes. Other causes more common in adults include infection following trauma, foreign body and dental problems.

HISTORY

Children with retropharyngeal abscess may present with a history of recent upper respiratory tract infection, fever, neck pain, sore throat, dysphagia, poor oral intake, trauma or other infective focus of the head and neck. In one study symptoms were present for a median of five days with 48% of cases presenting within three days and none after fourteen days.

EXAMINATIONS

Examination may reveal fever, a neck mass, lymphadenopathy, limitation of neck extension, torticollis, or displacement of the pharyngeal wall. There may be evidence of complications including respiratory compromise, dehydration or spread of infection.

INVESTIGATIONS

CT scanning is the investigation of choice. It is essential to ensure the patient is stable and safe for this procedure, especially the airway. Lateral soft tissue neck X-ray may reveal pervertibial swelling, gas, foreign body, air fluid level or bony erosion. Although MRI may give excellent soft-tissue resolution, it is not the suggested initial investigation due to greater time, expense, patient isolation and restricted availability. Ultrasound may be used but will not provide anatomical detail.

Laboratory studies typically reveal elevated white blood cell counts. Microbiology specimens, including blood cultures and pus at the time of surgery, are important in guiding subsequent antibiotic therapy. Common aetiological organisms include streptococci, staphylococci and Gram-negative organisms. Polymicrobial infection also occurs.

TREATMENT

The initial priority in treatment is to ensure an adequate and stable airway. If intubation is needed difficulty should be expected and planned for – although it is not usually required. If appropriate, intubation may best be performed in the operating theatre with surgical and anaesthetic assistance.

Once resuscitation is complete, antibiotics must be commenced as soon as possible. Initial cover must include streptococci, staphylococci and Gram-negative organisms. A recommended regimen includes a third-generation cephalosporin, flucloxacillin and metronidazole. Clindamycin is another option. Attention must also be given to fluid and metabolic resuscitation. Adequate analgesia is essential. Complications should be excluded and these include airway compromise, septic shock, aspiration, mediastinitis, vascular involvement including thrombosis, neurological involvement, septic emboli and osteomyelitis.

CONTROVERSIES AND FUTURE DIRECTIONS

❶ Current debate centres on the need for surgery or initial medical treatment with antibiotics and close observation.

FURTHER READING

Cmejrek RC, Coticchia JM, Arnold JE 2002 Presentation, diagnosis and management of deep-neck abscesses in infants. Archives of Otolaryngology-Head and Neck Surgery 128(12): 1361–1364

Craig FW, Schunk JE 2003 Retropharyngeal abscess in children: Clinical presentation, utility of imaging and current management. Paediatrics 111(6): 1394–1398

Gianoli GJ, Espinola TE, Guarisco JL, Miller RH 1991 Retropharyngeal space infection: Changing trends.

Otolaryngology-Head and Neck Surgery 105: 92–100

Goldenberg D, Goltz A, Joachims HZ 1997 Retropharyngeal abscess: A clinical review. Journal of Laryngology Otology 111: 546–550

Dawes LC, Bova R, Carter P 2002 Retropharyngeal abscess in children. ANZ Journal of Surgery 72(6):417

Sharma HS, Kurl DN, Hamzah M 1998 Retropharyngeal abscess: Recent trends. Auris, Nasus, Larynx 25: 403–406

14.5 FOREIGN BODIES AND CAUSTIC INGESTION

GERVASE CHANEY

ESSENTIALS

Nasal foreign bodies

1 Foreign body removal from the nasal passage requires good preparation and lighting.

2 The appropriate method of removal depends upon the type of object and its location.

Aural foreign bodies

1 Foreign bodies in the medial two-thirds of the ear canal are difficult to remove and frequently require general anaesthesia and ENT removal.

Caustic ingestion

1 Caustic ingestion is usually accidental in children.

2 The children are often asymptomatic and not at risk of complications such as stricture.

3 Airway management is the priority in resuscitation.

4 There is no proven treatment to prevent stricture formation.

NASAL FOREIGN BODIES

INTRODUCTION

Nasal foreign bodies are a relatively common presentation to a paediatric ED, although there is little published literature on the subject. They are not life threatening, but can cause significant morbidity.

HISTORY

Nasal foreign bodies predominately present in children from two to five years of age. Children with nasal foreign bodies are usually brought in within 24 hours of insertion/impaction. Delayed presentation is mostly with unilateral purulent nasal discharge, which is usually offensive. Other possible symptoms include foul breath, nasal pain, sneezing, snoring and mouth breathing.

EXAMINATION

The type of foreign body is extremely variable, although it is most commonly a plastic toy or bead. The foreign body is usually readily visible.

INVESTIGATIONS

Investigations are not usually required. Imaging is usually indicated for other possible causes such as tumour.

TREATMENT

Except for button batteries (see also Chapter 7.7), removal of the foreign body is not urgent and appropriate preparation should take place first. Most foreign bodies can be successfully removed in the ED. Prior to the attempted removal use of a topical anaesthetic nasal spray, such as lignocaine + phenylephrine, is recommended. Sedation and/or appropriate restraint of the child may be required. A good light source is essential.

The appropriate procedure for removal will depend upon the foreign body size, shape, consistency and location in the nares. These include:

- Right-angle hooked probes can be passed alongside and past larger objects, rotated and then drawn back gradually, removing the object.
- Forceps (alligator or bayonet) are useful for smaller objects near the anterior nares.
- Positive pressure ventilation using bag-valve-mask is effective particularly

for larger objects that occlude the nasal cavity. Air is expelled rapidly through the mouth while the unaffected nostril is occluded with a finger. There is an unreported theoretical risk of barotrauma.

- Suction catheters can be used. Generally a soft, pliable end is required, and this can be made up using soft tubing, although commercially available kits are now available.
- A balloon catheter can be used if passed beyond the foreign body, inflated and drawn back.
- Application of cyanoacrylate glue via a wooden swab stick or similar is described, but requires patience and a very steady hand. It may adhere to the mucosa.

General anaesthesia and removal by ENT staff is required for the failed removal and the unco-operative child.

COMPLICATIONS

Possible complications include epistaxis, local and more widespread infection. Uncommonly, septal perforation has occurred secondary to a button battery. Mucosal injury may occur within hours.

AURAL FOREIGN BODIES

INTRODUCTION

Aural foreign bodies in children are also a relatively common presentation to EDs. Again morbidity can be significant.

HISTORY

A greater proportion of children present beyond 24 hours from insertion compared with nasal foreign bodies and in many cases the time frame may not be determined. It may be a result of the event being witnessed, reported by the child due to irritation or pain, or as an incidental finding. The object may have been placed due to existing ear canal

irritation due to wax impaction or otitis. Live insects are a common finding, and may result in marked discomfort.

EXAMINATION

Visualisation of the foreign body is usually by otoscopy. The type and location of the object has a significant role in the difficulty of removal.

INVESTIGATIONS

Investigations are not indicated.

TREATMENT

Removal of foreign bodies from the lateral one-third of the external auditory canal is much easier and more successful than from the medial two-thirds. The latter is the osseous portion and is narrower, more vascular and very tender. Therefore removal is more likely to require general anaesthesia and ENT expertise.

- Appropriate, restraint of the child and a good light source are always necessary.
- Sedation may have a role in some children.
- Choice of method of removal will depend upon the object and its location:
- Irrigation is the simplest method, but is contraindicated if there is a tympanic perforation, or for soft objects or vegetable matter that may swell.
- Suction via a small catheter.
- Forceps – alligator, Hartmann.
- A right-angled hook passed beyond the object and pulled out.

Button batteries are again a risk (see also Chapter 7.7), causing necrosis of the ear canal or tympanic membrane and should be removed as soon as possible. A live insect should be killed or immobilised with microscopic immersion oil, mineral oil or local anaesthetic solutions (2% lidocaine). It can then be removed using irrigation or forceps. Putty is often very difficult to remove and may require otomicroscopic removal. Sharp objects

also usually require ENT removal.

Failure to remove in the ED will require ENT referral. Inspection following removal is advised to ensure there is no persisting foreign body and to assess for trauma or inflammation. Aural antibiotic drops with steroid are often recommended, particularly if there is evidence of trauma or inflammation.

COMPLICATIONS

Trauma to the ear canal is common as a result of the foreign body and/or its removal. More seriously trauma to the tympanic membrane or ossicles can occur. Otitis externa can occur as a result of trauma.

CAUSTIC INGESTION

INTRODUCTION

Caustic ingestion in children is an uncommon presentation and significant injury with stricture formation is rare because the volume ingested is usually small. The ingested agents are variable and include alkalis (more common) and acids in liquid, granule or solid form. The likelihood of significant injury is dependent upon how alkali or acidic the agent is (i.e. its pH). Strong liquid alkali is particularly dangerous.

HISTORY

In children, in contrast to adults, ingestion is largely accidental and, as a result, significant injury far less common. Most cases occur in children less than three years of age and, like accidents in general, occur in boys more frequently than girls. Most ingestions occur at the home of the child. The most common alkali agent ingested is dishwasher detergent and commonest acidic agent is acetic acid. Button batteries have a significant corrosive and burn risk if lodged or impacted in the oesophagus (see Chapter 7.7).

Many children are asymptomatic. If they do occur, symptoms include vomiting, drooling, pain on swallowing and dysphagia, chest pain and refusal to drink. Less commonly, stridor may occur secondary to upper airway burns and obstruction.

In one series, the most predictive symptoms of significant injury and scar formation were prolonged drooling and dysphagia (100% sensitivity and 91% specificity). In another, haematemesis and respiratory distress were always associated with severe injury.

EXAMINATION

Many children will have normal examination findings, but oral burns may be demonstrated by inflammation, oedema or white areas. In at least half of these, that will be the limit of injury. Occasionally significant burns occur beyond an unaffected oral cavity.

INVESTIGATIONS

Chest X-ray has demonstrated pulmonary irritation in up to 13% in some series. However, there is evidence that radiological investigations have little impact upon management and therefore cannot be recommended routinely, except to localise a button battery.

Oesophagoscopy may be performed according to symptoms, particularly ongoing drooling and dysphagia, vomiting/haematemesis and stridor. The type of caustic substance, its form and pH should be considered.

TREATMENT

Resuscitation, involving airway and breathing management, is the priority in severely

affected cases. Upper airway obstruction may warrant intubation. However, there is a case report of successful use of nebulised adrenaline (epinephrine) for acute marked stridor following hypochlorite ingestion.

Dilution using water or milk may be useful for solid or granule ingestions. Children who remain asymptomatic may be discharged. Button batteries should be removed endoscopically followed by a period of observation.

There is no proven effective treatment for oesophageal burns, especially in the prevention of stricture development. Antibiotics and corticosteroids have been commonly used, but have not been shown to be of any value.

COMPLICATIONS

Stricture formation is rare and in a combination of nine series giving a total of 1961 children, who had caustic ingestions, occurred in only 3.2%. This was despite a mean incidence of oesophageal burns of 21.4% and of deep burns of 4.7%. Upper airway obstruction has been mentioned and is potentially life threatening.

PREVENTION

Labelling, formulation, and child-proof containers and caps, have proved effective in prevention, when legislated. Storage of strong caustics should be in locked cupboards or similar, and handling should occur out of the reach of children. More hazardous caustics are available in developing countries and severe injury occurs more frequently.

CONTROVERSIES

❶ In caustic ingestion, acute oesophagoscopy has been advocated as critical to the early diagnosis and management of burns. This may help assess severity of injury and likelihood of stricture formation. However, as there is no clearly effective treatment and stricture formation is uncommon, it is difficult to recommend this routinely.

FURTHER READING

Anderson KD, Rouse TM, Randolph JG 1990 A controlled trial of corticosteroids in children with corrosive injury of the esophagus. New England Journal of Medicine 323(10): 637–640 [comment]

Ansley JF, Cunningham MJ 1998 Treatment of aural foreign bodies in children. Pediatrics 101(4): 638–641

Christesen HB 1994 Epidemiology and prevention of caustic ingestion in children. Acta Paediatrica 83(2): 212–215

Cox RJ 2001 Foreign bodies, nose. eMedicine

de Jong AL et al 2001 Corrosive esophagitis in children: A 30-year review. International Journal of Pediatric Otorhinolaryngology 57(3): 203–211

Karnak I et al 1996 Pulmonary effects of household bleach ingestion in children. Clinical Pediatrics 35(9): 471–472

Kiristioglu I et al 1999 Is it necessary to perform an endoscopy after the ingestion of liquid household bleach in children? Acta Paediatrica 88(2): 233–234

Lamireau T et al 2001 Accidental caustic ingestion in children: Is endoscopy always mandatory? Journal of Pediatric Gastroenterology & Nutrition 33(1): 81–84

Lovejoy FH Jr, Woolf AD 1995 Corrosive ingestions. Pediatrics in Review 16(12): 473–474

Mantooth R 2001 Foreign bodies, ear. eMedicine

Nuutinen M et al 1994 Consequences of caustic ingestions in children. Acta Paediatrica 83(11): 1200–1205

Samad L, Ali M, Ramzi H 1999 Button battery ingestion: Hazards of esophageal impaction. Journal of Pediatric Surgery 34(10): 1527–1531

Tong MC, Ying SY, van Hasselt CA 1996 Nasal foreign bodies in children. International Journal of Pediatric Otorhinolaryngology 35(3): 207–211

Ziegler DS, Bent GP 2001 Upper airway obstruction induced by a caustic substance found responsive to nebulised adrenaline. Journal of Paediatrics & Child Health 37(5): 524–525

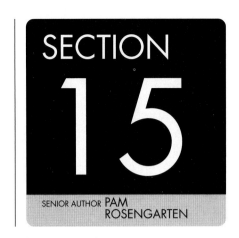

SENIOR AUTHOR PAM ROSENGARTEN

OBSTETRICS AND GYNAECOLOGY

15.1 PAEDIATRIC GYNAECOLOGY

PAM ROSENGARTEN • SHEILA BRYAN • SONIA GROVER

Essentials

Prepubescent girls

1 Vaginal examination is inappropriate in paediatric patients and usually provides little information. Ultrasound may provide further information or, if necessary, an examination under anaesthesia (EUA) is more appropriate.

2 Vulvovaginitis is the most common gynaecological problem in prepubertal girls and in most cases a specific infectious cause cannot be identified.

3 Vaginal bleeding in the prepubertal female is abnormal after 3–4 weeks of age.

Adolescents

1 Laboratory confirmation is required to make an accurate diagnosis of a vaginal discharge.

2 Pregnancy-related conditions need to be considered for all adolescents with pelvic pain or abnormal vaginal bleeding.

3 Abnormal vaginal bleeding may be secondary to an underlying haematological condition.

PREPUBESCENT GYNAECOLOGY

VAGINAL DISCHARGE

Introduction

Vaginal discharge in the prepubertal girl is abnormal except for two periods during development. In neonates a white mucoid vaginal discharge is present in most baby girls. This is normal and due to the effects of maternal oestrogens, it disappears by about three months of age. The second period where physiological discharge may occur is at the time of ovarian stimulation.

Other conditions that cause vaginal discharge in the prepubertal girl include vulvovaginitis, lichen sclerosis, foreign body, eczema and pinworms.

Vulvovaginitis

This is the most common gynaecological problem in childhood, usually occurring in girls aged between two years and puberty.[1] Most vulvovaginitis in this age group is non-infectious in origin and results from irritation of the vaginal and vulval skin.[2] Factors that contribute to genital inflammation include the vaginal and vulval skin of children being thin and atrophic due to low oestrogens and therefore easily irritated. In addition, lack of protective labial hair and fat pads as well as moisture from tight fitting synthetic underwear or clothing, wet swimming costumes, obesity and poor hygiene may play a role.[2,3] Additionally, the presence of bowel flora, which is the normal flora in the atrophic vagina, may contribute to skin irritation.

Infectious vulvovaginitis is less common and is due to an overgrowth of one organism, for example Group A *Streptococcus, Staphylococcus, enterococci* and *Escherichia coli*. In this instance profuse discharge is usually present with marked skin inflammation often beyond the contact surfaces of the labia.[2] Isolation of an organism that has strong sexual transmission, such as *Neisseria gonorrhoeae* or *Chlamydia trachomatis* generally indicates sexual abuse or sexual activity and therefore warrants further investigation.[2,3]

Lichen sclerosis is an uncommon condition of unknown aetiology. It may present in childhood with vulval irritation, pruritus, dysuria or bleeding.[1] Examination reveals pale atrophic patches on the labia and perineum. The patches can be extensive and coalesce, and with scratching lead to chronic inflammation and purpuric haemorrhage into the skin. The condition usually persists with intermittent exacerbations. Most resolve before puberty although some may continue to have problems into adult life.[4]

Eczema is usually present elsewhere on the body and can be superimposed on the irritation due to the discharge.

Foreign bodies are a potential cause for a persistent, unresolving, often blood-stained offensive discharge.

Candida is very uncommon in the prepubertal girl unless there has been significant antibiotic use or they are still in nappies.[3] (Thrush thrives in an oestrogenised environment, not in the atrophic setting.) In this age group recurrent or unexplained candida should have diabetes mellitus or other causes of diminished immune function excluded.

History

The child or parent/care giver usually describe:

- An offensive vaginal discharge.
- Erythema (redness)/irritation of the labia and perineal skin.
- Itch, dysuria and urinary frequency may also be present.

A general medical history is required with specific history of the symptoms and their duration including nature of discharge as well as any previous treatments. Also important is past history of urinary tract infection, encopresis, constipation, enuresis, the presence of skin disorders, and any other illness including antibiotic use in the previous four weeks. Although a history of perineal hygiene (e.g. wipe front to back, frequency of bathing, type of underwear/clothes, specific irritants, such as bubble baths or use of feminine hygiene sprays in the adolescent population, etc.) should also be established, there is limited evidence to support the role of this in the pathogenesis of vulvovaginitis.[2] Where itch is the dominant symptom pinworms should be considered and questions asked about family symptoms.

Although uncommon, the possibility of sexual abuse should always be considered in a child that presents with genital symptoms, and check for other signs that may be present including alterations in behaviour such as phobias, eating or sleeping disorders.

EXAMINATION

A general examination including sexual development is required. Perineal, vulval and introital examination may be required for the above conditions. Attempts must be made to ensure it is not a traumatic event for the child. The perineum is best examined either with the girl supine with heels together and knees flexed and hips abducted or in the lateral position with knees drawn up to the chest.[5] Vaginal examination is inappropriate in paediatric patients and usually provides little further information. Specific external examination of the perineum usually reveals mucoid discharge and reddened introitus, particularly on the contact surfaces between the labia.

The presence of a profuse discharge or marked skin inflammation especially if it extends beyond the contact surfaces of the labia suggests an infectious cause. An offensive discharge can occur with vulvovaginitis or foreign body. A bloody discharge can occur with vulvovaginitis (particularly with *Shigella* or Group A streptococci).[5] The presence of perianal excoriation suggests pinworm.

Investigations

Swabs are generally not required. If taken in mild cases usually reveal a growth of mixed coliforms.[2] If discharge is visible or profuse or marked erythema is present, introital swabs should be taken for culture. Vaginal swabs are painful and distressing and are not required.

If urinary symptoms are present the urine (mid-stream urine; MSU) should be checked to exclude urinary tract infection. A pinworm test should be taken if itch is a prominent symptom. This requires briefly placing clear sellotape on the perianal skin in the morning and viewing under a microscope for eggs. Otherwise worms may be seen in the perianal region at night.

Ultrasound may provide further information, especially if there is a possibility of foreign body, or if necessary an EUA may be more appropriate.

Management

Vulvovaginitis

Management consists of:

❶ Explanation and reassurance.
❷ Toileting/hygiene advice:
  - Avoidance of potential irritants such as soaps and bubble baths and other causal factors, such as tight/synthetic clothing and wet bathers.
  - Vinegar (add one cup white vinegar in a shallow bath and soak) or the use of a simple barrier cream to the labial area (e.g. zinc-castor oil or nappy rash cream) or both.

Rarely, if the problem persists, further action may be required. The natural history of vulvovaginitis is for recurrences to occur up until the age when oestrogenisation begins. If a primary bacterial cause is suspected, cultures should be taken and treatment commenced with the appropriate antibiotics, e.g. initial amoxicillin, and adjusted when culture results are available.

Where itch is a dominant symptom consider:

- Pinworms, especially if perianal excoriation is present, and treat the child and their family with pyrantel 10 mg kg^{-1} (maximum 500 mg) orally or mebendazole 50 mg (< 10 kg), 100 mg (> 10 kg) orally (contraindicated in pregnancy and < 6 months of age) as a stat. dose and repeat two weeks later.[6]
- Lichen sclerosis in the asymptomatic patient does not require treatment other than reassurance. In symptomatic patients, avoidance of irritants, improved hygiene, reduced trauma and barrier ointments, e.g. nappy rash creams. In more severe cases a brief course of topical steroid (1% hydrocortisone) and referral to a dermatologist or paediatric gynaecologist is required.
- Eczema, especially if skin disease is present elsewhere. Combined treatment of the vulvovaginitis (as above) and hydrocortisone or diprosone may be indicated.

Foreign body

If foreign body is suspected then an examination under anaesthesia with vaginoscopy is usually required. If the presence of a foreign body is questionable then an ultrasound may be beneficial to visualise the object. The most common foreign bodies are tiny pieces of tissue paper. The possibility of sexual abuse should be borne in mind.

Candidiasis

Treatment is with conventional topical antifungal creams. (Vaginal pessaries should never be administered to this age group).

VAGINAL BLEEDING

Introduction

Vaginal bleeding in the prepubertal child is abnormal after 3–4 weeks of age.[5]

Causes of vaginal bleeding in the prepubertal girl can be classed as hormonal and non-hormonal.

Hormonal causes

Neonates A withdrawal bleed from maternal oestrogens is common and does not require investigation or treatment. This will cease after approximately four weeks of age.[5]

Onset of menstruation Consider as premature (precocious puberty) if this occurs at less than eight years of age.[6]

Non-hormonal causes

Vulvovaginitis In prepubescent girls, vaginal bleeding in this age group is most commonly due to more severe vulvovaginitis (the most common pathogens are *Shigella* or Group A β-haemolytic streptococci).[5] The discharge is brown and often offensive (see above under vaginal discharge, vulvovaginitis).

Trauma Accidental injury usually results from straddle injuries where the girl falls on a narrow object (e.g. bicycle cross bar, jungle gym). Non-accidental injury/sexual abuse should be considered in trauma, especially where there is a hymenal tear without a history of accidental penetrating injury.

Foreign body Vaginal foreign body may also result in blood-stained discharge and should be considered if no infectious cause is identified or there is failure to respond to appropriate treatment. In bleeding secondary to excoriation from pinworms, lichen sclerosis or eczema, examination should demonstrate eczema and lichen sclerosis. The presence of anal and perineal excoriation suggests pinworms and treatment as previously described under vulvovaginitis.

Tumours Although rare, the possibility of a genital tumour should be considered when there is chronic genital ulceration, non-traumatic swelling, tissue protruding from the vagina or foul smelling, bloody, vaginal discharge . Vaginal bleeding associated with genital enlargement, premature sexual maturation or virilisation may be associated with hormonally active ovarian or adrenal tumour.

Non-vaginal causes of bleeding

Haematuria may stain the underwear or nappy and be reported as vaginal bleeding. This will become evident upon urinalysis. Urethral prolapse often presents with bleeding thought to be vaginal in origin. The peak age is five to eight years. Bleeding disorders are an uncommon cause of vaginal bleeding but should be considered when there are other systemic signs of a bleeding tendency, e.g. bruising and petechiae.

History

A general medical history including family and past history should be taken.

The history of vaginal bleeding should focus on the amount and circumstances of bleeding, the times of recurrences and the presence of associated pain. A history

regarding any perineal trauma should be elicited as well as the possibility of a foreign body. Other medical disorders and symptoms of blood dyscrasias, such as epistaxis and bruising should also noted.

Examination

Vital signs and haemodynamic stability should be established. General examination, including sexual development should be performed. On examination excessive bruising or petechiae and generalised skin disorders, such as eczema, should be noted.

Specific examination requires abdominal and vulval/perineal examination. Abdominal examination should note abdominal tenderness and the presence of a mass. Perineal examination should note the presence of vulvovaginitis, other skin disorders, such as eczema, or traumatic injury.

The common perineal injuries in trauma are bruising/haematoma of vulva and periclitoral folds and superficial lacerations of the labia minora and periurethral tissue. If a hymenal tear is present, a history of penetrating injury, e.g. broom handle or bed post should be sought. If there is no history of penetrating trauma then sexual abuse needs to be considered.

A foreign body in the vagina may be evident on examination of the perineum.

A urethral prolapse will be evident on examination of the perineum as a friable, red-blue (doughnut-shaped) annular mass.

Investigations

Bloods – full blood examination should be performed if the child appears clinically anaemic or bleeding has been prolonged. Coagulation studies may be indicated. Perineal swabs should be taken for microscopy and culture where there is evidence of severe vulvovaginitis.

In trauma, where there is a history of penetrating injury or where it is not possible to perform adequate perineal examination an examination under anaesthesia is required. Mid-stream urine for micro and culture should also be performed where haematuria is present.

In the child less than eight years of age who has signs of puberty evident referral to a paediatric endocrinologist or gynaecologist is required.

Management

Trauma

A warm bath several times a day to help voiding as well as assist in keeping the perineum clean is all that is required. The girl may be may find voiding in a bath more comfortable. Antibiotics are rarely required. Examination under anaesthesia is only required if there is persistent bleeding, uncertain origin of bleeding, massive bruising or history of a fall on a potentially penetrating object.

Urethral prolapse

The management is conservative as long as voiding is normal. Warm baths may be of assistance. Suspected sexual abuse must be referred.

Labial adhesions

Labial adhesions are seen in infancy, and usually resolve by about eight years, although they may occasionally persist through to puberty when they will resolve by the time of menarche. The adhesion is not congenital, but it is acquired from a secondary adherence of the atrophic surfaces of the labia minora, presumably as a result of irritation.[1]

Labial adhesions are usually asymptomatic in children and do not need to be divided as long as the child is able to void. When symptoms occur they usually relate to difficulty with urination or pooling of urine behind fused labia, which results in irritation.[1,4] Urinary tract infections are seldom a complication.[4] Parents should be reassured that separation of the labia will occur when oestrogenisation commences as the child grows. Although it is possible to divide the adhesions with lateral traction this is frequently distressing for the child and the parents, and unnecessary. There is a considerable recurrence rate after this approach.[4]

The use of topical oestrogen cream is likewise unnecessary, and is associated with significant failure and recurrence rates, but may occasionally be indicated when catheterisation is required for a micturating cystoureterogram.

Associated nappy rash or vulvovaginitis is managed as described above.

ADOLESCENT GYNAECOLOGY

VAGINAL DISCHARGE

Introduction

Vaginal discharge in an adolescent female may be physiological, a symptom of vaginal or cervical infection or secondary to a vaginal foreign body. Under the influence of oestrogen there is an increase in the glycogen production by the vaginal epithelial cells, which supports the growth of lactobacilli in the vagina, which leads to lowering of the vaginal pH to 3.8–4.5. The acidic environment helps to inhibit the growth of bacteria seen in the prepubertal female. Oestrogen also influences the cervix resulting in increased mucous production, which is largely responsible for the physiological vaginal discharge.[7]

Vaginal infections include candidiasis, bacterial vaginosis and trichomoniasis, with only the latter being sexually transmitted. Chlamydia and gonorrhoea are sexually transmitted infections of the cervix and/or the upper genital tract, which may also result in a vaginal discharge.

HISTORY

Diagnosis can often be suspected from the history and the appearance of the discharge.

- *Candida* infections typically present as a cheesy white discharge and are associated with vulval and vaginal itching, dysuria or superficial dyspareunia in sexually active girls. They are commonly associated with antibiotic use, stress and diabetes mellitus.
- Bacterial vaginosis generally presents as a homogenous white discharge associated with a fishy odour.

Symptoms of vaginal irritation are uncommon.
- Trichomoniasis is a sexually transmitted infection (STI) and typically presents with a frothy, green vaginal discharge.
- *Chlamydia* and gonorrhoea infections may present as vaginal discharge, intermenstrual or post-coital bleeding, urethritis or pelvic inflammatory disease (PID). *Chlamydia* and gonorrhoea may also be identified incidentally due to the high incidence of asymptomatic infections. The presence of lower abdominal pain and/or dyspareunia in the history increases the likelihood of PID with a positive and negative predicative value of 17% and 100% respectively.[8] STIs may be contracted by oral or digital contact and do not necessarily require penetrative intercourse for transmission.
- The most common vaginal foreign body in adolescent girls is a retained tampon. The presenting symptom is often a malodorous discharge.

Examination

Inspection of the external genitalia should be performed specifically looking for evidence of warts, herpetic lesions, the nature of the discharge and evidence of excoriation.

Adolescent girls who have never been sexually active and/or who have not used tampons should not be examined internally. If there is a suspicion of a vaginal foreign body, vaginal trauma or PID in a girl who is sexually active or uses tampons a gentle vaginal examination may be considered. However, even sexually experienced girls may be unable to proceed with the examination and alternative forms of assessment may need to be considered.

Investigations

Microscopy, culture and wet-preparation analysis of a vaginal discharge will help to confirm the diagnosis of candidiasis, bacterial vaginosis, and trichomoniasis.

The gold standard for diagnosis of both *Chlamydia* and gonorrhoea is culture

from a cervical sample. However, both infections can be detected with a high degree of sensitivity using a molecular replication technique (either PCR or LCR) performed on samples collected from either the cervix or a first catch-urine.

Management

- *Candida albicans* is the most common cause of vaginal thrush. One treatment option is clotrimazole 2% cream inserted vaginally at night for three days.[9]
- Bacterial vaginosis should be treated in symptomatic patients and in those at high risk of acquiring other STIs. Oral metronidazole 400 mg BD for five days is recommended in non-pregnant patients.[9]
- Trichomoniasis can be treated with oral metronidazole 2 g orally as a single dose.[9]
- *Chlamydia* treatment is with either a seven-day course of doxycycline (100 mg BD) or a single oral dose of 1 gm azithromycin.[9]
- Gonorrhoea has developed resistance to a number of antibiotics and therefore treatment should be based on local sensitivities. In urban Australia a single dose of 250 mg cefotaxime intramuscularly in combination with cover for *Chlamydia* is currently recommended.[9]
- A retained tampon can generally be removed in the ED. However, occasionally the swollen tampon cannot be extracted due to a hymenal ring and removal under general anaesthesia is required. If the tampon is removed in the ED it should be immediately placed into a container of water to limit exposure to the often offensive odour.

Disposition

Adolescents with a sexually transmitted infection should have a follow-up communicable disease consultation to discuss prevention of further STIs. Ongoing contraception and contact tracing should also be addressed.

Gonorrhoea and *Chlamydia* are notifiable diseases in some Australian states.

ABNORMAL VAGINAL BLEEDING

Introduction

Abnormal vaginal bleeding may be caused by a complication of pregnancy, trauma, infection or it may be secondary to contraceptive use. However, the most common causes are anovulatory bleeding or an underlying haematological condition.

Menstrual cycles in adolescents are often anovulatory due to the gradual maturation of the hypothalamic–pituitary–ovarian axis, which can take up to five years after the menarche.[10] Anovulatory or dysfunctional uterine bleeding generally presents as irregular, often heavy, blood loss. Anovulatory bleeding may result from a relative deficiency of either oestrogen or progesterone. Relative oestrogen deficiency is more common in thin young women who have just commenced their menstrual cycles. The relative oestrogen deficiency results in a thin, atrophic endometrium, which can bleed profusely.

In girls with higher endogenous oestrogen levels anovulatory menstrual cycles are more likely to result in a relative progesterone deficiency due to failure of the luteal phase. In this case the unopposed oestrogen results in thickening of the endometrial lining, which can bleed erratically.

Menorrhagia, whether associated with ovulatory or anovulatory cycles, may be a marker of systemic illness. Up to 20% of patients admitted with menorrhagia have been found to have an underlying haematological disease, the most common of which is a coagulopathy.[11]

Chronic untreated menorrhagia may also present with signs and symptoms of anaemia.

Examination

The haemodynamic status of the patient and the severity of the bleeding should be assessed. A general examination should be performed, particularly noting evidence of a haematological disorder or anaemia.

Investigations

A full blood count, iron studies and coagulation screen will assist in identifying anaemia, an underlying coagulopathy or haematological cause for the bleeding. A pregnancy test should also be performed.

Ultrasound may be helpful when ovarian pathology is suspected and can be used to assess the thickness of the endometrium. An STI screen should be obtained if clinically indicated.

Dilation and curettage is rarely indicated for a diagnosis and is not a recognised treatment for dysfunctional uterine bleeding.[12]

Management

Heavy bleeding either acute or chronic should be treated with fluid and blood products as clinically indicated.

Oestrogens and progestins are generally used in the management of anovulatory bleeding. Suggested regimens vary with respect to the route of administration, the dose and the type of hormone used. Currently there is no convincing evidence in favour of any particular regimen.[13]

If oestrogen deficiency is suspected on the basis of the history, treatment options include oral conjugated oestrogens 0.625–1.25 mg every 4–6 hours or oral estradiol 1–2 mg every 4–6 hours until the bleeding stops, which is usually about 24 hours. The dose is then reduced to once or twice daily. Acute severe blood loss may require treatment with intravenous conjugated oestrogens; a suggested dose is 25 mg every four hours for 24 hours or until the bleeding settles. High-dose synthetic oestrogens, such as ethinylestradiol, have been associated with thromboembolic complications, consequently oral regimens are generally preferred.[14]

If a progesterone deficiency is suspected treatment is often initiated with oral norethisterone 5–10 mg every two hours for four doses followed by 5 mg two to three times a day for fourteen days.[7]

Menorrhagia, in the absence of a coagulation disorder or other underlying pathology, can be treated with non-steroidal anti-inflammatory agents or tranexamic acid, which reduce the menstrual loss by 33% and 50% respectively.[15]

Disposition

The identification of a coagulation disorder will necessitate review by a haematologist. Pregnancy-related bleeding should be reviewed by an obstetrician/gynaecologist. Anovulatory bleeding and simple menorrhagia can be managed by either a primary care physician or a gynaecologist.

PELVIC PAIN

Introduction

The differential diagnosis of acute pelvic pain in an adolescent includes both gynaecological and non-gynaecological causes. Common gynaecological causes include pregnancy-related pain, dysmenorrhoea, ovulation pain (Mittelschmertz), ovarian cysts and their complications, torsion of the ovary, pelvic inflammatory disease (PID), endometriosis and congenital uterine abnormalities, such as imperforate hymen.

History

A general gynaecological history should be taken with particular note made of the relationship of the pain to the menstrual cycle. History should also include the nature of onset of the pain and a history of similar episodes. The pain of dysmenorrhoea, Mittelschmertz, endometriosis and imperforate hymen may be cyclical. However, they may also present during the first episode or as an unusually severe exacerbation. An ectopic pregnancy is not excluded by the history of a recent menstrual period.

- Primary dysmenorrhoea is common in the adolescent population, it refers to pain associated with menstruation in the absence of underlying pathology. The pain is generally described as crampy, occurring in the lower abdomen often with radiation to the back or to the inner thighs. Associated features may include nausea, vomiting, diarrhoea, headache and syncope. The symptoms have been attributed, in part, to an increased release of, or increased sensitivity to, prostaglandins. The diagnosis is generally made on the basis of history and limited physical examination findings.
- Mittelschmertz is pelvic pain related to ovulation. The pain is generally dull in

nature and located in either of the iliac fossae. The pain may last from a few hours to 2–3 days. The pathological basis of the pain is unclear but may be due either to distension of the capsule of the ovary prior to ovulation or to spillage of a small amount of follicular fluid at the time of ovulation.[7,16]

- Simple ovarian cysts are a normal physiological consequence of ovulation. They can be up to 6 cm in diameter. The pain may be from irritation of surrounding structures or stretching of the wall of the cyst. Corpus luteal cysts can reach up to 10 cm in size and may present as acute pain secondary to haemorrhage into the cyst. Both simple and corpus-luteal cysts can present as acute pain if they rupture. Although uncommon, a ruptured corpus-luteal cyst may continue to bleed and be associated with significant haematoperitoneum.[7]
- Complex ovarian cysts include dermoid cysts, which are often asymptomatic but may cause local pressure symptoms.
- Ovarian torsion is an uncommon condition and is almost exclusively seen in association with ovarian pathology. The history is typically an acute onset of colicky iliac fossa pain with the right being affected more than the left. There may be associated nausea, vomiting and a leucocytosis. Ultrasound has a high degree of sensitivity and specificity in making the diagnosis especially with the use of both arterial and venous Doppler studies.[17]
- Pelvic inflammatory disease can have a range of clinical presentations, depending on the location and the severity of the infection. The pain can range from mild to severe, systemic features of infection are not always present. Due to the significant complications associated with untreated PID the isolated finding of adnexal, uterine or cervical motion tenderness for which no other cause can be found have been suggested as a basis for the diagnosis and treatment of PID.[18]

- Endometriosis is reputed to cause a range of menstrual disorders and pain syndromes. However, the symptoms do not appear to correlate well with the degree of disease identified at laparoscopy. The diagnosis should be made with caution due to the risk of labelling a patient with what may be seen as a sentence for chronic pain and infertility.
- Congenital obstructive abnormalities include an imperforate hymen or obstruction of one side of a double uterine, cervical or vaginal system. An imperforate hymen may present as cyclical or irregular lower abdominal pain in a girl with well-developed secondary sexual characteristics and the absence of menstruation. Obstruction of a double system more typically presents with dysmenorrhoea that commences several days after the onset of menses and persists beyond the end of the menstrual period.

Examination

Examination should include vital signs and abdominal examination. Pelvic examination can give additional information regarding the location of the pain and its relationship to pelvic organs. Uterine, adnexal or cervical motion tenderness should be sought if pelvic examination is performed. The identification of an adnexal mass is clinically imprecise. However, it should prompt consideration of such conditions as ovarian torsion, tubo-ovarian abscess or ectopic pregnancy.

Investigations

A pregnancy test and a pelvic ultrasound are the most valuable tests for excluding pregnancy-related conditions. Ultrasound is the investigation of choice for the definition of masses and in the identification of ovarian cysts.[19]

Laparoscopy is reserved for pain that cannot be adequately explained or has failed to respond to appropriate treatments. Laparoscopy may be required to exclude torsion where a cyst is present combined with a suspicious history. It may also have a role in the investigation of chronic pelvic pain.

Management

- Dysmenorrhoea will generally respond to antiprostaglandin agents, such as mefenamic acid 500 mg orally eight-hourly or ibuprofen 400 mg orally eight-hourly. The response is improved by commencing treatment prior to the onset of symptoms. Lifestyle issues, such as increasing physical exercise and decreasing stress, may also improve symptoms.[20] For patients who fail to respond to treatment further investigation, such as ultrasound and laparoscopy, can be useful in identifying other pathology, for example significant endometriosis.
- Mittelschmertz and simple ovarian cysts can often be treated by reassurance. However, if this is not adequate, simple analgesia and NSAIDs may be required. If the pain is recurrent then consideration should be given to the use of the combined oral contraceptive pill in an attempt to suppress ovulation. Failure of resolution of a cyst after two months or a simple cyst greater than 8 cm diameter may require surgical exploration.[7]
- Complex ovarian cysts, including dermoids and endometriomas, are generally treated surgically.
- Ovarian torsion requires operative intervention.
- PID can be treated with either oral or parenteral antibiotics. However, there should be a low threshold for admission in adolescents.[21]

Disposition

Most forms of pelvic pain will require further management or investigation and should be referred accordingly.

CONTROVERSIES

❶ The management of anovulatory vaginal bleeding.

❷ The diagnosis and management of ovarian torsion.

❸ The diagnostic criteria and optimal management of PID.

REFERENCES

1. Mroueh J, Muram D 1999 Common problems in paediatric gynaecology: New developments. Current Opinion in Obstetrics and Gynaecology 11(5): 463–466
2. Jaquiery A, Styianopoulos A, Hogg G, Grover S 1999 Vulvovaginitis: Clinical features, aetiology, and microbiology of the genital tract. Archives of Disease in Childhood 81: 64–67
3. Farrington P 1997 Paediatric vulvo-vagitis. Clinical Obstetrics and Gynaecology 40(1): 135–140
4. Fischer G 2001 Vulval disease in pre-pubertal girls. Australasian Journal of Dermatology 42: 2 25–236
5. Quint E 1998 Vaginal bleeding and discharge in the paediatric and adolescent age groups. In: Pearlman M, Tintinalli J (eds) Emergency care of the woman. McGraw-Hill, New York 395–407
6. Grover S 2000 Gynaecological conditions In: Smart (ed) Paediatric handbook, 6th edn. Blackwell Science Asia, Melbourne 342–350
7. Mackay E, Beischer N, Pepperell R, Wood C 2000 Illustrated textbook of gynaecology, 2nd edn. WB Saunders, London
8. Blake DR, Fletcher K, Joshi N, Emans SJ 2003 Identification of symptoms that indicate a pelvic examination is necessary to exclude PID in adolescent women. Journal of Paediatric and Adolescent Gynecology 16(1): 25–30
9. Therapeutic Guidelines 2003 Antibiotic Version 12. VMPF. Therapeutics Committee
10. Apter D, Viinikka L, Vihko R 1978 Hormonal pattern of adolescent menstrual cycles. Journal of Clinical Endocrinology and Metabolism 47(5): 944–954
11. Claessens EA, Cowell CA 1981 Acute adolescent menorrhagia. American Journal of Obstetrics and Gynecology 139(3): 277–280
12. Duflos-Cohade C, Amandruz M, Thibaud E 1996 Pubertal metrorrhagia. Journal of Paediatric and Adolescent Gynecology 9(1): 16–20
13. Hickey M, Higham J, Fraser IS 2003 Progestogens versus oestrogens and progestogens for irregular uterine bleeding associated with anovulation. Cochrane Review. The Cochrane Library, Issue 3. Update software, Oxford
14. Richlin SS, Rock JA 2000 Abnormal uterine bleeding. In: Carpenter SEK, Rock JA (eds) Paediatric and adolescent gynaecology, 2nd edn. Lippincott Williams &Wilkins, Philadelphia, 207–224
15. Prentice A 1999 Fortnightly review: Medical management of menorrhagia. British Medical Journal 319: 1343–1345
16. Hann LE, Hall DA, Black EB, Ferrucci JT Jr 1979 Mittelschmerz. Sonographic demonstration. Journal of the American Medical Association 241(25): 2731–2732
17. Ben-Ami M, Perlitz Y, Haddad S 2002 The effectiveness of spectral and color Doppler in predicting ovarian torsion. A prospective stud. European Journal of Obstetrics, Gynaecology and Reproductive Biology 104(1): 64–66
18. Centers for Disease Control and Prevention 2002 Sexually transmitted diseases treatment guidelines. MMWR 51(NoRR-6): 32-36, 69–71
19. Arbel-Derowe Y, Tepper R, Rosen DJ et al 1997 The contribution of pelvic ultrasound to the diagnostic process in paediatric and adolescent gynaecology. Journal of Paediatric and Adolescent Gynaecology 10: 3–12
20. Bolton P, Del Mar C, O'Connor V 2003 Exercise for primary dysmenorrhoea (Protocol for a Cochrane Review). The Cochrane Library, Issue 3. Update Software, Oxford
21. Hemsel DL, Ledger WJ, Martens M, Monif GRG, Osborne NG, Thomason JL 2001 Concerns regarding the Centers for Disease Control's published guidelines for pelvic inflammatory disease. Clinical Infectious Diseases 32: 103–107

15.2 EMERGENCY CONTRACEPTION

ALASTAIR D. MCR. MEYER

Essentials

1 EC should be made available to an adolescent who has had unprotected sexual intercourse within 72 hours prior to presentation, regardless of the stage of her menstrual cycle.

2 Pregnancy must be excluded by urinary β-HCG testing.

3 Commonly prescribed treatment is with levonorgestrel (LNE) EC, two 0.75 mg tablets, twelve hours apart.

4 Follow-up is essential.

INTRODUCTION

Emergency contraception (EC) or post-coital contraception can be defined as preventing pregnancy after sexual inter-course. Every year over 3.5 million un-intended pregnancies occur in the United States alone, mostly to teenage mothers. It is believed that half of these un-intended pregnancies could be avoided by the judicious use of EC.[1] Indications for the provision of EC are shown in Table 15.2.1.

Many of these unintended pregnancies are later surgically terminated. Estimates of as many as 170 000 such terminations are performed in England and Wales an-nually.[2] These surgical terminations are not without clinical risk and cost, as well as a major social, religious and political issue.

Table 15.2.1   Indication for providing EC

- Unprotected intercourse
- Barrier contraception failure
- Intrauterine contraceptive device (IUCD) expulsion
- Missed contraceptive pills
- Sexual assault

CLINICAL ASSESSMENT

EC should be made available to an adolescent who has had unprotected sexual intercourse within 72 hours prior to presentation, regardless of the stage of her menstrual cycle. Pregnancy must be excluded by urinary β-HCG testing.

Depending on the age of the young person issues of child protection and consent to treatment may need to be explored.

AVAILABLE MEDICATIONS

Historically, the Yuzpe method of EC was commonly practiced in Australasia. This involved a high-dose oestrogen/progestogen preparation. Two doses of 100 µg of ethinylestradiol combined with 500 µg of levonorgestrel given twelve hours apart resulted in withdrawal bleeding within 21 days for 98% of women.[3]

Simple anti-emetics such as metoclo-pramide were routinely prescribed for nausea associated with the high oestrogen dose. This method of EC disrupted the natural hormone patterns necessary to sustain pregnancy. The high oestrogen and progestogen levels were believed to alter the endometrium thereby preventing implantation. The fertilised ovum had implantation prevented by blocking oestrogen and progestogen receptors, which made the endometrium hostile to implantation. Endometrial biochemistry and glandular and stromal development were affected such that the environment was hostile to the fertilised ovum. The therapy therefore prevents implantation and can consequently be described as a contraceptive rather than an abortifacient.

In June 2002, levonorgestrel (LNE) became the first drug licensed for use in Australia specifically as an EC agent. The first dose of 0.75 mg LNE is taken as soon as possible after unprotected sexual intercourse. This dose is repeated twelve hours later.

While the precise mechanism by which LNE prevents pregnancy is not clear, it is believed to work by preventing ovulation and by altering the tubal transport of sperm and ova. Fertilisation is thus prevented. When used within 72 hours of unprotected sexual intercourse, LNE EC prevents 85% of expected pregnancies. Efficacy falls with time (see Table 15.2.2).

Table 15.2.2   Efficacy of LNE EC[4,5]

Hours post-coital	Pregnancies prevented (%)
< 24 hours	95
24–48 hours	85
49–72 hours	58

LNE EC is contraindicated in unexplained vaginal bleeding, current breast cancer and pregnancy. Care should be taken with patients taking anticoagulants. Adverse reactions include fatigue, abdominal pain, gastrointestinal discomfort, dizziness, headache, breast tenderness and vaginal bleeding. LNE is primarily metabolised in the liver.

Conditions regarded as relative contraindications include: severe hypertension; diabetes with nephropathy; retinopathy; neuropathy; ischaemic heart disease; and past history of breast cancer.

LNE contraception has fewer side effects than the traditional Yuzpe method.[6] Only 20% of patients experience nausea, which usually responds to standard antiemetics. LNE EC results in 60% of women commencing their next menstruation within three days of their expected date. Fifteen percent of women can be up to seven days late with their period. It is essential that women have pregnancy testing if their period is more than seven days late.

If unprotected sexual intercourse has occurred more than 72 hours but less than five days before presentation, insertion of a copper-based IUCD should occur. These devices prevent implantation. IUCDs should be inserted in consultation with the gynaecology service.

If inserted up to five days after predicted ovulation, IUCDs can prevent 99% of expected pregnancies.[5] Relative contraindications are nulliparity and patients who are at high risk of sexually transmitted infection.

All women presenting to EDs following unprotected sexual intercourse should be counselled regarding sexually transmitted infections, ongoing contraception and the need for follow-up.

All patients receiving EC from EDs must have clear follow-up arrangements made. The patient's usual doctor or the hospital female health clinic are the most appropriate facilities.

CONTROVERSIES

❶ Is the ED an appropriate site for dispensing EC, as these patients are essentially well?

❷ There may be a place for non-medical providers of the EC, given its safety.

❸ The place of follow-up termination, should EC fail, is important to consider.

REFERENCES

1. Trussel J, Stewart F, Guest F et al 1992 Emergency contraceptive pills. Simple proposal to reduce unintended pregnancies. Family Planning and Prevention 24: 269–273
2. Anonymous 1993 Hormonal emergency contraception. Drug Therapeutics Bulletin 31(7): 27–28
3. Yuzpe AA, Percivalsmith R, Rademaker AW 1982 A multicentre clinical investigation employing ethinylestradiol combined with dinorgestrel as a post-coital agent. Fertility and Sterility 37: 508–513
4. Rodrigues I, Grou F, Joly J 2001 Effectiveness of emergency contraceptive pills between 72 and 120 hours after unprotected sexual intercourse. American Journal of Obstetrics and Gynaecology 84: 531–537
5. Bryan S 2003 Female sexual health. Emergency Medicine 15: 223–226
6. Task force on postovulatory methods of fertility regulation 1998 Randomised controlled trial of levonorgestrel versus the Yuzpe regimen of combined oral contraceptives for emergency contraception. Lancet 352: 428–433

RENAL

16.1 ACUTE RENAL FAILURE

BARRY WILKINS

ESSENTIALS

1 Acute renal failure is acute reduction in glomerular filtration rate.

2 A high or rising plasma creatinine is the hallmark, but this does not necessarily distinguish it from chronic renal failure.

3 A normal plasma creatinine does not exclude acute renal failure.

4 The commonest causes of acute renal failure presenting to the ED are haemolytic uraemic syndrome and post-streptococcal glomerulonephritis.

5 Not all ARF is oliguric or anuric.

6 Most cases of oliguria are not acute renal failure.

7 Most cases of elevated plasma urea are not acute renal failure.

8 The most important treatment areas are circulating volume, potassium, and blood pressure.

9 Hyperkalaemia in acute renal failure is not necessarily caused by potassium retention, especially when of short duration, but by potassium redistribution from cells.

10 Posterior urethral valves should be suspected in male infants with unexplained acute renal failure.

11 Do not continue diuretics if two IV doses of furosemide of 1 mg kg^{-1}, then 5 mg kg^{-1} (over one hour) produce no urine.

INTRODUCTION

Acute renal failure (ARF) means any acute reduction in glomerular filtration rate (GFR), i.e. in the excretory function of the kidneys, with oliguria (< 0.5 mL kg^{-1} h^{-1} in children or < 1 mL kg^{-1} h^{-1} in infants) or anuria, and a rise in plasma creatinine. Occasionally it is non-oliguric. It may evolve over hours (e.g. hypoxic-ischaemic cause) or days (e.g. glomerulonephritis). ARF caused by acquired renal disease presenting to the emergency department (ED) is rare (1 per 30000 children per year). However, it is common in hospitalised critically ill children where it is associated with significant mortality. The prognosis is more favourable if the ARF is non-oliguric. In a substantial proportion of cases ARF may be preventable and potentially may be totally reversible.

Classically, ARF has been divided into three broad categories:

❶ Pre-renal.
❷ Post-renal.
❸ Renal.

However, pathophysiological processes overlap, and the first and second groups can lead to the third when severe or prolonged.

❶ Hypovolaemia, hypotension and low cardiac output reduce renal blood flow and cause elevation of plasma urea and a mild reduction in GFR and elevation in creatinine. This is not true renal failure, but a normal physiological adaptation to reduced renal blood flow, which responds to rehydration or other treatment of the cause.

❷ Obstruction in the renal tract anywhere from the pelvicalyceal system to the urethra may lead to ARF or chronic renal failure (CRF). Crystalopathy (obstructing the tubules) is usually regarded as a 'renal' cause.

❸ Primary disease in the glomerulus, which may be intrinsic (e.g. glomerulonephritis (GN)) or imposed (e.g. hypoxia, ischaemia, toxins).

CAUSES

See Table 16.1.1.

There are many causes of oliguria other than ARF. Beware of urine retention or a blocked bladder catheter before assuming true oliguria (see Table 16.1.2).

There are many causes of polyuria other than ARF (see Table 16.1.3).

There are many causes of oedema other than ARF (see Table 16.1.4).

There are many causes of elevated plasma urea (P_{UREA}) other than ARF (see Table 16.1.5).

PATHOPHYSIOLOGY

Physiology

The kidney has three principal areas of function:

❶ Excretion of waste products of metabolism (e.g. urea and non-volatile acid) and excess ingested elements (e.g. potassium). This is effected by glomerular filtration, measured by the GFR.

❷ Regulation of the volume and mineral composition of body fluids. This is effected by tubular function, by absorption of $> 90\%$ of filtered water, $> 99\%$ of filtered sodium and 100% of glucose.

❸ Endocrine functions, e.g. erythropoietin, renin.

Normal GFR is around 1 mL kg^{-1} min^{-1} in newborn infants, rising to 2 mL kg^{-1}

Table 16.1.1   Causes of ARF

1. Reduced renal blood flow
- Severe shock from hypovolaemia or myocardial failure
- Rarely the following may cause acute tubular necrosis (ATN) or cortical necrosis, and is more common in children with pre-existing cardiac, renal or liver failure:
  Severe gastroenteritis
  Nephrotic syndrome[a]
  Burns
  Diuretic use
  Haemorrhage
  Salt-wasting tubulopathies
  Hypoaldosteronism
- Cardiogenic shock
- Pericardial tamponade
- Coarctation of the aorta or renal artery stenosis
- Septic shock
- Anaphylactic shock
- Systemic inflammatory response syndromes (e.g. severe trauma, pancreatitis)
- Hepatorenal syndrome (rare)
- Malignant hypertension
- Arterial or venous thrombosis
- Disseminated intravascular coagulation (DIC)
- Drugs (e.g. angiotensin converting enzyme (ACE) inhibitors, non-steroidal anti-inflammatory drugs (NSAIDs), tacrolimus, ciclosporin)

2. Intrinsic renal disease
- Haemolytic uraemic syndrome (HUS)[b]
- Thrombotic thrombocytopenic purpura (TTP)
- Acute proliferative glomerulonephritis (GN), including post-streptococcal and other post-infectious[c] glomerulonephritis
- Acute tubular necrosis (ATN) caused by hypoxia plus ischaemia; this has also been termed vasomotor nephropathy
- Systemic lupus erythematosus (SLE) or vasculitis
- IgA nephropathy
- Wegener's granulomatosis
- Anti-glomerular basement membrane (anti-GBM) disease
- Pyelonephritis
- Toxins (e.g. petrol, carbon tetrachloride, heavy metals)
- Drugs (e.g. aminoglycosides, vancomycin, cisplatin, tacrolimus, ciclosporin, ACE inhibitors, non-steroidal anti-inflammatory drugs (NSAIDs), amphotericin B)
- Acute tubulo-interstitial nephritis (TIN); drugs (e.g. furosemide, NSAIDs, penicillin, rifampicin, thiazides, allopurinol), immune-mediated diseases (e.g. IgA nephropathy, SLE) and infections (bacterial including *Yersinia*, viral, fungal, rickettsial) are causes
- HIV nephropathy
- Snake or arachnid envenomation
- Renal trauma
- Myoglobinuria from crush injury or rhabdomyolysis
- Haemoglobinuria (acute intravascular haemolysis, e.g. in G-6-PD deficiency)
- Sickle cell disease
- Leukaemic infiltration
- Shunt nephritis (ventriculo-peritoneal shunt infection)
- Radiographic contrast agents (rare in children)
- Renal dysplasia, hypoplasia, and agenesis in neonates (chronic but acute presentation)

3. Urinary tract obstruction
- Posterior urethral valves (chronic but acute presentation)
- Urethral stricture
- Ureterocele
- Pelvic or retroperitoneal tumours
- Neurogenic bladder
- Retroperitoneal fibrosis (rare)
- Stones, sludge (metabolic disease), pus, fungal ball, sloughed renal papilla, clots, proteinaceous material or crystals (uric acid, calcium oxalate, aciclovir, methotrexate, purines, sulphonamides) in the ureters or renal tubules

4. Acute presentation of end-stage renal failure

[a]Sometimes nephrotic syndrome caused by mesangio-capillary GN may present with features similar to acute post-streptococcal GN.
[b]In developed countries HUS and post-streptococcal GN are the commonest causes presenting to the ED, whereas in tropical countries 'pre-renal' causes predominate outside the hospital environment.
[c]Various infectious agents can produce nephritis similar to that of post-streptococcal GN (e.g. *Mycoplasma*, *Leptospira*, atypical *Mycobacterium*, *Varicella*, cytomegalovirus, Epstein-Barr virus, *Toxoplasma*, *Rickettsia*, hepatitis B and C).

Table 16.1.2   Causes of oliguria

- ARF
- Hypovolaemia
- Dehydration
- Low cardiac output
- Intrarenal vasoconstricting drugs when renal impairment is mild
- Syndrome of inappropriate antidiuretic hormone secretion (SIADH)

Table 16.1.3   Causes of polyuria

- ARF
- CRF
- Diuretics
- Obstruction of the urinary tract
- Nephrogenic diabetes insipidus (DI)
- Nephrocalcinosis
- Interstitial nephritis
- Renal tubular disorders, e.g. Bartter syndrome
- Hypoaldosteronism, e.g. Addison disease, congenital adrenal hyperplasia
- Cerebral salt wasting
- Sickle cell disease
- Psychogenic polydipsia

Table 16.1.4   Causes of water retention and oedema

- ARF
- CRF
- Nephrotic syndrome
- Chronic liver disease
- Other causes of hypoproteinaemia (e.g. protein-losing enteropathy)
- Inappropriate ADH secretion or administration (oedema rare)
- Congestive heart failure (congenital or acquired structural heart disease, tachyarrythmias, pericardial effusion)
- Excess sodium and water intake

Table 16.1.5   Causes of uraemia

- ARF
- Increased dietary protein load
- Catabolic states with fever, e.g. sepsis, rhabdomyolysis
- Gastrointestinal or internal haemorrhage
- Increased reabsorption by the renal tubules (hypovolaemia, dehydration, low cardiac output)

min^{-1} in adults, but there is wide variation between and within individuals, reflected in wide variations in plasma creatinine (P_{CR}) in normal children. Measurement of GFR is unhelpful in the acute situation. Creatinine clearance approximates to GFR. Plasma creatinine reflects GFR because creatinine production is remarkably constant, both within and between individuals, and is related to muscle mass. It is around 100 μmol kg^{-1} d^{-1} in infants rising to around 200 μmol kg^{-1} d^{-1} in adults. There is a little absorption from, or secretion into, the tubule and this is abolished by Histamine-2 (H2) receptor antagonists. In ARF with complete cessation of glomerular function plasma creatinine (P_{CR}) increases by up to 150 μmol L^{-1} d^{-1} in infants and 300 μmol L^{-1} d^{-1} in adults. In less severe ARF P_{CR} rises by > 50 μmol L^{-1} d^{-1}. In stable renal function GFR can be estimated by the formula: $70/P_{CR}$ mL kg^{-1} min^{-1} in infants or $140/P_{CR}$ mL kg^{-1} min^{-1} in adults, but this is an approximation. The formula does not hold true if GFR is changing.

Although there are published tables of P_{CR} and GFR according to age, gender and size, the variability and different P_{CR} assays in use preclude their being of much use in interpreting isolated creatinine results. A normal plasma creatinine does not exclude ARF. Generally any creatinine > 100 μmol L^{-1} is abnormal, but in infants > 50 should raise a suspicion of impaired GFR, in a five year old > 70, in a ten year old > 80, and in a fifteen year old > 100. More important is the rate of increase of plasma creatinine in ARF, which takes 24 hours to become evident.

Renal blood flow (RBF) is normally very high (one quarter of cardiac output) in order to effect glomerular filtration. It is auto regulated over a wide perfusion pressure range. Normally 20% of the renal plasma flow is filtered. There is only a small proportion of tubular reabsorption or secretion of creatinine; hence the plasma creatinine is an indication of glomerular function. Up to 50% of urea is reabsorbed, more in oliguric states; hence plasma urea may reflect dehydration more than GFR. The high metabolic rate (for tubular reabsorption) and high endothelial mass (greater than any other organ by weight) make the kidney vulnerable to hypoxia and ischaemia.

Pathogenesis of ARF

Most ARF presenting to EDs has a single identifiable cause, in contrast to hospital acquired ARF, which may be multifactorial.

In ATN there is a generalised hypoxic or ischaemic insult affecting the glomerulus and tubules. Tubular injury leads to failure of electrolyte absorption and a tendency to loss of extracellular fluid, which would be rapidly fatal if not limited by a reduction in GFR. ATN is a term that is not strictly correct. Rarely is there histological necrosis, though individual tubular cell apoptosis does occur. Acute tubular dysfunction (at a subcellular level) is a better term. Vasomotor nephropathy is another term that found brief favour in the 1980s, based on the tubulo-glomerular feedback causing afferent arteriolar vasoconstriction and mesangial cell contraction, reducing GFR and limiting massive tubular electrolyte loss. This process was once termed 'acute renal success' because of the saving of the patient's life by the kidney 'taking itself out'. Pre-existing haemodynamic compromise, CRF, age, hypovolaemia, diuretics, diabetes, or proteinuria favour the induction of ATN with any insult.

Vasoconstricting local mediators, including adenosine, angiotensin II, endothelin, thromboxane, leukotrienes, urotensin, platelet activating factor, heat shock proteins, oxygen free radicals and superoxides, together with deficiency of vasodilating mediators, including prostacyclin, atrial natriuretic peptide (ANP) and nitric oxide, are causes of the intense glomerular vasoconstriction in ATN. In future, endothelin A receptor antagonists may play a role in moderating renal injury.

Inflammatory infiltrate, interstitial oedema, up-regulation of adhesion molecules, tubule cell swelling, loss of epithelial surface area, loss of epithelial cell polarity, compression of peritubular capillaries, impaction of debris in tubules, increased intratubular pressure, back-leak of urea, aggregation of erythrocytes, leucocytes and fibrin in peritubular capillaries, all contribute to the established state of reduced GFR, which may take weeks to recover, if at all.

The following pathological processes may contribute to other causes of ARF:

- In snake and arachnid envenomation, haemolysis, disseminated intravascular coagulation (DIC) and the venom itself may contribute to renal injury.

- Sickle cell haemoglobinopathy causes papillary necrosis by red cell sickling in medullary blood vessels. This may cause gross haematuria. Sepsis and volume depletion may contribute to renal injury. Recurrent episodes often lead to a nephropathy with an irreversible urine concentration defect in teenagers. Approximately 10% of sickle cell crises have ARF.
- In hypovolaemia, hypotension and low cardiac output states the combination of decreased renal perfusion pressure and afferent arteriolar constriction reduces GFR.
- In ATN, increased tubular hydrostatic pressure due to obstruction caused by casts and injured tubular cell debris, and back leak of filtrate through injured tubular epithelium reduces effective GFR further. Influx of calcium into renal tubular cells may activate enzyme systems, leading to membrane and organelle dysfunction.
- Birth asphyxia may precipitate renal vein thrombosis in neonates commencing within the kidney, spreading into larger veins, but thrombogenic states (e.g. protein S or protein C deficiency) are rare causes. There are firm palpable kidneys with haematuria.
- Renal function may deteriorate suddenly in some patients without an oliguric phase. Obstruction, sepsis, hypercalcaemia and some drugs and other nephrotoxins may be causes. Functioning nephrons have reduced reabsorption capacity, thereby maintaining urine output. It has a better prognosis than oliguric renal failure.
- Although minimal change nephrotic syndrome rarely causes ARF, hypovolaemia, peritonitis, septicaemia, renal vein thrombosis and drug toxicity may precipitate ARF that is histologically ATN in 60% and may be reversible.
- HIV disease may first present as ARF, nephrosis or CRF. Minimal change, mesangial proliferation and focal segmental glomerulosclerosis (FSGS) may be seen.

After initiation of ARF by glomerular or tubular injury there is a maintenance phase where GFR remains relatively low for several days or weeks, then a recovery phase characterised by gradual and progressive restoration of GFR and tubular function.

PRESENTATION

See Table 16.1.6.

A careful history and examination may give clues to the cause of ARF. Ask about diuretic and other drug use, recent hospitalisation or radiographic investigations, diarrhoea or vomiting (may be the presenting symptom of UTI or HUS), weight change, musculo-skeletal symptoms, abdominal or flank pain, urinary dribbling, arthralgia and myalgia, recent URTI. Enquire for family history of renal disease or hypertension. Examine for signs of heart failure. Look for fever and rash that might be signs of GN or tubulo-interstitial nephritis (TIN), vasculitic signs, palpable bladder. Important

---

Table 16.1.6   Possible presenting features of ARF

- Oliguria
- Anuria
- Polyuria
- Haematuria
- Brown urine
- Hypertension
- Pulmonary oedema
- Water retention (but oedema less common)
- Recent weight gain or weight loss
- Acidosis
- Electrolyte abnormalities, especially hyperkalaemia, hyperphosphataemia
- Arrhythmias
- Pericarditis
- Gastro-intestinal symptoms (e.g. anorexia, nausea, vomiting, haemorrhage)
- Neuro-psychiatric manifestations (confusion, agitation, seizures, headache, visual disturbances)[a]
- Itching (uraemia)
- Generalised systemic illness with malaise, anorexia and fatigue
- Acute respiratory distress syndrome (ARDS)

[a]Neurological manifestations are usually late and may represent hypertensive encephalopathy.

---

features of hypovolaemia or low cardiac output include tachycardia (for normal pulse rates see Chapter 1.1), prolonged capillary refill time > 2 s (but beware of cold ambient temperature), postural hypotension (remember that supine blood pressure can be preserved until late in hypovolaemia and dehydration – for normal blood pressures, see Chapter 16.3) and possibly a gallop rhythm. Oedema, when present, can be hard to find – press firmly on the shin for at least one minute. Haematuria may suggest renal parenchymal disease. Poor urinary stream and palpable bladder points to obstruction but in the very young this can be only excluded by thorough investigation. Monitor cardiac electrical rhythm and oximetry.

INVESTIGATIONS

Tests in ARF include:

- Full blood count.
- Plasma Na, K, Cl, Ca, PO_4, Mg, osmolality.
- Plasma glucose.
- Plasma uric acid.
- Plasma urea and creatinine.
- Plasma albumin.
- Plasma pH, bicarbonate and lactate.
- Liver function tests.
- Coagulation screen.
- Blood cultures.
- Plasma creatine kinase (CK).
- Urinalysis for protein and blood by dipstick.
- Urine microscopy, Gram stain and culture.
- Urine chemistry (Na, K, urea, osmolality, creatinine). Only 1 mL is needed and can be aspirated from a cotton-wool ball placed in the nappy (calcium and phosphate may be falsely elevated).
- Urine protein (quantitative – protein:creatinine ratio > 20 mg mmol^{-1} is abnormal).
- Urine urate.

Examination of urine sediment by microscopy is often neglected. Normal urine indicates a pre- or post-renal cause of ARF. Cells, casts or protein suggests intrinsic renal pathology. In ATN there are granular and epithelial cell casts. White cell casts or eosinophils occur in acute TIN. Red blood cell casts and heavy proteinuria occur in GN or vasculitis. A dipstick positive for blood in the absence of red cells in urine is suggestive of hae-moglobin or myoglobin. Nitrite in urine may suggest UTI. Obstruction and UTI may cause pyuria.

Calculate the plasma anion gap, corrected for hypoalbuminaemia:

$$\text{Anion Gap (corr.)} = Na + K - Cl - Bicarbonate + \frac{(45 - Albumin)}{4}$$

NB. Albumin is in gm L^{-1}, the electrolytes in mmol L^{-1}.

Normal is 16 mEq L^{-1}.

Calculate the plasma osmolal gap:

$$\text{Osmolal Gap} = (Na + K) \times 1.86 + Urea + Glucose + 10 - Osmolality$$

NB. Electrolytes, urea and glucose are in mmol L^{-1}, osmolality in mosmol kg^{-1}.

If osmolal gap is >5 mosmol kg^{-1} then unmeasured solute such as ethanol or ethylene glycol may be present.

Chest X-ray will detect pulmonary oedema, pleural effusions or cardiomegaly.

Abdominal X-ray may detect nephro-calcinosis and spinal abnormalities.

All children with ARF should have a urinary tract ultrasound examination to check for two kidneys. This may diag-nose polycystic kidneys, renal vein throm-bosis, nephrocalcinosis, hydronephrosis or other causes of obstruction. The kidneys are likely to be normal in size or enlarged in ARF, but small in CRF. A non-dilated system does not necessarily exclude an obstructive uropathy in anuria; hence retrograde pyelography may be needed.

Further tests if there is any suspicion of GN or vasculitis include:

- ASOT.
- Complement C3, C4, CH50.
- Serology for hepatitis.
- Autoantibodies, especially anti-nuclear antibodies (ANA), anti-double-stranded DNA (anti-ds-DNA) antibodies, anti-neutrophil cytoplasmic antibodies (ANCA), anti-glomerular basement membrane (anti-GBM) antibody.

- Consider HIV serology.
- Consider isotope renal scans and angiography. Dimercaptosuccinic acid (DMSA) scan assesses functioning renal tubular mass and shows scars, while diethylene-triamine-penta-acetic acid (DTPA) and mercaptoacetyl glycylglycylglycine (MAG3) scans assess glomerular filtration and renal blood flow. They may be useful in distinguishing ATN from other causes of ARF.
- Echocardiography assists in assessing myocardial function or in excluding bacterial endocarditis.
- If the cause of renal failure still remains obscure the paediatric nephrologist will consider a percutaneous renal biopsy, generally after admission. This may show various types of acute GN, vasculitis or TIN that may need immunosuppression and/or plasmapheresis.

Urine chemistry is often neglected. Protein:creatinine ratio >20 mg $mmol^{-1}$ diagnoses significant proteinuria, but may be falsely elevated by fever, trauma, recent surgery, upright posture and exertion; early morning sample is best. Haematuria plus proteinuria strongly suggests a renal parenchymal lesion. Urate:creatinine ratio >1 mmol $mmol^{-1}$ suggests catabolic state, or tumour lysis, and uric acid nephropathy.

Urine electrolytes and osmolality are helpful in differentiating causes of uraemia. Always measure the urine creatinine. Calculate fractional excretion of sodium.

Fractional sodium excretion (FE_{Na}) is the fraction of filtered sodium that ends up in the urine, and is calculated by:

$$FE_{Na} = \frac{Urine\ Na}{Urine\ creatinine} \times \frac{Plasma\ creatinine}{Plasma\ Na}$$

NB. this formula *does* work even if the GFR is increasing or decreasing rapidly.

See Table 16.1.7

In health FE_{Na} is <1% except in high salt diet. In dehydrated patients, hypovo-laemia or low cardiac output it is <0.1% (representing normal renal physiology).

In general FE_{Na} >2% is seen in most cases of intrinsic renal failure. However, not all low FE_{Na} represents normal physiology; it may also be low in some causes of oliguric acute renal failure (e.g. cyclosporine toxicity). Not all high FE_{Na} with oliguria represents ARF with tubular injury. In pre-renal uraemia, FE_{Na} may be higher in the presence of glycosuria, bicarbonaturia or use of diuretics. Also, in SIADH there is oliguria with a high FE_{Na}. High FE_{Na} and polyuria suggest natriuresis, possible causes being a renal salt-wasting disorder, polyuric acute renal failure, diuretics (including osmotic di-uretics) and volume overload (mediated via natriuretic hormones). FE_{Na} is also unreliable in preterm newborns and in obstructive uropathy. Fractional urea ex-cretion (FE_{Urea}) may be more useful in distinguishing low renal perfusion forms of oliguria from ATN, especially after diuretics. FE_{Urea} is <35% in 'pre-renal' syndromes even after diuretic use, and >50% in ATN. FE_{Urate} is >15% in ATN and many tubulopathies, and <7% in 'pre-renal' states.

The urine calcium:creatinine ratio will help identify hypercalciuria as a cause of calculi or nephrocalcinosis (normal <0.7 mmol $mmol^{-1}$).

TREATMENT

The principles of treatment of ARF involve:

Treat established complications First, pay attention to the airway, breathing and circulation. Treat life-threatening complications (e.g. hypoxia, hypovolaemia, hyperkalaemia and seizures). Ventilation may be needed for pulmonary oedema not responsive to diuretic. Monitor con-tinuous ECG.

Minimise further renal injury Avoid excessive fluids and electrolytes (especially Na and K). Attempt to establish a diuresis to wash out intra-tubular debris. Use diuretics in small doses initially, because acute hypovolaemia can occur. Furosemide 1 mg kg^{-1} IV is appropriate, and then 5 mg kg^{-1} over 60 minutes if there is

Table 16.1.7   Using plasma and urine biochemistry to distinguish causes of oliguria

Cause	Plasma urea	Plasma creatinine	Plasma Na	Urine Na (FE_Na)	FE_Urea	Urine creatine	Urine Osmolality
Low cardiac output Hypovolaemia Dehydration Renal vasoconstriction (e.g. ciclosporin toxicity)	Moderate–marked increase	Mild–moderate increase	Normal, low or high	< 10 mmol L^{-1} (< 0.5%)	< 35%	> 4 mmol L^{-1}	> 400 mosmol kg^{-1}
ATN	High	Mild increase on 1st day, then progressive increase to high	Normal or low	> 20 mmol L^{-1} (> 3%)	> 50%	< 1 mmol L^{-1}	Similar to plasma osmolality
SIADH	Normal or low	Normal or low	Low	Often 100–200 mmol L^{-1} (> 1%)	—	Very high, often > 10 mmol L^{-1}	Inappropriately high for plasma osmo, > 300, often > 800 mosmol kg^{-1}

poor response. Give no more if there is no response. Remember that frusemide is itself nephro- and oto-toxic. Mannitol is not recommended as it may worsen the situation by acute intravascular expansion, especially if there is no diuresis.

Remove the cause   Treat sepsis. Remove nephrotoxic agents (e.g. drugs and poisons). Treat low cardiac output with inotropes, e.g. dopamine or dobutamine at 5–10 µg kg^{-1} min^{-1} IV, but note that there is no evidence that low-dose dopamine either improves prognosis or reduces the incidence of ARF in patients at risk. Avoid potentially nephrotoxic drugs, e.g. aminoglycosides, peptidoglycans, ACE inhibitors. Pure obstructive ARF is commonly reversible and always treatable. It is usual to treat urethral obstruction (posterior urethral valves) by urethral catheterisation (by urologist), or supra-pubic catheterisation, initially. In proven vascular thrombosis, tissue plasminogen activator (tPA) may be of benefit, but renal vein clot removal is unlikely to speed recovery.

Compensate for the reduced GFR and impaired tubular function   Avoid or reduce the dose of renally excreted drugs. Pay strict attention to water and electrolyte balance.

Remove accumulated water and minerals   Water and sodium input should

be reduced. Begin an accurate water balance chart. Replace each previous hour's urine output plus insensible losses (10–20 mL kg^{-1} d^{-1}). Refer early to the nephrology service for renal substitution therapy if diuretic is ineffective, for control of water, urea (plasma urea > 36 mmol L^{-1}), phosphate, metabolic acid and potassium retention, and to remove any toxic drugs or poisons. Oral calcium carbonate, calcium acetate (600–1800 mg elemental calcium per meal) or phosphate binding resin helps to control hyperphosphataemia. Aluminium is now avoided.

Optimise nutrition   Supply adequate energy.

DISPOSITION

All children with ARF should be admitted to a paediatric intensive-care or high-dependency facility under joint care of intensivist, nephrologist and any other relevant specialties. This may involve discussions with those specialties in a children's hospital and with an emergency retrieval service.

ACUTE PRESENTATION OF CRF

Occasionally a child with CRF (also called chronic kidney insufficiency), that may

have been previously undiagnosed, may present acutely with any of the symptoms of ARF. Anaemia, poor growth, clinical or radiological evidence of osteodystrophy, or small kidneys on ultrasound may suggest CRF (though polycystic kidneys are large). Elevated P_{CR} rising by < 40 µmol L^{-1} d^{-1} is also suggestive that the renal failure is chronic. ARF can occur in a child with CRF, which may be a flare of the original disease or genuine ARF. Most CRF patients will already be under the care of a nephrologist, who should be contacted early. Symptoms such as anorexia, nausea, vomiting, malaise and sleep disturbances are common, but be alert for acute deterioration in any of these.

History should be sought regarding medications (diuretics, antihypertensive agents, steroids, erythropoietin, salt supplements, alkali, vitamin D, calcium carbonate phosphate binder), type and frequency of renal support (if appropriate), other illnesses and usual follow-up. When CRF is previously undiagnosed a family history of Alport disease, haemophilia, polycystic kidney disease, sickling or stones should be sought. Ask for family history of 'kidney failure', 'dialysis machine', deafness, and blood or protein in urine.

The same investigations as in ARF are mandatory.

Acute problems in chronic renal failure include:

- Hypertensive crisis, possibly hypertensive encephalopathy with convulsions and coma.
- Salt depletion, especially with superimposed gastroenteritis.
- Dehydration can lead to irreversible deterioration in GFR caused by hypovolaemia. Urine output cannot be used to judge circulating volume. Hypertension may be normal for the child.
- Volume overload and heart failure.
- Hyperkalaemia. See hyperkalaemia protocol in Chapter 10.5.
- Arrhythmias.
- Acidosis. Chronic acidosis may be managed by oral alkali administration (2–$3\ \mathrm{mmol\ kg^{-1}\ d^{-1}}$).
- Hyper- or hypocalcaemia.
- Urinary tract infection.
- Urinary tract obstruction.
- Haemodialysis catheter or shunt, or peritoneal dialysis catheter malfunction.
- Haemodialysis catheter or shunt infection.
- Peritonitis in a child on continuous cycling or ambulatory peritoneal dialysis.
- Acute GI haemorrhage caused by platelet dysfunction. Desmopressin (DDAVP) is a therapeutic agent that may be useful, together with platelets, fresh frozen plasma or cryoprecipitate.
- Anaemia is often tolerated very well even down to haemoglobin levels of 30–$50\ \mathrm{g\ L^{-1}}$. Do not transfuse without consulting the nephrologist, except in emergency. Transfusion, especially of platelets, may actually worsen prognosis in HUS (see Chapter 16.5).
- Fractures secondary to renal osteodystrophy.

ARF IN THE RENAL TRANSPLANT RECIPIENT

The cause of a rising creatinine or sudden oliguria must be diagnosed without delay as a transplant carries high stakes. ARF in the transplanted kidney is often reversible with prompt management. Contact the transplant/nephrology service urgently

CONTROVERSIES AND FUTURE DIRECTIONS

❶ Acetylcysteine has been shown to ameliorate the acute progression of some causes of ARF, but its role is not yet defined.

❷ Low-dose vasopressin is being evaluated for a role in improving renal blood flow and GFR.

❸ Dopamine A1 receptor agonists, e.g. fenoldopam, are being evaluated for a role in improving renal blood flow and GFR.

❹ Adenosine A1 receptor agonists are being evaluated for a role in improving renal blood flow and GFR, especially in association with furosemide.

❺ Anaritide (atrial natriuretic peptide) may improve renal perfusion, particularly in oliguric renal failure.

❻ Melanocyte stimulating factor, insulin-like growth factor, epidermal growth factor and hepatocyte growth factor, anti-adhesion molecule compounds, free radical scavengers and antioxidants are also being evaluated.

❼ Endothelin A receptor antagonists may in future play a role in moderating renal injury.

❽ Stem cells to produce new renal tissue.

❾ More accurate markers of GFR may become available, e.g. cystatin C.

for all transplants presenting to the ED for any cause. Pre-renal uraemia must be excluded in any intercurrent illness.

Possible causes include:

- Volume depletion – the transplanted kidney compensates less well to dehydration.
- Delayed, antibody mediated rejection.
- Ciclosporin or tacrolimus toxicity (a glomerulopathy with hyaline arteriolar thickening).
- Urine leak at the ureteric-vesical anastomosis.
- Ureteric obstruction.
- ATN (rare in the child presenting to ED).
- Vascular thrombosis, including microangiopathic thrombosis diagnosed only on renal biopsy.
- Infection.
- Aciclovir.

FURTHER READING

Anderson RJ, Schrier RW 1993 Acute tubular necrosis. In: Schrier RW, Gottschalk CW (eds) Diseases of the kidney, 5th edn. Little Brown, Boston, 1287–1318
Andreoli SP 1999 Management of acute renal failure. In: Barratt TM, Avner ED, Harmon WE (eds) Pediatric nephrology, 4th edn. Lippincott, Williams & Wilkins, Baltimore, 1119–1134
Andreoli SP 2002 Acute renal failure. Current Opinion in Paediatrics 14: 183–188
Badr KF, Ichikawa I 1988 Prerenal failure: A deleterious shift from renal compensation to decompensation. New England Journal of Medicine 319: 623–629 [review]
Better OS, Stein JH 1990 Early management of shock and prophylaxis of acute renal failure in traumatic rhabdomyolysis. New England Journal of Medicine 322: 825–829 [review]
Bidani AK, Griffin KA 1995 Calcium channel blockers and renal protection: Is there an optimal dose? Journal of Laboratory & Clinical Medicine 125: 553–555 [review]
Chan JCM, Gill JR (eds) 1990 Kidney electrolyte disorders. Churchill Livingstone, New York
Cronan K, Norman ME 2000 Renal and electrolyte emergencies. In: Fleisher GR, Ludwig S (eds) Textbook of pediatric emergency medicine, 4th edn. Lippincott, Williams & Wilkins, Philadelphia, 811–858
Finney H, Newman DJ, Thakkar H, Fell JME, Price CP 2000 Reference ranges for plasma cystatin C and creatinine measurements in premature infants, neonates and older children. Archives of Diseases in Childhood 82: 71–75
Griffin KA, Bidani A 1989 Guidelines for determining the cause of acute renal failure. Journal of Critical Illness 4: 32
Mathew A, Berl T 1989 Fractional excretion of sodium: Use early to assess renal failure. Journal of Critical Illness 4: 45
Miller PD, Krebs RA, Neal BJ, McIntyre DO 1980 Polyuric prerenal failure. Archives of Internal Medicine 140: 907–909
Ronco C, Bellomo R (eds) 1998 Critical care nephrology. Kluwer Academic Publishers, Dordrecht
Siegel NJ, Van Why SK, Devarajan P, Gaudio KM 1999 Pathogenesis of acute renal failure. In: Barratt TM, Avner ED, Harmon WE (eds) Pediatric nephrology,

4th edn. Lippincott, Williams & Wilkins, Baltimore, 1109–1118

Siegler RL 1995 The hemolytic uremic syndrome. Pediatric Clinics of North America 42: 1505–1529 [review]

Stein JH 1992 Acute renal failure. Lessons from pathophysiology. Western Journal of Medicine 156: 176–182 [review]

Taylor CM, Chapman S 1989 Handbook of renal investigations in children. Wright, London

Thadani R, Pascual M, Bonaventre J 1996 Acute renal failure. New England Journal of Medicine 334: 1448–1460

Thurau K, Boylan JW 1976 Acute renal success. The unexpected logic of oliguria in acute renal failure. American Journal of Medicine 61: 308–315

Venuto RC 1992 Pigment-associated acute renal failure: Is the water clearer 50 years later? Journal of Laboratory & Clinical Medicine 119: 452–454

Wilkins BH, Goonasekera CDA, Dillon MJ 1999 Chapters 2.10 and 3.5. In: Macnab AJ, Macrae DJ, Henning R (eds) Care of the critically ill child. Churchill Livingstone, London

16.2 HAEMATURIA

FRANK WILLIS

ESSENTIALS

1 In children haematuria usually originates from the kidneys.

2 Haematuria can be caused by urinary infection, glomerular disease, tumours, congenital abnormalities and coagulopathies.

3 All paediatric haematuria should be investigated.

4 All patients with haematuria require follow-up.

INTRODUCTION

Blood in the urine (haematuria) may be visible to the naked eye (macroscopic) or be detected only on dipstick testing and/or urine microscopy (microscopic). It may be found in isolation or associated with other urine abnormalities such as proteinuria, crystals and casts. It is essential to consider urinary tract infection (UTI) as a possible cause and, if confirmed, to manage accordingly (see Chapter 16.4 on UTI).

Microscopic haematuria may be defined as > 10 red blood cells (RBCs) per high-power field, or > 50 RBCs mL^{-1} of urine (confirmed on three separate occasions).

Note that small numbers of red cells are normally excreted in urine.

Macroscopic haematuria exists when visible to the naked eye and confirmed on testing as being blood.

Haematuria can originate at any site in the urinary tract but, in contrast to adults, lower tract haematuria is relatively uncommon in children (and therefore cystoscopy is rarely indicated).

Remember:

❶ Microscopic haematuria in the setting of an acute febrile illness can be normal. UTI should be excluded by urine culture and the urine tested again after the acute illness has passed.

❷ Asymptomatic micro-haematuria in children without other signs of renal disease (hypertension, oedema, proteinuria, urinary casts, poor growth or renal impairment) is also relatively common.

❸ Consider idiopathic thrombocytopenic purpura (ITP), Henoch–Schönlein purpura (HSP) and coagulation disorders.

Causes of glomerular haematuria include:
- Glomerulonephritis (GN) (including nephritis in multisystem disorders, e.g. systemic lupus erythematosus (SLE).
- Familial nephritis (Alport disease).
- Thin basement membrane disease ('Benign' familial haematuria).
- IgA nephropathy.
- Polycystic kidney disease.

Causes for non-glomerular haematuria include:
- UTI.
- Idiopathic hypercalciuria.
- Stones.
- Anatomical abnormalities.
- Tumours.
- Trauma.
- Sickle cell disease (in relevant ethnic groups).

HISTORY

As in all cases attending the emergency department (ED), a relevant and thorough general and specific history should be taken.

Don't forget to obtain a family history of renal tract disease. In patients with isolated micro-haematuria, considerations include the possibility of familial haematuria. Check for a family history of renal tract stones (suggesting hypercalciuria) or sensorineural deafness and nephritis (with Alport Disease).

Ask about previous episodes of haematuria and/or features of HSP or SLE.

Historical features of upper tract haematuria include:
- Brown urine.
- Frothy urine, which may indicate proteinuria.

Features of lower tract haematuria include:
- Pink or bright red colour.
- Blood in the initial part of the stream suggests a urethral origin.
- Blood towards the end of the urine stream suggests bladder origin.

EXAMINATION

Physical examination should seek to elicit signs of renal disease. A thorough general examination is essential concentrating on the following in particular:

- *Cardiovascular status* (pallor, BP, hypovolaemia and/or fluid overload including gallop rhythm, pulmonary oedema, ascites, peripheral, scrotal/perineal oedema).
- *Abdominal examination* (loin tenderness, ascites, petechiae or purpura).
- *Neurologic status* (anaemia, hypertensive encephalopathy, uraemia).

INVESTIGATIONS

In children presenting to the ED with haematuria, investigations should focus on identifying the anatomical source of the haematuria as well as its clinical significance.

Urine dipstick testing, microscopy and culture should always be performed as part of the initial evaluation of a child with haematuria.

Features suggestive of upper tract haematuria include the following:

- Protein is often present.
- RBCs are often small and misshapen (dysmorphic).
- RBC casts and tubular casts may be seen.

Features suggestive of lower tract haematuria include:

- RBCs of normal shape (non-dysmorphic).
- No proteinuria.

NB. Urinary RBC morphology alone is an inaccurate method to determine the site of origin of haematuria and should not be relied upon in isolation.

The extent and type of other investigations done while in the ED will be determined by the clinical scenario. The following tests may be considered:

- Urine calcium:creatinine ratio > 0.7 mmol mmol^{-1} (hypercalciuria).
- Urine protein:creatinine ratio > 20mg mmol^{-1} (glomerulonephritides, chronic renal failure).
- Plasma urea, creatinine + electrolytes (abnormal renal function).
- Plasma calcium, PO$_4$, albumin (chronic renal failure).
- FBC, platelets, film (thrombocytopenia, anaemia).
- Coagulation screen (coagulopathy).
- Streptococcal serology (post-streptococcal GN).
- Pharyngeal swab culture (post-streptococcal GN).
- Complement C3, C4 (post-streptococcal GN, mesangiocapillary GN (MCGN), SLE).
- Antinuclear antibody (ANA), (screening for SLE).
- Abdominal X-ray (renal calculi, nephrocalcinosis).
- Renal ultrasound (structural abnormalities, stones, etc.).
- Sickle screen (sickle cell disease).
- Schistosomiasis serology (schistosomiasis infection).

DIFFERENTIAL DIAGNOSIS

It is important to remember that blood in urine may come from somewhere other than the urinary tract, e.g. vaginal haemorrhage, rectal fissure or contamination by the child or another person (such as in Münchausen syndrome by proxy).

Not everything staining the urine pink, brown or red is haematuria.

Urine dipstick tests for haematuria are very sensitive and will also be positive in the presence of haemaglobinuria and myoglobinuria. Dyes and foodstuffs (e.g. beetroot, blackberries) can colour the urine pink/red. Urates in the urine of neonates may also stain the nappy pink. Drugs (e.g. rifampicin, phenothiazines, phenolphthalein) and porphyria may also discolour the urine.

TREATMENT/ DISPOSITION

- Treatment of patients presenting to ED with haematuria will obviously depend on clinical factors such as the presence or absence of hypertension, anaemia, problems of fluid balance and fluid distribution and pain or discomfort. Biochemical, haematological and imaging results may also be important.
- Whatever the ED management, however, all cases of haematuria should be followed up by the family doctor, a paediatrician or paediatric nephrologist (as appropriate).

FURTHER READING

Andreoli SP 1999 Management of acute renal failure. In: Barratt TM, Avner ED, Harmon WE (eds) Pediatric nephrology, 4th edn. Lippincott, Williams & Wilkins, Baltimore, 1119–1134

Leticia UT, Fildes RD 1990 Hematuria and proteinuria. In: Barakat AY (ed) Renal disease in children – clinical evaluation & diagnosis. Springer-Verlag, New York, 133–156

Royal Children's Hospital – Melbourne Clinical Practice Guidelines – Haematuria. http://www.rch.unimelb.edu.au/clinicalguide/index.cfm?doc_id=S033. Last accessed 2004

Willis FR, Geelhoed GC 2002 Haematuria. In Management guidelines - Emergency Department. Princess Margaret Hospital for Children, Perth, Western Australia

16.3 HYPERTENSION

FRANK WILLIS

ESSENTIALS

1 Hypertension is blood pressure that is consistently above the 95th percentile.

2 Severe hypertension is blood pressure that is consistently above the 99th percentile (i.e. 1% of children).

3 All hypertension should be investigated.

4 The most common secondary cause is renal disease.

5 Accelerated hypertension with encephalopathy is an emergency.

6 In malignant hypertension blood pressure should be lowered slowly.

7 Borderline hypertension is of uncertain significance, but needs follow-up.

INTRODUCTION

In children, blood pressure (BP) is a continuous variable that is influenced by age, sex, body size, genetic, circadian and environmental factors.

Hypertension is defined as BP that is consistently above the 95th percentile for age, gender and height (nomograms are available with this data and should be present in both the emergency department (ED) and paediatric wards) (see Table 16.3.1).

Severe hypertension is BP consistently above the 99th centile with signs of end-organ damage such as retinopathy, nephropathy or left ventricular hypertrophy.

Accelerated hypertension occurs with severe hypertension and neurological signs and symptoms (hypertensive encephalopathy) plus severe hypertensive retinopathy.

Prevalence of hypertension is around 1–3% of children (note that this is a statistical issue related to use of BP centiles in defining hypertension). The most common secondary cause of hypertension in children is renal disease, though with increasing age (and the pandemic of childhood obesity) essential hypertension assumes more significance.

Ideally, all children presenting to ED should have a BP measurement.

Table 16.3.1 Upper limit of systolic blood pressure by age

Age	Upper limit for normal systolic BP (95th percentile)	
	Males	Females
1 month	104	102
2 months	109	106
3 months	111	108
4 months	110	109
6 months	110	110
1 year	110	110
2 years	110	110
3 years	111	110
4 years	112	111
5 years	113	112
6 years	115	114
7 years	117	116
8 years	118	117
9 years	120	119
10 years	122	121
11 years	124	123
12 years	127	125
13 years	129	128
14 years	130	129
15 years	133	130
16 years	136	131

Data obtained with permission from the National Heart, Lung and Blood Institute of the United States National Institutes of Health.

HISTORY AND EXAMINATION

History

Ask about signs or symptoms of underlying disease, urinary tract infection (UTI), drugs, family history of renal disease or hypertension (essential or otherwise).

Non-specific signs and symptoms of hypertension in infants may include vomiting, irritability, respiratory distress, failure to thrive and congestive heart failure.

In older children, also consider polyuria, polydipsia, fatigability, headache, epistaxis, chest pain, abdominal pain and neurological abnormalities such as Bell's palsy or impaired vision. Enquire regarding any noted deterioration in school performance and/or change in personality, as these can be seen in chronic hypertension.

Examination

Measurement of BP is 'classically' performed using a mercury sphygmomanometer, with the largest possible cuff (do not be misled by labels on cuffs). The inflatable part should encircle the arm and the width should cover 75% of the length of the upper arm.

Increasingly, oscillometric BP machines (e.g. Dinamap™) are routinely used in EDs and elsewhere. Automated devices need regular service and calibration. Elevated measurements should be confirmed with a mercury sphygmomanometer.

BP should be checked in both arms and at least one leg to exclude the possibility of aortic coarctation. BP should be repeated after an interval to exclude 'white coat' hypertension.

Ambulatory blood pressure monitoring is available for children and is a useful method of further evaluating BP as well as for monitoring treatment effects.

Feel all pulses. As well as a thorough general examination, physical assessment following identification of elevated BP should consider specifically: presence or absence of encephalopathy, growth, hydration, signs of chronic disease and presence of abdominal masses or bruits (cardiac, cranial and abdominal). The optic fundi must be visualised specifically looking for papilloedema and vascular changes.

INVESTIGATIONS

Investigations to be considered in ED

- Full blood count, electrolytes, urea and creatinine, liver function tests (LFTs), calcium, phosphate, magnesium, alkaline phosphatase.
- Urinalysis by dipstick for protein and blood.
- Urine microscopy and culture.
- Urine catecholamines.
- Chest X-ray, electrocardiogram (ECG) and echocardiography.
- Abdominal and renal ultrasound scan, including grey-scale sonography to identify parenchymal and collecting system disease and tumours, colour and duplex Döppler sonography to identify vessel disease.
- Plasma renin and aldosterone (refer to lab regarding collection).
- Complement C3, C4, anti-nuclear antibody (ANA).
- Drug screen, (e.g. amphetamines).
- Cranial CT scan.

Subsequent investigations will depend on results of preliminary investigations and on the underlying diagnosis.

CAUSES

There are many possible causes of hypertension:

Renal
- Reflux nephropathy.
- Obstructive uropathy.
- Glomerulonephritis.
- Haemolytic uraemic syndrome.
- Nephrotic syndrome.
- Renal artery stenosis.
- Renal vein thrombosis.
- Acute and chronic renal failure.
- Polycystic disease.
- Renal tumours.
- Renal dysplasia.

Endocrine
- Catecholamine excess (neuroblastoma, phaeochromocytoma).
- Corticosteroid excess (congenital adrenal hyperplasia).
- Hyperthyroidism.

Vascular
- Aortic coarctation.
- Arteriovenous fistula.
- Takayasu arteritis.
- SLE.

Metabolic
- Diabetes.
- Porphyria.
- Hypercalcaemia.

Neurological
- Guillain–Barré syndrome.
- Raised intracranial pressure.

Drugs
- Steroids.
- Oral contraceptives.
- Stimulant medications (methylphenidate and dexamphetamine).
- Recreational drugs.
- Liquorice.

Toxins
- Heavy metals.

Miscellaneous
- Anxiety and pain.
- Burns.
- Essential hypertension.

TREATMENT

Hypertensive encephalopathy

Treatment for encephalopathy/accelerated hypertension is urgent. The blood pressure should be treated before proceeding with investigation of the underlying cause. Such patients should be discussed with a paediatric intensivist and nephrologist and will generally be admitted to PICU.

Aim initially for 25% reduction towards target BP (upper limit of normal systolic – see Table 16.3.1) in the first 12–24 hours, then the reduction should be slow, over 24–48 hours. Neglecting to lower the blood pressure can lead to permanent disability or death. Lowering the blood pressure to normal acutely is also contraindicated, because a rapid drop in blood pressure to normal can produce tissue ischaemia. This may manifest as shock (despite normal to slightly elevated blood pressure values), encephalopathy leading to cerebral injury, retinopathy or optic nerve infarction leading to blindness, hypoventilation and apnoea.

Peripheral vasodilators
- IV nitroprusside infusion. Starting dose $1\ \mu g\ kg^{-1}\ min^{-1}$, increment by $1\ \mu g\ kg^{-1}\ min^{-1}$ every 5–10 minutes to maximum $5\ \mu g\ kg^{-1}\ min^{-1}$. Beware of cyanide toxicity above this dose, or with lower doses in renal failure. Check a plasma thiocyanate level every twelve hours. Half-life is very short.
- IV nitroglycerine infusion. Starting dose $1\ \mu g\ kg^{-1}\ min^{-1}$, increment by $1\ \mu g\ kg^{-1}\ min^{-1}$ every 5–10 minutes to maximum $5\ \mu g\ kg^{-1}\ min^{-1}$. Half-life is very short.
- IV hydralazine. $100–200\ \mu g\ kg^{-1}$ IV bolus followed by $4–6\ \mu g\ kg^{-1}\ min^{-1}$ infusion.
- IV clonidine. $3–6\ \mu g\ kg^{-1}$ as slow injection followed by $0.5–2\ \mu g\ kg^{-1}\ h^{-1}$ infusion. Clonidine is a centrally acting vasodilator acting on spinal cord α_2-receptors.

Avoid diazoxide because it has a too rapid, large and sustained effect.

Beta-blockers
- IV labetalol infusion. Starting dose $1\ mg\ kg^{-1}\ h^{-1}$, increment by $0.25–0.5\ mg\ kg^{-1}\ h^{-1}$ (to maximum $3\ mg\ kg^{-1}\ h^{-1}$) every 30 minutes until desired rate of reduction in BP is achieved. Monitor BP every fifteen

minutes initially. Half-life is approx four hours and not altered in chronic renal insufficiency. Be aware of negative inotropic and chronotropic effect in patients with cardiac failure or bradycardia, and risk of asthma exacerbation. Lower acceptable limit of heart rate is 120 in neonate, 100 in children up to three years, 80 in children 3–10 years, 60 in children > 10 years old.

- IV esmolol infusion. Starting dose 200 μg kg^{-1} min^{-1}, increment by 50 μg kg^{-1} min^{-1} every 5–10 minutes to maximum 1000 μg kg^{-1} min^{-1}. Half-life is very short – only a few minutes because of plasma esterase metabolism.

Beta-blockers and vasodilators may be used in combination. Beta-blockers and calcium channel blockers together are absolutely contraindicated. The combination is severely negatively inotropic.

Diuretics

In situations of clinical fluid overload, diuretics can be helpful. Furosemide 0.5–1 mg kg^{-1} IV bolus, which may be repeated after four hours, is first choice. If no response in patients with renal failure, try 2 mg kg^{-1}, then 5 mg kg^{-1} infusion over one hour once only. Avoid inducing hypovolaemia.

Less severe hypertension and oral management after control of malignant hypertension

When target blood pressure is reached, nitroprusside can be slowly withdrawn and other intravenous agents replaced by oral drugs as follows. Oral antihypertensive agents should be used to treat less severe hypertension because of their slower and more sustained effect. Drugs that may be used include:

Vasodilators

- Calcium channel blockers. Oral or sublingual nifedipine, initial dose 0.25 mg kg^{-1}, then 0.5–1.5 mg kg^{-1} d^{-1} in 3–4 doses. Amlodipine 0.05–0.3 mg kg^{-1} d^{-1}.
- Angiotensin converting enzyme (ACE) inhibitors. Captopril, initial test dose

---

CONTROVERSIES AND FUTURE DIRECTIONS

❶ Significance of borderline hypertension.

❷ Routine or selective BP measurement in paediatric EDs.

❸ Obesity and blood pressure in paediatric populations.

❹ Pharmacology and pharmacokinetics of antihypertensive drugs in children.

❺ Speed of reduction in hypertensive encephalopathy/accelerated hypertension.

❻ The role of ambulatory BP measurements.

❼ CT and MR angiography to identify small intrarenal vessel disease.

❽ Angiotensin converting enzyme inhibitor renography to identify small vessel disease.

❾ Assessment of the impact of rigorous treatment of hypertension in childhood on the later development of vascular disease, stroke, renal disease and congestive heart failure.

❿ Evaluation of the role of dietary salt intake in childhood on the development of hypertension.

⓫ Further evaluation of ambulatory BP monitoring in childhood.

⓬ Further evaluation of the genetic factors and the link with obesity and insulin resistance.

⓭ The role of newer angiotensin II inhibitor and angiotensin converting enzyme inhibitor drugs.

0.1 mg kg^{-1}, then 0.3–4 mg kg^{-1} d^{-1} Be aware that ACE inhibitors may decrease intrarenal blood flow and induce or worsen renal failure

- Angiotensin II receptor (AT$_1$) blockers, e.g. losartan 0.5–2 mg kg^{-1} as a once-daily dose.
- Clonidine, 1–6 μg kg^{-1} 8-hourly.

Beta-blockers

- Metoprolol, initial dose 1 mg kg^{-1} 12-hourly, incrementing to 2.5 mg kg^{-1}.
- Atenolol, initial dose 1 mg kg^{-1} 12–24-hourly, incrementing to 2 mg kg^{-1} 12-hourly.

NB. Where available, local guidelines should be referred to when using antihypertensive agents, especially when given by the IV route. Early consultation (as appropriate) with a paediatric intensivist or nephrologist is wise.

Treatment is less urgent in severe hypertension (without encephalopathy), but such patients should be admitted for

---

investigation and treatment. Early liaison with the admitting consultant is prudent.

What to do about borderline hypertension is less clear, though such children should be referred for follow-up by a paediatrician or paediatric nephrologist.

FURTHER READING

Flynn JT 2001 What's new in pediatric hypertension. Current Hypertension Report 3: 503–510

Julius S 1978 Clinical and physiological significance of borderline hypertension in youth. Paediatric Clinics of North America 25: 35–45

Mouin GS, Arant BS 1990 Hypertension. In: Barakat AY (ed) Renal disease in children – clinical evaluation and diagnosis. Springer-Verlag, New York, 307–328

Report of the second task force on blood pressure control in children 1987 Paediatrics 79: 1–25

Report of the task force on blood pressure control in children 1977 Paediatrics 59: 797–820

Rocchini AP 2002 Pediatric hypertension 2001. Current Opinion in Cardiology 17: 385–389 [review]

Sorof JM, Portman RJ 2000 White coat hypertension in children with elevated casual blood pressure. Journal of Paediatrics 137: 493–497

Vogt BA 2001 Hypertension in children and adolescents. Current Therapeutics Research Clinical Experiments 62: 283–297

Wells TG 1999 Trials of antihypertensive therapies in children. Blood Pressure Monitor 4: 189–192

APPENDIX

Age-specific percentiles of BP measurements

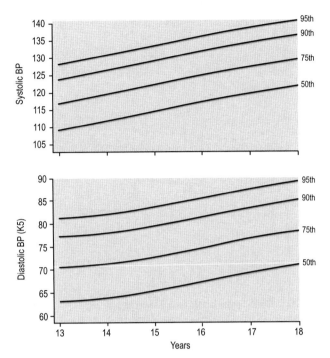

Fig. 16.3.1   Boys 13–18 years of age.

Fig. 16.3.2   Boys 1–13 years of age.

Fig. 16.3.3   Boys from birth to 12 months of age.

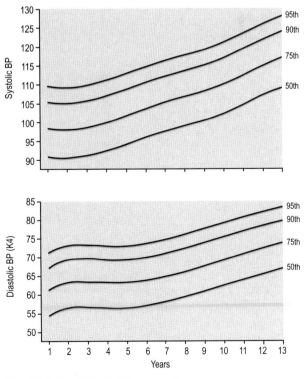

Fig. 16.3.4   Girls 1–13 years of age.

16.3.5   Girls 13–18 years of age.

16.3.6   Girls from birth to 12 months of age.

16.4 URINARY TRACT INFECTION IN PRE-SCHOOL CHILDREN

FRANK WILLIS

ESSENTIALS

1 Urinary tract infection is common and potentially serious.

2 Septicaemia may occur in babies.

3 Renal scarring is a serious and potentially preventable complication.

4 Urinary tract infection should be considered in all febrile infants and young children, as well as babies who are non-specifically unwell.

5 In young children, urinary tract infection cannot be diagnosed reliably or excluded on clinical grounds.

6 Dipstick urinalysis is an unreliable method of ruling out and ruling in urinary tract infection, especially in infants.

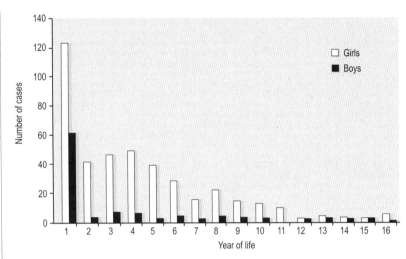

Fig. 16.4.1 Epidemiology of UTI in childhood. Cases recorded in Gothenburg 1960–1966. *Source*: Winberg J et al 1974 Acta Paediatrica Scandinavia Supplement.

INTRODUCTION

Bacterial infection of the urinary tract (UTI) is common in the paediatric age group. Its significance is greatest in young children, particularly in the first year or two of life, where the high incidence of upper tract infection (pyelonephritis) and the presence of immature kidneys lead to significant potential for renal scarring (reflux nephropathy). It is unlikely that new scarring occurs after age five years.

Data from Sweden suggest that in the first two years of life, up to 3% of infants may suffer UTI. Between 1–10 years of age 3–8% of girls and < 1% of boys will have at least one urine infection. It is important to remember that recurrences are common. UTI is more frequent in boys than girls in the first months of life, partly because of a higher incidence of obstruc-

tion including pelviureteric junction obstruction, thereafter occurring significantly more often in girls (see Fig. 16.4.1).

UTI is caused by organisms normally resident in the gut. It is thus an ascending infection that may affect the bladder (cystitis) or upper renal tract (pyelonephritis), which may in turn result in scarring. Neonates are unique in that they may also develop UTI following haematogenous dissemination of organisms.

Renal involvement is associated with:

- Young age (especially < 1 year).
- Symptoms > 5 days.
- Systemic upset, fever, leucocytosis.
- Presence of vesico-ureteric reflux (VUR) or other anatomical abnormality.

Long-term complications of renal scarring include: pregnancy-associated problems; hypertension; and, rarely, chronic renal insufficiency (see prognosis section below).

HISTORY AND EXAMINATION

In infants and young children with UTI, the clinical history is frequently non-

specific and may include irritability, jaundice (neonates), poor feeding or fever without apparent source. Symptoms and signs become more specific with increasing age (Table 16.4.1).

Don't forget to obtain a family history of renal tract disease, in particular regarding UTIs, VUR (probably an autosomal dominant condition) and renal impairment.

Physical examination of young children with UTI is often unremarkable or non-specifically abnormal. Septicaemia, however, does occur with UTI in infancy and must be considered in babies up to around six months of age. Fever is the best clinical marker of pyelonephritis in infants with UTI, but is non-specific.

DIAGNOSIS

A reliable urine sample is required to establish the diagnosis of UTI. In older children this is usually accomplished by obtaining a mid-stream sample. Difficulties arise in children too young to have been toilet trained, who are also the group at highest risk for pyelonephritis and renal scarring.

Table 16.4.1	UTI symptoms by age		
Age	0–2 years	2–5 years	5–12 years
Failure to thrive	✓		
Feeding problems	✓		
Screaming	✓		
Irritability	✓		
Diarrhoea	✓	✓	
Vomiting	✓	✓	
Fever	✓	✓	✓
Convulsions	✓		
Haematuria		✓	✓
Urinary frequency		✓	✓
Dysuria		✓	✓
Enuresis		✓	✓
Abdominal pain		✓	✓
Loin pain			✓

Table 16.4.2	Definition of significant bacteriuria
Method of collection	Colony forming unit count (CFU mL^{-1})
Clean catch	$> 10^5$
Catheter	$> 5 \times 10^4$
Suprapubic	> 0

In infants and toddlers, urine bag samples are unreliable (very high false-positive rate) and should not be used. Clean catch samples are more reliable and are the preferred method for non-invasive urine collection. If samples are required urgently, bladder catheterisation is the most reliable method, though those familiar with the technique can consider supra-pubic aspiration (SPA). The yield from SPA is markedly improved by using ultrasound to confirm a full bladder.

Samples should be sent to the laboratory for urinalysis, microscopy and culture. Findings on urinalysis and microscopy supportive of the diagnosis of UTI include presence of all of the following: leucocyte esterase; nitrites; and white blood cells. Organisms may be seen on Gram stain. In centres without 24-hour laboratory services, after-hours samples should be sent using a urine dip-slide.

Dipstick urinalysis may be helpful in making a provisional diagnosis of UTI. However, a negative result does not rule out UTI in infancy. One study showed that urinalysis was normal in 50% of infants < 8 weeks with confirmed UTI. Another study suggested that dipstick urinalysis was a reliable method of ruling out UTI only after age two years.

The traditional definition of pyuria is > 5 white blood cells (WBC) per high-power field (centrifuged urine). Another definition is > 10 WBC mm^{-3} (uncentrifuged urine).

The definition of significant bacteriuria is guided by the method by which the urine specimen was collected (Table 16.4.2) – interpret results in light of history and clinical findings.

TREATMENT

ED treatment recommendations for UTI vary. However, one approach is as follows:

Age < 6 months
- Admit all for IV/IM antibiotics (septicaemia occurs in this age group).
- Admit to medical ward (observation ward only if systemically well).
- If discharged from observation ward, arrange general practitioner (GP) or ED follow-up at 24–48 hours.
- Ensure urine culture and sensitivity results are checked at 48–72 hours.

Age 6–12 months
- If systemically unwell, admit to observation ward or medical ward for IV/IM antibiotics.
- If not systemically unwell, consider single IM/IV dose of ceftriaxone or gentamicin, followed by oral antibiotics.
- Arrange GP or ED follow-up at 24–48 hours.
- Ensure urine culture and sensitivity results are checked at 48–72 hours.

Age > 12 months
- Treat on clinical merits, i.e. admit or allow home, parenteral or oral antibiotics.
- Overnight admission to observation ward for IV/IM antibiotics may be worth considering if unwell.
- Ensure urine culture and sensitivity results are checked at 48–72 hours.

Which antibiotic?
Empirical antibiotic choice should be guided by local sensitivity patterns and antibiotic guidelines. However, consideration may involve the following:

Parenteral treatment (IV/IM)
- Ceftriaxone 25 mg kg^{-1} twice daily IV (may not cover enterococci in young infants);
  or
- Amoxicillin 10–25 mg kg^{-1} 8-hourly IV + gentamicin 7.5 mg kg^{-1} once daily IV/IM.

Oral treatment
- Ampicillin 20 mg kg^{-1} with clavulanic acid 8-hourly, or cefalexin 15 mg kg^{-1} twice daily.

- Co-trimoxazole (1.5–3 mg kg^{-1} trimethoprim) twice daily is generally less good.
- Amoxicillin is not recommended.

Duration of treatment?
- Infants up to 12 months: treat for 10 days at full dose.
- Older children: treat for 7–10 days at full dose.

Management after discharge from ED or observation wards

Arrange a 'proof of cure' urine culture at around ten days after stopping antibiotic.

In pre-school children (both sexes), following the first documented UTI (or if previous UTI not investigated), start low-dose nocturnal prophylactic antibiotics. Co-trimoxazole (because of its long shelf life) and nitrofurantoin are reasonable choices. The dose is 1–2 mg kg^{-1} at night for both drugs (expressed as the trimethoprim component in the case of co-trimoxazole). Trimethoprim suspension is unavailable commercially in Australia, but is a better choice than co-trimoxazole in countries where it is readily obtainable.

A practical note – after the full course of treatment, if any antibiotic is left over, continue this as a *nocte* dose until finished, and then change to a *nocte* dose of the chosen prophylactic antibiotic.

Arrange a renal tract ultrasound, and refer to medical out-patients, hospital UTI clinic or paediatric nephrology clinic (depending on local organisation) all those discharged home from ED/observation wards who have not previously been investigated.

It is generally not necessary to book other imaging studies as consultants will differ in the investigations that they prefer, e.g. micturition cysto-urethrogram (MCUG) and/or dimercapto-succinic acid (DMSA) isotope scan, though this can be expedited by speaking to the consultant or unit to whom the child has been referred.

PROGNOSIS

UTI in pre-school years is often associated with renal damage. Risk factors are

CONTROVERSIES AND FUTURE DIRECTIONS

❶ 'There is no subject in which there is so little uniformity of opinion and so much confusion.' This statement made in 1916 is seemingly just as pertinent in the early 21st century, with many questions about paediatric UTI management still the subject of debate and controversy. On the specific subject of VUR, one author, considering 'the effect of scientific evidence on clinical decision making in children with VUR during the past 40 years' (since its description), suggests that 'reported data have been overlooked in favor of unfounded speculation or clinical tradition'.[4]

❷ Current controversies and areas for potential investigation in paediatric UTI include:
- Parenteral or oral antibiotic treatment.
- Out-patient or in-patient management.
- Post-UTI imaging protocols.
- The role of antibiotic prophylaxis.
- Medical vs. surgical management of vesico-ureteric reflux.
- 'Complementary' therapies such as lactobacillus and bifidus consumption.
- Cranberry juice as prophylaxis.
- Recognition of dysfunctional voiding.
- Recognition of sphincter and detrusor dysynergia.

listed in the introduction to this section. While most children with UTI will not suffer any long-term sequelae, a not insignificant number will do so.

Examples include:
- 10–20% of children with VUR and scars develop hypertension during childhood.[1]
- 34% of adults with reflux nephropathy are hypertensive.[2]
- 30–50% of children with VUR have scarring at initial evaluation.[3]
- 5–15% of end-stage renal disease (ESRD) in adults < 50 years is due to reflux nephropathy.[3]

At least some of these consequences may be preventable by early and effective diagnosis and treatment of UTI in very young children.

PREVENTION

The 'basics' of good fluid intake, regular and complete voiding, avoidance of constipation and proper (front to back) bottom wiping (in toilet-trained females) should be encouraged in order to reduce the likelihood of repeat infections. There is also some evidence of benefit from the regular use of cranberry juice (which

acidifies urine and reduces bladder wall adhesiveness). Prophylactic antibiotics should be considered in cases of VUR in pre-school children, recurrent pyelonephritis, recurrent symptomatic UTI in older children and in pre-school children awaiting renal tract imaging.

REFERENCES

1. Smellie J, Edwards D, Hunter N, Normand IC, Prescod N 1975 Vesico-ureteric reflux and renal scarring. Kidney International Supplement 4: 65–72
2. Malek RS, Svensson J, Neves RJ, Torres VE 1983 Vesicoureteral reflux in the adult. III. Surgical correction: benefits. Journal of Urology 130: 882–886
3. Noe HN 1995 The current status of screening for vesicoureteral reflux. Paediatric Nephrology 9: 638–641
4. Arant BS 2001 Vesicoureteral reflux and evidence-based management. Journal of Paediatrics 139: 620–621

FURTHER READING

Bachur R, Caputo GL 1995 Bacteraemia and meningitis among infants with urinary tract infection. Paediatric Emergency Care 11: 280–284
Crabtree EG, Cabot H 1916 Colon bacillus pyelonephritis: Its nature and possible prevention. Transactions of the Section of Genitourinary Diseases of the American Medical Association 57: 209–217
Crain EF, Gershel JC 1990 Urinary tract infections in febrile infants younger than 8 weeks. Paediatrics 86: 363–367
Doley A, Neligan M 2003 Is a negative dipstick urinalysis good enough to exclude urinary tract infection in paediatric ED patients? Emergency Medicine 15: 77–80

Jakobsson B, Esbjorner E, Hansson S 2000 Minimum incidence and diagnostic rate of first urinary tract infection. Paediatrics 106: 620–621

Kinney AB, Blount M 1979 Effect of cranberry juice on urinary pH. Nursing Research 28: 287–290

Pollack CV, Pollack ES, Andrew ME 1994 Suprapubic bladder aspiration versus urethral catheterization in infants: Success, efficiency and complication rates. Annals of Emergency Medicine 23: 225–230

Shihab ZM. 1990 Urinary tract infection. In: Barakat AY (ed) Renal disease in children – clinical evaluation & diagnosis. Springer-Verlag, New York, 157–170

Sobota AE 1984 Inhibition of bacterial adherence by cranberry juice: Potential for treatment of urinary tract infections. Journal of Urology 131: 1013–1016

Willis FR, Geelhoed GC 2002 Urinary tract infection. In: Management guidelines – Emergency Department, Princess Margaret Hospital for Children, Perth, Western Australia.

16.5 HAEMOLYTIC URAEMIC SYNDROME

KAREN MCCARTHY

ESSENTIALS

1 Diagnosis is based on the presence of microangiopathic haemolytic anaemia, thrombocytopenia and renal impairment.

2 Diarrhoea associated haemolytic uraemic syndrome accounts for 90% of cases.

3 Cornerstone of treatment is careful attention to fluid and electrolyte balance.

4 Most patients with haemolytic uraemic syndrome have some degree of encephalopathy.

5 Hypertension is present in up to 50%.

6 Long-term follow up is necessary.

7 Use of antibiotics should be avoided in children infected with Shiga toxin *Escherichia coli*.

INTRODUCTION

Definition

Haemolytic uraemic syndrome (HUS) is the commonest cause of acute renal failure in infants and young children < 5 years of age in developed countries. There is multisystem involvement in this syndrome, which is characterised by sudden onset of non-immune microangiopathic haemolytic anaemia, thrombocytopenia and acute renal failure. Various degrees of severity occur. One-third of patients are anuric at presentation.

An inherited form, which is transmitted in an autosomal dominant manner, may present in the newborn period.

Epidemiology

The commonest form of HUS in children is the one that occurs following a prodromal illness of acute gastroenteritis with bloody diarrhoea. This diarrhoea-associated haemolytic uraemic syndrome (D+ HUS) accounts for 90% of cases. D+ HUS is most often caused by Shiga toxin (verotoxin) producing *Escherichia coli* (STEC, also called VTEC). Other cytotoxin-producing bacteria such as *Shigella dysenteriae* type 1, *Salmonella typhi* and *Campylobacter* are less common causes of HUS. *Streptococcus pneumoniae* also causes HUS but does so via a completely different mechanism, which involves neuraminidase rather than cytotoxin production.

D+ HUS occurs in epidemics as well as sporadically. Outbreaks can be traced to contaminated food especially under-cooked hamburger and contaminated water.

There are over 100 different serotypes of STEC with different phage typing and subtyping. STEC O157:H7 is the commonest subtype producing disease in North America, the British Isles and Japan. It is rare as a causative agent of HUS in Australia, where other types including O111:H are pathogenic. *E. coli* can be spread by person to person contact. The incubation period to onset of diarrhoea is 1–8 days.

Non-diarrhoeal associated HUS (D– HUS) cases account for 10% of cases. These are secondary to:

- Non-enteric infections, e.g. Streptococcal pneumonia.
- Immunosuppression: malignancy associated, following bone-marrow transplant, and drug-related, e.g. mitomycin, ciclosporin and FK-506 (tacrolimus).
- Immunodeficiency and pregnancy may also be associated with HUS.

Pathophysiology

The primary process in the pathogenesis of HUS is vascular endothelial cell injury. *E. coli* is ingested and colonises the gut. These bacteria attach to the epithelium of the distal ileum and large intestine by complex mechanisms. Cytotoxins are produced and they damage the microvasculature of the intestinal wall causing haemorrhagic and ulcerative intestinal lesions. Once the intestinal–blood barrier has been compromised, the toxins gain entry to the circulation. It is presumed that the toxin then initiates microvascular damage in the glomerular endothelium of the kidneys. Intravascular and intraglomerular fibrin clot is formed and at the same time there is activation of the coagulation system, which leads to occlusion of the vessels and glomerular loss. Erythrocytes passing through these vessels become damaged. Microvascular endothelial cell injury is central to the renal thrombotic microangiopathy that is characteristic of HUS. Thrombocytopenia results from intrarenal platelet adhesion and platelet survival is shortened. Renal dysfunction results from this process.

HISTORY

A child, who has previously been healthy, presents with a history of gastroenteritis within the previous two weeks. There is subsequent development of vomiting, bloody diarrhoea and crampy abdominal pain. The presentation may resemble an acute surgical abdomen. The child then becomes pale and develops haematuria and oliguria and is noted to become lethargic. Not uncommonly, the patient appears to be improving from his/her gastroenteritis but then deteriorates suddenly, becoming quite ill.

EXAMINATION

The child appears pale, lethargic and de-hydrated. Petechiae may be noted on the skin, which may also appear jaundiced.

Most patients have some degree of encephalopathy. Central nervous system involvement can range from irritability and restlessness to seizures or coma. Seizures can be present in up to 40%. Hemiparesis and cranial nerve dysfunction may be seen.

Hypertension is present in up to 50% and is likely secondary to increased renin levels. Evidence of cardiac involvement may present as myocarditis, cardiomyopathy or high-output failure. Oliguria occurs often. Hepatomegaly and oedema develop (reflecting fluid overload) if the oliguria is not recognised and fluid intake is not restricted. Splenomegaly is not as common as hepatomegaly.

INVESTIGATIONS

Diagnosis of HUS is based on the presence of microangiopathic haemolytic anaemia, thrombocytopenia and renal failure.

- Anaemia is usually severe and is normochromic normocytic in type with a haemoglobin level of 50–90 gm L^{-1}.

- White cell count is non-specific and often raised with increased number of immature forms.
- Platelet count is low in 95% and can be as low as 20×10^9 L^{-1}. Subsequent increase in platelet count may be the first indication of resolution of the microangiopathic process.
- Reticulocyte count is mildly elevated.
- Evidence of schistocytes, burr cells and helmet cells on blood film.
- Coombs test is negative – indicating anaemia is not immunologically mediated.
- Coagulation tests are usually normal but may show mild disseminated intravascular coagulation.
- Serum haptoglobin is low, lactic dehydrogenase (LDH) is elevated along with indirect bilirubin level – all indicators of intravascular haemolysis.
- Elevated serum blood urea, creatinine and phosphate reflect renal involvement, occurring at the same time as the urine output is declining and the haemolysis developing.
- High triglycerides.
- High lipase/amylase reflecting pancreatic involvement.
- Low albumin even without nephrosis.
- Electrolyte derangement may result from the renal abnormalities including hyponatraemia, hyperkalaemia, hypocalcaemia and metabolic acidosis (which can be severe).
- Urinalysis shows haematuria that can be gross and the red blood cells are dysmorphic. There can be evidence of proteinuria (mild to severe) and leucocytes. Granular and hyaline casts may be present.

Renal biopsy is rarely indicated in children who have the characteristic features of HUS.

DIFFERENTIAL DIAGNOSIS

- Intussusception.
- Disseminated intravascular coagulation (DIC) in patients with sepsis and multi-organ failure.
- Idiopathic thrombocytopenic purpura (ITP).

- Systemic lupus erythematosus (SLE) with nephropathy.
- Leukaemia.
- Toxic syndromes and encephalitis may have similar presentation.
- Post-infectious glomerulonephritis.

Findings on blood film, coagulation profile, urinalysis, stool and blood cultures assist in differentiating all these conditions from HUS. There is no evidence of haemolysis in intussusception. The complete blood count in leukaemia would reveal low haemoglobin, thrombocytopenia and a white cell count that was depressed or markedly elevated with the presence of blasts.

Patients with DIC have sepsis and prolongation of the prothrombin time and partial thromboplastin time. ITP has isolated thrombocytopenia with a normal coagulation profile.

TREATMENT

There is no specific therapy for Shiga-toxin-producing *E. coli* and prevention of the disease is therefore of utmost importance.

Supportive therapy may include dialysis, antihypertensive therapy, blood transfusions and management of neurological complications. With supportive therapy, 85% of children recover renal function.

Cornerstone of treatment is careful attention to electrolyte and fluid balance. Once intravascular volume has been restored, the amount and type of fluid administered should be limited to ongoing losses, i.e. insensible loss, urine output and gastrointestinal losses.

No added potassium is required unless serum levels are below normal values. Hyperkalaemia must be anticipated and treated in a timely fashion (refer to management of hyperkalaemia in Chapter 10.5 on electrolytes).

Anaemia should be treated with packed red blood cell transfusion (10 mL kg^{-1}) when anaemia is severe, the patient is symptomatic or the haematocrit is falling rapidly. In general an attempt is made to maintain Hb > 70 g L^{-1} when possible.

Platelet transfusion is avoided because of precipitous worsening of patient's clinical status. This results from the aggregation of platelets, which are a major constituent of microthrombi and thus induce further damage. Newly formed platelets in HUS function very well and platelet transfusion is not required, even prior to the surgical insertion of a central venous catheter or peritoneal dialysis catheter.

Hypertension responds well to treatment with short-acting calcium channel blockers, e.g. nifedipine. Intravenous nitroglycerine can be used if oral medication is not tolerated. Nitroprusside is not favoured because of the danger of cyanide poisoning in renal failure. Labetalol by intravenous bolus or continuous infusion can also be used to manage hypertension. See Chapter 16.3. Treatment of hypertension can prevent development of encephalopathy and congestive heart failure.

Seizures should be treated with short-acting benzodiazepines initially, followed by intravenous infusion of phenytoin or phenobarbital.

There is some evidence that early dialysis may improve outcome in HUS. Dialysis should be commenced in the following situations:

- Severe hyperkalaemia uncontrollable by medical means.
- Fluid overload and pulmonary oedema.
- Significant uraemic symptoms.
- Blood urea > 36 mmol L^{-1} even if electrolyte and water balances are satisfactory.
- Anuria.

Peritoneal dialysis is generally used in infants and pre-school age children unless there is evidence of severe colitis or abdominal tenderness is present. This management strategy is dependent on the resources and preferences of the managing team/unit.

There are no controlled clinical trials demonstrating efficacy of antibiotic therapy on the prevention and amelioration of HUS. In fact, the use of antibiotics should be avoided in children infected with Shiga toxin E. coli.

There are no controlled randomised studies on plasmapheresis as treatment for D+ HUS. Plasmapheresis may be beneficial in patients with drug-induced HUS. Vincristine and ciclosporin A are known to cause drug-induced HUS.

Nutritional requirements must be addressed aggressively, as these patients are catabolic and hypoalbuminaemic. Enteral feeds can be commenced once the diarrhoea has settled. Total parenteral nutrition is required in some cases.

No evidence exists for the use of aspirin, heparin, warfarin, streptokinase, urokinase, vitamin E or immunoglobulin G in the treatment of HUS.

PROGNOSIS

Overall prognosis for D+ HUS is better than that for D– HUS. However, long-term prognosis for those D+ HUS who recover, but have persistent proteinuria one year following recovery, is guarded. There is an early mortality rate of about 5%. Another 5% require lifelong dialysis because of the development of chronic renal failure and anuria.

The improved prognosis has resulted from careful correction of electrolyte abnormalities, judicious fluid management and earlier institution of dialysis.

The risk of renal sequelae in children is higher in males, and those with hypertension, prolonged anuria and haemoglobin < 100 g L^{-1} at onset of disease.

Other poor prognostic indicators include:

- Elevated white cell count ($> 20 \times 10^9$ L^{-1}) at presentation.
- Elevated white cell count at presentation, which remains elevated.
- Age < 1 year or > 5 years.
- Central nervous system involvement (seizures, coma, etc.).
- The degree and duration of renal dysfunction.

COMPLICATIONS

Children with D+ HUS should be followed for many years following full recovery as some long-term studies have shown late complications developing in patients who had fully recovered initially. These complications include hypertension, proteinuria, reduced glomerular filtration rate and late development of end-stage renal disease (ESRD). ESRD was shown to develop in 10–15% as late as 15–25 years following recovery.

CONTROVERSIES AND FUTURE DIRECTIONS

❶ In one study a strategy was developed in which a recombinant E. coli was generated that had on its surface a lipolysaccharide (LPS), which mimicked the Shiga toxin receptor. These recombinant E. coli bind to the Shiga toxin thus preventing the binding of Shiga toxin to target cells.

❷ Strategies for immunisation have been explored. The first steps in evaluation of development of a vaccine against Shiga-toxin-producing strains of E. coli have been undertaken in a preclinical study.

❸ An oligovalent water-soluble carbohydrate pentamer with five pairs of trisaccharide ligands linked to a central dendrimer, and called 'Starfish', neutralises all five B subunits of Shiga toxin and protects human cells from Shiga toxin in culture.

❹ Administration of intravenous γ-globulin IgG and gabexate mesilate, a synthetic serine protease inhibitor used as an anticoagulant resulted in amelioration of disease in five children with D+ HUS. The IgG itself has no proven benefit on the course of D+ HUS.

❺ The use of angiotensin-converting enzyme inhibitors in conjunction with controlled intake of protein (to recommended daily allowance) may help preserve renal function in children with persistent proteinuria during the chronic stages of Shiga toxin HUS.

The frequency of complications is higher in D– HUS patients.

HUS can recur in transplanted kidneys regardless of the aetiological agent. Recurrence of disease following renal transplant is infrequent in D+ HUS in comparison with D– HUS.

Occasionally children can be left with chronic sequelae due to HUS, which are not renal related. Almost any organ system can be involved. Stroke is the most serious sequela and occurs in 3–5% of patients. Colitis can result in bowel infarction leading to colostomy/colectomy or stricture formation.

Pancreatitis can develop, sometimes with diabetes, and hepatic involvement can occur.

PREVENTION

D+ HUS is an infectious disease and the most effective prevention strategy would be to prevent ingestion of the *E. coli*. Avoidance of undercooked meat can assist in this area. There are, however, other vectors for the transmission of the *E. coli* and these include contaminated water and beverages. Food handlers, vendors and consumers must be made aware of proper food-handling techniques.

FURTHER READING

Corrigan JJ Jr, Boineau F 2001 Hemolytic uremic syndrome. Pediatrics in Review 22: 365–368
Cronan K, Norman M 2000 Renal and electrolyte emergencies. In: Fleisher GR, Ludwig S (eds)
Textbook of pediatric emergency medicine, 4th edn. Lippincott, Williams & Wilkins, Philadelphia, Chapter 86, 847–848
Elliott EJ, Robins-Browne RM, O'Loughlin EV et al 2001 Nationwide study of haemolytic uraemic syndrome: Clinical, microbiological, and epidemiological features. Archives of Disease in Childhood 85: 125–131
Kaplan B, Meyers K 1998 The pathogenesis of hemolytic uremic syndrome. Journal of American Society of Nephrology 9: 1126–1133
Ray P, Liu X 2001 Pathogenesis of Shiga toxin-induced hemolytic uremic syndrome. Pediatric Nephrology 16: 823–839
Ring GH, Lakkis FG, Badr KF 2000 Microvascular diseases of the kidney. In: Brenner B (ed) The kidney, 6th edn. Vol. 2. WB Saunders, Philadelphia, Chapter 35, 1597–1603
Siegler RL 1995 The hemolytic uremic syndrome. Pediatric Clinics of North America 42(6): 1505–1522
Stewart CL, Tina LU 1993 Hemolytic uremic syndrome. Pediatrics in Review 14(6): 218–224
Trachtman H, Christen E 1999 Pathogenesis, treatment and therapeutic trials in hemolytic uremic syndrome. Current Opinion in Pediatrics 11: 162–168

16.6 NEPHROTIC SYNDROME

KAREN MCCARTHY

ESSENTIALS

1 Hypoalbuminaemia occurs in every child with nephrotic syndrome.

2 Despite the presence of oedema, shock still needs to be treated with 20 mL kg^{-1} 0.9% saline or albumin boluses.

3 Renal function is usually normal though serum creatinine may be slightly elevated at presentation.

4 There is 1–2% mortality despite good long-term prognosis.

5 The physical findings of peritonitis in nephrotic syndrome may be very subtle, thus the emergency physician must have a very high index of suspicion for peritonitis.

6 Death from peritonitis and thrombosis can occur despite very good care.

7 All non-immune children on steroid therapy, who are exposed to varicella, require prompt administration of zoster immune globulin.

INTRODUCTION

Definition

Nephrotic syndrome (NS) refers to the findings of hypoalbuminaemia, oedema and hyperlipidaemia, which result from a massive loss of protein in the urine sec-ondary to glomerular disease. All components of the disease do not need to be present for diagnosis. The protein lost in the urine includes plasma proteins of molecular weight up to and including albumin. Generalised glomerular leak to macromolecules does not occur in most cases, but can occur in severe disease. In severe disease, as there is progressive loss of glomerular permselectivity, renal clearance of IgG approaches that of albumin even though it is a larger molecule. Clearance of anionic macromolecules is increased whilst that of neutral macromolecules is unchanged. This, along with other evidence, suggests that this selective proteinuria results from a loss of the fixed negative charges of anionic glycosaminoglycans in the glomerular capillary wall. Protein selectivity is seen mainly in minimal change nephrotic syndrome. The determination of protein selectivity has little clinical value but does increase the likelihood of response to steroid therapy.

The hallmarks of nephrotic syndrome are hypoalbuminaemia (serum albumin < 30 g L^{-1}), heavy proteinuria (> 50 mg kg^{-1} body weight per 24 hours, or > 1000 mg m^{-2} per 24 hours), generalised oedema and hyperlipidaemia (triglycerides and cholesterol).

Primary nephrotic syndrome (idiopathic) represents disease limited to the kidney. Disease is classified by responsiveness to steroid therapy (steroid sensitive, steroid dependent or steroid resistant) and histology on renal biopsy (minimal change, mesangial proliferative GN and focal segmental glomerulosclerosis, FSGS).

Secondary nephrotic syndrome represents multisystem disease that has kidney involvement, e.g. lupus nephritis, hereditary nephritis and Henoch–Schönlein purpura.

Certain drugs and chemicals can cause nephrotic syndrome, e.g. phenytoin, non-steroidal anti-inflammatory drugs, and captopril.

Epidemiology

Minimal change nephrotic syndrome (MCNS) is more common in males. Mean age of onset is < 6 years for primary nephrotic syndrome, and > 6 years for secondary. It is usually sporadic. A congenital form, inherited in an autosomal recessive manner, presents in the newborn period.

Aetiology

The cause of primary nephrotic syndrome is unknown and hence is referred to as idiopathic. The commonest form is minimal change disease (85%). Renal biopsy findings in this form show no abnormality of the glomeruli on light microscopy. Electron microscopy shows effacement of the epithelial foot processes. Biopsy findings of focal segmental sclerosis (10%) reveal normal appearing glomeruli but may show some mesangial proliferation. Some biopsy specimens may demonstrate segmental scarring. Mesangial proliferative disease (5%) shows diffuse increase in mesangial cells and matrix on biopsy.

PATHOPHYSIOLOGY

An immune basis for MCNS was proposed in 1974 but no primary immune abnormality has been identified. Studies have shown increased levels of circulating soluble interleukin-2 receptor in patients with active MCNS and FSGS. This soluble interleukin-2 receptor is shed by activated lymphocytes and may therefore indicate generalised activation of the immune system. However, this circulating

soluble interleukin-2 receptor could serve as a neutraliser of circulating interleukin-2. It is unknown whether circulating levels represent evidence of activation or an attempt to down-regulate the immune responses.

There is hypercoagulability resulting from serum protein abnormalities introduced by renal protein wasting. All children with acute NS have increased platelet aggregation. Blood viscosity is increased and blood flow is reduced. Fibrinogen concentration is increased and antithrombin III is lost in the urine. All these factors contribute to this problem in NS.

Cause of cholesterolaemia and hypertriglyceridaemia remains uncertain. One theory is that reduced plasma oncotic pressure may stimulate lipoprotein synthesis and perhaps lipolytic factors may be lost in the urine.

Oedema reflects retention of salt and water. Reduced serum albumin causes a reduction in plasma oncotic pressure. When plasma oncotic pressure falls, intravascular volume is reduced, which stimulates proximal tubular reabsorption of sodium. The renin-angiotensin system is also stimulated, raising the serum aldosterone, which further increases distal tubular reabsorption of sodium. There is an increase in filtration capacity in patients with nephrotic syndrome along with an increase in glomerular permeability, resulting in proteinuria.

There is also evidence in some patients for primary salt and water retention by the kidney.

HISTORY

The presence of the following may be noted on history:

- Recent flu-like illness.
- Anorexia.
- Abdominal pain.
- Diarrhoea.
- Recent ant bites or bee stings.

EXAMINATION

Periorbital oedema is noted initially, but in time oedema becomes generalised.

Oedema of the lower extremities is usually 'pitting' in type and accumulates in dependent sites. The rate and degree of oedema formation is directly related to salt intake and to the degree of hypoalbuminaemia and therefore can vary from child to child. Ascites may be present. Pleural effusions or pulmonary oedema may develop. Scrotal or perineal oedema may be very distressing to the patient. Blood pressure may be decreased when hypovolaemia exists or may be elevated if there is significant renal disease by activation of the renin-angiotensin system or primary salt retention.

INVESTIGATIONS

- Hypoalbuminaemia (serum albumin < 30 g L^{-1}) occurs in every child with nephrotic syndrome.
- Reliably timed 24-hour urine collections are difficult to obtain in children (protein excretion exceeds 50 mg kg^{-1} per 24 hours or 1000 mg m^{-2} per 24 hours in nephrotic syndrome), so the proteinuria is generally quantified by the ratio of urine protein to urine creatinine. Spot urine protein:creatinine ratio is > 300 mg mmol^{-1} in nephrotic syndrome. Normal is < 20 mg mmol^{-1} and is mostly albumin.
- Microscopic haematuria is seen in < 15% but macroscopic haematuria is rare.
- Urinalysis by dipstick reveals + 3 or + 4 proteinuria.
- Urine specific gravity is usually high at > 1.020, but may be lower.
- Haematocrit is often elevated due to intravascular depletion and can be followed to assess fluid status.
- Hyperlipidaemia is present with elevated serum cholesterol and triglyceride levels.
- Serum sodium can be low but is rarely symptomatic and does not require treatment. Total body sodium is high.
- Hypocalcaemia is a common finding and reflects the low serum albumin. The ionized calcium is usually normal, however, and the hypocalcaemia is asymptomatic.

- Plasma urea and creatinine are elevated in approximately 25% of patients.
- Serum complement levels are normal in MCNS, FSGS and mesangial proliferative glomerulonephritis.

Steroids can be used as a diagnostic tool in the management of NS. The patient is said to be steroid responsive when the urine becomes free of protein. If the child continues to have proteinuria (> 2 +) after 4–8 weeks of compliance with continuous daily divided-dose prednisone, the nephrosis is termed steroid resistant and renal biopsy is indicated to determine the precise cause, e.g. FSGS.

Renal biopsy is not indicated during the initial episode of acute nephrotic syndrome. The need for, and timing of a renal biopsy is determined by the subsequent disease course, e.g. poor or no response of initial episode to steroid therapy after 4–8 weeks of treatment or if other signs or symptoms are present that indicate a systemic disease.

DIFFERENTIAL DIAGNOSIS

Other causes of oedema need to be excluded: congestive heart failure; starvation; protein-losing enteropathy; cystic fibrosis; hypothyroidism; vasculitis; and steroid therapy.

TREATMENT

- It can be difficult to assess volume status in patients with NS. The patient may be in shock despite the presence of oedema. Attention to detail on clinical examination can assist with the assessment. Clues to hypovolaemia are: tachycardia; peripheral vasoconstriction with poor capillary refill time; and orthostatic hypotension, i.e. positive tilt test. Other clues to volume status include a history of oliguria and evidence of renal insufficiency on laboratory investigations.
- Albumin infusions transiently increase plasma volume and are most useful in patients with profound volume depletion. Plasma volume is increased

using 4% albumin rather than 0.9% saline. It is important to note that this is only a temporising measure. The infused albumin is rapidly lost in the urine, especially when the original albumin level is very low because of high renal albumin clearance (rate of loss is proportional to albumin clearance and serum albumin level). The patient can develop acute pulmonary oedema requiring admission to an intensive-care unit.

- In a patient symptomatic from massive oedema, a trial of diuretics may be given, provided the patient is not hypovolaemic, and only after discussion with a nephrologist. Diuretics may induce hypotension, severe volume depletion, ARF and hyperkalaemia if there is already incipient hypovolaemia. An infusion of 20% salt-deficient albumin 0.5–1 g kg^{-1}, followed 30 minutes later by frusemide 0.5–1 mg kg^{-1} IV can be effective. In occasional circumstances, ultrafiltration or haemofiltration may be used to manage fluid overload.
- The natriuretic effect of furosemide is thought to be diminished in nephrotic syndrome. Increasing the dose or using furosemide in combination with a diuretic acting at another site such as a thiazide diuretic (hydrochlorothiazide 1 mg kg^{-1} d^{-1} in two divided doses) is recommended to overcome the hyporesponsiveness. Metolazone (diuretic activity on the distal tubule) is a powerful diuretic and is occasionally employed but must be used with caution. If serum albumin is < 15 g L^{-1}, diuretic therapy is ineffective.
- Oral fluids, when offered, should be given in small aliquots, especially in hyponatraemic patients in whom any free water will tend to lower the plasma sodium further.
- Therapeutic paracentesis may be indicated for acute respiratory distress but is rarely necessary. Respiratory distress is due to reduced lung capacity secondary to the increased abdominal pressure. Paracentesis should only be used when there is no other way to support respiration because of the

association of complications with the procedure, e.g. infection and the re-accumulation of the fluid.

- Prednisolone is started at 2 mg kg^{-1} d^{-1} (60 mg m^{-2} d^{-1}) in two divided doses. Divided dose is used in preference to single dose as some children who fail to respond to single daily dose, respond to divided doses. Disappearance of proteinuria is seen in 90% within 4–6 weeks.
- If the child is unwell or peritonitis is suspected, antibiotics are commenced after appropriate cultures are taken. Prophylactic antibiotics are generally recommended for all patients whilst nephrotic and on high-dose steroids.
- Some units advocate routine use of low-dose aspirin, though this is not commonly done.
- Angiotensin-converting enzyme (ACE) inhibitors are good antihypertensive drugs in those patients who have hypertension from their primary disease or as a result of steroid therapy. ACE inhibitors are useful as most of the hypertension is due to activation of the renin–angiotensin system. If the hypertension is a result of steroid therapy, the patient may respond better to a β-blocker.
- Some children with minimal change nephrotic syndrome (MCNS) who are steroid-responsive either relapse frequently or require high daily dose of steroids to maintain remission. These children are at risk of development of serious side effects from the steroids including growth failure, hypertension, osteoporotic bone disease and posterior sublenticular cataracts. The alkylating agents cyclophosphamide or chlorambucil can produce prolonged and sometimes permanent remission and are considered to be 'steroid-sparing'. These alkylating agents are not commonly needed in patients with MCNS but when needed they are very effective. Some patients with MCNS may not respond to the alkylating agents and will respond to ciclosporin (< 5.5 mg kg^{-1} per 24 hours or < 200 mg m^{-2} per

24 hours) if there is steroid responsiveness. Dependence on ciclosporin is common, the effect lasting only as long as treatment continues. Some nephrologists consider the limited risk of ciclosporin nephrotoxicity in this population to be preferable to the side effects of chronic steroid toxicity or the risk of sterility from a second alkylating agent when one course of an alkylating agent is insufficient therapy.

- In focal segmental glomerulosclerosis (FSGS) ciclosporin is more effective in steroid-dependent rather than in steroid-resistant disease and may even be more nephrotoxic in this latter group.
- Whilst on steroid therapy, non-immune children exposed to chicken-pox require prompt administration of zoster immune globulin.
- Immunisations: Live-virus vaccines should not be administered to children on high-dose corticosteroid therapy. Children receiving < 2 mg kg^{-1} per 24 hours of prednisolone or its equivalent, can be immunised. Those children receiving > 2 mg kg–1 per 24 hours daily or alternate daily prednisolone or its equivalent for more than 14 days, should have live-virus vaccine administration deferred for at least one month after discontinuation of the steroids.

DISPOSITION

Out-patient management is appropriate for children with the first presentation of nephrotic syndrome, if the oedema is not massive and there is no suspicion of infection or life-threatening complications and the physician can be assured of close follow-up. The rest are best managed as in-patients to permit further work-up and treatment and to provide education and support for the patient and family.

Admission is warranted in a child with known history of nephrotic syndrome if there are signs of severe dehydration, unexplained fever, renal insufficiency (i.e. elevation in serum creatinine), refractory oedema (e.g. respiratory distress) or suspected peritonitis. Discuss admission of frequent relapsers, or > 1st relapse, with the nephrologist.

PROGNOSIS

Long-term prognosis is good for children with steroid-responsive primary nephrotic syndrome, though 1–2% mortality is associated. Most deaths are due to peritonitis or sepsis (pneumonia), and thrombus, which may occur despite good care. Relapses may recur for many years, often until puberty, with a small number continuing to relapse through to adulthood. These relapses are not usually severe and can be treated with short courses of oral steroids. Though these children with steroid-responsive disease may require steroid therapy intermittently throughout childhood, serious sequelae of steroid toxicity are uncommon.

When in remission, the child should have unrestricted diet and activity.

Recovery is considered permanent if the child remains asymptomatic and has no requirement for medications for more than two years.

COMPLICATIONS

As MCNS is a self-limited disease in most children, a distinction must be made between the complications of the disease itself and those that are related to the treatment. Major complications of the disease itself are infection and thrombosis.

Acute complications occur in two groups of patients:

❶ Those who present de novo or in relapse but not taking steroids.
❷ Those who present in relapse or remission while still receiving pharmacological doses of steroids.

The tendency to develop infections is a true complication of the disease.

Hypogammaglobulinaemia Has been recognized as being a serious manifestation of NS and is a factor in the reduced defences against bacterial infections. IgG is the immunoglobulin most severely depleted. This may be a consequence of it being the smallest of the immunoglobulins and the one with the greatest renal excretion.

Bacterial infections Occur in both groups but are more common in the steroid-treated group.

Spontaneous bacterial peritonitis Is a major source of morbidity in children with nephrotic syndrome. Main causative organisms are *Streptococcus pneumoniae* and *Escherichia coli*. Diagnosis of peritonitis should always be considered in a child with nephrotic syndrome who complains of abdominal pain. The physical findings of peritonitis in NS may be very subtle. The patient does not necessarily have a rigid abdomen. The physician must have a high index of suspicion when assessing these patients. Steroid therapy, especially high dose (2 mg kg^{-1} d^{-1} of prednisolone) can mask the typical signs and symptoms of infection. Children with nephrotic syndrome can develop other infections such as pneumonia, cellulitis and sepsis.

Thromboembolism From hypercoagulability is the second major contributor to morbidity and mortality. The thrombus is usually venous and is located in the deep vessels of the extremities, renal vein, pulmonary venous system and cerebral cortical system. For this reason, it is recommended that femoral or deep venipuncture is avoided if possible in children with nephrotic syndrome. The risk of thromboembolus is real and exists even in the first acute presentation with nephrotic syndrome. This is due to increased platelet aggregation, and in part also due to the urinary loss of several proteins that inhibit blood coagulation, especially antithrombin-III, protein C and protein S. Increased blood viscosity and reduced blood flow also play a role. Renal vein thrombosis should be suspected if flank pain, haematuria and decreased renal function occur. Occlusion of the arterial system is uncommon.

Hyperlipidaemia Associated with nephrotic syndrome rarely gives rise to clinical complications as it usually reverses with steroid therapy. It may become problematic in patients with chronic nephrotic syndrome.

Symptomatic hypovolaemia Despite the presence of oedema, symptomatic hypovolaemia leading to shock can develop if fluids are restricted injudiciously with or without diuretic therapy.

Respiratory compromise Can rarely be caused by massive ascites, warranting emergency paracentesis in some cases.

Hypertensive encephalopathy Acute increase in blood pressure may occur in steroid-treated children at any stage of their illness. The diagnosis of hypertensive encephalopathy is based on the degree of change in the blood pressure and rate of increase rather than on a specific level of systolic and/or diastolic blood pressure.

Benign intracranial hypertension Can be precipitated by abrupt reduction in steroid doses.

Growth Can be impaired in nephrotic syndrome. Insulin-like growth factor (IGF-1)-binding protein is lost in the urine, which may account for the reduced serum levels of IGF-1 and IGF-2. Growth impairment is also a consequence of steroid therapy.

PREVENTION

As the primary causes of idiopathic nephrotic syndrome are unknown, there is no means of prevention.

CONTROVERSIES AND FUTURE DIRECTIONS

❶ The effect of co-administration of frusemide and albumin in the treatment remains controversial.

❷ The role and risks of albumin infusion.

❸ Angiotensin-converting enzyme (ACE) inhibitors and angiotensin-2 receptor antagonists (ARBs) reduce proteinuria in experimental models of NS as well as in some patients with NS.

❹ Cyclooxygenase inhibitors are a class of drugs that may be of assistance in reducing proteinuria in patients with NS, although unlike ACE inhibitors, they generally cause a reduction in GFR.

There is some evidence supporting a role of the immune system in paediatric minimal change disease. Relapses can be triggered by minor infections.

There is no clear data recommending against immunisation in general. Vaccination against varicella, influenza and pneumococcus would seem prudent, given the relapsing nature of nephrotic syndrome. Some susceptibility to infection may result from loss of opsonising factors in the urine so even if the child has been immunised, vigilance is warranted against the possibility of any bacterial infection.

FURTHER READING

Akcicek F, Yalniz T et al 1995 Diuretic effect of frusemide in patients with nephrotic syndrome – is it potentiated by intravenous albumin? British Medical Journal 310: 162–163

Bergstein J 2000 Conditions particularly associated with proteinuria. In: Behrman R, Kliegman R, Jenson H (eds) Nelson's textbook of pediatrics, 16th edn, WB Saunders, Philadelphia, 1592–1596

Chesney RW 1999 The idiopathic nephrotic syndrome. Current Opinion in Paediatrics 11: 158–161

Cronan K, Norman M 2000 Renal and electrolyte emergencies. In: Fleisher G, Ludwig S (eds) Textbook of pediatric emergency medicine, 4th edn. Lippincott Williams & Wilkins, Philadelphia, 832–835

Falk RJ, Charles Jennette J, Nachman PH 2000 Nephrotic syndrome. In: Brenner B (ed) The kidney, Vol. 2, 6th edn. WB Saunders, Philadelphia, 1266–1283

Fliser D, Zurbruggen I et al 1999 Co-administration of albumin and furosemide in patients with the nephrotic syndrome. Kidney International 55: 629–634

Grimbert P, Audard V et al 2003 Recent approaches to the pathogenesis of minimal-change nephrotic syndrome. Nephrology, Dialysis and Transplantation 18: 245–248

Haws RM, Baum M 1993 Efficacy of albumin and diuretic therapy in children with nephrotic syndrome. Pediatrics 91(6): 1142–1146

Kaysen GA 2003 Proteinuria and the nephrotic syndrome. In: Schrier RW (ed) Renal and electrolyte disorders, 6th edn. Lippincott, Williams & Wilkins, Philadelphia, 580–614

Roth KS, Amaker BH et al 2002 Nephrotic syndrome: Pathogenesis and management. Pediatrics in Review 23: 237–247

Schnapner HW 1996 Primary nephrotic syndrome of childhood. Current Opinion in Paediatrics 8: 141–147

Tune BM, Mendoza SA 1997 Treatment of the idiopathic nephrotic syndrome: Regimens and outcomes in children and adults. Journal of the American Society of Nephrology 8: 824–832

16.7 HENOCH-SCHÖNLEIN PURPURA

KAREN MCCARTHY

ESSENTIALS

1 There is no diagnostic laboratory test for the diagnosis of Henoch–Schönlein purpura.

2 A normal platelet count is required for diagnosis.

3 Urinalysis, serum creatinine and blood pressure should be measured at presentation.

4 Clinical hallmark of Henoch–Schönlein nephritis is haematuria.

5 Onset of nephritis may be delayed for weeks or months after onset of other symptoms.

6 All patients with Henoch–Schönlein nephritis need prolonged follow-up.

INTRODUCTION

Henoch–Schönlein purpura (HSP) is the most common acute vasculitis affecting children. It is a leukocytoclastic vasculitis that affects small vessels (arterioles and venules). The disease is more common in males with mean age of occurrence 4–7 years. Infants tend to have milder disease and those less than two years of age are less likely to have nephritis and abdominal pain in comparison with older children. With the exception of nephritis, it is generally an acute self-limited illness lasting from several days to several weeks.

Characteristic histological finding on skin biopsy is neutrophil infiltration in and around dermal vessels. Histological changes in the kidney range from minimal change to focal or diffuse mesangial proliferation that may be accompanied by glomerular crescent formation. Characteristic finding on immunofluorescence is diffuse mesangial deposition of immunoglobulin A (IgA) and complement 3 (C3). IgA plays a central role in the pathogenesis of HSP. In addition, properdin is present in some renal biopsy specimens.

IgA levels are elevated in 50% of patients. Complement 3 and 4 (C3 and C4) levels are usually normal.

The reported incidence of nephritis is 20-50% but may in fact be higher. Risk factors for renal progression are nephrosis, hypertension, renal impairment at presentation, C4 deficiency and haematuria.

HISTORY

There is usually a history of antecedent upper respiratory tract infection. The characteristic rash is the most frequent presentation. Arthritis is the second most frequent manifestation, occurring in approximately 80% and though it may be incapacitating, it is self-limiting and non-deforming. Gastrointestinal involvement occurs in 50–75% of patients and is potentially the most serious complication of HSP due to the possible development of gastrointestinal bleeding and intussusception.

The clinical hallmark of HSP nephritis is haematuria. In contrast to arthritis and abdominal pain, it is extremely uncommon for nephritis to precede the appearance of the rash. The onset of nephritis may in fact be delayed for weeks or months after the onset of other symptoms. Approximately 80% of patients manifest nephritis within four weeks and 95% within three months of the onset of other symptoms.

EXAMINATION

The clinical features of HSP may be atypical in the extremes of age. The characteristic rash consists of crops of palpable purpura and is symmetric in distribution and located on the extensor surfaces of the arms, legs and buttocks. It is worth noting that the rash is not restricted to these areas. The rash may begin with urticaria that progresses over 24 hours to palpable purpura. The arthritis involves the knees, ankles or feet and may result in refusal to weight bear. Asymptomatic microscopic haematuria occurs in most but up to 40% have gross haematuria. Proteinuria occurs in conjunction with haematuria in two-thirds of patients but the occurrence of proteinuria alone is rare.

INVESTIGATIONS

- Diagnosis of HSP is straightforward when the typical rash is present.
- Diagnosis of HSP requires a normal platelet count by definition.
- There is no diagnostic laboratory test for HSP – routine laboratory tests are neither specific nor diagnostic.
- Urinalysis should be performed to establish the presence of microscopic haematuria, with or without proteinuria.
- Serum creatinine should be checked when HSP nephritis is present.
- Blood pressure should be measured and recorded at presentation for baseline evaluation.

DIFFERENTIAL DIAGNOSIS

The differential diagnosis of a purpuric rash is broad. Purpura may be the initial manifestation of an infectious process.

Meningococcaemia Palpable purpura (as opposed to the usual non-palpable purpura) can occur if there are pre-existing coagulation abnormalities (such as protein S or protein C deficiency). This diagnosis must be considered in any child with purpura.

Kawasaki disease Considered in the patient with an unremitting fever with a maculopapular rash that is prominent on the lower extremities. This rash, however, does not appear in crops and is not associated with arthritis. The eye findings in Kawasaki disease are usually absent in HSP.

Bacterial endocarditis, infectious mononucleosis, rubeola and streptococcal infection may present with a purpuric rash. HSP can occur with other forms of vasculitis or autoimmune disease, such as inflammatory bowel disease or familial Mediterranean fever.

Rocky Mountain spotted fever should be considered in endemic areas when there is a history of tick exposure.

TREATMENT

Corticosteroids in usual doses (1–2 mg kg^{-1} d^{-1}) have no effect on established nephritis but may hasten resolution of the arthritis and abdominal pain.

Available data, though considered somewhat controversial, suggest that patients with severe nephritis (haematuria, nephrotic syndrome, decreased glomerular filtration rate (GFR) and crescent formation involving > 50% of the glomeruli) should receive a combination of high-dose intravenous methylprednisolone (30 mg kg^{-1} d^{-1}) for three days followed by oral steroids plus an immunosuppressive agent, either azathioprine or cyclophosphamide.

Plasmapheresis has been reported to be of benefit in a few patients with rapidly progressive HSP glomerulonephritis.

Hypertension – angiotensin blockade by use of angiotensin-converting enzyme (ACE) inhibitors like enalapril may decrease proteinuria and result in slower deterioration in renal function as well as providing effective control of blood pressure.

DISPOSITION

Out-patient management is appropriate for most patients with HSP. Urinalysis should be performed weekly whilst the disease is active. Provided there is no evidence of nephritis during this period, patients should have a urinalysis on a monthly basis for three months after all other manifestations have resolved.

Patients who develop nephritis at any time should have blood pressure and serum creatinine monitored periodically until the nephritis has resolved.

Patients with nephritis complicated by nephrotic syndrome, hypertension or significant renal insufficiency require a renal biopsy in order to predict prognosis more precisely.

With each recurrence of disease, patients should have urinalysis checked.

RECURRENCE

A recurrence rate of 40% has been reported for symptoms of HSP. In one study the recurrences tended to resemble the original episode but were usually milder and of shorter duration.

Recurrences appeared to be more common in those patients with nephritis.

HSP nephritis may recur in transplanted kidneys. Recurrence of the nephritis and extra-renal manifestations are more likely in recipients of living related-donor kidneys than of cadaveric kidneys.

COMPLICATIONS

- Acute renal insufficiency with elevation of serum creatinine can develop in patients with HSP nephritis.
- Patients can also develop nephrotic syndrome. In this situation the urine protein excretion is > 50 mg kg^{-1} per 24 hours with oedema and hypoalbuminaemia.
- End-stage renal disease (ESRD) is a possible complication of HSP nephritis.
- HSP nephritis may recur in transplanted kidneys. Nephritis and extra-renal manifestations are more likely to recur in recipients of living related-donor kidneys than recipients of cadaveric kidneys.
- Orchitis is a well-described complication of HSP and it may mimic testicular torsion.
- Testicular torsion can be an infrequent complication of scrotal oedema.
- Gastrointestinal bleeding and intussusception can complicate HSP.

PROGNOSIS

Though the overall prognosis is excellent for HSP, nephritis is the one manifestation that can become chronic. Prognosis depends on the severity and extent of renal involvement. In general, patients with isolated haematuria, with or without trivial proteinuria, have a uniformly good prognosis. However, up to 50% of children with nephritis associated with nephrotic syndrome may progress to renal insufficiency. Approximately 20–50% will have persistent urinary abnormalities on long-term follow-up but only 1% of patients progress to ESRD.

CONTROVERSIES AND FUTURE DIRECTIONS

❶ A number of studies have addressed the question of whether early corticosteroid treatment prevents the delayed appearance of nephritis but the results are conflicting.

❷ To date there have been no prospective, controlled studies on the use of corticosteroids in the treatment of HSP.

❸ Further work is needed to explore the role of cytokines in determining the exclusive involvement of IgA1 in the immunopathogenesis of HSP. IgA has two subclasses IgA1 and IgA2 but HSP is associated with abnormalities involving IgA1 rather than with IgA2.

❹ The fundamental abnormality responsible for HSP and IgA nephropathy needs to be elucidated.

❺ Role of other immunosuppressives?

Clinical presentation is helpful but is not a precise determinant of prognosis. Severity of renal disease and the ultimate outcome correlates more closely with histopathologic changes on renal biopsy and the degree of proteinuria at presentation. Poor prognosis is associated with crescent formation involving more than 50% of the glomeruli.

Regardless of clinical presentation or histological changes, all patients with nephritis need prolonged follow-up since deterioration in renal function may occur in some patients many years later.

PREVENTION

There appears to be no single pathogen or environmental agent that has emerged as an important precipitating cause of HSP, thus there is no means of preventing HSP.

FURTHER READING

Allen DM, Diamond LK, Howell DA 1960 Anaphylactoid purpura in children (Henoch–Schönlein syndrome). American Journal of Diseases of Childhood 99: 833–854

Cronan K, Norman M 2000 Renal and electrolyte emergencies. In: Fleisher G, Ludwig S (eds) Textbook of pediatric emergency medicine, 4th edn. Lippincott Williams & Wilkins, Philadelphia, 851

Levy M, Broyer M, Arsan A et al 1976 Anaphylactoid purpura nephritis in childhood: Natural history and immunopathology. Advances in Nephrology 6: 183–228

Meulders Q, Pirson Y, Cosyns JP 1994 Course of Henoch-Schönlein nephritis after renal transplantation. Transplantation 58: 1179–1186

Oner A, Tinaztepe K, Erdogan O 1995 The effect of triple therapy on rapidly progressive type of Henoch-Schönlein nephritis. Paediatric Nephrology 9: 6–10

Saulsbury FT 1999 Henoch-Schönlein purpura in children – Report of 100 patients and review of the literature. Medicine 78(6): 395–406

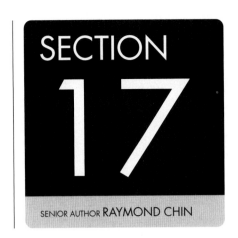

PSYCHIATRIC

17.1 PAEDIATRIC PSYCHIATRIC EMERGENCIES

RAYMOND CHIN • MICHAEL FAIRLEY

Essentials

1 Children with psychological problems often present with somatic complaints and at times of family crisis. The treating emergency physician should be aware of this.

2 Early identification of psychological illness can reduce prolonged investigations and expedite specific psychiatric treatment.

INTRODUCTION

Paediatric patients and, at times, their parents can provide complex diagnostic and logistic challenges to staff in a busy emergency department (ED). They often present in a time of life crisis. However, the complaint may be primarily emotional. The majority of cases have no clear diagnosis and may be complicated by multiple visits to previous medical practitioners.

Assessment requires time and patience and unique clinical skills. Intent listening with directed questioning is required. It is important to avoid drawing premature conclusions, and emotional factors should be considered, even when the problem appears predominantly organic.

GENERAL APPROACH

Assessment

In the case of children, parents generally initiate medical contact, so it is important to seek the child's opinion early. If possible, a history from both the parent and the child should be obtained. Reassurance needs to be provided that the

visit is not a punishment. Playing and drawing may put the child at ease.

In adolescents, self-referral for psychological problems is more likely, but is usually associated with reluctance to identify and discuss the problem.[1] Physical complaint may point to a psychological issue, e.g. headache and panic attack. As the patient is usually unco-operative, reassurance should be provided about confidentiality.

History

A thorough medical history is imperative. In addition the six Ps of collateral history should be explored.

Collateral history

❶ Pre-existing psychological disorders, life experiences, medical conditions, family vulnerability.

❷ Precipitants – trigger for presentation.

❸ Presentation – why now, who is most troubled by the symptom.

❹ Perpetuation – factors that operate to prevent recovery.

❺ Positives – strengths and resources, coping with previous problems.

❻ Preconceptions – belief system, expectations from medical consultation. What the child and parent really want.

Synthesis of assessment

It should be possible for the emergency physician to determine why the child is attending, who wants something done, and where the main pathology rests; in the patient, the parent or their relationship.

Examination

Examination includes obtaining vital signs, and a physical and mental state exam.

Investigations

Special tests should be confined to the differential diagnosis of assessment.

COMMON PAEDIATRIC PSYCHIATRIC PRESENTATIONS

THE ACUTELY DISTURBED CHILD

Acutely disturbed behaviour is often a response to fear, pain or anger. Such behaviour can consist of hitting, screaming, running, spitting and swearing.

Disturbed behaviour in children presenting to EDs is seen in the following situations:

- Unco-operative child (tantrums).
- Autistic or developmentally impaired child.
- Aggressive, violent adolescent (intoxication).
- Acute psychosis.

Initial assessment

This should include: assessment of whether the behaviour is an acute reaction; looking for precipitants; consideration of pre-existing conditions, such as attention deficit hyperactivity disorder (ADHD), drug abuse, or impaired parenting; and establishing what the patient needs.

Management

Patience is essential. Unfortunately both medical and nursing staff may lack time in a busy ED. The child should ideally be assessed in a safe and quiet area. Confrontation should be avoided, stimulation decreased and the number of people around minimised. The parents should be involved, although sometimes they are precipitants and it may be important to isolate them. A brief history and examination should be performed. Investigations need to be decided upon prior to blood collection, and extra help and sedation may be required. Sedation may include: midazolam, $0.1–0.2 \ mg \ kg^{-1}$ IV or IM up to 0.5 mg kg^{-1}; diazepam, 0.2 mg kg^{-1} per dose IV; or antipsychotics.

Olanzapine wafers Have revolutionalised management. They cannot be easily spat out and dissolve almost instantly and act in 30–60 minutes. The dose can be repeated after one hour. They are formulated in 5 mg or 10 mg, are difficult to overdose on, and the usual maximum dose is 30 mg for an adult, proportionately less for a child.

CLINICAL ASSESSMENT OF SUICIDAL PATIENTS

It is important to establish:

❶ Risk of suicide or repeat attempt.
❷ Nature of current crisis and meaning of the event.
❸ Presence of psychiatric disorder.
❹ Background history, personality style, coping mechanisms.
❺ Social supports.
❻ Source of appropriate help.

Introduction

The presentation of a child or adolescent with self-directed harm or injury, constitutes a medical and psychiatric emergency, even if the need for medical urgency appears low. The presentation of a child or adolescent with suicidal ideation but no apparent physical injury similarly constitutes a psychiatric emergency. More people die in Australia by suicide than by motor-vehicle accidents. The ratio of male to female suicides is currently approximately 4:1 and the figures representing ratios of male to female attempted suicides varies generally from being equal to up to 15:1 in favour of females.[2]

The rate of suicide in older teenagers has increased, especially over the past 30 years. Although rare in pre-pubertal children, it is always indicative of a severe disorder.

In young persons who commit suicide, up to 46% have made a prior threat or attempt, and of those who attempt suicide, some 10% eventually kill themselves, often within two years.

The most important contribution that can be made to the prevention of suicide is the recognition of the early signs of mental illness, in particular, depression and schizophrenia. Depression can present as school failure after normal achievement, hypochondriasis, social withdrawal and aggressive behaviour, more often than verbal complaints of depression and anxiety.

Energetic, persistent and effective treatment is required once a suicide attempt has been made.

Risk factors

Theories abound to explain these high suicide rates although many of the assumptions about causality are not proven but based only on occasions. Nevertheless, a thorough review of the literature[3] leads to the conclusion that the risk of suicidal behaviour is increased among young people who:

❶ Have previously attempted suicide.
❷ Have a mood disorder or are involved in harmful use of drugs (including alcohol).
❸ Have problems involving violence.
❹ Are from a socially disadvantaged background characterised by low socioeconomic status, limited educational achievements, low income, poverty and associated factors.
❺ Experience parental loss through separation and divorce.
❻ Have experienced physical or sexual abuse.
❼ Have experienced impaired parent-child relationships.
❽ Have parents with a mental illness such as mood disorders, harmful drug use (including alcohol) or problems involving violence.
❾ Experienced loss through suicide in their family or peer group.
❿ Experience a greater number of life stresses than normal.

Evaluation of the suicidal crisis

Suicidal act
- Intent (wish to die).
- Lethality (danger to life).
- Mitigating circumstances (factors interfering with the person's ability to assess the consequences of the act).

- Specific enquiry into:
  Degree of isolation, probability of intervention, precautions against discovery
  Actions to gain help during, or after, an attempt
  Degree of planning, level of impulsivity
  Communication of intent, suicide note
  Expectations of method's lethality
  Conception of reversibility with medical attention
  Use of alcohol or other drugs.

Circumstance of the act
- Precipitants – bereavement, separation, custody, disciplinary crisis.
- Immediate past history.
- Interpersonal relationships.
- Social support systems.
- Impact on others – e.g. rescue or rejection.
- Family diseases.

Mental state examination
Look for:

- Suicidal ideation.
- Ongoing depression.
- Psychotic features (delusions, hallucinations).
- Pervasive hopelessness.
- Quality of interaction with the interviewer.

Document:

- Appearance.
- Behaviour during interview.
- Communication (content, themes, structure).
- Affect (mood)
- Perception.
- Cognition (orientation level, formal thought disorder).
- Insight into present situation.
- Judgement.
- Rapport.

Hazards during assessment
❶ Use of denial by parents, doctors and nurses.
❷ Refusal to be interviewed.
❸ Lack of insight.
❹ Negative influence of relatives.
❺ Pressure and hostility from other staff.

Management following an attempt

❶ Comprehensive medical assessment for extent of injury as soon as possible. This should occur prior to psychiatric examination.

❷ Admission to a medical unit if outcome of assessment indicated that physical safety has been adversely affected.

❸ If medical status is stable, referral to psychiatry for assessment is required in all cases.

ANXIETY DISORDERS

Anxiety is a complex feeling of apprehension, fear, and worry often accompanied by pulmonary, cardiac, and other physical sensations. It is a ubiquitous condition that varies from the physiological to the pathologic in its presentation. Panic disorder has a lifetime prevalence of 1.5–3.5%.

In school refusal, the child often presents with a somatic complaint such as abdominal pain. Cases of syncopal collapse may manifest as a panic attack. Early identification can reduce the number of medical investigations and commence early psychiatric referral.

Acute anxiety can effectively be treated with a comprehensive approach utilising psychotherapy, counselling, and a wide spectrum of anxiolytics (e.g. benzodiazepines, buspirone, and antidepressants).

AUTISM

A syndrome of early childhood characterised by: abnormal social relationships; language disorder with impaired understanding, echolalia; rituals and compulsive phenomena; and uneven intellectual development with mental retardation in most cases.

Autism is two to four times more common in boys than girls.

Autism usually is manifest in the first year of life; its onset is not later than age three years.

Treatment

For the most severely impaired children, systematic application of behaviour therapy, a technique that can be taught to parents, helps manage the child in the home and at school. Butyrophenones provide limited benefit, mainly in controlling the most severe forms of aggressive and self-destructive behaviour – they do not resolve the psychosis. Fenfluramine, a serotonergic antagonist, is no longer available.

Speech therapy should begin early. For mute children, the value of learning sign language is not yet established. Children in the near-normal or higher IQ range often benefit from psychotherapy and special education.

CHILDHOOD SCHIZOPHRENIA

Psychotic states usually with onset after age seven years and with behavioural similarities to adult schizophrenia. Evidence suggests that environmental stress precipitates manifest illness in children with a genetic predisposition.

The prevalence of this disorder increases with age. Whereas autism and pervasive developmental disorder are distinctly different from the adult schizophrenias, childhood schizophrenia forms a continuum with the adolescent and adult forms.

It is characterised by withdrawal, apathy, flat affect, thought disorder (blocking and perseveration), ideas of reference, hallucinations and delusions, and complaints of thought control. Diagnosis is based on descriptive clinical phenomena.

Treatment

Combined psychotropic and psychotherapeutic treatment is required. Phenothiazines (e.g. thiothixene 0.10–0.40 mg kg^{-1} d^{-1}) and butyrophenones (e.g. haloperidol 0.05–0.15 mg kg^{-1} d^{-1}) may be effective in controlling acute psychotic symptoms, but relapse is common. Hospitalisation is useful in managing acute exacerbations; some children require continuing in-patient psychiatric care.

EATING DISORDERS

Anorexia nervosa occurs in approximately 1 out of 100 adolescent females and is most frequently found in middle-to-upper socioeconomic groups. Most recent studies have suggested no increased incidence of anorexia nervosa over the last four decades. A familial component appears to be present.

Mortality/morbidity The mortality rate for anorexia nervosa ranges from 5–10% and is greater (5–40%) among bulimic patients.

Race Anorexia nervosa is significantly more frequent in white populations than in people of other races. The co-existent effect of socioeconomic class, however, is difficult to isolate.

Sex Female to male ratio is 10–50:1 in developed countries.

Age Anorexia nervosa is primarily a phenomenon of puberty and early adulthood, although premorbid determinants and long-term outcomes are still being defined.

Anorexia nervosa is an eating disorder characterised by severe weight loss to the point of significant physiological consequences. Patients with anorexia nervosa generally fall into two categories: (1) those who practice extreme food restriction behaviours; and (2) those who display food binge/purge behaviour.

Complications

Complications of anorexia nervosa may result in ED presentation.

Cardiovascular effects include supraventricular and ventricular dysrhythmias, long QT syndrome, bradycardia, orthostatic hypotension, and shock due to congestive heart failure.

Renal disturbances include decreased glomerular filtration rate , elevated creatinine, oedema, acidosis with dehydration, hypokalaemia, hypochloremic alkalosis with vomiting, and hyperaldosteronism.

Gastrointestinal findings include constipation, delayed gastric emptying, gastric dilation and rupture, dental enamel erosion, palatal trauma, enlarged parotids, oesophagitis, Mallory-Weiss lesions, diminished gag reflex, and elevated transaminases.

Finally, bone marrow suppression may occur, leading to platelet, erythrocyte, and leukocyte abnormalities.

History

- Patients may present to the ED with extreme weight loss, food refusal, dehydration, weakness, or shock.
- Affect may be flat or nearly catatonic.
- Patients may be depressed and should be questioned to gauge risk of suicide.
- Obtain a mental history because there is a strong association with depression and substance abuse.
- Often, the family will bring in the patient because many patients may refuse to seek help or may have no insight into their problem.
- Recurrent patients may recognise their problem and present spontaneously for therapy.

Physical

- Physical examination may reveal hypothermia, peripheral oedema, thinning hair, and obvious emaciation.
- Behavioural, these patients often have a flat affect and display psychomotor retardation.

Care

ED care may include rehydration, correction of electrolyte abnormalities (e.g. hypokalaemia), and institution of appropriate disposition for continuing medical and psychiatric treatment.

Consultations

As appropriate, consult with psychiatry and adolescent medicine specialists in order to optimise in-patient care and facilitate out-patient follow-up care.

PROBLEM PARENTS

Parents with a mental illness
Depression
Mothers with postnatal depression may present frequently in a "cry for help".

Münchausen's syndrome by proxy
In 1977, Englishman Roy Meadow published[4] the first report of a new form of child abuse. He coined the term Münchausen's syndrome by proxy (MSBP) after the syndrome that first had been reported by Asher in 1951. This term is applied when an adult, usually the mother, presents a false history to the physician regarding a child who is not suffering from any of the fabricated symptoms. This history causes the physician to perform unnecessary diagnostic procedures that do not result in any specific diagnosis. (MSBP has also been called Polle syndrome, after Baron von Münchausen's only child, who died when aged one year.)

In 1994, the DSM-IV[5,6] included a definition for factitious disorder by proxy, which is now the accepted psychiatric category for MSBP. The definition includes the following:

❶ Intentional production or feigning of physical or psychological signs or symptoms in another person who is under the individual's care.
❷ The motivation for the perpetrator's behaviour is to assume the sick role by proxy.
❸ External incentives for the behaviour, such as economic gain, avoiding legal responsibility, or improving physical well being, are absent.

Children at risk for MSBP abuse are aged fifteen months to six years. The emergency physician often is confronted with baffling symptoms. Frequently, the child has been taken to many care providers before the diagnosis is finally established. Warning signs that are suggestive of MSBP include the following:

- Illness is multisystemic, prolonged, unusual, or rare.
- Symptoms are inappropriate or incongruent.
- Patient has multiple allergies.
- Symptoms disappear when parent or caretaker is absent.
- In children, one parent, usually the father, is absent during hospitalisation.
- History of sudden infant death syndrome in siblings is noted.
- Parent is overly attached to patient.
- Patient has poor tolerance of treatment (e.g. frequent vomiting, rash, and problems with intravenous lines).
- General health of patient clashes with results of laboratory tests.
- Parent shows inordinate concern for feelings of the medical staff.
- Seizure activity is unresponsive to anticonvulsants and is witnessed only by parent or caretaker.

Tests that emergency physicians may consider include the following:

- Urine toxicology screening.
- Chemistry panels.
- Electrocardiogram.
- Drug levels for suspected poisoning agents (e.g. aspirin, acetaminophen, anticonvulsants).
- Cultures.
- Coagulation tests.
- Head CT scan.

Parents with substance abuse
Parents with significant substance abuse, i.e. alcohol and other drugs have significant impact on the child's presentation. The parental behaviour can be inappropriate, threatening and aggressive towards the practitioner. This makes the assessment of the child much more difficult and unreliable.

MISCELLANEOUS

Night terrors
Sleep disruption is a parent's most frequent concern during the first two years of a child's life. Half of all infants develop a disrupted sleep pattern serious enough to warrant physician assistance. Night terror disorder is characterised by re-

current episodes of intense crying and fear, and by difficulty arousing the child. Children also can experience signs of autonomic arousal (e.g. tachycardia, tachypnoea, sweating) during episodes. Children do not recall a dream after a night terror and typically do not remember the episode the next morning. Night terrors are frightening episodes that disrupt family life and cause the child significant distress and impaired everyday function. Usually onset is in children aged 3–12 years; the disorder generally resolves during adolescence.

An estimated 1–6% of children experience night terror episodes. Recurrent night terror episodes accompanied by significant distress and impairment are less frequent

Peak frequency in children younger than $3\frac{1}{2}$ years is at least one episode per week; among older children, peak frequency is 1–2 episodes per month.

History

The most important step toward diagnosing this disorder is to obtain a detailed history.

- Approximately 90 minutes after falling asleep, the child sits up in bed and screams. Prominent autonomic activity (e.g. tachycardia, tachypnoea, diaphoresis, flushing) occurs. The child appears awake but confused, disoriented, and unresponsive to stimuli.
- Most episodes last 1–2 minutes, but the child may remain inconsolable for 5–30 minutes before relaxing and returning to quiet sleep.
- If the child awakens during the night terror, only fragmented pieces of the episode may be recalled.
- In the morning, the child typically has no memory of the experience.

Management

This consists of educating the family about the disorder and reassuring them that episodes are not harmful.

REFERENCES

1. Jureidini J 2002 Child psychiatry. In: Raftos J, Higgins M (eds) Paediatric handbook. Women's and Children's Hospital, Adelaide
2. Aghababian RV et al (eds) 1998 Emergency medicine: The core curriculum. Lippincott, Raven, Philadelphia, PA
3. Baeutrias A 1999 Risk factors for suicide and attempted suicide among young people.In: Setting the evidence-based research agenda for Australia: A literature review. National Health and Medical Research Centre, Commonwealth Department of Health and Aged Care, Canberra
4. Meadow R 1977 Munchausen syndrome by proxy. The hinterland of child abuse. Lancet 2(8033): 343–345
5. DSM-IV 1994 Diagnostic and statistical manual of mental disorders, 4th edn. American Psychiatric Association, Washington, DC
6. ICD-10-AM 2000 The international statistical classification of diseases and related health problems, 10th revision, Australian modification, 2nd edn. National Centre for Classification in Health, Lidcombe, NSW

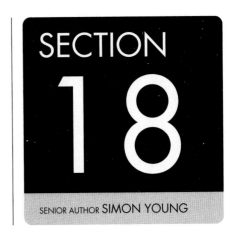

SECTION

18

SENIOR AUTHOR SIMON YOUNG

CRISIS INTERVENTION

18.1 SEXUAL ASSAULT

MATT RYAN

CRISIS INTERVENTION

ESSENTIALS

1 Sexual assault occurs when a child is engaged in sexual activity that the child cannot comprehend, for which the child is developmentally unprepared and cannot give consent, and/or that violates the law or social taboos of society.

2 Sexual assault includes a spectrum of activities ranging from rape to physically less intrusive sexual activity[1,2]

3 Assessment and management of children following alleged or suspected sexual assault is a highly specialised area and requires a multidisciplinary, multiagency team approach.

INTRODUCTION

Assessment of child sexual assault (CSA) requires a dedicated, well-trained and experienced doctor who is able to spend a significant amount of time making an unhurried and thorough assessment and detailed documentation of history and examination findings. The doctor must have an accurate knowledge of genital anatomy, experience in performing gynaecological examinations. Skills and experience in this field are developed through postgraduate studies, significant case numbers, a knowledge of current literature and involvement in peer-review pratices.[3]

Inexpert assessment of such cases may have a profound negative influence on the child and family. It may potentially lead to inappropriate removal of the child from the family or wrongful imprisonment.[4]

The roles of the emergency physician in this process are:

- Recognition of the *possibility* of sexual assault.
- Treatment of acute physical injury.
- Provision of emergency contraception and/or antibiotic and antiviral prophylaxis.
- Protection of the child and referral to local child protection agencies.
- Referral to a paediatrician.
- Ensuring appropriate psychological support is provided to the child and family.

In the majority of cases, determination of whether or not sexual assault has occurred is not possible within the ED. In the majority of cases, physical examination will neither confirm nor refute an allegation of sexual assault. The most important indicator of possible CSA is disclosure by the child.

DEFINITIONS

CSA is the use of a child for sexual gratification by an adult or significantly older child/adolescent.[5] It may involve a range of activities that vary from exposing the child to sexually explicit materials to anal or vaginal penetration of the child. Central to the definition is the limitation of the child to provide truly informed consent for sexual activity with adults.

Sexual play between children of similar age does not fit into this description.

The term 'assault' is preferred over 'abuse' as it highlights the criminal nature of the activity and avoids minimisation of such abusive acts.

ATTITUDES/MYTHS SURROUNDING CSA

The subject of CSA is an emotive one. Emergency physicians will often have strongly held opinions and attitudes on this subject. These attitudes may be shaped by past experience and/or social taboos. In order to approach CSA in a calm,

non-judgemental and objective manner it is important that emergency physicians are cognisant of their own opinions and emotional responses. In dealing with victims of CSA expressions of anger, sadness or surprise are not helpful and potentially stigmatising and harmful to the child. With emergency physicians infrequently encountering CSA it is useful to reflect on the following, sometimes poorly understood, statements:

- A broad range of sexual behaviours has been observed in 'normal' children.
- Most children are not abused by strangers.[11]
- As historians children are no less reliable than adults.
- CSA is not normally an isolated incident.
- CSA uncommonly produces severe genito-anal injury.[3,7–10]
- CSA often occurs in the context of other family problems, including physical abuse, emotional maltreatment and substance abuse.[6]

EPIDEMIOLOGY OF CSA

There has been a significant increase in the recognition of CSA,[3,11,12] which has been reflected by a substantial increase in the number of reports made to child protection services across Australia and overseas, particularly in the last five years.

Sexual assault has been documented as occurring on children of all ages and both sexes, and is committed predominantly by men, who are commonly members of the child's family, family friends or other trusted adults in positions of authority.[11]

Sexual abuse by family members or acquaintances usually involves multiple episodes over periods ranging from a week to years.

Victims of unknown assailants tend to be older than children who are sexually abused by someone they know and are usually only subjected to a single episode of abuse.

The estimated proportion of children exposed to some form of sexual assault varies depending on the definition of sexual abuse and methodology used. In the United States literature surveys provide estimates of 9–52% for females and 3–10% for males.[6] There is no comprehensive comparative Australian literature.

CSA AND EMERGENCY MEDICINE

Children who are victims of sexual assault may present to EDs in a variety of circumstances:

❶ They may be seen for an unrelated matter when routine history and physical examination produces information where sexual assault forms part of the differential diagnosis.

❷ They are brought by a parent or carer to the ED for evaluation of suspected abuse.

❸ They are brought to the ED by social services or the police for a medical evaluation for possible sexual abuse as part of an investigation.

❹ They are brought to an ED after a suspected acute sexual assault for evaluation, evidence collection, and crisis management.

RECOGNITION OF CSA

Recognition of the possibility of CSA is dependant on history and examination findings, both of which are normally non-specific.

History from the child remains the single most important diagnostic feature in coming to the conclusion that a child has been sexually abused.[13]

SIGNS AND SYMPTOMS

Non-specific

Children who have been sexually assaulted may develop a variety of emotional and physical complaints, often unrelated to the genital area these include:

- Developmentally regressive behaviour.
- Deterioration in school performance.
- Sleep disturbances.
- Abdominal pain.
- Enuresis, encopresis.
- Phobias.
- Sexualised behaviour.

Specific

- Disclosure by child.
- Genito-anal injury.
- Sexually transmissible disease.
- Pregnancy.

GENITO-ANAL INJURY

Only 4% of all children referred for medical evaluation of sexual abuse have abnormal examinations at the time of evaluation. Even with a history of severe abuse, such as vaginal or anal penetration, the rate of abnormal medical findings is only 5.5%.[13]

The physical examination of sexually abused children should not result in additional emotional trauma.

When the alleged sexual abuse has occurred within 72 hours, or there is bleeding or acute injury, the examination should be performed immediately. In this situation, protocols for CSA victims should be followed to secure biological trace evidence such as epithelial cells, semen, and blood, as well as to maintain a 'chain of evidence'. When more than 72 hours has passed and no acute injuries are present, an emergency examination usually is not necessary. An evaluation, therefore, should be scheduled at the earliest convenient time for the child, physician, and investigative team.[17]

In the child presenting with genito-anal injury or abnormality CSA is only one of a number of diagnoses that should be considered. The differential diagnosis of genito-anal injury includes:

- Accidental injury.
- Falls astride.
- Sexual assault.
- Medical/dermatological condition, e.g. lichen sclerosis/drug reaction.

Genital findings in children are difficult to interpret. Such interpretation is generally beyond the expertise of most emergency physicians.[14] Whilst acute trauma may be easily recognised, interpretation of such findings may be problematic for the occasional examiner.[14]

GENITO-ANAL ANATOMY

Knowledge of what constitutes normal and abnormal anatomy has evolved over recent years. This has been driven partly by several highly publicised cases where misinterpretation of normal findings led to inappropriate separation of children from parents and wrongful conviction.

Hymen

There is considerable variation in the shape of the hymen. In the pre-pubertal girl it is thin and relatively inelastic. In this age group blunt penetrating trauma to the vagina may result in tearing of the hymen. Such tears when healed may manifest as a notch or defect in the hymenal tissue.

As an oestrogen dependant/responsive tissue, at puberty the hymen becomes thick, irregular and elastic and distensible. It is less likely to sustain injury during penetration than in the pre-pubertal state.

SEXUALLY TRANSMITTED DISEASES

The diagnosis of a sexually transmitted disease in a child may be highly suggestive but is not diagnostic of sexual contact. Rectal and genital *Chlamydia* infections in young children may be due to a persistent perinatally acquired infection, which may last for up to three years.[15,16]

DIAGNOSTIC CONSIDERATIONS

The diagnosis of CSA can often be made based on a child's history. Physical examination is infrequently diagnostic in the absence of a history and/or specific laboratory findings. Physical findings are often absent even when the perpetrator admits to penetration of the child's genitalia. Many types of abuse leave no physical evidence, and mucosal injuries often heal rapidly.

On examination, findings which are suggestive, but not diagnostic, of CSA include:

- Abrasions or bruising of the inner thighs and genitalia.
- Scarring or tears of the labia minora.
- Enlargement of the hymenal opening.

Findings that are of greater concern include:

- Scarring, tears, or distortion of the hymen.
- A decreased amount, or absence, of hymenal tissue.
- Injury to, or scarring of, the posterior fourchette.
- Anal lacerations.[17]

Many cases of alleged sexual abuse involve parents who are in the process of separation or divorce and who allege that their child is being sexually abused by the other parent during custodial visits. Although these cases are generally more time-consuming they should not be dismissed because a custody dispute exists.

Allegations of abuse that occur in the context of divorce proceedings should either be reported to the child protective services agency or followed-up closely.

ROLE OF THE EMERGENCY PHYSICIAN

The emergency physician (EP) has many roles in CSA. The EP should ensure that any physical injuries are detected, accurately documented and correctly treated.

Medical issues, such as sexually transmitted diseases and emergency contraception, should be discussed and managed.

The EP should collect, or provide opportunity for collection of, forensic specimens, ensure appropriate psychological support is provided to the child and family, and report the case to protective agencies within the legislation of the local jurisdiction.

Documentation

Because the likelihood of civil or criminal court action is high, detailed records, and/or drawings should be kept.

Mandatory reporting legislation

Some form of mandatory reporting legislation exists in all Australian jurisdictions. Although this legislation varies from state to state the basic principles are similar. Doctors are mandated to report cases where there is reasonable suspicion that CSA will occur, or is occurring, and the guardian is unlikely to prevent such acts (see Table 18.1.1). The reporting practitioner has statutory protection from prosecution if a report is made in good faith.

REFERENCES

1. American Academy of Pediatrics 1994 Committee on Adolescence. Sexual assault and the adolescent. Paediatrics 94: 761–765
2. American Academy of Child and Adolescent Psychiatry 1997 Practice parameters for the forensic evaluation of children and adolescents who may have been physically or sexually abused. Journal of the American Academy of Child and Adolescent Psychiatry 36: 423–442
3. Donald T, Wells, D 2000 Graduate Diploma in Forensic Medicine Subject guide p. 253. Monash University Centre for Learning and Teaching Support, Melbourne
4. Butler-Sloss E 1988 Report of the Enquiry into Child Abuse in Cleveland 1987. HMSO, London

Table 18.1.1 Guidelines for decision making				
Data available				*Response*
History	Physical examination	Laboratory findings	Level of concern about sexual abuse	Report decision
None	Normal	None	None	No report
Behavioural changes	Normal	None	Variable depending upon behaviour	Possible report; follow-up closely (possible mental health referral)
None	Non-specific findings	None	Low (worry)	Possible report; follow-up closely
Non-specific history by child or history by parent only	Non-specific findings	None	Intermediate	Possible report; follow-up closely
None	Specific findings	None	High	Report
Clear statement	Normal	None	High	Report
Clear statement	Specific findings	None	High	Report
None	Normal, non-specific or specific findings	Positive culture for sexually transmissible disease, presence of semen, sperm acid phosphatase	Very high	Report
Behaviour changes	Non-specific findings	Other sexually transmitted diseases	High	Report

5. Kempe CH 1978 Sexual abuse, another hidden paediatric problem: The 1977 C. Anderson Aldrich lecture. Paediatrics 62: 382–389
6. Finkelhor D 1994 The international epidemiology of child sexual abuse. Child Abuse and Neglect 18(5): 409–417
7. Adams JA, Harper K, Knudson S, Revilla J 1994 Examination findings in legally confirmed child sexual abuse: It's normal to be normal. Paediatrics 94: 310–317
8. Finkel MA 1989 Anogenital trauma in sexually abused children. Paediatrics 84: 317–322
9. McCann J, Voris J, Simon M 1992 Genital injuries resulting from sexual abuse: A longitudinal study. Paediatrics 89: 307–317
10. McCann J, Voris J 1993 Perianal injuries resulting from sexual abuse: A longitudinal study. Paediatrics 91: 390–397

11. Tomison A 1995 Update on child sexual abuse National Child Protection Clearinghouse. Issues in child abuse prevention number 5. http://www.aifs.org.au/nch/issues5.html [accessed 12 June 2003]
12. Leventhal JM 1990 Epidemiology of child sexual abuse. In: Oates RK (ed) Understanding and managing child sexual abuse. Harcourt Brace Jovanovich, Sydney
13. Heger A, Ticson L, Velasquez O, Bernier R 2002 Children referred for possible sexual abuse: Medical findings in 2384 children. Child Abuse and Negligence 26(6-7): 645–659
14. Makoroff KL, Brauley JL, Brandner AM, Myers PA, Shapiro RA 2002 Genital examinations for alleged sexual abuse of prepubertal girls: Findings by pediatric emergency medicine physicians compared with child abuse trained

physicians. Child Abuse and Negligence 26(12): 1235–1242
15. Hammerschlag MR 1988 Sexually transmitted diseases in sexually abused children. Advances in Pediatric Infectious Diseases 3: 1–18
16. Hammerschlag MR, Doraiswamy B, Alexander ER et al 1984 Are rectogenital chlamydial infections a marker of sexual abuse in children? Paediatric Infectious Disease Journal 3: 100–104
17. American Professional Society on the Abuse of Children 1990 Guidelines for psychosocial evaluation of suspected sexual abuse in young children. American Professional Society on the Abuse of Children, Chicago, IL

18.2 CHILD ABUSE

SIMON YOUNG • RAYMOND CHIN • GERVASE CHANEY

ESSENTIALS

1 Child abuse occurs when an adult responsible for the care of the child either harms the child or fails to protect the child from harm.

2 Child abuse may consist of physical abuse, sexual abuse, emotional abuse or neglect.

3 Medical and nursing practitioners are often mandated by law to report suspicions of child abuse.

INTRODUCTION

Children and adolescents are, by virtue of their immature and developing intellectual, emotional and physical state, a vulnerable group in our society. The environment in which they develop is shaped by many factors outside their control. For example, the economic and social status of their family, the personality and values of family members and friends, and the extent of physical and intellectual stimulation that they receive may all have profound influence upon their development. The potential varia-bility in these factors and the recognition that negative experiences often have serious short- and long-term implications for the child has lead to a general acknowledg-ment that children and adolescents need protection.

The United Nations convention on the rights of the child recognises that: '... for the full and harmonious develop-ment of his or her personality, [a child] should grow up in a family environment, in an atmosphere of happiness, love and understanding ...'. The convention con-tinues, stating in Article 19 that govern-ments shall: '... take all appropriate legislative, administrative, social and edu-cational measures to protect the child from all forms of physical or mental viol-ence, injury or abuse, neglect or negligent treatment, maltreatment or exploitation, including sexual abuse, while in the care of parent(s), legal guardian(s) or any other person who has the care of the child ...'.

It is this philosophy that has driven the creation of the social and legal frame-work of child protection. Doctors, nurses and other healthcare workers who deal with children are an integral part of this system that acts to protect children and adolescents. Every health professional that has contact with children needs to be aware of the possibility of child abuse, must be able to detect when it is occurring and know how to act in the best interests of the child once it is suspected.

DEFINITION

Child abuse is not a medical diagnosis but rather a description of certain forms of behaviour displayed by adults respon-sible for the care of a child. Child abuse occurs when an adult responsible for the care of the child either harms the child or fails to protect the child from harm. Harm may be either physical (e.g. an injury or poisoning), psychological (e.g. terroris-ation or lack of stimulation), or both.

Child abuse is often categorised into four main areas:

❶ Physical abuse
❷ Sexual abuse
❸ Emotional abuse
❹ Neglect.

These are not exclusive groupings and clearly a child may be subjected to more that one type of abuse.

Physical abuse

Many thousands of children present to emergency departments (EDs) around Australia each year with a wide range of physical injuries, the vast majority of which are caused accidentally. It is a difficult, but vital, task to identify children within this group who have been injured as a consequence of abuse. While medical and nursing staff must be alert for the possibility of abuse in any injured child, specific circumstances that may raise suspicion include:

❶ A direct allegation of violence directed against the child made by the child or any other person.

❷ The type and pattern of injury observed at the examination.

❸ An explanation being offered for an injury that does not fit the type or pattern of injury.

❹ Delayed presentation for medical care with an injury that a reasonable person would have recognised as needing care sooner.

❺ Multiple presentations often to different healthcare providers seeking medical attention.

Once the possibility of abuse has been raised the priorities of the treating doctor are:

❶ To diagnose, treat and document the child's injuries.

❷ To interpret the pattern of injury or behaviour as to the possible causes.

❸ To notify and involve the agency responsible for ensuring safety of the child.

❹ To provide a written or verbal report and advice to that agency or the police.

Presentation

Physical abuse may present to the ED in many different ways. Most commonly it will present as a child with an obvious injury and a suggestive history but in some situations it will be more subtle, such as a younger child who presents not using a limb.

Children who present with a decreased conscious state with no obvious cause may have a head injury from a blow or a fall or may have been poisoned. If the child is very young the decreased conscious state may be a result of being shaken.

History

It is necessary to collect as much information as possible on the events that led to the child sustaining the injuries. Specifically enquire as to when, where and how the injury happened, who was present at the time and what happened after the injury. The child's medical, developmental and social history with specific information on past injuries, is important.

This history must be sought in an open and non-judgemental fashion, which encourages the participants to reveal all the important information. Unfortunately the ED is often not the ideal place to conduct a lengthy and in-depth forensic interview with the parents or carers and it may be prudent to limit the information gathering to items that will enable specific issues to be addressed. The interview can always be completed by trained investigators at a later time.

Physical examination

Prior to commencing the examination the doctor must ensure that the parents and, where appropriate, the child are informed of the nature and extent of the examination and that valid consent has been given. In addition it is ideal to have spent some time with the child, to gain their confidence and thus increase the chances of keeping their co-operation during the examination.

Consent from the parent or legal guardian is necessary to conduct a physical examination, to perform investigations (including photographs) and to release clinical information in the form of a report to a third party. If consent is refused the protective agency or police must seek a court order. If there is an urgent medical problem that needs intervention and such intervention is clearly in the best interests of the child then the examination and treatment should proceed and not be delayed by the lack of consent.

An adolescent may be able to give consent for their own examination as long as they are capable of understanding what the examination entails, what the results will be used for, and the implications that this may have for them.

A thorough physical examination of the child should be performed with inspection and palpation of skin, soft tissues, bones and joints. Specific attention should be given to the eyes, ears and mouth.

The examination should look for following physical findings:

Bruising of the skin Bruises are the commonest physical finding in child abuse. They provide evidence of blunt trauma and may provide some information on the implement or force of the blow. Specifically look for bruises in the mouth, behind the ears, on the inner aspect of the upper arm and around the buttocks. Look for a pattern of bruises that may suggest a blow from an open hand or other implement. Look for a pattern within the bruise that may suggest contact with a specific surface.

Whilst it is important to describe the appearance and colour of the bruising, it is not possible to be accurate about the age of a bruise. If a bruise is yellowing in colour then it is likely to be more than 18 hours old.

Accidental bruises are commonly found in children of all ages. Children of toddler age frequently have multiple small bruises on the anterior aspect of the lower legs or bruises on the bony prominences of the head from trauma associated with normal activity.

Laceration and abrasion of the skin Lacerations are the tearing of tissues caused by a blow from a blunt object. Abrasions are the disruption of the outer layers of the skin caused when the skin contacts a surface at an angle. They occur at or close to the site of impact and may occur after a blow with an object or after a fall on to a surface. They are frequently associated with bruising.

Examine the wound for neurovascular injury and for foreign bodies. The presence of foreign material such as glass, dirt or gravel should be noted. Lacerations of the frenulum may be seen when objects are forced into a child's mouth.

Burns or scalds Look at the site, shape and depth of the burn. Circumferential scalds of the hands or feet may be caused by forced immersion. Small round bruises above the burn may represent forcible gripping by a hand. Scalds of the buttocks extending on to the lower back or upper thighs with sparing of the natal cleft may indicate the child has been lowered into hot water. Although classically described as associated with child abuse, cigarette burns are extremely rare. These appear as small, deep, round burns usually on the limbs or back.

Healing burns can sometimes be difficult to diagnose and interpret. Inflammation can extend beyond the margins of the burn obscuring the shape and the healing area may become flaking and impetiginous.

Fractures Fractures of long bones, ribs and skull may occur when a child is intentionally struck, pushed, squeezed or dropped. While almost any fracture may be caused by child abuse, certain fractures have an association that warrants further attention. Specifically fractures in children under the age of 18 months, metaphyseal fractures, multiple fractures and fractures of differing ages should be carefully evaluated.

Eye injuries Direct blows to the face may cause subconjunctival haemorrhages or intraocular injuries such as retinal haemorrhages. A careful examination including visual acuity and fundoscopy is necessary.

Ear injuries Blows to the side of the face may cause bruising of and behind the pinna. The ear drum may rupture due to the air pressure changes.

Head injuries Head injuries are a major source of mortality and morbidity in child abuse. Young children have a large head to body size ratio, relatively weak neck musculature and compliant skull bones that predispose them to intracranial injuries. The child may be struck, dropped, thrown or shaken producing an open or closed head wound.

Skull fractures, cerebral contusion, intracerebral haemorrhages, extradural haematoma and subdural haematoma are all possible sequelae.

Intra-abdominal injury Blows to the abdomen may cause laceration or rupture of either solid abdominal organs, such as the liver or spleen, or of the hollow organs, such as the duodenum. There may or may not be accompanying bruising of the abdominal skin to alert you to this possibility.

Investigations The findings of the clinical examination dictate the type of investigations necessary. As would be the case in the investigation of any injured child, plain X-rays, CT scans, MRI, ultrasound and other imaging should be directed at areas where there is clinical suspicion of injury.

Other investigations, such as a skeletal survey and bone scan, are used in an attempt to detect injuries that may not be clinically apparent but which will assist in establishing the likelihood of child abuse. These are especially useful in children under the age of two.

In a child with multiple bruises the possibility of a bleeding disorder such as idiopathic thrombocytopenic purpura should be considered. A full blood examination and coagulation profile may be necessary in these circumstances.

Emotional abuse

Emotional or psychological abuse is difficult to define and even harder to detect, particularly in the ED, when frequently the child presents to a particular health worker on a single occasion. Five possible components of emotional abuse have been described. These are the following behaviours:

❶ Rejecting.
❷ Isolating.
❸ Terrorising.
❹ Ignoring.
❺ Corrupting.

The incidence of emotional abuse is unknown but it is likely to be common and under-diagnosed.

History and examination

Presentation is subtle and depends upon the age of the child. An infant may present with sleep or feeding problems, irritability or apathy. Older children may present with attention deficit, attention seeking, aggression, school failure, truancy, anxiety, depression and psychosomatic disease. It is likely that emotional abuse accompanies other forms of abuse, such as physical and sexual abuse. Consideration of its possible role is important in all assessments of child abuse.

As in all child abuse, detection, by all health workers looking after children, including emergency staff, requires a high index of suspicion and vigilance. Diagnosis is suggested by the consequences in the child as above.

Assessment should include that of behavioural, emotional and physical signs and the child-parent interaction. This will usually require time not available to emergency staff and therefore, when emotional abuse is suspected, referral is necessary. This may be to the hospital child protection/abuse unit and/or community social services.

Neglect

Neglect is another form of child abuse that can be difficult to define and diagnose. A broad definition is anything that individuals, institutions or processes fail to do, which directly or indirectly harms children or damages their prospects of a safe and healthy development into adulthood. Other definitions have tended to be narrower and therefore target more severe or persistent neglect. It is important to differentiate neglect from poverty or ignorance, as these will require a different intervention.

The true incidence of neglect is unknown and it is probably the most common form of child abuse. Its diagnosis usually only occurs when harm has occurred, but consideration should be made of potential for harm and long-term effects. Types of neglect include medical neglect, safety neglect, educational neglect, physical neglect and emotional neglect. Non-organic failure to thrive is likely to be due to a combination of a lack of calories and affection.

History and examination

Some possible features to look out for are frequent presentation and admission to hospital with accidents or illness, delay or failure to access health care, malnutrition, failure to immunise, poor physical presentation, poor compliance, behaviour disorders, developmental delay and, very importantly, failure to thrive. The assessment of growth and development is clearly an essential part of child health assessment, even in the emergency setting. Measurement of height, weight and head circumference and their plotting on standardised growth charts can be very useful in assessment and follow-up. Emotional and behavioural assessment is difficult in the emergency setting.

Treatment

The diagnosis of non-organic failure to thrive usually requires admission to hospital to assess the child's ability to grow with adequate nutrition and an interdisciplinary approach. Other forms of neglect may require admission or, if not, referral to child protection/abuse unit or community social services.

Münchausen's syndrome by proxy

Münchausen's syndrome by proxy (MSBP) is an unusual type of child abuse that may present to an ED. This condition occurs when an adult, usually the mother, presents a false history to the physician regarding a child who is not truly suffering from any of the reported symptoms. This history may cause the emergency physician to perform unnecessary diagnostic and therapeutic procedures that do not result in any specific diagnosis.

In 1995, the DSM-IV included a definition for factitious disorder by proxy, which is now the accepted psychiatric category for MSBP. The definition includes the following:

❶ Intentional production or feigning of physical or psychological signs or symptoms in another person who is under the individual's care.
❷ The motivation for the perpetrator's behaviour is to assume the sick role by proxy.
❸ External incentives for the behaviour, such as economic gain, avoiding legal responsibility, or improving physical well-being, are absent.

Children at risk for MSBP abuse are aged fifteen months to six years. The emergency physician is often confronted with baffling symptoms. Frequently, the child

has been taken to many care providers before the diagnosis is finally established. Warning signs that are suggestive of MSBP include the following:

- Illness is multisystemic, prolonged, unusual, or rare.
- Symptoms are inappropriate or incongruent.
- Patient has multiple allergies.
- Symptoms disappear when parent or caretaker is absent.
- In children, one parent, usually the father, is absent during hospitalisation.
- History of sudden infant death syndrome in siblings is noted.
- Parent is overly attached to patient.
- Patient has poor tolerance of treatment (e.g. frequent vomiting, rash, problems with intravenous lines).
- General health of patient clashes with results of laboratory tests.
- Parent shows inordinate concern for feelings of the medical staff.
- Seizure activity is unresponsive to anticonvulsants and is witnessed only by parent or caretaker.

THE COMMUNITY RESPONSE TO CHILD ABUSE

Responsibilities to report

For medical practitioners working in acute medicine often the first point of contact with a child at risk is when they present for treatment. Statistics suggest that doctors only diagnose cases of child abuse in about 2% of notifications.

Mandatory reporting legislation brought in across all states of Australia, have made it compulsory to report cases of child abuse and suspected cases of neglect to the State Child Protection Agency. For example in New South Wales under Section 22 of the Children (Care and Protection) Act 1987, medical practitioners were required to report child physical and/or sexual abuse of children under the age of 16 years. Mandatory notifiers who failed to notify under Section 22 of the Act were guilty of an offence.

All healthcare staff are now mandatory reporters under the Children and

Young Persons (Care and Protection) Act 1998. It is a criminal offence not to report.

Notification involves contacting the child protection authority relevant to the state. The Children (Care and Protection) Amendment (Disclosure of Information) Act 1996 extends voluntary reporting to any person who believes on reasonable grounds that a child who is aged 16 or 17 years has been, or is, in danger of being abused.

Once notification is made a process of risk management is commenced.

What to do as the medical practitioner, in suspected cases

❶ Take a concise history of events and physical examination.
❷ Document injuries and order appropriate investigations.
❸ Manage injuries as usual practice.
❹ Notify relevant child protection agency. (Clients consent is not required in child protection notification.)

This may be facilitated by social worker, nurses and paediatric specialists.

Legal responsibilities

❶ By law health services staff must provide all relevant information that they have available when asked (in writing) to do so by the child protection authority.
❷ Staff do not have to get permission of the client in order to forward the relevant information.
❸ Protection for notifier. The Children (Care and Protection) Act 1987 made provision for the safeguarding of the identity of the person who makes the report.
❹ Neither the report nor its contents are admissible as evidence in any proceedings against the person who made the report.
❺ If as a result of making a report a person is threatened or fears personal violence this should be reported to the police, who may apply for, and pursue on their behalf, an apprehended violence order.

What happens after notification?

❶ The Child Protection Agency must respond when someone reports that they think a child or young person under the age of 16 years has been, or is being, abused or neglected.

❷ When the agency receives information about child abuse, it makes decisions about how to go ahead with investigating the claims and how others may be able to help. For example, it may contact the child's teacher, child-care worker, relatives or the police.

❸ The police will be contacted and may become involved if the agency thinks the law has been broken.

Actions based on risk assessment

❶ If the child is in immediate danger, steps will be taken to reduce the level of risk or move the child to a safe place. This may mean admission to hospital or foster care.

❷ In many cases this might mean giving the family practical help, such as organising child care, emergency finance, providing a referral for counselling or information on health or other services.

❸ In some cases, the child protection agency takes the matter to the Children's Court. The court can order a child be placed in agency care for a period of time. The court can also order counselling and other types of support services including health services.

FURTHER READING

Browne K, Hanks H, Stratton P, Hamilton C 2002 Early prediction and prevention of child abuse: A handbook. Wiley, Chichester

Gabarino J, Guttman E, Seeley J 1988 The psychologically battered child. Jossey-Bass, San Francisco

Hobbs C, Hanks G, Wynne J 1999 Child abuse and neglect: A clinician's handbook. Churchill Livingstone, London

Oates KR 1996 The spectrum of child abuse: assessment, treatment and prevention. Brunner/Mazel, New York

SECTION

19

SENIOR AUTHOR RON CLARK

ADMINISTRATION AND EMS

19.1 MANAGING THE DEATH OF A CHILD IN THE ED: BEREAVEMENT ISSUES

ROGER BARKIN • PAT CLEMENTS

ESSENTIALS

1 The death of a child under any circumstances is likely to lead to a significant crisis and grief response in parents.

2 Emergency physicians should be prepared for parental presence in the resuscitation room, anticipate their high level of distress, and ensure that they are kept informed.

3 It is important that the family knows that everything that could have been done was done.

4 Parental questions should be answered honestly and directly, allowing humanity and empathy to show.

5 Personal, compassionate and individualised support should be provided for families, respecting their cultural, religious and social values.

6 Family members are likely to have impaired decision making and communication abilities, and this needs to be taken into consideration around informed consent issues.

7 The needs of the grieving family must be balanced with the legislative requirements of the Coroner's Act when this is relevant.

8 Relatives should be allowed to spend time with the deceased child if they want to, preferably in a quiet suite.

9 It is important to be available in the weeks following the death to clarify and answer any further questions from the family.

10 Team members need to be aware of their own likely emotional responses to the death of a child.

INTRODUCTION

Deaths occurring in the emergency department (ED) present unique challenges for the clinician, particularly if the patient is a child.[27,28]

The unexpected death of a child undoubtedly brings about the most severe and shattering grief response for the child's parents. Because the loss is unexpected and involves someone so young and so intrinsically a part of self, the grief response of parents may be very painful and prolonged. The death of a child must be viewed as a tragedy for the entire continuum of family and friends. Additionally, paediatric deaths are frequently personalised by ED staff, and hence have broad implications for the whole ED clinical team.

In large hospital EDs, particularly in urban areas, there is rarely a pre-existing relationship between the health professionals and the patient/family. While this facilitates the professional detachment needed for ED staff to function effectively, it creates inherent voids in the ability to support grieving relatives and friends. In smaller hospitals like those found in rural and regional communities, a pre-existing relationship may exist, potentially lowering communication barriers but bringing out other stresses and strains for ED staff.

THE RESUSCITATION PROCESS

Parents usually benefit from being present during the resuscitation process.[29] It is therefore unacceptable to discourage their presence unless they are interfering with, and compromising, the resuscitation itself. Family members watching monitors and seeing the trace 'go flat' experience much alarm and distress, but this should not be seen as a reason to exclude them.[1]

The resuscitation process can be traumatic for parents and family members, requiring ongoing communication and interpretation of events. It should be expected that parents will be visibly upset and distressed during this period. A staff member, often a social worker, should be assigned to support the family, to answer any questions about the procedures and responses, and to prevent distraught family members from impeding the resuscitation.[2] The ED medical officer in charge must communicate with this staff member and family members about the progress of the resuscitation. Viewing the resuscitation efforts allows the family to see a caring and competent staff, in control of their emotions, doing their best to save the child's life.

Where parents choose not, or feel unable, to be in the resuscitation room, it is essential that they be kept informed of progress. Panic, fear and a sense of isolation have been noted as the main responses of relatives who remain outside the resuscitation room.[1] Small, dull rooms with no windows or natural light were seen as heightening the sense of isolation, disconnectedness and fear for those family members unable to bring themselves to view the resuscitation.

It is important to be skilled in early recognition of the signs of trauma responses by parents, such as dissociation, as this can affect long-term adjustment. A social worker may provide support for parents and act as an advocate during what is likely to be an overwhelming and bewildering process. The social worker is also likely to be the main staff member to have an ongoing role after death has occurred and the family has left the hospital.

TALKING TO PARENTS AND FAMILIES

When talking with the family about the child's deteriorating condition, give details in a simple, straightforward and accurate manner. Provide the information using appropriate language. Answer questions and be responsive to needs and concerns.

When death has occurred, or is imminent, it is essential to have identified the relevant family members so that discussions are with the appropriate individuals. At the point of death, the medical officer in charge of the resuscitation should advise those family members present in the resuscitation room or in a private, quiet location. Research has indicated that families appreciated a high level of physician involvement.[3]

Clear, distinct and accurate information is essential, and medical jargon should be avoided. It is very important to state initially that the child has died. This is the piece of information that the parents will most want clarified. It is then desirable to provide a brief chronology of events, while reassuring the family that everything was done and that the child did not suffer pain.

Sometimes family members are not present at the time of death. If practicable it is best to delay notification of death until it can be done in person.[32] If the family cannot readily access the ED, telephone notification may be necessary. A survey of survivors suggested that if delay in personal notification was greater than one hour, telephone notification may be appropriate.[4] However, it is obviously difficult to be sensitive to the family's response via a telephone, and there may

be limited ability to provide immediate support. Ensure that the family is safe to transport themselves and that ongoing support options have been explored for those family members unable to make it to hospital.

If family members were not present at the hospital it is likely that they will have many questions related to the process, potential suffering, and any awareness by the child of the event. These may be asked either over the telephone or upon arrival. If parents arrive 'too late', this can create a further burden of guilt because they were not present.

Family members experiencing significant grief are likely to struggle with the integration of the information that they are being given and with the communication of any questions that they might have. They may need to revisit the same questions and information repeatedly in order to try to make sense of the event.[1]

It is important to allow parents and family members time to examine the implications of the loss, and to begin the process of searching for some answers and meaning in the midst of the event. It is also important to assist them to mobilise resources from their social, cultural and religious communities to help them to deal with their grief.

There can be a temptation to offer sedation to grief-stricken parents. This is often requested by relatives distressed by observing the parents' pain. Grief is a normal process, which is rarely helped by pharmacological intervention.

Junior medical staff are often involved in resuscitations, and it is essential that they have received some training/education to help them handle the unexpected death of a child. A number of programs have been described, which have been found to be useful in preparing staff to deal with loss in an effective manner, from the perspective of both the family and staff members.[5–8]

LAYING OUT OF THE CHILD

Where parents want to 'view' or spend time with their deceased child, it is im-

portant to facilitate their wishes (having due regard to the possibility that the death may need to be referred to the coroner). All tubes inserted during the resuscitation process (endotracheal tubes, intravenous cannulae, drains, etc.) should be removed, unless the medical officer in charge considers that the placement of a tube may have been associated with an adverse event. All wounds and cannula sites should be dressed to avoid leakage of bodily fluids. The child's face and exposed areas should be bathed/cleaned and any soiling removed.

The impact of the death can often cause an overwhelming sense of numbness and helplessness, diminishing the ability to self advocate. Therefore, it is important to be proactive with family members and ask how much they want to be involved with the bathing and laying out of the child, and about any specific cultural or religious practices that they would like observed.

It can often be useful to obtain mementos of the child. Photographs, a lock of hair, or a foot/hand print may become important mementos along the grieving journey. It is recommended that hospital EDs have access to such items as a camera, memento books and bereavement packs to give to families.

There are specific requirements in place for deaths that must be referred to the coroner. These may limit the process of 'laying out' the body, and require that family members may not be left unsupervised with the child. ED staff need to balance the needs of grieving family members with their legal responsibilities to the coroner.

VIEWING THE BODY – QUIET SUITE

Most available evidence strongly suggests that seeing the body of the deceased is an important part of accepting the reality of death.[9,10] This includes not only seeing, but also being able to touch and hold the loved one. It is helpful to describe to relatives what they are going to see prior to viewing the body, especially if there are trauma-related injuries.[1] Viewing the body can also relieve anxieties about mutilation, signs of trauma, or that the person was in pain when they died.[10] A parent or family member's preference not to spend time with the child should also be respected, particularly where severe trauma may have caused disfigurement.[1]

Most large paediatric hospitals have a 'quiet suite' or 'family room' to facilitate parents spending time with their deceased child. This can allow a private 'good bye' and time to reflect. It can also allow time to create an image of the child as dead, altered from the image of the living child.[10] The importance of the family/relatives room cannot be overemphasised – privacy and basic facilities are essential.

Subsequently, additional relatives/friends may arrive at the hospital. This can often lead to heightened distress for parents as they try to explain the events that have led to the child's death, hence taking them back to the initial traumatic stages. It can also be a useful process. By reviewing events parents may build a clearer picture and 'fill in the blanks' as they retell their story.

THE GRIEF RESPONSE

Grief is a normal reaction accompanying death. The severity of the grief response parallels the severity of the loss.

Perhaps the most well-known model of describing the process of grief is the 'stages' model with its clearly defined stages of shock, denial and isolation, anger and envy, bargaining, depression and acceptance.[11] These stages should not be seen as linear or rigid. Individuals can move back and forth between the stages or may appear 'stuck' in a stage. Although the 'stages' model is the most well known and can be a useful guide, there are a number of other models of grieving including psychodynamic,[12] attachment,[13,14] social constructionist,[15] cognitive/behavioural,[16,17] and personal construct.[18] Good practice requires being open and flexible, adapting to the needs of the grieving family as opposed to trying to fit the family into any particular model. It is important not to pathologise individuals whose grief response does

not fit neatly into a particular model of grief.[19]

The death of a child provokes the most intense form of bereavement. It is certain to alter the course of the parents' lives, their relationship with each other and with others. Losing a child is more than losing a relationship. For a parent it is losing part of their self, their present and their future. Many parents experience a loss of meaning in their lives and may never fully recover from the impact of their child's death.[14] A child's death is not a singular loss, but produces a ripple effect overwhelming all aspects of the family and environment. Parents, and even the extended family, may feel that they have failed, irrespective of the nature of the death and level of love, nurturing and caring that existed during the child's life.[10,20,30]

The parental relationship faces severe stress following the death of a child. It can pull a dysfunctional relationship further apart, or glue a functional one closer together. Adverse impacts on the relationship can occur through the real or perceived apportioning of blame by one parent to the other. This can occur where a child died while under the specific supervision of one parent, or one parent was simply not present when a critical event occurred.

Siblings of the deceased child will also experience a significant grief reaction. Not only must they manage the actual loss of their deceased sibling, but they must also cope with the loss of their normal family environment. Their parents will be struggling to cope with their own grief, and thus will be less emotionally available. The cognitive developmental level of a sibling has a significant bearing on their capacity to understand concepts of death like permanent, irreversible, inevitable, universal.[21] Regardless of how siblings understand and express their grief, it is critically important to remember that they are part of the social context in which the death has occurred. Their needs for explanation and support are just as important as the needs of their parents.

The death of a child does not occur in isolation, but rather it occurs in a social

context that includes many variables. The main ones are parental coping capacity and skills, family and relationship functionality, social networks, parental physical and mental health issues, education, socioeconomic status, and, importantly, any real or perceived parental responsibility in the death of the child. Thus the broader social context will have relevance on how parents and extended family members manage the impact of the child's death.[20] Any available psychosocial assessment or information, such as that provided by the ED social worker, should be factored into the management of the family.

SUPPORT OF THE FAMILY

Generally, parents are completely unprepared for the impact of their child's death as they have no prior knowledge or experience to draw on.[22] Arranging support is essential, and early social worker involvement is highly desirable. Parents and other family members must be provided with information about 'normal' grieving, and should be linked to appropriate resources. This can take the form of written information packs that parents can take away, and which they may choose to read at a later time.[23,24] Referral information should be readily available for support groups with particular expertise relating to the death of a child such as Sids & Kids,[33] SANDS Australia,[34] Compassionate Friends,[35] and other relevant organisations. The extent of involvement of support by ministers of religion will depend on the wishes of and the religious commitment of the family.

Practical assistance with arrangements at the time of the child's death, including organising family support, funeral and financial assistance, should be offered to families as appropriate, while being sensitive to the social and cultural environment of the family.

CULTURAL IMPLICATIONS

Many cultures have specific rituals and practices concerning death. It is critical to listen to the family members and be guided as much as possible by their requests. Some of these rituals may require modification when the death of a child has been referred to the coroner's office. Sensitivity is essential.

It is difficult to make broad statements about the cultural practices related to death and dying in indigenous (Aboriginal and Torres Strait Islander) communities, because across Australia there are different practices and rituals. Examples of the kinds of cultural practices and rituals to be aware of include:

- When a child is dying many families will want any extended family present to be in attendance.
- During the grieving process pre- and post-death, loud crying/wailing may need to occur as part of the community's customs. Privacy in these circumstances is desirable.
- Senior female or male figures may wish to take a lead role in mourning rituals after death has occurred. This can include ceremonial cleansing (washing the child's body), dressing and handling.
- Funeral arrangements may have to be organised by a specific extended family member or a senior member of the community.
- 'House smoking' (burning leaves in order to prevent the spirit from 'rising up') may need to occur relatively quickly after death has occurred. This can mean that the family will want to return to their community quickly.
- Many communities forbid the use of the deceased person's name after death (for up to one year). Nicknames or aliases may be used after death has occurred. A family member with the same name as the deceased may use their second name during the mourning period.
- After a year, there may be some ritual (i.e. tombstone opening) associated with the end of the mourning process, which requires community members to return home even if in hospital themselves.

The Maori culture of New Zealand traditionally has family members present with the body from the time of death through interment. This maintains the harmony of the child, assisting the decedent to join their ancestors. Family members will want to be part of the 'laying out' of the body, washing, dressing, etc.

Other practices reflecting different cultural belief systems that may need to be considered include parents needing to remain with the body 24 hours after the death, caring of the body by staff of the same gender as the deceased child, laying the body to face a certain direction (Mecca), special roles for specific religious/spiritual leaders, and the burning of incense/candles.

When working with families from different cultures following the death of a child, it is important to be guided by custom, ritual, experience, and the family's cultural environment.

LEGAL ISSUES

A life extinct form will need to be completed by one of the attending ED medical staff. However, it will also be necessary to decide whether or not a death certificate can also be completed. If the patient was known to the hospital and the death was not unexpected, the child's usual physician may be prepared to sign a death certificate. This physician may also discuss with the parents the option of performing a hospital-based autopsy.

Usually the death of a child in the ED is not anticipated, and hence becomes a coroner's case (see Chapter 19.2 on Forensic Paediatrics and The Law). For a coroner's case, only a life extinct form can be completed, laying out of the body will be restricted to spot cleaning, the local police must be notified, and parents must not be left unsupervised with the body. It is desirable for the family to formally identify the child's body in the presence of the police. Otherwise identification will have to be performed later and probably at the morgue, a process likely to increase family distress. All medical notes, investigations, observation sheets, etc., should be provided to the police when they depart with the child's body for the morgue. Full and accurate documentation of all events in the patient's hospital chart is essential.

ORGAN AND TISSUE DONATION

Organ donation (e.g. heart, lungs, liver, kidneys) requires intact cardiorespiratory function but brain death. Because of the preconditions required by Transplant Acts before brain death can be declared, organ donation discussions are commonly deferred until admission to the ICU.[31]

Tissue donation (e.g. corneas, heart valves) can occur from cadavers, and hence theoretically this issue could arise for children who die in the ED. However, deaths of children in the ED are usually coroner's cases. For parents faced with the extreme distress of the sudden death of a child and the need for coroner's-case status, it may be potentially too distressing to parents for ED staff to raise the further issue of tissue donation in this setting. This can come a little later at the Forensic Pathology Institute level, when parents have had a little time to regain some degree of composure and hence may be better able to give informed consent. On the rare occasion when the issue of tissue donation is spontaneously brought up by parents in the ED setting, contact with the transplant co-ordinator can be initiated if there are no potential medical contraindications to tissue donation. Consent by the coroner must be obtained prior to tissue removal.

DEBRIEFING AND SUPPORT FOR ED STAFF

Performing an operational debriefing of the resuscitative process with a view to clarifying events for attending staff and identifying areas for potential improvement is essential.

The same cannot be said for psychological debriefing sessions. It has become a popular and widespread practice to conduct single session psychological counselling for personnel attending traumatic critical incidents. ED staff in attendance at an unsuccessful resuscitation fit into this situation. A recent Cochrane Review concluded that single session psychological debriefings have not only failed to reduce the incidence of post-traumatic stress disorder but actually increased the risk of developing it.[25] In addition there was no evidence of reduction in general psychological disturbance, depression or anxiety.

Identifying abnormal psychological symptomatology in ED staff (flashbacks, sleep disturbance, bad dreams, absenteeism, detachment, intensified emotions, etc.) and making ongoing psychological counselling available to affected staff is clearly important. Such symptomatology may occur as a result of either a single exposure or cumulative exposures to traumatic situations. It is important for senior ED staff to promote the concept of self-care, to guarantee confidentiality to staff experiencing problems, and to ensure staff are made aware of counselling options available to them should they experience problems.[26]

CONCLUSION

The death of a child has the most profound effect on parents, family and friends. It can also have a profound effect on staff involved in the resuscitation process. It requires the sensitivity and strength of clinical staff to help relatives through this difficult time and to assist in the initiation of a healthy grieving process. A thoughtful and sensitive approach is likely to have profound and positive long-term implications for all those impacted upon by the death of a child.

Acknowledgements

The authors gratefully acknowledge the assistance of the Indigenous Liaison Service, Herston Hospitals Complex, Brisbane.

CONTROVERSIES

❶ There remains some controversy about actively encouraging parents to be in the resuscitation room.

❷ There is little evidence to support the widespread practice of mandatory single-session psychological counselling of distressed staff who attended the child.

❸ Raising the issue of tissue donation with parents in the ED setting is difficult.

REFERENCES

1. Wright B 1996 Sudden death: Intervention skills for the caring professions. Churchill Livingstone, New York
2. Tsai E 2002 Should family members be present during cardiopulmonary resuscitation? New England Journal of Medicine 346: 1019–1021
3. Scott JL, Sanford SM, Strong L, Gable K 1995 Survivor notification of sudden death in the emergency department. Academy of Emergency Medicine 2: 408–409
4. Leash RM 1996 Death notification: Practical guidelines for health care professionals. Critical Care Nursing Quarterly 19: 21–34
5. Schmidt TA, Norton RL, Tolle SW 1992 Sudden death in the ED: Educating residents to compassionately inform families. Journal of Emergency Medicine 10: 643–647
6. Bagatell R, Meyer R, Derron S et al 2002 When children die: A seminar series for paediatric residents. Paediatrics 110: 348–353
7. Swisher LA, Nieman LZ, Nilsen GJ, Spivey WH 1993 Death notification in the emergency department: A survey of residents and attending physician. Annals of Emergency Medicine 22: 1319–1323
8. Rutkowski A 2002 Death notification in the emergency department. Annals of Emergency Medicine 40: 521–523
9. Jones WH, Buttery M 1981 Sudden death. Survivors perceptions of their emergency department experience. Journal of Emergency Nursing 1: 7
10. Raphael R 1984 The anatomy of bereavement: A handbook for the caring professions. Hutchinson, London
11. Kubler-Ross E On Death and Dying. Tavistock, London
12. Freud S 1917 Mourning and melancholia. Standard Edition XIV. Hogarth Press, London
13. Bowlby J 1969 Attachment and loss. Vol. 1. Attachment. Hogarth Press, London
14. Parkes CM 1972 Bereavement: Studies of grief in adult life. Tavistock, London
15. Glick IO, Weiss RS, Parkes CM 1974 The first year of bereavement. Wiley, New York
16. Attig T 1994 The importance of conceiving of grief as an active process. Death Studies 15(4): 585–647
17. Worden JW 1983 Grief counselling and grief therapy: A handbook for the mental health professional. Routledge, London
18. Neimeyer RA, Neimeyer GJ 1997 Advances in personal construct psychology. Science & Technology Books. Jai Press, New York
19. Dubin WR, Sarnoff JR 1986 Sudden unexpected death: Intervention with the survivors. Annals of Emergency Medicine 15: 54–57
20. Murray J 2001 Loss as a universal concept: A review of literature to identify common aspects of loss in diverse situations. Journal of Loss and Trauma 6: 219–241
21. Murray J 2000 Understanding loss in the lives of children and adolescents: A contribution to the promotion of well being among the young. Australian Journal of Guidance and Counselling 10(1): 95–109
22. Heiney S, Hasan L, Price K 1993 Developing and implementing a bereavement program for a children's hospital. Journal of Paediatric Nursing 876: 385–391
23. Johnson L, Rincon C, Gober C, Rexin D 1993 The development of a comprehensive bereavement program to assist families experiencing paediatric loss. Journal of Paediatric Nursing 8: 3
24. Murray J 1993 An ache in their hearts. University of Queensland Press, Brisbane
25. Rose S, Bisson J, Wessely S 2002 Psychological debriefing for preventing post traumatic stress disorder (PTSD) The Cochrane Database of Systematic Reviews 2002, Issue 2
26. Everly GS, Flannery RB, Mitchell JT 1999 Critical incident stress management: A review of the literature. Aggression and Violent Behaviour 5(1): 23–40
27. ACEP 2002 Death of a child in the emergency department: A joint statement by the American Academy of Pediatrics and the American College of Emergency Physicians. Annals of Emergency Medicine 40: 409–410
28. Olsen JC, Buenefe ML, Falco WE 1998 Death in the emergency department. Annals of Emergency Medicine 31: 758–765
29. Doyle CJ, Post H, Burney RE, Maino J, Keefe M, Rhee KJ 1987 Family participation during resuscitation: An option. Annals of Emergency Medicine 16(6): 673–675
30. Murray J 2002 Children, adolescents and loss. Loss and Grief Unit, University of Queensland, Brisbane
31. Rivers EP, Buse SM, Bivins BA et al 1990 Organ and tissue procurement in the acute care setting: Principles and practice, part 1. Annals of Emergency Medicine 19: 78–85
32. Stewart AE 1999 Complicated bereavement and post-traumatic stress disorder following fatal car crashes: Recommendations for death notification practice. Death Studies 23: 289–321
33. Sids & Kids – www.sidsandkids.org
34. SANDS Australia – www.sands.org.au
35. Compassionate Friends – www.compassionatefriends. org.au

19.2 FORENSIC PAEDIATRICS AND THE LAW

MAREE CRAWFORD

ESSENTIALS

1 Emergency physicians will frequently overlap into the area of forensic medicine and hence require skills and knowledge of their responsibilities with regard to the legal system.

2 Thorough history, examination and documentation provide the basis for well-prepared legal reports. This, in turn, greatly assists in the presentation of evidence to courts.

3 Emergency physicians who deal with children must be aware of their legal obligations with regards to reporting of child abuse, reporting of criminal matters and management of deaths.

4 Doctors providing evidence in court must be seen to be independent, and competent within their level of expertise.

INTRODUCTION

The emergency department (ED) is the initial point of contact for the majority of children presenting with acute injuries. Within this large group will be a number of children with inflicted injury or with findings resulting from abuse or neglect, on whose behalf legal proceedings may be initiated in a variety of legal jurisdictions. Hence ED staff require some expertise in forensic medicine or medicine as it relates to the law.

The role of medical staff in the ED is carefully to assess and treat children with such injuries. A number will present with a clear history or findings to indicate that injury or abuse has been inflicted. Many others will present with non-specific injuries or findings that will not be flagged as abusive, but at a later date may evolve to require legal involvement. It is therefore essential that doctors in the front line adopt high standards of history, examination and documentation for all cases of injury, both to allow detection of abuse and also to meet standards required should a matter progress into the legal system.

Medical staff have a number of legal obligations in such matters. These include mandatory notification of suspected abuse or neglect, and a need to advise the police of a potential criminal matter and to assist police in their investigation of such an event. There are also obligations with regard to the management and notification of deaths to the state coroner.

By virtue of this front-line contact, emergency physicians will at times be required to provide evidence in a variety of legal jurisdictions. Familiarity with these systems, good preparation, and a neutral unbiased approach will allow doctors to discharge their duty to provide the courts with accurate representation of facts and balanced expert opinion.

FORENSIC MEDICAL ASSESSMENT

Forensic medicine, also known as medical jurisprudence, deals with the interaction of medicine and the law. All specialities or areas of medicine will have overlap with forensic matters at some time, and this is particularly so in paediatric emergency medicine. The aims of a forensic medical assessment are diagnosis and management that incorporates the requirements of the legal system. The qualities required include precision and thoroughness, objectivity, neutrality, clarity of thought and expression, and logical formulation of opinion.

Forensic paediatric medicine largely revolves around the assessment of trauma and the determination of whether an injury has been inflicted or imposed upon a child, or whether it is accidental or resulting from an unpredictable or unavoidable event.

As in all areas of medicine, a forensic medical opinion must be based on the information available to us as clinicians. This is obtained using standard clinical tools of history, examination and investigation, but also incorporates additional standards and procedures.

Accurate history and examination

The following points may assist in forensic matters.

❶ Key questions that should be asked and recorded in all cases of injury include:
- Who was present at the time of injury?
- When and where did it occur?
- How did it occur?
- What happened after the injury?

❷ Any explanation that the child gives for injury should be recorded.

❸ A child's developmental abilities should be evaluated to ensure that any actions the child has allegedly taken are within their developmental ability, e.g. standing and turning on hot-water taps.

❹ Any injury must be accurately described including site, colour, size and pattern.

❺ Accurate terminology for injuries should be used, e.g.
- Abrasion – superficial denuding of the skin confined to the epidermis, often called a graze or scratch.
- Bruise or contusion – extravasation of blood into surrounding tissue caused by blunt trauma.
- Laceration – tearing wound through the full thickness of skin caused by blunt trauma.

- Incised wounds – sharply cut injuries from any object with a cutting edge, e.g. stab wounds or slash wounds.

❻ If an injury or injuries are present, there must be careful examination for other abnormalities that might not be immediately obvious, e.g. a child with facial bruising should have careful examination of mouth and ears.

❼ This examination will extend on many occasions to further testing for occult injury, e.g. skeletal survey in infants with bruising, to look for occult fractures, or fundoscopy with dilated pupils in infants with rib fractures, looking for retinal haemorrhages.

❽ Whenever ED medical staff encounter injuries or findings that are suspicious of abuse or neglect they should in the first instance involve more senior staff, either a senior paediatric emergency physician or a child protection paediatrician, for guidance.

❾ Specific forensic sampling may be required, e.g. toxicology, or specimen collection in sexual abuse. Child protection or forensic physicians should be involved, and a clear 'chain of evidence' must be maintained from clinician to police to forensic pathologist.

Documentation

Both history and examination findings should be clearly recorded in detail. Accurate printed diagrams of body parts are an excellent aid and should be used. Any injury thought to be suspicious of being inflicted or of being caused by abuse should be photographed. This can be done using hospital photographic services or ED photographic equipment if available. However, if there are suspicions of abuse, staff will be notifying child protection agencies and the resources of the police may be used for photography. These are usually of higher quality, and police involvement overcomes problems of confirming a chain of evidence if the material is later used in a legal setting. Digital photography is unacceptable in a court because of the ability to alter images.

Notes made at the time of consultation will provide the doctor with information to prepare a statement or report for a court, if this is required at a later time (sometimes years later). They also will assist the doctor in providing evidence if asked to appear in court proceedings. For this reason documentation must be detailed and accurate.

Opinion formulation

The next step is to infer the mechanism of the injury, if possible, from the clinical findings, e.g. a patterned bruise is due to blunt trauma from contact with a specific object, and posterior rib fractures are due to chest compression. Frequently there are no discriminating features to assist with determining mechanism, e.g. child with multiple non-specific bruises. In all cases the adequacy of the parent or carer's explanation of the injury must be considered.

Any opinions as to causation and mechanism must be based on the medical findings and their compatibility with the history, and not on extraneous factors, e.g. adverse psychosocial history. Opinions must be logical and not based on speculation. An attempt should be made to differentiate whether injuries are truly accidental, accidental but with component of neglect, or inflicted. In many cases no definite conclusion can be drawn.

LEGAL OBLIGATIONS

Mandatory reporting of child abuse

Medical practitioners in all states of Australia except Western Australia are mandated to notify any suspicion of abuse or neglect to the relevant statutory authority in that state, e.g. Department of Child Safety in Queensland, or Department of Children's Services in NSW. Definitions of abuse commonly relate to the concept of harm, which, for example, under the Queensland Child Protection Act 1999 is defined as 'any detrimental effect of a significant nature on the child's physical, psychological or emotional wellbeing'. Practitioners should be familiar with the requirements and mechanisms for notification within their state and

locality. Doctors are free of any liability if such reports are made in good faith.

Notification of suspected criminal matters

In addition, if the medical officer considers that an injury is not accidentally caused or that a crime has been attempted or completed, there is obligation to notify the police. Individuals including medical practitioners are required to assist police in their investigations.

Notification to the coroner of deaths under certain circumstances

Medical practitioners are required to notify the coroner's office of deaths that occur in a variety of circumstances. These include, in broad terms, situations of any sudden, unexplained death, situations where cause of death is unknown, or whenever there are any suspicious circumstances surrounding the death. The coroner has the responsibility to investigate and report on these matters.

LEGAL JURISDICTIONS

At times, emergency physicians will be involved with children whose injuries or other findings will result from physical assault or abuse, sexual assault or abuse or emotional abuse or neglect. Some of these cases will end with involvement in the legal system in various jurisdictions.

Inflicted injury in which there is a single alleged offender may lead to criminal charges of assault or of torture. The child protection statutory agency may look to provide safety for a child or siblings via a range of orders in the Children's Court or information may be sought regarding a child's wellbeing by the Family Law Court in matters of contested custody or residency between parents.

To assist medical practitioners in their interaction with the legal system a brief outline of the different court systems follows.

Criminal court

In a criminal matter a person is charged with committing an offence under the criminal code of the state in which the offence occurred. Criminal courts are adversarial systems where the Crown must prove that the accused is guilty of the offence with which they have been charged. The level of proof required is *beyond reasonable doubt.*

Police are responsible for investigating any alleged crime and for laying charges against an individual if grounds exist. They are also responsible for assisting the Director of Prosecutions in obtaining witness statements. Initial evidence is heard in a committal proceeding before a magistrate. In this court the evidence is tested to ensure that there is sufficient for the matter to proceed to a higher court.

Whether the matter is heard in a higher court is determined by the nature of the offence. *Summary offences* (usually relatively minor offences, e.g. traffic offences, some assaults) are dealt with solely in the Magistrate's Court. *Indictable offences* proceed to a higher court before judge and jury in either District or Supreme Courts.

Doctors may be called to provide evidence either as a professional witness providing factual evidence of something that occurred in the clinical setting, or as an expert witness, a specialist or senior doctor who can provide expert opinion on certain facts.

The first involvement that a doctor may have with the proceedings is via a request from police for a statement of witness. This statement, which must be in a format acceptable to the court, will provide the basis for oral evidence to be provided. The report must be clear, truthful and unambiguous, should avoid the use of medical jargon and should clearly describe terminology in such a way that it may be understood by a lay person.

The statement should include details of professional qualifications and experience, a brief history provided to the doctor, and an accurate description of clinical findings. Reference should be made to any other documentation or investigation, e.g. photographs, so that they can be admitted as evidence. It is important to address whether the injuries found could produce effects consistent with the definition of the charges (see Table 19.2.1). This usually requires comments as to effects on the child with regards to pain and suffering, and prognosis assuming medical intervention had not occurred. It is not appropriate to describe injuries as, for example, constituting 'grievous bodily harm' as this is for the court to determine.

Children's court – child protection proceedings

Children's courts deal with criminal charges brought against children up to seventeen or eighteen years. They also handle matters related to children's welfare.

An ED medical officer who provides assessment and treatment of a child with inflicted injury or abuse may be required to provide information and expertise to assist this court in making decisions regarding a child's need for care and protection by the state or need for other protective orders. This court is conducted before a magistrate, is adversarial, but requires a lower standard of proof, i.e. *on the balance of probability.* The nature of evidence that can be admitted is more lenient than in criminal proceedings, allowing hearsay (second hand) information. As in criminal proceedings, a sworn report or affidavit will often be sought prior to appearance in court, and should follow the general principles for statements for criminal court.

Family law court

This is a federal court created to administer the Family Law Act 1975.

In this jurisdiction, medical practitioners may be required to provide evidence on behalf of children in contested matters between parents, related to guardianship and residency of children. Again the system is adversarial with legal representatives for both parental parties, and often a separate independent representative for the child or children, outlining a case before a judge for ruling. Proof is on the basis of the *balance of probability.*

Coroner's inquest

The coroner's role is to investigate and report on the circumstances surrounding a person's death. The coroner's powers are defined by state or territory legislation. This legislation also defines a medical practitioner's obligations to notify reportable deaths and to co-operate in any inquiry. The precise definition of reportable death varies between states but, in general, includes any death for which the cause is unknown or where the cause of death appears to be by violent, unnatural or accidental means or where there are suspicious circumstances.

Emergency physicians will sometimes encounter children dying or presenting dead to the ED and must be familiar with their state or territory requirements. The death should be notified to the coroner's office and also to the police. Police will assist the coroner in the investigation, and a forensic pathologist will conduct an autopsy and report back to the coroner.

At times doctors will be called to provide a statement and may be required to give evidence at a coronial inquest. This is not a trial but a fact-finding inquiry. A mix of inquisitorial and adversarial procedures is used and hearsay evidence can be accepted.

The Coroner will make public the findings of the inquest and may comment on inadequacies of systems and management. The coroner does not directly recommend criminal proceedings.

Table 19.2.1 **Terminology of criminal charges**
• *Bodily harm* – an injury which interferes with health or comfort (e.g. causes moderate pain or discomfort) but does not endanger life or cause permanent disability
• *Grievous bodily harm* – any bodily injury of such a nature as to endanger or be likely to endanger life or to cause or be likely to cause permanent injury to health if left untreated
• *Unlawful wounding* – an injury in which the true skin has been broken, e.g. laceration or incised wound
• *Torture* – an intentional infliction of severe pain or suffering on a person by an act or series of acts done on one or more than one occasion

Source: Derived from Queensland Criminal Code Act 1899.

PROVIDING EVIDENCE IN COURT

Doctors may be called to give evidence in any of the courts outlined. This will be either as a professional witness providing evidence in fact, related to what they saw or did as part of their work, or, alternatively, to provide an expert opinion on a matter.

Prior to attendance at court the doctor may have been requested to provide a statement of witness, affidavit, or medical report which will be composed from the doctors notes. The statement must include professional qualifications and, in the case of an expert witness, must establish that they have specialised skills and knowledge in their area of expertise.

The report should include a brief history of the reasons for seeing the child, the date, time and place the child was seen, and the person accompanying the child. Any spontaneous disclosures that the child has made to the doctor should be included. The general state and demeanour of the child, and detailed specific findings are important. Lastly, an opinion regarding mechanism of any injury, and the effects on the child of any injury with regards to pain and disability are important.

Court appearances can be stressful for doctors. However, it is important to remember that an individual's evidence is but a small part of any case. The doctor is there to assist the court in its deliberations, and is not personally on trial. The doctor must adopt an independent neutral role and be prepared to consider objectively any statements put to them. Doctors are not there to support a particular 'side'.

When appearing as an expert witness, a doctor will be asked initially to describe their qualifications and expertise. They will then be questioned by one counsel and cross-examined by the other. They should listen carefully to all questions and answer as accurately as possible. They should have their notes of the consultation available and ask leave of the court to refer to them. It is important to remain calm and professional in all ways and never be tempted to outsmart the lawyers in their domain. Careful preparation and a sound knowledge of the relevant medical problems will assist the doctor greatly in this whole process. If questioned about a matter outside their level of experience or expertise, a doctor should indicate that this is the case and not attempt to speculate.

Doctors providing evidence to a coronial inquest will normally be independent parties. However, if there are issues of possible medical negligence involved, prior contact with their medical indemnity organisation should be made.

FURTHER READING

Breen K, Plueckhahn V, Cordner S 1997 Ethics, law and medical practice. Allen & Unwin, St. Leonards, NSW
Dix A, Errington M, Nicholson K, Powe R 1996 Law for the medical profession in Australia, 2nd edn. Butterworth-Heinemann, Port Melbourne
Knight, B 1997 Simpson's forensic medicine, 11th edn. Arnold, London & Baltimore MD, USA
Queensland Child Protection Act 1999
Queensland Criminal Code Act 1899

ADMINISTRATION AND EMS

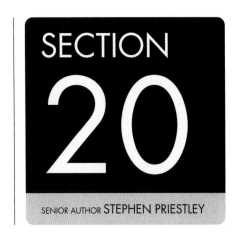

SECTION

20

SENIOR AUTHOR STEPHEN PRIESTLEY

ANALGESIA AND SEDATION

20.1 ANALGESIA AND SEDATION

STEPHEN PRIESTLEY • JASON ACWORTH • ANTHONY HARRINGTON

ESSENTIALS

1 Acute pain is one of the most common emergency department presenting problems.

2 Pain rating scales suitable to the age and development of the child are useful in establishing a child's level of pain and assessing the effect of analgesia.

3 Adopt a multimodal approach to pain management (pharmacological, cognitive, behavioural and physical therapies).

4 Involve families and tailor interventions to the individual child.

5 Minimise the number of drugs used and become familiar with dose, administration and potential complications.

6 Combining drugs without detailed knowledge and training risks serious adverse outcomes.

7 Establish educational programs and policies for procedural sedation.

INTRODUCTION

Acute pain in children is one of the most common reasons for presentation to the emergency department (ED).[1] Pain resulting from injury, illness and necessary medical procedures is associated with increased anxiety, avoidance behaviour, systemic symptoms and parental distress. Painful experiences involve the interaction of physiological, psychological, behavioural developmental and situational factors. Pain is a subjective multifactorial experience and should be treated as such.[2] Children with painful conditions can be difficult to assess and are often still under assessed and under treated. Children often receive less analgesia than adults and children younger than two years receive significantly less analgesia than older children.[3-5]

Early and appropriate analgesia may be achieved by developing a re-engineered system with well-developed pain management educational programs and policies and time-to-analgesia standards within the ED.[6] Definitions of terms are outlined in Table 20.1.1.

ASSESSMENT AND MEASUREMENT OF PAIN

Over the last twenty years many pain assessment and measurement tools have been developed that are suitable for the age and developmental stage of the child. A definitive review of pain measurement in infants and children has been published recently.[7]

Accurate assessment requires a detailed pain history and consideration of the complexity of the child's pain perception and the influence of situational, psychological and developmental factors. For older children pain is best assessed using the child's self-report. Four common ways of recognising pain in children are outlined in Table 20.1.2.

Observational assessment scoring is useful when the child is too young or self-report is not possible, e.g. child with cognitive impairment. Pain ratings provided by parents or regular carers may be useful[8] though whilst there is good correlation between the child's and the parent's assessment of pain intensity there is poor agreement. In particular, parents tend to underestimate and underscore more severe pain being experienced by their children[9] and this fact needs to be taken into consideration when assessing a child's level of pain. Physiological measures often reflect stress reactions. For example, the infant who is hungry, frightened or in need of a nappy change may give an inappropriately high score. Behaviour is observed for the following indicators: crying; facial expressions; body language and posture; sleeplessness; agitation; and appearance. Undue quietness

Table 20.1.2 Recognition of pain in children

1. The child's self-report of pain
2. Behavioural changes, e.g. crying, guarding, facial grimacing
3. Physiological changes, e.g. pallor, tachycardia, and tachypnoea
4. Pathophysiological process, e.g. fracture or burn

Table 20.1.1 Definitions of terms

Analgesia	Relief of the perception of pain without sedation
Anxiolysis	Relief of apprehension without sedation or analgesia
Sedation	Lessening of awareness of the environment and or pain perception
Anaesthesia (general)	Complete loss or awareness of the environment accompanied by loss of protective reflexes
Procedural sedation	A technique of administering sedative or dissociation agents, with or without analgesics, to induce a state that allows the patient to tolerate unpleasant procedures while maintaining cardiorespiratory function. Procedural sedation and analgesia is intended to result in a depressed level of consciousness but one that allows the patient to maintain airway control independently and continuously[39]

and blunted behaviour may be due to severe pain, fatigue, extreme illness or the overuse of sedatives. An understanding of the pathophysiological process can also give the clinician a surrogate indication of severity of pain.

Pain scores are typically standardised on a 0–10 scale. Pain scores are documented with other observations and vital signs. Some common pain rating scales appropriate to age are outlined in Table 20.1.3.[7]

NON-PHARMACOLOGICAL METHODS

A balanced multi-disciplinary approach using pharmacological and non-pharmacological strategies is essential to providing optimal analgesia and sedation for the child. Some useful non-pharmacologic strategies are outlined in Table 20.1. 4.

COMMONLY USED AGENTS

Some of the most commonly used agents are listed in Table 20.1.5.

Pure analgesics

Paracetamol is usually the first line of therapy for mild to moderate painful conditions. It can be given orally and rectally. NSAIDs, such as ibuprofen, are usually second-line therapy and have excellent analgesic and anti-inflammatory properties, which may enhance the effects of paracetamol.

Pure sedative agents

Sedative agents relieve anxiety but not pain. They may reduce the child's ability to communicate pain and discomfort

and a common side effect is paradoxical hyperexcitability. They are useful for painless diagnostic studies and, when used in combination with opioids or nitrous oxide, can produce a state of deep sedation.

Sedative analgesias

Opioid analgesics and nitrous oxide are the mainstay of treatment of severe pain. Infants and neonates require lower doses of opioid medication. Opioids are ideally administered intravenously in a dilute solution, e.g. morphine (1 mg mL^{-1}) given slowly over a few minutes and titrated against response. A further dose may be given after 5–10 minutes.

Fentanyl is a potent rapid acting analgesic with a shorter duration of action and used in combination with midazolam produces a state of dissociation and deep sedation. Intranasal fentanyl has been shown to give equivalent analgesia to intramuscular morphine in children with forearm fractures.[10] It offers a quicker onset, is less invasive, and its duration of action, although short, allows time for topical anaesthetic application prior to intravenous cannulation for ongoing analgesia.

Nitrous oxide mixed with oxygen has a potent analgesic action with rapid

Table 20.1.4 Supportive and distractive techniques

Environment
- Calm friendly non-clinical atmosphere
- Toys, mobiles, pictures and videos

Psychological
- Parental presence
- Age appropriate communication
- Clear confident instructions

Cognitive – Behavioural
- Distraction techniques
- Hypnosis
- Art/stories
- Music/video/TV
- Interactive computer games
- Guided imagery
- Relaxation therapy

Physical
- Massage/rubbing
- Comfort swaddling (infants)
- Heat/cold techniques
- Immobilisation and elevation (injured part)
- Comforter (favourite blanket/soft toy)

onset and offset. It is an excellent analgesic sedative for gaining rapid IV access, injecting local anaesthetics, performing a nerve block or splinting a fractured limb.[11,12] Entonox (50% nitrous oxide, 50% oxygen) is usually delivered via a demand-valve system. This limits its use in younger or uncooperative children. The use of machines that deliver variable concentration (30–70%) nitrous oxide via a continuous flow system allow the use of this very effective drug on a wider patient age range but have the potential for a higher adverse event rate if not used within strict guidelines. Oxygen should be administered for 3–5 minutes after cessation of nitrous oxide to prevent diffusion hypoxia. Nitrous oxide is contraindicated in conditions involving closed air spaces (e.g. pneumothorax, bowel obstruction).

Ketamine

Ketamine is a unique analgesic dissociative agent. Its action produces a near ideal state of sedation, amnesia, analgesia and motion control with few side effects. It has been extensively studied with safety and efficiency documented in over 11 000 children. Emergence reactions, common in adults during the recovery phase, are rare in children. Airway complications (including stridor, laryngospasm, respiratory depression, and apnoea) very rarely occur and may be associated with young age (under six months), rapid intravenous administration, and co-administration of other agents (e.g. opioids, benzodiazepines). Multiple routes of administration are available but IV and IM routes are preferred.[13–17]

Local anaesthetic agents

The expanded use of topical anaesthetics has revolutionised the management of simple lacerations in the ED and has also greatly improved conditions for intravenous cannulation and lumbar puncture. These agents provide a non-invasive means of producing local anaesthesia and can be applied at triage to facilitate timely management in the ED.[18]

EMLA™ (2.5% lidocaine, 2.5% prilocaine) is a well-established topical anaesthetic for intravenous cannulation

Table 20.1.3 Pain scoring

Age	Pain rating scale
0–3 years	Observer scores (parent and/or nurse)
3–8 years	Wong-Baker faces score
>8 years	Numerical rating score, Wong-Baker faces score

Table 20.1.5   Commonly used agents for sedation and analgesia

Classification	Doses	Comments
Pure analgesics		
Paracetamol	15–30 mg kg^{-1} PO/PR (< 3 months 10 mg kg^{-1})	30 mg kg^{-1} stat. only as a single dose (check no recent doses of paracetamol)
Ibuprofen (NSAID)	5–10 mg kg^{-1} PO	
Liquegesic Co paracetamol/codeine mixture (e.g. Painstop™)	Dose based on paracetamol content	
Pure sedatives		
Midazolam	0.05–0.15 mg kg^{-1} IV/IM; 0.5–0.75 mg kg^{-1} PO; 0.3–0.5 mg kg^{-1} IN	Paradoxical excitement reaction in 10% of children when used PO or IN
Chloral hydrate	0.2–0.5 mg kg^{-1} IV; 25–50 mg kg^{-1} PO/PR	Unreliable and prolonged onset of action
Sedative/analgesics		
Morphine	0.1–0.2 mg kg^{-1} per dose (>3 months) IV, IM 0.05–0.1 mg kg^{-1} per dose (<3 months) IV, IM Infusion (>3 months) 0.01–0.04 mg kg^{-1} hour^{-1}	Cardiorespiratory depression with IV/IM doses IV dose preferred
Fentanyl		IV recommended as more reliable and allows titration of small doses to achieve an end point
Nitrous oxide	50:50 mix inhalation agent (ENTONOX); N$_2$O:O$_2$ continuous flow variable mix 30–70% with oxygen	Rapid onset; continuous flow delivery system allows use in young children/short duration of action Vomiting can occur; contraindicated with pneumothorax/chest injuries
Dissociative agent		
Ketamine	1–2 mg kg^{-1} IV; 2.5–4.0 mg kg^{-1} IM; 5–10 mg kg^{-1} PO	Excellent safety profile in selected patients undergoing painful procedures; contraindicated in head injury, seizure disorders, ocular injuries
Local anaesthetic agents		
Injectable		
Lidocaine	1% or 2%; 3 mg kg^{-1} maximum dose without adrenaline (epinephrine); 7 mg kg^{-1} maximum dose with adrenaline	Pain of injection can be minimised by using small needles (e.g. 31G), slow infiltration, infiltrating through wound edges, pretreatment with topical LA, buffering and warming
Bupivacaine	3 mg kg^{-1} (maximum dose)	Slower onset, longer duration of action compared with lignocaine; useful for nerve blocks
Prilocaine	0.5% solution common; 2.5–3.0 mg kg^{-1}	Safe agent for intravenous regional anaesthesia (Biers blocks)
Topical		
• Surface EMLA™	Eutectic mix of lidocaine 2.5% and prilocaine 2.5%	Require 30–40 minutes post-application to achieve satisfactory dermal anaesthesia
AnGel/Ametop	Amethocaine 4%	
• Wound ALA	ALA solution is a mixture of 4% lidocaine, 0.5% amethocaine and adrenaline 1:1000	Contains adrenaline so cannot be used in end arteriole regions, e.g. digits, penis; requires > 20 minutes of good contact with wound to provide anaesthesia; may require supplementation with small doses infiltrated LA
AC Gel	Adrenaline 1:2000 and cocaine 4.7%	Cocaine content makes drug expensive and introduces storage issues; cocaine-containing topical anaesthetics have been associated with serious morbidity and mortality relating to rapid absorption of cocaine via mucosa, gel lessens this risk
Reversal agents		
Naloxone	10 μg kg^{-1} IV	May need to repeat doses
Flumazenil	0.02 mg kg^{-1} IV	

and lumbar puncture. Its use in the ED is, however, limited due to its long onset to peak effect (at least one hour) and its vasoconstrictive effect, which may make cannulation more difficult. AnGel™ (4% amethocaine) has a quicker onset of action (30–45 minutes) and its vasodilating effect may facilitate cannulation. It has been shown to be at least as effective as EMLA™ and has a good safety profile. Application may cause local itching and wheal formation as temporary side-effects.[19,20]

Topical wound anaesthetics, e.g. ALA (adrenaline [epinephrine] 1:1000, lidocaine 4%, amethocaine 0.5%) and AC Gel (adrenaline 1:1000, cocaine 12%) permit wound management with minimal to no discomfort.[21,22] ALA has a similar local anaesthetic efficacy to AC Gel and is less expensive. It does not require refrigeration or secure storage, may be used safely near mucous membranes and does not share the toxic effects of the cocaine-bearing compound. ALA instilled in a wound for 20–30 minutes provides sufficient anaesthesia for suturing 75–90% of scalp and facial lacerations[22,23] and 40–60% of extremity wounds.[24] Its vasoconstrictive effect is also useful prior to application of cyanoacrylate tissue adhesive.

Wound infiltration with injectable local anaesthetics can be carried out with lessened pain by buffering the local anaesthetic, warming the solution to body temperature, using fine-bore needles and slow administration techniques through the wound edges rather than through intact skin.[25-29]

Nitrous oxide and distraction techniques during the process of injection often provide good analgesia. Safe dosage regimes must be adhered to by the clinician.

SELECTION OF AGENTS BY PROCEDURE AND AGE

Pain management can be simplified by dividing pain into mild, moderate and severe categories and matching this with the appropriate analgesic agent(s) (Table 20.1.6).

Table 20.1.6 Analgesia options

Wong–Baker faces score			2		3		4	5		
Pain score	1	2	3	4	5	6	7	8	9	10
Mild pain				Moderate pain				Severe pain		
Paracetamol				Ibuprofen Codeine				Morphine Nitrous oxide		

It is best to minimise the number of agents used and to be familiar with doses, duration of action, adverse effects and contraindications. Choice of agent should be individualised for the child's level of pain and the procedure. Dissociative techniques using various combinations of agents are useful for very painful procedures or in infants and toddlers.

Ideally routes of administration should be non-invasive. Extensive knowledge and experience of the synergistic effects of analgesics and sedative agents can produce a 'balanced' state of sedation and analgesia (Table 20.1.7).

SOME COMMON PROCEDURES

Painless diagnostic study

Motion control for imaging procedures, such as CT scan or even plain X-ray, can be a challenge. Oral anxiolytics given prior may be useful. It is important to apply topical local anaesthetic (AnGel™ or EMLA™) 45–60 minutes prior to the procedure to facilitate intravenous cannula placement if adjunctive intravenous sedation becomes necessary.

Venepuncture and IV cannulation

Topical local anaesthetic agents are useful for semi urgent IV access. Rapid access is best gained using nitrous oxide analgesia/sedation and distraction techniques.

Small laceration

A pre-emptive approach using a combination of oral anxiolytics/analgesic medication will improve co-operation during the procedure. Topical wound anaesthetics (ALA, AC Gel) allow wound

Table 20.1.7 Balanced analgesia and sedation

The four components
1. Sedation
2. Analgesia
3. Amnesia
4. Motion control

cleaning and closure with minimal or no pain. Tissue adhesives are helpful for smaller wounds. Nitrous oxide and distraction are again useful.

Complex wound management

Infants and toddlers may require dissociative methods using a choice of ketamine IM or IV, fentanyl and midazolam IV, or nitrous oxide. With appropriate premedication older children can be managed with local or regional anaesthetic blocks.

Foreign body removal

Anxiolytic premedication may be all that is needed for the older child, however younger children usually require dissociative techniques.

Fracture, joint dislocation, splinting and manipulation

Severe pain associated with these injuries is best managed initially with nitrous oxide or intranasal fentanyl while IV access is gained for ongoing opioid analgesia. Regional local anaesthetic blocks, e.g. femoral nerve block, are useful to enable splints and traction to be applied. Intravenous regional anaesthesia (IVRA) is a useful technique for fracture manipulation in older children. Many children under the age of ten years are referred for general anaesthesia.

Multi-trauma

Children with severe multiple injuries often require many painful procedures during the initial assessment phase. A team approach is needed with special attention to analgesia and sedation. Rapid sequence intubation (RSI) is often the most humane option. This allows a more rapid approach to investigation and management. Other alternatives for managing ongoing pain relief include continuous opioid infusion during the initial phases of resuscitation and stabilisation and patient-controlled analgesia (PCA) once the patient is stable.

PROCEDURAL SEDATION: PATIENT SELECTION, RISK ASSESSMENT AND MANAGEMENT

The goal of procedural sedation in the ED is to provide a suitable level of sedation that enables successful completion of the procedure whilst minimising the risk of adverse events to the patient and enabling early safe discharge home from the department. In order to achieve this goal consideration needs to be given to the health status of the patient, the procedure to be performed – particularly the duration and likely amount of pain – selection of an appropriate drug or combination of drugs, provision of non-pharmacologic techniques, patient preparation and the informed consent and understanding of the parent(s) or carer(s).

Critical incident analysis of adverse sedation events in paediatrics have identified inadequate medical evaluation, inadequate monitoring during or after the procedure, inadequate skills in problem recognition and timely intervention and lack of experience of the practitioner with a particular age group or with an underlying medical condition as factors associated with adverse events in paediatric sedation.[30]

Development and implementation of ED sedation guidelines for children is associated with practice improvements and the lessening of adverse events and complications.[31,32]

Notably a survey of Australasian EDs conducted in 1998 found a wide variation of practice amongst the forty respondent departments with only 58% of mixed adult/paediatric departments reporting use of formal guidelines for paediatric sedation and only 52% of all departments surveyed reporting the use of formal discharge criteria.[33]

The formulation of a sedation plan and sedation policies can be divided into:

❶ Pre-procedure assessment.
❷ Procedure management.
❸ Post-procedure management.

Pre-procedure assessment

Health status of the patient is essential to identify elements of medical history or any current illnesses that may impact upon the safety of procedural sedation, choice of agent or consideration of alternative techniques.

Important factors to consider are listed in Table 20.1.8.

Though many of these factors are not absolute contraindications to many of the drugs used, their presence may prompt a change in drug used or dosage, a change in the level of both the patient monitoring used throughout the procedure and the experience level of the physician administering the sedation and, on occasion, may lead to referral for general anaesthesia or deferral of the procedure.

Children aged less than one year, and particularly the very young baby, have a higher incidence of hypoxic complications with procedural sedation and in very young infants consideration should be given to general anaesthesia with formal airway management.[34]

While the presence of active asthma or URTI is associated with a higher risk of complications, including laryngospasm, in patients undergoing general anaesthesia[35,36] it is unclear whether this increased risk also applies to procedural sedation. Most authorities assume that it does and tailor the sedation plans accordingly.

Further history that needs to be obtained includes current medications, allergies and fasting status.

The issue of necessary fasting status to minimise the risk of gastric aspiration for children undergoing procedural sedation remains unclear (see controversies). Many EDs use a general fasting guideline of two hours for clear liquids and four hours for solids or liquids that are not clear (including milk). The safe fasting state for patients with conditions associated with diminished airway protective reflexes or delayed gastric emptying should be adjusted.

Physical examination should include patient weight, baseline vital signs including oxygen saturation, assessment of conscious state, evaluation of the airway and examination of the cardiovascular and respiratory systems.

The ASA physical status categories developed for general anaesthesia[37] are not generally used for ED procedural sedation as it is unclear how they extrapolate to this setting.[38] Following risk assessment and generation of a sedation plan this plan should be discussed with the child's parent or carer to obtain informed consent. Clear explanation to the older child is often useful in an effort to allay anxiety and optimise co-operation.

The expected effects on the child, risks, benefits, alternatives and need for monitoring and observation during and after the procedure prior to safe discharge must be discussed with the parent or

---

Table 20.1.8   Patient factors to consider in procedural sedation

- Current illness URTI, active asthma, altered conscious state, haemodynamic compromise
- Age under 12 months (especially < 3 months)
- Airway abnormalities – craniofacial deformities, tracheomalacia, congenital anomalies
- Cardiac conditions – congenital heart disease, arrhythmias, cardiac failure
- Neurological conditions – seizure disorders, raised intracranial pressure
- Respiratory conditions – active asthma, upper or lower respiratory tract infections, respiratory failure
- Hepatic or renal disorders
- Prior history of failure of sedation
- Prior adverse event due to sedation, analgesia or anaesthesia

guardian. As the expected effects, risks and recovery times prior to discharge will vary greatly between different agents the use of a standardised consent form is suboptimal and consideration should be given to generating consent forms that reflect the individual features of the different agents to clearly identify that these issues have been discussed with the child's parent. An alternative to this involves standard documentation in the medical record that agent-specific issues were discussed with the parent(s)/ carer(s).

In most EDs there is a policy that informed consent for procedural sedation is obtained in written form unless it is employed in a life- or limb-threatening situation.

Procedure management

A number of recommendations and statements from clinical authorities have been published detailing particular aspects of required personnel, monitoring equipment, patient preparation for procedural sedation in children both inside and outside of the operating theatre.[39-42]

It is essential that the team administering procedural sedation are aware that it is impossible to reliably predict in advance the level of sedation that will occur in an individual patient given a sedative drug or combination of drugs. Regardless of the intended level of sedation or route of administration, the sedation of a patient represents a continuum, and may result in the loss of the patient's protective reflexes – a patient may move easily from a light level of sedation to deep sedation.[41] As a consequence it is imperative to plan for situations where the child becomes sedated to a far greater level than intended or experiences significant cardiorespiratory complications of sedation.

Accordingly, well-understood policies and procedures detailing the requirements for procedure management should be developed by EDs providing procedural sedation to children. Table 20.1.9 details the important elements of the conduct of procedural sedation management.

Personnel

There must always be at least two clinical staff involved in the procedure.

Table 20.1.9 Elements of safe procedural sedation management

1. Personnel
2. Environment
3. Monitoring
4. Medication
5. Patient preparation
6. Recovery
7. Documentation
8. Discharge criteria

Source: Adapted from ACEM policy on procedural sedation and analgesia in the ED.[39]

One acts as the 'sedationist' and is responsible for giving drugs and monitoring the patient – particularly from a respiratory and circulatory perspective. The sedationist should have no other responsibilities in the procedure thus enabling that person to be able to respond as rapidly as necessary to changes in the patient's vital signs or clinical state. If a nurse is not present this person should also be responsible for documenting observations, times and doses of drugs administered and recording specific interventions.

The sedationist should have formulated the sedation plan by taking a history and performing a physical examination of the child and should be knowledgeable about the drug or drugs being used. This person must be trained in the recognition and management of airway and ventilatory complications and be proficient in paediatric resuscitation.

The second person ('the proceduralist') is responsible for performing the procedure, e.g. fracture reduction or suturing.

In most cases there should be two further personnel. A nurse is valuable to perform the recording of observations and events and to liaise with the child's parent or carer who may often be present during the procedure.

Lastly, it is recommended that there is a supervising senior doctor – generally at specialist or advanced trainee level who has specific experience and competence in paediatric airway management and resuscitation. This person may be taking the role of sedationist but on other occasions it is appropriate that he or she is aware that the procedure is occurring and has guaranteed that they will be in the department and able to assist rapidly should complications arise.

Environment

Paediatric procedural sedation must be performed in a facility that is adequate in size and has equipment available for drug administration, clinical monitoring, airway management, vascular access and cardiorespiratory resuscitation.

Sedation in environments where the area does not meet these requirements is associated with an increased level of serious adverse events.[30]

Equipment

Equipment must be suitable for children of all the ages and sizes being treated. The ability to recognise respiratory or circulatory compromise early with the use of monitoring equipment is essential. Devices for airway management and techniques of advanced life support are recommended along with sedative drug-reversal agents and life-support drugs.

Recommended equipment and drugs are listed in Table 20.1.10.

Monitoring, observations and recording

The most important element of monitoring during sedation is close, continuous observation of the patient.[43]

Continuous oxygen saturation monitoring is recommended in all forms of procedural sedation as is continuous observation of colour and rate and depth of ventilation.

It is recommended that intermittent heart rate and blood pressure monitoring is used when the level of sedation is deep.

Observation and recording of heart rate, blood pressure, respiratory rate, conscious level should be recorded prior to the procedure, after sedative drug administration and at 5–10 minute intervals during the procedure, depending on the level of sedation achieved. Times of administration, drugs given, dosages and routes of administration of drugs should be clearly recorded on a time-based observation chart.

Interventions performed, such as provision of supplemental oxygen or basic airway management, should also be recorded.

There are a variety of quantitative sedation scores that can also be used to measure the level of sedation and guide administration of sedative drugs.[32,44] Use of these can assist in standardisation of terminology and classification of sedation depth, particularly for use in clinical audit and research.[45]

Medication

All sedative drugs to be used should be pre-measured, checked and labelled.

Reversal drugs and life-support drugs should also be available (see Table 20.1.10).

Intravenous access

In patients receiving intravenous sedation the intravenous access should be retained until the patient's conscious state has improved. Patients receiving sedation by a non-intravenous route may benefit from the safety of having an intravenous line placed, particularly when the level of sedation is deep or if there is a higher than usual probability of complications as a consequence of current illness or injury or comorbidities. Where an intravenous line is not established prior to sedation a practitioner with skills in establishing vascular access in children must be readily available.[40,43]

Post-procedure management

It is imperative that children are closely observed and monitored in an appropriate environment following procedural sedation. Children vary greatly in their speed of recovery from sedation. This is also influenced by the drug(s) used, the route of administration and the total dosage given.

The period immediately following the completion of the procedure – with cessation of the painful or unpleasant stimulus – is a period during which cardiorespiratory depressant effects of the sedation drugs may be most apparent and it is during this time that there is an increased risk of complications.[43]

If the child is moved to another area following the completion of the procedure they should continue to be closely observed and monitored by a suitably experienced nurse and resuscitation equipment should still be immediately available if needed. The frequency of vital signs observation can gradually lessen as the child awakens and the risk of cardiorespiratory complications diminishes. Generally, the frequency of vital signs observation will lessen from 5-minutely to 30-minutely as the child returns to their pre-sedation state.

Post-procedural observations should be recorded on the same time-based observation sheet as used during the procedure and evidence of improvement in conscious level and activity should also be recorded.

It is important to have standard discharge criteria, which must be met by the child prior to leaving the ED, and nursing staff caring for the child must be familiar with these. Suggested discharge criteria are listed in Table 20.1.11.

Development of a standard post-procedural sedation discharge instruction sheet, which includes advice regarding diet, activities, observation, and sleeping in the 24 hours after discharge along with specific signs to watch for and a direct ED contact number, is also valuable. The adult taking responsibility for the child after discharge should receive a copy prior to leaving and staff should both check that they understand it clearly and answer any questions about it that they may have.

Finally, follow-up arrangements relating to the procedure performed (e.g. review of wound, suture removal) should also be provided before discharge.

Table 20.1.10   List of drugs and equipment recommended for safe procedural sedation

Equipment*
- Oxygen source, masks and tubing
- Suction source and suckers
- Self-inflating bag mask device
- Oral and nasal airways
- Endotracheal tubes
- Laryngoscopes
- Defibrillator with paediatric paddles
- ECG monitor
- Non-invasive blood pressure measurement device
- Oxygen saturation monitor
- Delivery system and scavenger device for continuous nitrous oxide administration

Drugs**
- Adrenaline (epinephrine)
- Atropine
- Lidocaine
- Dextrose 10%
- Reversal agents – naloxone and flumazenil
- Hydrocortisone

*All equipment must be available in varying sizes appropriate to patient population.
**Correct weight-based dose information should be readily available.

Table 20.1.11   Discharge criteria post-procedural sedation

- Normal age-specific vital signs
- Child has regained pre-sedation conscious state and communication skills
- Child is able to ambulate independently (relative to age and pre-sedation ability)
- Child is able to tolerate oral food or fluids
- Post-procedure analgesia is satisfactory
- Parent or carer has been provided with post-discharge instructions, understands them and is capable of following them

COMPLICATIONS OF PAEDIATRIC PROCEDURAL SEDATION

Paediatric procedural sedation can be hazardous and both mortality and significant morbidity has been reported in the literature.[46–48]

Notwithstanding this, studies of procedural sedation in EDs with adherence to published guidelines and involvement of staff trained in sedation and paediatric resuscitation techniques has yielded rates of complications of 2.3–16.1%, with the incidence of significant complications

such as laryngospasm being extremely low.[17,49,50]

In a series of 1180 children undergoing procedural sedation in a paediatric ED with a wide variety of drugs and combinations of drugs 27 (2.3%) experienced adverse events.[34]

The majority (78%) of adverse events occurred in patients younger than eight years, with more than half (52%) occurring in children younger than four years.

The most common adverse event was oxygen desaturation less than 90% requiring supplemental oxygen[9] followed

CONTROVERSIES AND FUTURE DIRECTIONS

❶ Pre-procedure fasting guidelines are a feature of most protocols developed for procedural sedation in children and aim to minimise the risk of pulmonary aspiration. Both the American Academy of Pediatrics and the American Society of Anesthesiologists lists specific fasting times for solids and liquids that vary from two hours to 6–8 hours depending on the age of the child.[41,43]

❷ However, these recommended times were a result of expert consensus opinion and are not specifically directed at patients in the unique ED setting.

❸ In fact, aspiration associated with paediatric procedural sedation has not been reported in the literature and there is no compelling evidence to support specific pre-procedure fasting periods for either liquids or solids.[51]

❹ Two recent studies looking at over 3000 children examined the duration of fasting with adverse events rates in ED procedural sedation. No association between the length of pre-procedural fasting and adverse events was found leading investigators to question the necessity to apply prolonged fasting periods for this group of patients.[52,53]

❺ When making decisions regarding timing of procedures requiring sedation in the ED setting, the risks and benefits must be assessed for each child by balancing the potential for vomiting and aspiration with the urgency of the procedure and the target depth of sedation.

❻ The future for clinical practice in the area of analgesia and sedation for children is likely to centre on making our practices safer, more time efficient for the ED and less distressing for the child.

❼ Development of guidelines with greater attention paid to selection of appropriate patients, provision of adequate facilities and training of staff (as outlined earlier in this chapter) will further improve the safety profile of our practices. Clinical audit of sedation/analgesia practice should be routine.

❽ Our practices will be made more efficient by future research to help define the optimal agent(s) and route of administration for particular procedures and patient age groups. There is increasing interest in the use of ultra-short-acting intravenous agents, such as propofol, which have not previously been used outside the operating theatre. Initial studies of propofol in ED paediatric procedural sedation are promising with studies reporting that it is efficacious and safe for use in the ED under the guidance of a protocol.[54–56] Future large studies in different settings are required to identify its safety profile and applicability to paediatric procedural sedation.

❾ The role of capnography in children undergoing sedation is yet to be defined. Capnography provides a means of identifying respiratory depression resulting from sedative agents because early detection of respiratory depression by pulse oximetry is generally not possible as supplemental oxygen administration serves to mask hypoventilation. Futher studies correlating changes in capnography and their association with adverse events are necessary to define its place in the monitoring of children undergoing procedural sedation.

❿ Alternative routes of drug administration have already had a great impact on paediatric sedation and analgesia practices. The delivery of established drugs by innovative, less-invasive methods is an exciting area for future research.

⓫ The advent of bispectral index (BIS) monitoring to measure the depth of anaesthesia in patients in the operating room may potentially be a useful adjunct in procedural sedation in the ED. By utilising processed electroencephalographic data gathered from a non-invasive electrode the BIS may provide an objective measure of sedation level and assist in accurate drug titration to achieve a requisite level of sedation that will enable safe and successful completion of a procedure with minimal or no distress in the child. A small observational study measuring BIS in paediatric procedural sedation found that BIS monitoring was able to predict a sedation score.[57,58] Further studies using this index will better define what role an objective measure of sedation level may play in reduced complications of over sedation along with avoidance of inadequate sedation during procedures.

by paradoxical reactions[7] and emesis.[3] None of the children who vomited demonstrated clinical evidence of pulmonary aspiration of gastric contents.

The adverse events recorded in this study were described as transient, minor and easily managed with no patient requiring intubation, reversal of sedation, or hospital admission.

Adherence to published guidelines recommending minimum requirements for personnel, patient monitoring and assessment for safe discharge has been shown to reduce adverse events associated with procedural sedation in children.[32]

In particular, the generation of an individual sedation plan comprising an individual risk assessment with documentation of variables such as fasting status, quantitative sedation scoring, time-based recording of vital signs and pulse oximetry combined with standardised recovery and discharge criteria and use of a standardised record has been shown to progressively reduce risk in procedural sedation, particularly in those children requiring a deep level of sedation.[32]

The majority of significant adverse events are related to airway malpositioning, hypoventilation requiring supplemental oxygenation and degrees of paradoxical excitation or recovery agitation, which is associated with individual agents (see Table 20.1.12)

Table 20.1.12 Adverse events and complications in procedural sedation

- Sedation failure
- Paradoxical excitation
- Recovery agitation
- Vomiting with potential aspiration
- Airway malposition requiring suction or repositioning
- Hypoventilation requiring supplemental oxygenation and/or assisted ventilation
- Laryngospasm
- Bronchospasm
- Respiratory arrest
- Hypotension
- Bradycardia
- Allergic reactions
- Over sedation
- Seizures

REFERENCES

1. Maurice SC, O'Donnell JJ, Beattie TF 2002 Emergency analgesia in the paediatric population. Part 1, Current practice and perspective's. Emergency Medicine Journal 19(1): 4–7
2. American Academy of Paediatrics and American Pain Society 2001 The assessment and management of acute pain in infants and children. (1995) Paediatrics 108(3): 793–797
3. O'Donnell J, Ferguson LP, Beattie TF 2002 Use of analgesia on a paediatric ED following limb trauma. European Journal of Emergency Medicine 9(1): 5–8
4. Cassell EJ 1983 The nature of suffering and the goals of medicine. New England Journal of Medicine 306: 639–645
5. McGrath PA, Bingham MC 1992 Assessment of pain in children and adolescents. In: Turk DC, Melzark R (eds) Handbook of pain assessment. Guildford Press, New York
6. Lloyd-Thomas AR, Howard R 1994 A pain service for children. Paediatric Anaesthesia 4: 3–15
7. International Association for the Study of Pain 1998 Measurement of pain in infants and children. In: Finley GA, McGrath PA (eds) Progress in pain research and measurement, Vol. 10. IASP Press, Seattle
8. Wilson GA, Doyle E 1996 Validation of three paediatric pain scores for use by parents. Anaesthesia 51: 1005–1007
9. Kelly AM, Powell CVE, Williams A 2002 Parent visual analogue scale ratings of children's pain do not reliably reflect pain reported by child. Paediatric Emergency Care 18(3): 159–162
10. Younge P, Nicol M, Kendall J, Harrington A 1999 A prospective randomised pilot comparison of intranasal fentanyl and intramuscular morphine for analgesia in children. Emergency Medicine 11(2): 90–94
11. Burton JH, Auble TE, Fuchs SM 1998 Effectiveness of 50% nitrous oxide/50% oxygen during laceration repair in children. Academic Emergency Medicine 5: 112–117
12. Gamis AS, Knapp JF, Glenski JA 1989 Nitrous oxide analgesia in a paediatric ED. Annals of Emergency Medicine 18: 177–181
13. Priestley SJ, Taylor J, McAdam CM et al 2001 Ketamine sedation for children in the ED. Emergency Medicine 13(1): 7–8
14. Acworth JP, Purdie D, Clark RC 2001 Intravenous ketamine plus midazolam is superior to intranasal midazolam for emergency paediatric sedation. Emergency Medicine Journal 19(1): 39–45
15. Green SM, Nakamura R, Johnson NE 1990 Ketamine sedation for paediatric procedures. Part 1, A prospective series. Annals of Emergency Medicine 19: 1024–1032
16. Green SM, Johnson NE 1990 Ketamine sedation for paediatric procedures. Part 2, Review and implications. Annals of Emergency Medicine 19: 1033–1046
17. Green SM, Rothrock SG, Lynch EL, Ho M, Harris T, Hestdalen R et al 1998 Intramuscular ketamine for pediatric sedation in the ED: Safety profile in 1022 cases. Annals of Emergency Medicine 31: 688–697
18. Priestley SJ, Kelly AM, Chow L, Powell CVE, Williams A 2003 Application of topical local anesthetic at triage reduces treatment time for children with laceration: A randomized controlled trial. Annals of Emergency Medicine 42: 34–40
19. Arrowsmith J, Campbell C 2000 A comparison of local anaesthetics for venipuncture. Archives of Diseases in Childhood 82: 309–310
20. Molodecka J, Stenhouse C, Jones JM et al 1994 Comparison of percutaneous anaesthesia for venous cannulation after topical application of either amethocaine or EMLA cream. British Journal of Anaesthetics 72: 174–176
21. Dart C 1998 Comparison of lignocaine 1% injection and adrenaline-cocaine gel for local anaesthesia in repair of lacerations. Emergency Medicine 10: 38–44
22. Schilling CG, Bank DE, Borchert BA et al 1995 Tetracaine, epinephrine (adrenalin), and cocaine (TAC) versus lidocaine, epinephrine and tetracaine (LET) for anesthesia of laceration in children. Annals of Emergency Medicine 25: 203–208
23. Ernst AA, Marvez E, Nick TG et al 1995 Lidocaine adrenaline tetracaine gel versus tetracaine adrenaline cocaine gel for topical anesthesia in linear scalp and facial laceration in children aged 5 to 17 years. Paediatrics 95: 255–258
24. Zempsky WT, Karasic RB 1997 EMLA versus TAC for topical anesthesia of extremity wounds in children. Annals of Emergency Medicine 30(2): 163–166
25. Mader TJ, Playe SJ, Garb JL 1994 Reducing the pain of local anesthetic infiltration: Warming and buffering have a synergistic effect. Annals of Emergency Medicine 23: 550–554
26. Bartfield JM, Gennis P, Barbera J et al 1990 Buffered versus plain lidocaine as a local anesthetic for simple laceration repair. Annals of Emergency Medicine 19: 1387–1390
27. Scarfone RJ 1998 Pain of local anesthetics: Rate of administration and buffering. Annals of Emergency Medicine 31(1): 36–40
28. Kelly AM, Cohen M, Richards D 1994 Minimizing the pain of local infiltration anesthesia for wounds by injection into the wound edges. Journal of Emergency Medicine 12(5): 593–595
29. Davies RJ 2003 Buffering the pain of local anaesthetics: A systematic review. Emergency Medicine 15(1): 81–88
30. Cote CJ, Notterman DA, Karl HW et al 2000 Adverse sedation events in pediatrics: A critical incident analysis of contributing factors. Pediatrics 105: 804–814
31. Nicol MF 1999 A risk management audit: Are we complying with the national guidelines for sedation by non-anaesthetists? Journal of Accidental and Emergency Medicine 16: 120–122
32. Hoffman GM, Nowakowski R, Troshynski TJ, Berens RJ, Weisman, SJ 2002 Risk reduction in pediatric procedural sedation by application of an American Academy of Pediatrics/American Society of Anesthesiologists Process Model. Paediatrics 109: 236–243
33. Everitt I, Younge P, Barnett P 2002 Paediatric sedation in EDs: What is our practice? Emergency Medicine 14: 62–66
34. Pena BM, Krauss B 1999 Adverse events of procedural sedation and analgesia in a pediatric emergency department. Annals of Emergency Medicine 34: 483–491
35. Olsson GL, Hallen B 1984 Laryngospasm during anaesthesia – a computer-aided incidence study in 136,929 patients. Acta Anaesthesiology Scandinavia 28: 567–575
36. Cohen MM, Cameron CB 1991 Should you cancel the operation when a child has an upper respiratory tract infection? Anaesthesia and Analgesia 72: 282–288
37. Classification of Physical Status 2001 American Society of Anaesthesiologists. Manual for Anaesthesia Department Organization and Management. http://www.asahq.org/clinical/physicalstatus.htm Accessed 16 May 2005
38. Rodriguez E, Jordan R 2002 Contemporary trends in pediatric sedation and analgesia. Emergency Medicine Clinics of North America 20(1): 199–222
39. American College of Emergency Physicians 1998 Clinical policy for procedural sedation and analgesia in the ED. Annals of Emergency Medicine 31: 663–677
40. American Society of Anesthesiologists 1996 Practice guidelines for sedation and analgesia by nonanesthesiologists: A report by the American Society of Anesthesiologists Task Force on sedation and analgesia by nonanesthesiologists. Anaesthesiology 84: 459–471

41. American Academy of Pediatrics, Committee on Drugs 1992 Guidelines for monitoring and management of pediatric patients during and after sedation for diagnostic and therapeutic procedures. Paediatrics 89: 1110–1115

42. Australian and New Zealand College of Anaesthetists 2001 Policy Statement 9 – Guidelines on Conscious Sedation for Diagnostic, Interventional Medical and Surgical Procedures. http://www.anzca.edu.au/publications/profdocs/profstandards/ps9_2001.htm Accessed 16 May 2005

43. Krauss B, Green SM 2000 Primary care: Sedation and analgesia for procedures in children. New England Journal of Medicine 342: 938–945

44. Ramsay M, Savege T, Simpson B, Goodwin R 1974 Controlled sedation with alphaxalone-alphadolone. British Medical Journal ii: 6556–6559

45. De Jonghe B, Cook D, Appere-De-Vecchi C, Guyatt G, Meade M, Outin H 2000 Using and understanding sedation scoring systems: a systematic review. Intensive Care Medicine 26: 275–285

46. Yaster M, Nichols DG, Deshpande JK et al 1990 Midazolam-fentanyl intravenous sedation: Case report of respiratory arrest. Paediatrics 86: 463–467

47. Jastak JT, Pallasch T 1988 Death after chloral hydrate sedation: Report of case. Journal of American Dental Association 116: 345–348

48. Malviya S, Voepel-Lewis T, Tait AR 1997 Adverse events and risk factors associated with the sedation of children by nonanesthesiologists. Anaesthesia and Analgesia 85: 1207–1213

49. Dachs RJ, Innes GM 1997 Intravenous ketamine sedation of pediatric patients in the ED. Annals of Emergency Medicine 29: 146–150

50. Green SM, Rothrock SG, Harris T 1998 Intravenous ketamine for pediatric sedation in the ED: Safety profile with 156 cases. Academy of Emergency Medicine 5: 971–976

51. Green SM, Krauss B 2002 Pulmonary aspiration risk during ED procedural sedation – An examination of the role of fasting and sedation depth. Academy of Emergency Medicine 9: 35–42

52. Agrawal D, Manzi SF, Gupta R, Krauss B 2003 Preprocedural fasting state and adverse events in children undergoing procedural sedation and analgesia in a pediatric emergency department. Annals of Emergency Medicine 42: 636–646

53. Roback MG, Bajaj L, Wathen JE, Bothner J 2004 Preprocedural fasting and adverse evevents in procedural sedation and analgesia in a pediatric emergency department: Are they related? Annals of Emergency Medicine 44: 454–459

54. Bassett KE, Anderson JL, Pribble CG, Guenther E 2003 Propofol for procedural sedation in children in the emergency department. Annals of Emergency Medicine 42: 773–782

55. Havel CJ, Strait RT, Hennes H 1999 A clinical trial of propofol vs. midazolam for procedural sedation in a pediatric emergency department. Academy of Emergency Medicine 6: 989–997

56. Green SM, Krauss B 2003 Propofol on emergency medicine: Pushing the sedation frontier. Annals of Emergency Medicine 42: 792–797 [editorial]

57. Agrawal D, Feldman HA, Krauss B, Waltzman ML 2004 Bispectral index monitoring quantifies depth of sedation during emergency department procedural sedation and analgesia in children. Annals of Emergency Medicine 43: 247–255

58. Fatovich DM, Gope M, Paech MJ 2004 A pilot trial of BIS monitoring for procedural sedation in the emergency department. Emergency Medicine Australasia 16: 103–107

FURTHER READING

American College of Emergency Physicians 1998 Clinical policy for procedural sedation and analgesia in the ED. Annals of Emergency Medicine 31: 663–677

Cote CJ, Notterman DA, Karl HW et al 2000 Adverse sedation events in pediatrics: A critical incident analysis of contributing factors. Paediatrics 105: 804–814

Green SM, Krauss B 2002 Pulmonary aspiration risk during ED procedural sedation - An examination of the role of fasting and sedation depth. Academy of Emergency Medicine 9: 35–42

Green SM, Rothrock SG, Lynch EL et al 1998 Intramuscular ketamine for pediatric sedation in the ED: Safety profile in 1022 cases. Annals of Emergency Medicine 31: 688–697

Krauss B, Green SM 2000 Primary care: Sedation and analgesia for procedures in children. New England Journal of Medicine 342: 938–945

Krauss B, Shannon M, Damian FJ, 1998 Guidelines for paediatric procedural sedation, 2nd edn. American College of Emergency Physicians, Dallas, TX

National Health and Medical Research Council 1999 Pain in children. In: Acute Pain Management. http:www.nhmrc.gov.au/publications/pdf/cp57.pdr pp. 93–108

Pena BM, Krauss B 1999 Adverse events of procedural sedation and analgesia in a paediatric ED. Annals of Emergency Medicine 34: 483–491

Priestley SJ, Taylor J, McAdam CM et al 2001 Ketamine sedation for children in the ED. Emergency Medicine 13(1): 82–90

Rodriguez E, Jordan R 2002 Contemporary trends in pediatric sedation and analgesia. Emergency Medicine Clinics of North America 20(1): 199–222

Sachetti A, Schafermeyer R, Gerardi M et al 1994 Pediatric sedation and analgesia. Annals of Emergency Medicine 23: 237–250

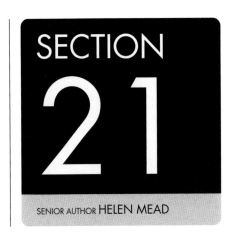

POISONING

21.1 GENERAL APPROACH TO POISONING

HELEN MEAD

ESSENTIALS

1 Most childhood poisonings are unintentional, involve a single known substance and result in minimal toxicity.

2 Poisoning in children is managed along the same guidelines as for their adult counterparts, with the usual priority of supporting the ABCs. Pharmacokinetic and/or pharmacodynamic differences in children may alter the manifestations after exposure to select toxins.

3 Management should be individualised, on the basis of a risk assessment. Treat the patient not the poison. A decision to prevent further absorption of the poison must be balanced against known risks. First, do no harm!

4 Most children require no investigations.

5 Most recover without treatment – observation is the mainstay of management.

6 Specific antidotes are rarely required.

7 Poisoning should be considered in 'non-specific' presentations, including altered mental state, behavioural disturbance and metabolic derangements.

8 Preventative strategies have greatly reduced mortality rates for child poisoning, but there is still scope for educational intervention to reduce accidental exposure to medicines and to prevent accidental and iatrogenic over-dosing.

9 Intentional poisoning is rare, but should be considered for repeatedly poisoned young children.

INTRODUCTION AND EPIDEMIOLOGY

Childhood poisonings occur most frequently in the under five years age group. They are usually related to the inquisitive, exploratory behaviour of preschool children and caused by a single agent that is found in the household. The time since ingestion is often known, the agents often have limited toxic potential and presentation to the ED occurs soon after exposure. The dramatic decline in paediatric poisoning deaths in the past few decades has been a result of altered prescribing habits, packaging legislation, heightened parental awareness of safe storage of medicines and household products and improved emergency and intensive-care management. Lapses in supervision are more liable to occur in the early evening and at times when the usual household routine is disrupted. Parents often underestimate the capabilities of young children and storage of household products and medications is often deficient. Most poisoning in neonates is iatrogenic. Adolescents may engage in recreational drug use/abuse or have self-destructive and suicidal intent. Poison information centres provide easy access to information for the community and health professionals.

STABILISATION

Most accidental ingestions in children are non-toxic, and therefore require minimal intervention. The priorities of childhood poisonings are the same as for adults. Vital functions may need to be supported whilst the poison is excreted or metabolised.[1]

Assess and secure the ABCs and measure blood glucose. Continuous and repeated monitoring of vital signs and mental state is required. Resuscitation antidotes include Digoxin-specific Fab fragments, naloxone, atropine, glucose and sodium thiosulfate.

Airway

An obstructed airway or inability to protect the airway is commonly due to CNS depression. Increased secretions due to cholinergic poisoning or mucosal oedema following corrosive exposure may also cause obstruction. Consider intubation in such cases.

Breathing

CNS depression with hypoventilation is the commonest cause of hypoxia. Ventilatory failure is most commonly due to CNS depression. Other causes include respiratory muscle weakness, pulmonary aspiration and pneumonitis, direct pulmonary toxicity, and increased secretions due to cholinergic poisoning. Cardiac and non-cardiogenic pulmonary oedema may also contribute to failure.

High-flow oxygen should be given via a Hudson mask.

Intubate and ventilate if hypoventilation or hypoxia persists. The addition of positive end-expiratory pressure (PEEP) may be required if pulmonary oedema is present.

Circulation

Circulation and tissue perfusion are assessed regularly with heart rate, BP, capillary return, conscious state and urinary output.

Causes of inadequate tissue perfusion include arterial vasodilatation (commonest), arrhythmias, hypovolaemia and the action of negative inotropes. A rapid heart rate and cool pale extremities may be the result of poisoning by a sympathomimetic agent rather than hypoperfusion.

Drug-induced asystole

Infusions of KCl are hazardous. Molar solutions of KCl are in common use in intensive care units especially after cardiac surgery. An inadvertent IV bolus of potassium can cause asystole. Note that a 1 mL bolus of molar KCl (1 mmol) in a 10 kg child will theoretically raise the serum concentration by 2.5 mmol L^{-1}.

Immediate-acting treatment (within seconds) is either 10% calcium chloride IV 0.2 mL kg^{-1} (or equivalent) or IV sodium bicarbonate 1 mmol kg^{-1} or both. Calcium antagonises the cardiac effects of potassium on the heart, while the bicarbonate lowers the serum concentration of potassium. Treatments of rapid onset (within minutes) are glucose 0.5 g kg^{-1} IV (e.g. 5 mL kg^{-1} of 10%) plus insulin 0.05 U kg^{-1} or salbutamol 0.25 mg kg^{-1} by aerosol. Slow treatment (within hours) is by resonium, oral or rectal, 0.5–1 g kg^{-1}.

Drug-induced bradycardia

Organophosphate and carbamate poisoning with bradycardia should be treated with atropine – repeated doses of 20–50 µg kg^{-1} every 15 minutes or until secretions are dry and an acceptable heart rate is restored. In organophosphate poisoning (but not carbamate), pralidoxime can reactivate cholinesterase. The dose is 25 mg kg^{-1} IV over 15–30 minutes then 10–20 mg kg^{-1} per hour for 18 hours or more.

Bradycardia induced by β-blocker poisoning is treated with glucagon 7 µg kg^{-1} IV then 2–7 µg kg^{-1} min^{-1}. This is the preferred antidote because it stimulates non-catecholamine cAMP. Isoprenaline 0.05–3 µg kg^{-1} min^{-1} by infusion may be used but it may cause β2-induced hypotension and should not be used if hypotension is pre-existing. Alternatively, an infusion of noradrenalin (norepinephrine) at 0.05–1 µg kg^{-1} min^{-1} may be infused.

Digoxin induced bradycardia may be treated with magnesium IV 25–50 mg kg^{-1} (0.1–0.2 mmol kg^{-1}) or with digoxin Fab antibody in a dose of ten vials per twenty-five 0.25 mg tablets or per 5 mg elixir ingested. At steady state, the number of vials is calculated as

$$\frac{\text{serum digoxin} \times \text{Body weight}}{100}.$$
$$(\text{ng mL}^{-1}) \quad (\text{kg})$$

Drug-induced tachyarrhythmias

The preferred treatment is a benzodiazepine such as diazepam or midazolam in doses that do not depress CNS function. Other treatments are the ultra-short-acting cardioselective β1-blocker esmolol IV 500 µg kg^{-1} over one minute and then 25–200 µg kg^{-1} min^{-1} by infusion. Treatments such as intravenous adenosine and DC shock are not likely to be effective because the toxic drug effect will be persistent. Calcium-channel blockers such as verapamil may cause severe hypotension and should not be given.

Drug-induced hypertension

Hypertension may occur with poisoning by cocaine, amphetamine and similar substances, which cause vasoconstriction, tachycardia and arrhythmias. Benzodiazepines are the preferred treatment. Another alternative is a smooth muscle dilator such as sodium nitroprusside IV 0.5–2 µg kg^{-1} min^{-1}, but its use mandates intra-arterial monitoring. Another choice is phentolamine IV 0.05–0.1 mg kg^{-1} and then an infusion of 5–50 µg kg^{-1} min^{-1}. Propranolol, a non-selective β-blocker is contraindicated because it may worsen hypertension when β2-adrenoreceptors are blocked.

Drug-induced ventricular tachycardia and fibrillation

Haemodynamically stable VT can be treated with antiarrhythmic agents. Typical drug causes are tricyclic antidepressants, cocaine and amphetamines. These cause a monomorphic VT by increasing the QRS interval. Treatment should be sodium bicarbonate, especially in cases of tricyclic poisoning. Both components of the sodium bicarbonate contribute to its antidotal effect – the sodium counters the sodium-channel blockade effect of the drugs and the alkalosis reduces bioavailability. Induction of respiratory alkalosis is also beneficial. The preferred antidysrrhythmic agent is lidocaine. Phenytoin is no longer recommended. Polymorphic VT (*torsades de pointes*) of any cause should be treated with magnesium 25–50 mg kg^{-1} IV.

Pulseless VT or VF require DC shock. The use of adrenaline (epinephrine) in this situation should be limited to 10 µg kg^{-1} boluses and higher doses avoided. Propranolol is contraindicated.

Drug-induced shock

Shock may result from drugs that cause depression of myocardial contractility, vasodilatation or loss of intravascular volume, or combinations of these. An extreme rise in peripheral vascular resistance may also lead to myocardial failure. Whenever possible preload, contractility and afterload should be measured.

Preload deficiencies (hypovolaemia) are corrected with volume administration, titrated against blood pressure, right-heart filling pressure and against pulmonary artery wedge pressure.

Infusion of dopamine is the preferred inotropic agent in doses of approximately 5–15 mg kg^{-1} min^{-1} although higher doses may be needed or other inotropic drugs added. If central access is not possible infusion of dobutamine in a similar dose may be given via a peripheral venous access, at least in the short term. Other inotropic agents are infusions of calcium (0.03–0.1 mL kg^{-1} h^{-1} of 10% $CaCl_2$, i.e. 3–10 mg kg^{-1} h^{-1}), milrinone (50 µg kg^{-1} loading dose then 0.375–0.75 µg kg^{-1} min^{-1}) and glucagon. It is desirable to measure cardiac output or to assess contractility with echocardiography.

Vasodilatation is treated with an α-adrenergic agent such as noradrenalin (norepinephrine) infusion (0.05–1 µg kg^{-1} min^{-1}) in the higher dose range. Other such agents are phenylephrine (1–5 µg kg^{-1} min^{-1}) and metaraminol (0.05–1 µg kg^{-1} min^{-1}). Vasoconstriction is also obtained with vasopressin infusion (0.002–0.01 U kg^{-1} min^{-1}).

In selected circumstances, cardiac output can be supported with ventricular assist devices, extra-corporeal membrane oxygenation (ECMO) or intra-aortic balloon pumping, although the last named requires intrinsic cardiac rhythm. These techniques are sometimes used in toxicological emergencies in centres that use these techniques for cardiac surgery. They are only indicated when standard supportive measures are insufficient but the situation is recoverable, and organ damage, particularly brain damage, has not occurred. The principal risks with these techniques are haemorrhage, infection and mechanical failure.

Disability – management of seizures and coma

Coma, delirium and seizures are common CNS manifestations of poisoning. Trends in the Glasgow coma scale are important and pupil size and light reaction should be documented. Airway protection is paramount because of the risk of pulmonary aspiration and mechanical ventilation may be required. Naloxone 0.1 mg kg^{-1} IV (maximum 2 mg) should be given if the history or examination (pinpoint pupils or hypoventilation) suggests a possibility of opioid intoxication.

Although CNS depression may be due to a direct toxic effect, consider other possible causes (head injury, hypoxia, hypoglycaemia, thiamine deficiency). Seizures may be subtle with minimal evidence of tonic-clonic contractions. Toxin-induced seizures are commonly brief and may be self-limited. Ensure adequate oxygenation and blood glucose. Benzodiazepines are the most appropriate agent for pharmacological management (midazolam or diazepam 0.1–0.2 mg kg^{-1} IV, repeated every ten minutes if required, with close monitoring of vital signs and airway reflexes). Intubation and mechanical ventilation may be required. Phenytoin has not been shown to be any more effective than benzodiazepines in treating toxic seizures. (Consider pyridoxine 0.5 g min^{-1} IV, up to 5 g IV (100 × 50 mg ampoules!) in a child with status epilepticus who has access to isoniazid. For known isoniazid ingestion give pyridoxine in a dose equal to the ingested dose).

Management of hypoglycaemia

Hypoglycaemia is treated with 2–4 mL kg^{-1} of 20% glucose.

Management of temperature extremes

Hypothermia occurs in poisoning in cool environments when cerebral depressants interfere with thermoregulation. Hypothermia can usually be managed with passive warming.

Treat toxin-induced hyperthermia aggressively. Paracetamol is usually ineffective. Remove all clothing. Tepid baths may not be practical if the patient is agitated or somnolent but options include spraying the patient with a water mist in front of a fan and the application of ice-packs to the groin, neck and axilla. If the patient is agitated sedate with diazepam 0.1 mg kg^{-1} IV, repeated as necessary to a maximum of 0.5 mg kg^{-1}. If a core temperature of over 40°C is not controlled with these measures the patient should be sedated, intubated and muscle relaxed. Dantrolene and bromocriptine have an unproven role in the treatment of severe toxin-induced febrile states, such as neuroleptic malignant syndrome, and should not take the place of supportive care.

DIAGNOSIS AND RISK ASSESSMENT

History

Children usually present with a history of known or suspected exposure to a specific substance. An accurate risk assessment depends on confirming the nature of the toxin and determining the degree of exposure. In childhood poisoning, the carer's history will usually give valuable information regarding the *what, when, how* and *why*. The potential for toxicity is determined by the nature of the agent and the nature of the exposure (amount ingested or duration of exposure) as well as host factors (age, body weight, pre-existing illnesses and usual medications). Whenever possible, examine the remainder of the suspected poison and its container to confirm the nature of the substance and the amount ingested. The type of formulation of the substance may determine the duration till onset of toxic symptoms. When evaluating the potential for toxicity, the worst case scenario should be considered.

At times the exact nature of the toxin cannot be easily determined and further information should be sought regarding the medications and substances to which the child may have had access (including medications of the patient, siblings, parents and grandparents), previously stored medications and chemicals and over-the-counter medications. Envenomation or plant ingestion may need to be considered.

The circumstances of exposure, including time of the incident, management already undertaken and possible intent of exposure should be explored. Most commonly the exposure is unintentional resulting from an inquisitive child or mistaken dosage or type of drug being given by the carer. Rarely there is the possibility of child abuse or Münchausen's syndrome by proxy and in older children there may be suicidal intent.

Physical examination

Suspect poisoning if there is a history of an ingested toxin with a clinical picture consistent with the known effects of the toxin or if the child presents with symptoms and signs that can be recognised as a toxicological syndrome or 'toxidrome' (see Table 21.1.1).

The possibility of poisoning should be considered in children with acute unexplained illness, especially if any of the following features are present:

- Vital sign abnormalities.
- Cyanosis.
- Cardiac dysrhythmia.
- Central nervous system depression.
- Convulsions.
- Unusual behaviour.
- Pupillary abnormality.
- Vomiting or diarrhoea.
- Metabolic disturbance, e.g. acidosis or hypoglycaemia.

Concentration should be on the following areas:

- Vital signs – HR, BP, core temperature.
- Respiratory – pattern and secretions.
- Neurological – Glasgow coma scale, eye signs (pupil size and reaction, nystagmus), ataxia, tremor/dystonias/abnormal movements.

Table 21.1.1   Common toxidromes

Description of toxidrome	Comments	Typical agents
Anticholinergic Some features are detailed in the phrase: Hot as a hare – fever Blind as a bat – spasm of accommodation Dry as a bone – dry mucous membranes and skin Red as a beet – flushed skin Mad as a hatter – central anticholinergic syndrome: disorientation, confusion, hallucinations (usually visual) agitation, seizures and coma	Additional peripheral signs include: Dilated pupils Ileus Urinary retention Mild hypertension, or hypotension Dysrhythmias or conduction blocks	Antihistamines Belladonna alkaloids Benztropine Carbamazepine Cyclic antidepressants Phenothiazines Some mushrooms
Cholinergic Signs of muscarinic over activity are described by the mnemonic 'SLUDGE': Salivation and sweating Lacrimation Urination Diarrhoea Gastrointestinal pain Emesis	Other muscarinic signs include: Bronchoconstriction Diaphoresis, bronchorrhoea Constricted pupils Bradycardia Signs due to excessive stimulation of nicotinic receptors: Fasciculations Weakness Paralysis Central cholinergic signs include: Agitation Seizures Coma	Carbamate insecticides Carbachol Edrophonium Lobeline Organophosphates Physostigmine Pilocarpine
Narcotic Coma Pin-point pupils Hypoventilation	In severe cases hypotension and non-cardiogenic pulmonary oedema may occur	Narcotic analgesics, including: Codeine Propoxyphene Abused narcotics Heroin Fentanyl derivatives Diphenoxylate (Lomotil®)
Phenothiazines Hypotension Dystonias – torticollis, oculogyric crisis, opisthotonus Constricted pupils Prolonged QT interval, widened QRS	Some phenothiazines have significant anticholinergic effects resulting in dilated pupils and other anticholinergic signs	Chlorpromazine Prochlorperazine Thioridazine
Tricyclic antidepressants Tachycardia, hypotension Anticholinergic signs CNS depression, seizures QRS widening, right axis deviation		Amitryptyline Imipramine Doxepin Dosulepin
Sympathomimetics Predominantly α-effects cause: Hypertension with bradycardia Dilated but reactive pupils Localised sweating (often palms and feet) Decreased GI motility Bladder contraction	Signs depend on the degree of α- and β-receptor stimulation. Predominantly β-effects present with: Tachycardia Vasodilation ± hypotension Miosis Decreased GI motility Bladder relaxation	Amphetamines Cocaine Ergot alkaloids Monoamine oxidase inhibitors Phenylpropanolamine Pseudoephedrine Salbutamol Yohimbine Xanthines – caffeine, theophylline
Barbiturates Coma Hypoventilation Hypotension Hypothermia	'Barbiturate blisters', bullous skin lesions over pressure points, are seen with a number of sedative drugs in overdose	Amylobarbitone Methylphenobarbitone Pentobarbitone Phenobarbital

• Other – skin dryness or sweating, state of hydration, odour (breath, blood, urine, vomitus), bowel sounds, urinary retention.

Examination is useful to exclude other causes for the presentation. In the case of intentional poisoning there may be other evidence of child abuse or neglect.

SCREENING AND SPECIFIC INVESTIGATIONS

Investigations are not required for the management of most childhood poisonings. Investigations should not delay treatment but may be helpful in defined circumstances:

• To provide a baseline to monitor changes in the symptomatic child and to exclude comorbidity (consider pre-existing renal or hepatic dysfunction or pregnancy as a trigger to deliberate self-harm).
• Occasionally to confirm a specific toxin.
• To monitor complications of toxic ingestions.
• Timed quantitative blood levels of specific toxins (e.g. paracetamol, iron, theophylline) to guide management.
• To exclude toxicological causes of an acute psychiatric presentation.
• For documentation in suspected intentional poisoning.

In the setting of a critically ill child, where poisoning is suspected, a toxicology screen may detect a toxin but qualitative screens of 'drugs of abuse' (which typically test for the presence of cannabinoids, cocaine, opioids, phencyclidine, amphetamines, lysergic acid diethylamide and benzodiazepines) are rarely of value in the seriously poisoned patient. Most drug screens are performed on urine, although blood is required for alcohols and solvents. The type of sample required should be discussed with the laboratory. Urine concentrations of drugs do not correlate with the severity of symptoms and high false positive rates make interpretation difficult. Few laboratories provide drug screens on a 24-hour basis

and results may not be available in time to be of use in the initial assessment and management.

Obtain a paracetamol level in all patients presenting with intentional overdose as paracetamol is a common and easily accessed drug with delayed toxicity, which requires early administration of an antidote. Screening for salicylates is unlikely to be helpful unless there are typical symptoms or acidosis.

Haemoglobin, white cell count and haematocrit, are significantly altered in acute iron poisoning.

An ABG can determine respiratory status and associated metabolic acidosis. If acidosis is present consider screening for:

• Iron.
• Ethylene glycol and methanol.
• Salicylates.
• Theophylline.
• Carbon monoxide.

An anion gap may be calculated for patients with acidosis [anion gap = Na − (Cl + HCO$_3$)]. An elevated anion gap (>8–12 mEq L^{-1}) is characteristic of certain poisonings (e.g. iron, salicylates, paraldehyde, methanol, isoniazid, theophylline).

If seizures are present screen for:

• Amphetamines.
• Cocaine.
• Tricyclic antidepressants (also venlafaxine).
• Carbamazepine.
• Isoniazid.

If a child has been recumbent for an extended period, serum CPK may exclude rhabdomyolysis.

Poisoning by opioids, hypoglycaemic agents and benzodiazepines can all be clinically diagnosed with a therapeutic trial of specific antidote.

An ECG may show a brady/tachycardia, broad complex, heart block or arrhythmia due to cardiotoxic poisons. If life-threatening arrhythmias are present, specific treatment based on clinical presentation and ECG findings may be necessary prior to results being available. If cardiac arrhythmias are present screen for:

• Amphetamines.
• Cocaine.
• Theophylline.
• Digoxin.
• Tricyclic antidepressants.

Radiological studies may be helpful in guiding management in specific circumstances. A CXR may be required for suspected pulmonary aspiration or for the investigation of respiratory and cardiac complications of toxic ingestions. Abdominal XR may confirm the presence of metallic foreign bodies and may show undissolved fragments of radio-opaque toxins (remembered by the mnemonic CHIPES):

• Chloral hydrate.
• Heavy metals.
• Iron.
• Phenothiazines.
• Enteric-coated preparations (salicylates).
• Sustained-release preparations (theophylline).

Examine the urine for crystalluria, protein, myoglobin, all suggesting actual or potential renal toxicity.

Table 21.1.2 lists some common poisons, which have specific antidotes, and discusses the utility of specific tests.

DECONTAMINATION

Surface decontamination

Skin contamination requires copious irrigation with water with special attention given to the hair, fingernails and skin folds. Soap and water washing should be used for hydrocarbons or oily substances. Staff should wear protective gloves and gown. For eye exposure flush with at least 1 L of sterile saline. Local anaesthetic drops may facilitate irrigation. If an acidic or alkaline chemical is involved, check the pH of tears five minutes after ceasing irrigation and recommence irrigation if pH is not neutral. Evert the lids and remove any particles. Ophthalmologic evaluation should be sought if pain persists despite thorough irrigation.

Inhalational poisoning may require oxygen administration and respiratory support.

Table 21.2 Specific antidotes

Toxins	Antidote or specific therapy	Need for qualitative test or drug level
Antiarrhythmics: Types Ia or Ic	Sodium bicarbonate 1–2 mmol kg^{-1} IV bolus to increase arterial pH to 7.45–7.55	**Yes** In some circumstances drug levels may help to differentiate between toxicity and primary cardiac disease. If no cardiac disease suspected administer as per cyclic antidepressants
Anti-psychotics: Butyrophenones and phenothiazines	Benztropine 0.02 mg kg^{-1}, IM or IV, repeat in 15 minutes, if required	**No** Administer for dystonic reactions
Benzodiazepines	Flumazenil 0.01 mg kg^{-1}, each dose not exceeding 0.2 mg, repeated if necessary to total dose of 2 mg	**No** Administer if airway is unprotected and intubation not desirable, provided no contraindications – suspected cyclic antidepressant use (look for ECG changes) or benzodiazepine dependence
β-Antagonists	Glucagon 0.05–0.1 mg kg^{-1}	**No** Indicated if hypotension or bradycardia in suspected β-blocker overdose
Calcium-channel blockers	Calcium gluconate 10%, 0.2–0.3 mL kg^{-1} Calcium chloride 10%, 0.1–0.2 mL kg^{-1}	**No** Administer for hypotension
Carbon monoxide	Hyperbaric oxygen	**Maybe** Some hyperbaric units use a COHb > 20–25% as an indication for hyperbaric poisoning. COHb levels correlate poorly with severity of poisoning and clinical indicators are usually more relevant.
Cyanide	Amyl nitrate, sodium nitrate, sodium thiosulfate, dicobalt edetate, hydroxocobalamin	**No** Administer antidote based on history and symptoms or if severe lactic acidosis and potential for cyanide exposure
Cyclic antidepressants	Sodium bicarbonate 1–2 mmol kg^{-1} IV bolus to increase arterial pH to 7.45–7.55	**No** Administer if wide QRS, arrhythmias or hypotension. ECG changes are better indicators of toxicity than drug levels
Digoxin	Digoxin Fab fragments If doses of digoxin unknown give 200–400 mg in acute overdose, 100–200 mg if chronic	**Maybe** Administer for life threatening arrhythmias or hyperkalaemia > 5.0 mmol L^{-1} Digoxin level may be indicated to differentiate between toxicity and primary cardiac disease. Blood for level should be taken prior to administration of Fab
Ethylene glycol	Ethanol 750 mg kg^{-1} as loading dose, then 100–150 mg kg^{-1} h^{-1} to maintain blood ethanol of 100 mg dL^{-1}	**Maybe** While an ethylene glycol level is required to confirm exposure and the need for continuing an ethanol infusion rapid levels may be difficult to obtain Give loading dose of ethanol if a reliable history of ingestion and: Metabolic acidosis Unexplained elevated osmolar gap
Insulin	Dextrose 2–4 mL kg^{-1} of 25% solution	**No** Monitor blood glucose
Iron	Desferrioxamine up to 15 mg kg^{-1} h^{-1}, to maximum daily dose of 6 g	**Yes** Administer if serum iron is greater than 75 μmol L^{-1} or systemic toxicity present Monitor serum iron levels
Isoniazid	Pyridoxine administer gram for gram amount of isoniazid ingested.empirical dose 5 g	**No** Administer if seizures and suspected isoniazid toxicity
Metoclopramide	Benztropine 0.02 mg kg^{-1}, IM or IV, repeat in 15 minutes, if required	**No** Administer for dystonic reactions

(Continued)

Table 21.2   Specific antidotes (Continued)

Toxins	Antidote or specific therapy	Need for qualitative test or drug level
Methaemoglobinaemia	Methylene blue 1–2 mg kg^{-1}, repeat in 1 hour if necessary	**Maybe** Methaemoglobin levels may be useful to confirm the diagnosis but the administration of methylene blue should not be delayed in the ill child with features of hypoxia and exposure to a known oxidant
Methanol	Ethanol 750 mg kg^{-1} as loading dose, then 100–150 mg kg^{-1} h^{-1} to maintain blood ethanol of 100 mg dL^{-1}	**Maybe** While a methanol level is required to confirm exposure and the need for continuing an ethanol infusion rapid levels may be difficult to obtain Give loading dose of ethanol if a history of ingestion and: 　Metabolic acidosis 　Unexplained elevated osmolar gap 　Visual symptoms ('snowstorm')
Narcotics	Naloxone 0.1 mg kg^{-1}, repeat to maximum dose of 2 mg	**No** Administer for sedation and any of the following: 　Constricted pupils 　Hypoventilation 　History of narcotic exposure 　Consider use if unknown cause of sedation
Oral hypoglycaemics	Dextrose 2–4 mL kg^{-1} of 25% solution	**No** Monitor blood glucose
Organophosphate or carbamate insecticides	Atropine 0.02–0.05 mg kg^{-1}, repeat every 5–10 minutes until secretion dry	**No** Administer if bronchorrhoea or excessive secretions
Organophosphate insecticides	Pralidoxime 20–50 mg kg^{-1}, to maximum of 1 g	**No** Administer for suspected organophosphate poisoning if more than 0.05 mg kg^{-1} of atropine is required to control secretions
Paracetamol	N-Acetylcysteine 150 mg kg^{-1} over 15–30 min, 50 mg kg^{-1} over 4 hours, 100 mg kg^{-1} over 16 hours	**Yes** Paracetamol should be routinely screened for in intentional ingestions. If present, a serum concentration is required to determine therapy
Salicylates	Sodium bicarbonate 50–100 mmol L^{-1} NaOH in 1000 mL of dextrose-saline at 2–3 mL kg^{-1} h^{-1} and titrate to urine pH	**Yes** Urinary alkalinisation can enhance clearance Monitor salicylate levels
Theophylline	Charcoal haemoperfusion	**Yes** While an absolute level is rarely an isolated indication for extracorporeal drug removal, a theophylline level may be necessary for diagnosis in the child with unexplained vomiting, arrhythmias, seizures or metabolic acidosis
Warfarin and other coumarin anticoagulants	Vitamin K$_1$ 1–2 mg, IV or IM	**Yes** Vitamin K is not indicated unless PT (INR) is elevated Prophylactic administration is not indicated and may obscure the severity of the poisoning

Gastrointestinal decontamination

Preventing the absorption of the ingested poison is a desired outcome but there are no controlled studies of poisoned patients that demonstrate the effectiveness of any gastrointestinal decontamination procedure. Significant absorption is likely to have taken place prior to the presentation to the ED. No method of gastric decontamination should be used routinely. A consensus is evolving regarding the role of gastrointestinal decontamination in the management of potential poisoning.[2–6]

Gastric emptying procedures

Methods may be chemical such as induction of vomiting or mechanical like gastric lavage.

Emesis

Emesis has no place in the hospital management of patients presenting with poisoning. The role of induction of emesis in the home is controversial. After a dose of ipecacuanha (1–2 mL kg^{-1}, to a maximum of 30 mL) vomiting is induced in the majority of children within 20–30 minutes. This delay may permit the onset of toxic effects such as altered conscious state or seizures, increasing the risk of aspiration pneumonitis. At best, following emesis within 60 minutes of ingestion, 'ipecac' removes less than 40% of an ingested substance. Complications of therapy are infrequent but protracted vomiting, Mallory–Weiss tears, gastrointestinal haemorrhage, diarrhoea and pneumomediastinum have been reported. Use of 'ipecac' is contraindicated in children less than six months of age and for ingestions of corrosive agents, sharp objects and hydrocarbons with potential for pulmonary aspiration. Administration is dangerous if the patient has ingested toxins that may cause depressed conscious state, seizures or cardiovascular compromise. 'Ipecac' may delay the administration of activated charcoal by one to two hours, increase the risk of aspiration pneumonitis, and may prolong the time spent in the ED. There is no evidence that use of 'ipecac' improves clinical outcome.[2]

Gastric lavage

The role for lavage is probably limited to patients with potentially life-threatening ingestion of a substance in whom the procedure can be undertaken within one hour.[3] There may be some benefit in performing the procedure after one hour in toxic ingestions of a substance not absorbed by charcoal, especially if the toxin impairs gastric emptying, e.g. tricyclic antidepressants.

The procedure involves positioning the child head down on the left side, pointing the pylorus up. A large-bore orogastric tube is inserted, correct position is confirmed and gastric contents aspirated prior to instilling aliquots of warm water or saline (1 mL kg^{-1}) then aspirating completely and repeating till the effluent is clear.

Lavage recovers 42–90% of a substance if used within one hour, however no controlled clinical studies have confirmed that gastric lavage improves outcome. Gastric lavage should only be performed with appropriate airway protection if conscious state is impaired or likely to become impaired. The procedure may compromise cardiac and respiratory function (hypoxia, dysrhythmias, inadvertent tracheal intubation). The procedure is technically difficult in children. Gastric lavage is ineffective for large tablets, such as iron, and of no use in alcohol ingestion. Absolute contraindications for lavage include hydrocarbons with a high potential for aspiration, corrosive agents and the child with a bleeding diathesis. Traumatic complications to the nasopharynx, oesophagus, larynx, lungs and stomach may occur. Lavage may actually enhance toxicity by pushing the tablets beyond the pylorus and increasing absorption.

Activated charcoal

Activated charcoal (AC) is more effective than 'ipecac' and gastric lavage in reducing absorption for most toxins but has not been shown to improve clinical outcomes in poisoned patients. There is evidence that it will decrease absorption and possible side effects of many toxins. Complications in children are rarely documented but aspiration of charcoal may be fatal. It is reasonable to use AC for toxic ingestions with potentially serious consequences.[4]

Substances *not* bound by charcoal include:

- Acids.
- Alkalis.
- Cyanide.
- Essential oils.
- Alcohols, e.g. ethanol, methanol.
- Metals, e.g. iron, lithium, lead, mercury.
- Petroleum distillates.
- Some pesticides, e.g. malathion, DDT.

AC is a finely ground powder, with a huge surface area, which is made into a slurry with water. It is not systemically absorbed. The dose is ten-times the weight of the ingested drug, or 1–2 g kg^{-1}. Before administration check for bowel sounds. Certain drugs may become trapped in an acid pH, so are less likely to bind to activated charcoal. Co-ingestants and a full stomach may also affect adsorption.

If administration is delayed more than 60 minutes post-ingestion the toxin may not be available to adsorb to activated charcoal. Charcoal may be useful beyond this period where the ingestant delays gastric emptying (e.g. tricyclic antidepressants), for sustained-release substances (e.g. theophylline) or for substances that may form concretions within the stomach (e.g. aspirin).

Multiple-dose activated charcoal

This theoretically provides a greater total adsorptive capacity, and can prevent drug availability by preventing resorption through the enterohepatic or enteroenteric circulations, enhancing gut elimination by the process of 'intestinal dialysis'. It is generally given in a dose of 0.25–0.5 g kg^{-1} every 4–6 hours. Drugs with improved elimination kinetics include phenobarbitone, cyclic antidepressants, theophylline, carbamazepine, digoxin, phenytoin and salicylates.

Catharsis

This is a technique used to eliminate toxin from the gastrointestinal tract by causing diarrhoea. Sorbitol may improve the palatability of charcoal but may exacerbate the tendency for vomiting. Sorbitol, magnesium citrate and magnesium sulphate have previously been popular but may cause fluid and electrolyte abnormalities. Studies have not shown charcoal to be constipating and cathartics alone or in combination with charcoal have not been shown to decrease the bioavailability of the ingestant.[5]

Endoscopy

This method can be used where gastric lavage and activated charcoal are contraindicated. It may be necessary in the assessment of alkali or acid ingestion. It may be used to extract undissolved agents for which activated charcoal is likely to be ineffective (e.g. a massive ingestion of iron). It is also used to extract foreign bodies such as button batteries from the stomach and sharp objects from the gastrointestinal tract.

Surgical removal

This may be used in rare circumstances for removal of extremely toxic substances, which may potentially erode the gut, especially if they have formed concretions (e.g. aspirin, iron) or in massive overdose to prevent further absorption from the GI tract (e.g. iron, slow-release calcium-channel blockers).

Whole-bowel irrigation

This technique is occasionally advised for potentially severe poisoning with very toxic substances.[6] Iso-osmolar polyethylene glycol-electrolyte solution (Glycoprep®, Golytely®) is used at a dose of 30 mL kg^{-1} h^{-1} for 6–8 hours until faecal effluent is clear. The technique has been very effective in human volunteer studies with reduced bioavailability of 67–73% at one hour post-ingestion. Clinical studies are descriptive, with iron being the most described. This technique is most useful where there has been a delayed presentation of a significant quantity of potentially toxic agent that is not adsorbed by charcoal, e.g. iron, or for sustained-release or enteric-coated preparations or for foreign bodies such as lithium button batteries. It is messy and labour intensive. It is contraindicated in the presence of gastrointestinal ileus.

ENHANCED ELIMINATION

Extracorporeal techniques are rarely used and are generally reserved for severe toxicity and deterioration of vital functions despite maximal supportive therapy, for those with impaired clearance and those with pre-existing disease that may make them more susceptible to the effects of the toxin.[7] Early referral to a paediatric intensive care unit of selected patients may significantly reduce morbidity and mortality.

The efficacy of these techniques for general renal support has been clearly demonstrated but there are numerous limitations to enhancing drug elimination.

The technique must be able to remove clinically significant amounts of the toxin and the potential benefits must outweigh the risks. Complications include those related to vessel cannulation and heparinisation, infection and abnormalities of fluid, electrolyte and glucose balance.

Haemodialysis and haemofiltration may be useful for elimination of toxins with low molecular weight, high water solubility, protein binding < 90% and a small volume of distribution. Haemodialysis may be technically difficult in small children but may be considered for lithium, salicylates, ethanol and methanol. Haemofiltration has been used for theophylline.

Charcoal haemoperfusion is less dependent on the physical properties of the toxins and may be an option for water-soluble toxins that are adsorbed by activated charcoal, have low fat and protein-binding and low endogenous clearance.

Urinary alkalinisation enhances excretion of drugs filtered at the glomerulus that are unable to be reabsorbed at the collecting tubule when in an ionised form at alkaline pH. Urinary alkalinisation is as effective as forced alkaline diuresis for salicylate poisoning.[8]

ANTIDOTES

Pharmacological antagonists (e.g. naloxone) and chelating agents (e.g. desferrioxamine) are useful in only a small minority of poisonings. Specific antidotes are listed in Table 21.1.2.

DISPOSITION

Most children can be discharged home after a short period of observation, especially where the risk assessment is low for that particular child. Where there is physical evidence of a significant toxi-drome or suspicion of a serious ingestion, admission to a monitored area for observation is essential. Observation entails repeated assessment of airway and vital signs and cardiac monitoring if cardiotoxins or unknown substances have been ingested. Further investigation and a longer period of observation should be instituted if the ingested substance has the following characteristics:

- Delayed onset of toxicity, e.g. modified release preparations.
- Slow intestinal absorption, e.g. carbamazepine, digoxin.
- Tendency to form gastric concretions, e.g. heavy metals, salicylates.
- Slow tissue distribution, e.g. lithium, digoxin.
- Undergo metabolic activation, e.g. paracetamol, chlorinated hydrocarbons.
- Inhibit metabolic pathways, e.g. colchicine, neoplastic agents.

Psychiatric assessment and mobilisation of additional support services may be required in the management of deliberate self-harm. Consensus guidelines for managing these young people have recently been released.[9]

The carers should be informed of any possible delayed sequelae that might prompt review after the child has been discharged.

Every opportunity should be taken to educate the community in the safe supervision of children and the proper use and storage of medications.

CONTROVERSIES AND FUTURE DIRECTIONS

❶ There is little clinical evidence for the use of any gastric decontamination technique. Activated charcoal is currently the preferred method of gastrointestinal decontamination because it has a theoretical benefit and a low side-effect profile. Further multi-centre trials are needed to establish an evidence-based approach to this treatment. There may be specific subgroups that might benefit from particular GI decontamination techniques.

❷ There is little evidence for the safest and most efficient approach to observation in the ED. The incidence of life-threatening complications is extraordinarily low in the child with no toxidrome or history suggestive of life-threatening ingestion. Prospective validation of decision rules should be studied in a large population.

RESOURCES

The Australian Poisons Information Centre (Tel: 131126) is a 24-hour national resource that provides current information on constituents of products, potentially toxic doses and can advise on the appropriate management of a particular child. The services of a toxicologist can be accessed through the centre. Similar regional services exist in the UK and the USA.

REFERENCES

1. American College of Emergency Physicians 1995 Clinical policy for the initial approach to patients presenting with acute toxic ingestion or dermal or inhalation exposure. Annals of Emergency Medicine 25(4): 570–585
2. American Academy of Clinical Toxicology and European Association of Poison Centres and Clinical Toxicologists 1997 Ipecac syrup. Journal of Toxicology and Clinical Toxicology 35: 699–709
3. American Academy of Clinical Toxicology and European Association of Poison Centres and Clinical Toxicologists 1997 Gastric lavage. Journal of Toxicology and Clinical Toxicology 35: 711–719
4. American Academy of Clinical Toxicology and European Association of Poison Centres and Clinical Toxicologists 1997 Single-dose activated charcoal. Journal of Toxicology and Clinical Toxicology 35: 721–741
5. American Academy of Clinical Toxicology and European Association of Poison Centres and Clinical Toxicologists 1997 Cathartics. Journal of Toxicology and Clinical Toxicology 35: 743–752
6. American Academy of Clinical Toxicology and European Association of Poison Centres and Clinical Toxicologists 1997 Whole bowel irrigation. Journal of Toxicology and Clinical Toxicology 35: 753–762
7. Pond SM 1991 Extra-corporeal techniques in the treatment of poisoned patients. Medical Journal of Australia 154: 617–622
8. Prescott LF et al 1982 Diuresis or urinary alkalinisation for salicylate poisoning? British Medical Journal 285: 1385–1386
9. Australasian College for Emergency Medicine, Royal Australian and New Zealand College of Psychiatrists 2000 Guidelines for the Management of Deliberate Self-harm in Young People. Australasian College for Emergency Medicine, Royal Australian and New Zealand College of Psychiatrists, Melbourne

FURTHER READING

Bates N, Edwards N, Roper J, Volans G (eds) 1997 Paediatric toxicology. Handbook of poisoning in children. Macmillan Reference, London
Riordan M, Rylance G, Berry K 2002 Poisoning in children. Archives of Disease in Childhood 87: 392–410

21.2 SPECIFIC POISONS

HELEN MEAD • NICHOLAS CHENG

INTRODUCTION

The most common calls to the Australian National Poisons Centre and the ten most common poisons to which children are exposed are shown in Table 21.2.1.

There is a vast number of substances that can be ingested by children. The best way of classifying these is to think of a potential ingestant as coming from one of four major groups of agents. Within each of the groups in Table 21.2.2. are some common and very important poisons. Many have a range of toxicities and specific clinical effects. The most commonly encountered or medically important of these agents will now be discussed in detail.

SPECIFIC POSIONS

The overall mortality of patients reaching hospital alive following drug overdose is exceedingly low. Supportive care is the mainstay of management. In some circumstances specific antidotes or treatments will improve outcome. It is important for the emergency physician to have a good knowledge of these poisons.

PAINKILLERS

Paracetamol

Paracetamol is by far the commonest poisoning presentation to the ED, but the large majority will have no toxic effects. Absorption from the GI tract is rapid ranging from thirty-nine minutes after ingesting elixir formulation to four hours after tablets (possibly with concomitant ingestion of other drugs that may delay gastric emptying). Uniform distribution occurs throughout most body fluid compartments. The volume of distribution is approximately $0.75\ L\ kg^{-1}$. Most of the paracetamol is conjugated by the hepatic pathways of sulfation and glucuronidation to inactive metabolites, which are excreted in the urine. Children under the age of 9–12 years have a more active sulfation pathway. Less than 5% is excreted unchanged by the kidney and 5–15% is oxidised by the hepatic cytochrome P450 enzyme system to form a highly reactive electrophile NAPQI, which binds to cells and induces oxidation of enzymes, leading to cell death. When there are inadequate glutathione reserves NAPQI binds to hepatocytes, causing hepatotoxicity. The literature has cited impaired hepatic function, depleted glutathione stores and cytochrome P450-inducing drugs as predisposing to toxicity, but this was based on an incomplete understanding of the complexities of the P450 enzyme system. Concerns regarding increased toxicity in children with malnourishment, anorexia or failure to thrive are anecdotal, and acute toxicity from accidental ingestion is extremely rare. Concomitant alcohol ingestion may alter metabolism and be protective. Paracetamol toxicity is more likely to be problematic in children taking standard

Table 21.2.1   The ten most common childhood poisons

- Paracetamol
- Antidepressants
- Benzodiazepines
- Detergents
- Cough and cold preparations
- Cleaners – all purpose
- Alcohol, ethanol (beverage)
- Silica gel
- Rodenticides
- Antihistamines

Table 21.2.2   Classification of possible ingestants

1. Painkillers
- Paracetamol
- Non-steroidal anti-inflammatory drugs (NSAIDs)
- Salicylate

2. Common medicines
- Benzodiazepines
- Anticholinergics
- Antidepressants
- Serotonin reuptake inhibitors
- Cough and decongestant medications
- Oral contraceptive pill
- Antibiotics
- Vitamins
- Topical preparations
- Asthma medications
- Antihistamine
- Iron
- Clonidine

3. Household products, plants and mushrooms
- Hydrocarbons
- Corrosive ingestions
- Alcohols and glycols
- Essential oils
- General household cleaning products
- Perfumes and mouthwash
- Rodenticides
- Mushroom poisoning

4. Rare and dangerous poisons
- Digoxin
- Calcium-channel blockers
- β-Blockers
- Clonidine
- Carbamazepine
- Iron
- Lithium
- Opioids
- Organophosphates and carbamates
- Oral hypoglycaemics
- Carbon monoxide
- Cyanide
- Ecstasy
- Cocaine
- Nicotine
- Isoniazid

---

doses of paracetamol chronically or repeated supra-therapeutic dosing than after a single accidental ingestion.

Children usually ingest the elixir formulation rather than tablets. Absorption of elixir occurs within minutes of the dose so minimal paracetamol is available to bind to charcoal. Nomograms exist to predict toxicity in acute overdose in adults but the validity of extrapolation to children is questionable. Nomograms were developed from blood levels in adults taken at four hours after ingestion of tablets, possibly in association with co-ingestants, which may have delayed gastric emptying. Children appear less sensitive to the hepatotoxic effects of paracetamol than adults. This may be related to metabolic differences, age-related clearance rates and to the increased propensity for children to vomit after acute paracetamol ingestion. The peak serum concentration is reached in < 2 hours in the majority of children having a single ingestion of paracetamol elixir.

N-acetylcysteine (NAC) is metabolised in the liver to form cysteine (a glutathione precursor) and acts as a substrate for hepatic sulfation, reducing the amount of paracetamol undergoing microsomal metabolism.

The clinical course is divided into four stages. In the early phase, < 24 hours, a child may be totally asymptomatic or complain only of mild abdominal pain, nausea and vomiting. After an extremely large ingestion lethargy and coma may be present, although this is extremely rare. In the second phase (24–48 hours after the ingestion) clinical and biochemical manifestations of hepatotoxicity and hepatocellular necrosis may be evident (increased hepatic enzymes, bilirubin, AST and ALT and elevated prothrombin time). The third phase at 48–96 hours is associated with clinical hepatotoxicity with right upper quadrant abdominal pain, marked abnormality of biochemical markers and possibly renal failure with back pain, proteinuria and haematuria. Death from fulminant hepatic failure may occur or the patient may enter the recovery phase with return to normal hepatic function within four weeks. Rare consequences of paracetamol toxicity include myocardial necrosis, haemolytic anaemia, methaemoglobinaemia, skin rashes and pancreatitis.

Obtain a serum level four hours post-ingestion in all children with potential ingestions of greater than 200 mg kg^{-1} paracetamol. Activated charcoal can be administered for potentially toxic doses if given within one hour but should not be given after ingestion of liquid preparations, which are very rapidly absorbed. The treatment line is the lowest paracetamol level at a given time for which patients without additional risk factors should be given NAC. Treat all children with blood levels in the hepatotoxic range on the Matthew–Rumack nomogram (serum paracetamol concentration > 1300 μmol L^{-1} [> 200 μg mL^{-1}] at four hours to > 170 μmol L^{-1} [> 250 μg mL^{-1}] at sixteen hours) with *N*-acetylcysteine but it is also common practice to use the 'safety line' (1000 μmol L^{-1} [> 150 μg mL^{-1}] at four hours to 125 μmol L^{-1} [> 160 g mL^{-1}] at sixteen hours) for those thought to be at higher risk. The dose is 150 mg kg^{-1} as an IV loading dose over fifteen minutes, 50 mg kg^{-1} over four hours then 100 mg kg^{-1} over sixteen hours. NAC should be commenced within sixteen hours, and is most effective if given within eight hours, but has been documented to be successful in adult patients when given up to forty-eight hours after a serious ingestion. Anaphylactoid reactions, including rash, bronchospasm, vomiting, hypotension and tachycardia, occur in up to 15%, and are more likely in asthmatics. Reduce or temporarily stop the infusion if any allergic features develop.

Children who present with established hepatic failure must receive prompt resuscitation and stabilisation. Pay attention to fluid volume loading and give inotropes early if necessary. Correct any coagulopathy. Admit all of these children to intensive care for continued monitoring and therapy and assessment for possible liver transplantation.

Chronic over-dosing or repeated supra-therapeutic over-dosing is a significant problem and may arise due to confusion regarding different formulations. The treatment nomogram is not applicable to these situations and cases should be discussed with a toxicologist.

Children with paracetamol levels that fall below the possible hepatotoxicity line do not need treatment and can be discharged. A child who has an equivocal result should have a further level within the next 2–4 hours and if this again is not within the hepatotoxic range that child may be discharged. Those with intentional ingestion should have psychosocial factors addressed.

NSAIDs

There are many different types of non-steroidal anti-inflammatory drugs (NSAIDs) available. Many are now obtainable as over-the-counter medicines without prescription. Of these, ibuprofen is the most significant NSAID ingested by children. As a group NSAIDs are generally of low toxicity, exceptions to this being mefenamic acid and phenylbutazone. NSAID ingestion may produce gastrointestinal upset, headache, dizziness, tinnitus, and visual disturbance. Hypotension, tachycardia, and hypothermia have been reported when NSAIDs were consumed in large amounts. Prolongation of the prothrombin time is common. In even larger quantities, electrolyte disturbances, metabolic acidosis, central nervous system depression, and respiratory failure can occur.

Some NSAIDs have additional idiosyncratic effects in overdose. Ibuprofen may cause bradycardia or hepatic dysfunction, mefenamic acid is associated with convulsions while phenylbutazone can cause hepatic failure, arrhythmias, and bone-marrow suppression.

Children who have consumed more than 100 mg kg^{-1} of ibuprofen should receive activated charcoal. If they remain asymptomatic, they can be discharged at four hours post-ingestion. Sustained release preparations will require a minimum period of twelve hours of observation. Children who have consumed more than 25 mg kg^{-1} of mefenamic acid should receive activated charcoal. They should be observed for twelve hours post-ingestion.

Symptomatic children require hospital admission. Oral fluids should be encouraged and dehydration corrected. Electrolytes, creatinine, prothrombin time, and acid–base balance should be monitored. Diazepam is very effective in the management of convulsions.

In the case of phenylbutazone ingestion, elimination may be enhanced by the use of repeated doses of activated charcoal as well as haemoperfusion.

Salicylates

The incidence of acute salicylate poisoning has declined due to improvements in medication packaging, removal of aspirin from oral paediatric formulations and due to paracetamol now being the favoured over-the-counter analgesic. Methyl salicylate and salicylic acid are common in many topical medications. Choline salicylate is a constituent of many teething gels.

Aspirin is rapidly absorbed from the upper gastrointestinal tract with peak plasma concentrations at 1–3 hours after therapeutic doses. An ingestion of 150–300 mg kg^{-1} may result in mild to moderate toxicity. Ingestions over 300–500 mg kg^{-1} may be lethal. Oil of wintergreen is 100% methylsalicylate and extremely small amounts may be lethal.

Aspirin is hydrolysed to form salicylic acid (salicylate). Pharmacobezoar formation in the stomach may occur and the absorption characteristics in overdose are erratic and delayed. Peak serum levels may be delayed till 24 hours after overdose of sustained-release or enteric-coated preparations. In therapeutic doses salicylate is 85–95% plasma bound, but in overdose, free salicylate concentration rises as plasma protein binding is saturated. As metabolic pathways in the liver become saturated, the kidney becomes the main route of elimination. Clearance is markedly enhanced by an alkaline urinary pH.

Salicylate poisoning leads to the uncoupling of oxidative phosphorylation and inhibition of the enzymes of the Krebs cycle, resulting in anaerobic metabolism and deranged metabolism of carbohydrates, lipids and amino acids. The resulting metabolic acidosis is more prominent in young children. Hyperthermia and rhabdomyolysis may occur. Salicylate intoxication causes stimulation of the respiratory centre of the medulla. Adults compensate with a respiratory alkalosis (large tidal volumes, often normal rate) but respiratory alkalosis is rare in children under four years of age. The kidney compensates by excreting large amounts of bicarbonate, sodium and potassium ions and water, resulting in dehydration, electrolyte imbalances and development of an anion gap acidosis, which facilitates transfer of salicylate ion across the blood–brain barrier, causing agitation, coma and seizures. Vomiting, increased insensible losses and osmotic diuresis lead to dehydration. Nausea, vomiting and abdominal pain usually occur early. Hyperglycaemia often occurs. Hypoglycaemia may be seen late. Hypocalcaemia with tetany and paresthesias may occur due to respiratory alkalosis and administration of alkali. Acidaemia with plasma pH less than 7.35 is a late and ominous sign. Coagulopathy may result from competitive inhibition of synthesis of vitamin-K dependent factors. Atopic children may have wheezing. Non-cardiogenic pulmonary oedema has been reported, but the mechanism is unclear.

Serial serum salicylate levels and repeated clinical and biochemical evaluation are more reliable than an isolated serum salicylate level.

Young children are more susceptible to serious toxicity and quickly develop a metabolic acidosis. Symptoms of mild toxicity (serum salicylate level usually less than 200 mg L^{-1}) include nausea, vomiting, epigastric pain and tinnitus. With moderate toxicity, sweating, hyperventilation and metabolic acidosis may occur. Respiratory alkalosis may occur in children over four years of age. Severe toxicity is manifest by altered blood chemistry including hypo- or hyperglycaemia, hypo- or hypernatraemia and hypokalaemia. CNS effects of drowsiness, coma and seizures may occur. Hyperthermia and coagulopathy may occur. Rarely, there may be hepatic, renal, cardiovascular collapse and pulmonary oedema and death due to cardiorespiratory arrest.

Assess and secure the ABCs. Secure IV access. Serum salicylate level, plasma glucose and electrolytes should be taken on presentation, at 4–6 hours and at 2–4-hourly intervals subsequently. GI decontamination with activated charcoal should be given to prevent further absorption, even when presentation is delayed by several hours. Repeat-dose charcoal may inhibit ongoing absorption in symptomatic patients with rising serial serum salicylate levels and whole bowel irrigation with polyethylene-glycol electrolyte solution (Golytely®) should be considered for sustained-release and enteric-coated formulae. There is no specific antidote. Catheterise the bladder and carefully monitor fluid balance.

Correct dehydration and metabolic disturbances. Glucose administration is mandatory even if plasma glucose is normal to avoid neuroglycopenia. In patients with serious toxicity, serum salicylate levels must be interpreted in conjunction with the clinical state and biochemical status. Intravenous potassium supplementation is usually required after establishing urine output. Alkalinisation of the urine will enhance salicylate ion excretion 10–20 fold and is as effective as forced diuresis or forced alkaline diuresis (which is no longer recommended due to complications of fluid and electrolyte abnormalities). Urinary alkalinisation is recommended for patients with ingestions of > 300 mg kg^{-1}, peak salicylate concentration > 300 mg L^{-1} or those with symptoms. Alkalinise the urine with an IV bolus of sodium bicarbonate (2 mEq kg^{-1}) then a bicarbonate infusion (150 mEq sodium bicarbonate in 1 L of 5% dextrose, run at 2–4 mL kg^{-1} h^{-1}, titrating to a urinary pH greater than 7.5).

Seizures indicate a serious prognosis and should be treated with anticonvulsants and correction of any hypoglycaemia, hypocalcaemia and other electrolyte abnormality. If seizures do not respond immediately to anticonvulsants consider using glucose and calcium, even if plasma levels are normal.

Haemodialysis is rarely required but may be indicated for normalisation of acid–base status, fluid balance and electrolyte abnormalities and can remove salicylates in severe toxicity. Indications for haemodialysis include rising serum salicylate levels above 500 mg L^{-1} despite aggressive decontamination and urinary alkalinisation, serum salicylate greater than 1000 mg L^{-1} at any time, CNS manifestations (coma, seizures), acidaemia with pH < 7.35 with mixed respiratory acidosis and metabolic acidosis, impaired elimination due to renal failure, cardiovascular instability, hyperthermia or pulmonary oedema not responding to the usual supportive treatment.

Admit children who are symptomatic and those with an ingestion of > 150 mg kg^{-1}. Most patients will require admission for 6–12 hours for observation of clinical state and serial serum salicylate levels.

Patients with acid–base abnormalities or significant clinical symptoms should be admitted to an intensive care unit. All patients with deliberate self-poisoning should be assessed for co-ingestants and psychiatric status.

COMMON MEDICINES

Benzodiazepines

Benzodiazepines are commonly available agents with low toxic potential. They are often taken by adolescents as part of a mixed overdose.

Benzodiazepines bind predominantly to the GABA-A receptor complex in the CNS, enhancing GABA binding and opening chloride channels to produce sedative, hypnotic, anxiolytic and anticonvulsant activity. They are rapidly absorbed orally with peak levels between 0.5–3 hours with marked variability in elimination half-life depending on the agent. The duration of sedation ranges from 12–36 hours. Flumazenil is a competitive antagonist to benzodiazepines.

Drowsiness, slurred speech and ataxia are the most common manifestations. This may progress to coma and hypotension, hypothermia and respiratory depression in more significant ingestions. Death is rare unless other CNS or respiratory depressants have been taken as well.

Management is usually supportive. Hypotension usually responds to fluid administration. GI decontamination is not indicated due to the low toxic potential. Clinical effects correlate poorly with serum levels. Assess the child for co-ingestants. A qualitative urine test for benzodiazepines may provide reassurance as to the aetiology of drowsiness in the setting of an unconscious patient without a clear history of ingestion. On rare occasions, the antagonist flumazenil may avert the need for intubation and mechanical support but it has been implicated in precipitating seizures in patients on long-term benzodiazepine treatment. The dose is 5 μg kg^{-1} repeated every 60 seconds to a maximum of 40 μg kg^{-1} then 2–10 μg kg^{-1} h^{-1}.

Most children can be discharged after 4–6 hours if vital signs are satisfactory and the child can walk unaided.

Anticholinergics

Anticholinergic poisoning can result from a diverse range of therapeutic substances including antihistamines and decongestants, many of which can be bought over the counter. Drugs with prominent anticholinergic properties include anti-Parkinson agents, antipsychotics and tricyclic antidepressants. Some plants, e.g. Jimson weed, deadly nightshade and mushrooms produce alkaloids with similar effects.

Anticholinergics competitively inhibit the muscarinic effect of acetylcholine in the autonomic nervous system. Atropine is well absorbed from the GI tract, skin, eye and lung and crosses the blood-brain barrier. Elimination occurs through hepatic metabolism and renal excretion.

The classic anticholinergic toxidrome describes a combination of central and peripheral manifestations:

- *Hot as a hare* – fever.
- *Blind as a bat* – dilated, unreactive pupils with loss of accommodation.
- *Dry as a bone* – hot, dry skin and mucous membranes.
- *Red as a beet* – erythematous skin.
- *Mad as a hatter* – CNS toxicity ranges from excitation manifest by agitation, delirium, hallucinations (often visual), dystonic movements and seizures to sedation with lethargy and subsequent coma.

Cardiovascular manifestations include hypotension or hypertension, sinus tachycardia, conduction blocks with prolonged QT interval or QRS widening and ventricular arrhythmias. There may be gastrointestinal ileus or urinary retention.

The management of anticholinergic poisoning includes attention to the ABCs with appropriate supportive therapy and monitoring of vital signs and mental state. Symptomatic patients should have IV access, a 12-lead ECG and continuous cardiac monitoring.

For potentially serious ingestions, gastric lavage followed by gastrointestinal decontamination with charcoal may be performed in the patient with airway protection. Lavage may be useful several hours after ingestion due to impaired gastric motility.

Benzodiazepines may be useful in treating agitation or seizures. Physostigmine functions as an anticholinesterase and should probably be reserved for severe CNS toxicity in patients with pure anticholinergic poisoning. The dose in children is 0.02 mg kg^{-1} (maximum 2 mg) slow IV push, repeated every five minutes till response then 0.5-2 µg kg^{-1} min^{-1}.

Aggressive cooling measures may be required. Patients with protracted seizures and hyperthermia should have creatine phosphokinase measured to exclude rhabdomyolysis.

Urinary catheterisation is required for patients with urinary retention.

Dysrhythmias are treated by standard measures. Sodium bicarbonate is the most appropriate agent for treating wide complex tachycardias including *torsades de pointes* associated with tricyclic antidepressant toxicity.

Patients with no or minimal symptoms may be discharged after six hours. Patients with moderate or severe toxicity should be admitted to an intensive-care facility.

Antidepressants

This group of medications includes tricyclic antidepressants (TCAs), monoamine oxidase inhibitors and the newer selective serotonin reuptake inhibitors (SSRIs) and noradrenaline (norepinephrine) reuptake inhibitors. TCAs are still widely used in the treatment of major depression, obsessive-compulsive disorder, panic disorder and bulimia nervosa and occasionally for nocturnal enuresis in children. The efficacy and favourable side effect profile of the newer agents has led to the increased use of these drugs. They are less toxic than the older tricyclics and monoamine oxidase inhibitors, but can cause adverse effects in overdose. Venlafaxine may cause seizures.

Tricyclic antidepressants

Despite the declining prescription of TCAs the low therapeutic index and potential for lethal toxicity remain a concerning cause of paediatric morbidity and mortality.

TCAs are rapidly absorbed. TCAs have a high degree of protein binding and a large volume of distribution. Although different TCAs have different pharmacokinetic parameters, the effects in overdose are similar. Dosulepin is associated with the greatest lethality. Minor TCA toxicity is generally manifest by central and peripheral anticholinergic signs and the antiadrenergic effect of vasodilatation. More serious toxicity results from fast sodium-channel blockade in the myocardium, causing a wide variety of atrial and ventricular dysrhythmias, impaired contractility and impaired conduction with ECG changes of prolonged QT interval and widened QRS complexes.

Tricyclic ingestions of < 5 mg kg^{-1} result in minimal toxicity and no treatment is required. Ingestions of 5–10 mg kg^{-1} may cause mild anticholinergic symptoms of drowsiness, ataxia, dilated pupils, ileus and urinary retention but life-threatening toxicity is unlikely. Ingestions over 10 mg kg^{-1} may cause life-threatening coma, seizures and cardiac dysrhythmias. There may be acidosis, hypokalaemia and inappropriate ADH secretion. Onset of symptoms is usually within two hours and persists for less than 12–24 hours.

The management of TCA poisoning includes attention to the ABCs, good supportive therapy and GI decontamination for potentially serious ingestions. Continuous cardiac monitoring, serial 12-lead ECGs and close observation of vital signs and mental state are required for all ingestions of > 5 mg kg^{-1}. Secure IV access. Airway protection should precede administration of charcoal if the patient is less than fully conscious. There may be a role for gastric lavage prior to administration of charcoal in intubated patients with severe toxicity.

Depressed conscious state is the best predictor of serious toxic complications (seizures, ventricular arrhythmias, hypotension and the need for mechanical ventilation) and the ECG limb lead QRS duration of 100 ms or greater is associated with an increased incidence of seizures and cardiotoxicity. Early intubation and hyperventilation to a serum pH of 7.45–7.55 may attenuate or prevent seizures and ventricular dysrhythmias. Intubate and mechanically ventilate all patients with rapidly decreasing conscious state, seizures and ventricular dysrhythmias. Hypotension should be treated with volume replacement and adrenaline (epinephrine) or noradrenaline (norepinephrine) infusion if required.

Sodium bicarbonate is regarded as a specific antidote in the treatment of the cardiovascular effects of TCA toxicity. It competitively overcomes sodium channel blockade and its effect on serum pH appears to improve sodium channel function. Ventricular dysrhythmias will usually respond to treatment with sodium bicarbonate (1–2 mEq kg^{-1} IV bolus, repeated till the QRS narrows or serum pH reaches 7.45–7.55). Refractory ventricular arrhythmias should be treated according to standard ACLS protocols avoiding type 1a and 1c antiarrhythmics. Lidocaine is safe. There is no documented evidence to support the use of phenytoin, which may aggravate hypotension and conduction problems due to its effect on fast sodium channels.

Seizures may be averted or attenuated by bicarbonate therapy. Benzodiazepines are the preferred agents to treat seizures but barbiturates may be required to treat refractory seizures. TCAs are not amenable to removal by extracorporeal methods due to their large volume of distribution. Quantitative analysis of TCA levels does not aid management but screening for other drugs should be considered in deliberate self-harm.

Patients who ingest > 5 mg kg^{-1} TCA should be admitted for observation for at least six hours, but may be discharged at that time if the ECG remains normal and the child is well. TCA ingestions with significant CNS depression, seizures or significant cardiotoxicity should be admitted to an intensive-care facility.

Selective serotonin reuptake inhibitors (SSRIs)

The efficacy and favourable side-effect profile of the newer agents has led to the increased use of these drugs. They are less toxic than the older tricyclics and monoamine oxidase inhibitors, but can cause adverse effects in overdose. Venlafaxine may cause seizures.

SSRIs desensitise presynaptic serotonin autoreceptors, leading to a rise in synaptic serotonin concentration and stimulation of serotonin receptors. Agitation may occur. Venlafaxine and nefazodone are inhibitors of both serotonin and noradrenalin uptake. Venlafaxine is potentially more toxic than other SSRIs.

Serotonin syndrome can occur as a result of interaction of two classes of drugs that increase serotonin levels synergistically, but has been reported after overdose of a single agent.

Serotonin syndrome is a clinical diagnosis. There may be alteration of behaviour/cognition, with anxiety, agitation and confusion. Seizures may occur. Increased neuromuscular activity with hyperthermia, rigidity, hyperreflexia, resting tremor and rhabdomyolysis may occur. Diarrhoea and sweating are common.

Treatment of serotonin syndrome is supportive. Benzodiazepines are effective in relieving the agitation and muscle rigidity and for treatment of seizures. Resistant severe hyperthermia may warrant treatment with neuromuscular paralysis. Anecdotally, oral cyproheptadine (a 5-HT$_3$ antagonist) 4–8 mg 8-hourly has been reported to be effective in treating manifestations of serotonergic excess.

Patients with agitation or symptoms of serotonin excess should be admitted for observation and supportive treatment.

Cough and decongestant medications

Proprietary preparations for the treatment of coughs, colds, and nasal congestion are frequently ingested accidentally. Most preparations are made up of more than one active ingredient, sympathomimetic agents being most frequently used. Adverse effects are unusual and occur fairly soon after ingestion. There are case reports in children of hypertension, reflex bradycardia, arrhythmias, convulsions, and coma. The key to management is good supportive care.

Paracetamol and aspirin are commonly found in ingredients. Their presence should not be overlooked as measurement of blood concentration may be required, depending on the dose consumed. Opioid analgesics are found in a number of preparations.

As the presence of several active ingredients in a single preparation may produce a confusing clinical picture, poison-centre advice should be sought if the maximum daily therapeutic dose of any preparation is exceeded.

Oral contraceptive pill

Accidental ingestion of oral contraceptive pills although common in children rarely produces any toxic effect other than transient gastrointestinal upset on the following day. Parents should be advised that vaginal bleeding could occur, in girls of all ages, during the first few days following ingestion.

Antibiotics

Accidental overdose of most commonly prescribed antibiotics is associated with little in the way of toxic effects. Transient gastrointestinal disturbance may occur. No treatment is required.

Vitamins

Vitamin preparations are in general of low toxicity in overdose. Some of these products may contain iron and this must be determined as a mater of urgency.

Topical preparations

Topical medicines are of low toxicity with ingestion commonly resulting in nausea, vomiting, and diarrhoea. A few exceptions exist, such as salicylates in wart and callus treatments. If consumed in small quantities, hair removal creams cause oropharyngeal irritation and burning as they contain thioglycolate as an active ingredient. Larger amounts may cause corrosive injury or systemic toxicity.

Asthma medications
Salbutamol

Salbutamol is the most common asthma medication to be accidentally ingested by children. In overdose salbutamol can induce tremor, tachycardia, agitation, metabolic acidosis, hyperglycaemia, and hypokalaemia. Symptomatic ingestion is uncommon in children and mostly associated with doses in excess of 1 mg kg^{-1}. Under these circumstances activated charcoal should be administered. Asymptomatic children can be discharged at four hours post-ingestion. Symptoms are generally minor, short lived and resolve spontaneously.

Theophylline

Theophylline has a narrow therapeutic index and is available in many dose formulations. The most common causes of acute severe toxicity are inadvertent iatrogenic parenteral overdosing, especially in neonates, and deliberate selfharm in adolescents. Chronic toxicity may result from repeated excessive dosing, often due to confusion as to the strength of formulation or associated with drug–drug or drug–disease interaction.

Theophylline is a methylxanthine, structurally related to caffeine, which relaxes smooth muscle. Proposed mechanisms of action include inhibition of phosphodiesterase leading to prevention of cyclic AMP breakdown, competitive antagonism of adenosine receptors, inhibition of prostaglandins, changes in intracellular calcium transport and inhibition of cyclic guanosine monophosphate metabolism. Theophylline is rapidly absorbed with peak concentrations within 1–3 hours but peak levels after overdose of sustained-release formulations may be delayed till 24 hours, with prolonged effects. It is metabolised by the liver, with only 10% excreted unchanged in the urine. It has a relatively low volume of distribution, constant even in overdose. Metabolism is strongly influenced by other drugs, disease states and age, with non-linear kinetics occurring in children < 6 years old. The medullary vomiting centre and respiratory centre are stimulated. Stimulation of β$_2$-adrenergic receptors leads to hypotension and tachyarrhythmias. There may be diuresis due to increased renal blood flow. Electrolyte disturbances include hypokalaemia, hyperglycaemia, hypophosphataemia and hypercalcaemia. Rhabdomyolysis has been reported. Gastric acid and pepsin secretion is stimulated.

The toxic serum theophylline level is > 20 mg L^{-1} (110 μmol L^{-1}), whilst the therapeutic range is 10–20 mg L^{-1} (55–110 μmol L^{-1}). Potentially lifethreatening toxicity with serum theophylline levels of 100 mg L^{-1} (550 μmol

L^{-1}), can be expected after ingestions of 50 mg kg^{-1} of standard formulation or 100 mg kg^{-1} of sustained-release theophylline.

The main manifestations of acute toxicity are gastrointestinal, neurological and cardiovascular. Nausea and vomiting may be severe and lead to dehydration. Gastrointestinal bleeding is not likely to be clinically significant. CNS manifestations include hyperventilation, headache and altered mental state with agitation and seizures. Seizures are an ominous sign and are common at levels > 80 mg L^{-1} (440 µmol L^{-1}). Coma is usually a postictal event rather than a direct effect of theophylline. Hypotension and tachyarrhythmias (characteristically multifocal atrial tachycardias) are common.

Acute-on-chronic theophylline toxicity presents similarly to acute toxicity, but seizures and death may occur at levels as low as 20–30 mg L^{-1} (220–330 µmol L^{-1}). It should be suspected in patients on maintenance therapy who develop hypotension, multi-focal atrial tachycardia or hypokalaemia.

Good supportive management is vital. Administer activated charcoal if conscious state is normal and check theophylline levels on all patients with potential ingestion of > 10 mg kg^{-1}, ingestions whilst on maintenance theophylline and those with symptoms. Antiemetics such as metoclopramide or ondansetron may be required for successful administration of charcoal. Airway protection is required before administering charcoal to patients with altered conscious state. Cardiac monitoring is required. Arrhythmias are treated with β-blockers. Ventricular arrhythmias are uncommon and are treated according to standard guidelines. Electrolytes, renal function and glucose should be measured on all admitted patients. Treat dehydration and hypotension with intravenous fluids but cellular shifts of electrolytes are often transient, so correction should be cautiously monitored. Serial theophylline levels should be taken every two hours (4-hourly for slow release preparations) until levels are declining. Benzodiazepines may be useful in treating agitation or seizures. Multiple-dose charcoal enhances drug elimination and is useful for toxic ingestions and those with ingestion of sustained-release preparations. Whole bowel irrigation may be considered for patients with very large ingestions and patients with persistently high theophylline levels at 24 hours (suggestive of gastrointestinal concretions). Extracorporeal removal (charcoal haemoperfusion or haemodialysis) may be required for levels > 100 mg L^{-1} (550 µmol L^{-1}).

Observation for four hours is warranted for those with ingestions of an unknown amount of standard-release theophylline. Those with symptoms, history of > 10 mg kg^{-1} ingestion or ingestion of sustained-release preparations should be admitted for serial theophylline levels and observation for twelve hours (after standard formulations) to twenty-four hours (after sustained-release formulations).

Antihistamines

Antihistamines cause central nervous system depression and anticholinergic side effects in overdose. Hypotension, muscle weakness, paradoxical central nervous system stimulation, and convulsions can also occur.

Antihistamine overdose can produce a variety of cardiac arrhythmias. For the majority of antihistamines this effect is mediated by myocardial sodium-channel blockade (quinidine-like effect). Two of the newer non-sedating antihistamines, terfenadine and astemizole, cause delayed cardiac repolarisation by potassium-channel blockade resulting in prolongation of the QT interval. This may predispose to the development of ventricular tachyarrhythmias.

Children should be observed for a minimum of four hours following ingestion. Symptomatic children, and those who have ingested terfenadine, astemizole, or slow-release preparations, even in the absence of symptoms, require admission. Activated charcoal should be considered up to four hours post-ingestion as gut motility is impaired. The key to good outcome in children is good supportive care. The anticholinergic effects of antihistamines while unpleasant are not generally life threatening.

Hypotension should be treated with intravenous fluids. Where inotropes are considered necessary, adrenaline (epinephrine) should be avoided as paradoxical hypotension has been reported. Convulsions and paradoxical excitement are best managed with a benzodiazepine. Phenothiazine-based sedatives should be avoided because of their anticholinergic side effects. Continuous ECG monitoring is advised for symptomatic children and those who have ingested terfenadine or astemizole. The management of arrhythmias in antihistamine poisoning can be problematic. Sinus tachycardia is the most frequent abnormality and this should be managed conservatively. For other arrhythmias care must be taken in the choice of antiarrhythmic drugs. Sodium bicarbonate is the first drug of choice for QT prolongation with sodium-channel blocking antihistamines. Class Ia and III antiarrhythmic drugs should be avoided in this situation. Magnesium sulphate may be of value for arrhythmias caused by terfenadine or astemizole.

HOUSEHOLD PRODUCTS AND MUSHROOM POISONING

Hydrocarbons

Hydrocarbons, such as petrol, diesel, turpentine substitutes, lubricating oils and kerosene are frequently available in the home. Hydrocarbons defat mucous membranes. Most straight-chain hydrocarbons (e.g. petrol, diesel, kerosene, solvents) are poorly absorbed across the GI tract and large amounts (up to 5 mL kg^{-1}) have to be ingested before CNS toxicity occurs. However, the halogenated hydrocarbons in this group include carbon tetrachloride and trichloroethylene, which are particularly dangerous as they are well absorbed across the GI tract and the lung. Death due to hepatic failure has occurred with an ingestion of 3 mL of carbon tetrachloride.

The cyclic or aromatic hydrocarbons (including toluene and xylene) contain a benzene ring and are well absorbed by the gut. Ingestion of 15 mL of benzene has caused death.

Turpene compounds contain cyclic turpene rings and have clinical effects similar to hydrocarbons.

Toxic hydrocarbons can be remembered by the mnemonic CHAMP:

- Camphor
- Halogenated hydrocarbons
- Aromatic hydrocarbons
- Metals (i.e. heavy-metal additives) and
- Pesticide additives.

The physicochemical properties of volatility, viscosity and surface tension determine the type and extent of toxicity. Volatile hydrocarbons (butane and methane) are associated with a high risk of CNS toxicity, due to absorption across the lung, compounded by secondary hypoxia caused by displacement of alveolar gases. Compounds with low viscosity and low surface tension also may cause pulmonary toxicity. Agents with low volatility and high viscosity, e.g. mineral oils, tars, asphalt, diesel fuel and motor oil may cause gastrointestinal irritation, but absorption across the GI tract is poor.

Petrochemicals are of low systemic toxicity and ingestion is usually manifest by gastrointestinal irritation. Central nervous depression may occur following ingestion of large quantities. Gastrointestinal irritation is common with nausea and vomiting. A high fever can occur within 30 minutes of ingestion. Aspiration may occur during ingestion or following vomiting. Although pulmonary effects may be delayed up to 24 hours, most children who develop chemical pneumonitis will show effects before six hours. The onset of respiratory distress can be rapid and severe.

Hydrocarbons are also found in combination with other chemical groups, e.g. insecticides, camphor, nitrobenzene and eucalyptus oil. Some of these agents are extremely dangerous when ingested or inhaled.

Petrochemicals including paraffin, kerosene, petrol, diesel and lubricating oils commonly cause gastric irritation, and large amounts may cause CNS depression. Inhalation may cause headaches, nausea and vomiting but seizures, coma and cardiac arrhythmias do not occur from brief accidental inhalation. A history of

coughing and gagging is consistent with aspiration. Respiratory distress and hypoxaemia may be present. About 80% of children with respiratory crackles, wheeze, tachypnoea and coughing will develop a chemical pneumonitis. CXR changes may include increased peribronchial markings and pulmonary infiltrates. Pleural effusions, pneumothorax and pneumomediastinum are uncommon. A CXR is not indicated for asymptomatic children.

Adolescents with frequent volatile substance abuse may have a facial dermatitis. These patients may present with fatal arrhythmias due to the myocardium being hypersensitised to sympathetic stimuli.

Closely monitor respiratory function and mental state. Treatment of aspiration pneumonitis is supportive.

Gastric lavage is not recommended and induced emesis is absolutely contraindicated due to the low risk of GI absorption and the potential risks of aspiration. Activated charcoal or whole bowel irrigation (after airway protection) may be appropriate for a patient who has ingested a significant amount of toxic hydrocarbon (e.g. associated organophosphate).

Asymptomatic children can be discharged after six hours' observation. Patients with impaired conscious state or respiratory distress on presentation should be admitted for intensive monitoring with serial CXR, blood gases and respiratory support if required.

Corrosive ingestions

Most serious caustic ingestions involve strong acids and alkalis which account for a high number of presentations to the ED. The initial presentation and treatment are similar to other burns. Domestic bleaches and ammonia products generally cause minor injuries. Serious injuries result most often from the ingestion of drain and oven cleaners (NaOH, KOH). Dishwashing powder residue left in the dispenser of machines is a commonly accessed alkali that may cause serious injury.

The severity of burn depends on the nature, volume and concentration of the agent and the duration of contact. Stomach contents may afford some

protection from injury, but pylorospasm, oesophageal reflux and vomiting may exacerbate injury. Liquids may cause a circumferential injury and powders/granules or tablets may cause prolonged contact with a mucosal surface, with potential for linear burns, deep erosion and penetration. Acids cause superficial corrosion and a coagulative necrosis, and the extent of tissue penetration is limited by eschar formation. Alkalis start to burn immediately on contact and cause a liquefaction necrosis of fat and protein, penetrating deeply into tissues. Acids typically injure the stomach while alkalis damage the oropharynx and lower oesophagus.

Many children will be asymptomatic, especially if low-concentration household products are involved. Pain, drooling, dysphagia, vomiting and abdominal pain and haematemesis may occur. Airway compromise with laryngeal oedema, cough and bronchospasm may be seen after ingestion of high-concentration agents. Endoscopy provides the best guide to prognosis and management. The extent of injury is graded by the depth of ulceration and the presence of necrosis. Typically, after ingestion the mouth or oesophagus is red and ulceration follows within 24 hours. One-third of patients with oral burns have associated oesophageal lesions, whereas 10–15% of patients with oesophageal lesions have no oropharyngeal burns. Asymptomatic patients with no oral burns may have significant oesophageal injuries. Drooling and dysphagia persisting beyond 12–24 hours are reliable predictors for oesophageal scar formation and suggest the need for upper GI endoscopy.

Oesophageal perforation and mediastinitis may be suspected by chest pain, fever, pleural rub, dyspnoea. Abdominal pain, fever, peritonism and ileus may indicate gastric or abdominal oesophageal perforation. These signs may progress to septic shock, multi-organ failure and death. Large acid ingestions may be associated with hypotension, metabolic acidosis, haemolysis, nephrotoxicity and pulmonary oedema.

Late complications are infection, achlorhydria and stricture formation in

1–3%. All patients with full-thickness and 70% with deep ulceration will develop strictures. Eighty percent of all strictures occur within two months of ingestion and 99% within one year.

The management of caustic ingestions is aimed at limiting the extent of injury and preventing strictures and other complications. Immediate management consists of rinsing the skin with water or drinking water unless respiratory distress is notable or visceral perforation is suspected. Alkalis do not bind to charcoal. Attempts to neutralise the substance are contraindicated, but dilution with water may possibly be helpful for acids and may reduce mucosal contact time in ingestion with particulate alkalis. Early treatment focuses on ensuring an adequate airway, intravenous fluid replacement, monitoring fluid balance, avoiding vomiting and adequate analgesia. Oesophagoscopy in the symptomatic patient guides further management. Patients with deep, especially circumferential burns of the oesophagus should be admitted to an intensive care unit and may require prolonged parenteral feeding and repeated endoscopic stricture dilatations. Early surgical intervention and prophylactic antibiotics are required if perforation or penetration is suspected clinically, on endoscopy or contrast radiography. Steroids have no proven benefit and may possibly increase the risk of perforation.

Asymptomatic patients should be advised to return if they develop respiratory difficulty, pain or dysphagia. All symptomatic children should be admitted for observation and endoscopy. Symptomatic patients must always have adequate follow-up.

Alcohols and glycols

Alcohols are widely available in household products and acute ingestion of colognes, aftershave and cleaning products should be considered in intoxicated children and in children with a metabolic acidosis. Large volumes of dilute solutions are usually more available to young children than the more concentrated form.

All the alcohols, especially isopropanol, produce drunkenness. Gastrointestinal complaints, a sweet ketotic breath and acetonuria suggest isopropanol intoxication. Severe metabolic acidosis with a large anion gap is a feature of methanol and ethylene glycol poisoning. Visual impairment suggests methanol poisoning. Back pain with renal failure, hypocalcaemia and oxaluria often occur with ethylene glycol poisoning.

Alcohols do not bind to activated charcoal.

Ethanol

Ethanol is available in numerous household medicinals, mouthwashes and perfumery products as well as alcoholic drinks. Methylated spirit is 95% ethanol. Although frequently ingested by children, serious toxicity is uncommon.

Ethanol is well absorbed across gastrointestinal mucosa and respiratory tract, most within 30–60 minutes. The volume of distribution in children is 0.7 L kg^{-1}. Ingestion of large amounts of concentrated alcohol, e.g. spirits, ingestion with food, and ingestion with drugs that depress GI motility may delay gastric emptying and slow absorption.

Ethanol is metabolised by three pathways:

❶ Alcohol dehydrogenase is the major method of breakdown to acetaldehyde, the rate-limiting step.
❷ Microsomal oxidising system located in the endoplasmic reticulum.
❸ Peroxidase catalase system in the peroxisomes.

Children metabolise alcohol faster than adults. Only very small amounts are excreted unchanged in the urine and the breath. Hypoglycaemia is caused by depressed gluconeogenesis. The potentially fatal dose of alcohol for children is 4 mL kg^{-1} of absolute alcohol (e.g. 10 mL kg^{-1} for a 40% alcohol spirit), about half the dose required for adults. Quite low serum levels (> 10 mmol L^{-1}, > 0.05% or > 500 mg L^{-1}) may produce clinically significant effects in children.

Ethanol acts on the reticular activating system to cause CNS depression. Low concentrations result in alterations of mood and thought processes, whereas higher concentrations affect cerebellar function causing ataxia and slurred speech. Higher levels still depress all cortical function and brain-stem activity, depressing respiratory drive and protective airway reflexes. Respiratory arrest or aspiration is a frequent cause of death.

Facial flushing, excessive sweating and vomiting are common. Lactic acidosis can occur with a high anion gap.

Management depends on the time elapsed since ingestion. Assess and secure the ABCs and correct electrolyte abnormalities and dehydration. Patients with severe CNS depression are at risk of aspiration and require airway protection. Respiratory depression may require ventilatory support. Blood glucose should be monitored. A blood alcohol level should be taken at least one hour post-ingestion if symptoms are present, although management is generally determined by the clinical state. Hypoglycaemia should be corrected with 5 mL kg^{-1} 10% dextrose. Hypotension will usually respond to intravenous fluids and acidosis usually responds to correction of hypovolaemia and hypoglycaemia. Hypothermia should be corrected. Activated charcoal does not bind ethanol but may be considered if co-ingestants are suspected. Gastric lavage is likely to be ineffective due to the rapid absorption from the stomach but may be considered (after appropriate airway protection) for severe intoxications resulting in coma.

Haemodialysis may be indicated in the extremely intoxicated child who is haemodynamically unstable, but this is uncommon.

Admit all children who are clinically intoxicated until asymptomatic.

Methanol and ethylene glycol

These agents are encountered in antifreeze compounds and radiator additives. Methanol is a rapidly absorbed from the GI tract with peak levels occurring within 30–60 minutes. The volume of distribution is 0.6 L kg^{-1}. The highest concentrations are found in the kidney, liver, GI tract, vitreous humour and optic nerve. Methanol is oxidised to formaldehyde by the rate-limiting enzyme alcohol dehydrogenase, and then aldehyde dehydrogenase converts the formaldehyde to formic acid (formate). Approximately

2% of methanol is excreted unchanged by the kidneys and a small amount is excreted via the lungs. Methanol has a serum half-life of 14–20 hours in mild toxicity and 24–30 hours in severe toxicity, increasing to 30–35 hours with concurrent ethanol ingestion. Half-life is reduced in children. Formaldehyde is approximately thirty-times, and formic acid six-times, more toxic than methanol. Formaldehyde does not accumulate, but formic acid becomes the major contributor to toxicity causing metabolic acidosis with increased anion gap. The optic nerve is particularly susceptible to the toxic effects of formic acid. Lactate is produced from anaerobic glycolysis as a result of tissue hypoxia and a formate-induced inhibition of mitochondrial respiration.

Ingestion of 1.5 mL of 100% methanol in a child weighing 10 kg would produce a potential peak plasma level of 6 mmol L^{-1} (0.02%, 20 mg dL^{-1}), so a single mouthful is potentially lethal.

Ethylene glycol is rapidly absorbed in the GI tract with the peak level at 1–4 hours. It is highly water soluble and it distributes evenly throughout body tissues. Ethylene glycol has a plasma half-life of 3–5 hours. Minimum lethal dose is approximately 1–1.5 mL kg^{-1}. Ethylene glycol is converted to glyco-aldehyde by alcohol dehydrogenase. Ethylene glycol depresses the CNS, but the hepatic metabolites glyco-aldehyde, glycolic acid, glyoxylate and oxalate are responsible for toxicity. Formation of glycolic acid and some lactic acid is the primary cause of the delayed metabolic acidosis, which can occur 4–12 hours after ingestion. Oxalate is highly toxic causing myocardial depression and acute renal tubular acidosis. Calcium oxalate crystals may be noted on examination of the urine. Ethanol has a 100-fold greater affinity for alcohol dehydrogenase than ethylene glycol, hence its use in the treatment of acute ethylene glycol poisoning.

Symptoms of methanol poisoning may be delayed with a 12–24 hour latent period because of the slow metabolism to formate. The most common presentation of intoxication consists of a triad of findings related to the GI tract, eyes and metabolic acidosis. Nausea and vomiting, epigastric abdominal pain, pancreatitis and GI bleeding may occur. Visual disturbance including blurred vision, central scotoma, yellow spots and complete blindness offer an important diagnostic clue. Fixed and dilated pupils, retinal oedema and constricted visual fields may be noted. If visual function is to return to normal it will occur in the first six days. Children presenting with normally reactive pupils do not suffer permanent visual loss. CNS depression may occur. Papilloedema may be seen.

The initial symptoms of an acute ethylene glycol poisoning include those of alcohol intoxication with lethargy, slurred speech, nystagmus, ataxia and vomiting. Papilloedema occurs less frequently than with methanol poisoning. An elevated anion osmol gap acidosis may occur. Seizures, myoclonic jerks and tetanic contractions reflect hypocalcaemia. At 12–36 hours post-ingestion, progressive pulmonary oedema and congestive heart failure occur and may be followed by death due to cardiovascular collapse. If the child survives, renal insufficiency may ensue over the next 2–3 days.

Early suspicion of methanol intoxication and the initiation of therapy are the keys to survival and avoidance of long-term disability. Aggressive gastrointestinal decontamination with gastric lavage may be indicated for children presenting in the first hour. Acidosis may require treatment with bicarbonate.

Fomepizole and ethanol block alcohol dehydrogenase, which is involved in the metabolism of the parent compounds of methanol and ethylene glycol to their toxic metabolites. These antidotes do not replace supportive therapies with bicarbonate therapy or dialysis in patients with established toxicity. Fomepizole is very expensive but easier to prepare and monitor than IV ethanol, without the complications of profound hypoglycaemia, hepatotoxicity and inebriation that may occur with ethanol infusions. Indications for treatment with ethanol of fomepizole are ethylene glycol/methanol concentrations > 200 mg L^{-1} (> 0.02%), presence of acidosis or an osmolar gap > 10 mOsm kg^{-1} H_2O.

Serum formate levels of > 10 mg L^{-1} may be a better predictor of potential toxicity than methanol concentration alone.

Maintaining a serum ethanol concentration of 20 mmol L^{-1} (100 mg dL^{-1}, 0.1%) will fully inhibit alcohol dehydrogenase, and formic acid production, because ethanol has approximately 9-20-times greater affinity for alcohol dehydrogenase compared with methanol. This is difficult to achieve in children. An IV loading dose of 7.5–10 mL kg^{-1} of 10% ethanol in 5% glucose water should be administered over 30 minutes followed by a maintenance dose of 1.4 mL kg^{-1} h^{-1}. Serum ethanol and glucose levels should be monitored after the loading dose and frequently thereafter. Haemodialysis enhances elimination and is indicated for renal failure, visual impairment, metabolic acidosis not corrected with bicarbonate therapy and peak levels > 15 mmol L^{-1} (> 50 mg dL^{-1}, > 0.05%). Haemodialysis may also be used to reduce the duration of therapy.

Management of ethylene glycol poisoning includes resuscitation and good supportive care. Correct hypoglycaemia and hypocalcaemia, maintain body temperature and treat seizures. Start ethanol therapy for signs and symptoms of severe poisoning or where levels are > 3 mmol L^{-1} (> 20 mg dL^{-1}, > 0.02%). Haemodialysis may be required if these therapies have failed to control the acute poisoning.

Asymptomatic children should have blood taken for determination of the serum level of the relevant alcohol and the metabolic products, acid-base status and electrolytes. Admit all children who are clinically intoxicated until asymptomatic.

Isopropyl alcohol

Isopropanol may be found in some antifreezes, rubbing alcohols and in the manufacture of acetone and window cleaners. Severe toxicity in children is uncommon.

Isopropyl alcohol (isopropanol) is rapidly absorbed from the intestine. Significant toxicity has been reported from dermal absorption in animal studies. Isopropyl alcohol is oxidised in the liver to acetone by alcohol dehydrogenase and about 20% is excreted unchanged by the kidneys. The elimination half-life of acetone is up to 31 hours so the CNS effects may be prolonged. Isopropanol-induced hypotension and the accumulation of the metabolites of acetone may contribute to the development of acidosis. Hyperglycaemia or hypoglycaemia may occur.

Significant clinical effects may be seen after ingestion of 0.5–1 mL kg^{-1} of 70% isopropanol solution. Blood concentrations > 21 mmol L^{-1} (> 125 mg dL^{-1}, > 0.125%) have produced coma.

Clinical effects occur within thirty minutes to one hour. Gastrointestinal manifestations include abdominal pain, vomiting and haemorrhagic gastritis. CNS depression occurs rapidly and is due to the potent inebriant effects of the metabolite acetone. Ketosis and ketonuria, with or without acidosis, may occur and a significant osmolal gap may be noted. The respiratory elimination of acetone causes a fruity acetone odour on the breath.

Management involves general supportive therapy and follows the general lines of the other alcohols. Treat hypotension with intravenous fluids. As the toxicity of isopropanol is predominantly due to the parent compound, there is no advantage is blocking the action of alcohol dehydrogenase. Isopropanol does not bind to charcoal. Haemodialysis may be required for severe toxicity.

Asymptomatic children can be discharged after observation for two hours.

Essential oils

Essential oils are complex aromatic mixtures of alcohols, esters, aldehydes, ketones and turpenes widely used in perfumery, food flavourings, massage and alternative remedies. Eucalyptus oil is an agent commonly implicated in hospitalisations for poisoning. Incidents usually involve vaporiser solutions, eucalyptus oil preparations and other medicinal preparations, which are freely available over the counter. Citronella oil is used as an insect repellent. Oil of turpentine has been largely replaced by white spirit and turpentine substitutes, which are less toxic.

Essential oils are complex mixtures of substances distilled from plant species including oil of cloves, eucalyptus, citronella, lavender, peppermint, melaleuca (tea tree) and turpentine. The oils probably differ in the degree of toxicity but comparative data is lacking. The irritant effects are manifest by the GI tract after ingestion and aspiration causes a chemical pneumonitis.

Essential oils are potentially very toxic. The breath, vomitus, urine and faeces smell strongly of the oil. Skin irritation may occur. Oil of turpentine has been reported to cause gastrointestinal irritation, central nervous system toxicity, hepatic and renal failure and metabolic acidosis. Eucalyptus oil toxicity has been reported to involve all major body systems and death has been reported in an adult after ingestion of 4 mL. CNS depression, seizures and gastrointestinal effects generally occur soon after ingestion and respiratory complications including respiratory depression, bronchospasm, aspiration pneumonitis and pulmonary oedema have been reported. In a retrospective hospital-based series of 41 paediatric cases of eucalyptus ingestion, 80% remained asymptomatic, eight children had transient symptoms prior to attendance at ED (vomiting in seven patients, respiratory distress in one patient) but only two children remained symptomatic on presentation to ED (one with drowsiness, hypertonia and hyperreflexia and another with drowsiness and rash). Both children were discharged the following day.

Assess and secure the ABCs and give supportive therapy. Gastric lavage should only be attempted in the patient with appropriate airway protection.

Reports of significant toxicity after small ingestions of eucalyptus oil have led to a cautious approach to management, with children being admitted for observation after gastric decontamination with activated charcoal. Charcoal administration soon after ingestion may be useful, but airway protection is required in the presence of CNS depression. Treatment is supportive. A CXR is indicated only if respiratory symptoms are apparent. Aspiration pneumonia is treated with respiratory support if required. Benzodiazepines are preferred for managing seizures.

Asymptomatic children can be discharged after 4-6 hours' observation. Patients with impaired conscious state or respiratory distress on presentation should be admitted to an intensive-care unit.

General household cleaning products

The main products ingested in this group are disinfectants, detergents, toilet blocks, and carpet cleaners.

Disinfectants contain a variety of potentially toxic constituents. However, in most household products, these substances are present in very small quantities and severe adverse effects are unusual. Symptoms are usually limited to transient gastrointestinal upset and irritation of the oral mucosa. Oral fluids should be encouraged and asymptomatic children, who have consumed small quantities (< 10 mL) of domestic disinfectant, may be discharged.

Non-ionic and anionic detergents are of low toxicity. Observation is only required if respiratory symptoms, suggestive of aspiration, are present. Cationic detergents are less frequently encountered in domestic cleaners. They may produce corrosive effects if a concentrated solution is consumed. Oral fluids should be encouraged and asymptomatic children may be discharged after a short period of observation.

Perfumes, and mouthwash

Ethanol is the main concern in mouthwash, perfumes, and aftershaves. Most serious cases of poisoning involve ingestion of large quantities of products containing a lower concentration of ethanol. Children who have ingested the equivalent of 0.4 mL kg^{-1} of pure alcohol should be observed for four hours. If ingestion is considered to be significant then appropriate treatment should be instituted.

Rodenticides

Domestic rodenticides are widely available in almost every household. The majority of products available use warfarin a long-acting anticoagulant as their base.

Anticoagulant-based products cause no immediate effects and urgent medical assessment is not necessary. Prothrombin time should be measured at 24 and 48 hours if more than 0.5 mg kg^{-1} of warfarin, or 0.01 mg kg^{-1} of any other anticoagulant, has been consumed.

Asymptomatic children should be observed for four hours.

Children ingesting a unidentifiable domestic poison should be treated as if they had consumed a mixture of both poisons. That is, activated charcoal should be administered if more than two tablespoons of product have been ingested, children should be observed for four hours, and all children should have prothrombin time measured at 24 and 48 hours.

Mushroom poisoning

Serious cases of mushroom poisoning are very rare. Symptoms that occur within six hours of ingestion are unlikely to be a result of consumption of the most poisonous species. Mushrooms growing in lawns are unlikely to be seriously toxic; the most poisonous mushrooms are largely confined to woodland areas. Mushrooms with very pale, or white gills should be regarded with particular suspicion.

Amanita phalloides is the most deadly fungus known and is responsible for the majority of cases of mushroom poisoning in children. A delay of 6–24 hours in the onset of symptoms following ingestion is characteristic. Violent vomiting, diarrhoea, and abdominal pain are the first symptoms. Then there is an apparent recovery followed a few days later by hepatic and renal failure, leading to death.

The main toxins responsible are the amatoxins, which inhibit nuclear RNA polymerase B, interrupting protein synthesis. The toxins are excreted in the urine and bile and undergo extensive enterohepatic circulation.

A high index of suspicion is required if *Amanita* poisoning is to be recognised early. Management includes gastric lavage, repeated doses of activated charcoal, and continuous duodenal aspiration. Of the drugs advocated for the management of amatoxin poisoning, high-dose benzylpenicillin is probably the most effective. Benzylpenicillin possibly acts by inhibiting hepatocyte toxin uptake or dis-

placing protein-bound toxin. Other therapies to be considered include the use of forced diuresis or haemoperfusion.

RARE AND DANGEROUS POISONS

Digoxin

Digoxin is a cardiac glycoside used for management of heart failure and supraventricular arrhythmias. Many plants contain digitalis glycosides (e.g. foxglove, oleander) and ingestions of these plants should be managed in the same manner as digoxin ingestion.

Digoxin is well absorbed from the gastrointestinal tract and has a relatively large volume of distribution. Digoxin is predominantly excreted unchanged by the kidney, with an elimination half-life of about 36 hours. Digoxin inhibits the action of the cardiac Na/K ATPase pump and accumulation of sodium and calcium ions leads to intracellular depletion of potassium and hyperkalaemia. The slowing of conduction, as well as increased refractory period, through the AV node, enhanced automaticity of the Purkinje fibres and enhanced vagal tone leads to a multitude of arrhythmias including sinus bradycardia, sinoatrial arrest, conduction blocks, ventricular tachycardia and fibrillation. Digibind® (digoxin-specific antibodies) is a specific antidote, which has a higher capacity for binding digoxin than have the cardiac receptors.

Gastrointestinal effects of nausea, vomiting and diarrhoea are common. Hypotension, cardiac dysrhythmias and hyperkalaemia are the major concerns.

Chronic toxicity may occur due to inadvertent over-dosing, drug interactions or impaired renal function. Chronic digoxin toxicity often causes nausea, vomiting, arrhythmias and neurologic manifestations such as fatigue and visual disturbances. Diuretic-associated hypokalaemia and hypomagnesaemia are more common than hyperkalaemia in these patients. Tachyarrhythmias occur more commonly in patients with underlying cardiac disease.

Patients can deteriorate suddenly. Assess ABCs, secure IV access and continuously

monitor BP and ECG. Although digoxin is well bound by activated charcoal, repeated vomiting may reduce its effectiveness. Repeated doses may be considered. Obtain a serum digoxin concentration and serum electrolytes. Children with underlying cardiac disease (especially if on maintenance digoxin therapy) are more susceptible to toxicity and serum digoxin concentrations in these children and in patients with chronic overdosing are difficult to interpret.

A serum digoxin six hours post-ingestion above 15 μg L^{-1} indicates severe toxicity (upper therapeutic range is 2 μg L^{-1}). Lesser levels do not correlate well with toxicity.

Serum potassium concentration should be monitored frequently. Hyperkalaemia should be corrected with ion exchange resins, sodium bicarbonate, glucose/insulin or dialysis rather than salbutamol infusions or calcium, which may destabilise the myocardium.

Bradycardia and AV block may require treatment with atropine and occasionally cardiac pacing may be required. Amiodarone has been effective in reversing refractory ventricular fibrillation in acute poisoning of adults. Cardioversion may precipitate asystole and should only be used as a last resort. Tacharrhythmias may respond to lignocaine, amiodarone or phenytoin.

Intravenous Fab fragments of digoxin-specific antibodies should be considered for patients with symptomatic hyperkalaemia (>6 mmol L^{-1}) and cardiac arrhythmias not responding to the above measures or for ingestions > 300 μg kg^{-1}. The dosage is based on total body load, estimated from the serum digoxin concentration or from the ingested dose. Alternatively, one vial of 40 mg will bind 0.6 mg of digoxin and a clinical response is seen in 20–30 minutes, with maximum effect at 2–4 hours. An empiric dose of 20 vials, given IV over twenty minutes should be given for severe toxicity.

Acute overdoses should be observed for twelve hours. Children on digoxin therapy for pre-existing disease should be treated for any ingestion above their usual dose. Other children require treatment for ingestions exceeding 100 μg kg^{-1}.

Symptomatic patients should be monitored in an intensive-care facility. Patients treated with Fab fragments should be monitored for subsequent hypokalaemia and for deterioration of pre-existing cardiac disease.

Calcium-channel blockers

Calcium-channel blockers (CCBs) are widely used in the treatment of hypertension, coronary artery disease and atrial fibrillation.

CCBs are rapidly absorbed from the gastrointestinal tract and have peak plasma concentrations ranging from thirty minutes (nifedipine) to ninety minutes (verapamil), but sustained-release preparations are associated with longer times to peak concentration and clinical effect. These agents inhibit the entry of calcium into the cells of cardiac and smooth muscle, decreasing the activity of the calcium-dependent actin-myosin ATPase. The three main classes of CCBs (represented by the prototypes nifedipine, verapamil and diltiazem) differ structurally, acting on a different subset of calcium channels and have differing therapeutic and toxic profiles. Excretion is predominantly by the renal route for nifedipine, hepatic route for diltiazem and both hepatic and renal for verapamil. All may cause reduced myocardial contractility, peripheral vasodilatation and decreased AV conduction and cerebral hypoperfusion.

The features of overdose include bradyarrhythmias, such as sinus bradycardia, varying degrees of AV block, asystole and ventricular escape rhythms. Myocardial depression may cause congestive failure or cardiogenic shock. Dose-dependent peripheral vasodilatation with hypotension may occur. Other manifestations include nausea and vomiting, lethargy, coma, seizures, hyperglycaemia and lactic acidosis.

Good supportive management is essential. Intravenous access should be secured, and blood glucose and electrolytes measured. ECG and BP should be continuously monitored. Activated charcoal is the decontamination method of choice. Repeated dose charcoal should be considered for sustained-release formulations but whole bowel irrigation with electrolyte-polyethylene glycol should be considered for ingestions with these preparations. Further fluids after an initial IV load are unlikely to be helpful and may contribute to pulmonary oedema.

Calcium is the drug of choice for hypotension and bradycardia (10% calcium chloride 0.2 mL kg^{-1} to maximum 10 mL or 10% calcium gluconate 0.5 mL kg^{-1} to a maximum of 20 mL per dose, given as a slow IV injection over several minutes). Atropine is likely to be ineffective. Catecholamine infusions (e.g. adrenaline (epinephrine), commencing at 1 μg kg^{-1} min^{-1}) may be required. Glucagon (0.1 mg kg^{-1} IV bolus over one minute then as an infusion 0.3–2 μg kg^{-1} min^{-1}) may be of some use in treating cardiovascular compromise. Transvenous pacing may be required if response to glucagon is inadequate.

Symptomatic children should be monitored in an intensive-care setting. Observation for 24 hours is warranted for ingestion of sustained-release formulations.

β-Blockers

β-Blockers have wide clinical use in the treatment of cardiac conditions, hypertension, thyrotoxicosis and prophylaxis for migraine.

β-Blockers are class II antiarrhythmics, which act by competing with catecholamines at β-receptor sites. Different β-blockers have differing cardioselectivity, membrane-stabilising activity, partial agonist activity and lipid solubility. They are well absorbed from small intestine with peak serum levels within 1–4 hours. The elimination half-life is less than twelve hours. They have a moderate to large volume of distribution. Highly lipid soluble drugs, such as propanolol, cross the blood-brain barrier more readily than water-soluble drugs and thus have more potent CNS effects.

The major clinical effects are the cardiovascular effects. Bradycardia may be sinus, junctional or ventricular and may progress to cardiac arrest. Hypotension results from bradycardia, myocardial depression and vasodilatation. Deterioration can be sudden. Lipid-soluble β-blockers (e.g. propanolol) may cause delirium, coma and seizures. Hypoglycaemia may occur due to impaired gluconeogenesis and glycogenolysis. Bronchospasm is more likely in atopic subjects, and more prominent with non-selective agents.

Good supportive management is essential. Activated charcoal is the decontamination method of choice. Intravenous access should be secured, and blood glucose and electrolytes measured. ECG and BP should be continuously monitored. Atropine should be administered for bradycardia and prior to procedures that may increase vagal tone (e.g. intubation). Unnecessary vagal stimulation should be avoided. Cardiovascular effects should be treated with atropine, volume expansion and catecholamines. IV Glucagon (0.1 mg kg^{-1} bolus over one minute then as an infusion 0.3–2 μg kg^{-1} min^{-1}) may be useful in treating cardiovascular compromise. Glucagon enhances heart rate, myocardial contractility and atrioventricular conduction by increasing cyclic AMP and activating myosin kinase independently of β-receptors. Transvenous pacing may be required if response to glucagon is inadequate. Hypoglycaemia should be treated in the usual manner with 2.5-5 mL kg^{-1} 10% dextrose. Seizures may respond to IV dextrose, even if blood glucose is normal. Benzodiazepines are the preferred anticonvulsant. Bronchoconstriction should be treated with inhaled β$_2$-agonists. Symptomatic children should be monitored in an intensive-care setting.

Clonidine

Until recently clonidine was used primarily as an anti-hypertensive agent and accessibility to children was limited. The drug is now widely prescribed in the treatment of ADHD, conduct disorders, Tourette syndrome and for narcotic and alcohol withdrawal symptoms. Children with behavioural disorders are possibly at increased risk of accidental ingestion. The increased availability of the drug has been reflected in the increasing number of childhood poisonings with this substance.

Clonidine is an imidazole derivative with central and peripheral actions. It is a central α-adrenoceptor agonist that acts on brain-stem receptors, causing inhibition of sympathetic outflow. The peripheral effects result from action on pre-synaptic receptors, reducing noradrenaline output from adrenergic nerve endings. Uncommonly, stimulation of peripheral α_1-receptors may cause transient hypertension but hypotension usually occurs subsequently. The effectiveness of clonidine in controlling behavioural disorders may be due to reduced γ-amino-butyric acid levels in the brain. It is rapidly absorbed and distributed, with peak plasma concentrations 60–80 minutes postingestion. The elimination half-life is 6–24 hours.

Clinical effects are seen 30–60 minutes after ingestion. Depression of the CNS with lethargy and impaired conscious state is the most frequent manifestation. Miosis and hypothermia may be observed. Symptoms are minimal with ingestions of under 10 μg kg^{-1}, but cardiovascular compromise with hypotension and bradycardia may occur after ingestion of 10–20 μg kg^{-1}. Respiratory depression and apnoea may be seen after ingestions of 20 μg kg^{-1}. There have been no reports of in-hospital paediatric deaths.

Treatment is largely supportive. Activated charcoal is only useful if given soon after exposure. Hypotension should be treated with volume expansion and vasopressors. Hypertension is usually transient and, if treatment is required, a shortacting agent such as nitroprusside should be used. Atropine may be useful in the treatment of bradycardia. There may be inconsistent reversal of the neurological, cardiovascular and respiratory effects after administration of naloxone.

Maximal toxicity is expected in the first six hours and children who show no symptoms at that stage can be discharged. Children with significant respiratory and cardiovascular compromise may require admission to an intensive-care unit for up to 24 hours.

Carbamazepine

The physical findings of carbamazepine poisoning involve the central nervous, gastrointestinal and cardiovascular systems. Plasma concentrations of > 50 μmol L^{-1}

usually cause behavioural symptoms such as confusion, excitation and aggression, dizziness, ataxia with nystagmus and pupil deviation. Nausea and vomiting occur. After some hours CNS depression is evident, with altered consciousness, and respiratory depression.

In severe toxicity cardiac rhythm disturbances occur including loss of P-waves, QRS prolongation, premature ventricular contractions and complete heart block. Dysrhythmias usually occur with relatively high plasma concentrations. In severe poisoning the patient may present in coma with fixed, dilated pupils. Reflexes may vary from initially hyper-reflexic to progressive hyporeflexic. Anticholinergic symptoms of decreased bowel motility and sinus tachycardia are commonly seen. Patients may also present with seizures or brain-stem dysfunction.

Management is primarily supportive. Clearance is enhanced by repeated doses of activated charcoal.

Iron

Iron tablets are commonly available in the homes of toddlers but severe poisoning is uncommon.

The amount of elemental iron varies according to the formulation. Initial toxicity is due to the corrosive effects on the gastrointestinal tract. Iron is absorbed in the ferrous state and after oxidation to the ferric state becomes bound to ferritin. Toxicity occurs when ferritin and transferrin are saturated and serum iron exceeds the total iron-binding capacity (TIBC). High concentrations of intracellular iron cause mitochondrial dysfunction, interfering with mitochondrial processes, causing metabolic acidosis and cell death.

Ingestions of less than 20 mg kg^{-1} elemental iron usually remain asymptomatic. At doses of 40–60 mg kg^{-1} abdominal pain, vomiting and diarrhoea may be marked and these symptoms may be more severe at doses greater than 60 mg kg^{-1} when systemic symptoms may also occur. Potentially lethal systemic toxicity may follow ingestions of greater than 100 mg kg^{-1} elemental iron. Serum iron peaks at 4–6 hours but may be delayed to 8–12 hours for slow-release

preparations. Serum iron levels should be considered in conjunction with the clinical state.

Iron is a gastric irritant and vomiting and abdominal pain are common even after doses not associated with systemic toxicity. Radio-opaque tablets demonstrated on abdominal XR can help formulate the risk assessment but a negative XR does not exclude significant iron ingestion.

Although four stages of iron poisoning are classically described, distinct phases may not be apparent with severe poisoning. In the initial six hours the gastric irritant effects predominate with vomiting, diarrhoea and haematemesis or melaena. Circulating free iron may damage blood vessels and cause a transudate of fluid and hypotension. There may be a quiescent phase when the patient may appear to be improving, but about 12–24 hours after ingestion the physiologic processes of cells are disrupted leading to metabolic acidosis, gastrointestinal haemorrhage, altered mental state, pulmonary oedema, cardiovascular, hepatic and renal failure. The liver is particularly vulnerable and fulminant hepatic failure may cause hypoglycaemia, coagulopathy and death. At 4–6 weeks there may be stricture formation in the gastrointestinal tract due to scarring.

Assess ABCs. Asymptomatic patients with a potential ingestion of less than 60 mg kg^{-1} of elemental iron do not require laboratory or radiographic evaluation and gastrointestinal decontamination is not required. Patients with 20–60 mg kg^{-1} of elemental iron ingestion with gastrointestinal symptoms should have an XR to further refine the risk assessment, and serum iron levels may be deferred if symptoms are transient. Iron does not bind well to activated charcoal. Patients with ingestions potentially in excess of 60 mg kg^{-1} of elemental iron should have IV access, a blood glucose level and a gastric emptying procedure. IV fluid resuscitation may be required and electrolytes and glucose should be monitored. Gastric lavage is technically difficult in children and gastroscopic removal may be considered in the young child with a large number of gastric radio-opacities seen on AXR. Whole bowel irrigation with polyethylene glycol at 30 mL kg^{-1} h^{-1} via a nasogastric tube is generally the favoured option. A venous bicarbonate level should be performed and serum iron concentration is indicated at 4–6 hours after ingestion (which may be repeated at 6–8 hours post-ingestion if a sustained release preparation has been ingested) or earlier if chelation therapy is to be given. TIBC does not assist acute management. The peripheral blood white cell count greater than 15×10^9 L^{-1} and hyperglycaemia are suggestive of systemic toxicity.

Desferrioxamine (desferoxamine) binds unbound iron in the intravascular and extracellular space and the chelate complex is eliminated in the urine, imparting a pink-brown colour (vin-rose). The decision to use chelation therapy should be based on the combination of the patient's clinical condition and serum iron concentration. IV desferrioxamine (15 mg kg^{-1} h^{-1} to a maximum of 80 mg kg^{-1} per 24 hours) is urgently required for patients with hypotension, shock, coma, convulsions or a serum iron concentration of greater than 90 µmol L^{-1}. Infusion rate may be limited by desferrioxamine-induced hypotension or by allergic reactions. Infusions of more than 24 hours duration have been associated with non-cardiogenic pulmonary oedema. Acid-base and electrolyte balance should be maintained and hepatic and renal function monitored. The chelate complex can be removed with haemodialysis should renal function be significantly impaired.

Children with less than 20 mg kg^{-1} elemental iron ingested do not require any intervention and can be discharged. Symptomatic patients with ingestions of less than 60 mg kg^{-1} of elemental iron require further evaluation and symptomatic therapy and an admission of 12–24 hours. Early evaluation and aggressive management is required for ingestions of greater than 100 mg kg^{-1} of elemental iron and any child requiring chelation therapy should be admitted to an intensive-care unit. Gastrointestinal stricture formation is a late manifestation and care-givers should be advised of the warning symptoms.

Lithium

Lithium is a monovalent cation with chemical and physical properties similar to sodium and potassium. Lithium is commonly used for treating bipolar depression. Although an uncommon ingestion in children it can be fatal.

Lithium toxicity most commonly involves the central nervous, gastrointestinal, renal, haematopoietic and metabolic systems. Nausea, vomiting, diarrhoea and abdominal pain are common early side effects. In children severe toxicity includes nystagmus, worsening tremors, myoclonus, seizures, paralysis and coma. Toxicity may progress to death or permanent neurologic sequelae, especially of the cerebellum. Cardiovascular effects may also be life threatening and include T-wave changes and/or cardiac conduction disturbances. The renal (polyuria, polydipsia) and endocrine effects are rarely seen in children except in chronic overdose.

Management must focus on removing the lithium from the body and restoring and maintaining fluid and electrolyte balance and providing supportive medical care. Lithium is poorly adsorbed by activated charcoal so for large ingestions (especially of the sustained-release formulation) consider gastric lavage and/or whole bowel irrigation. Patients with lithium toxicity are often salt and water depleted and this requires rehydration before the kidneys will begin excreting significant amounts of lithium. After initial rehydration with saline, 0.45% saline with 2.5–5% glucose can be used to maintain a urine output of 2–3 mL kg^{-1} h^{-1}. Early dialysis in patients with a decreased level of consciousness, malignant dysrhythmias or seizures may be worth consideration.

Opioids

Opioids are frequently available where family members suffer chronic pain, abuse drugs or are on drug-rehabilitation programs. The opioids are a common agent of intentional substance abuse. Iatrogenic intravenous overdosing of children is a common result of ten-fold errors in dose calculation.

Morphine and codeine are natural opium alkaloids. Other opioids are synthetic or semi-synthetic analogues. The opioids act on various receptors on the brain, spinal cord and gastrointestinal tract as full or partial agonists or antagonists. Opioids are well absorbed by all routes except skin, are metabolised by the liver and are renally excreted. Some opioids (e.g. pethidine and diphenoxylate) have potent metabolites. Opioids vary in their duration of action. Toxicity is enhanced by co-ingestion of other sedative medications, which may be found in some cough remedies or analgesic preparations. Children are especially sensitive to the depressive effects of opioids.

Young children appear markedly sensitive to the toxic effects of Lomotil® (diphenoxylate with atropine), the onset of symptoms is often delayed and numerous childhood deaths have been reported. Dextropropoxyphene has a membrane-stabilising effect on cardiac conducting tissue and may induce ventricular arrhythmias and heart block. A major metabolite of diphenoxylate is more potent than the parent compound and undergoes enterohepatic circulation.

Naloxone is a competitive antagonist, which acts to a variable degree on most opioid receptors.

The classic features are of nausea and vomiting, drowsiness, pinpoint pupils, respiratory depression, decreased gut motility, urinary retention, constipation, bradycardia and occasionally hypotension. Respiratory depression may lead to hypoxia and respiratory arrest. Dextropropoxyphene may cause cardiac arrhythmias. The histamine-releasing effects of some opioids may cause urticaria and hypotension.

Assess and secure the ABCs. Activated charcoal should be considered for large doses, or for sustained-release or for long-acting preparations. There may be a role for repeat-dose activated charcoal for large ingestions of sustained-release opioids and for diphenoxylate ingestions, but therapy may be limited by impaired gastrointestinal motility.

Naloxone (IV 0.1 mg kg^{-1}, maximum 2 mg, as a bolus, repeated every few minutes till appropriate response) may be useful to reverse the neurologic and respiratory depression. The short therapeutic half-life of 30–80 minutes may necessitate a continuous infusion (at an hourly infusion rate of two-thirds the initial effective bolus dose) to maintain the reversal and obviate the need for mechanical ventilation. For habituated opioid users, small doses of naloxone can be used to avoid precipitating withdrawal. Naloxone may only be partially effective in reversing the effects of agonist-antagonist drugs.

All patients should be observed for a minimum of six hours. Methadone, dextropropoxyphene and slow-release morphine may cause symptoms persisting for 24–48 hours so prolonged observation is necessary after ingestion of these agents.

Organophosphates and carbamates

These insecticides are uncommon poisons, more likely to be seen in rural emergency departments. They both act as cholinesterase inhibitors preventing breakdown of acetylcholine. The carbamate–cholinesterase bond is reversible and the clinical effects of carbamate poisoning last 8–24 hours and blood-brain barrier penetration is poor, so CNS symptoms are mild. Organophosphates bind irreversibly to the cholinesterase molecules resulting in phosphorylation and inactivation. This inactivation leads to a rapid accumulation of acetylcholine at the nerve endings at both parasympathetic and sympathetic ganglia and neuromuscular junctions. Because the amount of available acetylcholine at the synapse cannot be measured practically, the laboratory measures the concentration of cholinesterase in erythrocytes or plasma. The level is well below the normal range if there are clinical effects due to poisoning.

Delayed neurotoxicity can occur primarily in large myelinated fibres, resulting in distal axonal death in organophosphate poisoning resulting in peripheral neuropathy. Toxic amounts vary. Detoxification occurs via hydroxylation, hydrolysis and liver conjugation. The mnemonics 'DUMBELS' or 'SLUDGE' can be helpful in describing the effects of cholinergic excess (see Table 21.2.3).

Stimulated parasympathetic muscarinic receptors lead to miosis, bronchocon-

Table 21.2.3 Effects of cholinergic excess

- Diarrhoea
- Urination
- Miosis
- Bronchospasm
- Emesis
- Lacrimation
- Salivation
- Salivation and sweating
- Lacrimation
- Urination
- Diarrhoea
- Gastrointestinal pain
- Emesis

striction, nausea, vomiting, diarrhoea, tenesmus, faecal incontinence, increased frequency of urination and urinary incontinence and excessive lacrimation, salivation, bronchorrhoea and sweating. Bradycardia, hypotension and ventricular tachycardia may occur. Nicotinic motor effects include sympathetic and skeletal muscle stimulation causing muscle twitching, fasciculation and weakness. Other nicotinic effects include pallor, tachycardia, hypertension and hyperglycaemia.

In children lethargy, coma and stupor are common early features of organophosphate toxicity. Other features, such as odour of garlic from the skin or breath and contact dermatitis are uncommon. The CNS symptoms of organophosphates include emotional lability, restlessness, tremors, headaches, withdrawal, depression, drowsiness, lethargy and depressed mental state. In severe cases this can progress rapidly to ataxia, generalised weakness, coma, convulsions, respiratory depression and cardiovascular instability.

The main treatment of organophosphate and carbamate intoxication is anticholinergic therapy. Assess and secure the ABCs. GI decontamination should be performed being careful to decontaminate the skin before touching the child. Give the antidote atropine immediately in suspected serious intoxication to alleviate the peripheral muscarinic and CNS effects. The dose of atropine in children up to age twelve years is 0.05 mg kg^{-1} by slow IV injection followed by a maintenance dose of 0.02–0.05 mg kg^{-1} repeated every 20–25 minutes until the child is atropinised, with warm, dry, flushed skin, dilated pupils, dry mouth, decreased bowel sounds and a rapid heart rate. Children older than twelve years may be

given the adult dose of 1–2 mg repeated as necessary. Pralidoxime, although an effective antidote for some nicotinic effects, should only be used in children for organophosphate intoxication after adequate atropinisation and consultation with the poisons centre. A cholinesterase reactivator at the neuromuscular junction, pralidoxime restores skeletal muscle responses to normal making it especially effective in re-establishing respiratory muscle and diaphragmatic action. CNS dysfunction is unaffected by pralidoxime as it does not cross the blood-brain barrier. The usual dose is 25–50 mg kg^{-1} (maximum 2 g) infused IV over 15–30 minutes. The dose should be repeated in 1–2 hours and then at 6–12-hourly intervals if cholinergic effects persist. Severe poisoning and highly lipophilic organophosphates may require more frequent dosing.

All children with possible or potential organophosphate or carbonate ingestion should be admitted for prolonged observation. Patients who remain asymptomatic in the ED after several hours may be discharged home for observation.

Oral hypoglycaemics

Sulfonylurea poisoning is uncommon in children, but even ingestions of a single tablet have led to significant morbidity and mortality, and the onset of symptoms may be delayed and prolonged. Children may access the tablets in the home of elderly relatives. Chlorpropamide, glipizide and glibenclamide are responsible for the majority of poisonings.

Sulfonylureas stimulate endogenous insulin secretion by producing a depolarisation of the pancreatic islet β-cell membrane, leading to release of preformed insulin into the circulation. They are rapidly absorbed, subject to extensive hepatic metabolism, and some have active metabolites. Children are more susceptible to hypoglycaemia than adults because of their increased metabolic rate and limited ability for gluconeogenesis.

Hypoglycaemic manifestations occur with palpitations, shaking, hunger, sweating, weakness and with increasing neuroglycopenia, confusion, coma, and seizures occur. Long-term neurologic disability and death may occur.

Assess and secure the ABCs. A blood-glucose level should be performed immediately and checked hourly till stable for at least four hours. An initial serum insulin level may be helpful in guiding subsequent management. Gastric decontamination with activated charcoal is warranted. Documented hypoglycaemia should be treated with dextrose 10% 5 mL kg^{-1} IV bolus, followed by infusion of 10% dextrose (commencing at 1–2 mL kg^{-1} h^{-1}). Glucagon is not recommended for sulfonylurea-induced hypoglycaemia. Dextrose and glucagon lead to stimulation of insulin and may lead to rebound hypoglycaemia, which may be recurrent and prolonged.

Octreotide, a long-acting synthetic somatostatin analogue, inhibits secretion of insulin from the pancreas and may be the most appropriate method of stabilising blood glucose levels. Patients who remain hypoglycaemic despite 1 g kg^{-1} dose of dextrose should be given 25 µg IV stat. then commenced on an octreotide infusion (250 µg in 250 mL 5% dextrose at 1 µg kg^{-1} h^{-1}, to maximum of 25 µg h^{-1}). A serum level of insulin should be taken one hour after commencing octreotide. Octreotide is continued at least four hours after cessation of a dextrose infusion and serum insulin is checked four hours after ceasing octreotide.

Asymptomatic children should be observed for 24 hours. Symptomatic children require intensive monitoring of blood sugar and clinical condition.

Carbon monoxide

Carbon monoxide (CO) is most frequently encountered as a product of incomplete combustion. In children with carbon monoxide poisoning there are often associated injuries, such as burns or smoke inhalation. The affinity of haemoglobin for carbon monoxide is 210-times its affinity for oxygen. Once bound to haemoglobin, carbon monoxide dissociates very slowly. In addition, the binding of a single CO molecule to haemoglobin increases the strength with which oxygen molecules are attached, making oxygen dissociation in the tissues harder. The amount of carboxyhaemoglobin (COHb) formed depends on the concentration in inspired air and the duration of exposure. Carbon monoxide dissolved in the plasma acts as a direct cellular poison reacting with other haem proteins, such as mitochondrial cytochromes, to disrupt cellular metabolism.

Patients with up to 20% of haemoglobin affected complain of headaches and nausea. At 20–40% involvement, patients tire and become confused. Involvement of more than 40% haemoglobin results in ataxia, collapse, and coma. Cardiac arrhythmias, cerebral oedema, and acidosis can occur. Oxygen saturation monitors are very unreliable in the presence of COHb with saturations of 100% occurring in the presence of significant hypoxia. Conventional blood gas analysers can also be misleading.

Children considered at risk of carbon monoxide poisoning should be treated with high concentrations of inspired oxygen immediately as this will hasten the dissociation of COHb. The classical sign of 'cherry red' lips and nail beds is uncommon. More importantly the clinician should look for signs of cardiovascular or neurological toxicity. Blood should be taken for acid–base balance, electrolytes, and muscle enzymes. Metabolic acidosis is common and should not be over corrected, as a mild metabolic acidosis will enhance oxygen dissociation in the tissues. Measurements of CO are best made as soon as possible following exposure; however, the half life of CO is five hours, in patients breathing air, and measurements may still be of value after considerable delay. Unconscious patients should undergo early cranial imaging and may require aggressive management to control cerebral oedema.

Cyanide

Cyanide poisoning is most frequently encountered following inhalation of smoke containing the combustion products of nitrogen-containing polymers natural (wool and silk) and synthetic (polyurethane and polyacrylnitrile), which are used extensively in domestic furnishings. Cyanide and carbon monoxide poisoning frequently coexist in those patients involved in house fires.

Cyanide binds to ferric iron (Fe^{3+}) in the cytochrome a–a$_3$ complex, inhibiting its action and blocking the final step in oxidative phosphorylation. Aerobic metabolism is halted and carbohydrate metabolism is diverted to the production of lactic acid.

Cyanide poisoning requires a high index of suspicion; signs are very hard to detect with co-existing CO poisoning. Cardinal features are the presence of a profound, refractory acidosis and a massively increased anion gap. There may be little difference between venous and arterial PO_2, because of impaired cellular respiration. Patients who have been exposed to fumes from burning plastics, are profoundly unconscious, or have persistent myocardial ischaemia in the absence of elevated COHb should be considered at high risk.

Rapid treatment is essential. Blood levels are useful in confirming toxicity, but therapeutic intervention is usually necessary before the level is available.

Patients should receive high concentrations of inspired oxygen. Specific antidotes such as hydroxocobalamin (vitamin B$_{12}$) should be administered as soon as possible.

Ecstasy

Ecstasy is widely available as a drug of abuse. Ecstasy, 3,4-methylenedioxymethamphetamine or MDMA, is an amphetamine derivative. The mechanism of action is uncertain but appears to relate to increased 5-hydroxytryptamine (5-HT) release accompanied by a decreased 5-HT uptake by nerve terminals.

It produces typical amphetamine effects, such as locomotor stimulation, euphoria, excitement, and stereotyped behaviour. Ecstasy has additional psychotomimetic effects that alter perception and mood.

Severe idiosyncratic reactions have been reported to ecstasy following doses that have previously been well tolerated. Reactions include coma, convulsions, arrhythmias, malignant hyperthermia, rhabdomyolysis, hypertension, and multiorgan failure.

Patients who are asymptomatic should receive activated charcoal if ingestion has occurred within one hour. Blood pressure, temperature, and ECG monitoring should occur. In the absence of symptoms patients can be discharged after 24 hours' observation, provided that adequate parental supervision is available. Patients with symptoms require a minimum of 48 hours' observation. Adverse effects, related to psychomotor stimulation or hallucination, require only supportive treatment. These effects usually last for 4–6 hours, but can occur for up to 48 hours.

Patients with signs of cardiac or central nervous system toxicity require admission to the paediatric intensive-care unit. Careful monitoring of haematological and biochemical parameters is essential. Hyperthermia may respond to simple cooling measures but, should these fail, patients should receive dantrolene 1 mg kg^{-1} intravenously over 10–15 minutes. If there is no response this dose may be repeated at fifteen-minute intervals to a cumulative maximum of 10 mg kg^{-1} in 24 hours. Hypertension responds well to labetalol. Convulsions and agitation should be treated with benzodiazepines. Chlorpromazine and haloperidol are best avoided as they may decrease seizure threshold. Vigorous fluid replacement is often necessary to rehydrate patients, promote a diuresis to clear myoglobin, and allow for increased insensible losses. However, care is necessary as self-induced water intoxication has been described in these patients. Fluid therapy should be guided by regular blood tests and invasive monitoring.

Cocaine

Cocaine is a psychomotor stimulant and may be frequently consumed by adolescent patients. Cocaine is supplied as a salt or, more recently, as a free base known as crack. Crack cocaine is favoured as it can be smoked, producing an effect equivalent to intravenous injection of the salt. Cocaine acts by inhibiting the uptake of dopamine, noradrenaline (norepinephrine), and 5-HT from synapses.

The effects of acute overdoes include agitation, hallucinations, convulsions,

hypertension, myocardial ischaemia, and cerebral infarction. Cardiac arrhythmias may pose a particular problem. Patients who are asymptomatic should receive activated charcoal if ingestion has occurred within one hour together with close monitoring of blood pressure and ECG. Patients who are symptomatic require intensive monitoring. Agitation, hallucinations, and convulsions can be controlled with benzodiazepines. Acidosis exacerbates cardiac toxicity and should be corrected; resistant arrhythmias may respond to calcium antagonists. Hypertension and chest pain can be treated with diazepam, nitrates, and calcium antagonists.

Drugs to be avoided are those acting on noradrenergic or dopaminergic systems, such as, β-blockers or phenothiazines due to potential interactions. If myocardial infarction occurs it should be managed in the usual way.

Nicotine

Children most frequently encounter nicotine in the form of cigarette or cigarette butt ingestion. Nicotine is a toxic alkaloid found in a range of plants, most notably tobacco. Nicotine stimulates nicotinic acetylcholine receptors throughout the central and autonomic nervous systems. With significant ingestion, confusion and convulsions are accompanied by arrhythmias and parasympathetic over stimulation.

Vomiting is the commonest symptom following cigarette ingestion and tends to limit toxicity. Asymptomatic children who have ingested less than one cigarette or two cigarette butts should merely be observed for two hours as no specific treatment is required. Children who have consumed more than this amount, should receive activated charcoal, close monitoring and hospital admission if there is significant concern.

Isoniazid

Isoniazid is widely used in the treatment of tuberculosis. With the resurgence of this disease in many countries over the last decade overdose with isoniazid is now more frequently reported in children. Isoniazid reacts with pyridoxine to

form a compound which is rapidly excreted in the urine in overdose. Pyridoxine is requkred for the production of the inhibitory neurotransmitter γ-aminobutyric acid (GABA). A deficiency of GABA results in intractable seizures, resistant to most conventional anticonvulsant therapies.

The effects of isoniazid toxicity generally appear within two hours of ingestion with neurological symptoms predominating. Seizures may occur if more than 30 mg kg^{-1} has been ingested. Lactic acidosis, hyperglycaemia, hypokalaemia, and ketonuria are common.

Children who are asymptomatic should receive activated charcoal. Children who are symptomatic should receive intravenous pyridoxine at a dose equivalent to the amount of isoniazid ingested in milligrams. This dose may be repeated at ten-minute intervals to control seizures. Aggressive supportive treatment is often required in these children. Other therapies to consider in the child who has failed to respond include urinary alkalinisation or haemodialysis to enhance isoniazid clearance.

FURTHER READING

General
Riordan M, Rylance G, Berry K 2002 Poisoning in children 1: General management. Archives of Diseases in Childhood 87: 392–396
Riordan M, Rylance G, Berry K 2002 Poisoning in children 2: Painkillers. Archives of Diseases in Childhood 87: 397–399
Riordan M, Rylance G, Berry K 2002 Poisoning in children 3: Common medicines. Archives of Diseases in Childhood; 87: 400–402
Riordan M, Rylance G, Berry K 2002 Poisoning in children 4: Household products, plants, and mushrooms. Archives of Diseases in Childhood 87: 403–406
Riordan M, Rylance G, Berry K 2002 Poisoning in children 5: Rare and dangerous poisons. Archives of Diseases in Childhood 87: 407–410

Specific poisons
American Academy of Clinical Toxicology 1997 European Association of Poisons Centres and Clinical Toxicologists. Position statement: whole bowel irrigation. Journal of Toxicology and Clinical Toxicology 35: 753–762
Anderson BJ, Holford NHG, Armishaw JC, Aicken R 1999 Predicting concentrations in children presenting with acetaminophen overdose. Journal of Paediatrics 135: 290–295
Anderson KD, Rouse TM, Randolph JG 1990 A controlled trial of corticosteroids in children with corrosive injury of the esophagus. New England Journal of Medicine 323: 637–640
Anis N, Namasonthi V, Ginsburg CM 1981 Criteria for hospitalising children who have ingested products

containing hydrocarbons. Journal of American Medical Association 246: 840–843

Antman EM, Wenger FL, Butler VP et al 1992 Treatment of 150 cases of life threatening digitalis intoxication with digoxin specific Fab antibody fragments: Final report of multicenter study. Circulation 81: 1744–1752

Borys DJ, Setzer SC, Ling LJ et al 1992 Acute fluoxetine overdose: A report of 234 cases. American Journal of Emergency Medicine 10: 115–120

Boyer EW, Shannon M 2001 Treatment of calcium-channel-blocker intoxication with insulin infusion. New England Journal of Medicine 344: 1721–1722 (letter)

Brent J 2001 For the Methylpyrazole for Toxic Alcohols Study Group (University of Colorado, Denver) et al. Fomepizole for the treatment of methanol poisoning. New England Journal of Medicine 344: 424–429

Buckley N, Dawson AH, Howarth D, Whyte IM 1993 Slow release verapamil poisoning. Use of polyethylene glycol whole bowel lavage and high dose calcium. Medical Journal of Australia 158: 202–204

Buckley NA, Dawson AH, Whyte IM, Henry DA 1995 Greater toxicity of dothiepin in overdose than of other tricyclic antidepressants. Lancet 343: 159–162

Burns MJ, Lindon CH, Graudins A et al 2000 A comparison of physostigmine and benzodiazepines for the treatment of anticholinergic poisoning. Annals of Emergency Medicine 35: 374–381

Chan BC, Graudins A, Whyte IA, Dawson AH, Braitberg G, Duggan GG 1998 Serotonin syndrome resulting from drug interactions. Medical Journal of Australia 169: 523–525

Chyka PA, Butler AY 1993 Assessment of acute iron poisoning by laboratory and clinical observations. American Journal of Medicine 11: 99–103

Dahlqvist R 1984 Non-linear metabolic disposition of theophylline. Therapeutic Drug Monitor 6: 290–297

Day LM, Ozanne-Smith J, Parsons BJ, Dobbin M, Tibballs J 1997 Eucalyptus poisoning among young children: Mechanisms of access and the potential for prevention. Australian and New Zealand Journal of Public Health 21: 297–302

Dugandzic RM, Tierney MG, Dickinson GE et al 1989 Evaluation of the Done nomogram in the management of acute salicylate intoxication. Annals of Emergency Medicine 18: 1186–1190

Dziukas LJ, Vohra J 1991 Tricyclic antidepressant poisoning. Medical Journal of Australia 154: 344–350

Erickson SJ, Duncan A 1998 Clonidine poisoning - an emerging problem: Epidemiology, clinical features, management and preventative strategies. Journal of Paediatric Child Health 134: 280–282

Fiser DH, Moss MM, Walker W 1990 Critical care for clonidine poisoning in toddlers. Critical Care Medicine 18: 1124–1128

Flanagan RJ, Meredith TJ 1991 Use of N-acetylcysteine in clinical toxicology. American Journal of Toxicology 91: 131S–139S

Fraser NC 1980 Accidental poisoning deaths in British children 1958-1977. British Medical Journal 280:1595–1598

Gill M, LoVecchio F, Selden B 1999 Serotonin syndrome in a child after a single dose of fluvoxamine. Annals of Emergency Medicine 33: 457–459

Gorman R, Khin-Maung-Gyi MT, Klein-Schwartz W et al 1992 Initial symptoms as predictors of esophageal injury in alkaline corrosive ingestions. American Journal of Emergency Medicine 10: 189–194

Graudins A, Linden CH, Ferm RP 1997 Diagnosis and treatment of sulfonylurea-induced hyperinsulinemic hypoglycemia. American Journal of Emergency Medicine 15: 95–96

Graudins A, Vossler C, Wang R 1997 Fluoxetine-induced cardiotoxicity with response to bicarbonate therapy. American Journal of Emergency Medicine 15: 501–503

Haddad L, Shannon MW, Winchester JF (eds) 1998 Clinical management of poisoning and drug overdose, 3rd edn. WB Saunders, Philadelphia

Hulten B, Adams R, Askenasi R et al 1992 Predicting severity of tricyclic antidepressant overdose. Clinical Toxicology 30: 161–170

Kerns W et al 1994 Beta-blocker and calcium channel blocker toxicity. Emergency Medicine Clinics of North America 12(2): 365–390

Lacouture PG 1981 Emergency assessment of severity in iron overdose by clinical and laboratory methods. Journal of Paediatrics 99(1): 89–91

Leung AKC 1986 Ethanol alcohol ingestion in children. A 15-year review. Clinical Paediatrics 25: 617–619

Mayer AL, Sitar DS, Tenenbein M 1992 Multiple-dose charcoal and whole bowel irrigation do not increase the clearance of absorbed salicylate. Archives of International Medicine 152: 393–396

McLaughlin SA, Crandall CS, McKinney PE 2000 Octreotide: An antidote for sulfonylurea-induced hypoglycemia. Annals of Emergency Medicine 36: 133–138

Mofenson HC, Caraccio TR 1987 Continuous infusion of intravenous naloxone. Annals of Emergency Medicine 16(3): 374–375

Nuutinen M, Uhari M, Karvali T et al 1994 Consequences of caustic ingestions in children. Acta Paediatrica 83: 1200–1205

Penna A, Buchanan N 1991 Paracetamol poisoning in children and hepatotoxicity. British Journal of Clinical Pharmacology Therapeutics 32: 143–149

Peterson RG, Rumack BH 1981 Age as a variable in acetaminophen overdose. Archives of International Medicine 141: 390–393

Prescott. LF, Balali-Mood M, Critchley JA, Johnstone AF, Proudfoot AT 1982 Diuresis or urinary alkalinisation for salicylate poisoning? British Medical Journal 285: 1385-1386

Quadrani DA, Spiller HA, Widder P 1996 Five-year retrospective evaluation of sulphonylurea ingestion in children. Clinical Toxicology 34: 267–270

Reid D, Hazell W 2003 Paracetamol poisoning: Which nomogram should we use? Emergency Medicine 15: 486–496

Rumack BH, Peterson RG 1978 Acetaminophen overdose: Incidence, diagnosis, and management in 416 patients. Paediatrics 62: 898–903

Shann F 2003 Drug doses, 12th edn. Collective Pty Ltd, Melbourne

Shannon M 1992 Effect of acute versus chronic intoxication on clinical features of theophylline poisoning in children. Journal of Paediatrics 121: 125–130

Tibballs J 1995 Clinical effects and management of eucalyptus oil ingestion in infants and young children. Medical Journal of Australia 163: 177–180

Webb NJA, Pitt WR 1993 Eucalyptus oil poisoning in childhood: 41 cases in south-east Queensland. Journal of Paediatric Child Health 29: 368–371

Wiley JF, Wiley CC, Torrey SB et al 1990 Clonidine poisoning in young children. Journal of Paediatrics 116: 654–658

Woolf AD et al 1992 The use of digoxin-specific Fab fragments for severe digitalis intoxication in children. New England Journal of Medicine 26: 1739–1744

Woolf AD, Wenger TL, Smith TW et al 1991 Results of multicenter studies of digoxin-specific antibody fragments in managing digitalis intoxication in the pediatric population. American Journal of Emergency Medicine. 9(suppl): 16–20

Yip L, Dart RC, Gabow PA 1994 Concepts and controversies in salicylate toxicity. Emergency Medicine Clinics of North America 12: 351–364

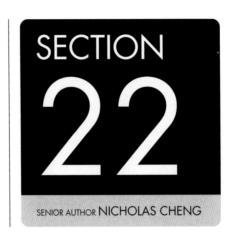

SENIOR AUTHOR NICHOLAS CHENG

ENVIRONMENTAL

22.1 ENVENOMATION

JULIAN WHITE

INTRODUCTION

Envenoming is a significant global problem, particularly in the rural tropics, but more temperate and urban environments are not immune. Children represent 25% or less of all cases, but because of their lower body mass, are disproportionately represented in cases of severe envenoming. In general, early diagnosis and treatment is required to optimise outcomes, but diagnosis is not always easy and specific treatments frequently unavailable. With estimates as high as several million cases of envenoming worldwide each year it is not surprising that deaths may exceed 100 000 per year. For most major causes of envenoming, antivenom remains the definitive treatment, when available. Dosage is based on extent of envenoming, not patient size, so there is no paediatric dosage – children receive the same dose as adults.

SNAKEBITE

Introduction

Snakebite is the single most important cause of envenoming. Some experts have estimated more than 2.5 million venomous snakebites per year, with more than 125 000 deaths. Accurate data to confirm such estimates is unavailable, but small regional studies point to the broad veracity of such statements. It is not just the number of fatalities that are concerning in snakebite, many survivors are left with permanent physical impairment, sometimes severe. Paediatric cases represent 20–25% of the total, but a higher proportion of fatalities.

Snakes are ectothermic ('cold-blooded') reptiles, comprising around 3000 species. Venomous snakes are restricted to just four families; Colubridae, Elapidae, Atractaspididae, Viperidae (Table 22.1.1). Fang structures and venom types vary between families, but the common theme is a bite resulting in injection or inoculation of venom through a break in the victim's skin. In most cases, venom is injected by fangs, paired teeth evolved to deliver venom, usually through a venom groove or enclosed channel, exiting near the tip. The act of biting can leave a variety of bite marks, which may be highly visible or almost invisible. Venom need not be injected ('dry bites').

Venom varies between snake families, within families, between genera, within genera, between species, within species, between individual snakes, and even over time for a particular snake. It follows that while broad patterns of envenoming can be stated, there is always the possibility of an atypical pattern of effects eventuating, because of venom variability. This is just one aspect of the potential difficulties in diagnosing and treating snakebite.

Venom has evolved from digestive juices. It has a variety of functions, that vary between species, but in broad terms, venom has evolved to fulfil one or more of the following:

- Assist prey capture by promoting immobilisation.
- Assist prey death, to avoid injury to the snake.
- Assist prey digestion.
- Act as a deterrent to predators, by causing rapid, unpleasant effects.

As humans, we tend to focus on the last function, but it is the other three functions that cause major medical problems.

Venom actions are diverse. Some major actions are listed in Table 22.1.2. From a clinical perspective, venom effects can be divided into three major groups:

❶ Local effects.
❷ Non-specific general effects.
❸ Specific systemic effects.

For many snakebites, in most regions of the world, local effects are a major, often the principal, medical problem. In these cases there may be local pain, swelling, which may be severe, involving much or all of the bitten limb, resulting in fluid shifts, secondary hypovolaemic shock and the risk of compartment syndrome. There may be local blistering, bruising or development of skin necrosis. Systemic coagulopathy may manifest locally as persistent oozing or bleeding from the bite or damaged areas of the affected limb. The extent of local necrosis may be significant, with potential, often realised, for long-term tissue injury and dysfunction. Secondary infection may develop in the injured limb. For some species (e.g. lance headed vipers, such as *Bothrops* spp. in South America) there may be local abscess formation. Long-term disability is a frequent outcome. In some cases, amputation is required. In cases with ongoing skin damage, never fully healed, skin tumours can develop after some years. This range of major local effects and secondary systemic effects can be seen following bites by many, but not all, species of viper and atractaspids but not colubrids and only selected African and Asian cobras amongst the elapids. Such severe local effects are generally absent from snakebite in New Guinea and Australia, where the only medically important venomous snakes are all elapids.

The non-specific general effects of envenoming vary between species, but usually include one or more of the following:

- Nausea or vomiting.
- Abdominal pain or cramps.
- Headache.
- Dizziness.
- Non-paralytic blurred vision.
- Tender or enlarged draining lymph nodes.
- Brief period of collapse.
- Hypertension (occasionally hypotension).

As most of these can be the result of anxiety as well as envenoming, they may not be reliable indicators of systemic envenoming.

Table 22.1.1   Families of venomous snakes and their principle characteristics

Family	Fang type	Common names of selected medically important species	Geographic range of Family
Colubridae (colubrids)	Back-fanged (opisthoglyphs) (see Fig. 22.1.1) OR No-fangs (aglyphs)*	Boomslang (Africa) Vine snakes (Africa) Yamakagashi and red-necked keelbacks (Asia)	Global
Elapidae (elapids)	Front-fanged (proteroglyphs) (see Fig. 22.1.2) Fangs fixed or with minimal rotation	Cobras (Africa, Middle East, Asia) Coral snakes (Americas, Asia) Kraits (Asia) Mambas (Africa) Tiger snakes (Australia) Brown snakes (Australia and New Guinea) Taipans (Australia and New Guinea) Death adders (Australia, New Guinea, and eastern Indonesia) Mulga and black snakes (Australia and New Guinea) Small-eyed snake (New Guinea) Sea snakes (Pacific and Indian Oceans)	Global
Atractaspididae (atractaspids)	Front-fanged (proteroglyphs) (see Fig. 22.1.3) Fang placed to exit mouth through side ('side-fanged')	Side-fanged and mole vipers (Africa and Middle East)	Africa and Middle East
Viperidae Subfamily Viperinae (viperids) Subfamily Crotalinae (crotalids)	Front-fanged (proteroglyphs) (see Fig. 22.1.4) Fangs on mobile maxilla, with considerable rotation possible	Common vipers and asps (Europe) Puff adders and Gaboon vipers (Africa) Night adders (Africa) Carpet or saw-scaled vipers (Africa, Middle East, and western Asia) Russell's vipers (Asia) Rattlesnakes (Americas) Lance-headed vipers (Americas) Bushmasters (Americas) Green tree vipers (Asia) Mamushis (Asia)	Global, except New Guinea and Australia

*The absence of fangs in most colubrids does not exclude the possibility of at least local envenoming from toxic salivary secretions inoculated into the wound in the act of biting.

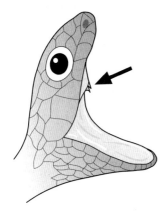

Fig. 22.1.1   Diagramatic representation of the head of an opisthoglyph (back fanged) snake. Reproduced with permission of Dr Julian White.

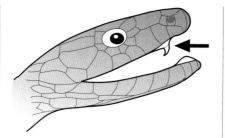

Fig. 22.1.2   Diagramatic representation of the head of a proteroglyph (front fanged) snake of the cobra type. Reproduced with permission of Dr Julian White.

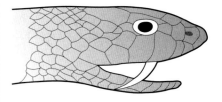

Fig. 22.1.3   Diagramatic representation of the head of a side 'fanged' atractaspid snake. Reproduced with permission of Dr Julian White.

The specific systemic effects of snake venoms are the most intensely studied, partly because they can usually be ascribed to particular venom components that can be isolated and studied in detail. An overview of these components is listed in

Table 22.1.2. Specific clinical findings for the effects of these components will be discussed in the sections on 'history', 'examination' and 'investigations'.

History

There may be a clear history of snakebite, or an encounter with a snake, where an actual bite is uncertain, or no history of a snake or bite. Particularly in young children, there may be no possibility of obtaining a history. Listen carefully to the story from young children, because

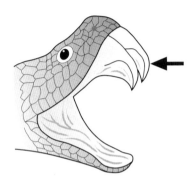

Fig. 22.1.4 Diagramatic representation of the head of a proteroglyph (front fanged) snake of the viper type, with maxillary rotation to allow folding of the fang against the mouth. Reproduced with permission of Dr Julian White.

relevant information may be disguised by rudimentary language. Some key points are listed in Table 22.1.3.

The environment and circumstances can be of great importance in deciding if a snakebite is likely. Do not assume that bites are unlikely indoors; snakes do enter houses, commonly in the rural tropics, but even in temperate urban areas such as Australian cities.

If there is a history of an encounter with a snake, note if the snake struck, how many times, if bites were through clothing, as well as noting the apparent length and colouration of the snake. For selected cobra attacks in Africa and Asia, the snake may spit first, particularly aiming for the eyes, before either retreating or pressing home an attack with actual bites. A chewing bite, where the snake hangs on is also important, as there is more opportunity for venom injection. Similarly, multiple bites are associated with higher rates of major envenoming.

A description of the snake and geographic location may help narrow the range of possible culprit species. This can be combined with clinical features to assist in identifying the most likely culprits using diagnostic algorithms (see Figs 22.1.5 and 22.1.6).

It is important to ask about any local, general or specific symptoms that might indicate developing significant envenoming (see Table 22.1.3).

In children it may prove difficult, even impossible, to obtain any history from the child, however, parents, siblings or bystanders may have useful information. For instance, a small child seeking a parent because they are upset, then collapsing, having a convulsion, then recovering, but remaining miserable is a classic presentation for significant snakebite in some regions (e.g. Australia).

Examination

While examination must be thorough, time is of the essence in major envenoming. Therefore, if snakebite is suspected, examination should be directed initially to determine if there is evidence for snakebite and the extent of any envenoming.

It is clearly important to look at the bite site, or look for a bite, if no site is indicated from the history. Snakebites may result in single or paired fang punctures, multiple teeth punctures or even scratches, as fangs are dragged through the skin during release (Figs 22.1.7, 22.1.8, 22.1.9, 22.1.10). If there is a bandage over the

Table 22.1.2 Broad overview of major clinical actions of snake venoms			
Type of venom action	*General site of action*	*Type of venom component*	*Clinical effects*
Local toxins	Bite site and bitten limb	Necrotoxins, cytotoxins, etc.	Local effects; may include pain, swelling, blistering, bruising, necrosis
Paralytic toxins	Specific systemic (neuromuscular junction)	Neurotoxins (presynaptic, postsynaptic, dendrotoxins, fasciculins)	Progressive flaccid paralysis of skeletal muscle and diaphragm
Myolytic toxins	Specific systemic (skeletal muscle)	Myotoxins	Destruction of skeletal muscle throughout body (or locally in bitten limb only for some crotalids)
Haematologic toxins	Specific systemic (interfere with haemostasis in a variety of ways, or may damage vessel walls, promote bleeding)	Procoagulants Fibrino(geno)lytics Anticoagulants Haemorrhagins Various other toxins affecting haemostasis	Varies, depending on type of toxin; may cause consumption coagulopathy, complete defibrination, active haemorrhage promoting, or even thrombosis and infarction or embolism (Martinique vipers only)
Nephrotoxic toxins	Specific systemic (kidneys)	Nephrotoxins	Renal damage, failure, or necrosis
Cardiotoxic toxins	Specific systemic (heart)	Cardiotoxins	Cardiac arrhythmias, failure or arrest

Table 22.1.3 Summary of principal points in history for snakebite

Broad category	Question	Significance
Details of bite	Was snake seen?	Increases likelihood of snakebite
	Description of snake?	May assist identifying type of snake, so possible problems can be anticipated
	Size of snake?	May indicate potential for severe bite if large specimen, but beware, even juvenile snakes can inflict a severe bite
	Geographic location?	May limit types of snake to be considered
	Environment?	May indicate likelihood of snake encounter, if no clear history of snake being seen
	Number of bites?	Multiple bites increase the likelihood of severe effects
	Was bite through clothing?	Clothing may soak up some venom, reduce the chance of an effective bite. This may also be a source for venom detection (Australia)
Details of first aid	Was first aid used?	If no first aid then nothing to impair development of effects of venom
	What type of first aid?	Some types of first aid (e.g. tourniquets, cut and suck, suction devices, snake stones, electric shock/stun guns) may make matters worse or be ineffective. Effective first aid (e.g. immobilisation of the bitten limb, or full pressure immobilisation bandage) may delay onset of envenoming, thus the patient may present well, yet deteriorate after removal of first aid.
	When was first aid applied?	If applied promptly, it may be effective, delaying envenoming. If applied late or after physical activity (e.g. chasing snake, running for help) it may be ineffective
Local effects of bite	Were any bite marks, etc., noted prior to application of first aid	If bite marks present, snakebite more likely, but absence of visible bites does not exclude snakebite (especially for some Australian elapids, notably brown snakes)
	Is there any local pain, swelling, bleeding, blistering, skin discolouration or other local effect?	May indicate likelihood of effective bite and possibly even type of bite
General symptoms	Headache, nausea, vomiting, abdominal pain?	Non-specific indicators of possible systemic envenoming (or anxiety)
	Collapse?	If in association with a definite bite, is suggestive of systemic envenoming
	Convulsion?	If in association with a definite bite is strongly suggestive of major systemic envenoming
	Blurred or double vision experienced within a few minutes of the bite?	Common effect, not likely to indicate developing paralysis
Specific systemic effects		
Paralytic effects	Presence and time of onset of paralytic symptoms? (Early ptosis may be described as heavy or sleepy eyes/eyelids)	Cranial nerves affected first, usually ptosis. Important to pick this up, before paralysis advances too far. May also help indicate the most likely type of snake
Myolytic effects	Presence and time of onset of myolytic symptoms? (muscle pain, tenderness, weakness; urine becoming pink, red, brown or black)	Usually takes several hours to manifest. May indicate most likely type of snake
Coagulopathic and haemorrhagic effects	Presence of coagulopathy effects, such as persistent bleeding from bite site or cuts, gums, or bruising, haemoptysis, haematemesis, haematuria?	Indicates coagulopathy likely and probably significant. May indicate most likely type of snake
Renal effects	Presence of anuria or oliguria or polyuria	Indicates likely significant renal damage
General history		
Medications	Anticoagulants or NSAIDS?	May affect coagulation test results or increase likelihood of a major bleed if coagulopathy present
	Antihypertensives?	Though not proven for antivenoms, it is suspected that β-blockers and ACE inhibitors may increase the chance of and severity of anaphylactic reactions to antivenom
Past history	Past bites requiring antivenom?	Past exposure to antivenom may increase the likelihood of reactions to subsequent antivenom therapy
	Past renal problems?	May increase the likelihood of envenoming causing renal damage
	Other past medical history?	Evaluate as appropriate

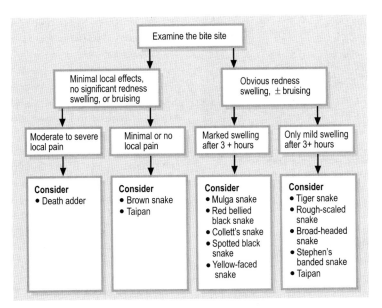

Fig. 22.1.5   Diagnostic algorithm for Australian snakes, using the bite site effects. Reproduced with permission of Dr Julian White.

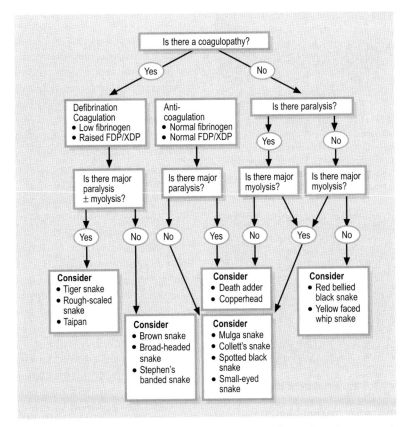

Fig. 22.1.6   Diagnostic algorithm for Australian snakes using the systemic effects of the bite. Reproduced with permission of Dr Julian White.

bite site, as first aid, cut a window only to inspect. Keep the removed bandage portion, if in Australia, for possible venom detection later. If venom detection is available (Australia, New Guinea), swab the bite site with the stick provided in the test kit. Do not allow anyone to clean the bite area until it has been swabbed for venom. Look for bite marks and particularly for multiple bites. Observe for local bruising, bleeding, blistering, swelling or necrosis. If there is significant local tissue injury or swelling, check pulses, etc., to exclude compartment syndrome in affected compartments.

Check draining lymph nodes; if they are tender or swollen it may indicate venom absorption and movement.

Examine for specific effects, notably neurotoxicity (flaccid paralysis; check for cranial nerve paralysis first, starting with ptosis; Figs 22.1.11, 22.1.12), myolysis (muscle tenderness and weakness), coagulopathy (persistent bleeding from bite site, needle punctures, etc.; Fig. 22.1.13) or thrombosis (DVT, pulmonary embolism; Martinique crotalids only), cardiotoxicity (arrhythmias), 'allergy' (angioneurotic oedema; particularly European vipers).

Investigations

The most specific investigation is venom detection, but currently this is only routinely available in Australia (most reliable sample is bite site swab; urine can be tested if there is systemic envenoming; blood is unreliable). However, venom detection will not always provide a useful answer, even if available, so it is important to be aware of other diagnostic tools in determining the type of bite and clinical effects. These are discussed further under 'differential diagnosis'.

Laboratory or similar investigations are often crucial to the management of snakebite. The key areas are coagulation, renal function and muscle integrity.

Many snakes, especially vipers but also some colubrids and many Australian elapids, can cause coagulopathy, which in many cases is potentially lethal. Coagulopathy can develop early or gradually over many hours. The type of coagulopathy is determined by the type of venom components, but just a few tests are adequate

**Fig. 22.1.7   Brown snake bite.
Note scratches rather than punctures
and lack of local reaction.** Reproduced
with permission of Dr Julian White.

**Fig. 22.1.8   Tiger snake bite.
Multiple bite with two sets of marks
and local bruising.** Reproduced with
permission of Dr Julian White.

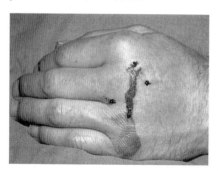

**Fig. 22.1.9   Persistent bleeding from
bite site, a sign of coagulopathy.**
Reproduced with permission of Dr Julian
White.

**Fig. 22.1.10   Extensive bruising of
bitten limb.** Typical of viper bites causing
coagulopathy (green pit viper bite).
Reproduced with permission of Dr Julian
White.

**Fig. 22.1.11   Early stage flaccid
neurotoxic paralysis with mild
ptosis.** An important early sign, easily
missed (tiger snake bite). Reproduced with
permission of Dr Julian White.

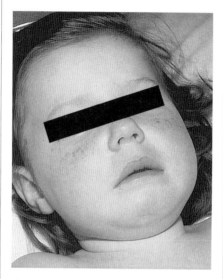

**Fig. 22.1.12   Flat facial
appearance.** Caused by progressive
involvement of cranial nerves in flaccid
neurotoxic paralysis. Ptosis is also present
(tiger snake bite). Reproduced with
permission of Dr Julian White.

**Fig. 22.1.13   Persistent blood ooze
from IV site indicative of
coagulopathy (taipan bite).**
Reproduced with permission of Dr Julian
White.

in most situations to determine the extent
of pathology. For rural areas or hospitals
without laboratory facilities, including out-
back Australia, the whole blood clotting
test (WBCT) is the only practical test.
5–10 mL of venous blood is placed in a
glass test tube or similar and allowed to
clot. If possible, the time to clot is
measured. Normal blood should clot in
under ten minutes. If there is minimal or
no clot at twenty minutes, this strongly
suggests a coagulopathy. If possible, perform a parallel test on blood from a normal control (e.g. relative or staff member).
If laboratory facilities are available, the
key tests are prothrombin time (PT) or
INR, aPTT, fibrinogen titre, fibrin (ogen)
degradation products (or d-dimer) titre,
and platelet count.

Renal function tests are usually urea
and creatinine levels. In the absence of a
laboratory, monitoring renal output is all
that is practical.

Muscle integrity relates to myolytic
venoms, the best measure being creatine
phosphokinase level (CK, CPK). In the
absence of a laboratory, the presence of
red, brown or black urine is suggestive of
myolysis and myoglobinuria. However, red
urine can also be caused by haematuria.
If in doubt, spin down the urine and
examine under a microscope, looking for
evidence of red cell casts. Both haemoglobin and myoglobin test positive for
blood with dipstix testing of urine.

If there is evidence of infection around
the bitten area, culture and sensitivity
should be performed on wound swabs.

In cases where there is clinical evidence of cardiovascular effects of envenoming, primary or secondary, or for bites
by snakes known to be cardiotoxic, ECG
monitoring is appropriate, but in other
cases it may be unnecessary.

Chest X-ray is only required if there
are clinical grounds to suspect respiratory
pathology. Similarly, arterial blood gas
examination is not routinely required,
but could be considered if there is respiratory impairment, particularly if there
is respiratory paralysis developing. In the
later stages, after extensive IV fluid therapy, secondary pulmonary oedema is a
risk, especially in young children; if suspected, a CXR may be diagnostic.

Envenoming does not always manifest early. It is therefore appropriate to retest for coagulopathy, renal impairment and elevated CK, if the initial tests are normal. In general, a useful protocol is to retest 2–3 hours and 5–6 hours after the initial test, or earlier if symptoms or signs of envenoming develop.

Differential diagnosis

A full discussion of all possible differential diagnoses for snakebite is beyond the scope of this chapter. It is important to include snakebite in the differential diagnosis for patients with unexplained collapse, convulsions, bleeding, coagulopathy, thrombosis (in Martinique, specifically), myolysis, flaccid paralysis, muscle fasciculation (mamba bites in Africa), renal failure or impairment, or local tissue injury.

Differential diagnosis can also be applied within snakebite, in determining the type of snake most likely to have caused the bite. Diagnostic algorithms have been developed for Australia (Figs 22.1.5 and 22.1.6) and South East Asia (Figure 22.1.14). These are based on cases with significant envenoming and will not function if the patient is not envenomed, though this hardly matters, as such a patient will not require antivenom therapy. In some regions, notably Australia, it is important to know the type of snake involved, because antivenom therapy can be targeted appropriately. A similar situation applies in some other regions, where specific antivenoms are available. In regions such as North America, this is less important, because there is only one polyvalent antivenom covering all venomous species, except coral snakes.

Treatment

Snakebite treatment can be divided into several areas: first aid; diagnosis; and treatment, the latter further divided into specific (antivenom) and non-specific treatment.

First aid for snakebite is controversial. Many techniques have been advocated and are in use throughout the world. Almost none meet the critical criteria of safety and effectiveness. For snakes not likely to cause major tissue injury in the bitten area, the Australian-developed 'pressure immobilisation' method is appropriate.

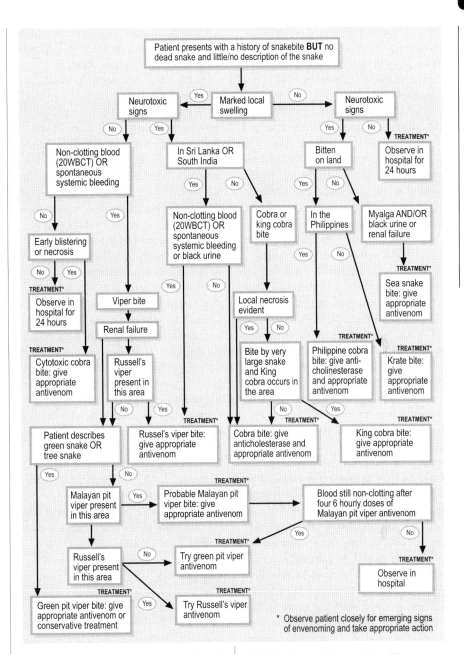

Fig. 22.1.14   Diagnostic algorithm for snakebite in southeast Asia. After Warrell et al. Reproduced with permission of Dr Julian White.

A broad bandage is applied over the bite site, then the rest of the bitten limb, at the same pressure as used for a sprain, that is firm but not occlusive. The limb is then immobilised using a splint. Correctly and promptly applied, this method is both safe and effective. However, for snakes likely to cause local tissue injury, even the pressure of this technique may cause further tissue damage, at least theoretically. For this reason, the pressure immobilisation method has not been recommended for all snakebites. The theoretical danger from this method has been challenged by recent research and it may be that extension of this research will show that the pressure immobilisation method is safe and effective for all snakebites.

Other popular first aid methods enjoy no such success and are either unsafe or ineffective, or both, and should never be used. Amongst these are tourniquets, 'cut & suck', patent venom extraction devices (suction), application of chemicals to the bite, snake stones and 'witch doctor' treatments. The application of certain plant extracts is still undergoing evaluation.

Diagnosis of snakebite has been discussed earlier.

Definitive treatment for snakebite will vary depending on the type of snake, but some general principles apply.

First, not every bite will result in envenoming, but the extent of envenoming, if any, may not be immediately apparent, therefore all bites should be treated with caution.

Second, in many regions, the bulk of snake fauna is non-venomous, so many snakebites may be trivial. However, it is necessary to be sure of the snake's identity as non-venomous, before dismissing the case and identification is rarely easy, especially in paediatric cases where history is scant. An exception is Australia, where almost all snakes causing bites are potentially lethal.

Third, if significant envenoming has occurred, with few exceptions, antivenom, if available, is the treatment of choice and should always be given IV. Choice of antivenom will be determined by the type of snake and the availability of methods to determine snake identity. Thus in Australia, specific antivenoms are available, together with venom detection and diagnostic algorithms, so polyvalent antivenom is often not required. In contrast, in North America the only available snake antivenom is polyvalent, covering all endemic pit-viper species, so identifying the snake is less important. In general, antivenom will be more effective than any other therapeutic agent at reversing envenoming. Used appropriately it is life saving and the old 'wisdom' that 'the antivenom is more dangerous than the venom' is outdated, inappropriate and dangerous.

Fourth, if antivenom is indicated, always give IV in sufficient dose and be prepared to give more if the response is inadequate.

Fifth, antivenom is generally disappointing as therapy for local effects of envenoming, but is still better than other therapies in most cases. Equally, do not overlook adjunctive therapies, in particular adequate IV hydration if there is massive local or limb swelling following the bite, as untreated hypovolaemic shock secondary to such fluid shifts is potentially lethal, especially in children.

Sixth, for coagulopathy caused by venom, antivenom is the best treatment to reverse effects, and factor replacement therapy, including even whole blood, is best reserved for those cases with catastrophic bleeding, or no available antivenom, or where sufficient antivenom has already been given to neutralise all venom. Giving factor replacement therapy while active venom is still circulating is to invite worsening of the coagulopathy. Heparin is generally ineffective in these cases and should be avoided.

Finally, for cases with flaccid paralysis, consider anticholinesterase therapy as an adjunct to antivenom, if a Tensilon test has shown benefit (there is likely benefit for cobra bite causing paralysis, also death adders, possibly some kraits, sea snakes, possibly some coral snakes). Venoms with presynaptic neurotoxins will not show response to anticholinesterase therapy (most Australian snakes causing paralysis; exception is the death adder).

From the above it will be clear that antivenom is the key treatment for snakebite, when available. The latter is a real issue, because for many species and substantial areas of the rural tropics, antivenom is not available.

Prognosis

The majority of all snakebites globally prove non-fatal, but with an estimated global fatality of more than 100 000 per year, death is clearly a significant risk. This is especially true for children. Their lower body mass and often delayed application of appropriate first aid puts them at greater risk. With such a wide variety of snake species, it is beyond the scope of this chapter to define prognosis for all snakes. However, some general principles apply.

The more rapid and severe the onset of envenoming, the more grave the prognosis, but this is not absolute. For instance, in Australia, a small child (under five years) may show early irritability, collapse, even convulsions following a snakebite (especially bites by brown snakes, tiger snakes, taipans), yet will usually spontaneously recover consciousness. Such a presentation is indicative of major envenoming, but with correct treatment, is survivable. Thus prognosis is determined by several factors, not just the type and toxicity of the snake, but also the treatment response. It is likely that if high standard treatment were universally available, the global toll from snakebite would be far lower.

For local effects of envenoming, after bites by snakes causing local tissue injury (most vipers, many African and Asian cobras), the more rapid the swelling, the more extensive blistering, the more serious the bite. Similarly, development of discolouration of the skin with a well demarcated edge often indicates an area of impending necrosis.

For general systemic effects, the more severe the symptoms, such as vomiting, abdominal pain, headache, often, though not universally, the more severe the envenoming.

For specific systemic effects, rapid onset often indicates severity. Early development of progressive flaccid paralysis is usually indicative of severe envenoming, while paralysis of very limited extent after six hours is often indicative of a less severe bite. However, this may not always be the case. Occasionally flaccid paralysis may not be evident, even just as ptosis, until 24 hours post bite, yet without treatment may progress to severe paralysis. This may occur with many snakes causing paralysis, but notably Australian death adders. This is an important reason why early discharge of an apparently well patient is ill advised. Once flaccid paralysis is extensive, with respiratory failure, the patient can still survive if ventilation is supported. However, for snakes with presynaptic neurotoxins, reversal of paralysis will not occur until the damaged terminal axons at neuromuscular junctions have recovered, which may take days to weeks. Antivenom will not reverse such paralysis. In contrast, paralysis caused by snakes with purely postsynaptic neurotoxins will usually reverse with adequate antivenom therapy. The Tensilon test will generally predict such responses.

For coagulopathy, rapidity of onset and presence of signs such as persistent oozing from the bite site and bleeding gums indicate significant coagulopathy.

With appropriate treatment, this does not imply a poor prognosis, but is a warning that more critical haemorrhaging is possible. Any bleeding into a vital organ, most commonly the brain, indicates a poor prognosis, with a fatal outcome most likely with intracranial bleeds. For Russell's viper in Myanmar (Burma), there may be haemorrhagic infarction of the anterior pituitary gland, with resulting Sheehan's syndrome developing, though this may not be rapidly apparent.

Myloysis is most often measured as profoundly elevated CK levels, and may progress to secondary renal failure and hyperkalaemia, the latter indicating a poor prognosis, as cardiac complications may ensue. In general, the more rapid the rise in CK levels, the more severe is the myolysis, but this is not always the case. In some cases the CK rise may initially be slight, but become more significant after 24 hours, rising to high levels over several days. Early muscle pain and myoglobinuria is also suggestive of more severe myolysis.

Renal damage may be primary or secondary, but irrespective of which, can prove lethal if untreated. Rapid development of anuric renal failure indicates a poor prognosis, unless dialysis can be instituted. A slower rise in creatinine levels, without anuria, usually indicates less severe renal damage, but still may take a week or more for return of normal renal function. In most cases, even acute renal failure after snakebite is reversible, over days to weeks. A small minority of cases will develop more lasting renal failure, generally because bilateral renal cortical necrosis has occurred. This severe complication with a poor prognosis is not easily predicted and is generally only discovered at renal biopsy in patients who have failed to recover from early renal failure. It has been reported after bites by only a few species, such as the Australian taipan and South American lance headed pit vipers (jararacusu, jararaca), but other species could potentially cause this outcome.

Prevention

Prevention of snakebite can be considered in two ways. First, there is prevention of bites, by educating the population about ways to avoid contact. These will vary from region to region and are beyond the scope of this chapter. Second, there is prevention of the more severe effects or complications of envenoming, by prompt diagnosis and appropriate treatment. This commences with early application of appropriate first aid pre-hospital, to minimise the chance of severe envenoming developing before treatment can be instituted. Once in hospital, urgent triage and assessment will permit prompt IV rehydration, for cases where there is a major fluid shift into the bitten limb, or rapid commencement of IV antivenom, if indicated, before more delayed forms of envenoming (e.g. flaccid paralysis, myolysis) have progressed too far, as well as instituting any life-support measures required.

Many deaths or cases with long-term morbidity after snakebite are the result of either delays in commencing treatment, or inadequate or inappropriate treatment. The latter may be the result of poor training of health personnel. It follows, therefore, that adequate training of staff will be preventative.

Controversies

Possibly the most controversial area of snakebite is the recommended type of first aid. Many types of first aid have been advocated and remain in widespread use, but only immobilisation, or pressure bandaging and immobilisation have consistently enjoyed both scientific and medical expert support (see earlier discussion on first aid).

The role of antivenom in treatment should no longer be considered controversial as where available, if of reasonable quality, it is the treatment of choice. Less certain is the role of antivenom in treating purely local effects of envenoming, especially in preventing necrosis. Recent clinical experience suggests that high-quality antivenoms, particularly Fab' antivenoms, are at least able to lessen the extent of local tissue injury, if used promptly. No antivenom can be expected to reverse established local necrosis. However, debate continues on the relative merits of different types of antivenom. The most recent Fab' antivenoms have proven clinically effective, but are rapidly cleared, requiring higher and repeat doses. F(ab')2 antivenoms are less rapidly cleared and are effective. Whole IgG antivenoms have the highest rate of adverse reactions, but are cheaper and may be the most potent. The choice of animal is also contested. Horses, while traditional and easy to use in most regions, produce an antivenom with higher rates of adverse reactions than sheep, but sheep can only be used safely if raised in regions free from prion diseases, essentially limiting them to Australia and New Zealand. IgY antivenoms from egg yolk, produced by immunising chickens, are potentially easy and cheap to produce, but their safety and effectiveness is not yet established.

There remains debate on the value of premedication prior to antivenom therapy to reduce the likelihood of acute adverse reactions, especially 'anaphylaxis'. Antihistamines have been shown to be ineffective at preventing such reactions. They have adverse side effects (drowsiness and occasionally hyperexcitability) and should not be used. Hydrocortisone carries no proven benefit, but no great risk. Adrenaline (epinephrine) remains the most controversial, as it can reduce the incidence of reactions for poor-quality antivenoms, but has a significant risk profile, so for most antivenoms its use is not recommended. It is particularly dangerous for bites likely to cause coagulopathy (e.g. many Australian snakebites). The practice of pre-testing for allergy to antivenom, using a small subcutaneous dose of the antivenom is to be deprecated. It has been shown to have no reliable predictive value, but carries a significant risk, without benefit, and will delay commencement of antivenom therapy.

The treatment of coagulopathy remains contentious, though most experts agree antivenom is the best therapeutic choice, if available. Factor replacement therapy is often the only option if no antivenom is available, as for some colubrid snakes, but is not without hazard. Heparin has been advocated, but most evidence suggests that it is both ineffective and dangerous in this setting.

The treatment of local swelling should be standard, with fasciotomy reserved for

FUTURE DIRECTIONS

❶ Even for many common species of venomous snakes, known to cause significant numbers of bites, reliable clinical studies of envenoming are scant or lacking. The medical literature on snakebite is replete with epidemiological studies that fail to relate bite effects to particular species of snakes, rendering these studies almost useless. It is essential that accurate profiles of the clinical spectrum of envenoming be documented for every species biting humans, preferably in controlled prospective studies.

❷ Controlled studies to establish antivenom effectiveness and dosage are required. Use of modern techniques to measure venom and component levels in serial patient blood samples should greatly assist in such research. Antivenoms need to become safer, more effective and much more widely available, particularly in the rural tropics.

those few cases with proven compartment syndrome (intracompartmental pressure measurement). However, early fasciotomy is still practiced in some areas, often with distressing and unacceptable functional and cosmetic sequelae.

SCORPION STINGS

Introduction

Scorpion stings are the second most important form of terrestrial envenoming, after snakebite, with global cases probably exceeding one million per year, and deaths numbered in the many hundreds, to possibly as high as 5000 per year, nearly all in children. Scorpion envenoming is unpleasant for adults and occasionally is severe enough to threaten life. In children, however, it can be a rapidly severe and lethal disease, with some centres still reporting paediatric fatality rates in excess of 10%.

Scorpions vary in size, with over 1200 species known. All have a sting in the 'tail' (telson) with associated venom glands. Most scorpions either rarely sting humans, or are too small to cause envenoming, or have venom of little potency in humans. Unfortunately, a small number of scorpions do possess potent venoms and these species predominate in parts of the world where humans exist in large numbers, often in less than affluent conditions. The combination of warm to hot evenings, sandy soils, a tendency to walk around barefoot and dwellings that do not exclude scorpions leads to the large number of stings. Major risk areas include South and Central America, particularly Brazil (*Tityus* spp.), Mexico and adjacent USA (*Centruroides* spp.), North Africa and the Middle East (*Leiurus quinquestriatus*, *Androctonus* spp., *Buthus* spp.), and Western Asia and India (*Buthus* spp., *Mesobuthus* spp.).

In general, it is not the larger scorpions with robust front 'pincers' that are most concerning, but the smaller, more delicate species with unimpressive front 'pincers', because they rely on the toxicity of their venom.

Scorpion venoms contain a wide array of ion-channel toxins of great potency, causing an excitatory neurotoxic reaction (not paralysis), not dissimilar to an autonomic storm. Only a matter of minutes, not hours, may elapse from the time of the sting to major systemic envenoming. Once the systemic toxicity is established, antivenom therapy has less chance of success, though it may still save lives. In Mexico, with > 100 000 cases per year, death rates in children following scorpion sting have fallen from thousands per year to a hundred or less following the introduction of antivenom.

Scorpion venoms do not contain paralytic neurotoxins, myolysins, components affecting coagulation or renal function, nor do they contain local necrotic toxins (except for one species in the Middle East).

History

Often a scorpion will have been seen. There will usually be a clear history of an immediately painful sting, followed by development of systemic envenoming with effects that may include some of the following:

- Tingling of the lips
- Nausea, vomiting
- Abdominal pain
- Collapse
- Convulsions
- Hypertension or labile blood pressure
- Increased sweating, salivation or lachrymation
- Piloerection
- Dyspnoea
- Pulmonary oedema
- Cardiac collapse
- Multiple organ failure.

Symptoms appropriate to each of these effects may be described. It is important to note the time of onset for symptoms – a rapid onset and escalation in severity indicates a severe sting.

Examination

The local effects of the sting are not generally impressive, though there may be local sweating and piloerection. It is the systemic effects that will be most important, so particularly check blood pressure, look for signs of neuroexcitation, pulmonary oedema and cardiac collapse. In small children there may be a nystagmus.

Investigations

There are no specific tests for scorpion venom, nor specific indicators of envenoming, but in severe cases it is important to exclude secondary effects of envenoming and multiple organ failure.

Differential diagnosis

Full differential diagnosis of scorpion sting is beyond the scope of this chapter. The 'autonomic storm' clinical picture seen in severe scorpion envenoming can also be caused by some other venomous animals, particularly funnel web spiders (in Australia, where major scorpion stings do not occur), banana spiders (in Brazil; typically also cause priapism in boys), and some jellyfish (irukandji type). Accidental or deliberate exposure to certain pesticides and pharmaceuticals should also be considered.

Treatment

Treatment of major scorpion envenoming is controversial, particularly centering around the role of antivenom. Most evidence suggests that antivenom use has resulted in greatly reduced fatality rates in children, but a few doctors argue that pharmacotherapy is more effective than antivenom, particularly focusing on the cardiac failure seen in fatal cases. Prazosin, in particular, has enjoyed success and should be considered, both as an adjunct to antivenom and as first-line therapy in the absence of antivenom (i.e. in India). If antivenom is available it should be used IV without delay. Dose will vary depending on product.

Prognosis

The prognosis in scorpion envenoming depends on several factors. More severe envenoming is likely in smaller children, with more rapid development of effects and a shorter window for effective antivenom therapy. If multiple organ failure develops then prognosis is generally poor.

Prevention

Most scorpion stings occur because of the patterns of human living, and thus are theoretically avoidable. It is possible to 'scorpion-proof' houses, by use of tiles around the lower walls, preventing scorpion entry. Use of enclosed footwear and avoidance of sitting down or lying down outside after dusk can also reduce sting incidence.

SPIDERBITE

Introduction

Spiderbite is probably very common, but most bites are trivial, with only a few species likely to cause major harm to humans (Table 22.1.4). For these species, morbidity can be significant, but mortality is low, with global deaths directly related to spiderbite probably measuring twenty or less per year. Even the world's most

dangerous spider, the Australian funnel web spider, has only caused one known fatality in the last twenty years. As with other venomous animals, spiderbite is more likely to be severe in small children.

History

Spiderbite is not always initially painful, and spiders are small and easily misidentified, so most commonly there will be no certainty from the history about the species involved. However, particular spiders cause quite specific envenoming syndromes, making diagnosis possible even without a spider being available. The common presentations for the medically important spiders are listed below. In general, however, it is important to note the circumstances of definite or possible exposure to spiderbite, a description of the spider, if seen, and the timing of onset for any symptoms that develop.

Australian funnel web spiders

These large mygalomorph spiders are robust in appearance (Fig. 22.1.15), generally ground dwelling (there are tree-dwelling species) and are found only in eastern Australia (Fig. 22.1.16). Their large fangs and acidic venom generally cause immediate local pain on biting and they may hang on, being difficult to dislodge. Apart from pain, other local effects are not prominent. In about 10% of cases, systemic envenoming will develop, often rapidly, and can be lethal in less than sixty minutes in children. First symptoms are tingling of the lips and twitching of the tongue, followed by non-specific symptoms, which may include headache, nausea, vomiting

CONTROVERSIES AND FUTURE DIRECTIONS

❶ The major controversy in management of scorpion sting is the issue of antivenom effectiveness, as discussed earlier. Of the various types of antivenom, animal studies have indicated that Fab' antivenoms are not more effective than F(ab)2 or IgG antivenoms.

❷ Among non-antivenom therapies, the most controversy has surrounded the proposal to use insulin, suggested by an Indian doctor (where no antivenom is available). This technique is not favoured by most experts, considering it both highly risky and of most uncertain theoretical and practical benefit.

❸ Despite the frequency of scorpion stings, there are still few published studies of series of stings by particular species and few trials of various methods of treatment. There is a need for more intensive systematic study of scorpion envenoming and controlled trials of treatment alternatives.

Table 22.1.4	Medically important spider groups			
Family	Genera	Common name	Distribution	Clinical effects
Hexathelidae	Atrax Hadronyche	Australian funnel web spiders	Eastern Australia, from Cape York to Tasmania	Severe neuroexcitatory ('autonomic storm') envenoming; about 10% of cases develop major envenoming, which untreated, carries a significant risk of fatality
Theriidae	Latrodectus Steatoda	Red back or widow spiders	Global	Moderate, generally non-lethal neuroexcitatory envenoming
Ctenidae	Phoneutria	Banana spiders	Central and South America, especially Brazil	Moderate to severe neuroexcitatory envenoming, rarely lethal
Loxoscelidae	Loxosceles	Recluse or fiddleback spiders	Global, particularly the Americas	Severe local tissue injury, with occasional major, potentially lethal systemic effects

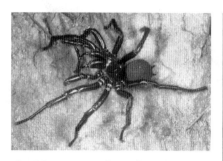

Fig. 22.1.15   Male Sydney funnel web spider (*Atrax robustus*).
Reproduced with permission of Dr Julian White.

and abdominal pain. There is frequently evidence of neuroexcitation, with sweating, salivation, lachrymation and piloerection. Hypertension is usual and dyspnoea secondary to pulmonary oedema can develop rapidly. Without treatment this can progress to hypoxia, coma and death.

Widow spiders including Australian redback spiders

Widow spiders have a classic appearance (Fig. 22.1.17) with a globular abdomen, comparatively small cephalothorax and long thin legs. They utilise a drop-line web structure to capture prey. Humans most often receive bites when they either come in contact with the web or occasionally when touching a wandering spider (i.e. caught in footwear, clothing or similar). Widow spider venom, though neuroexcitatory, is rarely lethal in humans. A typical significant bite causes local pain, becoming more severe, sometimes with local sweating, then progressive proximal movement of pain and sweating, ultimately becoming severe regional or generalised pain, sweating, plus hypertension, nausea and malaise. Envenoming can mimic acute abdomen and cardiac chest pain. Untreated, pain may take days or weeks to resolve and often gravitates to the lower limbs, causing burning pain in the feet and legs, often with associated sweating. Rarely, severe systemic envenoming can cause pulmonary oedema or a secondary rise in creatine kinase. In infants, a generalised rash is common, the infant presenting as highly distressed and irritable, not consolable, erythematous, but with no obvious cause apparent. A widow spider may be found in the bedding or underneath the bed. Less than 20% of bites cause major envenoming.

Banana spiders

Banana spiders are large aggressive spiders, well known within their range. They are active hunters and invade houses, with bites occurring year round, but especially in autumn. They are a common cause of bites in Brazil, accounting for 20% of all presentations in some hospitals. The neuroexcitatory venom has effects similar to widow spider bites in many ways, with pain being a predominant feature, as is sweating, hypertension and nausea. However, unlike widow spiders, there is often local swelling of the bite area and piloerection is a classic feature of envenoming in boys. Death is a rare outcome, but severe cases can develop pulmonary oedema or cardiac arrhythmias.

Recluse or fiddleback spiders

These small, delicate spiders are generally brown with long spindly legs and a darker brown pattern on the cephalothorax in the

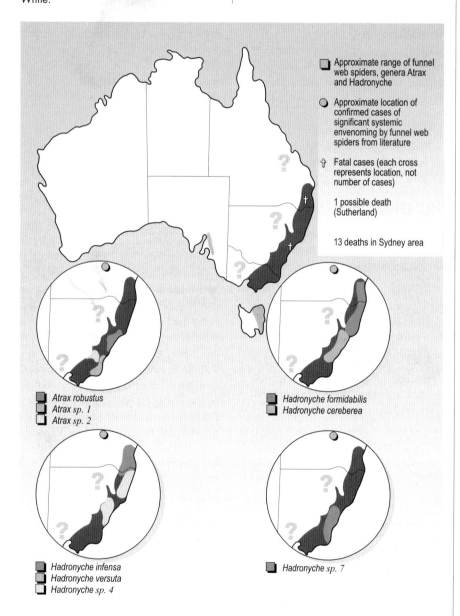

Approximate range of funnel web spiders, genera Atrax and Hadronyche

Approximate location of confirmed cases of significant systemic envenoming by funnel web spiders from literature

† Fatal cases (each cross represents location, not number of cases)

1 possible death (Sutherland)

13 deaths in Sydney area

Atrax robustus
Atrax sp. 1
Atrax sp. 2

Hadronyche formidabilis
Hadronyche cereberea

Hadronyche infensa
Hadronyche versuta
Hadronyche sp. 4

Hadronyche sp. 7

Fig. 22.1.16   Distribution of Australian funnel web spiders (*Atrax* spp. and *Hadronyche* spp.).
Reproduced with permission of Dr Julian White.

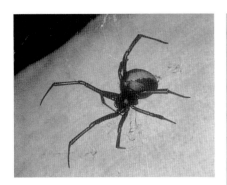

Fig. 22.1.17   Female widow (red back) spider.
Reproduced with permission of Dr Julian White.

Fig. 22.1.18   Recluse spider, with violin-shaped marking on the cephalothorax.
Reproduced with permission of Dr Julian White.

rough shape of a violin (Fig. 22.1.18). They have a venom that is predominantly dermonecrotic. The most common effect of bites is 'cutaneous loxoscelism'. The bite is rarely noticed and often occurs in bed at night. However, hours later the area becomes red, painful, may blister or bruise and darken as necrosis develops over the following 4–7 days. The area finally involved can be local to extensive, with skip lesions, and is usually painful. There is commonly an associated non-specific, self-limited, systemic illness. In a few cases, a more severe systemic illness can occur, potentially lethal, with haemolysis, shock, coagulopathy, or renal failure. This is 'viscero-cutaneous loxoscelism'.

Examination
Initial examination may show little locally at the bite site, depending on the type of envenoming involved. For those spiders causing predominantly regional or systemic effects, these will dominate examination findings.

Investigations
There are no clinical diagnostic tests specific for spiderbite. Most bites will result in leukocytosis. For suspected loxoscelism, it is important to look for haemolysis, DIC and renal failure, especially in children.

Differential diagnosis
Detailed differential diagnosis is beyond the scope of this chapter, but the geographic location and pattern of local and systemic effects makes differentiation between these types of spiderbite straightforward. For severe neuroexcitatory envenoming, as seen with Australian funnel web spiders, consider pesticide or pharmaceutical poisoning in the differential. Widow spiderbite should be considered in the differential for selected cases of apparent unexplained acute abdomen or chest pain, before laparotomy is scheduled.

Treatment
Treatment for Australian funnel web spiderbite is principally the use of specific IV antivenom, available in Australia only. Initially 2–4 vials are needed, but severe cases require more. All cases with any evidence of venom spread require antivenom urgently, before life-threatening envenoming develops, which may occur rapidly in children.

Widow spiderbite only requires treatment in those cases with significant local, regional or systemic envenoming, which is a minority of cases. Antivenom is the most effective treatment and may be given IM (in Australia), but is more rapidly effective if used IV (even in Australia). Experience has shown that only antivenom reliably reverses envenoming and is more effective than narcotic analgesics in treating pain. It can be effective for up to days post-bite. It is usually given as single vials, waiting 2 + hours before giving a further dose, if symptoms warrant.

Banana spiderbite is most often managed without use of antivenom, the latter reserved for severe cases, where it should be given IV, most of these cases being children under seven years of age. In the less severe cases, local anaesthetic block is usually adequate.

Loxoscelism is difficult to treat. Specific antivenom is only available in Brazil and its place in management is controversial. In general, patients present late, after tissue injury has commenced, requiring good wound care. Secondary infection requires appropriate antibiotic therapy. Early surgical debridement can extend the area of injury and should be avoided. Steroids have not been shown to be effective. Dapsone, given early, can reduce injury, but is toxic and not widely favoured as therapy. Hyperbaric oxygen therapy is controversial. It may benefit some patients, but is unsuitable for most children.

Prognosis
Prognosis varies depending on the type of spider, but only for Australian funnel web spiders is death a likely outcome unless specific treatment is urgently instituted.

Prevention
Spiders are ubiquitous and it is not practical to avoid human contact. In areas where the potentially deadly funnel web spiders are common, such as parts of Sydney, residents should avoid walking barefoot, leaving clothes on the ground or putting on footwear without first checking for spiders.

TICK BITE PARALYSIS

Introduction
Tick bite is probably common in some regions, but rarely causes major harm to humans. However, a few species of ticks have toxic saliva, containing paralytic neurotoxins, which can cause potentially lethal flaccid paralysis, especially in children. In Australia, for instance, paralysis ticks (*Ixodes* spp.) have caused more deaths than funnel web spiders.

History
There may be a clear history of a tick being found, but often in children presentation is as an unexplained progressive flaccid paralysis, first manifesting as an ataxic gait.

CONTROVERSIES AND FUTURE DIRECTIONS

❶ Major controversies for spiderbite centre around adequate treatment, particularly the role of antivenom, with attendant risks, in envenoming unlikely to prove lethal. This concern has held sway in North America for widow spiderbites, with few cases offered antivenom therapy. As a result countless patients probably suffer prolonged periods of eminently treatable major discomfort. The opposite situation occurs in Australia where widow (red back) spiderbites routinely receive antivenom, with good results and little risk.

❷ Bites by most spiders remain poorly documented and, even for major species, treatment is controversial. For these latter, controlled trials are required to establish best treatment practice.

Occasionally the paralysis may be purely local, notably a Bell's palsy. Without treatment, the envenoming may cause complete respiratory paralysis. For Australian paralysis ticks only, the paralysis may worsen for up to 48 hours after removal of all ticks. It is important to ascertain if the patient had exposure to ticks, such as walking in scrubland in eastern Australia.

Examination
Examination is crucial, both to document the extent of paralysis and to locate every attached tick. These may be hiding in the scalp, behind or in the ears or in body skin folds.

Investigations
There are no specific investigations for tick envenoming.

Differential diagnosis
Apart from ticks, at least in Australia, flaccid paralysis can be caused by snakebite. Ataxia only can also be caused by exposure to pesticides or some pharmaceuticals.

Treatment
The principal treatment for tick envenoming is prompt removal of all ticks. Care must be taken to lever the tick off, including mouthparts, and not squeeze it between fingers, which forces in more saliva and often leaves the head embedded, when secondary infection can ensue. For cases with severe flaccid paralysis, an antivenom is available (in Australia), but its role is uncertain. The paralysis resolves after several days, during which time ventilatory support may be needed.

Prognosis
With removal of all ticks and respiratory support, the prognosis should be optimistic. The more rapid the onset of paralytic features, the more likely is major paralysis.

Prevention
If visiting tick-infested areas, it may be difficult to exclude all tick contact risk, so routine checking for ticks after departure and their removal is advisable.

JELLYFISH STINGS

Introduction
Jellyfish are numerous in all seas and oceans and stings, mostly trivial, are common. A few jellyfish can cause more severe stings and an even smaller number can cause potentially lethal envenoming. Of the many species that cause some effects, only the three groups of most medical significance will be discussed here. All jellyfish have a common mechanism of envenoming, using individual sting cells (nematocysts) that both produce and inject the venom. This can result in some venom directly entering small blood vessels in the skin, causing rapid envenoming. In the case of large jellyfish, like the box jellyfish, with millions of nematocysts discharging simultaneously through the skin, very rapid and severe envenoming can develop.

Box jellyfish
The Australian box jellyfish, *Chironex fleckeri*, is found in northern Australian

CONTROVERSIES AND FUTURE DIRECTIONS

❶ The major controversy concerns the value of tick antivenom. This will not be resolved until a controlled trial of effectiveness is undertaken. This is unlikely, given the sporadic and infrequent nature of cases with major envenoming.

marine waters and areas to the north, including Borneo. It is the most dangerous of all jellyfish and can even kill an adult human in less than five minutes, from cardiac arrhythmia and arrest. Most stings are minor, not a threat to life, and cause local pain only. In cases with extensive and severe stings, there is immediate excruciating pain, with a ladder mark present, often with adherent tentacles. Collapse may follow rapidly, either due to the pain or to cardiac effects. Respiratory failure can develop, but it is cardiac toxicity that is most likely to prove lethal.

Irukandji syndrome
This is caused by envenoming by a variety of jellyfish, including *Carukia barnesii*, some of which are very small. The initial sting may be trivial and may be from the bell rather than tentacles. However, 20–40 minutes later systemic envenoming develops, with muscle and back pain, often severe, hypertension and malaise and pulmonary oedema, consistent with an 'autonomic storm'. While death is very rare, it has been recorded as a result of intracranial haemorrhage associated with severe hypertension, though the actual contribution of envenoming is controversial.

Portuguese-man-o-war
Blue bottles or Portuguese-man-o-war are global oceanic 'jellyfish' (actually hydrozoan colony organisms), which swarm and can cause stings from their tentacles. In most cases the stings are minor, with local pain and wheal formation, but rarely more severe envenoming is reported, with a very few cases of vascular injury locally. More common is an allergic reaction to

stings, occasionally resulting in lethal anaphylaxis.

History

For most jellyfish there will be a clear history of being stung while in the sea and tentacles may still be adherent. These may still be active, so caution is advisable on removal. For box jellyfish only, the first aid application of copious amounts of vinegar may inactivate the tentacles, so they may be removed safely. The geographic location is important, as is the time of day and season, as this affects the likely local jellyfish fauna.

For stings by Irukandji-type jellyfish, the presentation may be one of unexplained severe pain following a swim in the sea, at any time of the year (but only in northern Australian waters and adjacent areas). It is important to note pre-existing medical conditions and medications that might increase the risk from envenoming.

Examination

The sting area should be examined and the extent determined. For box jellyfish, stings covering half or more of one limb or an equivalent area on the trunk should be considered as potentially lethal. Such a sting area is easily achieved in small children, who are those most often involved in fatal envenoming. Evidence of systemic effects should be sought.

Investigations

There are no specific tests for jellyfish envenoming.

Differential diagnosis

Except for Irukandji syndrome, which can be confused with non-envenoming illness, jellyfish stings are usually easily diagnosed, the major differential diagnosis being other types of marine envenoming, particularly stings from venomous fish, but these usually show only a few spine penetration points, not the widespread tentacle tracks of jellyfish.

Treatment

Most jellyfish stings require either no treatment or simple symptomatic relief of pain. A cold pack applied locally is often effective. For box jellyfish stings, where either an extensive area has been stung or systemic envenoming is evident, then box jellyfish antivenom is required urgently, either IM if pre-hospital, or preferably IV in hospital, 1–3 vials. In addition full cardiorespiratory support should be instituted, where needed. Local infection of the tentacle tracks can occur, requiring antibiotic therapy. Many cases develop delayed 'allergic' reactions locally, responding to antihistamines and topical corticosteroids.

Irukandji envenoming cannot be treated with antivenom (there is none suitable), so treatment should be supportive and symptomatic. Narcotic analgesia (excluding pethidine) is often required, with hypertension most often treated with glyceryl trinitrate (beware hypotension) and pulmonary oedema managed with oxygen, dopamine, adrenaline (epinephrine) and positive pressure ventilation.

Bluebottle envenoming is treated with supportive and symptomatic care only.

Prognosis

For box jellyfish envenoming, the larger the area of sting, the more severe the envenoming, with half or more of one limb involved being potentially lethal. For Irukandji, the prognostic indicators are less clear.

Prevention

The only sure way of preventing jellyfish stings is to avoid using the sea. Stinger suits can greatly reduce the chance of contact and will prevent potentially lethal box jellyfish stings, by limiting the area stung, but since only a small contact area is required for Irukandji jellyfish, exposed face, hands or feet may permit major envenoming. Similarly, stinger exclusion nets on beaches will prevent large box jellyfish from entering, so preventing major stings, but do nothing to prevent Irukandji stings.

VENOMOUS FISH STINGS

Introduction

There are numerous species of fish, in both marine and fresh-water environ-ments, both bony and cartilaginous, capable of inflicting venomous stings, but envenoming, though often distressing, is rarely likely to be lethal, even in children. More concerning, in the case of cartilaginous fish, specifically stingrays, is the potential for major, even lethal, mechanical injury during the act of stinging. Stingray spines on the muscular tail can inflict major trauma, with cases of transection of vessels, nerves, tendons and direct penetration of the chest and abdomen, including direct cardiac puncture. Such mechanical wounds can pose a great threat to life, but are beyond the scope of this chapter, as envenoming is not the significant problem in such cases.

Venomous fish exist in many families, representing hundreds of species, with venomous spines in a number of different locations, depending on species, including on the back (dorsal as in stonefish), pectoral, behind the head (particularly catfish) and even on the tail. A primitive venom gland surrounds the spine and as the spine is forced into the skin by mechanical pressure (such as by stepping on a stonefish or handling a fish) the gland is compressed, forcing venom up groves in the spine and into the victim.

Most venomous fish species have never had their venom studied. For those few that have been investigated, notably the stonefish, while the venom may contain a variety of components, in the clinical setting it is toxins causing pain and swelling that predominate. There is no evidence that the neurotoxin found in stonefish venom has any clinical effect in humans.

History

There is always a history of definite or likely exposure to a stinging fish, in a marine or fresh-water environment, or of handling a fish out of water. This includes sudden pain in a foot after walking in water, such as reef walking, usually indicative of stepping on a fish, notably stonefish. The pain may be very severe, sufficient to cause collapse, but systemic symptoms are related principally to local pain, not general toxicity. There are very rare reports of pulmonary oedema following stonefish stings (in Madagascar).

CONTROVERSIES AND FUTURE DIRECTIONS

❶ There are a number of current controversies for jellyfish sting management. For box jellyfish, while vinegar is widely accepted as first aid to inactivate unfired nematocysts, the use of pressure immobilisation bandages in severe cases has been questioned, research showing that this technique may actually increase envenoming. As a consequence, most authorities now do not recommend using pressure immobilisation bandages for any box jellyfish stings, though official recommendations are yet to reflect this change in practice.

❷ The role of antivenom for box jellyfish stings remains clouded in uncertainty, but most authorities still recommend its use. Verapamil, once suggested for treating severe cardiotoxic box jellyfish envenoming, is no longer recommended by most authorities and has never undergone clinical testing in this setting.

❸ Irukandji envenoming remains problematic. There are still calls for antivenom development, but the delayed nature of envenoming and the increasing and varied range of the species of jellyfish involved make development of an effective antivenom problematic and economically unviable.

❹ Research is required into the mechanisms of major jellyfish envenoming in humans, as these are still not fully understood, mirroring the difficulties in collecting and studying jellyfish venom.

❺ Research is required to determine most effective treatment strategies for jellyfish envenoming. Irukandji syndrome, in particular, requires more research at all levels, starting with a concerted effort to identify and describe all likely culprit species.

Portions of the sting may have been seen in the wound.

Examination
For venomous fish stings, there may be sting present in the wound(s). The number of wounds can be significant (i.e. for stonefish, as it determines antivenom dose). For stingray wounds, apart from residual sting left in the wound, careful examination to determine the extent of any mechanical trauma is essential.

Investigations
There are no specific investigations for fish sting envenoming.

Differential diagnosis
The sharp and localised pain of a fish sting is distinctive and can be separated from jellyfish stings due to the tentacle tracks caused by the latter.

Treatment
With the exception of stonefish, for which there is an antivenom, fish stings must be treated symptomatically and supportively. Both for first aid and in-hospital care, hot water immersion appears effective at reducing pain in the short term. The contralateral limb should first be immersed in water that is hot, but not so hot that thermal injury might occur. The

affected limb is then immersed, usually bringing rapid relief of pain. Unfortunately, pain may recur on removal from the water and if this persists, other analgesia must be considered, often a local or regional anaesthetic block in more severe cases. The wound must be examined for remnants of stings, which should be removed. The wound should be allowed to heal by secondary intention and the temptation to surgically close the wound resisted. For any wound that is extensive (i.e. many stingray injuries) a course of antibiotics should be considered. For stingray injuries with extensive trauma, surgical input on managing this injury should be paramount.

For stonefish, there is a specific antivenom in Australia, which can be given IM or IV, the dose depending on the number of stings. It is effective at reducing the severe pain and should be considered in all cases of stonefish sting with more than trivial symptoms.

Prognosis
With the exception of severe mechanical trauma from stingray injuries, the prognosis for fish stings is generally optimistic, with recovery likely. The greater the number of stings, the more likely that symptoms will be severe and possibly prolonged.

Prevention
Avoidance of contact with stinging fish is the obvious preventative measure. When reef walking or on sandy bottoms where stingrays may hide, avoid sudden movements, running into water, wear strong-soled reef shoes and observe and choose carefully when placing feet. Despite all such precautions, stings may occur, particularly if reef walking, by stepping on larger stonefish.

VENOMOUS MARINE MOLLUSCS

Introduction
There are two groups of marine molluscs (snails) that are able to inflict major, even lethal, envenoming on humans. These are the blue-ringed octopus, from Australian and adjacent waters and selected cone snails, found widely in the Indo-Pacific area. Neither are a common cause of envenoming, surprisingly, since both groups are common – the blue-ringed octopus particularly, with its various species common all around the Australian coast.

The blue-ringed octopus has a potent paralysing neurotoxin, tetrodotoxin, in its saliva. Bites, which usually occur when the octopus is removed from the water and placed in contact with skin, are often

CONTROVERSIES AND FUTURE DIRECTIONS

❶ There are no major controversies for fish stings. There is uncertainty if stonefish antivenom is useful for stings by other types of fish. There is no formal study to validate such non-specific use, but anecdotal clinical experience suggests that this antivenom may work for some related species, including the bullrout.

❷ There is great scope for studies on fish sting venoms and for research into more targeted treatment strategies.

painless and may go unnoticed until 5–20 minutes or so later when paralytic features start to develop. These may rapidly progress to respiratory paralysis and collapse, with death possible in under an hour. The paralysis is a general flaccid paralysis.

Cone snails fire poisoned 'darts' at their prey, or human victims, the venom being both complex and incredibly potent, immobilising fish prey in a few seconds. In humans the sting may be painless or quite painful. Systemic envenoming, with collapse and flaccid paralysis, rapidly follows.

History

There is usually a clear history of picking up and handling a blue ringed octopus or cone snail. In significant cases, which are rare, envenoming is rapid, with neurotoxic symptoms quickly evident. The earliest feature of envenoming is often tingling of the lips.

Examination

The sting or bite site may not be readily evident. The key effects to exclude are those of progressive flaccid paralysis and cardiovascular collapse, notably hypotension.

Investigations

There are no investigations specific to envenoming by molluscs.

Differential diagnosis

The onset of progressive flaccid paralysis after a marine sting or bite is uncommon and apart from mollusc envenoming, the likely differential is sea snake bite, which may manifest as either paralysis and/or myolysis. However, the development of paralysis is much less acute than with mollusc envenoming.

Treatment

There are no antivenoms for venomous molluscs, so both first aid and treatment is supportive and symptomatic. Pressure immobilisation bandaging may reduce the rate of development of systemic envenoming, if applied early enough. The key requirement is to support respiratory function and blood pressure. The latter may require pressor therapy. The former may require intubation and mechanical ventilation, but this may not be for a prolonged period, often only for 6–12 hours, unlike snakebite, where ventilation may be needed for days, weeks, even months.

Prognosis

If respiratory support is instituted early, before irreversible hypoxic organ injury occurs, ultimate prognosis is good. Cases without evidence of significant systemic envenoming six hours post-exposure are unlikely to develop envenoming.

Prevention

The principal preventative measure is abstinence from contact with and certainly handling these molluscs. This may require local education programmes, particularly directed at children, who will find these small and attractive animals tempting to pick up.

FURTHER READING

- While there are numerous papers on various aspects of envenoming, covering different regions, there are few texts giving a detailed overview of snakebite or other types of specific envenoming or clinical toxicology. Some recent key texts are noted here. A major source of information is the Clinical Toxicology Resources Website (www.toxinology.com), a detailed site, initially

CONTROVERSIES

❶ There are no major controversies in managing marine mollusc envenoming, in part reflecting the rarity of this clinical problem.

developed with public funds, global in scope, supported by subscription income.
Chippaux J-P 2002 Venins de Serpent et Envenimations. IRD Editions, Paris, 288 pp [French handbook on global snakebite]
Covacevich J, Davie P, Pearn J 1987 Toxic plants and animals: A guide for Australia. Queensland Museum, Brisbane, 501 pp [a comprehensive textbook with a clinical focus]
Gopalakrishnakone P, Chou LM 1990 Snakes of medical importance (Asia-Pacific Region). National University of Singapore, Singapore, 670 pp [covers snakes in the designate region]
Goyffon M, Heurtault J 1995 La Fonction Venimeuse. Masson, Paris, 284 pp [French handbook covering many aspects of toxinology]
Junghanss J, Bodio M 1996 Notfall-Handbuch Gifttiere: Diagnose, Therapie, Biologie. Georg Thieme Verlag, Stuttgart, 646 pp [this German textbook covers a global spectrum of envenoming with a focus on management in EDs]
Mebs D 2002 Venomous and poisonous animals. Medpharm/CRC Press, Boca Raton, FL, 339 pp [this textbook, beautifully illustrated in colour, covers the broad scope of venoms, the animals that produce them and their clinical effects and treatment – the focus is more on toxinology than detailed medical advice, but it is a valuable source of information]
Meier J, White J (eds) 1995 Handbook of clinical toxicology of animal venoms and poisons. CRC Press, Boca Raton, FL, 752 pp [this is the standard textbook for clinical toxicology and contains chapters covering all aspects of envenoming, especially snakebite, scorpion stings, spiderbite, tick envenoming and marine envenoming – the coverage is global, but with considerable detail for most regions and animal types]
Sutherland SK, Tibballs J 2001 Australian animal toxins. Oxford University Press, Melbourne, 856 pp [a major work covering the Australian venomous fauna]
Warrell DA 1999 WHO/SEARO guidelines for the clinical management of snake bites in the Southeast Asian region. SE Asian Journal of Tropical Medicine and Public Hygiene 30(Suppl 1): 1–85
Warrell DA et al 1996 Oxford textbook of medicine. Oxford University Press, Oxford [this standard medical text includes an extensive chapter on envenoming]
White J 2002 CSL Antivenom handbook. CSL, Melbourne, 69 pp [a concise handbook on the diagnosis and treatment of envenoming by Australian fauna, which is available in its entirety on the toxinology website: www.toxinology.com]
Williamson JA, Fenner PJ, Burnett JW, Rifkin JF 1996 Venomous and poisonous marine animals: A medical and biological handbook. University of NSW Press, Sydney, 504 pp [this is the major textbook covering marine toxinology]

22.2° DROWNING

SIMON WOOD

Essentials

1 Drowning is a leading cause of accidental death in Australian children. Children aged 0–4 years are the most vulnerable. The most common site of drowning in this age group is the domestic swimming pool.

2 There is no current consensus regarding terms used to describe death or survival following submersion. The terms *near-drowning* and *secondary drowning* should be avoided.

3 There is no clinical or therapeutic difference between submersion in fresh or salt water.

4 The major pathophysiological consequence of submersion is hypoxic brain injury.

5 Pulmonary injury due to aspiration of water is an important clinical consideration in all submersion victims.

6 The mainstay of treatment is early effective oxygenation.

7 Whilst hypothermia may be protective in small children who suffer a submersion event, it does not reliably predict good outcome.

8 Response to resuscitation is the single most important predictor of outcome in children who have suffered submersion.

9 Isolation pool-fencing with a self-locking gate has been shown to effectively reduce submersion incidents in pre-school-age children.

INTRODUCTION

Definition

Traditionally *drowning* has been defined as death due to suffocation within 24 hours of submersion in a liquid medium and *near-drowning* as survival for 24 hours or more following such an incident.[1,2] The term *secondary drowning* has been used to describe death from respiratory failure occurring after a period of recovery following a submersion event.[3] The term *submersion* is generally accepted to indicate an incident in which the victim is totally covered by water, while the term *immersion* refers to an incident in which the victim is only partially covered by water, although distinguishing between the two has little clinical relevance.[1]

Considerable confusion surrounds the use of these terms. In part this is because the distinction between drowning and near-drowning often cannot be made before 24 hours, making the terms clinically irrelevant.[2] In addition it has been suggested that the use of a time limit for survival is not a scientific concept and is not in accordance with outcome parameters as used in the internationally accepted Utstein style.[1]

At present there is no universally agreed terminology applicable to death or survival following submersion. There is reasonable consensus, however, that the terms *near-drowning* and *secondary drowning* should no longer be used.[1,2]

The Guidelines 2000 Conference, pending the future recommendations of an ILCOR Task Force revising the Utstein Guidelines, has recommended the following terms:

Water rescue A person who is alert but experiences some distress while swimming and who displays minimal, transient symptoms, such as coughing, which clear quickly.

Submersion A person who experiences some swimming-related distress that is sufficient to require support in the field plus transportation to an emergency facility for further observation and treatment.

Drowning Refers to death following submersion. The victim may be pronounced dead at the scene of rescue, in the ED, or within 24 hours of the event. Death occurring after 24 hours should be termed a 'drowning-related death', up until which time the victim should be referred to as a *submersion victim*.[2]

EPIDEMIOLOGY

In Australia drowning is a leading cause of accidental death in children. Its incidence peaks in early childhood and again in adolescence. Males outnumber females in both groups. Children under five years of age are the most vulnerable to drowning in Australia.[4] Twenty-two percent of all drowning victims are in the 0–4 years age group.[4] The rate of drowning in this group is 4.6 in 100 000 population per year and has changed little since 1986–1990.[4]

Risk groups for childhood drowning are children aged 0–4 years, children living in cities with high swimming pool to population ratios, children living in hot climates, children living in areas with lack of isolation pool fencing, and Indigenous children.[5] More toddlers drown in swimming pools than from any other cause.[6] Most children who drown in pools are out of sight for less than five minutes and are in the care of one or both parents.[7] Around the home small children can also drown in baths, buckets, and garden ponds. Up to 8% of cases of submersion in small children in the domestic setting may be secondary to non-accidental injury.[8]

While pool-fencing legislation has proven to be effective in reducing the incidence of drowning in small children it has had little impact on rates of drowning in older children and adolescents. In this group alcohol, suicide, and risk-taking behaviours are important factors that lead to increased risk of drowning.[8]

AETIOLOGY

Drowning is most commonly a primary event. In children it most often occurs when the victim is unable to rescue him or herself after entering the water, as in the case of a toddler falling into a swimming pool, or an infant drowning in a bath whilst unattended. In older children and adolescents fatigue while swimming may play a role, but drowning in these age groups is more likely to be secondary to other causes.

Drowning can occur secondarily to a number of underlying causes. These should be considered during assessment of the submersion victim. Individuals with seizure disorders have a 4–13-times higher risk for submersion accidents regardless of age.[3,8] Prolonged QT-syndrome leading to dysrhythmia has been implicated as significant cause of drowning, although the true incidence of this condition in drowned children is unknown. Ethanol is an important risk factor for submersion injury, particularly in adolescents. Elevated serum ethanol levels are documented in 10–50% of adolescent drownings.[8] Head and cervical trauma from diving and boating-related accidents may also lead to drowning as a secondary event. Non-accidental injury is an important cause of drowning in infants and smaller children, particularly in events that occur in the home, such as in baths and buckets. Up to 8% of drownings presenting to tertiary paediatric centres may be attributed to child abuse.[8]

The immersion syndrome is sudden loss of consciousness secondary to a bradycardia, or tachyarrhythmia induced by contact with water at a temperature of at least 5°C below body temperature. This can lead to secondary drowning. The immersion syndrome can occur in water with temperatures as warm as 31°C, although it is more likely to occur in much colder water. Wetting the face before entering the water may reduce its incidence.[1]

PATHOPHYSIOLOGY

The two most significant pathophysiological consequences of submersion are hypoxia from asphyxiation during the submersion itself, and aspiration of water into the lungs. It is the severity of the initial hypoxic insult that is the major determinant of outcome.[2] If the initial hypoxic event is survived, the degree of hypoxic organ injury and pulmonary injury secondary to aspiration, become the clinically important factors.

Much that is known about the sequence of events following submersion has come from animal models. Aspiration of water initially causes breath-holding or laryngospasm and the resultant asphyxiation leads to progressive hypoxia. Active and passive swallowing of water follows and, as hypoxia worsens, breath-holding and laryngospasm are terminated, resulting in aspiration of water into the lungs.[1]

Anoxia lasting 1–3 minutes can shut down both the brain and the heart, causing loss of consciousness and hypoxic cardiac arrest. Rescue and early institution of cardiopulmonary resuscitation can salvage myocardial function, but the brain is more sensitive to hypoxic injury and it is the severity of this injury that determines outcome. Effects of hypoxia on other organ systems are delayed. Profound hypoxia can cause an acute respiratory distress syndrome, which develops within hours and further worsens hypoxic injury. Post-hypoxic cerebral oedema is a major complication and can develop 6–12 hours following successful initial resuscitation from a serious submersion event. Most paediatric drowning deaths in hospital are due to hypoxic cerebral injury rather than pulmonary complications.[8]

The average volume of water aspirated in human drownings is 10–15 mL kg^{-1}. Aspiration of volumes as little as 1–3 mL kg^{-1} of water can cause profound alterations in gas exchange and subsequent ventilatory abnormalities.[9] Laryngospasm is thought to occur in 10–15% of drowning victims and a subset of patients who drown without evidence of significant aspiration of water at post-mortem, so-called *dry-drowning*, has been described. This concept has recently been ques-

tioned and it has been suggested that in these cases death has occurred prior to submersion.[1] Regardless of whether dry-drowning is a true clinical entity, or whether laryngospasm has occurred at the time of submersion, aspiration of water into the lungs remains a clinically important consideration in the management of all submersion victims.

Despite the large literature dedicated to the subject, there are no clinically or therapeutically important differences between drowning in fresh or salt water.[1,8] Pulmonary injury is related more to the amount of water aspirated than to the composition of the water itself. Both fresh and salt water cause loss of pulmonary surfactant, non-cardiogenic pulmonary oedema, impaired alveolar-capillary gas exchange, and increased intrapulmonary shunting with the potential for profound hypoxia.[1,3] Aspiration of water that is contaminated with particulate matter or bacteria can lead to complications from obstruction of small airways or increased risk of pulmonary infection, although neither is seen in the majority of patients.[10] If present, evidence of significant pulmonary injury due to aspiration will usually manifest or progress within hours of rescue. Delayed onset of respiratory distress and hypoxia, the so-called 'delayed immersion syndrome' or 'secondary drowning' has been refuted by recent evidence.[8]

Clinically significant electrolyte and fluid volume abnormalities are rarely seen in cases of drowning in humans despite being demonstrated in animal models.[1,3,8,10] Occasionally a mild hyponatraemia, which self-corrects without specific therapy, is observed.[8] Theoretical exceptions are submersions occurring in hypertonic solutions, such as the Dead Sea, or water contaminated with industrial waste.

Hypothermia is an important issue following submersion, particularly in small children who have a large body surface area to weight ratio. Cooling can occur at the time of submersion, but can also continue following rescue and during attempted resuscitation due to heat loss through evaporation. Hypothermia can confer some degree of protection from cerebral hypoxia, particularly in small children. Multiple case reports in the literature attest to intact survival of both children and adults following prolonged (> 15 minutes) submersions in icy water (water temperature < 10°C).[11] Profound hypothermia and subsequent intact survival has also been documented in children suffering submersion in non-icy water and in temperate climates.

The mechanisms of temperature drop and cerebral protection remain unclear. Surface cooling at the time of submersion is thought to be insufficient on its own to provide central cooling of a degree that confers cerebral protection. Other mechanisms of heat loss, such as via ingestion and/or aspiration of cold water, are not supported by quantitative evidence. Some authors suggest that core temperature drop is insufficient on its own to explain the cerebral protection afforded by hypothermia.[12] The diving reflex, in which blood is shunted from the limbs and splanchnic circulation to the brain and heart alongside slowing of the heart rate and reduction of the basal metabolic rate, has been suggested as being an important mechanism for cerebral protection in children.[12] There is little clinical evidence to indicate that the diving reflex is sufficiently active in humans, even small children, to confer any benefit on its own.[1,8] It is most likely that a combination of the effects of the diving reflex initially, followed by rapid and continued cooling, is what underlies the cerebral preservation that is sometimes seen in small children who suffer submersion and who are profoundly hypothermic.

By whatever mechanism cooling occurs, and whether the diving reflex plays a significant role in cerebral protection or not, hypothermia in the submersion victim, particularly if the victim is an infant or young child, should be considered to be an indication for aggressive and prolonged resuscitation efforts. This issue is discussed further in Chapter 22.4 on cold injuries.

HISTORY

Key points in history are summarised in Table 22.2.1. Broad areas in history include details of the submersion event itself, details of rescue and resuscitation, response to resuscitative efforts, possible underlying causal factors, and medical conditions that may influence recovery. Features of history that alert to the possibility of non-accidental injury should be recognised. These include a history that is inconsistent or a history that is incompatible with the victim's developmental level.

EXAMINATION

Examination is dictated by the clinical condition of the victim on arrival in the ED and is mainly directed at assessing the degree of neurological impairment due to hypoxic cerebral injury, the severity of respiratory embarrassment due to aspiration, and cardiovascular instability due to a combination of the initial insult and/or ongoing hypoxia. In broad terms submersion victims arriving in the ED will fall into two categories: (1) those

who respond to minimal resuscitation and who will generally do well with minimal complications; and (2) those 'high risk' patients who fail to respond to resuscitation and who will require ongoing resuscitation and or monitoring.[8]

Vital signs, including oxygen saturation, a bedside blood glucose estimate, and a temperature should be recorded on all patients. It is important to detect hypothermia, particularly in patients who have failed to respond to resuscitation efforts. Small children may rapidly become hypothermic due to evaporative heat loss during resuscitation efforts and transfer to the hospital. Apparent lifelessness and severe bradycardia due to profound hypothermia needs to be distinguished from asystole and brain death. Assessment of cardiac rhythm requires observation of the continuous electrocardiograph (ECG) monitor for up to a minute to detect very slow heart rates that can occur in profound hypothermia. Similarly, lack of response to painful stimulus along with fixed and dilated pupils should not be interpreted as brain death in the presence of profound hypothermia.

Depending on the clinical condition of the victim at arrival, neurological evaluation may range from an assessment of level of responsiveness as graded by the 'AVPU' or Glasgow coma score and pupillary reaction, to a focused neurological examination looking for focal deficit or spinal-cord injury. An assessment should always be made for the possibility of cranial or cervical spine trauma, particularly in diving-related accidents. Trauma to other areas of the body should also be sought.

In the awake child, examination of the respiratory system can establish a clinical baseline against which subsequent deterioration can be measured. Work of breathing should be assessed, and abnormalities found on auscultation, such as crackles and wheezes, should be noted. The finding of signs on an initial examination indicates the possibility of significant aspiration and dictates close observation to identify deterioration. A clear chest initially does not exclude aspiration and a period of observation and re-examination is necessary in all

---

Table 22.2.1 Key points in history

- The circumstances leading to the submersion
- The location of the submersion
- Water and environmental temperatures
- Duration of submersion
- Time from when the victim was last seen to the time when found (if the submersion was unwitnessed)
- Time from rescue to effective CPR
- Time to first gasp or return of spontaneous circulation
- Elements of basic and advanced life support employed
- Symptomatology following successful resuscitation
- Medical history particularly with regard to possible predisposing factors (i.e. neurological disorders, such as epilepsy)
- Factors that may complicate recovery (i.e. respiratory illness, such as asthma)

children who have been symptomatic following submersion.

INVESTIGATIONS

Investigations will also be dictated by the clinical condition of the patient on arrival in the ED. A child who has suffered a submersion injury and who is alert and asymptomatic on arrival requires little in the way of laboratory or radiological evaluation. The more symptomatic or seriously unwell child may benefit from further evaluation with laboratory and radiological investigations.

Useful investigations include arterial blood gas (ABG) analysis, serum glucose, and chest radiography. ABG analysis may demonstrate a metabolic acidosis, which confirms a significant submersion.[8] The severity of the acidosis reflects the severity of the hypoxic insult as well as ongoing hypoxic injury. Profound acidosis (pH < 7.10) implies a poorer prognosis but needs to be interpreted in the clinical context.[13] ABG analysis can be used to guide decisions regarding oxygenation and ventilation, and serial determinations may be useful in monitoring and quantifying deterioration of pulmonary function due non-cardiogenic pulmonary oedema secondary to hypoxia or aspiration. Determination of the blood glucose level is important in any critically ill child as hypoglycaemia can complicate physiological stress and should be actively treated. Hyperglycaemia in a comatose child, although not requiring treatment, implies a poor prognosis.[8] Initially the chest X-ray (CXR) may be normal, may demonstrate pulmonary infiltrates, or may display frank pulmonary oedema. Abnormalities detected on an early CXR mandate close observation and the patient should be monitored for clinical deterioration. Repeated CXR may be required but should be dictated by the patient's clinical condition.

Other investigations that may be helpful include baseline electrolytes and full blood count, although rarely are any clinically or therapeutically significant abnormalities found on initial determinations. Blood ethanol levels may be relevant depending on the age of the patient. A 12-lead ECG may be helpful in excluding prolonged QT syndrome as a cause for the submersion event.[9] Cervical spine films should be considered if cervical injury is suspected or the submersion event is secondary to a diving accident.

DIFFERENTIAL DIAGNOSIS

The major issues in differential diagnosis relate to the cause of the submersion event. Underlying medical conditions, such as epilepsy, should be considered. Trauma, either leading to or as a consequence of the submersion, should be recognised. Non-accidental injury should be suspected when there are inconsistencies in the history.

Severe hypothermia (core temperature less than 29°C) can mimic irretrievable cardiorespiratory arrest and brain death. The profound bradycardia associated with very low core body temperature can easily be confused with brady-asystole secondary to hypoxic injury and will not respond to usual resuscitation measures until hypothermia is corrected. Similarly, severe hypothermia can cause depression of cerebral function leading to unresponsiveness and fixed, dilated pupils, indistinguishable from irreversible hypoxic cerebral injury.[14] Failure of the core temperature to rise despite aggressive, active rewarming may be the only indication that death has occurred.

TREATMENT

Treatment of the submersion victim occurs in three major phases: (1) rescue and resuscitation at the scene; (2) initial assessment and stabilisation in the emergency department; and (3) subsequent observation and supportive care in the hospital ward, intensive-care unit (ICU), or after discharge.

Early institution of effective cardiopulmonary resuscitation with an emphasis on providing adequate ventilation is the key task in pre-hospital management. Manoeuvres to drain the lungs of water have not been shown to be clinically effective and may increase the risk of aspiration of gastric contents. The Heimlich manoeuvre should be reserved for cases in which repeated attempts to position the airway and provide ventilation have been unsuccessful or when foreign body aspiration and obstruction is suspected.[1] Emesis is common in submersion victims, both spontaneously and as a complication of resuscitation, and aspiration of gastric contents is a major potential complication following rescue. Spontaneously breathing patients should be managed and transported in the right lateral decubitus position. Cricoid pressure may reduce the risk of gastric distension and aspiration during cardiopulmonary resuscitation but requires an additional rescuer.[1]

Hypothermia can be exacerbated by ongoing evaporative heat loss during resuscitation efforts following rescue. Wet clothing should be removed and the patient should be dried if possible. Exposure during cardiopulmonary resuscitation (CPR) should be minimised as much as is practicable. If hypothermia is severe at the scene (< 30°C) rewarming should probably be delayed until adequate ventilation and oxygenation has been instituted.[14] Invasive rewarming techniques should be reserved for the hospital phase of management.

Treatment in the ED involves provision of adequate oxygenation, stabilisation of the body temperature, prevention of complications such as aspiration, and assessment of the patient's clinical status in order to make decisions regarding ongoing management and disposition.

Supplemental oxygen should be administered at concentrations and via delivery systems appropriate to the patient's oxygen requirement. Continuous pulse oximetry and serial estimations of respiratory rate and work of breathing should be undertaken during observation in the ED to determine worsening or improvement of the patient's respiratory status. If available, non-invasive ventilation techniques, although not extensively evaluated in paediatric submersion victims, may be considered if the oxygen requirement outstrips conventional mechanisms of oxygen delivery. Intubation to isolate the airway and provide ventilation with positive end-expiratory pressure (PEEP) may be required in patients with depressed neurological status or if respiratory compromise progresses despite supplemental oxygen therapy. Failure to maintain an SaO_2 of greater than 90% with an FiO_2 of 0.50 or higher, a $PaCO_2$ of more than 35mmHg, an abnormally high respiratory rate (> 50 bpm) or inadequate spontaneous ventilation, are all indications that mechanical ventilation is likely to be required.[1,9] Passage of a nasogastric or orogastric tube, if cranial trauma is suspected, should be performed following intubation to decompress the stomach and facilitate mechanical ventilation.

Diuretics are not recommended in the management of non-cardiogenic pulmonary oedema.[1,8,9] Steroids have not been shown to be useful in the management of aspiration pneumonitis and the role of antibiotics in this setting remains controversial.[1,8,9] Prophylactic antibiotics are generally not recommended, although they are sometimes used when there is a history of submersion in heavily contaminated or polluted water. In general, antibiotics should be reserved for patients who develop signs of pulmonary infection, such as fever or leukocytosis.[1] Fluid therapy should be judicious and should be aimed at maintaining adequate circulatory status and euglycaemia without overloading the patient.

Hypothermic patients should be warmed once adequate ventilation and oxygenation has been assured. Awake and spontaneously breathing patients with mild to moderate hypothermia (core temperature > 32°C) require passive or external active rewarming techniques only. Patients with severe hypothermia (core temperature < 32°C) who are obtunded or in cardiorespiratory arrest will require invasive active rewarming techniques. These are discussed fully elsewhere in this text (see Chapter 22.4 on cold injuries).

In the setting of cardiorespiratory arrest and severe hypothermia, resuscitation efforts should be continued until the core temperature has risen to around 32°C before a decision to cease resuscitation is made. Although there are no clear guidelines to determine how long efforts at rewarming should be continued, failure to affect rewarming despite maximal invasive efforts may be an indication that continuing resuscitation is futile. The decision to cease resuscitative efforts in the presence of persistent severe hypothermia should follow a multidisciplinary approach involving the emergency physician, paediatrician and/or paediatric intensivist and other members of the resuscitation team, together with the parents and family. Cardiorespiratory arrest on arrival in the ED in a patient with a core temperature above 32°C carries a uniformly poor prognosis and prolonged efforts at resuscitation are generally not indicated.

Treatment in the ICU involves provision of ventilatory support to ensure adequate oxygenation, maintenance of cardiovascular stability, minimisation of secondary brain injury due to cerebral oedema, management of hypoxic organ injury, and management of the complications of pulmonary aspiration. The use of PEEP in submersion victims ventilated in the ICU is controversial. Although PEEP may be necessary to maintain adequate oxygenation some authorities express concern regarding the potential reduction in cerebral venous outflow and subsequent increase in intracerebral pressure associated with its use. PEEP may have unfavourable effects on cardiovascular status and may increase the risk of barotrauma in already insulted lungs.[8] Other ventilation strategies to minimise non-cardiogenic pulmonary oedema and barotrauma, such as pressure-control ventilation with low-peak airway pressure and prolonged expiratory time, and permissive hypercapnia have been suggested, although again the trade-off is the risk in adversely influencing intracerebral pressure.[8] Various measures to provide cerebral resuscitation and control intracranial pressure have been evaluated in the literature and have generally been found to be not helpful in influencing outcome.[1] In general the aim should be to maintain adequate cerebral oxygenation and to minimise causes of secondary cerebral injury such as hypotension, hypercapnia, and hypo/hyperglycaemia.

DISPOSITION

Disposition is dictated by the clinical condition of the patient in the ED, the nature of the submersion event, the need for resuscitation, and the presence or absence of other factors, such as trauma, suspicion of non-accidental injury, and underlying or complicating medical conditions. In general, all victims of submersion will require some period of observation.

The alert, otherwise healthy, patient who is asymptomatic or who has suffered only mild, transient symptoms following a brief submersion can be safely discharged if they remain well after 6–8 hours of observation.[8] Patients with a history of submersion for longer than one minute, a period of cyanosis or apnoea, or who required pulmonary resuscitation, should be admitted for observation for 24 hours, or at least overnight, even if they are well in the ED. Although recent evidence discredits the idea of the 'delayed immersion syndrome', cases of fulminant pulmonary oedema up to twelve hours after submersion have been reported as occurring in patients who appear well and display normal chest radiography in the ED.[1] Any child discharged from the ED following a submersion event should be in the care of a reliable and responsible adult. Instructions should be given to represent for further medical assessment in the event of any change in the child's respiratory status.

Patients who have suffered trauma may require admission for the management of their injuries. Children with underlying cardiac or respiratory disorders, those who suffer submersion secondary to a pre-existing illness, and victims of suspected non-accidental injury also warrant in-patient evaluation.

Asymptomatic children and children with mild symptoms who are admitted for observation can be managed in a general ward environment, provided that there is the facility to increase the level of monitoring and care should it be required. Children who have required CPR, who have abnormal chest radiography or ABGs on arrival in the ED, or who have required ventilatory support, should be admitted to a high-dependency unit or ICU for observation and management.[1] Transfer to a facility that provides paediatric ICU should be considered for all such patients prior to clinical deterioration.

PROGNOSIS

Most children who suffer submersion injury will either survive intact or die. Death occurs in 30–50% of submersion victims, most of these not surviving to treatment in the ED. A small proportion of victims will be left with severe neurological deficit, either persistent vegetative state or spastic quadraplegia. Mild learning deficits may occur in apparently intact survivors, although the extent of these and the impact on subsequent function have not been clearly quantified.[8] In general, however, the prognosis of children who suffer submersion events and survive to hospital admission is excellent.[15]

Despite a large body of literature dedicated to the subject, the factors that predict prognosis in the ED following childhood submersion injury remain poorly defined. There are no prospectively validated scoring systems and most of the literature is based on retrospective data. Individual case reports of children surviving prolonged resuscitative efforts with good outcome continue to arise in the popular press and medical literature.

Factors elicited in history that influence prognosis are duration of submersion, time to institution of effective CPR, and time to first spontaneous gasp, all three reflecting the duration of the hypoxic cerebral insult. Duration of submersion can often be difficult to determine but submersion for longer than five minutes is associated with a poorer prognosis.[13] Although time to institution of effective CPR can be similarly difficult to ascertain accurately, delays of longer than 10–20 minutes are also associated with poorer outcomes, while early effective CPR has been shown to be an important factor in improving survival after rescue.[13]

As already discussed, hypothermia may be protective in small children who suffer submersion, particularly, but not exclusively, if the submersion has occurred in cold or icy water. However, neither hypothermia nor water temperature can be reliably used to predict outcome.[16]

Response to resuscitation following rescue and prior to arrival in the ED is the single most important indicator of outcome in children who have suffered submersion. Children who arrive conscious in the ED after successful resuscitation have almost universally excellent outcomes.[9] Similarly, lack of response to early resuscitation efforts and coma on arrival in the ED are associated with a poor outcome. In a classification system based on the neurological status of the patient on arrival in the ED, it was discovered that less than 15% of patients who were unresponsive and flaccid to painful stimulation had intact survival.[17] This is supported by the findings of other investigators that a GCS of 5 or less on arrival in the ED is associated with a dismal outcome, either death or severe neurological disability.[1,18] Lack of pupillary response in the ED has similarly been identified as a predictor of dismal outcome.[19] The caveat concerning the use of level of responsiveness and pupillary reaction to predict poor prognosis and withdraw treatment applies to the child who presents with severe hypothermia, which may mimic brain death. In these patients lack of response to aggressive rewarming and resuscitation becomes a surrogate indicator of poor outcome. In non-hypothermic patients who are in cardiorespiratory arrest, a lack of response to 25 minutes of effective advanced life support measures is almost universally associated with poor outcome.[8] It should be noted, however, that studies of outcome following out-of-hospital cardiac arrest in children indicate that children who suffer cardiac arrest secondary to submersion have significantly better outcomes than those who suffer cardiac arrest from other causes.

PREVENTION

Drowning remains a leading cause of accidental death in toddlers and adolescents in Australia. Most drowning-prevention strategies are aimed at the small child who drowns after falling into the domestic swimming pool, with few or none aimed at older children and adolescents.

Programmes to prevent drowning by teaching children under the age of four to swim remain unproven. Public-education programmes outlining the need to provide adult supervision when children are near water may be helpful. Pool alarms, pool covers, and fencing that does not isolate the pool from the home are probably not effective, although evidence is lacking.[6] Isolation or four-sided fencing with a self-locking or dynamic gate, on the other hand, has been shown to effectively reduce submersion incidents by up to 50%, in both Australia and New Zealand, and in the United States.[8] Pool-fencing legislation exists in Australia, but is not uniform across states. Compliance with legislation remains incomplete. Further research is required to aid in establishing uniform pool-fencing requirements based on Standards Australia specifications.[6]

CONTROVERSIES AND FUTURE DIRECTIONS

❶ Consensus is needed regarding terminology related to survival and death following submersion events.

❷ Prospective collection of data on submersion victims is needed to generate more useful information regarding prognosis. Scoring systems for prognosis should also be prospectively validated.

❸ Further research regarding preventative strategies is required to develop standardised and uniform legislation pertaining to pool fencing in Australia.

❹ Preventive educational programmes aimed at older children and adolescents are lacking, and are an area of possible future development in public health.

REFERENCES

1. Orlowski JP, Spilzman D 2001 Drowning: Rescue, resuscitation, reanimation. Paediatric Clinics of North America 48(3): 627–646
2. Guidelines 2000 for Cardiopulmonary Resuscitation, International Consensus on Science. Part 8, Section 3: Advanced challenges in resuscitation, submersion or near-drowning. Circulation 102(Suppl I): I-233-I-236
3. DeNicola LK, Falk JL, Swanson ME, Gayle MO, Kissoon N 1997 Submersion injures in children and adults. Critical Care Clinics 13(3): 478–502
4. Mackie IJ 1999 Patterns of drowning in Australia, 1992-1997. Medical Journal of Australia 171: 587–590
5. Edmond KM, Attia JR, D'Este CA, Condon JT 2001 Drowning and near-drowning in Northern Territory children. Medical Journal of Australia 175: 605–608
6. Pitt WR, Cass DT, 2001 Preventing children drowning in Australia. Medical Journal of Australia 175: 603–604
7. Moon RE, Long RJ 2002 Drowning and near-drowning. Emergency Medicine 14: 377–386
8. Quan L 1999 Near-drowning. Paediatrics in Review 20(8): 255–260
9. Sachdeva RC 1999 Environmental emergencies. Near drowning. Critical Care Clinics April 15(2): 81–96
10. Modell JH 1993 Drowning. New England Journal of Medicine 328(4): 253–256
11. Orlowski JP 1987 Drowning, near-drowning, and ice-water submersions. Paediatric Clinics of North America Feb 34(1): 75–92
12. Gooden BA 1992 Why some people do not drown. Hypothermia versus the diving response. Medical Journal of Australia 157: 629–632
13. Orlowski JP1979 Prognostic factors in pediatric cases of drowning and near-drowning. Journal of the American College of Emergency Physicians 8(5): 176–179
14. Theilade D 1977 The danger of fatal misjudgement in hypothermia after immersion. Successful resuscitation following immersion for 25 minutes. Anaesthesia 32: 889–892
15. Pearn J 1977 Neurological and psychometric studies in children surviving freshwater immersion accidents. Lancet 1(8001): 7–9
16. Suominen PK, Korpela RE, Silfvast TGO, Olkkola KT 1997 Does water temperature affect outcome of nearly drowned children? Resuscitation 35: 111–115
17. Conn AW, Montes JE, Barker GA, Edmonds JF 1980 Cerebral salvage in near-drowning following neurological classification by triage. Canadian Anaesthetic Society Journal 27(3): 201–209
18. Dean JM, Kaufman ND 1981 Prognostic indicators in pediatric near-drowning: the Glasgow coma scale. Critical Care Medicine 9(7): 536–539
19. Graf WD, Cummings P, Quan L, Brutaco D 1995 Predicting outcome in pediatric submersion victims. Annals of Emergency Medicine 26(3): 312–319

22.3 HEAT-INDUCED ILLNESS

MIKE RAGG

ESSENTIALS

1 Most heat-induced illness in children is due to overheating from exogenous sources.

2 The syndrome of heatstroke is made when hyperpyrexia occurs in association with altered mental state.

3 Aggressive cooling methods should be instituted for heatstroke.

4 Prevention in the form of public education about the dangers of heat-induced illness in children may be an effective measure.

INTRODUCTION

Hyperthermia in the paediatric patient differs physiologically from fever. Fever is caused by an elevation of body temperature secondary to regulation by the hypothalamus. High body temperature not caused by hypothalamic thermo-regulatory mechanisms is usually caused in children by one of the following:

- prolonged exposure to high ambient temperature (overheating)
- increased heat production
- reduced heat loss.

In the neonate and small infant, overheating is almost always the cause.

In children, heat-induced illness is the second most common cause of non-traumatic death after heart disease.[1] Children are particularly at risk because of their greater body surface area relative to mass.

Overheating

Overheating is usually seen in settings of high ambient temperature and humidity. Examples are with athletics, with summertime sporting events, and during heatwaves. Young children left in cars are also particularly at risk.

Increased heat production
- Metabolic (e.g. hyperthyroidism).
- Drugs (e.g. anticholinergics such as atropine, sympathomimetics, aspirin, neuroleptic agents, and selective serotonin reuptake inhibitor, SSRI, drugs).
- Seizures.

Decreased heat loss
- Over-wrapped babies.
- Excess clothing on hot and humid days.
- Disease states (e.g. cystic fibrosis).
- Heart disease.
- Drugs (e.g. phenothiazines and anticholinergics).

CLINICAL FEATURES

Heat-induced illness in children can be conveniently divided into a number of syndromes. It should be noted that over-heating syndromes represent a continuum of pathophysiological derangement in which cerebral dysfunction is at the extreme end of the spectrum. A consideration also needs to be given to child safety and neglect issues.

The neonate and infant
Overheating is the most common cause of hyperthermia in the neonate and infant. It is important to distinguish the healthy infant who is overheated from the febrile infant (Table 22.3.1).[2]

Mild overheating is usually not dangerous to infants, although there may be some association with apnoeic episodes in premature babies.[2] Hyperthermia from

Table 22.3.1   The overheated and febrile infant

Overheated infant	Febrile infant
High rectal temperature	High rectal temperature
Warm hands and feet	Cool hands and feet
Pink skin	Pale skin
Extended posture	Lethargic
Healthy appearance	Looks unwell[3]
Abdominal temperature exceeds hand temperature by less than 2°C	Abdominal temperature exceeds hand temperature by more than 3°C

overheating, however, is dangerous and has been linked with sudden death,[4] particularly in families with a history of malignant hyperthermia.

Heat syncope

Heat syncope commonly involves children who have been standing for prolonged periods in hot and humid weather or who have undergone strenuous exertion.

Heat cramps

Heat cramps occur in the setting of strenuous exercise in hot and humid conditions. A relative lack of body salt plays a part. Heat cramps can be very painful. However, most last for less than 1 minute. Abdominal muscle cramps have been known to simulate an acute abdomen.[5]

Heat exhaustion

Heat exhaustion in children presents as hyperpyrexia, vomiting, headache, lethargy, and weakness, with *a normal mental state*. The major problem is body water depletion. However, in some paediatric patients (e.g. those with cystic fibrosis, in whom greater amounts of salt are lost in their sweat) heat exhaustion may occur predominantly due to salt depletion.[5]

Heatstroke

Heatstroke is defined as a core body temperature greater than 40.5°C in association with acute mental state changes. There are two types: exertional and classic.

In the paediatric population, exertional heatstroke is most likely to occur in the adolescent who is exercising vigorously in a hot and humid environment. Sweating is usually present in this group. Classic heatstroke typically occurs during heat-waves or when children are left in cars in hot weather.

Common symptoms are irritability, confusion, and ataxia. Seizures may be seen, particularly during cooling. Coma is a common finding at presentation. However, the child's conscious state may improve in the pre-hospital environment.

Other serious complications of heat-stroke include cerebral oedema, liver injury, renal failure secondary to rhabdomyolysis, non-cardiogenic pulmonary oedema, and disseminated intravascular coagulation.

Other heat-induced syndromes

Malignant hyperthermia

Malignant hyperthermia is usually seen in the paediatric patient after general anaesthesia. Seventy-five per cent of victims have no family history, and 20.9% have had a previous 'normal' anaesthetic.[6] Initially, an increase in heart rate is followed by an elevation of blood pressure. Because these children are often paralysed, tachypnoea may not be seen. Elevation of the end tidal CO_2 is also an early sign. Muscle rigidity or increased tone may become apparent, and the body temperature rises at a rate of 1–2°C every 5 minutes. When succinylcholine is used, an acceleration of the syndrome may occur. Hyperkalaemia,

hypercalcaemia, metabolic acidaemia, and myoglobinuria follow.

The condition of masseter muscle rigidity is said to be associated with malignant hyperthermia. The peak age group is 8–12 years. It occurs after administration of succinylcholine. In approximately 50% of patients, malignant hyperthermia occurs after masseter muscle rigidity is first seen. The rigidity can usually be overcome with effort and resolves after 2–3 minutes. Repeated doses of succinylcholine do not help.

The association between malignant hyperthermia and skeletal abnormalities such as osteogenesis imperfecta is unclear.[6]

Serotonin syndrome and neuroleptic malignant syndrome (NMS)

Both syndromes are rare in children. When they do occur, they are seen in the context of an adolescent taking certain medications. Serotonin syndrome usually occurs when a combination of medication is used (e.g. monoamine oxidase inhibitors with an SSRI). NMS is usually a reaction to a single drug (e.g. haloperidol). Some commonly used drugs, for example promethazine and methylphenidate (Ritalin) have been implicated in NMS.

Other drug-related heat-induced syndromes

Amphetamine use (e.g. ecstasy at rave parties) and other drugs (e.g. salicylates and anticholinergics) can cause heat-induced illnesses in the adolescent group. Vigorous activity, high ambient temperatures, lack of hydration, and ingestion of amphetamine compounds contribute to the risk of hyperthermia at rave parties.[7]

INVESTIGATIONS

Heat-induced illness in children is diagnosed on clinical criteria and rectal temperature measurements. Investigations are directed at the complications of heat-induced illness in the paediatric patient.

Children who present with heat syncope or heat cramps usually do not require any investigations. Those children with more severe heat-induced illness, however, do require further investigations. In heat exhaustion, basic blood tests including full blood count, electrolytes and urea, serum creatine kinase, and glucose should be performed. Urinalysis to exclude myoglobinuria is also indicated.

The paediatric patient with heatstroke or another life-threatening hyperpyrexial illness requires full investigation. In addition to the above investigations, liver function tests, coagulation studies, arterial blood gases, and a 12-lead ECG should be performed.

TREATMENT

Heat syncope and heat cramps

For children with heat syncope and heat cramps, external cooling and oral fluids (such as oral rehydration fluids) are usually sufficient. These patients usually do not require admission.

Heat exhaustion

Children with heat exhaustion need fluids (oral if tolerated, otherwise the nasogastric or intravenous route should be used) and rest in a cool environment. Admission should be considered.

Heatstroke

Heatstroke in children is a medical emergency. The ABC approach is important, and all children with heatstroke should be triaged to a resuscitation environment. Rapid external cooling is the next immediate goal. Convection methods are probably the most effective. Initial cooling should aim for a core temperature of 38.5°C. Removing the child's clothes; spraying with water, with fanning (the 'wet and windy' approach); and applying ice packs to the neck, groin, and axillae are all indicated. It is important to prevent shivering, which can generate heat, by the administration of diazepam or chlorpromazine. Antipyretics such as paracetamol or ibuprofen have no role. More aggressive lavage cooling methods may be considered in extreme cases.

All children with genuine heatstroke require intravenous fluids, an indwelling urinary catheter, and admission to an intensive care unit. Complications such as shock, non-cardiogenic pulmonary oedema, cerebral oedema, consumptive coagulopathy, renal failure, and hepatic failure should be treated in the manner described in other chapters of this book.

Malignant hyperthermia

The suspected agent should be stopped immediately, especially if it is an inhalational anaesthetic. A specific antidote, dantrolene, is available. Dantrolene inhibits the release of calcium into muscles. The dose is 2.5 mg kg^{-1} given intravenously and repeated every 10 minutes to a maximum of 10 mg kg^{-1}.[6] Other manoeuvres include hyperventilation with 100% oxygen, bicarbonate in fulminant cases (2–4 mEq kg^{-1}), lidocaine to treat arrhythmias, and aggressive cooling of the child. The principles of cooling in malignant hyperthermia are similar to those of heatstroke.

Serotonin syndrome and neuroleptic malignant syndrome

In most patients with serotonin syndrome, symptoms will resolve within 24–48 hours after the drugs are stopped. In NMS, dantrolene may have a role. Benzodiazepines are useful in mild cases. Chlorpromazine (0.25–1.0 mg kg^{-1}) has been used as an antiserotonergic drug.[8] Other drugs that have been used include methysergide, cyproheptadine, and beta-blockers.

PROGNOSIS AND DISPOSITION

The decision to admit in heat syncope, cramps, and exhaustion will depend on a number of factors, including the severity of the presentation and the ongoing safety of the paediatric patient at discharge. If safety cannot be guaranteed, then admission for in-patient evaluation is warranted.

However, most children with mild heat-induced illness (i.e. heat syncope, heat cramps, and mild heat exhaustion) can be treated in the emergency department. All children with more severe forms of heat-induced illness should be admitted to hospital. Any child with suspected heatstroke should be admitted to an intensive care unit.

The mortality rate for heatstroke and for malignant hyperthermia is approximately 10% and 7%, respectively. Prognosis in heat-induced illness is related both to the absolute temperature level reached and to the duration of hyperpyrexia.[9] Persistent coma and multiorgan failure are poor prognostic signs. As prognosis correlates with duration of hyperthermia, immediate cooling is critical.

PREVENTION

Prevention, particularly in babies and infants, centres on educating new parents about the risks of sun exposure; clothing; and leaving children in cars, even for brief periods. Sports medicine guidelines regarding older children taking part in sporting activities in hot, humid weather need to be established.

CONTROVERSIES

Controversies relevant to heat-induced illness in children include:

❶ There is no high-level evidence for the most efficacious form of cooling in children.

❷ The association between malignant hyperthermia and masseter muscle rigidity has not been fully explored.

❸ The occurrence of NMS with methylphenidate (Ritalin) use is somewhat controversial.

❹ There is still a lack of public education about the susceptibility of infants and young children to heat-induced illness compared with that of adults. Issues of child neglect are also important.

REFERENCES

1. Behrman RE et al 1996 Textbook of Paediatrics. Saunders, London, 2106
2. Roberton NRC 1999 Temperature control and its disorders. In: Rennie JM, Roberton NRC (eds) Textbook of Neonatology. Churchill Livingstone, London, 229
3. Hewson P, Oberklaid F 1994 Recognition of serious illness in infants. Modern Medicine July: 89–96
4. Denborough MA, Galloway GJ, Hopkinson KC 1982 Malignant hyperpyrexia and sudden infant death. Lancet 2(8307): 1068–1069
5. Thompson A 1996 Environmental emergencies. In: Fleisher GR et al (eds) Synopsis of Pediatric Emergency Medicine. Williams & Wilkins, Philadelphia, 452–456
6. Rosenberg H et al 2001 Malignant hyperthermia and other pharmacogenetic disorders. In: Barash PG et al (eds) Clinical Anaesthesia Textbook. Lippincott William & Wilkins, Philadelphia, Chapter 20
7. Rieder MJ 2000 Some light from the heat: Implications of rave parties for clinicians. Canadian Medical Association Journal 162(13): 1829–1830
8. Gillman P 1996 Successful treatment of serotonin syndrome with chlorpromazine. Medical Journal of Australia 165: 345
9. Cameron P et al 2000 Textbook of Adult Emergency Medicine. Churchill Livingstone, London, 610

22.4 COLD INJURIES

SIMON CHU • NICHOLAS CHENG

ESSENTIALS

1. Hypothermia is defined as a core body temperature less than 35°C.

2. Cold injury is uncommon in Australia, but when cold injuries do occur it is more significant in children than in adults.

3. The major complications of hypothermia are altered mentation and arrhythmias.

4. Hypothermia is treated with passive external, active external, active internal, and/or extracorporeal rewarming, depending on severity. In addition, hypothermia should be rigorously prevented in any patient with a severe illness.

5. The major complications of rewarming are an 'after-drop' in temperature and vasodilatory shock.

6. Severe local cold injuries are treated with rapid immersion rewarming, then care given as for burns.

7. No patient is dead until they are warm and dead.

INTRODUCTION

Cold injury is uncommon in Australia due to its warm climates. However, its significance is more important in children, as they have:

- a larger surface area:weight ratio[1]
- underdeveloped behaviour responses to cope with extreme cold (young children can't put on more clothes).

When cold injuries do occur, they can be subdivided into generalised injury (namely accidental or environmental hypothermia) and localised injury. Cold injury is also a common problem potentially com-plicating any other severe illness (especially trauma) and must be prevented.[2]

NORMAL PHYSIOLOGY: A REVIEW

Heat production is from basal metabolism, digestion, and muscular activity, which may be voluntary (exercise) or involuntary (shivering). Emotional factors and hormonal fluctuations influence heat production. The main mechanisms by which the body compensates for low core body temperature are by increasing its metabolic rate, primarily through shivering, and by shunting blood away from non-essential organs to preserve vital organs. The capacity to shiver is dependent on local glycogen stores and the rate of change of core and external temperature.[1,3]

Neonates are the patients most prone to hypothermia. They are unable to shiver and have limited stores of energy. Because of this, newborn children utilise catabolism of brown fat to generate heat. This is an inefficient process that consumes oxygen, thus exacerbating hypoxia. In addition, the large surface area to weight ratio, due to a relatively large head, contributes to heat loss. At birth, neonates are covered in amniotic fluid, and evaporative losses are significant. An overhead radiant heater is not adequate to compensate for this evaporative loss.[4,5]

Heat loss from the human body is by four methods:

- radiation
- conduction
- convection
- evaporation.[1]

Radiation occurs when heat energy leaves the skin at the speed of light. Patients with more fat become more hypothermic than thinner patients, due to the former's larger surface area for radiation heat loss. In children, who have a higher surface area to weight ratio, it accounts for up to 50% of all heat loss; indeed, up to 75% in neonates. This higher number in neonates is due to a proportionally larger head increasing the

Table 22.4.1 Compensatory mechanisms at different severities of hypothermia

Mild (32–35°C)	Moderate (28–32°C)	Severe (< 28°C)
• Increased basal metabolic rate by shivering • Vasoconstriction peripherally, leading to fluid shifts • Mild tachycardia • Cold diuresis (see text) • Apathy, ataxia, amnesia, dysarthria	• Limits of increasing basal metabolic rate reached • Shivering stops • Decreasing cerebral blood flow, causing delirium and gradual decreased level of consciousness • Decreased rate of neural impulse transmission, causing clumsiness and numbness • Falling blood pressure • Muscle rigidity due to increasing acidosis	• Complete loss of thermoregulation • Stupor, coma • Pulseless • Fixed dilated pupils • Absent reflexes • Dysrhythmias, initially slow atrial fibrillation then ventricular fibrillation • Appearance of death at < 25°C with asystole See text for more specific changes

surface area:weight ratio.[1,4] Radiation losses decrease when a patient is clothed.

Conduction of heat is poor in air and therefore does not contribute much to hypothermia in normal circumstances. However, water-conductive heat loss is 24 times more than that of air. It is this method by which patients suffering from water immersion become profoundly hypothermic, and how patients in wet clothes become hypothermic quickly. The surface on which the patient is lying also contributes to conduction heat loss. For instance, a patient lying on snow is likely to become more hypothermic than a person lying on sand.

Convection occurs as warm air next to the skin is replaced by cool air. This can contribute to 25% of total body heat loss in still air. In a wind of 63 km hour^{-1}, this increases by 14 times. This is described as the 'wind chill factor'.

Evaporation from the skin accounts for only 7% of heat loss at rest. This may be increased in cold, dry conditions and by sweating. Evaporation from the respiratory tract removes another 7%. This can increase by breathing faster (such as at high altitude or during exercise).

Temperature is perceived through central and peripheral mechanisms. Heat sensors in the central hypothalamus receive input from the skin, central arteries, and viscera. It is this central thermostat that is reset, which causes fever. Skin receptors respond to a change in skin temperature but do not themselves indicate the patient's core temperature. A result of all this input is that the body responds by those autonomic reflexes listed below to increase or decrease core body temperature.[3]

Table 22.4.2 Findings at low body temperatures

Temperature (°C)	Findings
27	Reflexes absent, no response to pain, comatose
25	Cerebral blood flow one-third of normal, cardiac output one-half of normal
23	No corneal reflex, ventricular fibrillation risk is maximal
19	Asystole, flat EEG
15	Lowest temperature survived from accidental hypothermia

HYPOTHERMIA

This is defined as a core temperature of < 35°C.[1] Hypothermia is classified on the basis of severity. The reason for the classification is that it roughly determines the rewarming mechanisms that are most often employed. It is also related to the physiological ability of the patient to compensate for hypothermia. An easy way to remember these temperature ranges is:

- Acceptable low temperature: 2°C below 37°C (> 35°C).
- True mild hypothermia: 3°C below that (32–35°C).
- Moderate hypothermia: 4°C below that (28–32°C).
- Severe hypothermia: anything below that (< 28°C).

Tables 22.4.1 and 22.4.2 show the main consequences of hypothermia at a given temperature.[1,3,6] Much of our understanding of this pathophysiology comes from controlled hypothermia in cardiac surgery. Note that there is a huge variation of the onset of certain clinical signs based on temperature level. For instance, some patients may exhibit confusion at higher temperatures compared with others.

Note that only during severe hypothermia does protection from hypoxia occur, due to decreased demand for oxygen by tissues, and even then only at extremely low temperatures (patients <20°C can tolerate anoxia for up to 60 minutes). Metabolic processes slow by approximately 6% for each 1°C drop in body temperature.[1] Thus at 28°C the basal metabolic rate is about 50% of normal. This leads to hypoventilation and hypoxia. However, at this temperature the decreased cellular metabolism affords some protection against hypoxia.

Cold diuresis is an initial brisk diuresis; this is due to decreased tubular reabsorption and also a decreased production of antidiuretic hormone. There is also an increased central blood circulating volume as blood is shunted away from the periphery, thus presenting the kidneys with an apparent increased blood volume for filtration.[1]

History

Important points in history are:

- approximate time of exposure, if known
- environment in which patient was found
- resuscitation at the scene
- pre-existent illnesses (e.g. thyroid disease)
- drugs, medications, allergies, and immunisation status

Examination
- Full primary and secondary assessment of patient.
- Accurate measurement of core body temperature.

Diagnosis
This requires only two essentials:[1]

- a thermometer able to record low core temperatures accurately
- a high index of suspicion.

Core temperatures can be measured best with oesophageal or rectal probes.[1] The most direct method of measurement is with a cardiac catheter such as a Swan–Ganz, but this is impractical in the emergency setting. Rectal probes are often used,[7] but care must be taken when using these. The probe must be at least 10 cm into the rectum in older children (more than 8 years old) and 5 cm in younger children. Inaccuracies may occur due to the presence of faecal material,[1] and the probe must be left in until the temperature equilibrates. Tympanic measurements are well known to be unreliable in the very young,[7] but they are a good indicator of therapy progression in the older child. Oral and axillary temperature probes are unreliable and impractical in the setting of true hypothermia.

Treatment
Pre-hospital treatment
This is mainly the realm of passive external rewarming methods (see below). Patients should be carefully removed from the precipitant cold environment to a dry, sheltered area. If clothes are wet, they should be removed, and the patient dried and covered with a warm dry blanket. All patients should be gently handled, especially during transport, as there is evidence that sudden movements to the body in severe hypothermia can

precipitate arrhythmias, particularly ventricular fibrillation.[6] While this is occurring, one should attend to the patient's airway, breathing, and circulation, as per any resuscitation.

Active rewarming should be avoided until the patient reaches the emergency department. This is because of the complications of rewarming, namely 'after-drop' and shock.[1,6,8]

Treatment in the emergency department
Once in the emergency department, the patient should be triaged to an appropriate area, which is warm. In the very young, a radiant warmer bed and heating lamps should be available when the patient presents.[4,9] Patients should have their airway, breathing, and circulation reassessed and appropriate resuscitation commenced. Appropriate monitoring should be instituted, including ECG, and core temperature, either by rectal or oesophageal means. Oxygen saturation monitoring should be attempted, knowing that initial vasoconstriction will give inadequate readings. Urine output should be monitored. Gentle handling should be continued to avoid precipitation of arrhythmias.[6] Patients should continue 100% oxygen on arrival in emergency.

Blood tests taken should include arterial blood gas (ABG); full blood count; electrolyte, urea, creatinine (EUC); liver function tests; amylase; comprehensive metabolic panel (CMP); glucose; thyroid function tests (TFTs); coags; tests for infection; and, if suspected, a screen for sedative drugs and ethanol. Hypothermia causes measured pH to fall and pO_2 and pCO_2 to be higher. It is recommended that these ABG values should not be corrected for temperature to better reflect the physiological state of the patient.[6]

A 12-lead ECG should be taken. Classic changes include the presence of a J (Osborn) wave, interval (PR, QRS, QT) prolongation, atrial dysrhythmias, and ventricular dysrhythmias.[10] Other less well-known changes include changes similar to myocardial infarction. Hypothermia can also blunt the ECG changes with hyperkalaemia.[6] Note that all these are not present in all hypothermic patients.

Once temperature is measured, the severity of hypothermia determines the methods of rewarming. Specific methods of rewarming are classically divided into four categories:[6,8,11]

- passive external rewarming
- active external rewarming
- active internal (core) rewarming
- extracorporeal rewarming.

Passive external rewarming These are methods used to prevent excessive endogenous heat loss and promote the patient to self-warm to normal core temperature. They include placing the patient in a warm room to prevent excessive convection, evaporation, and conduction heat losses. Sheets of foil (foil space blankets) are placed over the patient to decrease loss of heat through radiation.

Active external rewarming These are methods used to transfer heat energy to the patient from the external environment. They include:

- warmed blankets
- chemical hot packs and warm water bottles
- forced warm air blankets
- radiant heaters and lights
- warm-water body immersion.

Active internal rewarming These are methods used to transfer heat energy to the patient that deliver heat internally. They can be subdivided into simple methods (the first two methods below) and invasive methods. They include:

- warmed IV fluids (normal saline 40°C)
- inhalation of humidified warm oxygen (40°C)
- gastric lavage
- bladder lavage
- colonic lavage
- pleural and peritoneal lavage ($10–20$ mL kg^{-1} of 40°C saline)

Extracorporeal rewarming These are methods by which the patient's blood is removed, rewarmed outside the body, and replaced. They include:

- haemodialysis
- veno-venous transfer of blood

- extracorporeal (coronary bypass) circulation.

Due to the child's larger surface area to weight ratio,[1,5] emergency physicians should start to institute limited active external rewarming methods, such as radiant light warmers and forced warm air blankets, even in mild hypothermia.[11] If the child is unable to produce extra heat, then the institution of simple active internal rewarming methods (warm humidified oxygen and warmed IV fluids) is appropriate.

In older children, asking them to drink some warm liquids (hot chocolate or soup) will in effect give them the effects of a warm gastric lavage. However, patients should only have warmed fluids if they are fully conscious, can protect their airway, and have no evidence of gastroparesis.

Moderate hypothermia (28–32°C) should have all active external rewarming techniques instituted except immersion in warm bath therapy, which is limited to localised cold injury in the emergency setting (see frostbite later in the chapter). It is almost impossible to adequately monitor patients while they are in an immersion bath. Forced air warming blankets can increase core temperature by up to 1.5°C hour^{-1}. Patients should also have warmed IV fluids and heated humidified oxygen for inhalation. Together, they can increase core temperature by 1–2°C hour^{-1}.[6] Normal saline bags can be safely warmed in a microwave oven. The optimum operating system for warming 500-ml bags of crystalloid is 400-W microwave for 100 seconds or 800-W microwave for 50 seconds.[12] Alternatively, if a heat infusion pump is available, this should be used. Intravenous infusion tubing should be as short as possible, as longer tubing loses more heat to the atmosphere.

Severe hypothermia requires institution of invasive core-rewarming techniques. All can raise core temperature by 2°C every 5 minutes.[6] In cardiac arrest, cardiopulmonary resuscitation (CPR) should be commenced until core temperature has reached 35°C, and then a further assessment of the patient done (see

Controversies). Note that, according to criteria for diagnosing brain death as quoted from the Australian and New Zealand Intensive Care Society,[13] the patient must have a core temperature above 35°C, whereas other sources say 32°C.[14]

The decision of who to rewarm continues to evolve. There is a case report of a 26-month-old patient with a core temperature of 15°C who, after rewarming, recovered neurologically intact.[15] For patients without submersion, extreme duration of exposure is not incompatible with life. In immersion patients, successful recovery is very rarely seen unless patients are immersed in ice-cold water (< 10°C) for long periods of time (see *Drowning* chapter). However, further attempts to resuscitate after failure to restore a circulating cardiac rhythm within 30 minutes of rewarming to above 32°C are likely to be ineffective.[14]

Neonatal resuscitation

In neonatal resuscitation, every attempt should be made to provide a warm ambient environment for the newborn child. A heated room with an overhead warmer is required. Warmed towels and blankets are used to rapidly dry the newborn to prevent evaporative heat loss. Unwell neonates should be admitted to special care nurseries or neonatal intensive care within humidicribs or transport cribs with radiant heat. If ventilated, humidified warm gases should be used.[4,5]

Complications

Complications can be classified as due to the hypothermia itself and complications as a result of rewarming.

Complications from hypothermia include:[1,3]

- Cardiac: arrhythmia
- Haematological:
  platelet dysfunction
  hrombocytopenia
  disseminated intravascular coagulopathy
- Pulmonary:
  pneumonia
  pulmonary oedema
  acute respiratory distress syndrome

- Infection:
  immune complex suppression
- Renal:
  acute tubular necrosis
  rhabdomyolysis
- Neurological:
  cerebral oedema
  prolonged coma
  slow neurological recovery (up to 6 months)
- Gastrointestinal:
  pancreatitis
- Biochemical and metabolic derangements, including glucose, sodium, potassium

There are two main complications that result directly from the rewarming of patients: after-drop and shock.[1,6,8] After-drop is a drop in core temperature after rewarming therapies have commenced. There are two proposed mechanisms for after-drop:

❶ Cold peripheral blood re-enters the circulation once peripheral vasodilatation occurs with rewarming.

❷ After-drop is due to ongoing conduction of heat from the warmer core into colder peripheries and surface layers of the body.

In reality, after-drop is most probably a combination of the two mechanisms described. This can be minimised by ensuring that rewarming only occurs over the core of the body, while the peripheries of the body are not actively rewarmed. For instance, a forced warm air blanket is placed over the patient's body, but their hands and feet are left outside the blanket.

Shock occurs from the same mechanism, where peripheral vasodilatation increases the intravascular space to be filled, and one sees a consequent drop in blood pressure and rise in heart rate. In addition, the cold diuresis experienced has already decreased the circulating blood volume (up to 35%). In immersion patients, there is also a hydrostatic squeeze effect, which further decreases blood volume. Rewarming should therefore occur only once vascular access is established and warmed normal saline is instituted if active rewarming occurs, starting with usual shock doses of 20 mL kg^{-1}. Insertion of a central venous pressure (CVP) line would be useful; however, this needs to be balanced against the increased rough handling of the body during insertion.

Medications in hypothermia behave unpredictably. Metabolism of most drugs will be slowed due to hypothermia. Some drugs have decreased effectiveness; others, such as morphine, have increased effects. Drugs not used in treatment include sodium bicarbonate, insulin, corticosteroids, empirical antibiotics, and ethanol (contrary to popular belief).[3,6]

Electrical defibrillation and antiarrhythmics may be administered at any temperature, but most efforts do not succeed until the temperature reaches above 28–30°C.[3]

Disposition

A patient with mild hypothermia, once treated, may be observed in the emergency department for a few hours before discharge if the patient is well. Moderate and severe hypothermia are an indication for ward or intensive care unit admission, depending on if cardiac abnormalities are present during assessment. Discharge should include education to patients on prevention of further occurrences, for example the proper use of clothing, checking weather reports, etc.[1]

LOCALISED COLD INJURIES

Frostbite is the most severe of the injuries, but others include chilblain (perniosis), cold-induced fat necrosis (panniculitis), frost nip, and trench foot.[16,17]

Frost nip is transient blanching and numbness of peripheries that resolves with rewarming. Only the skin surface is damaged. No ice crystals form within tissues, as opposed to frostbite (see below).

Trench foot, also known as immersion foot, is historically the most interesting, with the most famous occurring at Napoleon's failed invasion of Russia. It is due to prolonged exposure to wet cold, most common in the feet when poorly ventilated cold shoes are worn. There is

peripheral neurovascular damage, but no ice crystal formation within tissues.

Perniosis or chilblain is injury due to repeated exposure to dry cold. Bullae form 12 hours post injury. These bullae burst to form ulcers, which are painful and itchy. It is possibly due to repeated vasoconstriction.

Panniculitis consists of red lesions due to cold. Treatment is with non-steroidal anti-inflammatory drugs (NSAIDs), and the lesions resolve in 10–21 days.

FROSTBITE

Frostbite is the most dangerous of the local cold injuries. It is caused by freezing and ice crystal formation within the interstitial and cellular spaces due to prolonged exposure to freezing temperatures. It tends to occur more if the skin is directly exposed to temperatures less than −10°C. Several pathogenic phases evolve, called the frostbite injury cascade:[8,17]

❶ Pre-freeze phase. Superficial tissue cooling occurs, which leads to increased blood viscosity, microvascular constriction, and endothelial plasma leakage.
❷ Freeze phase. Ice crystals form in the extracellular space, leading to disruption of endothelium, disruption of cell anatomy, and hyperosmolality within cells due to crystals osmotically drawing water out of cells. This leads to protein denaturation and DNA synthesis inhibition.
❸ Vascular stasis. There is arteriovenous shunting within damaged tissue, leading to stasis coagulopathy and thrombus formation.
❹ Late progressive ischaemic phase. The thrombus induces inflammation, distal hypoxia, and anaerobic metabolism, which eventually leads to tissue necrosis.

Clinical features and diagnosis

Symptomatically, frostbite begins as an initial coldness of the skin. It then progresses to a stinging or burning pain, then to an anaesthetic limb, loss of fine

motor function, loss of gross motor function, and finally severe joint pain. Examination of the affected limb will reveal varying degrees of frostbite.[17] In the past, they have been classified similarly to burns, from first-degree to fourth-degree injury. It is much easier to classify them as superficial or deep.[8] Superficial injuries go only to the skin and subcutaneous tissues, whereas deep frostbite also affects bones, joints, and tendons.

Most investigations are unhelpful. However, a full blood work-up with full blood count, EUC, liver function tests, glucose, and creatine kinase to look for rhabdomyolysis should be done. Urinary myoglobin should be checked. Imaging is unhelpful initially; however, there is some evidence that a bone scan will help surgeons later determine how much limb is still viable, and whether superimposed osteomyelitis has developed.[8,17,18]

Treatment

Pre-medical treatment involves preventing further hypothermia and initiating resuscitation. As for hypothermia, removing the patient from the cold environment is paramount. Rubbing the limb to try to warm it should be avoided, as this increases tissue damage.[8,17]

Once in emergency, the mainstay of treatment is rapid immersion rewarming.[8,17] The affected limb should be placed in a whirlpool of water about 40°C for 20–40 minutes for superficial frostbite, 1 hour for deep frostbite. This procedure will be painful, so narcotic and NSAID analgesia should be started before treatment is commenced. Rewarming is complete when the distal area of the limb is flushed, soft, and pliable. The patient should start to move the limb during rewarming to encourage blood flow in the limb. The main reason for suboptimal results is premature cessation of rewarming. After rewarming, the limb is dried and placed in a splint and elevated, and dressings applied four times a day.

Blistering of the limb will occur. The blisters are usually clear in superficial frostbite, and haemorrhagic blisters in deep frostbite. Controversy exists as to whether to aspirate these blisters. Haemorrhagic blisters should not be aspirated,

Cause	Details
Metabolic or endocrine	• Hypoglycaemia • Diabetic ketoacidosis • Hypopituitarism • Hypothyroidism • Addison's disease • Uraemia • Malnutrition
Toxicological	• Alcohol • Barbiturates • Anaesthetic agents • Carbon monoxide • Cyclic antidepressants • Narcotics • Phenothiazines
CNS disorders	• Head trauma • Spinal trauma • Subarachnoid haemorrhage • Degenerative diseases • Cerebrovascular accidents • Intracranial neoplasm
Infections	• Sepsis • Meningitis • Encephalitis • Pneumonia
Vascular or skin	• Shock • Gastrointestinal tract haemorrhage • Pulmonary embolism • Burns • Erythrodermas
Iatrogenic	• Cold fluid infusion • Exposure during treatment • Prolonged extrications • Exposure during transport • Exposure post birth

Table 22.4.3 Hypothermia not due to environmental causes

as this increases trauma to the wound. Clear blisters are not as well defined with regard to treatment.

All patients should have their tetanus status updated and, as 30% of wounds become infected, IV prophylactic antibiotics may be of use. IV penicillin G is most commonly used.[17]

Disposition

All patients should be admitted under a specialised (burns) unit.[8,17] Patients are observed for up to 6 weeks, which is usually the time the gangrenous parts of the limb are fully delineated so that safe amputation, if necessary, will occur. Good prognostic factors are patients with superficial injuries only, clear blisters, and sensation still present after rewarming.[17]

HYPOTHERMIA NOT DUE TO ENVIRONMENTAL CAUSES

There are many other causes of hypothermia,[1,3] as seen in Table 22.4.3.

Once the hypothermia is treated, then non-environmental causes should be investigated and, if found, appropriate treatment instituted. Iatrogenic causes need to be prevented. Always prevent hypothermia in trauma patients after full assessment, as hypothermia worsens the diagnosis.

REFERENCES

1. Corneli HM 1992 Accidental hypothermia. Journal of Pediatrics 120(5): 671–679

CONTROVERSIES

❶ In certain countries, active rewarming is commenced prior to arrival in the emergency department.[8] This is due to well-organised emergency medical systems catering for such emergencies, like in Canada. In Australia, this is more of a contentious issue, as we don't see hypothermia as often.

❷ Controversy exists regarding CPR causing arrhythmias when a patient loses spontaneous circulation.[1] However, the evidence that CPR causes ventricular fibrillation in hypothermic patients is at best circumstantial, and therefore the general consensus is that, to promote brain perfusion, CPR should be continued till the core body temperature reaches 35°C.[13]

❸ Continuing CPR in the absence of cardiac output in a hypothermic patient has traditionally been mandatory. However, as survival occurs only in patients who have been immersed in water < 5°C prior to cardiac arrest,[1] it is more likely that patients arrest in Australia before they become hypothermic. Therefore when to stop cardiac resuscitation is an issue.

❹ The use of hypothermia in treatment, particularly in trauma and head injury, has always been of some debate.[11] Hypothermia causes a reduction in oxygen consumption and is theoretically cerebroprotective. This contradicts the results that trauma patients presenting with hypothermia have a worse prognosis.[2]

2. Kirkpatrick AW, Chun R, Brown R et al 1999 Hypothermia and the trauma patient. Canadian Journal of Surgery 42(5): 333–343
3. Strange G, Cooper M 1996 Cold illness. In: Strange G, Ahrenf W, Lelyveld S et al (eds) Pediatric Emergency Medicine, A Comprehensive Study Guide, 1st edn. McGraw-Hill, New York, 616–622
4. Phillips B, Zideman D, Wyllie J et al 2001 European Resuscitation Council Guidelines 2000 for Newly Born Life Support. A statement from the Paediatric Life Support Working Group and approved by the Executive Committee of the European Resuscitation Council. Resuscitation 48(3): 235–239

5. Bissinger RL 2001 Neonatal resuscitation. eMedicine Journal 2(11). Online. Available: http://author.emedicine.com/ped/topic2598.htm 11 Sep 2003

6. Danzl DF, Pozos RS 1994 Accidental hypothermia. New England Journal of Medicine 331(26): 1756–1760

7. Riddell A, Eppich W 2001 Should tympanic temperature measurement be trusted? Archives of Disease in Childhood 85(5): 431–434

8. Biem J, Koehncke N, Classen D et al 2003 Out of the cold: Management of hypothermia and frostbite. Canadian Medical Association Journal 168(3): 305–311

9. Day SE 1993 Intra-transport stabilization and management of the pediatric patient. Pediatric Clinics of North America 40(2): 263–274

10. Mattu A, Brady WJ, Perron AD 2002 Electrocardiographic manifestations of hypothermia. American Journal of Emergency Medicine 20(4): 314–326

11. Bernardo LM, Henker R, O'Connor J 2000 Treatment of trauma-associated hypothermia in children: Evidence-based practice. American Journal of Critical Care 9(4): 227–234

12. Lindhoff GA, Mac G, Palmer JH 2000 An assessment of the thermal safety of microwave warming of crystalloid fluids. Anaesthesia 55(3): 251–254

13. Australian and New Zealand Intensive Care Society 1998 Recommendations on brain death and organ donation, 2nd edn. Australian and New Zealand Intensive Care Society, Melbourne. Online. Available: http://www.anzics.com.au/files/brain_death_organ_donation.pdf 11 Sep 2003

14. Wijdicks EFM 2001 The diagnosis of brain death. New England Journal of Medicine 344: 1215–1221

15. Kelly K, Glaeser P, Rice T et al 1990 Profound accidental hypothermia and freeze injury of the extremities in a child. Critical Care Medicine 18(6): 679–680

16. Herrin J, Antoon A 1996 Cold injuries. In: Behrman R, Kliegman R, Arvin A (eds) Nelson's Textbook of Pediatrics, 15th edn. Saunders, Philadelphia, 277–278

17. Cheng D, Hackshaw D 2003 Frostbite. eMedicine Journal Jan. Online. Available: http://www.emedicine.com/ped/topic803.htm 11 Sep 2003

18. Cauchy E, Chetaille E, Lefevre M et al 2000 The role of bone scanning in severe frostbite of the extremities: A retrospective study of 88 cases. European Journal of Nuclear Medicine 27(5): 497–502

FURTHER READING

Adnot J, Lewis CW 1994 Immersion foot syndromes. In: James WD (ed) Textbook of Military Medicine: Military Dermatology. United States Government Printing Office, Washington, 55-68. Online. Available http://www.vnh.org/MilitaryDerm/Ch4.pdf 11 Sep 2003 – *a comprehensive text on military dermatology, part of a large tome on military medicine; unlikely to be specifically useful in a paediatric sense, but this chapter is useful to round out understanding of localised cold injury*

Douwens R 2003 Hypothermia prevention, recognition and treatment. Online. Available: http://www.hypothermia.org 11 Sep 2003 – *an excellent web site with up-to-date insight on hypothermia and future directions in management*

Meteorological Service of Canada 2002 Wind chill charts and tables. Meteorological Service of Canada, Ottawa. Online. Available: http://www.msc.ec.gc.ca/education/windchill/charts_tables_e.cfm 11 Sep 2003 – *an excellent article with excellent graphical depictions of wind chill effects; the reader should also peruse the rest of the web site*

22.5 ANAPHYLAXIS

ANDREW KEMP

ESSENTIALS

1 Adrenaline (epinephrine) is the treatment of choice and should be administered if there are any respiratory symptoms.

2 Biphasic reactions occur, with relapse 4–10 hours after initial successful treatment.

3 A full history should be obtained with the aim of identifying the triggering factor.

4 If repeated exposure is considered possible, consider provision of an anaphylaxis action plan and instruction in use of an EpiPen.

5 An allergy referral is indicated for definitive diagnosis of precipitating factors.

INTRODUCTION

There is no clear medical consensus on the definition of anaphylaxis. Acute allergic reactions resulting from the degranulation of mast cells present as a continuum of responses from mild cutaneous erythema and urticaria to severe hypotension, collapse, and death. Different authorities include varying components of the reaction along the continuum within the definition of anaphylaxis. From the perspective of paediatric emergency medicine, anaphylaxis may be defined as a severe acute allergic reaction that involves the respiratory tract and/or results in circulatory compromise with hypotension. An alternative definition proposed with broader manifestations is that exposure to an allergen within 1 hour produces one or more systemic signs (hypotension, upper or lower respiratory tract compromise, or increased gastrointestinal motility), and one or more of these signs is accompanied by urticaria or angioedema.[1]

The epidemiology of anaphylaxis is not well defined, because cases of sudden or acute death secondary to anaphylaxis may be misclassified or diagnosed as due to another cause, such as severe asthma. An additional factor is that there is no standard definition of anaphylaxis.

Along with the increasing incidence of allergic diseases, anaphylaxis has also increased. Hospital admissions for anaphylaxis in England more than doubled during the 1990s. A study in the UK identified eight deaths in a population of 13 million children over a period of 10 years from food anaphylaxis. This indicates that death from food anaphylaxis is an uncommon event but does not address the issue of the prevalence of anaphylaxis not resulting in mortality. In addition, it is uncertain whether all cases of anaphylactic death were identified as such, or indeed recorded as another diagnosis, such as asthma.

In the USA, there are approximately 1500 annual deaths from anaphylaxis. It has been calculated that from 1 to 15% of the US population are at risk of anaphylaxis.[2] Fatalities due to food-induced anaphylaxis usually occur in adolescents and young adults, and are due to peanut or tree nut in more than 90% of cases.[3]

553

A survey of South Australian children reported a rate of anaphylaxis of 1:170 children.[4] In Canada over a 5-year period, 0.9% of the population had injectable adrenaline (epinephrine) dispensed, with the highest rate, of 1.4%, being in individuals younger than 17 years. However, the prescription of adrenaline does not necessarily equate to the occurrence of anaphylaxis, particularly as there is an increasing tendency to provide prophylactic adrenaline for milder cases of allergic reaction.

Food-induced anaphylaxis has become the leading cause of anaphylaxis reactions occurring outside a hospital setting, particularly in the paediatric age group. An important feature of paediatric anaphylaxis is that more than half of the reactions occur in the home.

PATHOPHYSIOLOGY

Anaphylaxis is due to mast cell mediator release and causes profound changes in the cardiovascular and respiratory systems. Those mediators with vasoactive and/or bronchoconstrictive activities (histamine and the sulphidopeptide leukotrienes) are principal factors in the development of anaphylaxis. There are additional contributions from platelet activating factor, adenosine, prostaglandin D_2 and interleukin-6.

An increase in vascular permeability causes loss of fluid from the circulation into the interstitial space. The relative contributions of the mediators to the various clinical features are not completely defined. Animal models suggest that histamine contributes primarily to respiratory symptoms and hypothermia, with lesser effects on cardiac dysfunction and hypotension. However, in sting-induced anaphylaxis in humans, the rise in histamine correlated inversely with the arterial blood pressure. Mediators may directly compromise cardiac muscle function, and the intravascular volume depletion and haemoconcentration further compromise the cardiac output. Secondary cardiac arrhythmias can occur.

Both upper and lower airways are affected. Laryngeal oedema results in a variable degree of upper airway obstruction, and bronchospasm and increased mucus secretion compromise the lower airways. Bronchospasm is more marked in asthmatic patients or in those taking beta-blockers.

AETIOLOGY

The causative agent can be identified in about three-quarters of patients presenting to emergency departments.[5] In children, the percentage of cases due to a known trigger are:[6]

- Food: 50%
- Medications: 25%
- Insect bites: 10%
- Immunotherapy: 1%
- Immunisations: 1%

CLINICAL FEATURES

Symptoms occur along a continuum, from acute allergic reactions that are primarily cutaneous in nature plus or minus ocular and nasal symptoms, through mild to moderate anaphylactic reactions that may have respiratory symptoms but without tachypnoea or hypotension, to severe life-threatening anaphylaxis with hypotension and hypoxia.

In children, cutaneous (90% of cases) and respiratory (80% of cases) manifestations occur earlier and are more common than gastrointestinal and cardiovascular manifestations. In 'food' anaphylaxis, gastrointestinal symptoms are more frequent, whereas cardiovascular symptoms are rare. Gastrointestinal symptoms include abdominal discomfort and vomiting. In contrast, in anaesthetic anaphylaxis, which is commonly due to muscle relaxants, cardiovascular collapse is the common presenting problem and in 10% of cases the only manifestation.

The cutaneous features of pruritus, erythema, local or generalised urticaria, and angioedema occur in nearly all children. These are commonly the first symptoms experienced, occurring within minutes following allergen exposure. Occasionally, other symptoms of anaphylaxis occur in the absence of cutaneous features.

Life-threatening symptoms and signs include loss of consciousness, syncope, dizziness, light-headedness, cerebral dysfunction, hypotension, hypoxia, stridor, cyanosis, and laryngeal oedema.

Table 22.5.1 lists the frequency of the presenting symptoms and signs in children admitted to hospital for anaphylaxis.

Biphasic anaphylactic reactions are defined as worsening of symptoms, requiring new therapy, after the resolution of anaphylaxis, and occur in approximately 5% of children with anaphylaxis.[6] The reaction usually occurs 4–10 hours after the initial event; however, it has been described up to 48 hours later. Biphasic reactions are not readily predicted from the initial clinical features. The delayed administration of adrenaline (epinephrine) is associated with an increased occurrence of biphasic reactions, and patients with biphasic reactions have required higher doses of adrenaline to control their initial symptoms.

Table 22.5.1 Presenting features of children with anaphylaxis[6]

Presenting feature	Per cent
Cutaneous (urticaria, angioedema, flushing, or warmth	90
Upper airway (throat tightness or itchiness, drooling, stridor, oropharyngeal swelling)	80
Lower airway (chest tightness, wheezing)	60
Gastrointestinal (abdominal discomfort, vomiting)	40
Cardiovascular (arrhythmias, hypotension, poor capillary refill, weak pulses)	30
Neurological (confusion, decreased conscious state)	25
Generalised (diaphoresis, tingling, an impending sense of doom)	15

INVESTIGATION

Anaphylaxis is a clinical diagnosis, and investigations do not have a role in the acute management.

On occasions, it may be difficult to differentiate anaphylaxis from other cardiac, respiratory, or neurological episodes. In this situation, determination of plasma levels of mast cell mediators (histamine and mast cell tryptase) may provide additional diagnostic help.[7] Mast cell tryptase occurs in an alpha form that is constitutively released and a beta form that is released only following mast cell activation. In anaphylaxis, mediators are elevated in approximately 50% of patients presenting to emergency departments and in approximately 80% of fatal cases. Histamine elevation is better correlated than tryptase with the severity of the symptoms. However, histamine and tryptase may also be elevated in milder cases of acute allergic reactions with cutaneous reaction alone.

It is necessary to collect blood for histamine within 10 minutes to 1 hour following the reaction, as histamine levels peak at 5–10 minutes and decline rapidly to baseline by 15–60 minutes. Tryptase should be collected not later than 6 hours after the initial reaction. Peak levels of beta-tryptase occur at 1–2 hours and decline with a half-life of approximately 2 hours. If blood is collected in the initial 30 minutes after a reaction, tryptase elevation may not be detected. Tryptase is stable and can be identified in plasma or serum stored at room temperature for several days. Interpretation of tryptase levels is often difficult and is improved if baseline levels are available; however, in the majority of cases this is unlikely to be present. Comparison with a baseline may be helpful in cases with recurrent presentation where the diagnosis is uncertain.

The reliability of measuring mast cell tryptase post mortem has been questioned, because elevation of tryptase may be seen in control cases where death has occurred from other causes. Constitutionally raised levels of mast cell tryptase in the non-acute phase have been associated with an increased incidence of severe reactions following insect stings, suggesting that the patients most likely to develop anaphylaxis may have either an increased mast cell mass or an increased mast cell releasability.

The investigation of allergic triggers requires referral to a consultant allergist for performance of appropriate skin prick and RAST tests to determine the presence of specific IgE antibodies. It is essential that the results be interpreted in the light of the clinical history.

TREATMENT

Adrenaline (epinephrine)

Adrenaline is the cornerstone of treatment and should be given via the intramuscular rather than the subcutaneous route, due to better absorption from muscle.[8] The vasoconstriction associated with adrenaline, plus the relatively avascular nature of the subcutaneous fat, results in reduced circulating levels following subcutaneous administration. In children, peak adrenaline levels are reached 8 minutes after intramuscular and 34 minutes after a subcutaneous injection, and the peak levels are 20% higher after intramuscular injection. The preferred injection site for intramuscular administration is the upper outer side of the thigh, which gives significantly better absorption as compared with the deltoid muscle. Adrenaline does not always initially help the symptoms of anaphylaxis. In one out-of-hospital study, the conditions of one-quarter of patients were not improved by adrenaline.

- The dose of adrenaline is 0.01 mL kg^{-1} of 1 in 1000 intramuscular injection. Improvement should be seen within minutes. The dose should be repeated after 10–15 minutes if the effect is incomplete. Approximately one-third of patients will require more than one dose of adrenaline.
- In situations where there is severe circulatory compromise, adrenaline 1 in 10 000 0.1 mL kg^{-1} should be given by a slow intravenous injection over 10 minutes. Patients given intravenous adrenaline require cardiac, respiratory, and blood pressure monitoring.

- If there is an inadequate response, administer continuous intravenous adrenaline using a 1:100 000 (0.01 mg ml^{-1}) dilution at a rate of 0.1 µg kg^{-1} per minute, to a maximum of 1 µg kg^{-1} per minute, titrated according to the response.
- For refractory cardiorespiratory arrest, the initial intravenous dose is 10 µg (0.01 mg) per kg body weight of a 1 in 10 000 (wt/vol) dilution. Subsequent doses are 100 µg kg^{-1} (1 mL of 1 in 10 000) (wt/vol) every 3–5 minutes and, if still refractory, the dose may be increased to 200 µg kg^{-1}.
- Adverse effects of adrenaline include transient pallor, tremor, anxiety, palpitations, cardiac arrhythmias, headache, and nausea.

Airway and breathing

- Give high-flow oxygen by mask.
- For bronchospasm, give continuous nebulised salbutamol (0.5%).
- Nebulised adrenaline (epinephrine) 0.5 mL of 1% may be used in conjunction with systemic administration or alone for isolated mild upper airway obstruction.
- Intubate if obstruction is severe.

Circulation

- Achieve intravascular access with large-bore cannula.
- Treat hypotension with normal saline 20 mL kg^{-1}.
- If hypotension continues, give further colloid boluses of 10 mL kg^{-1} and repeat adrenaline (epinephrine) dose.
- In unrelenting hypotension, pressors such as dopamine or isoproterenol may be indicated.

Supplemental treatment

- The rationales for supplementary treatment with steroid and antihistamines are less well defined.
- If steroid is used, give methylprednisolone 1 mg kg^{-1} intravenously.
- Antihistamine: promethazine 1.0 mg kg^{-1} per dose (maximum 25 mg) orally or intravenously (slow) is given for symptomatic relief of urticaria.

Duration of treatment

- Duration of treatment is determined by clinical response. Repeated doses of adrenaline (epinephrine) are often required.

Admission

Admit or observe for at least 12 hours all patients with significant anaphylaxis, as a biphasic reaction with deterioration may occur following the initial episode.

The role of H₁ and H₂ blockers

The role of antihistamines is unclear. Antihistamine prophylaxis does not prevent subsequent anaphylactic reactions to antivenom but has a role in drug-induced and radiocontrast anaphylaxis. Addition of H_2 to H_1 antagonists produces no differences in blood pressure and symptoms; however, there is less urticaria at 2 hours in patients treated with combined H_1 and H_2 blockers.

Patients on beta-blockers

Glucagon 0.02 mg kg^{-1} intravenously has been used in an attempt to reverse beta blockade.

DIAGNOSIS

It is important to determine the cause of the anaphylactic reaction whenever possible.

Types of anaphylaxis

Common

Foods Severe life-threatening reactions are predominantly due to peanut and tree nut. In pre-school-age children, they may be due to egg and cow's milk proteins.

Drugs Many reactions, in particular those due to antibiotics, are IgE-mediated. Non–IgE-mediated anaphylactoid reactions due to drug-induced release of mast cell mediators are clinically indistinguishable from anaphylaxis. Drugs that can cause anaphylactoid reactions include opiates, muscle relaxants, radiocontrast media, and quinolone and vancomycin antibiotics. Non-steroidal anti-inflammatory drugs may induce anaphylaxis by interference with arachidonic acid metabolism, resulting in inhibition of prostaglandin synthesis and enhanced generation of bronchoconstrictive leukotrienes.

Stings Stings are most commonly due to bees and less often wasps. In Australia, jumper ant (*Myrmecia* spp.) stings are a common cause of anaphylaxis in endemic areas.

Latex Sensitisation occurs particularly in children with multiple exposure to latex-containing items during medical procedures. Children with spina bifida are particularly at risk due to multiple exposures following surgery and urinary tract catheterisation.

Less common

Idiopathic No triggers are identified, despite full investigation. Cases may present with laryngeal oedema as the only manifestation. The episodes can usually be controlled by regular antihistamine and, if necessary, the addition of alternate day steroids.[9] Psychogenic anaphylaxis has been classified as a variant of idiopathic anaphylaxis and should be considered in the differential diagnosis.[10]

Uncommon

Exercise-induced Symptoms of urticaria, angioedema, and stridor plus or minus hypotension develop during or soon after cessation of vigorous exercise.

Food-dependent exercise-induced In this situation, exercise induces symptoms only following ingestion of the relevant foodstuff, which has included wheat, celery, shellfish, oranges, and peaches. In some but not all cases, IgE sensitisation to the relevant food can be demonstrated.

Recurrent anaphylaxis

Anaphylaxis is frequently multiple, and in one series two-thirds of patients had three or more anaphylactic episodes. Failure to identify a definite cause is common, occurring in a third of individuals. Efforts should be made to identify unrecognised triggers. In children, this is often due to foods (generally peanut or tree nut products) contained in manufactured or processed foods. Some cases without an identifiable cause are due to idiopathic anaphylaxis.

Differential diagnosis

Anaphylaxis should be distinguished from other presentations that may cause confusion. These include:

- acute asthma
- vasovagal syncope
- urticaria or angioedema
- psychogenic stridor
- cardiovascular events
- seizure disorders
- mast cell mediator release in mastocytosis
- hereditary angioedema.

PREVENTION

Avoidance of the triggering allergen is critical. This will usually require referral to a consultant allergist for a definitive diagnosis and provision of appropriate instructions on avoidance.

The provision of emergency treatment in the form of self-injectable adrenaline (EpiPen) should be considered for all children who have presented with an anaphylactic reaction. This involves an assessment of the severity of the presenting reaction and the likelihood of re-exposure to the triggering allergen. Inadvertent re-exposure is most likely in the case of insect stings and foods, and least likely for drugs. The prescription of an EpiPen alone is not a satisfactory response to the risk of anaphylaxis. This is highlighted by the Australian evidence that less than a third of Epipens prescribed were used appropriately in a subsequent anaphylactic reaction.[11] Instruction in the indications for EpiPen use, demonstration of use with an EpiPen trainer device, and the provision of a clear and simple anaphylaxis action plan are essential.

Epipens are available in two fixed-dosage forms: EpiPen Junior (0.15 mg of adrenaline) for children 15–30 kg and EpiPen Adult (0.3 mg of adrenaline) for children greater than 30 kg. Although the manufacturer states that EpiPen

CONTROVERSIES

An unresolved question is which food-allergic children should be prescribed an EpiPen. Community concerns concerning the risk of food-induced anaphylaxis and death in children have multiplied in recent years. The provision of EpiPen Junior increased by 300% in Australia over the 5 years from 1998 to 2002, which is considerably greater than the increase in food allergy. Concurrent with the marked increase in EpiPen prescription has been controversy in the medical literature concerning benefits and risks, with some authorities expressing the opinion that these are over-prescribed and challenge to this by others.

Currently, there are no clear guidelines on which children should be prescribed an EpiPen. The great majority of fatalities are recorded in children over 5 years of age, despite the fact that food-allergic reactions are more common in pre-school children and frequently lessen with time. As the prescription of an EpiPen is primarily concerned with risk management, it is necessary to consider the factors that point to the likelihood of developing a severe life-threatening reaction.[13] These are:

- age over 5 year
- a history of respiratory tract involvement with the initial or subsequent reactions
- a history of asthma requiring preventive medication
- peanut or tree nut sensitivity
- reactions induced by traces or small amounts of allergen
- a strongly positive skin prick test (>8 mm).

Each factor should be considered, and the greater the number that are positive, the lower the threshold for prescribing an EpiPen. In addition, these factors need to be weighed in the light of the parental wishes and environmental circumstances. Providing the parents with a rational perspective on the remote risk of death is essential.

FUTURE DIRECTIONS AND RESEARCH

❶ Humanised monoclonal anti-IgE antibodies increase the threshold dose of food required to trigger symptoms in food-induced anaphylaxis. Regular administration is required. Unlike desensitisation, the treatment is not allergen-specific, and therefore offers promise in individuals with life-threatening reactions to multiple allergens.

❷ Characterisation of the molecular structure of allergenic epitopes may allow the construction of peptides for immunotherapy that trigger T-cell responses without binding IgE, thus significantly reducing the risks and increasing the efficacy of immunotherapy.

Adult is to be used for children greater than 30 kg, the American Academy of Asthma Allergy and Immunology recommends an EpiPen Adult for children >20 kg.[12]

Desensitisation should be considered for life-threatening reactions to bee stings. This will involve a series of injections with bee venom for a duration of 3 or more years. In general, bee venom desensitisation is not recommended for generalised cutaneous reactions in the absence of respiratory or cardiovascular involvement. If this form of therapy is considered, referral to a consultant allergist is indicated.

REFERENCES

1. Apter AJ, LaVallee HA 1994 How is anaphylaxis recognized? Archives of Family Medicine 38: 717–722
2. Neugut AI, Ghatak AT, Miller RL 2001 Anaphylaxis in the United States: An investigation into its epidemiology. Archives of Internal Medicine 1611: 15–21
3. Bock SA, Munoz-Furlong A, Sampson HA 2001 Fatalities due to anaphylactic reactions to foods. Journal of Allergy and Clinical Immunology 1071: 191–193
4. Boros CA, Kay D, Gold MS 2000 Parent reported allergy and anaphylaxis in 4173 South Australian children. Journal of Paediatrics and Child Health 361: 36–40
5. Kemp SF, Lockey RF 2002 Anaphylaxis: A review of causes and mechanisms. Journal of Allergy and Clinical Immunology 1103: 341–348
6. Lee JM, Greenes DS 2000 Biphasic anaphylactic reactions in pediatrics. Pediatrics 1064: 762–766
7. Lin RY, Schwartz LB, Curry A et al 2000 Histamine and tryptase levels in patients with acute allergic reactions: An emergency department-based study. Journal of Allergy and Clinical Immunology 106(1 Part 1): 65–71
8. Simons FE, Roberts JR, Gu X et al 1998 Epinephrine absorption in children with a history of anaphylaxis. Journal of Allergy Clinical Immunology 101(1 Part 1): 33–37
9. Ditto AM, Krasnick J, Greenberger PA et al 1997 Pediatric idiopathic anaphylaxis: Experience with 22 patients. Journal of Allergy and Clinical Immunology 1003: 320–326
10. Choy AC, Patterson R, Patterson DR et al 1995 Undifferentiated somatoform idiopathic anaphylaxis: Nonorganic symptoms mimicking idiopathic anaphylaxis. Journal of Allergy and Clinical Immunology 96(6 Part 1): 893–900
11. Gold MS, Sainsbury R 2000 First aid anaphylaxis management in children who were prescribed an epinephrine autoinjector device (EpiPen). Journal of Allergy and Clinical Immunology 106(1 Part 1): 171–176
12. AAAI Board of Directors 1994 The use of epinephrine in the treatment of anaphylaxis. Journal of Allergy and Clinical Immunology 944: 666–668
13. Kemp AS 2003 EpiPen epidemic: suggestions for rational prescribing in childhood food allergy. Journal of Paediatrics and Child Health 39(5): 372–375

FURTHER READING

Joint Task Force on Practice Parameters, American Academy of Allergy, Asthma and Immunology, American College of Allergy, Asthma and Immunology, and the Joint Council of Allergy, Asthma and Immunology 1998 The diagnosis and management of anaphylaxis. Journal of Allergy and Clinical Immunology 101(6 Part 2): S465–S528

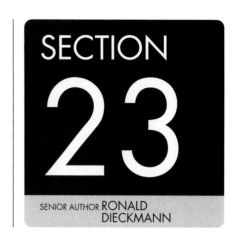

COMMON PROCEDURES

23.1 LENGTH-BASED PAEDIATRIC DRUG DOSING AND EQUIPMENT SIZING

RONALD DIECKMANN

BACKGROUND

Emergency treatment of infants and children is sometimes difficult because children of different ages require different sizes of equipment, doses of medications, and volumes of fluids. Errors are common when selecting appropriate equipment and medications in critical paediatric emergencies, and mistakes are especially frequent with doses of drugs that are powerful cardiovascular agents, such as adrenaline (epinephrine).

Length-based drug dosing and equipment sizing is an effective method for rapid selection of emergency treatments. Using length as a basis for ordering drugs and equipment is at least as accurate as weight, and length may be more accurate than weight for equipment sizing. It is also less likely to cause error in high-stress circumstances.

There are two methods of rapid drug dosing and equipment sizing: 1) a software paediatric decision support program; 2) a length-based resuscitation tape. Software decision support programs for desktop, or laptop computes or PDA are now available: by imprinting a child's length, the programs provide exact drug doses or equipment sizes for a vast range of medications and equipment.

The paediatric resuscitation tape or length-based resuscitation tape is a simple visual tool to measure lengths and to approximate weights in children. There are several commercial products available. One type of tape utilises colour-zones to cluster closely matched sizes of children into categories that have the same drug and equipment requirements. A disadvantage of the resuscitation tape is that only a few drugs are listed on the tape. Hence, a current additional comprehensive drug reference is imperative to address the multiple pharmacologic needs of children.

INDICATION

- Children requiring equipment, medication, or fluids, weighing 3–34 kg body weight (about age 10–12 years).

CONTRAINDICATIONS

- Premature infant weighing less than 3 kg.
- Child older than 10–12 years of age or weighing more than 34 kg body weight (use adult equipment and drug dosages).

EQUIPMENT

❶ Computer or PDA based paediatric decision support software (Fig. 23.1.1).

❷ Colour-coded paediatric resuscitation tape (Fig. 23.1.2). Store the tape in a place that is easily accessible, such as in the paediatric equipment kit, on the paediatric code cart, or on a wall hook. Lamination of the tape may preserve longevity. There are several different brands of length-based paediatric resuscitation tapes, and these have not been compared for speed, accuracy, or safety.

PREPARATION

❶ Place the patient in a supine position.
❷ Extend the patient's legs.
❸ Measure the child in centimeters.

Fig. 23.1.1   Decision support software allows instantaneous calculations of drug doses and equipment sizes, based upon patient length.

Fig. 23.1.2   Colour-coded paediatric resuscitation tape.

PROCEDURE DECISION SUPPORT SOFTWARE

After measuring the child's length, input into computer program and read drug doses and equipment sizes (Fig. 23.1.1).

TAPE

❶ Measure child's length – from head to heel – with the tape. Note and say weight in kilograms that corresponds to the child's measured length at the heel.

❷ If the child is longer than the tape, use adult equipment and medication doses.

❸ From the tape, identify appropriate equipment sizes (Fig. 23.1.2).

❹ From the tape, identify appropriate medication doses (Fig. 23.1.2).

COMPLICATIONS

- None.

TIPS

- Use the decision support software or resuscitation tape instead of attempting to estimate weight or calculate equipment sizes or drug doses.
- Measuring to the child's toes (instead of heel) will add a number of kilograms to the estimated weight and may result in over-sized equipment and over-large drug doses.

FURTHER READING

Black K, Barnett P, Wolfe R, Young S 2002 Are methods used to estimate weight in children accurate? Emergency Medicine (Fremantle) 14(2): 160–165

Davis D, Barbee L, Ririe D 1998 Paediatric endotracheal tube selection: A comparison of age-based and height-based criteria. American Association of Nurse Anesthetists Journal 66(3): 299–303

Hofer CK, Ganter M, Tucci M, Klaghofer R, Zollinger A 2002 How reliable is length-based determination of body weight and tracheal tube size in the paediatric age group? The Broselow tape reconsidered. British Journal of Anaesthetics 88(2): 283–285

Lubitz DS, Seidel JS, Chameides L, Luten RC, Zaritsky AL, Campbell FW 1988 A rapid method for estimating weight and resuscitation drug dosages from length in the paediatric age group. Annals of Emergency Medicine 17(6): 576–581

Luten RC, Wears RL, Broselow J, Zaritsky A, Barnett TM, Lee T, Bailey A, Vally R, Brown R, Rosenthal B 1992 Related articles, links abstract length-based endotracheal tube and emergency equipment in paediatrics. Annals of Emergency Medicine 21: 1454–1460

23.2 BAG-MASK VENTILATION

MICHELLE LIN

BACKGROUND

Bag-mask (BM) ventilation is the most important skill in paediatric airway management. This non-invasive manoeuvre for assisted, positive-pressure ventilation is effective treatment for most children with hypoventilation and hypoxia. A child with respiratory insufficiency may require only temporary assisted ventilation with BM. Some children in respiratory failure who require prolonged ventilation or airway protection may need tracheal intubation (Chapter 23.3).

In the BM setup, oxygen flows into a bag reservoir, through a pop-off valve, and into a mask, which forms a tight seal around the child's nose and mouth. Squeezing the bag administers oxygen under positive pressure to the lungs. While this manoeuvre does not fully protect the airway, as tracheal intubation, BM ventilation adequately provides emergent airway support during the acute decompensation period (Table 23.2.1). Additionally, Gausche et al[1] demonstrated that BM ventilation is as effective as tracheal intubation in the pre-hospital setting for airway management, regardless of the underlying aetiology. Thus, both pre-hospital and in-hospital practitioners must be comfortable and proficient in performing BM ventilation.

INDICATIONS

- Hypoventilation or apnoea.
- Respiratory failure.
- Hypoxia despite high-flow oxygen administration via a non-rebreather mask.

CONTRAINDICATIONS

- Do not perform BM ventilation in the setting of a complete airway obstruction. If this exists, first perform airway clearance and basic life-support manoeuvres. Then attempt foreign-body removal of the obstruction, if necessary, under direct laryngoscopy with Magill forceps.

Relative contraindication

- In the presence of a congenital diaphragmatic hernia or a tracheo-oesophageal fistula, BM can cause insufflation of the stomach and subsequent extra-pulmonary compression of the lungs. This may compromise adequate oxygenation and ventilation.

EQUIPMENT

❶ Appropriately-sized mask (Fig. 23.2.1).

❷ Self-inflating bag reservoir (Fig. 23.2.2).

❸ Oxygen saturation monitor.

PREPARATION

❶ Select an appropriately-sized mask and ventilation bag.

❷ Connect the oxygen tubing to the ventilation bag, and attach to the face mask.

❸ Begin 15 litres of oxygen per minute.

POSITIONING

Patient positioning is essential for successful BM ventilation. Maintain a supine, neutral neck position to keep the airway patent. Because of their large occiputs, infants and toddlers are prone to hyperflexion of the neck and consequently benefit from a small towel roll under their shoulders to achieve a neutral 'sniffing' position. Both hyperflexion and hyperextension of the neck may worsen airway obstruction, compromise ventilation, and increase risk of spinal injury.

PROCEDURE

❶ Perform the head-tilt and chin-lift manoeuvre to open the airway and lift the tongue away from the soft palate of the oropharynx. Proper positioning and suctioning of excess secretions will often relieve the respiratory compromise without BM ventilation.

❷ In the setting of trauma where spinal injury is a consideration, do not perform the head-tilt/chin-lift manoeuvre. Instead, provide in-line spinal immobilisation and perform a jaw-thrust manoeuvre to create a patent airway.

❸ If airway patency is still suboptimal, reposition and suction the patient. If

Table 23.2.1 Choosing BM ventilation versus tracheal intubation		
Sample patient case	BM	Intubation
Hypoventilation during procedural sedation	•	
Hypoventilation during post-ictal stage	•	
Hypoxia during asthma exacerbation despite non-rebreather oxygen mask	•	
Persistent hypoxia or hypoventilation despite BM		•
Partial airway obstruction (laryngeal burn, angio-oedema)		•
Cardiopulmonary arrest	•	•

Fig. 23.2.1 **Choosing the appropriately sized bag-mask.** Variously-sized, clear masks are available for all ages, ranging from neonates to adults. These masks have an inflated circumferential rim, which provides a tight seal to the patient's lower face. With an appropriately-sized mask, the superior aspect of the mask should rest over the patient's nasal bridge and the inferior aspect should rest over the cleft of the chin. Too large a mask may compress the patient's eyes, and too small a mask may occlude the nostrils and impede adequate oxygenation and ventilation.

Fig. 23.2.2 **Paediatric oxygen bag.** Supplemental, high-flow oxygen flowing into a bag serves as the oxygen reservoir for BM ventilation. A paediatric bag, which has a volume of 450–750 mL, is adequate to oxygenate and ventilate a small child. Alternatively, if a paediatric bag is not readily available, an adult bag, which has a volume of about 1200 mL, can also provide adequate oxygenation and ventilation. Be careful not to administer excessive tidal volumes with this larger bag.

still inadequate, insert an oropharyngeal or nasopharyngeal airway underneath the mask to lift the tongue from the posterior oropharynx (Chapter 23.3).

❹ In the *one-person BM technique*, place the mask on the patient's face and achieve an airtight seal over the mouth and nose. Using the non-dominant hand, place the thumb and index finger on the superior and inferior parts of the face mask, respectively. Cradle the tips of the other three fingers along the mandible and lift the jaw up toward the mask to create the seal. This is the 'E–C clamp' manoeuvre, based on the E-shape of the three fingers along the jaw and the C-shape of the thumb and index finger along the face mask (Fig. 23.2.3). In creating the seal, pull the jaw anteriorly rather than push the mask posteriorly into the patient's face. To ventilate, squeeze the oxygen reservoir bag using the dominant hand. For prolonged BM ventilation, use the little finger of your non-dominant hand (used for the E–C clamp) and apply cricoid pressure to reduce gastric air insufflation.

❺ In the *two-person technique*, place the mask on the patient's face and achieve an airtight seal over the mouth and nose. For operator #1, place the thumb and index finger of both hands on the superior and inferior parts of the face mask, respectively. Cradle the tips of the other three fingers of both hands along either side of the mandible and symmetrically lift the jaw up toward the mask to create a seal. This is a double 'E–C clamp' manoeuvre (Fig. 23.2.4). Again, pull the jaw anteriorly rather than push the mask posteriorly into the patient's face. Operator #2 ventilates the patient by squeezing the oxygen reservoir bag, and applies cricoid pressure for prolonged BM ventilation to reduce gastric air insufflation.

❻ Provide BM ventilation at a rate of 20, 30, and 40 inspirations per minute for the child, infant, and neonate, respectively. Squeeze and release the bag at an inspiratory-to-expiratory

Fig. 23.2.3   E-C clamp BM technique.

ratio of 1:2. A common error is to over-ventilate the patient with too rapid a rate.

❼ Provide a BM tidal volume of 8 mL kg^{-1} to oxygenate and ventilate the patient. As an equally effective alternative measure of appropriate ventilation volume, watch for bilateral chest rise and fall.

❽ In addition to visualisation, auscultation of bilateral breath sounds in the mid-axilla and improvement of the oxygen saturation both corroborate with adequate ventilation.

❾ With prolonged BM ventilation, decompress the likely over-distended stomach with an orogastric (OG) or nasogastric (NG) tube. This reduces the risk of emesis and consequent aspiration.

COMPLICATIONS

- Incorrect mask sizing causing inadequate ventilation or trauma to the eyes.
- Gastric insufflation and distension.
- Aspiration from emesis.
- Pneumothorax from poor lung compliance or excessive tidal volumes.
- Hypoxia.

TIPS

- In paediatric trauma cases requiring in-line spinal immobilisation, perform BM ventilation with the two-person technique. One operator focuses on providing an adequate mask seal, while the other operator focuses on squeezing the bag and maintaining spinal alignment. In comparison, a one-person BM technique often inadvertently extends the patient's neck while trying to achieve an adequate mask seal.
- When elevating the jaw anteriorly to form a mask seal with the third, fourth and fifth fingers, be sure to lift up along the bony mandible rather than the submandibular soft tissue. In addition to trauma, compressing the submandibular soft tissue may inadvertently occlude the airway.
- Some BM reservoir bags have a pop-off valve to prevent excessive positive pressure ventilation. This may inadequately ventilate a patient with low lung compliance. Occlude this valve to allow higher positive pressures during inspiration, while watching for chest rise.
- For the neonate and infant, assessing chest rise and fall for adequate BM tidal volume is subtle. The optimal viewing angle is from the patient's side at the level of his or her bed.
- In order to prevent the common complication of over-ventilating a patient, say aloud 'squeeze – release – release' repeatedly while correspondingly squeezing and releasing the bag. This approximates the correct ventilatory rate and inspiratory-to-expiratory ratio for the patient.

REFERENCES

1. Gausche M et al 2000 Effect of out-of-hospital paediatric endotracheal intubation on survival and neurological outcome: A controlled clinical trial. Journal of American Medical Association 283(6): 783–790

FURTHER READING

Brown RE 1997 Bag and mask ventilation. In: Dieckmann RA et al (eds) Paediatric emergency and critical care procedures. Mosby, St Louis, MO
Chameides L, Hazinski MF (eds) 1997 Paediatric Advanced Life Support. American Heart Association, Dallas, Texas
Dieckmann RA et al (eds) 2000 Paediatric Education for Prehospital Professionals. Jones & Bartlett Publishers, Sudbury, MA
Lee BS, Gausche-Hill M 2001 Paediatric airway management. Clinical Paediatric Emergency Medicine 2(2): 91–106
Zideman D et al 2001 Airways in paediatric and newborn resuscitation. Annals of Emergency Medicine 37(4 Suppl): S126–S136

Fig. 23.2.4   Double E–C clamp BM technique.

23.3 NASOPHARYNGEAL AND OROPHARYNGEAL AIRWAYS

MICHELLE LIN

BACKGROUND

Children have relatively large tongues, which may fall back and cause airway obstruction when there is loss of nasopharyngeal muscle tone, for instance, in patients who are post-ictal or overly sedated by drugs. Hypoxia and hypercarbia may develop. Non-invasive airway adjuncts, such as nasopharyngeal (NP) and oropharyngeal (OP) airways, can maintain a patent airway even when the tongue falls back against the posterior pharyngeal wall.

Structurally, an NP airway is hollow, made of latex or a latex-like substance, and has a slight curvature to approximate the curvature of the nasopharynx. The distal end has a bevel, which helps to tunnel through the nasopharyngeal soft tissue, but which may also cause inadvertent shearing trauma to the nasal septum. The proximal end of the NP airway has a wide flange to anchor the tube in place at the nostril orifice. Patients tolerate this airway adjunct better than an OP airway because it does not trigger the gag reflex.

In comparison, the OP airway is hollow, made of plastic, and has a slight curvature to approximate the curvature of the oropharynx. The distal end rests along the posterior tongue, which would trigger the gag reflex in an awake patient, and the proximal end has a wide flange to anchor the tube in place at the lips.

Airway adjuncts may allow adequate spontaneous ventilation and avert the need for bag-valve-mask ventilation or the more invasive technique of tracheal intubation.

INDICATIONS

- Airway obstruction.
- Respiratory decompensation.
- Seizures.

CONTRAINDICATIONS

NP airway

- Age less than one year old – the nares diameter is too small to introduce an NP airway.
- Nasal obstruction – attempting to introduce an NP airway into a nasal passage that is obstructed will be

unsuccessful and may cause traumatic epistaxis.
- Severe facial injury or suspicion for basilar skull fracture – a fractured cribriform plate may allow an NP airway to traverse incorrectly into the intracranial space rather than into the posterior oropharynx.

OP airway
- Intact gag reflex – because the OP airway tip rests on the posterior tongue, a patient with an intact gag reflex will likely vomit and aspirate gastric contents.

EQUIPMENT

❶ Lubricating jelly (for NP airway).
❷ Tongue blade (optional for OP airway).
❸ NP airway (Fig. 23.3.1).
❹ OP airway (Fig. 23.3.2).

PREPARATION

NP airway
Determine the correct NP airway size by one of three methods:

❶ Follow the recommendations on a length-based resuscitation tape.
❷ Choose an NP airway the length of which is equivalent to the distance from the patient's nasal tip to the tragus of the ear (Fig. 23.3.3).
❸ Choose an NP airway the outer diameter of which is equivalent to the nostril's inner diameter. Cut the length of the tube according to the length-measurement guide in Method 2.

OP airway
Determine the correct OP airway size by one of two methods:

❶ Follow the recommendations on a length-based resuscitation tape.
❷ Choose an OP airway the length of which is equivalent to the distance from the corner of the patient's mouth to the mandibular angle, as measured from the side of the patient's face (Fig. 23.3.4).

POSITIONING

❶ Place the patient in a supine, neutral 'sniffing' position.
❷ To prevent the patient's tongue from worsening the airway obstruction, perform a chin-lift manoeuvre. Use a jaw-thrust manoeuvre for the trauma patient in whom spinal immobilisation is crucial.

Fig. 23.3.1   Nasopharyngeal airway.

PROCEDURE

NP airway
❶ Pre-lubricate the NP airway before insertion.
❷ When inserting the NP airway in the *right nostril*, the bevel already points toward the septum and is of minimal risk for nasal septal trauma. Gently introduce the NP airway directly posteriorly into the patient's nostril until the flange rests just external to the nostril orifice.

Fig. 23.3.2   Oropharyngeal airway.

Fig. 23.3.3   Sizing the NP airway: nasal tip to tragus of ear.

❸ When inserting the NP airway in the *left nostril*, the bevel is pointed away from the septum. To avoid septal trauma, rotate the NP airway 180 degrees so that the bevel now points towards the septum. Insert the airway approximately 2 cm so that the tip

passes the septal border. When resistance is felt, re-rotate the NP airway 180 degrees into its original, correct orientation. Finish inserting the NP posteriorly into the nostril until it rests just external to the nostril orifice.

Fig. 23.3.4   Sizing the OP airway: corner of mouth to mandibular angle.

Fig. 23.3.5   Tracheal tube cut into an NP airway.

OP airway

The most common mistake in OP airway insertion is pushing the tongue further back while inserting it and thus worsening airway obstruction. Two methods will prevent this:

❶ With tongue blade – after pushing the tongue inferiorly with a tongue blade, slide the OP airway directly over it with the tip pointed inferiorly. Continue until the flange gently rests against the lips.

❷ Without tongue blade – rotate the OP airway 180 degrees such that the tip points superiorly and insert it into the mouth. When it contacts the hard palate, depress the tongue with the OP airway curvature. Insert the OP airway completely until the flange reaches the lips. Then re-rotate the airway 180 degrees so that the tip correctly points inferiorly and rests along the posterior tongue.

COMPLICATIONS

- Emesis and aspiration.
- Laryngospasm.
- Local trauma and bleeding.
- Worsening airway obstruction – when the OP airway is inappropriately long, it may directly occlude the posterior oropharynx; when it is inappropriately short, it may push the tongue further back, causing more airway obstruction.
- NP airway plug – the relatively small diameter of the NP airway makes it easily prone to occlusion with mucus, secretions, and blood.
- Intracranial placement of the NP airway.

TIPS

❶ Insert the NP airway directly posteriorly along the floor of the nose and not superiorly.
❷ Do not select too wide an NP tube, which may cause pressure necrosis to the nasal ala.

❸ If an NP airway is not immediately available, an alternative is to use a tracheal tube, normally used for intubations. First, choose the tube where the outer diameter is equivalent to the inner diameter of the patient's nostril. Second, trim the tube from the proximal end to the appropriate length as measured from the patient's nasal tip to the tragus of the ear. Leave the proximal ventilator adapter on the tracheal tube in place so that the tube is anchored at the nasal tip and does not accidentally slip beyond the nares (Fig. 23.3.5).

❹ Be sure the patient does not have a gag reflex before placing an OP airway.

FURTHER READING

Chameides L, Hazinski MF (eds) 1997 Paediatric advanced life support. American Heart Association, Dallas, Tx

Dieckmann RA et al (eds) 2000 Paediatric education for prehospital professionals. Jones & Bartlett Publishers, Sudbury, MA

Greenberg RS 2002 Facemask, nasal and oral airway devices. Anesthesiology Clinics of North America 20(4): 833–861

Shifrm SW 1997 Insertion of oral and nasal airways. In: Dieckmann RA et al (eds) Paediatric emergency and critical care procedures. Mosby, St Louis, MO

23.4 ENDOTRACHEAL TUBE AND ENDOTRACHEAL INTUBATION

MICHELLE LIN

BACKGROUND

Endotracheal intubation (TI) provides a definitive airway. Insertion of a tube between the vocal cords and into the trachea allows optimal management of the patient's oxygenation and ventilation, while also protecting the airway from aspiration. Depending on the preparation and skill of the practitioner, this procedure can be either life saving or life compromising. TI is the standard rescue procedure when BM ventilation is ineffective or insufficient.

The anatomy of the paediatric airway creates unique considerations during intubation as compared to adult intubation. Specifically, the differences are as follows:

❶ A paediatric patient has a relatively larger tongue, making visualisation of the vocal cords more difficult. Hence, pre-intubation positioning of the patient plays a crucial role in TI success.

❷ A paediatric patient has a wider and floppier epiglottis. Thus, in neonates and infants, use a straight laryngoscopic blade to achieve the best visualisation of the vocal cords. The blade moves the posteriorly-hanging epiglottis anteriorly, exposing the vocal cords.

❸ A paediatric patient has more anterior and cephalad vocal cords. A straight laryngoscopic blade provides the best direct line-of-sight to the anteriorly-positioned cords.

❹ The cricoid ring is the narrowest part of the airway in patients less than eight years old. This anatomical narrowing naturally secures the tracheal tube in place at the cricoid ring level without an air leak. Tracheal tubes therefore do not need to be cuffed. In contrast, adolescents and adults have a cylindrical-shaped rather than a funnel-shaped airway, and they do require cuffed tracheal tubes to help secure the tube and prevent an air leak.

❺ A paediatric patient has large adenoidal tissue and relatively small nares. Consequently, nasotracheal intubation in the paediatric population is technically difficult and has a high complication rate from traumatic bleeding, aspiration, and oesophageal intubation. These intubations also generally take a longer time to perform and require a patient who is awake and cooperative. The orotracheal route is the preferred approach.

In addition to proper positioning and equipment selection, successful emergent intubation often requires the administration of rapid sequence induction (RSI) medications. These medications provide transient sedation and neuromuscular relaxation during the procedure. Induction agents include ketamine, fentanyl, and midazolam, and neuromuscular paralysing agents include succinylcholine, rocuronium, and vecuronium. The advantages of RSI are two-fold. First, the patient will not instinctually struggle against noxious stimuli, such as the laryngoscopic blade and tracheal tube insertion. This optimises the chances of visualising the vocal cords. Second, the induction agents blunt the following autonomic reflexes.

❶ Bradycardia – patients less than five years old have a higher risk for bradyarrhythmias with direct laryngoscopy because of vagal nerve stimulation. Consequently they may require atropine prophylactically in their RSI drug regimen.

❷ Tachycardia and hypertension – induction medications attenuate this catecholamine response to laryngoscopy and intubation.

❸ Gag reflex – patients requiring emergency intubation benefit from RSI medications because they assumedly may have a full stomach the contents of which may regurgitate during intubation. By blunting the gag reflex by RSI, the risk of oesophageal reflux and pulmonary aspiration decreases.

The advantages of RSI agents, however, balance the primary disadvantage of persistent apnoea after a failed intubation. The practitioner must be aware that when patients receive these drugs, unsuccessful intubations may cause the patient to drop their oxygen saturation precipitously.

INDICATIONS

- Cardiopulmonary arrest.
- Respiratory failure or obstruction.
- Excessive work of breathing refractory to BM ventilation.
- Loss of the gag reflex.
- Need for prolonged ventilation or hyperventilation.

CONTRAINDICATIONS

- Adequate response to BVM ventilation with anticipated short requirement for assisted ventilation.
- Structural abnormalities, such as a large tongue haematoma, or massive facial injuries that require a tracheostomy or cricothyrotomy.
- Functioning tracheostomy.

EQUIPMENT

❶ Cardiopulmonary and oxygen saturation monitor.
❷ Rigid-tip suction catheter.
❸ BM and self-inflating bag.
❹ Laryngoscope (Figs 23.4.1, 23.4.2).
❺ Tracheal tube (Fig. 23.4.3).
❻ Tracheal tube stylet.
❼ Syringe for cuffed tracheal tube.

❽ Device for confirmation of intubation (Chapter 23.5).

❾ Strong adhesive tape for securing the tracheal tube.

❿ Bite block or oropharyngeal (OP) airway.

PREPARATION

Because many pieces of equipment require preparation, the 'SOAP ME' mnemonic is a helpful checklist reminder for the provider (Table 23.4.1).

Laryngoscope There are two types of blades to visualise the vocal cords – straight and curved. For the neonate or infant, use a straight blade to more easily visualise the anteriorly located vocal cords. For older patients, whose anatomy more resembles that of adults, use either a straight or a curved laryngoscopic blade.

Additionally, the laryngoscopic blades come in different sizes. To determine the correct size to use for a specific patient, either (1) use the length-based resuscitation tape (Chapter 23.1) or (2) use an age-based table (Table 23.4.2).

Endotracheal tube Cuffed endotracheal tubes serve to prevent an air leak around the tube. Because of the relatively funnel-shaped airway in patients less than eight years old, an uncuffed tube should be used. Conversely, for older patients and adults, cuffed tubes are essential because of their cylindrical-shaped airway. Without a balloon cuff, this airway shape is susceptible to significant air leaks. After choosing a cuffed or uncuffed tracheal tube, select the appropriate size of the tube for the patient (Table 23.4.3). The tubes sizes range from 1.0 to 9.0, representing the tube inner diameter in millimetres.

POSITIONING

The patient should be placed in a supine, neutral 'sniffing' position. For infants and small children, placing a small towel roll under the shoulders prevents the occiput from hyperflexing the neck and occluding the airway.

PROCEDURE

❶ Provide in-line spinal immobilisation, if necessary. Have an assistant stand at the side of the bed, and maintain the neutral position of the head and neck by cupping the patient's ears with both hands (Fig. 23.4.4).

Fig. 23.4.1 Curved (top) versus straight (bottom) laryngoscopic blades.

Fig. 23.4.2 Insertion of laryngoscopic blades. Laryngoscopes are available with either a straight blade end (A) or a curved blade end (B). The straight laryngoscopic blade should slide just 'under' or posterior to the epiglottis and elevate the tongue and epiglottis as a unit to visualise the vocal cords. Because of their floppy and large epiglottis, neonates and infants less than five years old require this straight blade for better visualisation of the cords. For older patients, both straight and curved blades are acceptable. When the curved laryngoscopic blade is used, the blade should rest in the vallecular space just anterior to the epiglottis and posterior to the base of the tongue. Lifting the laryngoscope up towards the ceiling elevates the vallecular space and the tongue as a unit, which indirectly lifts the epiglottis anteriorly to allow visualisation of the vocal cords.

Fig. 23.4.3   Tracheal tubes, uncuffed (top) and cuffed (bottom).

Table 23.4.1	Preparing the equipment - 'SOAP ME' mnemonic

1. Suction – turn the suction apparatus on and test the suction catheter.
2. Oxygenation equipment – test the self-inflating reservoir bag and bag-valve-mask (BVM) setup.
3. Airway equipment – select the appropriately sized tracheal tube and insert a stylet. Check the tracheal tube cuff integrity with a syringe, if applicable. Also obtain tube sizes slightly larger and smaller than expected, in case of unexpected anatomy. Obtain largyngoscopic blades slightly larger and smaller than anticipated, and test the blade lights. Finally, check the rescue airway devices in case of a failed intubation.
4. Pharmacologic agents – prepare rapid sequence intubation drugs.
5. Monitoring equipment – turn on the cardiopulmonary monitor, oxygen saturation monitor, and tracheal confirmation device.

Table 23.4.2	Laryngoscope size selection
Age	Blade type and size
Premature infant	Straight blade 0
Newborn to 2 years	Straight blade 1
2–6 years	Straight blade 2
6–12 years	Straight blade 2, Curved blade 2
Adolescent	Straight blade 2 or 3, Curved blade 3

Table 23.4.3	Tracheal tube size selection

- Option 1 – use a length-based resuscitation tape.
- Option 2 – the inner diameter of the tracheal tube should equal the patient's fifth fingernail.
- Option 3 – the tube size should equal the sum of the patient's age in years divided by four and added to four. For instance, an eight-year-old child requires a $(\frac{8}{4}) + 4$ tube, or a 6.0 tube.

❷ Pre-oxygenate the patient by BVM ventilation with 100% oxygen for 1–2 minutes. Be aware that the smaller the child, the faster rate of oxygen desaturation during the intubation procedure. If time permits, fully pre-oxygenate the patient.

❸ During pre-oxygenation and intubation, have an assistant apply gentle posterior pressure to the cricoid cartilage. This reduces oesophageal reflux of gastric contents and the risk of aspiration.

❹ Administer RSI medications and continue BVM ventilation until neuromuscular paralysis occurs.

❺ Grasp the laryngoscopic handle with the left hand and engage the blade so that the attached light bulb illuminates.

❻ Gently insert the laryngoscope starting from the patient's right side of the mouth and 'sweep' the tongue towards the left.

❼ Continue inserting the blade deep while lifting the laryngoscope anteriorly and inferiorly, trying to visualise the vocal cords.

❽ Suction any excessive secretions or gastric contents that are obscuring adequate visualisation of the epiglottis and vocal cords.

❾ Once the vocal cords are identified, use the right hand to insert the tracheal tube into the ride side of the mouth, aiming between the vocal cords.

❿ Watch the tube actually pass between the vocal cords and enter the trachea. The best way to determine whether a TI is successful (i.e. not an oesophageal intubation) is by direct visualisation. Other confirmatory modalities may provide false and misleading information.

⓫ Insert the tube to the appropriate length (Table 23.4.4).

⓬ Inflate the cuff, if applicable.

⓭ Attach the oxygen bag to the tracheal tube and ventilate the patient, watching for equal chest rise with each bag insufflation.

⓮ Listen for equal breath sounds in bilateral axilla and the absence of breath sounds in the epigastrium.

⓯ Check for successful placement of the tracheal tube by a confirmatory device (see Chapter 23.5).

⓰ Obtain a post-intubation chest radiograph to check for successful tube placement and adequate depth of tube insertion. The tube should end 1–2 cm above the carina.

⓱ Secure the tube in place with adhesive tape.

⓲ Insert a bite block or OP airway to prevent the patient from chewing off the tracheal tube.

COMPLICATIONS

- Traumatic injury to lips, teeth, oropharynx, larynx, vocal cords and oesophagus.
- Incorrect insertion of tube into oesophagus or intracranially.
- Emesis and aspiration.

COMMON PROCEDURES

Fig. 23.4.4   Spinal immobilisation by assistant.

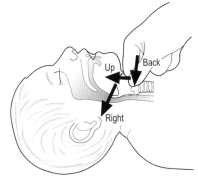

Fig. 23.4.5   Improving vocal cord visualisation – BURP manoeuvre.
Using your right hand (non-laryngoscope hand), manipulate the external cricoid cartilage with Back (posterior), Up (superior), and Rightward Pressure. This essentially moves the vocal cords towards the right and out from 'under' the overhanging epiglottis.

Table 23.4.4   Determining the correct tracheal tube insertion depth

- Option 1 – insert the tracheal tube (3 × tracheal tube size) centimetres as marked at the patient's teeth. For instance, a 5.0 tube correlates with a 15 cm insertion depth.
- Option 2 – there exists a black double line drawn circumferentially about 2–5 cm from the tube's distal tip. Insert the tracheal tube until this double line rests at the level of the vocal cords.

- Increased intracranial, intra-ocular, and intragastric pressures.
- Cervical spinal injury.
- Dysrhythmia.
- Hypertension or hypotension.
- Hypoxia and/or hypercarbia.
- Pain and anxiety.
- Dislodgement of tracheal tube during movement.

TIPS

- Equipment failure is an unnecessary complication with potentially devastating consequences. Be sure to test the functionality of the suction apparatus, the brightness of the laryngoscope light bulb, and the integrity of the tracheal tube cuff prior to intubation.
- Anticipating a failed initial intubation reduces the complication rate in tracheal intubation. Prepare variously-sized laryngoscopes, slightly larger and smaller tracheal tubes, and failed-airway alternatives at the bedside.
- During pre-oxygenation and intubation, applying cricoid pressure too aggressively may not only occlude the oesophagus but also the airway.
- While looking for the vocal cords with the laryngoscope, a common mistake is to use the patient's teeth as a fulcrum for the blade. Beware of fracturing the patient's teeth.
- To help visualise a patient's vocal cords, which are being obscured by a floppy epiglottis, use the BURP manoeuvre (Fig. 23.4.5).
- Because of the short trachea in the paediatric population, a common mistake during intubation is inserting the tracheal tube too deep, resulting in a right mainstem intubation.
- Also, because of the short trachea in paediatric population, the tracheal tube may easily dislodge from its position in the airway. Be vigilant about securing the tube at all times, but especially during transport or with any movements. Frequently recheck its position.

FURTHER READING

Chameides L, Hazinski MF (eds) 1997 Paediatric advanced life support. American Heart Association, Dallas, Tx
Dieckmann RA et al (eds) 2000 Paediatric education for prehospital professionals. Jones & Bartlett Publishers, Sudbury, MA
Gnauck K et al 1994 Emergency intubation of the paediatric medical patient: Use of anesthetic agents in the ED. Annals of Emergency Medicine 23(6): 1242–1247
Knill RL 1993 Difficult laryngoscopy made easy with a BURP. Canadian Journal of Anaesthetics 40(3): 279–282
Lee BS, Gausche-Hill M 2001 Paediatric airway management. Clinical Paediatric Emergency Medicine 2(2): 91–106
McAllister JD, Gnauck KA 1999 Rapid sequence intubation of the paediatric patient. Fundamentals of practice. Paediatric Clinics of North America 46(6): 1249–1284
Moynihan RJ et al 1993 The effect of cricoid pressure on preventing gastric insufflation in infants and children. Anesthesiology 78(4): 652–656
Stoelting RK 1977 Circulatory changes during direct laryngoscopy and tracheal intubation: Influence of duration of laryngoscopy with or without prior lidocaine. Anesthesiology 47(4): 381–84
Thompson A 1997 Paediatric emergency airway management. In: Dieckmann RA et al (eds) Paediatric emergency and critical care procedures.: Mosby, St Louis, MO
Tintinalli JE, Claffey J 1981 Complications of nasotracheal intubation. Annals of Emergency Medicine 10(3): 142–144

23.5 CONFIRMATION OF INTUBATION

MICHELLE LIN

BACKGROUND

Confirming correct placement of the tracheal tube is crucial because of the high morbidity and mortality of an inadvertent and unrecognised oesophageal intubation. The most accurate means of assuring success is by visualising the tracheal tube between the vocal cords and into the trachea. A successful tracheal intubation (TI) is also highly likely when condensation appears in the plastic tracheal tube during assisted-ventilation, when breath sounds are heard in both axillae but not in the epigastrium, when the pulse oximetry is 100%, and when the chest cavity rises and falls with positive-pressure ventilation. At times, however, these findings can be equivocal especially in children. The clinical exam is notoriously deceptive in determining correct tracheal tube placement, and it is imperative to use at least one of the following techniques for every intubated patient.

❶ Oesophageal aspiration. An oesophageal aspirator is a large syringe or a self-inflating bulb (Fig. 23.5.1), which attaches to the proximal end of the tracheal tube. The aspirator differentiates between an oesophageal versus a tracheal placement because the oesophagus is a collapsible structure under negative pressure, while the trachea is not. Successful air aspiration is highly associated with trachea placement. It has been determined that the oesophageal aspiration modality has a sensitivity of 99% and specificity of 100% in confirming endotracheal tube placement in patients weighing more than 20 kg.

- Oesophageal intubation. When air is aspirated from the tracheal tube, significant airflow resistance suggests an oesophageal intubation, because of oesophageal wall collapse. The large syringe or self-inflating bulb will not fill with air to full capacity.
- Tracheal intubation. When air is aspirated from the tracheal tube, there will be no resistance to 30–40 mL of airflow if the tube indeed lies in the trachea.

❷ End-tidal colorimetric capnometry (Fig. 23.5.2): The capnometer attaches to the proximal end of the tracheal tube and detects the presence of CO_2 within the tube. The capnometer will display a yellow (CO_2 present) or purple (CO_2 absent) colour in the indicator window, which generally correlates with a tracheal or oesophageal intubation, respectively. Multiple studies find that a yellow colour change has a 100% positive predictive value for correct tracheal tube placement. When used for a poorly-perfused patient (e.g. cardiac arrest), however, there will often be no yellow colour change because of expected low CO_2 levels. This is the primarily limitation when using this modality. Table 23.5.1 provides a mnemonic to help remember the colour scheme.

❸ Digital capnography (Fig. 23.5.3). This latest technology continuously detects and displays the partial pressure of CO_2 at the proximal end of the tracheal tube. In adult cardiac arrest patients, a $PCO_2 < 5$ mmHg correlates with an extremely poor prognosis. Digital capnography will be the standard for all intubations confirmations in the near future.

- Tracheal intubation. With each exhalation and inhalation, a characteristic waveform, showing the rise, plateau, and fall of CO_2 levels, confirms correct positioning of the tube in the trachea.
- Oesophageal intubation. With each exhalation and inhalation, an unchanging, flat waveform demonstrates the absence of CO_2 and thus the misplacement of the tracheal tube into the oesophagus.

INDICATIONS

- All intubated patients.

CONTRAINDICATIONS

- Do not use an adult-sized colorimetric capnometry device on intubated patients weighing less than 15 kg, because the device adds a significant dead-space volume for the neonate to rebreathe CO_2. Instead, attach a paediatric-sized capnometer for these patients.
- Use caution with oesophageal aspiration on patients weighing less than 20 kg. Several studies, however, suggest that oesophageal aspiration

Fig. 23.5.1   Oesophageal bulb (left) and aspirator (right).

COMMON PROCEDURES

Fig. 23.5.2   Colorimetric capnometer.

Table 23.5.1   End-tidal colour capnometer – interpreting the colour

(Presenting complaint)

- If you see Yellow, then 'Yes' – there is CO_2 return. At least 20 mmHg of CO_2 is detectable. Several studies show a 100% positive predictive value of a yellow indicator colour with a tracheal space intubation (rather than an oesophageal).
- If you see Purple, then there is a 'Problem' – there is no CO_2 return. A TI is unlikely, unless the patient has extremely poor perfusion, such as during asystole. If a purple colour is displayed, less than 4 mmHg of CO_2 is detectable.
- If you see an intermediate 'Tan' colour, then 'Think about it', because the tube could be sitting in the trachea or the oesophagus. The capnometer is sensing between 4–15 mmHg of CO_2. This equivocal finding requires direct laryngoscopy re-visualisation of the tube's placement to help determine placement.

Fig. 23.5.3   Digital capnography instrument (A) and typical waveform reading (B).

may still be safe at a lower weight limit of 4 kg, because the resting lung volume is still greater than 50 cc, which is the typical volume in an oesophageal aspirator.

EQUIPMENT

1. Oesophageal aspiration syringe or bulb (Fig. 23.5.1).
2. End-tidal colorimetric capnometer (Fig. 23.5.2).
3. Digital capnography (Fig. 23.5.3).

PREPARATION AND POSITIONING

- Prepare at least one confirmation device for bedside use before the patient is intubated so that immediate confirmation is available.

- Specific for the colorimetric capnometer, open the packaging for this disposable device. Check that the unit is dry and initially displays a purple colour in the indicator window to ensure proper functioning.
- Specific for digital capnography, be sure that the device is plugged in and turned on. Blowing across the capnography tubing tests the monitoring and sensing function.

PROCEDURE

Oesophageal aspiration

1. Expel all the air out of the oesophageal syringe or bulb, and attach it to the proximal end of the tracheal tube just after intubation. Inadvertently instilling air into the tracheal tube with the syringe or bulb may cause a falsely reassuring aspiration result.
2. Slowly aspirate air over five seconds.
3. If the tracheal tube is correctly positioned in the trachea, there will be no resistance during aspiration.
4. If the tracheal tube is incorrectly positioned in the oesophagus, there will be resistance during aspiration. Reposition the tube under direct laryngoscopy.

End-tidal colorimetric capnometer

1. Attach the capnometer in series with the entire ventilation system between the tracheal tube and the bag-valve device. Ventilation can continue through the capnometer.
2. After ventilating the patient over six times, check the colour of the capnometer indicator window during the exhalation phase. Initially purple in colour when attached, exhalation phases correlate with a yellow colour change.
3. Recall that a yellow colour confirms correct TI because it indicates the presence of CO_2.
4. Secure the capnometer in place for continuous monitoring while the patient transfers to the intensive-care unit.

Digital capnography

❶ Connect the digital capnography tubing to the distal end of the bag-valve device. The air in the tracheal tube is now contiguous with the air in this tubing.

❷ Ventilate the patient and observe the live-time waveforms of CO_2 return during exhalation. The absence of CO_2 indicates a failed intubation.

COMPLICATIONS

• There are no direct complications to the patient by using these devices. Indirectly, however, the misinterpretation of their findings may cause the practitioner to incorrectly change patient management.

TIPS

❶ Check tube placement after every intubation and after any patient movement, such as during transport, because the tracheal tube can easily shift into the oesophagus.

❷ Use a paediatric-sized colorimetric capnometer for patients less than 15 kg to decrease the volume of dead space in the ventilatory circuit.

❸ When intubating a poorly perfused patient, using an oesophageal aspirator is more accurate than the end-tidal colorimetry capnometer or digital capnography, because the tracheal tube's CO_2 level is extremely low. In this case, the latter instruments, which rely on CO_2 levels, may only equivocally confirm tracheal tube placement. The oesophageal aspirator, however, functions based on the anatomical differences between the collapsible oesophagus and the semi-rigid trachea, independent of expired CO_2 levels. Thus, with low perfusion states, the aspirator provides a more accurate confirmation of correct tracheal tube placement.

FURTHER READING

Anderson KH, Schultz-Leban T 1994 Oesophageal intubation can be undetected by auscultation of the chest. Acta Anaesthesiology Scandinavia 38: 580–582

Bhende MS et al 1992 Utility of an end-tidal carbon dioxide detector during stabilization and transport of critically ill children. Paediatrics 89: 1042–1044

Bhende MS et al 1992 Validity of a disposable end-tidal CO_2 detector in verifying endotracheal tube placement in infants and children. Annals of Emergency Medicine 21: 142–145

Burnett YL et al 1995 Efficacy of the self-inflating bulb in verifying tracheal tube placement in children. Anesthetic Analg 80: S63 [abstract]

Dieckmann RA et al (eds) 2000 Paediatric Education for Prehospital Professionals. Jones & Bartlett Publishers, Sudbury, MA

Marley CD Jr et al 1995 Evaluation of a prototype oesophageal detection device. Academic Emergency Medicine 2(6): 503–507

Sharieff GQ et al 2003 The self-inflating bulb as an oesophageal detector device in children weighing more than twenty kilograms: A comparison between two techniques. Academic Emergency Medicine 41(5): 623–629

Ward KR, Yealy DM 1998 End-tidal carbon dioxide monitoring in emergency medicine. Part 1. Basic principles. Academic Emergency Medicine 5(6): 628–636

Wee MYK 1998 The oesophageal detector device: Assessment of a new method to distinguish oesophageal from tracheal intubation. Anaesthesia 43(1): 27–29

Zideman D et al 2001 Airways in paediatric and newborn resuscitation. Annals of Emergency Medicine 37(4 Suppl): S126–S136

23.6 THE SURGICAL AIRWAY

JUDITH KLEIN

BACKGROUND

The paediatric airway is distinct from that of the adult. The epiglottis is floppy and the larynx is shorter, more anterior, and more cephalad. The larynx is narrower and therefore more prone to obstruction by oedema, scarring, fluids, or foreign bodies. The cartilage of the larynx is also softer, which makes palpation of landmarks on the skin more difficult. The cricoid ring is the only spot where cartilage encircles the paediatric trachea, and it is also the narrowest portion of the airway (Fig. 23.6.1)

The vast majority of paediatric airway emergencies can be readily managed with bag-valve-mask (BVM) ventilation and/or tracheal intubation (TI). Rarely, a child presents with complete airway obstruc-tion or anatomic abnormalities, and ventilation with BVM or TI is impossible. In these situations, a surgical airway may be necessary to provide life-saving oxygenation and ventilation to avoid anoxic brain injury. Surgical airways in children include: needle cricothyroidotomy; surgical crico-thyroidotomy; and, rarely, tracheostomy. Placing a needle, catheter or tube directly into the trachea through the neck will temporarily relieve airway obstruction or bypass anatomic abnormalities.

In children under the age of five years, the membrane between the thyroid cartilage and the cricoid cartilage, the cricothyroid membrane (Fig. 23.6.1), is extremely small. For this group, needle cricothyroidotomy is easier than surgical cricothyroidotomy. While the needle technique will provide emergency oxygenation,

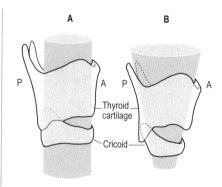

Fig. 23.6.1 Locating the cricoid membrane. Comparison of adult (A) and paediatric (B) airways. Note funnel shape of paediatric airway with narrowest portion at cricoid ring.

it may not provide adequate ventilation, especially over time. Even a jet 'ventilator', a rescue device that attaches to the needle and provides intermittent bursts of high-pressure oxygen to simulate the normal respiratory cycle, may not allow for adequate ventilation and clearance of CO_2.

In children five years and over, surgical cricothyroidotomy is easier and more effective, because it creates a larger conduit and allows both immediate oxygenation and ventilation via a bag-valve device. Tracheotomy in a young child is extremely difficult to perform emergently and is rarely indicated in the ED.

INDICATIONS

- Failure to ventilate with BVM and/or TI.
- Obstructed or disrupted larynx.

Table 23.6.1 lists situations in which these indications occur. The most common circumstances in which intubations fail are the presence of massive nasopharyngeal haemorrhage, large tongue haematoma, laryngeal spasm, laryngeal stenosis, or obstruction of the airway by a foreign body that cannot be removed.

Table 23.6.1   Situations requiring cricothyroidotomy

Trauma
- Laryngeal fracture
- Airway burns
- Massive haemorrhage
- Foreign body
- Subglottic stenosis (late)
- Burn contractures (late)

Congenital abnormalities
- Laryngeal atresia/stenosis/clefts
- Tracheoesophageal fistula
- Pierre-Robin syndrome
- Treacher-Collins syndrome

Cervical spine abnormalities
- Trisomy 21 syndrome
- Klipel-Feil malformation
- Torticollis

Inflammatory/infectious
- Severe croup
- Epiglottis
- Bacterial tracheitis
- Retropharyngeal abscess
- Cricoarytenoid arthritis

Laryngeal spasm

CONTRAINDICATIONS

- Presence of a secure airway.
- Traumatic destruction of the cricothyroid membrane.
- Transection of the trachea with retraction of the distal segment.
- Surgical cricothyroidotomy is relatively contraindicated in children under the age of five years. In this group, perform needle cricothyroidotomy.

NEEDLE CRICOTHYROIDOTOMY

EQUIPMENT

Table 23.6.2 lists the equipment for this procedure, which can be divided into three categories:

❶ Oxygen source. A transtracheal jet ventilator device is ideal. It provides high-pressure 100% oxygen (50 psi) in intermittent bursts, which allows *more* time for passive CO_2 exhalation (Fig. 23.6.2). Alternatively, use a bag-valve device connected to 15 L min^{-1} of wall oxygen.

❷ Adaptors. The jet ventilator device connects directly to the catheter at the neck. To use the bag-valve system, attach a 3 mm paediatric tracheal tube adapter with one end connected to the bag-valve device and the other to the end of the cricothyroidotomy catheter. Alternatively, set up a ventilation

Table 23.6.2   Equipment for needle cricothyroidotomy

Oxygen source
- Jet ventilator (50 psi)
- Bag-valve-mask device attached to 15 L min^{-1} wall oxygen

Adaptor
- 3 mm endotracheal tube adaptor
- 3 cm^3 syringe barrel and 8.0 mm endotracheal tube

Catheter
- 14-gauge catheter over a needle
- 3 cm^3 syringe

system with a 3 mL syringe and an 8 mm tracheal tube that attaches to the bag-valve device (Fig. 23.6.3).

❸ Needle/cannula. A 14G over the needle catheter.

PREPARATION

❶ Since children have relatively large occiputs, place a shoulder roll transversely to prevent hyperflexion of the neck and improve visualisation of the anterior neck anatomy.

❷ If time allows, prepare the skin with povidone-iodine solution.

PROCEDURE

❶ Palpate the hyoid bone high in the neck and move caudally to identify the thyroid and cricoid cartilages (Fig. 23.6.4A).

❷ Stabilise the cartilage using the thumb and index finger of the non-dominant hand.

❸ Insert a 14G over the needle catheter attached to a 3 cm^3 syringe just superior to the cricoid cartilage (Fig. 23.6.4B). Angle the catheter caudally at about a 45° angle to the skin.

❹ Apply continuous backpressure to the syringe barrel. A rush of air into the syringe confirms entry into the

Fig. 23.6.2   Transtracheal jet ventilator device.

Fig. 23.6.3   Using a 3.0 mm tracheal tube or an 8 mm tracheal tube into a 3 mL syringe hub as a connector.

Cricothyroid membrane

Fig. 23.6.4   Inserting the needle through the membrane.

trachea. Alternatively, fill the syringe with saline to use as an indicator. The marker of entry into the trachea is the presence of air bubbles in the syringe.

❺ Advance the catheter into the trachea and remove the needle and syringe. Do not let go of the catheter until it

is secured or an alternative airway is obtained.

❻ If a jet ventilator device is available, attach it directly to the catheter. If this device is not available, attach a bag-valve system to high-flow (15 L min^{-1}) wall oxygen. Place an adaptor

between the catheter and the bag-valve device. Either attach a 3 mm endotracheal tube adaptor directly onto the catheter or attach an 8 mm endotracheal tube in a 3 mL syringe barrel.

❼ With a jet ventilator, administer 100% oxygen at 20 bursts per minute with an approximate I:E ratio of 1:4 to allow for passive exhalation. If a bag-valve device is used, provide 20 'breaths' per minute with the same I:E ratio.

COMPLICATIONS

- Bleeding, but it is rarely massive.
- Inappropriate placement of a needle can cause injury to:
  The larynx and vocal cords
  Great vessels of the neck
  Nerves
  Oesophagus.
- High-pressure oxygen can also cause significant barotrauma resulting in extensive subcutaneous emphysema, pneumothorax, and pneumomediastinum.

TIPS

- Needle cricothyroidotomy is a temporising measure that may provide enough ventilation for about thirty minutes. Immediately consider other airway options.
- Remember to allow adequate time for passive exhalation to prevent barotrauma.
- Do *not* let go of the catheter until an alternative airway is established.

SURGICAL CRICOTHYROIDOTOMY

EQUIPMENT

Table 23.6.3 lists the equipment for surgical cricothyroidotomy.

Several commercial kits contain all equipment for a cricothyroidotomy tube using the guidewire or Seldinger technique. Other useful instruments include a tracheal hook and a tracheal dilator.

PREPARATION

❶ Expose the thyroid and cricoid cartilage by placing a roll under the child's shoulders.

❷ If time permits, prepare the skin with povidone-iodine solution and infiltrate the skin with lidocaine with adrenaline (epinephrine) to provide local anaesthesia and hemostasis.

Table 23.6.3   Equipment for surgical cricothyroidotomy

- Frazier tip suction
- Scalpel
- Haemostat
- Tracheostomy or endotracheal tube
- Oxygen delivery system
- Tracheostomy suction

Optional
- Povidone-iodine solution
- Lidocaine with adrenaline (epinephrine)
- Tracheal hook
- Tracheal dilator

Fig. 23.6.5   Making the surgical incision in the skin.

PROCEDURE

❶ Palpate the hyoid bone high in the neck and move caudally to identify the thyroid and cricoid cartilages (Fig. 23.6.4A).

❷ Stabilise the larynx by placing thumb and forefinger of the non-dominant hand on either side of the thyroid cartilage.

❸ Make a midline vertical incision in the skin from thyroid cartilage to cricoid cartilage (Fig. 23.6.5). Expose the cricothyroid membrane via blunt dissection with haemostats.

❹ Make a horizontal incision in the cricothyroid membrane carefully avoiding inserting the scalpel too far and lacerating the posterior aspect of the larynx.

❺ Insert the haemostat into the airway next to the scalpel to hold the space and widen the opening.

❻ Use a tracheal hook, if available, to maintain the opening and provide traction cranially while inserting the tube caudally (Fig. 23.6.6).

❼ If a tracheostomy tube of the appropriate size is not available, use an endotracheal tube of the same calibre. Trim the length of the tube to $\frac{3}{2}$ of its diameter in centimetres (e.g. 4.0 ETT (cut to $\frac{3}{2} \times 4 = 6$ cm).

❽ Attach a bag-valve device and ventilate the patient. Do not let go of the tube until it has been secured to the patient's neck.

The guidewire or Seldinger technique is an alternative to surgical placement of a cricothyroidotomy tube.

❶ Position the patient for surgical cricothyroidotomy.

❷ Identify the cricothyroid membrane and prepare the skin with povidone-iodine solution.

❸ Insert the needle mounted on a syringe through the cricothyroid membrane.

❹ Angle caudally at 45° to the skin with the bevel of the needle up.

❺ Once air rushes into the syringe, pass the J-tipped guidewire through the needle and remove the needle.

❻ Make a stab incision over the needle through the skin and membrane.

❼ Insert the catheter and dilator over the guidewire into the trachea and remove both the wire and the dilator.

❽ Provide ventilation via a bag-valve device.

COMPLICATIONS

- Bleeding.
- Tube misplacement, resulting in hypoxia and subcutaneous emphysema.
- Laryngeal, oesophageal, or neurovascular injury.
- Barotrauma, which can result in pneumothorax or pneumomediastinum.
- Significant late complications include voice change due to vocal cord damage and subglottic stenosis.

TIPS

- If the cricothyroid membrane is not visible with the initial vertical incision, extend it.

Fig. 23.6.6   Inserting the cricothyroidotomy tube.

- Do not cut into the larynx blindly as this will increase the rate of complications.
- Have suction readily available for any bleeding into the trachea.
- Avoid using too large a tube. This can lead to laryngeal fracture.
- Size the catheter by using a length-based resuscitation tape.
- If a child requires prolonged ventilation, establish a definitive airway (tracheal intubation or tracheostomy) as soon as possible.

FURTHER READING

Bower CM 1997 The surgical airway. In: Dieckmann RA, Fiser DH, Selbst SM (eds) Paediatric emergency and critical care procedures. Mosby, St Louis, MO
Granholm T, Farmer DL 2001 The surgical airway. Respiratory Care Clinics North America 7(1): 13–23
Mace SE 1998 Cricothyrotomy and translaryngeal jet ventilation. In: Roberts JR, Hedges JR (eds) Clinical procedures in emergency medicine, 3rd edn. WB Saunders, Philadelphia, PA
Peak DA, Roy S 1999 Needle cricothyroidotomy revisited. Paediatric Emergency Care 15(3): 224–226
Yealy DM, Plewa MC, Steward RD 1991 An evaluation of cannulae and oxygen sources for paediatric jet ventilation. American Journal of Emergency Medicine 9(1): 20–23

23.7 NEEDLE THORACOSTOMY

JUDITH KLEIN

BACKGROUND

Normally, the visceral and parietal pleura are closely adherent to one another. However, if either surface is violated, air enters into the potential space between visceral and parietal pleura, creating a simple pneumothorax (Fig. 23.7.1). This typically occurs in the setting of blunt or penetrating trauma. Occasionally, spontaneous pneumothorax occurs, as with excessive air trapping in an asthmatic child. If enough air collects, a tension pneumothorax can develop in which pressure in the space shifts the mediastinum, impedes venous return to the heart, and decreases cardiac output (Fig. 23.7.2). Another pathophysiologic mechanism for tension pneumothorax occurs when a patient with a simple pneumothorax is intubated – positive pressure ventilation will force air into the pleural space resulting in a tension pneumothorax. Tension pneumothorax can progress to shock and cardiopulmonary arrest.

The typical clinical scenario for tension pneumothorax is the child who experiences a penetrating injury to the chest wall or back. A sucking chest wound (open pneumothorax) may be present. The classic adult clinical findings of unilateral decreased air movement and trachea shift may not be readily detectable in children. More commonly, the clinical signs are tachypnea, oxygen desaturation, retractions, flaring, grunting and shock. Once tension pneumothorax develops, progression to shock and cardiopulmonary arrest can be rapid.

Needle evacuation of the air between the visceral and parietal pleura and conversion of the tension pneumothorax to an open pneumothorax will re-expand the lung and improve venous return and cardiac output. Needle thoracostomy is a temporising procedure. Immediately after needle thoracostomy, insert a chest tube to provide ongoing drainage in a closed system (Chapter 23.8). The risk of not performing needle thoracostomy in a child spiralling towards death from a tension pneumothorax is far greater than the risk of performing the procedure in a child without a pneumothorax.

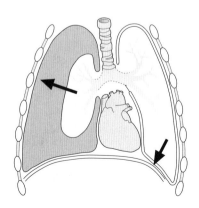

Fig. 23.7.1   Simple pneumothorax.

INDICATIONS

- Blunt or penetrating trauma with signs of tension pneumothorax.
- Chest X-ray evidence of a tension pneumothorax in a child in respiratory distress for any reason.

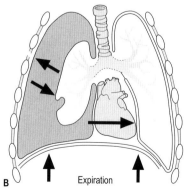

Fig. 23.7.2   Tension pneumothorax.
(A) Inspiration, (B) Expiration.

- Suspected tension pneumothorax in an intubated patient who is rapidly deteriorating (e.g. hypotension, hypoxia).
- Pulseless electrical activity (PEA) in the setting of trauma or asthma.

CONTRAINDICATIONS

- A stable child with a simple pneumothorax, not under tension.
- There is no absolute contraindication to needle thoracostomy in a child with possible tension pneumothorax and shock. While preparing for open thoracotomy in the ED, placing a needle in the pleural space will not cause further deterioration.
- If a skin infection is present at the preferred needle site, select an alternative location.

EQUIPMENT

❶ 14-gauge catheter over a needle.
❷ 30 mL syringe.
❸ Povidone-iodine solution.

Fig. 23.7.3 Anatomy of the ribs and intercostal neurovascular bundle.

Parietal pleura

Vessels and nerves

PREPARATION

❶ Inspect the anatomy of the ribs and select an entry site above the rib that avoids injuring the intercostal neurovascular bundle (Fig. 23.7.3).
❷ Identify a site to insert the needle over the rib.
❸ Position the child supine with the head of the bed angled up at 30 degrees. Have an assistant gently restrain the conscious child.
❹ Use a local and/or intravenous analgesic if time allows and if the child is conscious.
❺ Identify the 2nd intercostal space (above the 3rd rib) at the mid-clavicular line. This space is ideal since air in the pleural space rises and typically collects toward the top of the lungs. A lateral approach is an alternative, but may have more complications including lung penetration and subsequent adhesions.
❻ Prepare the skin of the entry site with povidone-iodine solution.

PROCEDURE

❶ Attach the catheter over the needle to the 30 cm^3 syringe.
❷ Insert the catheter into the chest wall at a 90° angle above the 3rd rib (2nd intercostal space) at the mid-clavicular line (Fig. 23.7.4A).
❸ Provide back pressure on the syringe. Once there is a free flow of air in the syringe, continue to pull back on the plunger to evacuate the air.

Fig. 23.7.4 Inserting the thoracostomy needle.

❹ Remove the syringe and the needle, and leave the catheter in place (Fig. 23.7.4B).
❺ Place a chest tube immediately.

If there is an open connection between the chest wall and the pleural space from a penetrating injury – an open pneumothorax or sucking chest wound – cover with a petrolatum gauze, extending 6–8 cm from the wound edges on all sides and taped on three sides, to stop further air entry during inspiration (Fig. 23.7.5). Leave one side free to allow for the ongoing egress of air from the pleural space.

COMPLICATIONS

- Performing needle thoracostomy in a patient without a pneumothorax who is subsequently intubated can cause a pneumothorax or injury to the lung parenchyma. Under positive pressure ventilation, this pleural penetration can result in an ongoing air leak, which can then lead to a tension pneumothorax. Always place a chest tube after needle thoracostomy to prevent this complication.
- Placing the needle below the rib can cause laceration of an intercostal artery and subsequently, a haemothorax.
- Placing the catheter lower in the chest or closer to the mediastinum can result in diaphragm penetration, bowel penetration, haemopericardium or coronary vessel.
- If the catheter becomes occluded and fails to drain air, the tension pneumothorax can reoccur.

Fig. 23.7.5   Treating a sucking chest wound.

FURTHER READING

Barton ED, Epperson M, Hoyt DB, Rosen P 1995 Prehospital needle aspiration and tube thoracostomy in trauma victims: A six-year experience with aero medical crews. Journal of Emergency Medicine 13(2): 155–163

Bliss D, Silen M 2002 Paediatric thoracic trauma. Critical Care Medicine 30(11 Suppl): S409–S415

Wright SW 1998 Tube thoracostomy. In: Roberts JR, Hedges JR (eds) Clinical procedures in emergency medicine, 3rd edn. WB Saunders, Philadelphia, PA

Zimmerman KR 1997 Needle thoracostomy. In: Dieckmann RA, Fiser DH, Selbst SM (eds) Paediatric emergency and critical care procedures. Mosby, St Louis, MO

23.8 TUBE THORACOSTOMY

RONALD DIECKMANN

BACKGROUND

Traumatic pneumothorax and haemothorax are the most frequent paediatric indications for tube thoracostomy. Pneumothorax is a serious sequela of major chest trauma in children and may occur as a result of blunt injury without rib fractures or chest penetration. Sometimes, spontaneous pneumothorax occurs without trauma, from rapid increase in intraluminal pressure, especially with patients who have pre-existing bronchopulmonary disease. Air or fluid in the pleural space can cause significant impediments to oxygenation/ventilation and drastically reduce cardiac output, usually when the haemothorax is large or the pneumothorax is under tension. Tension pneumothorax and large haemothorax are potentially lethal emergencies that require immediate chest decompression. Rarely, large pleural fluid collections from non-traumatic aetiologies, such as empyemas, that are causing respiratory distress require tube thoracostomy for drainage.

The typical clinical presentation for tension pneumothorax and/or large haemothorax is the child who experiences a penetrating injury to the chest wall or back. A sucking chest wound may be present. Sometimes, these conditions result from penetrations below the nipple line or tip of the scapula that may also involve penetration into the abdomen, or from remote penetrations with gunshots that traverse multiple anatomic regions. Less frequently, blunt trauma is the mechanism. The classic adult clinical findings of unilateral decreased air movement and trachea shift are rarely present in children. More commonly, the clinical signs are tachypnea, oxygen desaturation, retractions, flaring, grunting and shock.

Tube thoracostomy is the insertion of an intra-pleural tube to evacuate air and/ or fluid from the pleural space. The procedure is a time-honoured evacuation technique for all age patients, and it may be life saving. The technique is effective for removal of most pleural air or fluid collections and has a good safety record in children. The main differences in the procedure between adults and children are the need for more meticulous patient preparation and smaller catheters in children. Sometimes, detection of pleural air or fluid is more difficult in children, requiring CT imaging to localise and quantify.

In the setting of tension pneumothorax, needle thoracostomy (Chapter 23.7) may precede tube thoracostomy, but tube thoracostomy must always follow needle thoracostomy. Stable, small pneumothoraces not under tension (e.g. < 20%), may sometimes be managed with observation alone, without a chest tube. Massive haemothorax occurs when a large vascular structure under systemic pressure bleeds into the pleural space. This is usually the internal mammary artery or an intercostal artery. In this setting tube thoracostomy is the only treatment likely to salvage the child. Occasionally re-circulation or autotransfusion of evacuated blood from the pleural space is indicated to treat massive haemothorax. In the overwhelming majority of children with significant chest-wall penetrations, tube thoracostomy is the only treatment indicated.

INDICATIONS

- Tension pneumothorax.
- Haemothorax.
- Rapid pleural fluid accumulation with respiratory distress.

CONTRAINDICATIONS

- Need for immediate open thoracotomy.

EQUIPMENT

❶ Chest tube tray (Table 23.8.1).
❷ Chest tube sizes French 12–36.
❸ Pigtail chest tubes.
❹ Chest tube drainage device.
❺ Wall suction.

PREPARATION

❶ Identify the presence of pneumothorax/haemothorax and the effected side by clinical examination and/or chest X-ray.

❷ Establish secure vascular access and apply cardiac monitor and pulse oximetry.
❸ If the child is conscious, provide parenteral sedation/analgesia.
❹ If the child is stable, consider an intercostal nerve block.
❺ Explain the procedure to the verbal child.
❻ Place a nasogastric tube to decompress the stomach, when there is abdominal distension.
❼ Place the child in the supine or upright position with the arm raised on the affected side.
❽ Identify the entry site (Fig. 23.8.1), on the middle-anterior axillary line between the fourth and fifth rib, at the nipple level.
❾ Drape the area and prepare the area widely between the fourth and sixth ribs with providone-iodine solution.
❿ Infiltrate the entry site above the sixth rib generously with lidocaine in conscious patients, and also infiltrate along the insertion site superiorly to the fourth interspace.
⓫ Select a properly-sized standard chest tube or pigtail catheter (Table 23.8.2).

PROCEDURE

Inserting the tube

❶ Incise the skin above the sixth rib 1–3 cm horizontally.
❷ Insert a curved Kelly into the incision, with tips away from the chest, and dissect the track superiorly to the fourth interspace (Fig. 23.8.2).

Table 23.8.1	Chest tube tray
• Kelly clamps (2) • Mayo scissors • Suture scissors • Needle holder • Scalpel • Forceps • Silk suture • 10 mL syringe • 25-gauge needle • 20-gauge needle	• Sterile towels • 4 × 4 sterile gauze • Vacuum device • Drainage apparatus with water seal • Plastic connectors (straight and Y type) • Chest tubes • Petrolatum • Lidocaine or bupivacaine for local injection • Antiseptic prep solution • Wide cloth tape

Second intercostal space midclavicular line

Fourth intercostal space anterior axillary line

Needle at 60°angle

Nipple

Fig. 23.8.1   Entry site for chest tube.

Table 23.8.2	Sizing chest tubes
Age	Chest tube size (Fr)
Newborn	8–12
Infant	14–20
Child	20–28
Adolescent	28–36

Formula: chest tube size (in Fr) = 4 × endotracheal tube size (mm)
Use larger tube size for haemothorax

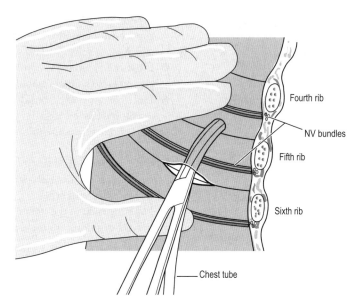

Fig. 23.8.2 Inserting the chest tube.

❸ Rotate the Kelly and puncture through the chest wall.

❹ Enter over the rib to avoid the neurovascular bundle.

❺ Widen the hole with the Kelly then insert a gloved finger into the hole to assure the track is clear to the pleura.

❻ Insert the appropriately-sized thoracostomy tube into the hole and direct the tube posteriorly.

❼ Facilitate tube entry by grasping the tube with the Kelly to guide tube entry into the pleural space. Assure the tube is inserted beyond the last hole.

❽ Attach the tube to the drainage system.

Securing the tube

❶ Use 2–0 silk to secure the tube.

❷ Employ a purse string suture, and wrap the suture material around the tube (Fig. 23.8.3). This will allow removal of the tube and closing of the incision without additional suturing.

❸ Place a gauze, slit in half and coated with petrolatum jelly over the tube and entry site.

❹ Secure all tube connections with tape.

❺ Obtain an X-ray to confirm tube placement and decompression of air or fluid.

COMPLICATIONS

- Haemopericardium.
- Tension pneumothorax.
- Haemothorax.
- Myocardial injury.
- Diaphragm perforation.
- Solid organ injury.
- Viscus injury.
- Cardiopulmonary arrest.

TIPS

- Sizing a chest tube involves estimation of the size of the child. If an exact size is not known, use the following formula: Chest tube size = 2 × nasogastric tube size or 4 × endotracheal tube size.
- Use a larger tube for haemothorax.
- Monitor for air leak for evidence of system air leak or tracheobronchial injury.
- Avoid trocars in children, to minimise lung lacerations.
- If a child with a penetrating chest injury is in shock or respiratory failure, do not wait for a chest X-ray before performing tube thoracostomy.
- Use of CT or video imaging may assist chest-tube placement.

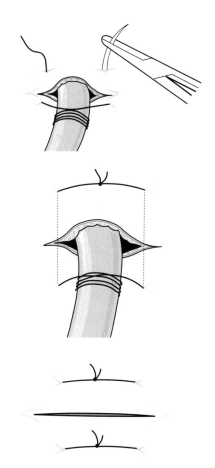

Fig. 23.8.3 Securing the chest tube.

FURTHER READING

Cullen ML 2001 Pulmonary and respiratory complications of paediatric trauma. Respiratory Care Clinics North America 7(1): 59–77

Dieckmann RA, Fiser D, Selbst S 1997 Illustrated textbook of paediatric emergency and critical care procedures. Mosby, St Louis, MO, 579–583

Dull KE, Fleisher GR 2002 Pigtail catheters versus large-bore chest tubes for pneumothoraces in children treated in the ED. Paediatric Emergency Care 18(4): 265–267

Genc A, Ozcan C, Erdener A, Mutaf O 1998 Management of pneumothorax in children. Journal of Cardiovascular Surgery (Torino) 39(6): 849–851

Sarihan H, Cay A, Aynaci M, Akyazici R, Baki A 1998 Empyema in children. Journal of Cardiovascular Surgery (Torino) 39(1): 113–116

Wilcox DT, Glick PL, Karamanoukian HL, Allen JE, Azizkhan RG 1995 Spontaneous pneumothorax: A single-institution, 12-year experience in patients under 16 years of age. Journal of Paediatric Surgery 10: 1452–1454

23.9 REMOVING AND REPLACING A TRACHEOSTOMY TUBE

RONALD DIECKMANN

BACKGROUND

Children with tracheostomy tubes are increasingly common in out-of-hospital and ED settings. Laryngeal trauma, cervical cord injury, subglottic stenosis, and conditions requiring prolonged ventilation often need short- or long-term tracheostomy-tube placement. Most of these children live at home and have trained caregivers, often parents. Because the tracheostomy tube may be the primary airway for the child, if the tube comes out (decannulation) or becomes obstructed (mucus plugging), immediate action is necessary to secure the airway and preserve gas exchange.

Treatment of most tracheostomy problems requires only simple techniques to establish a patent airway, such as suctioning of the existing tube, or removal of the old tracheostomy tube and replacement with a new tube. The child's major ongoing risk is airway obstruction from clogging of the old tube with secretions or foreign bodies. Occasionally, it is impossible to ventilate a child through an existing tracheostomy tube because of frank decannulation or complete tube obstruction. Under these conditions, ventilating through the nose and mouth with a bag-valve-mask (BVM) device, or inserting a new tracheostomy tube or another temporary airway will save the child's life.

INDICATIONS FOR EMERGENT REPLACEMENT

Respiratory distress or failure in the presence of:

• Decannulation.
• Tube obstruction.

CONTRAINDICATIONS

• Inadequately sized tract or stoma for insertion of a new tracheostomy tube. In this case, insert an endotracheal tube or replacement tracheostomy tube that is smaller in diameter than the original tracheostomy tube.

EQUIPMENT

❶ Suction device.
❷ Sterile suction catheters.
❸ Oxygen.
❹ BVM, standard paediatric and adult mask sizes.
❺ Tracheostomy cannulas, appropriately sized for patient (see Fig. 23.9.1).
❻ Endotracheal tubes, standard paediatric and adult sizes.
❼ Laryngoscope handle with blades.
❽ Tape or tracheostomy ties.
❾ Gauze pads.
❿ Syringes, 5 mL or 10 mL.
⓫ Water-soluble lubricant.
⓬ Scissors.

Fig. 23.9.1   Tracheostomy cannulas.

⓭ Sterile saline.
⓮ Stethoscope.

PREPARATION

❶ Ask the caregiver if there are any special problems with the child's trachea or special requirements involving the child's tracheostomy.
❷ If the child has an obstruction of the airway as a reason for tracheostomy placement, rescue breathing with a BVM may be difficult or impossible.
❸ Ask the caregiver if a replacement tracheostomy tube is available.
❹ Speak directly to the child about what to expect and attempt to enlist co-operation.

PROCEDURE

Removing an old tracheostomy tube:

❶ Position the child with the head and neck hyper-extended to expose the tracheostomy site.
❷ Apply oxygen over the mouth and nose, and occlude the stoma or tracheostomy tube. Most children with tracheostomies have an intact airway from the moth and nose to the trachea.
❸ If the existing tube has a cuff, deflate it:
  • Connect a 5–10 mL syringe to the valve on the pilot balloon.
  • Draw air out until the balloon collapses.
  • Cutting the balloon will not deflate the cuff.
❹ Cut or untie the cloth ties that hold the tracheostomy tube in place.
❺ Withdraw the tracheostomy tube using a slow, steady, outward and downward motion.

❻ Assess airway for patency and adequate ventilation.

❼ Provide oxygen and ventilation through the stoma as needed.

Replacing the tracheostomy tube

Option 1. Using a new tracheostomy tube

Insert a tracheostomy tube of the same size and model whenever possible. If the tube uses an insertion obturator, place this in the tube. If the tube has an inner and outer cannula, use the *outer* cannula and obturator for insertion.

❶ Moisten or lubricate the tip of the tube (and obturator) with water, sterile saline, or a water-soluble lubricant.

❷ Hold the device by the flange (wings) or hold the actual tube like a pencil.

❸ Gently insert the tube with an arching motion (follow the curvature of the tube) posteriorly then downward. Slight traction on the skin above or below the stoma may help (Fig. 23.9.2).

❹ Once the tube is in place, remove the obturator, attach the bag, and attempt to ventilate. If the tube has an inner cannula, insert to allow mechanical ventilation with a BVM device.

❺ Check for proper placement by watching for bilateral chest rise, listening for equal breath sounds, and observing the patient. Signs of improper placement include lack of chest rise, resistance to assisted ventilation, air in the surrounding tissues, and patient agitation.

❻ If the tube cannot be inserted, withdraw the tube, administer oxygen, and ventilate as needed.

❼ Use a smaller size tracheostomy tube for the second attempt.

Option 2. Using an endotracheal tube

If a replacement tracheostomy tube is not available, use an endotracheal tube of the same outer diameter as the tracheostomy tube.

❶ Check the length of the original tracheostomy tube, note the markings on the endotracheal tube, and advance it to the same depth as the original tube.

- The inserted portion of the endotracheal tube will be approximately half the distance needed for oral insertion.
- Do not advance the tube too far, or it may go into the right main-stem bronchus.

Option 3. Using a suction catheter as a guidewire

If unsuccessful with the initial replacement attempt, use a suction catheter as a guide:

❶ Insert a small, sterile suction catheter through the tracheostomy tube.

❷ Without applying suction, insert the suction catheter into the stoma.

❸ Slide the tracheostomy tube along the suction catheter and into the stoma, until it is in the proper position.

❹ Remove the suction catheter.

❺ Assess ventilation through the tracheostomy tube.

Option 4. Endotracheal intubation

❶ If still unsuccessful, consider either orotracheal intubation or ventilation through the stoma, using a stoma mask or newborn mask.

❷ Alternatively, do BVM over the nose and mouth while covering the stoma with a sterile gauze.

Securing the tracheostomy tube

❶ After proper placement, cut the ends of the tracheostomy ties or tape diagonally (allows for easy insertion), pass through eyelets (openings) on the flanges, and tie around the patient's neck, so that only a little finger can pass between the ties and the neck.

COMPLICATIONS

- Creation of a false lumen.
- Subcutaneous air.
- Pneumomediastinum.
- Pneumothorax.

Fig. 23.9.2 Inserting a new tracheostomy tube.

- Bleeding at insertion site.
- Bleeding through tube.
- Right main-stem intubation with endotracheal tube.

TIPS

- Talk to the caregiver about the size and type of tracheostomy tube and about known problems with the stoma, trachea or tube before proceeding.
- Most children who have lost a tracheostomy tube can be ventilated by BVM over the nose and mouth, with the stoma occluded.

- If unable to reinsert a tracheostomy tube, use a similarly sized endotracheal tube.
- Do not force a large tracheostomy tube through a new stoma site.
- Do not advance an endotracheal tube too far through the stoma, or it may intubate the right main-stem bronchus.

FURTHER READING

Bahng SC, VanHala S, Nelson VS, Hurvitz EA, Roloff DW, Grady EA, Lewis CC 1998 Parental report of paediatric tracheostomy care. Archives Physiology of Medical Rehabilitation 79(11): 1367–1369

Bosch JD, Cuyler JP 1987 Home care of the paediatric tracheostomy: Our experience. Journal of Otolaryngology 16(2): 120–122
Dieckmann RA, Fiser D, Selbst S 1997 Illustrated textbook of paediatric emergency and critical care procedures. Mosby, St Louis, MO, 121–122
Dieckmann RA, Brownstein D, Gausche M 2001 Textbook for paediatric education for prehospital professionals. Jones & Bartlett, Sudbury, MA, 300–302

23.10 CENTRAL AND PERIPHERAL INTRAVENOUS LINES

JUDITH KLEIN

BACKGROUND

Most children who present to an ED do not need vascular access for drug or fluid therapy. Medications can usually be administered orally, transmucosally, intramuscularly or by inhalation. Even fluid administration in dehydrated children does not ordinarily require vascular access. Oral rehydration, performed slowly and methodically, is often successful in children with vomiting and/or diarrhoea. However, when oral rehydration is unsuccessful or when a child presents critically ill or injured, IV or IO access (Chapter 23.11) becomes essential.

Finding veins to cannulate in infants and small children can be quite a challenge. The higher ratio of subcutaneous fat and smaller vessel size in young patients pose significant barriers to rapid venous cannulation. A peripheral venous site, rather than a central site, offers the highest benefit:risk ratio of any vascular access option. Fig. 23.10.1 illustrates common sites for peripheral intravenous (IV) line insertion.

When a peripheral site is unavailable, an IO site provides a second option

(Chapter 23.11). When peripheral venous and IO access cannot be obtained or if central venous pressure monitoring is required, consider cannulating central veins, such as the femoral vein, subclavian vein, or internal jugular vein. Avoid saphenous vein cutdowns in children, because they are technically difficult to perform and

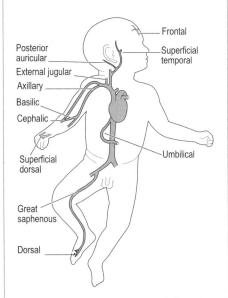

Fig. 23.10.1   Common peripheral IV sites.

the technique is time consuming in infants and young children, even for experienced operators. Make every effort to provide the least invasive form of access required by the degree of the child's illness.

INDICATIONS

- Peripheral IV access is indicated if oral, transmucosal, intramuscular or inhalation routes are not adequate to meet the patient's needs for fluids and/or medications.
- Use a central IV for:
  Central venous pressure monitoring.
  Administration of hypertonic solutions.
  Essential access when peripheral and IO attempts have failed.

CONTRAINDICATIONS

- Peripheral IV catheters are contraindicated if other, non-invasive, routes can meet the child's needs.
- Central venous catheters are contraindicated if peripheral venous

access sites are available and there are no special indications for central venous catheter placement.

- If possible, do not pass peripheral IV catheters:
  Through cellulitic skin.
  In an extremity that has a wound, e.g. burn or laceration.
  Distal to unstable fractures or injured veins.
- Avoid placing central lines in non-compressible sites in patients with bleeding diatheses.

PERIPHERAL VENOUS LINE PLACEMENT

EQUIPMENT

Table 23.10.1 lists peripheral IV equipment. Determine appropriate sizing of IV catheters by consulting a length-based resuscitation tape.

❶ If time permits, consider anaesthetising the skin with an anaesthetic drug or by iontophoresis. To anaesthetise skin, apply a topical anaesthetic, such as the eutectic mixture of local anaesthetics (EMLA) cream, under an occlusive dressing at the selected entry site at least 45 minutes prior to any IV attempt. The alternative technique of iontophoresis requires specialised equipment for delivery of a low amperage, painless electrical charge to the skin. The technique is safe, non-invasive and usually quite effective. Iontophoresis takes

Table 23.10.1 Equipment for peripheral IV insertion

- Gloves
- Arm or leg board
- Tourniquet
- Alcohol pads
- Gauze pads
- 22–24-gauge venous catheters
- Saline flush
- IV tubing, solution and pump
- Protective covering for IV (small plastic cup, roller gauze)
- Tape

10–20 minutes to numb skin for peripheral IV insertion.

❷ Use over-the-needle catheters whenever possible. Butterfly needles are far less stable but are acceptable for short-term infusions. Use armboards/legboards and a plastic container to cover the IV to avoid unintentional (or deliberate!) dislodgement of the catheter. Prime the tubing, and set up the IV fluid chamber with microdrip and an infusion pump in advance. Carefully monitor infusions in infants and small children to prevent over-administration of fluids. Select the smallest sized catheter that will meet the patient's needs for drug and fluid administration.

PREPARATION

❶ Prepare all equipment and place near the child. Avoid using the bed as an equipment table as the equipment may find its way quickly to the floor with an active child.
❷ Flush the catheter with saline solution if diagnostic blood samples are not necessary during IV insertion. This will reduce the risk of air embolisation.

Fig. 23.10.2   Restraining an infant.

❸ Remove any topical anaesthetic at the IV site or the apparatus for iontophoresis.
❹ Have an assistant restrain an infant or toddler with a sheet (Figs 23.10.2 and 23.10.3).
❺ Attempt to talk an older child through the procedure with a parent or caregiver present.
❻ Have the assistant gently restrain the extremity/body part selected for IV access. Use padded boards to stabilise arm or leg access sites in infants and young children.
❼ Locate landmarks and determine insertion sites first with an ungloved hand that is more sensitive in detecting surface veins and palpating landmarks than the gloved hand.

PROCEDURE

There are a number of possible sites for placement of peripheral IV lines in infants and children. The easiest sites are the dorsum of the hands and feet, the antecubital fossa and, in infants < 1 year, the scalp. In non-emergent situations, start distally and move proximally when initial attempts fail. Consider using a warm compress to dilate constricted veins and make them more visible. In emerg-

Fig. 23.10.3   Restraining a child.

Fig. 23.10.4   Securing the catheter to the skin.

ent situations, cannulate the largest vein available and consider less commonly used peripheral sites, such as the external jugular vein and deep brachial vein.

❶ Make sure that the child is well immobilised.

❷ Don gloves and clean the insertion site with isopropyl alcohol or povidone-iodine solution.

❸ Apply a tourniquet just proximal to the insertion site. Use a rubber band around the scalp caudad of the insertion site to cannulate scalp veins.

❹ Locate a straight segment of the vein and provide in-line traction away from the direction of catheter insertion.

❺ Insert the catheter at about a 10–20° angle to the skin. Once there is a flash of blood in the hub of the catheter, advance the catheter with the needle in place another 1-2 mm. Then advance the catheter over the needle into the vein.

❻ Draw any blood samples needed, remove the tourniquet, and connect the IV line.

❼ Secure the catheter and IV line to the patient with tape and a plastic container over the IV (Fig. 23.10.4).

If insertion is unsuccessful at traditional peripheral IV, consider two alternative sites prior to moving to a central line: the external jugular vein and the deep brachial vein. To cannulate the external jugular vein, place the patient in Trendelenburg position to dilate the vein. Restrain the patient well and turn his/her head slightly away from the cannulation site (Fig. 23.10.5). Do not use a tourniquet for placement of an IV at this site. Clean the area with isopropyl alcohol or povidone-iodine solution and use an 18G needle to make a nick in the skin at the catheter site. This will facilitate passage of the catheter through the skin. Use the peripheral insertion technique but apply firm counter-traction at the entry site to help stabilise the vessel. Secure the needle carefully to avoid dislodgement.

The second alternative site is the deep brachial vein. In contrast to the other sites, identify the likely location of the deep brachial vein by anatomic landmarks, not by visualisation or by palpation. Ultrasound can assist in localisation of the vein. Consider this option in older children. Palpate the brachial artery medial to the biceps just proximal to the antecubital fossa (Fig. 23.10.6). Place a tour-

niquet and prepare the skin with isopropyl alcohol or povidone-iodine solution. Insert the catheter at a 30° angle approximately the patient's finger breath medial to the brachial artery. Angle the catheter parallel to the course of the brachial artery and slowly advance the catheter. If arterial blood appears or the patient complains of hand paraesthesiae (median nerve irritation), remove the catheter and hold pressure at the site. There is anatomic variability in the position of the vein, so try marginally different slightly medial insertion sites if initial attempts are unsuccessful.

COMPLICATIONS

Local complications
- Phlebitis.
- Site infection.
- Infiltration.
- Bleeding.
- Pressure necrosis due to IV stabilisation methods.

To avoid these complications, clean insertion sites well prior to passing the needle through the skin. Make sure blood can be easily withdrawn from and fluids easily infused through the IV. Avoid infusing irritant or hyperosmolar solutions through peripheral lines. Tape IV lines securely but do not create a tour-

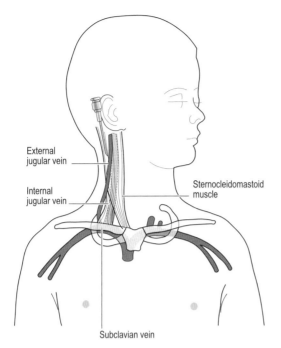

External
jugular vein

Internal
jugular vein

Sternocleidomastoid
muscle

Subclavian vein

Fig. 23.10.5   Positioning for external jugular vein puncture.

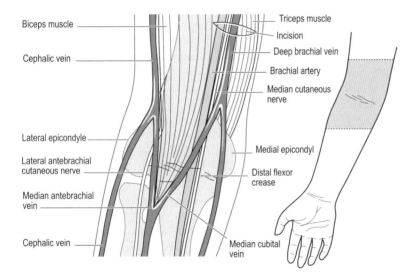

Biceps muscle

Cephalic vein

Triceps muscle

Incision

Deep brachial vein

Brachial artery

Median cutaneous
nerve

Lateral epicondyle

Lateral antebrachial
cutaneous nerve

Median antebrachial
vein

Cephalic vein

Medial epicondyl

Distal flexor
crease

Median cubital
vein

Fig. 23.10.6   Cannulating the deep brachial vein.

niquet with tape and remember to pad all joints. Replace peripheral lines every 48–72 hours.

Systemic complications
- Thrombosis.
- Air embolism.
- Catheter tip embolisation.

Flush catheters regularly but not force-fully. Do not re-insert the needle stylet into the catheter once it has been removed. Doing this can shear the catheter and cause catheter fragment embolisation.

TIPS

- Whenever possible, use a topical anaesthetic at several possible IV sites at least 45 minutes prior to line placement, or consider iontophoresis.

Table 23.10.2 Sizing central IV catheters		
Weight (kg)	Age	Catheter size (French)
< 5	Newborn to 6 months	3, 4
5–15	6 months to 5 years	5, 7
15	> 5 years	5–11

- Avoid joint surfaces and the patient's dominant hand. If a large-bore catheter is required, use more proximal sites, such as those at the antecubital fossa or external jugular vein.
- Do not let go of recently-placed IV catheters until they are well-secured.
- Monitor newly-placed IVs closely, particularly in infants and small children with persistent crying. A swollen extremity may be the only marker of an infiltrated catheter.

CENTRAL VENOUS LINE PLACEMENT

EQUIPMENT

The equipment for placement of a central venous line is usually in a pre-packaged kit. The simplest and most-straightforward technique for central-line placement is the guidewire or Seldinger technique. Pre-packaged kits will contain, among other things, a needle, syringe, J-wire, scalpel, dilator and catheter. Determine appropriate catheter sizes by measuring the child next to a length-based resuscitation tape or by consulting Table 23.10.2. Estimate insertion distance by measuring from the insertion site externally to the desired tip position.

PREPARATION

❶ If time allows, sedate the child prior to insertion of a central venous catheter and/or use a topical anaesthetic such as EMLA cream. If the situation is emergent, use a sheet wrapped around the child and an assistant to restrain the child. Excessive patient movement will increase the rate of complication and decrease the likelihood of procedure success.

❷ Prepare all equipment on the tray so that items can be easily located. Do not use the child's bed as an instrument table as the instruments will soon find their way to the floor.

❸ Flush the catheter with saline solution in advance unless diagnostic blood specimens are required.

PROCEDURE

Sites for central venous line placement in children include: the femoral vein, the internal jugular vein, and the subclavian vein. The external jugular vein is also a possible central venous insertion site. Passage of the catheter centrally via the external jugular vein is difficult because of the acute angle of entry of the external jugular into the subclavian vein. It is, therefore, the least desirable site.

Fig. 23.10.7 illustrates the essential anatomy for placement of a femoral venous catheter.

❶ Place the patient supine in a mild reverse Trendelenburg position. Maintain the hip in slight external rotation and abduction.

❷ Palpate the femoral artery at the inguinal ligament. The insertion site is about a patient's finger breath medial to the artery and 2–3 cm distal to the inguinal ligament. The right side is easier for a right-handed operator.

❸ Measure from insertion site to the umbilicus to estimate catheter insertion distance.

To cannulate the internal jugular vein, place the patient in Trendelenburg position with the neck extended and the head turned slightly away from the insertion site. A roll placed under the ipsilateral shoulder will facilitate neck extension, particularly in infants. Fig. 23.10.8 illustrates the relevant anatomy and landmarks.

❶ Identify the triangle formed by the sternal and clavicular heads of the sternocleidomastoid muscle and the clavicle.

❷ Palpate the carotid artery just medial to the triangle.

❸ The insertion site is either at the apex of the triangle or half-way (from mastoid to sternum) along the medial border of the sternal head. In either case, aim towards the ipsilateral nipple and away from the carotid artery. The right side is preferable because of the straighter course to the superior vena cava, the lower pleural dome, and the absence of the thoracic duct.

❹ Place the catheter tip at the junction of the superior vena cava and the right atrium.

Positioning and anatomy relevant for placement of a subclavian central venous line is similar to that for placement of an internal jugular venous line (Fig. 23.10.9).

❶ Sedate conscious patients before attempting a subclavian line, as patient movement can result in a high rate of complications. Place the patient in Trendelenburg position with a towel roll underneath the ipsilateral shoulder to help keep the neck in extension.

❷ Mentally divide the clavicle into thirds.

❸ The insertion site is just inferior to the junction of the middle and medial thirds of the clavicle aiming towards the sternal notch. Aim the J curve of the guidewire caudally during insertion. Also, turn the patient's head toward the site of insertion while advancing the wire to avoid passage of the wire up the internal jugular vein.

❹ Place the catheter tip at the junction of the superior vena cava and the right atrium.

The general procedure for placement of a central venous catheter is the same regardless of location.

❶ Clean the skin with a povidone-iodine or chlorhexidine solution.

❷ Anaesthetise the site with 1% lidocaine.

❸ Attach a syringe to the insertion needle so that the bevel lines up with the numbers on the syringe. This allows for identification of bevel direction even when the needle is inside the patient.

❹ Insert the needle at the selected insertion site with the bevel pointed anteriorly (femoral), medially (internal jugular), or caudally (subclavian).

❺ Angle the needle at approximately 30° to the skin, except when placing a subclavian line. With subclavian line placement, use the shallowest angle possible that allows insertion of the needle underneath the clavicle aiming towards the sternal notch.

Maintain constant negative pressure on the syringe while inserting or withdrawing

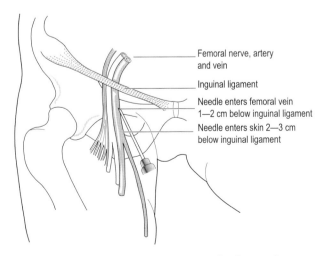

Femoral nerve, artery and vein

Inguinal ligament

Needle enters femoral vein 1—2 cm below inguinal ligament

Needle enters skin 2—3 cm below inguinal ligament

Fig. 23.10.7 Essential anatomy for placement of a femoral venous catheter.

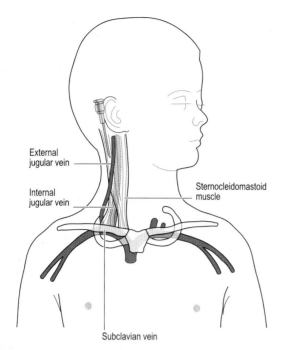

External jugular vein

Internal jugular vein

Sternocleidomastoid muscle

Subclavian vein

Fig. 23.10.8   Cannulating the internal jugular vein.

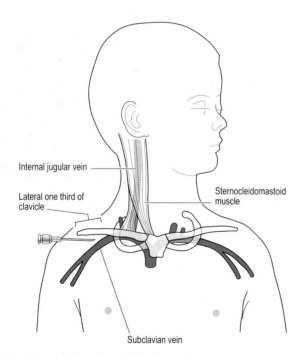

Internal jugular vein

Lateral one third of clavicle

Sternocleidomastoid muscle

Subclavian vein

Fig. 23.10.9   Cannulating the subclavian vein.

the needle as vessel entry may occur during withdrawal. Once blood flows freely into the syringe, stabilise the needle with a hand resting on the patient. Remove the syringe carefully, trying not to alter the position of the needle. Insert the J-wire through the needle, J end first (Fig. 23.10.10). Point the J of the guide-wire in the direction the catheter is intended to go. The wire should pass easily. Do not force it if it does not. Removing the wire and repositioning the needle can often resolve gentle resistance. If strong resistance is met, remove the needle and wire together to avoid shearing off the wire into the vein.

Table 23.10.3   Complications of central venous line placement
• Bleeding
• Arterial puncture/cannulation/laceration
• Infection
• Catheter thrombosis
• Pneumothorax
• Haemothorax
• Thoracic duct laceration

Once the wire is passed to the pre-marked distance, remove the needle. Never let go of the wire. Make a small stab incision with a scalpel over the wire. Insert a dilator over the wire, once again, remembering to hold onto the wire at all times. Remove the dilator and insert the catheter over the wire to the pre-measured distance (Fig. 23.10.11). Remove the wire. Draw off any diagnostic blood specimens. If the catheter has not been flushed in advance, withdraw blood from all lumens of the catheter prior to infusing any fluids or medications to avoid air embolisation. Suture the catheter in place and apply a sterile dressing. Verify location of the catheter tip with an X-ray.

COMPLICATIONS

Table 23.10.3 lists the most common complications of central venous line placement.

- Bleeding can occur during traumatic line placement or after arterial puncture. Patients with bleeding diatheses are at great risk for bleeding complications. Compress bleeding sites from femoral or internal jugular sites. These sites are safer than the subclavian route where the internal bleeding site is non-compressible. Avoid subclavian catheterisation in patients who are moving around or who have clotting problems.
- Pneumothorax can occur with internal jugular or subclavian line insertion. A shallow angle of insertion with subclavian lines can help prevent this complication. Obtain an X-ray after all line placements not only to verify catheter position but also to detect a pneumothorax.

Fig. 23.10.10   Inserting the J-wire through the needle.

Fig. 23.10.11   Inserting the catheter over the wire to the pre-measured distance.

- Suspect catheter thrombosis if withdrawal of blood or infusion of fluids becomes difficult. Eventually pain and swelling of the extremity will tip the clinician off to the presence of the clot. Manage thromboses expeditiously with catheter removal.
- Infection is equally likely to occur at any of the central venous sites. Remove infected catheters as soon as possible and treat with antibiotics. If possible, avoid insertion of a new central catheter for 24–48 hours.

TIPS

- In the awake patient, restraint and proper sedation and analgesia will improve procedural success and avoid complications.
- Use ultrasound, if possible, to identify vessels prior to line placement.
- If the patient is moving and there is no time for sedation, the femoral site is the safest and most easily compressible vein if bleeding occurs.

- If central venous pressure monitoring is required, use an access site above the diaphragm. While the internal jugular vein is larger, the subclavian site is more comfortable for the patient in the long term.
- If the patient is pulseless, the subclavian vein is the preferred site for central venous catheterisation as it does not require a pulse for localisation and can be used for central venous pressure monitoring.

FURTHER READING

Bagwell CE, Salzberg AM, Sonnino RE, Haynes JH 2000 Potentially lethal complications of central venous catheter placement. Journal of Paediatric Surgery 35(5): 709–713

Chiang VW, Baskin MN 2000 Uses and complications of central venous catheters inserted in a paediatric emergency department. Paediatric Emergency Care 16(4): 230–232

Cunningham FJ, Engle WA 1998 Paediatric vascular access and blood sampling techniques. In: Roberts JR, Hedges JR (eds) Clinical procedures in emergency medicine, 3rd edn. WB Saunders, Philadelphia, PA

Fernandez EG, Sweeney MF, Green TP 1997 Central venous catheters. In: Dieckmann RA, Fiser DH, Selbst SM (eds) Paediatric emergency and critical care procedures. Mosby, St Louis, MO

King D, Conway EE Jr 1996 Vascular access. Paediatric Annals 25(12): 693–698

Macnab AJ, Macnab M 1999 Teaching paediatric procedures: The Vancouver model for instructing Seldinger's technique of central venous access via the femoral vein. Paediatrics 103(1): E8

Stoyroff M, Teague WG 1998 Intravenous access in infants and children. Paediatric Clinics North America 45(6): 1373–1393

Webster PA, Salassi-Scotter MR 1997 Peripheral vascular access. . In: Dieckmann RA, Fiser DH, Selbst SM (eds) Paediatric emergency and critical care procedures. Mosby, St Louis, MO

23.11 INTRAOSSEOUS INFUSIONS

LINDSAY BRIDGFORD • RONALD DIECKMANN

BACKGROUND

Peripheral intravenous cannulation in a critically ill or injured child can be difficult, time consuming, and sometimes impossible. Small veins collapse or disappear during shock, and increased body fat may camouflage superficial skin veins. Central venous access and surgical cutdown are also technically difficult procedures that may be risky or impossible in critical situations. Although the endotracheal route is an alternative to vascular access in cardiopulmonary arrest, endotracheal intubation may be delayed, drug absorption may not be reliable, and large fluid administration is contraindicated by this route.

The intraosseous (IO) or intramedullary route for the delivery of resuscitation fluids and medications has been used for over fifty years in children and adults. Many studies have confirmed that the highly vascularised IO space is an excellent route for medications and fluids. The only technical problem is successfully piercing the bony cortex in older children. The bones of neonates and infants are usually soft and the IO space is relatively large, so needle insertion is easy in children of youngest age. Good equipment, preparation, and effective technique are especially important for success in IO needle insertion. While IO access is easy, quick, and safe, it is painful in a conscious child and therefore is only practical in a critically ill or injured child.

The IO space functions as a non-collapsible vein. There are several possible sites for insertion; but the easiest location in children is the proximal tibial. The emissary veins of the IO space absorb all parenteral medications, crystalloid fluids, or blood products – which move quickly into the central circulation. Complications are minor and infrequent. Out-of-hospital emergency-care professionals have also employed the IO technique with a high rate of success.

INDICATIONS

- Cardiopulmonary arrest.
- Any critical emergency when a peripheral cannulation site is unavailable and oral, transmucosal, intramuscular or inhalation routes are not adequate to meet the patient's needs for fluids and/or medications.

CONTRAINDICATIONS

- Do not use an IO infusion if the child is stable.
- Do not place an IO needle below a fracture site. Use the other side.
- Avoid placement of an IO below any open injury on an extremity. Use the other side.

Relative contraindications

- Avoid IO needle insertion in children with osteoporosis and osteogenesis imperfecta, due to the high fracture potential.

- Recent prior use of the same bone for IO infusion, due to the potential for extravasation from previous IO sites.

EQUIPMENT

❶ A variety of needles will work. Butterfly needles and spinal needles may be effective, especially in neonates and infants, but these needles bend too easily in the more calcified bones of children and adolescents.

❷ Commercially available IO needles have more durable parts intended for penetration of bone. There are several styles (Fig. 23.11.1). A central stylet is universal. There are short, 2.5 cm, needles for neonates and infants and longer, 3.0 and 3.5 cm, needles for older children. Some needles have stylets with multi-faceted cutting edges intended for a rotary insertion, and others have bevels. The shaft may have side ports.

❸ 10 mL syringe.

Fig. 23.11.1   IO needles.

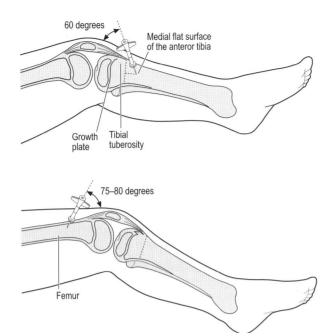

60 degrees

Medial flat surface of the anterior tibia

Growth plate

Tibial tuberosity

75–80 degrees

Femur

Fig. 23.11.2   IO needle entry sites.

❹ Normal saline.
❺ Stopcock (optional).

PREPARATION

Identification of the entry site

The best site in children is the antero-medial aspect of the proximal tibia lateral to the tibial tuberosity. Alternative sites are the distal end of the femur 2–3 cm above the patella in the midline, and the medial malleolus at the ankle (Fig. 23.11.2). The sternum is not recommended in children. In adults, the medial malleolus may be the best site, although studies are lacking.

Positioning the child

Place the child supine with the knee slightly flexed and a small towel roll or other bulky material under the popliteal fossa. Make sure the conscious child is well immobilised.

Selecting the correct side

A right-handed operator will more easily insert the needle in the child's right leg, and visa versa for the left-handed operator.

PROCEDURE

❶ Introduce the IO needle in the skin, directed slightly away from the growth plate. Grasping the limb with the non-dominant hand beside the insertion site (e.g. behind the knee for proximal tibia insertion) helps to steady the bone during placement.

❷ Pierce the bony cortex with a firm, twisting motion from a position directly above the entry site. A 'pop' may be felt as the needle passes through the bony cortex and into the marrow cavity. Do not push too hard on the needle. Too much force may push the needle all the way through the bone and into the soft tissues.

❸ Remove the stylet and aspirate marrow contents with a 10 mL syringe. Keep any bone marrow aspirate for glucose check or for other tests in the ED. Sometimes, marrow cannot be aspirated.

❹ Confirm correct placement by infusing 10 mL of normal saline without resistance. Once the IO needle has been placed, attach a stopcock (if available) to the end of the needle before attaching the IV line.

❺ Attach IV line to the hub and infuse fluids or drugs directly into IO space. Pushing the fluids too hard may force the fluids out of the IO space. The rate of fluid infusion may be limited by the small marrow space.

❻ Secure the needle to the overlying skin with tape.

❼ Monitor the calf to ensure that there is no swelling to indicate leakage of fluid.

COMPLICATIONS

- Compartment syndrome.
- Failed infusion.
- Growth-plate injury.
- Bone infection.
- Skin infection.
- Skin necrosis.
- Bony fracture.

TIPS

- If the child is conscious, provide generous local anaesthesia at the entry site.
- In addition to serving as a route for drug and fluid administration, blood samples drawn from the site can be used for culture, haematological, and biochemical analysis, but there are limitations. Emergency type and crossmatch is reliable with an adequate sample. A complete blood cell count may not be reliable, as it reflects the marrow cell count rather than the cell count in the peripheral circulation, and also because blood aspirated from the marrow usually clots rapidly, even if it is placed in a tube that contains heparin. Blood chemistry determinations are possible, but they may not correlate with blood samples taken from central veins.
- All commonly used intravenous fluids and drugs can be administered via the IO route.
- The rate of infection from IO needle placement is low and comparable to IV cannulation.

- A slow infusion rate does not mean the IO needle is misplaced, and pressure infusion may be necessary to maintain flow.

FURTHER READING

Brunette DD, Fischer R 1988 Intravascular access in paediatric cardiac arrest. Annals of Emergency Medicine 6: 577

Fiser DH 1990 Intraosseous infusion. New England Journal of Medicine 322: 1579
Johnson L, Kissoon N, Fiallos M et al 1999 Use of intraosseous blood to assess blood chemistries and haemoglobin during cardiopulmonary resuscitation with drug infusions. Critical care medicine 27: 1147–1152
Phillips B, Zideman D, Garcia-Castrillo L et al 2001 European Resuscitation Council guidelines 2000 for advanced paediatric life support. Resuscitation 48: 231–324
Vidal R, Kissoon N, Gaylor M 1993 Compartment syndrome following intraosseous infusion. Paediatrics 91: 1201–1202

Wenzel V, Lindner KH, Augenstein S et al 1999 Intraosseous vasopressin improves coronary perfusion pressure rapidly during cardiopulmonary resuscitation in pigs. Critical care medicine 27: 1565–1569

23.12 RECTAL DRUG ADMINISTRATION

RONALD DIECKMANN

BACKGROUND

Status epilepticus is a major paediatric medical emergency that requires emergency treatment. Although the first priority is airway and breathing, additional therapy includes termination of the seizure. Cannulating a peripheral vein in a child in status epilepticus limits timely delivery of essential advanced life support (ALS) drugs, especially in infants and toddlers. However, IV, IM, or IO drug administration is not necessary because rectal benzodiazepine administration is probably as effective and has no added complications. Rectal drug administration is a time-honoured drug-delivery technique in children and is useful for many medications, including antipyretics and anticonvulsants. The rectum is highly vascularised, and lipid-soluble drugs are rapidly absorbed when correctly administered (Fig. 23.12.1). Diazepam is a lipid-soluble benzodiazepine that is reliably absorbed through the rectum and will terminate most seizures without further treatment. Lorazepam is an effective alternative drug choice.

Rectal drug administration is a technique that allows delivery of an absorbable benzodiazepine in the setting of status epilepticus. The relative effectiveness and safety of rectal diazepam versus IM midazolam, lorazepam or other benzodiazepines for treatment of status epilepticus are not known. Rectal diazepam or lorazepam administration may take a

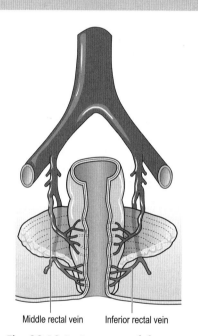

Middle rectal vein   Inferior rectal vein

Fig. 23.12.1 Anatomy of the rectum.

few minutes longer to stop the seizure, compared to IV administration, and drug levels may be more variable. Occasionally, as with the IV diazepam preparation, more than one dose of rectal diazepam is necessary.

INDICATIONS

- Repetitive seizures.
- Status epilepticus.

CONTRAINDICATIONS

- Newborn age (a month or less).
- Recent prior rectal surgery (e.g. for Hirschsprung's disease, imperforate anus).

EQUIPMENT

❶ Diazepam gel preparation or IV solution of diazepam or lorazepam.
❷ Lubricant.
❸ Tuberculin syringe, or 14–20-gauge over-the-needle catheter with 3–5 mL syringe.
❹ Tape (optional).

PREPARATION

❶ Determine the weight of the child using a decision support software program or paediatric resuscitation tape or other accurate estimate of size. Or obtain the patient's weight from the caregiver.

Option 1. Diazepam gel preparation
❶ Remove the rubber-tipped gel container from the sterile package.

Option 2. IV diazepam preparation
❶ Draw up the calculated dose of IV medication into a disposable tuberculin syringe or into a 3–5 mL syringe.

Lubricate the syringe or catheter:
   a. If using the tuberculin syringe as the administration device, remove needle and apply lubricant to the tip of the syringe.
   b. If using a 3–5 mL syringe, remove needle, attach over-the-needle catheter (plastic portion only), and lubricate catheter.

PROCEDURE

❶ Position the patient in the decubitus position, knee-chest position, or supine position (Fig. 23.12.2) and have a second person hold the legs apart.

❷ Carefully introduce the rubber tip of the gel container, or the syringe or over-the-needle catheter approximately 5 cm (2 inches) into the rectum.

❸ Inject the gel or solution into the rectum. Remove the syringe.

❹ Hold buttocks closed for ten seconds.

❺ Tape buttocks closed (optional).

COMPLICATIONS

• The most serious potential complication of rectal diazepam is respiratory depression, which is usually from the drug, but may be from the prolonged seizure, or the underlying cause of the seizure.

• Administration of diazepam too high or too proximal into the rectum may decrease its anticonvulsant effect. When

Fig. 23.12.2   Administering rectal drugs.

the drug is delivered too proximal in the rectum, absorption may occur into the superior haemorrhoidal veins, which drain into the portal system instead of the middle and inferior haemorrhoidal veins, which drain into the systemic venous system. The drug will then undergo hepatic metabolism, which will significantly reduce brain concentrations.

• Rectal tearing.

TIPS

• The rectal dose of diazepam is 0.5 mg kg^{-1}, or five-times the intravenous dose, to a maximum dose of 10 mg. Onset of action for rectal diazepam is slower.

• Do not give additional rectal diazepam until approximately five

minutes after the first dose, to avoid 'stacking' doses and increasing the risk of respiratory depression.

• Rectal lorazepam may be at least as effective as rectal diazepam in status epilepticus.

• Do not perform endotracheal intubation on every child with diminished breathing after rectal diazepam. Most will not need it if BVM is effectively performed for a few minutes until the child begins breathing again spontaneously.

• Do not use the benzodiazepine reversal agent flumazenil when respiratory depression occurs after diazepam administration. The drug may precipitate seizures by interfering with the effect of the diazepam in the brain.

FURTHER READING

Appleton R, Martland T, Phillips B 2002 Drug management for acute tonic-clonic convulsions including convulsive status epilepticus in children. Cochrane Database System Review 4, CD001905

Dieckmann RA, Brownstein D, Gausche M 2001 Textbook for paediatric education for prehospital professionals. Jones & Bartlett, Sudbury, MA, 291–292

Dieckmann RA, Fiser D, Selbst S 1997 Illustrated textbook of paediatric emergency and critical care procedures. Mosby, St Louis, MO, 274–278

Dieckmann RA 1994 Rectal diazepam for prehospital paediatric status epilepticus. Annals of Emergency Medicine 23(2): 216–224

Fitzgerald BJ, Okos AJ, Miller JW 2003 Treatment of out-of-hospital status epilepticus with diazepam rectal gel. Seizure 12(1): 52–55

Mitchell WG, Conry JA, Crumrine PK, Kriel RL, Cereghino JJ, Groves L, Rosenfeld WE 1999 An open-label study of repeated use of diazepam rectal gel (Diastat) for episodes of acute breakthrough seizures and clusters: Safety, efficacy, and tolerance. North American Diastat Group. Epilepsia 40(11): 1610–1617

COMMON PROCEDURES

23.13 UMBILICAL VESSEL CANNULATION

JUDITH KLEIN

BACKGROUND

During fetal life, two umbilical arteries transport nutrients and oxygen from the placenta and one umbilical vein helps dispose of fetal waste. During delivery, these vessels are cut and clamped and the newborn is separated from the placenta. However, the umbilical vessels can be re-cannulated and utilised for emergent vascular access in ill neonates for up to seven days after birth. This is an excellent method of central drug and fluid delivery, because peripheral venous access in infants in the first week of life is quite difficult, particularly in the ill or intra-vascularly depleted neonate. The other alternative for emergency vascular access in newborns is the insertion of an IO needle (Chapter 23.11).

While either of the umbilical arteries and the umbilical vein is available for vascular access, the umbilical vein is tech-nically easier to cannulate. Therefore, use the vein in an emergent situation. Can-nulate one of the umbilical arteries if blood pressure monitoring and arterial blood gas sampling are important for patient management.

INDICATIONS

- Emergent vascular access for resuscitation.
- Central access for delivery of fluids, medications, or exchange transfusion.
- Frequent blood gas sampling.
- Haemodynamic monitoring.

CONTRAINDICATIONS

- Do not place an umbilical vessel line if a peripheral intravenous line is available and adequate for the infant's needs.

EQUIPMENT

Table 23.13.1 lists the equipment for cannulation of either the umbilical artery or vein.

PREPARATION

❶ Prepare all equipment in advance.
❷ Flush the umbilical catheter with saline or heparin flush and attach the stopcock.
❸ Place the infant supine under a radiant warmer with all extremities restrained.
❹ Utilise cardiorespiratory and pulse oximetry monitors for the duration of the procedure.
❺ Don a mask, sterile gown and sterile gloves.

PROCEDURE

Umbilical vein catheterisation

❶ Have an assistant to hold the umbilical stump up, scrub the umbilicus with povidone-iodine solution from xiphoid to pubis.

Table 23.13.1 Equipment for cannulation of the umbilical artery or vein

- Sterile gown, gloves and mask
- Povidone-iodine solution
- Sterile gauze
- Sterile drapes
- Umbilical tape
- 3.0 Silk suture with needle
- Scalpel
- Haemostats
- Smooth, curved iris forceps
- Iris scissors
- Needle holder
- Umbilical catheter (3.5 or 5.0F)
- Heparinised saline/syringes
- Three-way stopcock

❷ Apply a sterile drape.
❸ To provide haemostasis, loosely tie umbilical tape at the base of the umbilical cord at the junction with the skin and cut the cord approximately 1–2 cm from the skin.
❹ Identify the two thick-walled arteries and the larger, thin-walled umbilical vein (Fig. 23.13.1).
❺ Holding the umbilical cord with a haemostat, insert the flushed 3.5F (preterm) or 5F (term) catheter into the umbilical vein (Fig. 23.13.2).
❻ Use gentle, but steady, pressure while inserting the catheter and provide gentle traction on the cord if resistance is met. Insert the catheter so that the tip is in the inferior vena cava below the diaphragm at a depth of approximately 4–5 cm or above

Fig. 23.13.1 Identifying the umbilical arteries and vein.

Fig. 23.13.2 Inserting the catheter into the umbilical vein.

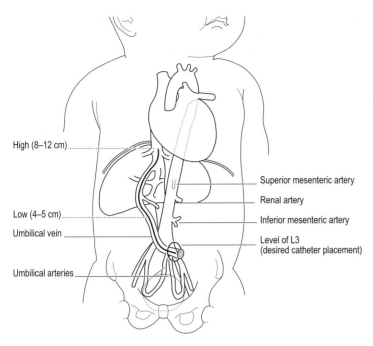

Fig. 23.13.3 **Location of tip of catheter.**

High (8–12 cm)

Superior mesenteric artery

Renal artery

Low (4–5 cm)

Inferior mesenteric artery

Umbilical vein

Level of L3
(desired catheter placement)

Umbilical arteries

Fig. 23.13.4 **Stabilising the vessels.**

Umbilical
arteries

Umbilical vein

Fig. 23.13.5 **Inserting the iris forceps into the artery.**

Umbilical
arteries

Umbilical vein

Fig. 23.13.6 **Advancing the catheter.**

Umbilical arteries

Umbilical vein

the diaphragm (via the portal system) at a depth of 8–12 cm (Fig. 23.13.3).

❼ The deeper line allows for administration of higher concentration fluids as well as central venous pressure monitoring. Confirm that blood returns freely through the catheter prior to infusion of any fluids or medications.

Umbilical artery catheterisation

❶ Prepare and drape the umbilical cord as with umbilical vein catheterisation.

❷ Loosely tie umbilical tape at the base of the umbilical cord at the junction with the skin and cut the cord approximately 1–2 cm from the skin.

❸ Identify the two thick-walled arteries and attach two haemostats to either side of the umbilical cord to stabilise the vessels (Fig. 23.13.4).

❹ Do not place the haemostats on the arteries.

❺ Insert the smooth-curved iris forceps into the artery selected, and gently dilate the artery (Fig. 23.13.5).

❻ Continue dilating until the forceps can be inserted about 1 cm. Gentle introduce and advance the pre-flushed catheter (3.5 preterm; 5.0 term) towards the patient's feet with gentle cephalad traction on the cord (Fig. 23.13.6).

❼ Overcome any resistance with gentle steady pressure, but do not force the catheter. Place the catheter either 'low' at the level of the L3 vertebra or 'high' between the T6 and T9 vertebrae (Fig. 23.13.7). Low catheter insertion distances are based on patient weight and are available on graphs. High catheter insertion distance is approximately 60% of the distance between the infant's umbilicus and either shoulder.

❽ Anchor the catheter to the umbilical cord with a purse string suture then secure the catheter to the abdomen with tape (Fig. 23.13.8).

❾ Verify placement of the radio-opaque catheter by thoraco-abdominal X-ray.

COMPLICATIONS

• Haemorrhage.
• Infection.
• Air embolism.

Fig. 23.13.7 Placing the catheter.

Fig. 23.13.8 Anchoring the catheter to the umbilical cord.

- Vessel dissection.
- Perforation.
- If umbilical venous catheters are left in the liver, sclerosing substances injected via the catheter can cause hepatic damage.
- Thromboembolic events, particularly to kidneys, intestines and the lower extremities. If blanching or cyanosis of the lower extremities occurs, remove the catheter immediately.

TIPS

- Always advance catheters slowly and use only gentle pressure if resistance is encountered.
- Aggressive catheter insertion can result in creation of a false lumen or perforation of a vessel.
- Always confirm catheter position radiographically.
- If an umbilical venous catheter is needed emergently prior to radiographic confirmation of position, place it 'low' to avoid accidental injection of sclerosing medications directly into the liver. However, if time

allows for radiographic confirmation of catheter position, place the umbilical artery catheter 'high' since that position appears to be associated with fewer complications.

FURTHER READING

Barrington KJ 2000 Umbilical artery catheters in the newborn: Effects of catheter materials. Cochrane Database Systems Review 2, CD000949

Barrington KJ 2000 Umbilical artery catheters in the newborn: Effects of position of the catheter tip. Cochrane Database Systems Review 2, CD000505

Cohen RS, Ramachandran P, Kim EH, Glasscock GF 1995 Retrospective analysis of risks associated with an umbilical artery catheter system for continuous monitoring of arterial oxygen tension. Journal of Perinatology 15(3): 195–198

Cunningham FJ, Engle WA, Rescorla FJ 1998 Paediatric vascular access and blood sampling techniques. In: Roberts JR, Hedges JR (eds) Clinical procedures in emergency medicine, 3rd edn., WB Saunders, Philadelphia, PA

Green C, Yohannan MD 1998 Umbilical arterial and venous catheters: Placement, use, and complications. Neonatal Network 17(6): 23–28

Kim JH, Lee YS, Kim SH et al 2001 Does umbilical vein catheterisation lead to portal venous thrombosis? Prospective US evaluation in 100 neonates. Radiology 219(3): 645–650

McAneney C 1997 Umbilical vessel catheterisation. In: Dieckmann RA, Fiser DH, Selbst SM (eds) Paediatric emergency and critical care procedures. Mosby, St Louis, MO

Weber HS 2001 Transumbilical artery interventions in the neonate. Journal of Invasive Cardiology 13(1): 39–43

23.14 ELECTRICAL COUNTERSHOCK

RONALD DIECKMANN

BACKGROUND

When a child's heart deteriorates into ven tricular fibrillation (VF) or pulseless ventricular tachycardia (VT), there is usually a severe systemic insult, such as profound hypoxia, ischaemia, acidosis, electrocution, or myocarditis. Sometimes the child has a congenital heart defect such as idiopathic hypertrophic subaortic stenosis or long QT syndrome. Any detectable ventricular rhythm, even fibrillation, suggests that there is still some perfusion of the heart – therefore VF or pulseless VT is a survivable presenting rhythm. Another important childhood dysrhythmia, supraventricular tachycardia (SVT), may also present with pulselessness, and has a high survival rate with appropriate treatment. This is in distinction to the clinical circumstances with asystole or bradyasystole, the most common paediatric cardiopulmonary arrest rhythms. In these rhythm presentations, the degree of hypoxia is usually so severe that treatment of any kind is unlikely to work. Ventricular dysrhythmias represent approximately 5–10% of presenting paediatric cardiopulmonary arrest rhythms. SVT represents < 1%. Resuscitation from such pulseless rhythms also includes ventilation, oxygenation, and effective chest compressions.

Electrical countershock for tachydysrhythmias is a common life-saving procedure in adult emergency cardiac care and is the most effective treatment for sudden cardiac arrest from ventricular dysrhythmias in all age groups. The concept behind electrical countershock is that if a properly delivered electrical dose is applied to the heart in a magnitude that does not damage the myocardium, all electrical activity will be momentarily ablated through depolarisation, and the intrinsic pacemaker of the heart will resume rhythm control (automaticity). When the child is *pulseless* and has a ventricular dysrhythmia or SVT, the most effective treatment is immediate electrical asynchronised countershock (defibrillation) performed as quickly as possible with the appropriate technique. In contrast, if a child has a pulse, and the rhythm is either SVT or VT, use synchronised countershock.

Electrical countershock is frequently effective in children with ventricular dysrhythmias or SVT, but it will not provide benefit in asystole, bradyasystole or pulseless electrical activity (PEA). Essential treatments for VF, such as CPR, improved gas exchange, correction of acidosis and vasopressor support of perfusion may change the type of VF from fine, low amplitude VF to coarse, high amplitude VF. Coarse, high amplitude VF is more responsive to electrical countershock than fine, low amplitude VF. After electrical countershock for a ventricular dysrhythmia, administer lidocaine or amiodarone to reduce recurrence. In addition, in children with *torsades de pointes* VT, give magnesium.

In certain clinical scenarios, other interventions in addition to countershock may also improve survival, e.g. fluids for hypovolaemia, potassium-lowering treatment for hyperkalaemia, calcium for hypocalcaemia, pericardiocentesis for pericardial tamponade and needle thoracostomy for tension pneumothorax.

INDICATIONS FOR ASYNCHRONOUS COUNTERSHOCK (DEFIBRILLATION)

- VF.
- Pulseless VT.

INDICATIONS FOR SYNCHRONOUS COUNTERSHOCK

- SVT with shock and pulse but no vascular access rapidly available.
- VT with shock and pulse but no vascular access rapidly available.
- Atrial fibrillation or atrial flutter with shock.
- Stable VT or SVT with specialist present.

CONTRAINDICATIONS

- Conscious patient with good perfusion.

EQUIPMENT

❶ Standard defibrillator.
❷ AED.
❸ Newer models feature lower power outputs to deliver lower energy countershocks.

STANDARD PREPARATION

❶ Open airway and ventilate by BVM while assembling equipment.
❷ If child is pulseless, begin closed chest compressions.
❸ Turn *on* the defibrillator but do *not* activate the synchronised mode.
❹ Select the proper paddles size. Use the 8 cm adult paddles if these will fit on the chest wall; otherwise, use the 4.5 cm paediatric paddles (Table 23.14.1).
❺ Prep paddles or skin electrodes with electrode jelly, paste, or saline-soaked gauze pads, or use self-adhesive defibrillator pads. Do not let jelly or paste from one site touch the other and form an 'electrical bridge' between sites, which could result in ineffective defibrillation or skin burns.
❻ Establish appropriate electrical charge (Table 23.14.2).
❼ Stop CPR, verify rhythm and ascertain good chest contact with paddles.
❽ Select synchronised or asynchronised mode.

Table 23.14.1   Paddle size

- Use the largest paddles that will fit!
Attempt to decrease transthoracic impedance to electrical delivery to heart by using the largest paddle size that allows good skin contact

- 8 cm adult paddles on chest wall anterior-posterior
Use in children over twelve months of age or weighing > 10 kg and > 77 cm in length

- 4.5 cm paediatric paddles on the chest wall
Use in infants up to twelve months of age or weighing < 10 kg and < 77 cm in length

Table 23.14.2   Appropriate electrical charge for countershock

Dysrhythmia	Mode	Charge
VF Pulseless tachycardia	Asynchronised (defibrillation)	2 J kg^{-1}, then 4 J kg^{-1}, then 4 J kg^{-1}, as needed Then 4 J kg^{-1} 30–60 seconds after each medication
VT with pulse SVT Atrial fibrillation and atrial flutter with shock	Synchronised	0.5–1.0 J kg^{-1} Repeat as needed

Fig. 23.14.1   Placement of paddles on the child's chest.

STANDARD PROCEDURE

❶ Apply the paddles directly to the skin of the chest wall with firm pressure. Place one paddle on the anterior chest wall on the right side of the sternum inferior to the clavicle and the other paddle on the left midclavicular line at the level of the xiphoid process (Fig. 23.14.1).

❷ As another option, use the anterior-posterior position (Fig. 23.14.2).

❸ Clear the nearby area of personnel so that no one is in contact with the patient, gurney or equipment. Announce, 'I am going to shock on three. One, I am clear. Two, you are clear. Three, everybody is clear'.

❹ Begin recording rhythm.

❺ Deliver the countershock by depressing the discharge buttons simultaneously, or by activating the discharge button when the equipment has hands-off pads.

❻ Assess the patient for evidence of reperfusion and check the monitor for the rhythm.

❼ If the first electrical shock is unsuccessful, deliver additional electrical countershocks, depending on specific rhythm.

❽ Either deliver countershocks in clusters of three to decrease chest wall impedance, then give drugs and 30–60 seconds of CPR before next cluster of three countershocks, in shock-shock-shock-drugs-CPR sequence, or use sequence of shock-drugs-CPR.

❾ Give specific drug treatment with adrenaline (epinephrine).

❿ If there is no rhythm response with countershocks after three sequences, do CPR for one minute, and administer a vasopressor. If no response with an additional countershock, consider administering lidocaine, or amiodarone.

⓫ Treat reversible causes.

⓬ Treat other rhythms that develop such as PEA or asystole.

AED PROCEDURE

❶ In out-of-hospital setting, use device on any aged child, although effectiveness in children <12 months of age is not known.
  – Open airway ventilate while preparing equipment
  – If child is pulseless, begin chest compression

Fig. 23.14.2   Placement of paddles on the child's chest and back.

❷ Turn AED *on*.

❸ Attach AED electrodes to chest wall (right upper sternal border, left chest in axilla, left chest under nipple).

❹ Allow the device to analyze rhythm.

❺ If countershock indicated, clear the area and deliver electricity.

❻ Repeat countershocks times three or until AED indicates that no countershock is indicated.

❼ Do CPR and check airway, breathing and circulation for one minute, then re-analyse rhythm and deliver additional countershocks as indicated.

COMPLICATIONS

- Ineffective delivery of countershock because of failure to charge, improper positioning on the chest, incorrect paddle size, or improper conduction medium (e.g. alcohol swabs).
- Burns on the chest wall.
- Failure to 'clear' before voltage discharge, leading to electrical shock of a team member or bystanders.
- Tachydysrhythmias.
- Bradycardia.

- Myocardial damage or necrosis.
- Cardiogenic shock.
- Embolic phenomena.

TIPS

- If the child has SVT or VT *and* is in shock and unresponsive, give electrical countershock at 0.5–1.0 J kg^{-1}.
- Use sedation with analgesia for conscious children receiving countershocks.
- Assure the device is in the synchronised mode (SYNC) before every countershock.
- For a child with VF or pulseless VT, use the asynchronised mode – the defibrillator will not discharge in the synchronised mode.
- Do not forget chest compressions and adrenaline (epinephrine) treatment in pulseless patients.
- Failure to apply paddles firmly to the chest wall, using too small paddles or

too low energy, and failure to deliver countershocks rapidly and in sufficient numbers will decrease effectiveness.

FURTHER READING

American Academy of pediatrics, American Heart Association 2002 PALS Provider Manual. American Heart Association, Wallingford, CT

Cecchin F, Jorgenson DB, Berul CI, Perry JC, Zimmerman AA, Duncan BW, Lupinetti FM, Snyder D, Lyster TD, Rosenthal GL, Cross B, Atkins DL 2001 Is arrhythmia detection by automatic external defibrillator accurate for children? Sensitivity and specificity of an automatic external defibrillator algorithm in 696 paediatric arrhythmias. Circulation 103(20): 2483–2488

Deboer S, Sicilia MR, Seaver M, Hood JR, O'Neill KA 2002 Paediatric defibrillation: Concerns and opportunities. Paediatric Emergency Care 18(6): 466–468

Dieckmann RA, Brownstein D, Gausche M 2001 Textbook for paediatric education for prehospital professionals. Jones & Bartlett, Sudbury, MA, 283–285

Dieckmann RA, Fiser D, Selbst S 1997 Illustrated Textbook of paediatric emergency and critical care procedures. Mosby, St Louis, MO, 323–336

Silka MJ, Kron J, Walance CG, Cutler JE, McAnulty JH 1990 Assessment and follow-up of paediatric survivors of sudden cardiac death. Circulation 82(2): 341–349

23.15 PERICARDIOCENTESIS

RONALD DIECKMANN

BACKGROUND

The pumping heart is extremely sensitive to rapid accumulation of pericardial fluid. Small amounts of fluid acutely increase intrapericardial pressure and may significantly impede venous return and cardiac output. Haemopericardium is the most common fluid collection – blood collects between the visceral and parietal pericardium after a penetrating injury in the high risk zone formed by the triangle of the two nipples and the sternal notch. The risk of death from a penetrating injury to the heart is higher from the haemopericardium than from direct injury to the myocardium, coronary arteries or cardiac valves.

The classical presentation of paediatric cardiac tamponade is a child with a penetrating anterior chest-wall injury who has distant heart sounds, neck vein distension and hypotension (Beck's triad). However, because other blood loss may concurrently reduce central venous pressures, and because audible intensity of heart sounds may be difficult to distinguish in children, suspect tamponade in any child with a high-risk chest-wall penetration in the triangle, even tiny, with signs of a possible perfusion deficiency – tachycardia, poor skin colour or temperature, delayed capillary refill or diminished pulses.

In contrast to haemopericardium, slow fluid accumulation in the pericardium, from other aetiologies, such as viral, bacterial or mycobacterial infection, or from immunological/collagen vascular disease or malignancy, has a minimal effect on cardiac function. The distensible pericardium readily accommodates slow fluid collections and the presentation of such patients often does not involve perfusion abnormalities. In this setting, needle pericardiocentesis is best accomplished with echocardiographic guidance.

Pericardiocentesis is a needle procedure for either life-saving decompression of acute cardiac tamponade, or for diagnostic evaluation of a non-emergent pericardial effusion. Rapid removal of acute haemopericardial fluid by needle pericardiocentesis is sometimes life saving. The decompression of the pericardium will temporarily restore myocardial performance in a perfusing patient, until reaccumulation occurs. Hence, needle pericardiocentesis is a temporising measure that precedes open surgical decompression. Sometimes, it is a heroic intervention in cardiopulmonary arrest. In non-emergent settings, an indwelling catheter may be necessary to prevent fluid reaccumulation. The procedure can be done with or without electrocardiographic or echocardiographic guidance, depending on the urgency of the clinical situation. Because the majority of needle pericardiocentesis procedures are performed on children in cardiopulmonary arrest, who have low probability of survival, the efficacy and safety of the procedure are poorly understood.

INDICATIONS

- Cardiac tamponade.
- Pericardial effusion of unknown aetiology.

CONTRAINDICATIONS

- There are no contraindications in the child presenting emergently with shock or cardiopulmonary arrest and evidence of acute tamponade. If equipment and appropriate personnel are present, open thoracotomy may be preferred over needle pericardiocentesis.
- In the non-emergent situation, an uncorrected bleeding diathesis is a contraindication.

EQUIPMENT

Emergent procedure
❶ Providone-iodine solution.
❷ 30–50 mL syringe.
❸ 2.5 or 3.5 inch 18–20-gauge spinal needle.

Non-emergent procedure
❶ 1% lidocaine.
❷ 25-gauge needle.
❸ Two 5 mL syringes.
❹ Two 2.5 or 3.5 inch 18–20-gauge spinal needles.
❺ Three-way stopcock.
❻ 30–50 mL syringe.
❼ 18 and 20-gauge over-the-needle catheters.
❽ Cable with alligator clip at each end.
❾ Sample containers.
❿ ECG machine.
⓫ Echocardiograph (desirable).

Indwelling catheter
❶ Flexible guidewire or J-wire.
❷ Plastic over-the-wire catheter.

STANDARD PREPARATION

❶ Place the child in a semi-reclining position (30–45 degrees).
❷ Establish secure vascular access and apply cardiac monitor.
❸ Secure the airway if necessary.
❹ If the procedure is non-emergent, administer sedation.
❺ Identify the subxiphoid entry site (Fig. 23.15.1), below and to the left of the xiphoid process.
❻ Prepare the area widely with providone-iodine solution.
❼ Infiltrate the entry site with lidocaine in conscious patients.

Non-emergent procedure
In addition to the preparation:

❶ Attach the correctly-sized spinal needle to a stop cock and 30 mL syringe.
❷ Attach one clip of the cable to the hub of the spinal needle and one clip to the V-lead of the ECG machine (Fig. 23.15.2).
❸ Turn the ECG to the V-lead position.

PROCEDURE

❶ Aim the needle to the left shoulder and enter at a 30–45 degree angle (Fig. 23.15.1) toward the anatomic location of the right ventricle.
❷ Apply continuous negative pressure and advance the needle until there is a 'pop' as the needle enters the pericardium.
❸ When blood flows into the syringe, place a haemostat at the skin surface to prevent further advancement of the needle.
❹ Aspirate until blood is evacuated from the pericardium.
❺ If prolonged drainage is necessary, advance the guidewire or J-wire through the needle, remove the spinal needle, and place the larger catheter with side holes over the wire.

Non-emergent procedure
After the preparation:

❶ Do constant ECG monitoring to detect myocardial puncture.
❷ If the needle punctures the ventricular epicardium, ST segment elevation or a dysrhythmia may occur (Fig. 23.15.3).
❸ If an injury pattern develops, withdraw the needle slightly or reposition more medially.

Right auricle
Right coronary artery
Left circumflex coronary artery
Left ventricle
Left anterior descending coronary artery
Right ventricle

Fig. 23.15.1 Subxiphoid entry site.

Fig. 23.15.2   Using the ECG for guidance.

❹ If echocardiography is available, use the ultrasound to guide the needle to the area of largest fluid accumulation.

COMPLICATIONS

• Ventricular puncture.
• Atrial puncture.
• Coronary artery laceration.
• Cardiac dysrhythmia.
• Haemopericardium.

• Pneumothorax.
• Haemothorax.
• Diaphragm perforation.
• Bowel or stomach perforation.
• Infection.
• Cardiac arrest.

TIPS

• If the effusion is not causing tamponade, identify the size and

Fig. 23.15.3   Injury current with needle in myocardium.

location of the effusion with echocardiography, CT or MRI before doing pericardiocentesis.
• Use echocardiographic guidance if possible.
• If there is a large volume of aspirated blood, the needle may be in the ventricle. The presence or absence of clotting does not reliably indicate needle location.

FURTHER READING

Dieckmann RA, Fiser D, Selbst S 1997 Illustrated textbook of paediatric emergency and critical care procedures. Mosby, St Louis, MO, 592–595

Lee C, Mason LJ 2001 Paediatric cardiac emergencies. Anesthesiology Clinics of North America 19(2): 287–308

Tsang TS, El-Najdawi EK, Seward JB, Hagler DJ, Freeman WK, O'Leary PW 1998 Percutaneous echocardiographically guided pericardiocentesis in paediatric patients: Evaluation of safety and efficacy. Journal of the American Society of Echocardiography 11(11): 1072–1077

23.16 TRANSURETHRAL CATHETERISATION AND SUPRAPUBIC BLADDER ASPIRATION

JUDITH KLEIN

BACKGROUND

Obtaining an uncontaminated specimen of urine is essential to diagnose urinary tract infection (UTI). In the last several years, UTIs have become a common aetiology of fever and serious bacterial infection in infants, particularly young females and uncircumcised males less than six months of age. In children who cannot provide clean-catch urine specimens, the diagnosis of UTI involves obtaining a urine sample directly from the bladder. Urine specimens obtained via bags attached temporarily on to the perineum are frequently contaminated samples, particularly with infant girls. Waiting for bagged urine specimens is also time-consuming and frustrating in the ED setting. Hence, urinary bag specimens frequently confuse diagnosis of UTI, and often result in false positive specimens and unnecessary treatment.

Obtaining an appropriate urine specimen requires either transurethral catheterisation or suprapubic aspiration. Unfortunately, in very young females and circumcised males with small foreskins, the urethra can be difficult to find and even more difficult to cannulate. In these cases, perform suprapubic aspiration of urine directly from the bladder, whenever possible under ultrasound guidance. This is an easy procedure that requires minimal equipment. Suprapubic aspiration provides a sterile urine specimen with less trauma to the infant than repeated, failed attempts at urethral catheterisation.

Transurethral catheterisation and placement of an indwelling bladder catheter, is also useful in the management of critically ill and injured children, to monitor urine output in the setting of shock or trauma. Urine output is one of the best measures of core perfusion and can help guide fluid resuscitation of a child in shock. The combination of heart rate and urinary bladder output are two excellent measurements of intravascular volume and response to treatment.

INDICATIONS

Indications for transurethral catheterisation
- Collection of a diagnostic urine specimen.
- Intermittent bladder decompression for neurogenic bladder.
- Urological study.
- Measurement of urine output in critically ill or injured child.
- Acute urinary retention.

Indications for suprapubic bladder aspiration
- Collection of a clean diagnostic urine specimen when transurethral catheterisation is impossible or unsuccessful.

CONTRAINDICATIONS

Urethral catheterisation
- Obvious pelvic trauma.
- Blood at the urethral meatus.
- Upward displacement of the prostate in males following trauma.
- Perineal haematoma.

In these circumstances, perform a retrograde urethrogram prior to cannulation of the urethra. Placement of a catheter without such a study could convert a partial urethral tear into a complete transection. Urethral injuries are uncommon in females because of the relatively short distance between the urethral meatus and the bladder. Bladder injuries, however, are more common in females and children in general because of the higher abdominal location of the organ in children versus adults. If blood appears following urethral catheterisation in trauma, perform a retrograde cystogram to search for bladder injury.

Suprapubic aspiration
- Coagulopathy.
- Thrombocytopenia.
- Significant abdominal distension.
- Recent abdominal surgery.

In addition, if ultrasound is available, do not perform suprapubic aspiration if the bladder diameter is less than 3.5 cm or if a volumetric scan demonstrates less than 10 mL of urine (Fig. 23.16.1). Under these circumstances, delay the procedure because it is unlikely to be successful.

TRANSURETHRAL CATHETERISATION

EQUIPMENT

The equipment required for transurethral catheterisation is often available in pre-packaged trays to which only the appropriately sized catheter need be added. Determine the appropriate catheter size either by using a length-based resuscitation tape, by using the formula 2 × (endotracheal tube size), or by using a table listing equipment sizes by age (Table 23.16.1). Remember to use lidocaine jelly in a syringe, particularly when catheterising the male urethra.

PREPARATION

❶ Review the male and female anatomy of the perineum.
❷ Have all equipment readily near the child.

Fig. 23.16.1   Using ultrasound for suprapubic aspiration.

Table 23.16.1   Catheter sizing for children

	Male (French)	Girl (French)	Type
Newborn	3	3–5	Straight
1–2 years	5	5 or 8	Straight
3–5 years	8	8	Balloon-tipped
6–10 years	8 or 10	8 or 10	Balloon
10–12 years	10 or 12	12	Balloon
13 years and older	12	12 or 14	Balloon

❸ Place the appropriately sized catheter and the syringe with lidocaine jelly (Lidojet®) on to the sterile field.

❹ Have an assistant gently restrain the child in a frog-leg position to prevent disruption of the sterile field and unnecessary trauma due to patient movement.

❺ If the child is older, discuss the procedure, clearly relate the steps of the procedure to the child, and move slowly.

PROCEDURE

❶ Use sterile procedure.

❷ With a male patient, use the non-dominant hand and a gauze to retract the foreskin and expose the meatus. In the circumcised male, the gauze is still useful to maintain a firm grasp on the penis during catheterisation.

❸ With a female patient, use the thumb and forefinger of the non-dominant hand to spread the labia majora and expose the urethra. Clean the urethral meatus three times with povidone-iodine solution, making sure to swab from front to back in females to avoid contamination.

❹ Insert a few millilitres of lidocaine jelly using a syringe device to provide topical anaesthesia particularly in male patients.

❺ Lubricate the catheter with the same jelly and insert the catheter into the urethra. Do not force the catheter against resistance. Once urine flows through the catheter, stop advancing.

❻ Discard the first 1 mL of urine, which may be contaminated, and collect a specimen.

Table 23.16.2   Complications of urethral catheterisation

- Urinary tract infection
- Urethral or bladder trauma
- Haematuria
- Paraphimosis
- Vaginal catheterisation
- Urethral strictures

❼ If the catheter is being left in, inflate the balloon, if there is one, and pull back until resistance is met. Inflate the balloon with the amount of fluid listed on the catheter itself.

❽ Connect the catheter to a sterile closed drainage system. With a balloon-tipped catheter, secure the catheter or tubing to the inner thigh with tape. With non-balloon catheters, tape the tube to the shaft of the penis in a spiral fashion or to the proximal inner thigh next to the labia majora in females.

❾ Remember to return the foreskin to its original position in uncircumcised males to prevent paraphimosis and penile constriction.

COMPLICATIONS

Table 23.16.2 lists the complications of urethral catheterisation.

- The most common complication of urethral catheterisation is infection, particularly if a catheter is left indwelling for a prolonged period of time. Single urethral catheterisations for collection of diagnostic specimens are rarely complicated by infections.
- Urethral or bladder trauma can also occur with urethral catheterisation particularly with oversized catheters or when a catheter is placed in a child with urethral trauma.
- Urethral strictures can also occur if catheters are left indwelling for a prolonged period of time.

TIPS

- There are circumstances in which urine specimens can be obtained non-invasively using urinary bags.

Fig. 23.16.2   Equipment for suprapubic aspiration.

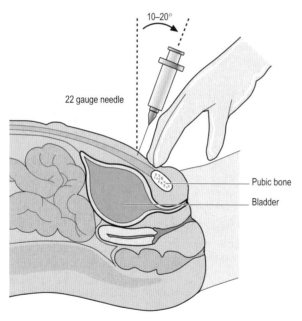

Fig. 23.16.4   Inserting the suprapubic needle.

- For example in the setting of trauma, microscopic haematuria (UA > 10–25 RBC per high powered field) can help detect occult intra-abdominal and genitourinary trauma in children.
- In uninjured children, a bag urine specimen is acceptable if the intent of diagnostic specimen collection is not the detection of infection.

SUPRAPUBIC ASPIRATION

EQUIPMENT

Fig. 23.16.2 illustrates the equipment required for suprapubic aspiration. Use an ultrasound to improve the likelihood of success.

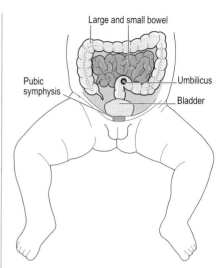

Fig. 23.16.3   Anatomy of the lower abdomen.

PREPARATION

❶ Review the anatomy of the lower abdomen (Fig. 23.16.3).
❷ Restrain the child in a frog-leg position using an assistant who can help soothe the child.
❸ Have all equipment near the patient's abdomen including the ultrasound.

PROCEDURE

❶ Locate a spot approximately 1 cm cephalad of the pubic symphysis in the midline.
❷ Use ultrasound to determine if the bladder is full enough. If the bladder diameter is 3.5 cm or if 10 cm^3 of urine is present on a volumetric bladder scanner, the procedure is likely to be successful.
❸ Prepare the skin at this spot with povidone-iodine solution.
❹ In males, provide gentle penile compression prior to skin cleansing to prevent voiding prior to the procedure.
❺ Using a 3 cm^3 syringe attached to either a 23-gauge butterfly or 22-gauge 1.5 inch needle, insert the needle at an angle approximately 10–20 degrees cranially (Fig. 23.16.4). Remember that the bladder lies higher in the abdomen in children than in adults.

❻ Provide constant backpressure on the syringe.

❼ Aspirate the urine specimen, remove the needle, and place a small bandage on the site.

COMPLICATIONS

- Bowel perforation. This is a rare complication. The only reports of bowel penetration are in children with markedly distended abdomens. Even if needle penetration of the bowel occurs, there is no treatment and infection is extremely unusual.
- Infections around the puncture site can occur, but are unusual with a sterile technique.
- Microscopic haematuria (< 10 RBC per high powered field) can occur transiently following aspiration.

TIPS

- Suprapubic aspiration is not often required in the ED. However, when urethral catheterisation is unsuccessful, it is a straightforward and safe procedure that provides diagnostic specimens with a contamination rate approximately half that of transurethral catheterisation.
- Use ultrasound in the ED to guide suprapubic aspiration.

FURTHER READING

Bell LM 1997 Transurethral bladder catheterization. In: Dieckmann RA, Fiser DH, Selbst SM (eds) Paediatric emergency and critical care procedures. Mosby, St Louis, MO
Bell LM 1997 Suprapubic bladder aspiration. In: Dieckmann RA, Fiser DH, Selbst SM (eds) Paediatric emergency and critical care procedures. Mosby, St Louis, MO
Garcia-Nieto V, Navarro JF, Sanchez-Almeida E, Garcia-Garcia M 1997 Standards for ultrasound guidance of suprapubic bladder aspiration. Paediatric Nephrology 11(5): 607–609
Liso JC, Churchill BM 2001 Paediatric urine testing. Paediatric Clinics of North America 48(6): 425–440
Pollack CV, Pollack ES, Andrew ME 1994 Suprapubic bladder aspiration versus urethral catheterization in ill infants: Success, efficiency and complication rates. Annals of Emergency Medicine 23(2): 225–230
Schneider RE 1998 Urologic procedures. In: Roberts JR, Hedges JR (eds) Clinical procedures in emergency medicine, 3rd end. WB Saunders, Philadelphia, PA

23.17 PENILE ZIPPER INJURY

MICHELLE LIN

BACKGROUND

The most common cause of penile entrapment is an unintentional zipper injury. Most commonly seen in boys aged 2–6 years, this injury occurs while the child is zipping up his pants. In addition to being painful, this condition is a tremendous anxiety-inducing injury for the child.

The patient usually presents for medical attention only after failed attempts at self-extrication. There are two patterns of entrapment for the often-macerated and oedematous soft tissue. First, the movable zipper head may 'catch onto' the external genitalia tissue. Second, the interlocking teeth along the zipper path may entrap some soft tissue. In order to disassemble a zipper, one must understand its anatomy. Specifically, a thin median bar is the only structure separating the two tracks on the zipper-sliding device, interlocking them.

INDICATIONS

- Soft-tissue entrapment in a zipper.

CONTRAINDICATIONS

- None.

EQUIPMENT

❶ Bone or wire cutters.
❷ Mineral oil.
❸ Local anaesthesia (1% lidocaine without adrenaline (epinephrine), syringe, 30-gauge needle).

PREPARATION AND POSITIONING

❶ Carefully position the patient supine or semi-supine in the caregiver's lap, being careful not to jostle the pants or zipper.

❷ In a child whom you anticipate is going to be too agitated or fearful of the procedure, consider procedural sedation.

PROCEDURE

❶ Soak the exposed external genitalia in mineral oil for ten minutes to lubricate the contact points. Occasionally, this manoeuvre alone will allow the zipper to easily retract so that the tissue is freed.

❷ Anaesthetise the entrapped tissue using 1% lidocaine without adrenaline (epinephrine).

❸ For the external genitalia entrapped *in the zipper sliding device*, use the bone or wire cutter to break the thin median bar that separates the two

Fig. 23.17.1 Diagram of zipper separation after cutting median bar.

sliding tracks. The front and back plates will fall apart, releasing the entrapped skin (Fig. 23.17.1).

❹ For the external genitalia entrapped *in the interlocking teeth*, cut the zipper just inferiorly to the entrapment site. The two interlocking rows of teeth will, with gentle manipulation, slowly separate from one another and release the skin.

❺ Provide supportive wound care to the injury site using warm soaks and apply a dressing. In severe soft tissue injuries, however, suture repair and/or debridement of the wound may be necessary under the guidance of a consulting urologist.

COMPLICATIONS

• The primary complication in penile zipper removal is pain. This occurs most commonly during the positioning and preparation of the patient. Gentle manipulation and positioning are essential for this procedure.

TIPS

• Cutting off the pant legs (and possibly even the rest of the pants around the zipper) can provide significant pain relief.

• Because pain is a significant fear in these patients, a compromise between local anaesthesia and procedural sedation is a regional block. A dorsal penile block will anaesthetise the entire penis.

FURTHER READING

Kanegaye JT, Shonfeld N 1993 Penile zipper entrapment: A simple and less threatening approach using mineral oil. Paediatric Emergency Care 9(2): 90–91

Lundquist ST, Stack LB 2001 Diseases of the foreskin, penis, and urethra. Emergency Medicine Clinics of North America 19(3): 529–546

Nolan JF et al 1990 Acute management of the zipper-entrapped penis. Journal of Emergency Medicine 8(3): 305–307

Woodward GA 1997 Penile zipper injuries. In: Dieckmann RA et al (eds) Paediatric emergency and critical care procedures. Mosby, St Louis, MO

Wyatt JP, Scobie WG 1994 The management of penile zip entrapment in children. Injury 25(1): 59–60

23.18 LUMBAR PUNCTURE

RONALD DIECKMANN

BACKGROUND

Lumbar puncture (LP) is a time-honoured method for obtaining cerebrospinal fluid (CSF) for diagnostic evaluation of suspected central nervous system (CNS) abnormalities. LP is an essential procedure in children with suspected meningitis, and represents the only simple method of obtaining fluid for rapid diagnosis and appropriate pathogen analysis for specific treatment. While LP is most commonly performed to diagnose meningitis, it is also a useful procedure to help identify encephalitis, CNS haemorrhage, malignancy, and other rare metabolic and degenerative conditions of childhood. Occasionally, LP is a therapeutic procedure in treatment of such conditions as pseudotumour cerebri, or for administration of intrathecal antibiotics or chemotherapeutic agents.

LP is a relatively simple procedure in infants and children but has a known complication rate, with both minor and major sequelae. Appropriate patient selection, preparation and patient positioning, and aseptic technique will avoid most complications. Do not do LP immediately on haemodynamically unstable patients, who first require meticulous management of airway, breathing and circulation, or on patients with clinical signs of focal CNS processes or significantly elevated intracranial pressure. In such patients, obtain blood cultures and administer antibiotics first, then perform LP after stabilisation and brain imaging, when indicated.

INDICATIONS

• Clinical symptoms and signs of meningitis or encephalitis in neonate, infant or child.

• Evaluation of sepsis in infant < 3 months of age.

• Seizure with fever in child < 12 months of age.

• Intrathecal drug administration.

CONTRAINDICATIONS

• Haemodynamic instability.

• Active seizure activity.

• Focal neurologic signs.

• Significant intracranial pressure elevation (hypertension, bradycardia, and apnoea).

In children with possible significant intracranial pressure elevation from oedema or space-occupying brain lesions, brain herniation after LP is an important consideration. Obtain a computerised axial tomography (CT) brain scan before the LP.

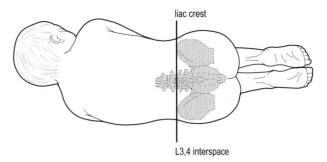

Fig. 23.18.1 Lateral decubitus position.

EQUIPMENT

Pre-packaged LP trays are available in most hospitals.

❶ 18-, 20- or 22-gauge styleted spinal needles:
  1.5 inch for neonates, infants, young children
  2.5 inch for older children and adolescents
  3.5 inch for large patients.
❷ Providone-iodine solution.
❸ 1% lidocaine.
❹ 25-gauge needle.
❺ 20-gauge needle.
❻ 3–5 mL syringe.
❼ Four capped sterile specimen tubes.
❽ Manometer (for children aged two years).
❾ Stopcock.

PREPARATION AND POSITIONING

❶ In most patients, establish secure vascular access, obtain blood cultures × 2 and appropriate blood tests, administer oxygen and begin cardiac monitoring and pulse oximetry.
❷ Secure the airway if necessary.
❸ Place the child in a lateral recumbent (Fig. 23.18.1) or sitting position (Fig. 23.18.2) at the edge of the gurney.
❹ If the child is conscious, consider sedation.
❺ Identify the entry site at the L3–L4 interspace.
❻ Don sterile gloves and prepare the area widely with providone-iodine solution.
❼ If the child is conscious, infiltrate the entry site with 1% lidocaine and a 25-gauge needle, then the deeper

tissue to the level of the paraspinous ligaments with a 20-gauge needle.

Lateral decubitus position
❶ Flex the child's knees and torso, but do not over-flex the neck and compress the airway.
❷ Have an assistant hold the child firmly in the decubitus position.

Sitting position
❶ Have an assistant hold the child upright with the hips flexed. Hold the child's right elbow and knee with the left hand and the left elbow and knee with the right hand.
❷ Put the thighs against the abdomen and flex the trunk.
❸ Keep the craniospinal axis perpendicular to the transverse plane of the line connecting the iliac crests.

PROCEDURE

❶ Drape the area.
❷ Grasp the needle with the thumbs and index fingers.
❸ Position the needle with the bevel up.
❹ Aim the needle into the interspace at 90 degrees, just above the L4 spinous process and advance slowly until there is resistance at the paraspinous ligaments.
❺ Advance the needle until there is a 'pop' as the needle enters through the dura, into the subarachnoid space.
❻ Remove the stylet.
❼ If CSF does not appear at the hub, replace the stylet and advance further.
❽ If the child is two years old, attach a three-way stopcock and manometer

Fig. 23.18.2   Sitting position.

to the hub, and measure opening pressure. Normal opening pressure for a child in the lateral decubitus position is 5–20 cm, but a struggling child may artificially elevate this number. Do not attempt an opening pressure in a sitting child, because it is unreliable.
❾ Limit CSF withdrawal to 2 mL in neonates, or 3–6 mL in infants and older children. Put the CSF in 3–4 separate tubes, labelled #1, #2, #3, and #4.
❿ Replace the stylet and remove the needle.
⓫ Bandage the entry site and encourage the child to remain prone for 3–4 hours to minimise CSF leak.
⓬ Send CSF for WBC count and differential, glucose, protein, Gram stain, other pathogen studies (e.g., viral, AFB or fungal cultures, antigen studies, VDRL). If the CSF is bloody, ask for a cell count on both tubes #1 and #4. Clearing of blood suggests a traumatic tap, whereas no clearing suggests subarachnoid haemorrhage.
⓭ Interpret CSF findings (Table 23.18.1).

Table 23.18.1   Interpretation of CSF

Condition	WBC mm^{-3}	Protein (mg dL^{-1})	Glucose (mg dL^{-1})	Gram stain	Opening pressure (cmH$_2$O)
Normal	< 6	< 45	60–70% peripheral	Negative	5–20
Bacterial meningitis	100–10 000 (PMN predominance)	50–100	< 50% peripheral	Positive (80% of cases)	Elevated
Partially treated	10–100 (PMNs or lymphs)	50–100	< 50% peripheral	Negative or positive	Elevated
Viral meningitis	20–100 (early PMNs, late lymphs)	< 100	Normal	Negative	Normal or slightly elevated
TB meningitis	20–500 (usually ymphs)	50–200	< 40%	Negative	Elevated
Crypto meningitis	Few–100s	100s	< 40%	Negative	Elevated
Brain abscess	10–100s	50–100s	Normal	Negative	Elevated

COMPLICATIONS

Local
- Puncture-site pain.
- Backache.
- Headache (uncommon < 10 years of age).
- Vomiting.
- Temporary paralysis.
- Epidermoid tumours.
- Discitis.
- Epidural haematoma.
- Epidural abscess.
- Osteomyelitis.
- Traumatic LP.

CNS
- Subarachnoid haemorrhage.
- Subdural haemorrhage.
- Brain-stem herniation.
- Cardiopulmonary arrest.

TIPS

- Positioning and restraining the infant or child properly will greatly facilitate the procedure.
- If no CSF appears in the hub after initial penetration, rotate the needle 90 degrees and withdraw the stylet.
- If there is no success with multiple attempts, try a paramedian approach a few millimetres off the midline.
- Use latex agglutination or another bacterial antigen test for partially treated or Gram-stain negative CSF.
- If the child appears ill, administer empiric antibiotics after blood cultures are obtained.
- If the LP is traumatic and CSF is bloody, calculate a WBC:RBC ratio and 'Observed: Predicted' CSF WBC to help predict probability of bacterial infection. The WBC:RBC ratio is calculated as a simple ratio on CSF fluid. The Predicted CSF WBC is calculated using the formula Predicted CSF WBC = CSF RBC × blood WBC/blood RBC. A WBC:RBC ratio <0.01 (1:100) and an O:P ratio <0.01 makes bacterial infection unlikely.

FURTHER READING

Al-Eissa YA 1995 Lumbar puncture in the clinical evaluation of children with seizures associated with fever. Paediatric Emergency Care 11(6): 347–350

Barnett ED, Bauchner H, Teele DW, Klein JO 1994 Serious bacterial infections in febrile infants and children selected for lumbar puncture. Paediatric Infectious Disease Journal 13(11): 950–953

Dieckmann RA, Fiser D, Selbst S 1997 Illustrated Textbook of Paediatric Emergency and Critical Care Procedures. Mosby, St Louis, MO, 533–537

Grant T 1994 Paediatric meningitis. Annals of Emergency Medicine 24(1): 118

Ward E, Gushurst CA 1992 Uses and technique of pediatric lumbar puncture. America Journal of Diseases in Childhood 146(10): 1160–1165

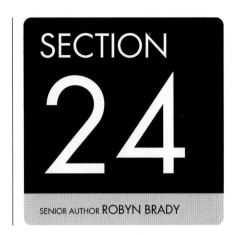

ORTHOPAEDICS AND RHEUMATOLOGY

24.1 ORTHOPAEDICS AND RHEUMATOLOGY

ROBYN BRADY • TREVOR JACKSON

INTRODUCTION

The child who has pathology of the bones and joints may present in a variety of ways. Acute paediatric orthopaedic conditions range from the many infective, inflammatory and other causes of limp and limb pains, to the isolated acute limb fracture as a result of moderate trauma, which is among the top ten paediatric emergency department (ED) presentations in Australia.[1] Risk management in paediatric orthopaedics and rheumatology is also an important consideration.

THE CHILD WITH ACUTE MUSCULOSKELETAL PAIN OR DYSFUNCTION

GENERAL APPROACH

The spectrum of orthopaedic pathology occurring in the paediatric population, with the exception of some fractures and

Essentials

1 Painful dysfunction of limb, posture, or gait may be caused by trauma, infection, or occasionally inflammatory or neoplastic developments.

2 Hip, knee, abdominal and spinal pathology must be considered with each presentation.

3 Careful attention to history and close assessment of posture and response to palpation are required to delineate focal pathology.

adolescent injury, is entirely different from that seen in the adult population.

Infant and child development have extensive influence on the musculoskeletal pathology seen and its manifestations, as well as the techniques used in assessment. These differences are outlined up in Table 24.1.1. The most important differences are:

- The *developing skeleton*, with its relative plasticity and physeal vulnerability, which changes the mechanics of energy dissipation in injury, causing a completely different spectrum of fracture patterns to the adult. This plasticity also offers less protection to the underlying structures, so significant damage to the underlying organ (brain, lungs, liver, etc.) for a given external force is more likely, and may not be accompanied by actual fracturing of the overlying bone.
- The *vulnerability* of the growing child to infective, psychological, and physical trauma, the latter either from external dangers which he or she does not yet recognise, such as traffic, or from local environmental dangers including his own care-givers.
- The *communication difficulties* as a consequence of emotional and intellectual immaturity, which call upon a range of different assessment techniques and skills.

It is particularly important to recognise that these differences manifest differently at different stages during maturity, resulting in varying pathologies of neonates, infants, toddlers, primary-school-age children, and adolescents.

THE LIMPING CHILD

The wide spectrum of causes of limp in children is illustrated in Table 24.1.2. In terms of frequency, common causes in

different age groups are outlined in Table 24.1.3.

Diagnoses that require specific treatment to avoid further damage or danger are primarily displaced or unstable fractures (including slipped upper femoral epiphysis), non-accidental injury (as a presenting feature or incidental finding), bone or joint infection, and neoplastic processes, principally bone tumours and leukaemia.

Assessment

The most useful characteristics of a child with an acute limp or painful limb dysfunction are the following:

- Age.
- Trauma history.
- Well-being.
- Pain magnitude.
- Pain localisation.

Age

The neonate or infant with focal pain or dysfunction should not be discharged without a specific diagnosis, (most of which, with the specific exception of pulled elbow, warrant admission), and should generally be assessed by someone experienced in this area. Adolescents with a limp or knee or hip pain must have slipped upper femoral epiphysis (SUFE) specifically ruled out.

Trauma history

The history is less sensitive or specific than in adult medicine because:

- Children are often poor historians.
- Minor injuries are very frequent.
- There is always a possibility of non-accidental injury and inadequate or erroneous history.

However, a clear history of completely normal function prior to a specific event that precipitated crying and subsequent pain and dysfunction should prompt a search for a fracture.

Table 24.1.1   How children differ: Impact of development on musculoskeletal pathology

Body proportions
- Large, heavy head: higher fulcrum for spinal disruption
- Low centre of gravity
- Relatively short legs

Physiology of developing bone
- Zone of calcification: weakest point of muscle/tendon/ligamentous/bony continuum
- Increased plasticity means increased susceptibility to plastic deformation, e.g. torus, bowing fractures
- Physeal vulnerability predisposes to specific pathological responses to subacute or chronic micro-trauma, e.g. avascular necrosis of ossification centres, slipped upper femoral epiphysis
- Physeal damage from fracture or ischaemia produces long-term complications
- High blood flow to physeal zones increases risk of vascular dissemination of bacterial disease, e.g. osteomyelitis

Joints and ligaments
- Increased flexibility means less brittleness and fewer fractures in response to arcuate deformation, e.g. carpal, tarsal, rib, vertebral fractures less common
- Ligaments generally stronger than bones: sprains uncommon and complete ligamentous tears rare

Exposure to mechanisms
- Infant-abuse mechanisms especially shearing/shaking forces
- Pre-school children fall on average four times a day (same-level falls)
- Highly active pre- and school-age children have frequent, relatively low-force impactions from falls (monkeybars, trees)
- Pedestrian vs. car causes classical femoral or tibial/fibula injuries from fender, plus head injury from secondary impact
- High-force MVA/MBA/high energy sports injuries increase from adolescence

Immunology
- Increased incidence of bacterial and viral infection
- More rapid dissemination of, and destruction from, bacterial infection

Psychology
- Fear and pain make young children difficult to examine and increase importance of observation and gentle handling
- Immature intellectual development means poor verbalisation of symptoms, incomplete self-other differentiation, and other blocks to symptom communication
- Medical management of traumatic experiences, such as injuries, may influence future psychological responses to trauma
- Altered body perception increases susceptibility of adolescents (particularly females) to unconsciously exaggerated dysfunction in response to minor injuries

Healing
- Rapid healing of most fractures (e.g. femoral fractures: infants three weeks!)
- Enormous remodelling potential of deformation within arc of use
- Great ability to compensate, physically and psychologically, for loss of function
- Minimal stiffness after immobilisation

Well-being

The following key points should be sought:

- History of fever/malaise.
- Eating and activity level, which is unlikely to be normal in sepsis.
- Minor illnesses are also common and can co-exist with injury.

Pain magnitude

- Septic arthritis is painful to the slightest movement.

- Subacute arthritides and Perthes disease present fluctuating disability and pain.
- Disruption of night sleep needs further assessment.

Pain localisation

This is the foundation of acute orthopaedic diagnosis and efficient investigation use. A suggested sequence of examination for young children with musculoskeletal pain is shown in Table 24.1.4.

Other useful features in assessment include:

History
- Details of onset.
- Whether symptoms are constant or intermittent.
- Exacerbations.
- Daily pattern.
- History of previous limp or similar pains.
- Physical activities, such as elite sport.
- Bullying or school/home problems.

Observation and examination
- Gait if ambulant.
- Posture and symmetry.
- Activity level.
- Well-being – fever, heart rate.
- Bones, joints, soft tissues.
- Abdomen and spine.
- Lymphadenopathy and lymphadenitis.
- Focal pathology, e.g. warts, bites, and callosities.

At the conclusion of the history and examination the emergency physician should have established the site and severity of musculoskeletal pain, identified practical precipitants, and considered the likelihood of traumatic, neoplastic, or septic processes. In patients with minimal physical findings, or findings out of keeping with other aspects of history and examination, the environmental and psychological context of the limp should be explored further. Clues to possible neoplastic illness are discussed later in this chapter.

The child whose examination findings suggest an irritable hip is likely to have one of the pathologies outlined in Table 24.1.5. A suggested pathway for investigation is shown in the algorithm in Fig. 24.1.1. This algorithm incorporates the findings of a number of studies of the prognostic significance of various features of the limping child with respect to septic arthritis,[2-4] which are further discussed below.

Investigations

A number of recent research findings have allowed for more selective and meaningful investigation of the limping child.

Inflammatory markers

Traditional blood investigations for inflammatory markers include full blood

Table 24.1.2   Causes of acute limp in children

Trauma:
- Fractures – accidental and non-accidental

Infection (point focus):
- Septic arthritis
- Osteomyelitis
- Inguinal lymphadenitis
- Muscle abscess, e.g. psoas

Post-infective:
- Rheumatic fever/post-streptococcal reactive arthritis
- Serum sickness
- Lyme disease
- Post-immunisation inflammation

Inflammatory:
- Transient synovitis
- Vasculitis, e.g. Henoch–Schönlein purpura
- Juvenile inflammatory arthritis
- Enthesitis/ankylosing spondylitis
- Associated with, e.g. systemic lupus erythematosis, inflammatory bowel disease, cystic fibrosis
- Dermatomyositis/polymyositis

Primary bone disorders:
- Slipped upper femoral epiphysis (SUFE)
- Perthes
- Osteochondroses, e.g. Osgood-Schlatter disease, Sever disease
- Unicameral bone cyst/aneurysmal bone cyst/fibrocystic disease/eosinophilic granuloma
- Blount disease
- Tarsal coalitions

Neoplastic:
- Leukaemia
- Neuroblastoma
- Bony tumours, e.g. Ewing's sarcoma, osteosarcoma
- Non-malignant tumours, e.g. osteoid osteoma

Haematological:
- Haemophilia
- Sickle cell disease

Practical:
- Splinter/foreign body
- Compensatory, e.g. footwear
- Soft-tissue injury
- Plantar warts/calcaneal spurs
- Insect bites

Psychological:
- Pain amplification syndromes, including reflex sympathetic dystrophy and hypermobility
- Conversion reactions

Abdominal:
- Appendix
- Infective and inflammatory bowel disease

Spine:
- Scoliosis
- Discitis
- Transverse myelitis
- Spondylolisthesis
- Scheurman's disease
- Guillain–Barré syndrome

count (FBC), erythrocyte sedimentation rate (ESR) and C-reactive protein (CRP).

FBC is useful primarily to flag bone-marrow dysfunction. Each cell line (haemoglobin, white cells and platelets) should be individually assessed. The sensitivity of a raised white-cell count (WCC) ($> 12 \times 10^9$ L^{-1}) for the identification of septic arthritis has been assessed as 60–75%[5,6] with some authors finding no significant association.[7] The absence of an elevated white-cell response should never be used to rule out septic arthritis. ESR has shown higher sensitivity (90–95%) in identifying the subgroup with septic arthritis, however this may miss early infection.[5] C-reactive protein has shown superior sensitivity and specificity in the early identification of invasive bacterial infection in general and septic arthritis in particular.[8] CRP rises within 24 hours of acute illness, and also falls rapidly and can be used to monitor effectiveness of treatment.[9]

In an award-winning study, researchers at Harvard calculated the usefulness of different parameters in distinguishing between culture proven septic arthritis and transient synovitis.[2] They found four variables to give a predicted probability of septic arthritis in a given child with the clinical syndrome of irritable hip. These factors are:

- Non-weight-bearing.
- Febrile > 38.5°C.
- WCC $> 12 \times 10^9$ L^{-1}.
- ESR > 40 mm h^{-1}.

The predicted probability of septic arthritis is 0.2% in the presence of zero predictors, 3% if one, 40% if two, 93.1% if three, and 99.6% if four predictors are present.

Radiology
X-ray

X-rays are usually non-contributory in children under ten years of age with acute onset limp without a specific trauma history. In septic arthritis an increased head to teardrop distance (the closest distance between the medial femoral neck metaphysis and the opacity representing the ileo-ischio-pubic interface at the acetabulum) may suggest lateral displacement of the femur by an effusion, although

Table 24.1.3 Common causes of acute limp/single-limb dysfunction in children of various ages presenting to the ED with no specific history of trauma

Infants	Young children	Primary-age children	Adolescents
Occult fracture*	Occult fracture**	Transient synovitis	SA/OM
Septic arthritis	Transient synovitis	SA/OM	SUFE
Osteomyelitis	SA/OM Perthes disease	Perthes disease Psychogenic pain	Osteochondroses Tumour

*Includes pulled elbow, accidental and non-accidental injury.
**Includes pulled elbow, toddler fracture.

Table 24.1.4 Tips for assessing young children

- The foundation of acute orthopaedic diagnosis is precise localisation of pain and dysfunction
- The foundation of a productive paediatric examination is a relaxed, non-fearful child
- Personality and parental factors aside, a gentle, slow-moving, highly observant examiner whom the child senses has the trust of the parent, will be most successful in gaining meaningful information

1. Make friends with the parent
2. Ask parents for clues about site of pain, e.g. is it worse during nappy changes or being picked up under arm, etc. If the child is old enough, ask them to tell or show you exactly where it hurts
3. Where possible, observe child at free play before attempting palpation
4. Visually scan child for alterations of posture, symmetry, or function
5. Record any other clues, such as temperature, dysmorphic features, bruising, psychological state
6. Examine the infant or child in parent's arms (under six months and over five years they may often be assessed on the couch without concern)
7. Introduce a washable or disposable toy, such as light, name-badge, or 'funny face'
8. Make your first touch very gentle and at a site distant from the target limb! Keep some touch continuous so the rhythm is reassuring. Verbal soothing, such as a hum, may settle anxiety
9. Palpate the limb in question from one end to the other, watching the child's face continuously
10. The first sign of discomfort may be an eyebrow flicker (i.e. a pre-frown) or a flinch
11. If discomfort is sensed, move touch to another area immediately and slowly move back in even more gently for confirmation and further information
12. Put all joints through their full range of movement unless discomfort is noted
13. Examine the spine, groin, and abdomen of all lower limb or gait-disturbed children
14. Areas of focal tenderness or limited range of motion can be further assessed by radiology or ultrasound

this demonstration is not reliable, influenced as it is both by degree of abduction and by relative pressure/traction on the joint.[55] Radiological findings in osteomyelitis are usually not present for up to ten days from the onset of illness, at which time there may be periosteal elevation outlined by new bone formation and or lucent areas.[3] The increasing public awareness of the risks of radiation exposure to bone marrow and gonads alters ED X-ray ordering behaviour, particularly with respect to films with high exposure requirements, such as the pelvis.[7] Whole-limb requests and comparison views are only rarely indicated, and many units do initial hip or pelvis screening as a single frog-leg view, with AP or further views as requested to delineate particular anatomical regions. X-rays of hip or pelvis are necessary in any child presenting with occult acute hip pain or limp in whom acute fracture (including non-accidental injury) or SUFE are possibilities, or in whom persistent unexplained limp (> 1 week's duration) warrants evaluation for possible Perthes disease or less commonly bony disorders.

Ultrasound

Ultrasound is a sensitive, non-invasive assessment tool for evaluation of the irritable hip. It will detect even small hip effusions, may show a subperiosteal pus collection in some cases of osteomyelitis, and may be diagnostic for Perthes disease and SUFE,[38, 41] although it is not usually the first line investigation for these pathologies. Disadvantages of ultrasound include variations in quality from different operators, and difficulties in after-hours access. An ultrasound cannot distinguish between reactive and infective effusions. There is controversy over the place of ultrasound-guided hip aspiration in the evaluation of the irritable hip with an effusion.[11] The majority of Australian paediatric orthopaedic units favour orthopaedic evaluation of irritable hips with selective aspiration and arthrotomy under general anaesthesia. However ultrasound guided diagnostic hip aspiration has a role in some units.[3,4,12]

Bone scan

Isotope bone scans with three-phase technetium-99m MDP are sensitive early and well tolerated by children, but lack specificity.[13] Confusion may arise particularly in relation to physeal sites where uptake is already above base-line. 'Hot' scans indicate increased osteoblastic uptake and generally relate to a response to infection or injury. A 'cold' scan suggests infarction, which in severe cases may be a consequence of osteomyelitis.

MRI

Magnetic resonance imaging (MRI) is excellent for detailed delineation of soft-tissue and bony pathology, particularly when surgery is planned.[14] Limitations include cost, access limitations, and the need to remain still for a longer time period, necessitating general anaesthetic in most small children.

Transient synovitis

Transient synovitis is a self-limited inflammatory disorder of uncertain aetiology, occurring particularly in boys (70%) in the age group 3–10 years. The onset of pain is generally gradual and initially may be localised to hip, knee, groin, or thigh. The child may be mildly unwell or have had a recent non-specific upper respiratory tract illness, although this is not

Table 24.1.5   Comparative features of paediatric hip-joint pathology

Diagnosis	Transient synovitis	Septic arthritis	Femoral neck osteomyelitis	Perthes	SUFE	Inflammatory mono-arthritis	Bone tumour
Age	≈3-6	Any	Any	≈3–10	≈9–15	Any	Any
Joint	Hip	Hip, knee	Hip	Hip	Hip	Any	Not joint
Pain (0–3)	1	3	≈1	0–1 early	≈1–3	0–1	≈1
Illness (0–3)	0	≈1-3	≈1–3	0	0	0–1	Variable
ROM	> 80%	< 50%	< 80%	60–80%	Flexes into external rotation	Usually > 70%	Normal unless spasm
Inflammatory markers	Normal	Elevated	Elevated	Normal	Normal	Variable	Normal except leukaemia
Ultrasound	Effusion	Effusion	?Reactive effusion, ?sub-periosteal collection	Diagnostic changes	Diagnostic changes	?Effusion	n/a
Plain X-ray	?HTDD up	?HTDD up	Bony changes late only	Diagnostic changes	Diagnostic changes (Klein line)	May be normal	May be diagnostic

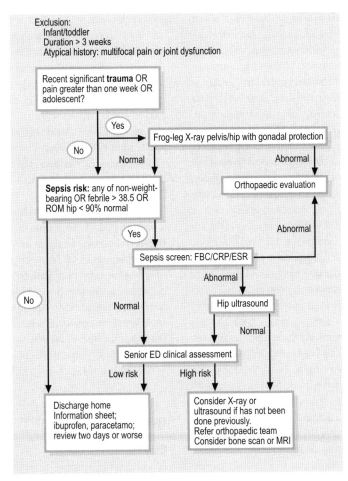

Fig. 24.1.1   Algorithm for management of children > 2 years presenting with acute irritable hip.

uniformly present. Range of movement at the hip joint is usually mildly diminished, with discomfort at the endpoints of the range. A hip effusion is present. Transient synovitis is a diagnosis of exclusion, the major differential being septic arthritis. Children with localised hip pain should be managed according to the algorithm in Fig. 24.1.1, and non-weight bearing children with a hip effusion who do not have needle aspiration to rule out septic arthritis should be admitted under the close observation of the orthopaedic team.

Management

Rest is the key to management of the irritable hip. Non-steroidal anti-inflammatory medications may be used,[15] if not contraindicated, until the hip is painless and normal range of motion has returned. The acute phase may last 3–7 days, with total recovery expected within three weeks.

Prognosis

Various authors have noted that 0.5–10% of children given a diagnosis of irritable hip later develop evidence of Perthes' disease.[16] All children discharged with this presumptive diagnosis should have orthopaedic follow-up.

Essentials

1 Delayed or inadequate treatment can lead to irreversible joint damage.

2 Diagnosis of septic arthritis is based on clinical features, and confirmed by blood and synovial fluid culture. Imaging techniques have an important role in localising osteomyelitis.

3 *Staphylococcus aureus* is the most frequent pathogen, via haematogenous spread or direct extension from infected joint to bone.

4 Successful treatment requires parenteral antibiotics and complete drainage of pus from the joint, or surgical clearance of necrotic bone.

SEPTIC ARTHRITIS AND OSTEOMYELITIS

INTRODUCTION

Septic arthritis is infection of the synovial lining and fluid of a joint. Bacteria are the usual pathogens having seeded the joint haematogenously. Direct spread from adjacent bone infection may also occur, particularly where the metaphysis is intracapsular as in the proximal femur. Phagocytic and neutrophil responses to the bacteria result in proteolytic enzyme release and cytokine production, with synovial abscess formation and cartilage necrosis.[17] Pus under pressure may also reduce epiphyseal blood flow.

Most infections in children are community acquired and in normal joints, but comorbidity or deficient host defences, if present, predispose to infection that may be more rapidly progressive.[18] Infants and young children are at particular risk, comprising one-third and on-half, respectively, of a large recent series.[19] These may present with occult infection, pseudo-

Table 24.1.6   Risk factors for septic arthritis

Relative immune deficit
- Neonates
- Malnourished
- HIV infection
- Immunosuppressive therapy
- Corticosteroid therapy

Injury mechanism
- Penetrating trauma

Joint disease
- Chronic arthritis
- Sickle cell disease

paralysis or generalised sepsis. Risk factors for septic arthritis are shown in Table 24.1.6.

Joints of the lower limb, especially hip and knee, account for the majority of infections, with multifocal septic arthritis less common in children.

Most cases of osteomyelitis in children are initiated via haematogenous spread of *Staphylococcus aureus*, but direct extension of contiguous joint infection or direct inoculation during trauma also occur. Associated comorbidity is rare in the paediatric setting. Bacteria enter metaphyseal bone initially, then typically extend to the subperiosteal space forming an abscess. New bone deposition results with later necrosis of cortical bone. Bone fragments or sequestra may be formed over time, which harbour bacteria. Successful treatment must combine eradication of the bacteria and complete removal of any necrotic infected bone. However, in recent times earlier diagnosis and aggressive antibiotic therapy has limited the degree of bone destruction present.[10]

The disorder of chronic recurrent multifocal osteomyelitis (CRMO) has been recognised in infants and children.[19,20] This is an inflammatory process of unknown origin, which demonstrates culture negative bony inflammation with histological evidence of necrosis and chronic inflammatory cell infiltrates. Biopsy and culture are mandatory to diagnose the disorder, but antibiotics may be discontinued if pathology is consistent with CRMO. Treatment is with non-steroidal anti-inflammatory agents, or steroids in resistant cases.[21]

PRESENTATION

History

Cardinal features are recent onset of a painful, red or swollen joint or limb, limp or refusal to bear weight. Pseudo-paralysis or refusal to move a limb may occur in neonates and young infants. Infants may presents non-specifically with poor feeding, vomiting, lethargy or fever. Infrequently, a vertebral or pelvic infection will be the cause of an abnormal gait or abdominal pain. The immunisation status should always be ascertained in respect to *Haemophilus influenzae*.

Examination

Typical findings include a warm tender joint with marked limitation of passive or active movement due to pain. Children with a painful hip will usually maintain the joint in flexion and external rotation. An effusion will be evident in most distal joints, but in general, fever is low grade and most patients will not appear 'toxic' or unwell. Osteomyelitis may be suggested by an area of maximal tenderness next to a joint, with a greater range of movement of that joint than would be expected with septic arthritis. Deep or chronic infections may be clinically 'silent' with minimal or absent examination findings. Careful examination of the skin may reveal areas of infection or trauma.

Differential diagnosis

The differential diagnosis of septic arthritis is discussed in detail in the section on the limping child. Non-septic arthritis or synovitis, fractures and osteomyelitis all share a similar presentation. Non-accidental injury and neoplastic disease must always be considered. The differential diagnosis of the child presenting with polyarthralgia/polyarthritis is considered in the section on acute arthritides.

INVESTIGATION

Blood tests

Blood cultures should always be taken, and will be positive in up to 50%. The sensitivity and utility of various inflammatory markers (WCC, ESR, CRP) is discussed earlier in this chapter. These have predictive value only and cannot be used to exclude the diagnosis, but aid in monitoring response to therapy.

Imaging studies

As discussed in the previous section, ultrasonographic demonstration of an effusion can be useful in confirming a joint as abnormal, but cannot usually differentiate between septic arthritis, transient synovitis, or a reactive effusion from a nearby osteomyelitis.

Isotope bone scans are very sensitive early, but not specific for sepsis. X-rays may remain normal for 10–14 days after infection. Thereafter the findings reflect bony destruction manifested by cortical rarefaction and new bone formation beneath a raised periosteum. Chronic osteomyelitis may show involucrum formation or sequestrae. In subacute infection, a bone abscess, known as Brodie's abscess, may appear as a lucent lesion with sclerotic margins at the metaphysis. CT and MRI are excellent for displaying the extent of established infection or, in difficult sites (e.g. the spine), soft-tissue involvement

Microbiology
Synovial fluid examination and culture

Aspiration of affected joints should be performed promptly to confirm the diagnosis and obtain culture specimens. Most young children will require general anaesthesia or conscious sedation for these procedures, and in the majority of units in Australia, arthrotomy with washout is the procedure of choice in probable septic arthritis of the hip. The overriding principles are early accurate diagnosis, and minimal delay or exposure of joint to the chondrolytic enzymes of bacterial joint infection.[22]

Orthopaedic consultation is required in all cases.

Typical synovial fluid findings in septic arthritis are shown in Table 24.1.7.[23]

Initial Gram stain results will guide empiric antibiotic therapy, with definitive therapy based on final cultures. Positive cultures occur in up to 60% of aspirates. Causative bacteria generally relate to the age of the child, but *Staphylococcus aureus* will account for the large majority of cases in both septic arthritis and osteomyelitis (Table 24.1.8).[22] Non-bacterial pathogens occur rarely. Tuberculosis is still a cause of chronic bone and spine infection, particularly in Northern Australia.[24]

Culture of infected bone obtained by needle aspiration or surgery provides definitive evidence in up to 80% of cases of osteomyelitis.[25]

MANAGEMENT

Joint drainage and empiric parenteral antibiotic therapy are the mainstays of treatment for septic arthritis and should take place without delay. Early diagnosis and modern antimicrobial therapy and monitoring have reduced the necessity for curettage in osteomyelitis in some units to under 40%.[10] Antibiotic therapy is initiated after culture specimens have been obtained, with clinical presentation and Gram stain guiding the choice of agents. All regimens should include an antistaphylococcal agent and/or Gram-negative cover.

Suggested regimen:

- Di(Flu)cloxacillin 5 mg kg^{-1} per dose to 8 g d^{-1}, 6-hourly.

For children under five not immunised against *Haemophilus influenzae*, or when Gram-negative infection is suspected, add:

- Cefotaxime 50 mg kg^{-1} per dose to 2 g IV, 8-hourly
  OR
- Ceftriaxone 50 mg kg^{-1} to 2 g IV, daily.[26]

Community-acquired methicillin resistance is becoming an increasing problem world-wide. Specific populations at high risk of community acquired MRSA include Aboriginal and Torres Strait Islanders in Western and Northern Australia, and Pacific Islanders in Eastern Australia and the parts of New Zealand.[27] Suspicion of methicillin resistance will require consultation with infectious-disease units and addition of vancomycin or clindamycin. Therapy will be fine-tuned once the organism and its sensitivities are known.

In view of the range of possible organisms and destructive potential, management of neonatal septic arthritis or osteomyelitis should be by a team of orthopaedic, neonatal, and infectious-disease specialists.

Because of earlier diagnosis and other aspects of modern care, in most cases

Table 24.1.7 Synovial fluid characteristics

Characteristic	Septic arthritis	Non-septic arthritis	Non-inflammatory effusion
Colour	Yellow–green	Yellow	Colourless
Turbidity	Purulent, turbid	Turbid	Clear
Leucocytes mm^{-3}	10–100 000	5–1 000	< 1000
Predominant cell	PMN*	PMN*	Monocyte

*PMN = polymorphonuclear leucocyte.

Table 24.1.8 Bacterial causes of septic arthritis and osteomyelitis

Age	Typical bacteria
Neonates/infants	Group B streptococci Staphylococcus aureus Kingella kingae Haemophilus influenzae Gram-negative rods*
Children	Staphylococcus aureus Group A streptococci
Young adults	Neisseria gonorrhoeae Staphylococcus aureus

*Pseudomonas sp. and Enterobacteriaceae.

beyond the neonatal period combined in-patient/out-patient treatment can occur with length of treatment guided by clinical and inflammatory markers.[3,8,28]

General care, with joint rest, appropriate analgesia and physical therapy, is important.

PROGNOSIS

This depends upon the organism, patient comorbidity, age of patient and the adequacy and rapidity of treatment. Remarkable remodelling of bony deformity can occur in the young child providing treatment has been adequate. Out of a thirty-year series of 332 infants and children with osteomyelitis, with documented follow-up of 170 cases, complications were described in 19%.[19] These related largely to joint complications, but some 8% demonstrated epiphyseal damage. However, more recent series showed many fewer complication rates.[10] Patients at highest risk of complication include neonates, septic arthritis in which diagnosis has been delayed, complicated osteomyelitis (involucrae, sequestrum or sinus formation) or epiphyseal involvement, which may cause subsequent limb length discrepancy or deformity. All cases should have close orthopaedic follow-up.

PREVENTION

Thorough debridement, wound cleansing and antibiotics are essential in the setting of bone trauma.

CONTROVERSIES

❶ The role of ultrasound-guided hip aspiration: most orthopaedic surgeons prefer open arthrotomy on selected patients.

❷ Extent and timing of surgery in suspected osteomyelitis.

❸ Duration and route of antimicrobial therapy for bone and joint infections.

PERTHES DISEASE

Essentials

1 Perthes disease is a chronic disorder of the femoral head in children, causing limp and usually low-grade pain.

2 Operative intervention is necessary in the minority of cases in which progressive femoral head deformation and loss of acetabular coverage are significant.

3 Early X-ray changes may be subtle and children with persisting undiagnosed limp should have orthopaedic follow-up.

PATHOPHYSIOLOGY

Legg–Calve–Perthes disease is a disorder of unknown aetiology principally affecting boys (M:F 5:1) in the 4–8-year age group. It is bilateral in approximately 10%. The pathophysiology affects articular cartilage, where synovitis results in oedema, hypermetabolism, hypertrophy, and deterioration of the cartilaginous mechanical properties. Cartilaginous ischemia is thought to be the active mechanism, although Doppler-measured feeding artery resistive indexes appear normal[29] and only a minority of children are shown to have a pro-coagulant disorder.[30] It is more prevalent in malnourished children,[31] those with delayed bone age, and those exposed to passive smoking.[32–34] The end result may be subchondral fracturing, anterolateral deformation and joint incongruence, although the majority of children have spontaneous gradual remission of their disease process. Four stages are recognised:[16]

❶ Initial – ischaemia causes cartilage hypertrophy and synovitis; X-ray smaller femoral head, increased joint space.

❷ Fragmentation – X-ray shows fragmented epiphysis and subchondral radiolucency ('Caffey's crescent line').

❸ Reossification – altered shape of femoral head with increased radiopacity.

❹ Healing – resolution or persistence of deformity.

ED PRESENTATIONS

Hip pain in Perthes disease is usually mild, chronic and dull, increasing with physical activity, often with a history of pain for weeks to months. There are no systemic symptoms. Because of the gradual onset of Perthes disease, acute presentations to the ED usually represent either an early (stage 1) Perthes and fall within the 'irritable hip' differential, as discussed previously, or a flare-up in a child with known Perthes disease in whom coincidental comorbidity must be excluded.

EXAMINATION

Children with Perthes syndrome have limited range of hip movement, particularly in abduction and internal rotation, from synovial thickening and adductor muscle spasm. Those with longstanding disease may have muscle atrophy, leg-length discrepancy, and a positive Trendelenburg test on the affected side.

DIFFERENTIAL DIAGNOSIS

In the early stages of disease, X-ray changes will mimic that of transient synovitis, and children should be managed according to the irritable hip outline suggested earlier.

Children with less-acute irritable hips and non-specific X-ray or ultrasound evaluations should be referred for orthopaedic evaluation if symptoms persist longer than three weeks.

INVESTIGATION

The plain hip X-ray is diagnostic in established Perthes disease, although findings may be subtle in early disease. Recent studies have refined the diagnostic use of ultrasound even in the early phases of this disease. Measurement of capsular depth, cartilage thickness and muscle atrophy, compared with controls, allowed a sensitivity of 71% and a specificity of 99%.[35] Magnetic resonance imaging can demonstrate decreased epiphyseal signal intensity and bone-marrow oedema and is useful for the diagnosis and the prognosis where available,[36] although prognosis is better evaluated beyond the initial stages of disease.[17]

TREATMENT AND PROGNOSIS

Treatment of Perthes disease depends on the age of patient, stage of disease, and grading. Extensive head involvement, loss of the femoral head 'lateral pillars', subluxation of head beyond the acetabular margin, and late age at presentation are all poor prognostic indicators.[16] Orthopaedic management goals are restoration of range of hip movement and containment of the hip within the acetabulum. These goals are sought through a variety of methods including traction, surgery, orthotics and physiotherapy. Although three quarters of patients with Perthes disease are pain-free and active in 10–20 year follow-up studies, longer follow-up suggests some predisposition to early osteoarthritis.[16]

SLIPPED UPPER FEMORAL EPIPHYSIS (SUFE)

EPIDEMIOLOGY AND PATHOPHYSIOLOGY

SUFE is common in males, with a peak age of 10–16 years in males and 9–15 years in females, although it has been reported in children as young as eight years. SUFE is related to puberty (80% occurring during the adolescent growth spurt), and obesity (two thirds are > 90th centile weight-for-height), with genetic and endocrine factors playing a role.[16] Mechanical failure occurs at a widened zone of hypertrophy within the physeal plate. It is important to note that

Essentials

1 Delay in stabilisation of SUFE increases the risks of avascular necrosis, chondrolysis, deformity, and long-term poor hip outcomes.

2 All adolescents with undiagnosed acute hip or knee pain should have AP and frog-leg lateral hip X-rays or ultrasound performed by competent operators. A history of trauma is not required.

3 ED doctors must be able to recognise early SUFE and must refer all patients with SUFE to orthopaedics immediately.

although traditional Salter–Harris proximal femoral physeal fractures can occasionally occur in adolescence from high-energy injuries, these differ from classical SUFE both in the amount of force involved and in the histological plane of cleavage, i.e. the SUFE can be thought of as a 'pathological fracture' occurring as a result of minor torsional or low-energy injury in a weakened physeal plate with a high-sheer stress load.[16]

CLINICAL PRESENTATION

The classical child with SUFE will be an obese adolescent with pain either in the groin or referred to knee (femoral) or medial thigh (obturator nerve). They may have some leg-length discrepancy and hold the leg in external rotation. Range of motion depends on degree of slip and chronicity. A classical feature of the chronic slip is that passive flexion is accompanied by external rotation.

Initial presentation of SUFE may take one of four patterns:

❶ Pre-slip. This is usually a retrospective diagnosis, relating to an episode of intermittent pain and evidence of synovitis but without radiological evidence of epiphyseal shift.

❷ Chronic slip. Pain greater than three weeks, ambulant, mild to moderate

Normal AP

Trethowan's sign

Frog leg lateral

Fig. 24.1.2 Slipped upper femoral epiphysis (SUFE). Look for Trethowan's sign in the AP, where a line drawn up the superior femoral neck fails to cut into the head.

pain with decreased range of motion. X-ray shows SUFE ± evidence of remodelling.

❸ Acute-on-chronic slip. Increased pain and radiological evidence of slip following a period of lower-grade symptoms. Acute slip and evidence of remodelling are present on X-ray.

❹ Acute slip (≈10%). Acute, severe hip pain and diminished range of movement with less than three weeks' prodrome and no radiological evidence of remodelling.

SUFE is also graded as stable or unstable depending on the ability to weight-bear at the time of presentation, and as mild, moderate or severe depending on the percentage of epiphyseal translation.

The radiological findings in SUFE are outlined in Fig. 24.1.2. It is essential that the emergency physician be aware of the clinical and radiological features of SUFE so that they can recognise at-risk presentations, and actively seek Trethowan's sign (a Klein line intersecting the lateral femoral head).

Ultrasound has also been shown to have high sensitivity and specificity for epiphyseal displacement, even in the early stages, in the right hands.[38]

DIFFERENTIAL DIAGNOSIS

The differential diagnosis of SUFE is discussed earlier. A normal Klein line on a frog-leg pelvic X-ray rules out all but the pre-slip phase of SUFE. In high-risk clinical situations, MRI may be helpful.

TREATMENT

Once an unstable SUFE has been diagnosed patients should be treated as at risk of avascular necrosis. Admission under the orthopaedic team pending surgical fixation should be expedited. Bed-rest with toilet privileges is usual, with pain relief as required. The acutely slipped femoral head is usually fixed by percutaneous or minimal-incision internal fixation.

COMPLICATIONS

Avascular necrosis may occur in up to 50% of unstable slips, with an overall incidence in SUFE of ≈5%. Other complications include chondrolysis and leg-length discrepancy.

CONTROVERSIES

❶ The necessity or danger of attempted reduction prior to fixation (which may precipitate avascular necrosis).

❷ The value of pinning the contralateral hip (asymptomatic bilateral SUFE evolves in up to 40% of children but represents AVN danger in much fewer) as fixation in itself can cause avascular necrosis or chondrolysis.

Delays in diagnosis and referral are common and avoidable.[39] Causes of delay include:

- Failure to X-ray (particularly with low-grade and/or referred pain).
- Failure to interpret X-ray correctly (this should be visually accessible in every ED).
- Failure to refer appropriately (immediate telephone contact with orthopaedic team).

GENERALISED OR MULTI-FOCAL BONE/JOINT PAIN

INTRODUCTION

The child presenting with generalised or multi-focal acute musculoskeletal disturbance represents a different diagnostic spectrum. This is outlined in Table 24.1.9. As might be expected, infective and inflammatory disorders predominate and the 'risk profile' relates to the possible consequences of the generalised disease process, such as rheumatic fever, nephritis, leukaemia, or juvenile arthritis.

Table 24.1.9 Causes of acute multifocal limb or joint pain in children presenting to the ED ([†]more common causes highlighted)

Infection:
- Acute viral illness[†]
- Streptococcal disease
- Other bacterial illness, e.g. *Neisseria*
- Kawasaki disease

Post-infectious (immune-mediated):
- Serum sickness[†]
- Reactive arthritis[†]
- Rheumatic fever

Inflammatory/vasculitic:
- Henoch-Schönlein purpura
- Juvenile inflammatory arthritis
- Associated with SLE/IBD/other

Neoplastic:
- Leukaemia[†]
- Neuroblastoma

Haematological:
- Sickle cell
- Haemophilia

In assessing the child with multifocal joint or bone pain, or with arthralgia or arthritis in a setting of a febrile illness, the following features should be explored:

History
- Antigen exposure – drugs, infections, insects, animals.
- Previous infection or autoimmune dysfunction.
- Features suggestive of infection – fever and its pattern and duration, other symptoms.
- Features suggestive of metabolic drain – lethargy, weight loss, anorexia, night sweats.

Examination
- Skin and mucosae.
- Eyes (visual acuity mandatory).
- Bones (including spine), joints, and surrounding soft tissues.
- Lymph nodes.
- Liver and spleen.
- Heart and lungs.
- Kidneys and urine.

Investigation
- Urinalysis and microscopy for casts.
- Inflammatory markers – FBC, CRP, ESR.
- Serology, e.g. antistreptolysin O test (ASOT), parvovirus, Barmah Forest alphavirus, Ross River fever.
- Rheumatological investigations – antinuclear antigens, rheumatoid factor.

JUVENILE INFLAMMATORY ARTHRITIS (JIA)

This spectrum of disorders is outlined in Table 24.1.10.[40] With the exception of systemic arthritis, these children have a chronic disease process that is generally gradual in onset. The pain of juvenile inflammatory arthritis is generally less acute than that of infective arthritis, and for that reason these children usually present to their local medical practitioner with a longer history of pain and stiffness. Difficulties may occasionally arise

Table 24.1.10   Juvenile idiopathic arthritis (JIA)

- Systemic arthritis: fever two weeks plus at least one of rash, LN, HS megaly, serositis
- Polyarthritis, RF pos: at least five joints in first six months, RF pos
- Polyarthritis, RF neg: at least five joints in first six months, RF neg
- Oligoarthritis: no more than four joints in first six months
- Enthesitis related arthritis: enthesitis and/or arthritis, plus two of
  SI/spine inflammation, or
  HLA B27, or
  family history HLAB27-associated disease in first- or second-degree relative, or
  anterior uveitis, or
  boy arthritis onset over age eight years
- Psoriatic arthritis: arthritis and psoriasis or two of dactylitis, nail abnormalities, FH psoriasis first-degree relative

early in the development of a juvenile arthritis in which a child may have a single joint that is painful and limited in range of movement. Risk management dictates that these children be evaluated as possible septic arthritis, however follow-up may show them to be evolving juvenile idiopathic arthritis.

The child with systemic arthritis will present as an ill child with a history of prolonged daily or twice-daily high fever (generally > 39°C) and debility. Characteristically the child with systemic juvenile arthritis is aged between two and five years, has an evanescent macular erythematous rash, generalised lymphadenopathy, and may have hepatosplenomegaly or evidence of serosal inflammation, i.e. pleuritis, pericarditis, or abdominal pain. In severe cases pericarditis can manifest as tamponade. Arthritis or arthralgia may be minimal in the early stages of disease.[41]

Depending on the duration of fever at the time of ED presentation, and the clinical features present, differential diagnosis for these children may include acute viral or bacterial infection, Kawasaki disease and other vasculitides, malignancy, and autoimmune disorders. Investigations must include blood culture, inflammatory markers, (FBC, CRP, ESR), viral serology, coagulation studies, and investigations as appropriate to the clinical findings and differential, e.g. CXR, ECG, echocardio-

gram, abdominal ultrasound. Anaemia of chronic disease is usual, with elevated inflammatory markers and thrombocytosis, which may exceed 1 million mm^{-3}.[42] Coagulation abnormalities may be present and may correlate with disease activity.[43]

In general, juvenile idiopathic arthritis is managed with supportive therapy and non-steroidal anti-inflammatory agents. Corticosteroids may be required for systemic arthritis with pleural or pericardial complications.

MACROPHAGE ACTIVATION SYNDROME

This rare disorder presents as a systemic arthritis but with an evolving coagulopathy and encephalopathy secondary to macrophage activation and haemophagocytosis.

Laboratory investigations reveal hepatic dysfunction, disseminated intravascular coagulation, hypofibrinogenaemia, lowered haematological indices without classical leukaemic features, and a falling ESR. High-dose steroids, ciclosporin and ICU can be life-saving.[44]

URTICARIA AND SERUM SICKNESS

The young child presenting with low-grade fever and urticarial rash, plus or minus arthralgia, represents a different end of the 'febrile child' differential. Toddlers and pre-school children may present with dramatic skin signs of urticaria, with migratory wheals plus or minus target lesions suggestive of erythema multiforme. Low-grade temperature may be present and there may be significant soft-tissue swelling and arthralgias. The most common single trigger identified with this symptom complex in Australia is cephalosporin use, although no specific trigger is identified in up to 50% of cases.[45] In the absence of atypical features (mucosal lesions, non-weight-bearing, toxicity, haematuria or organomegaly) this may be managed expectantly with removal of any unnecessary medication and rest. Anti-histamines and non-steroidal anti-

inflammatory medication may be useful for itch and joint pains.[46]

POST-STREPTOCOCCAL IMMUNE-MEDIATED DISEASE: REACTIVE ARTHRITIS

In the differential of the young child presenting with a rash and joint swelling, but generally with less florid wheals than in urticaria, is post-infectious reactive arthritis. This may occur after a number of viral or bacterial triggers, alone or in immunogenic combination with antibiotics. Children must be carefully examined, as outlined above. However, the child with limited joint and skin involvement may be managed conservatively by stopping any possible contributory triggers and providing symptom relief with non-steroidal anti-inflammatory agents.

In the setting of recent sore throat and positive ASOT, some researchers believe this to be part of the immune-mediated spectrum of acute rheumatic fever.[47] Children may also have other clinical manifestations, including erythema nodosum or vasculitis. The reactive arthritis pattern is more persistent than the migratory arthritis of rheumatic fever, tenosynovitis is often present, and there are no cardiac manifestations. Post-streptococcal reactive arthritis also lacks the characteristic aspirin sensitivity of rheumatic fever.[48] However, the association mandates investigation of these children with FBC and ASOT, and referral for follow-up by a paediatrician or rheumatologist.

RHEUMATIC FEVER

Rheumatic fever has become rare amongst Caucasians in Australia and New Zealand but still occurs and causes preventable morbidity and mortality in the Aboriginal and Pacific Islander populations of both countries, particularly in the South Auckland region.[49] Modified Jones criteria are shown in Table 24.1.11 and the condition is discussed in more detail in another section (see Chapter 5.5).

Table 24.1.11 Modified Jones criteria for diagnosis* of acute rheumatic fever

Major manifestations	Minor manifestations
Carditis	Fever
Polyarthritis	Arthralgia
Subcutaneous nodules	Prolonged PR interval
Erythema marginatum	Increased ESR or CRP
Chorea	—

*Diagnosis requires the presence of two major criteria, or one major and two minor criteria with supporting evidence of preceding streptococcal infection.

HENOCH–SCHÖNLEIN PURPURA

This vasculitic disorder of uncertain aetiology is among the more frequent diagnoses presenting as joint pain and rash in the paediatric population. Characteristically there are four potentially affected systems:

❶ Skin – lower limb and buttock, extensor surface petechiae and maculopapules.

❷ Joints – with acral arthritis and/or limb swelling.

❸ Kidney – micro-or macroscopic haematuria may be present or there may be frank nephritis.

❹ Gastrointestinal system – submucosal vasculitis may present as intussusception, PR bleed or melaena, or peritoneal irritation.

Risk management involves ruling out other causes of petechial illness, including leukaemia, idiopathic thrombocytopenic purpura and partially treated meningococcal illness, and watching for renal complications. Children must be followed-up with urinalysis for twelve weeks for delayed renal complications.[50]

MALIGNANCY

Bone or joint pain is frequently the presenting symptom in children with leukaemia and other bone-marrow-related

Table 24.1.12 Features suggestive of malignancy in infants/children presenting with bone/joint pain or limp

- Non-articular bone pain or tenderness
- Systemic illness (fever, weight loss, anorexia, night sweats)
- Back pain
- Abnormal neurology
- Abnormal masses
- Bruising
- High ESR (cf. joint findings)
- Low platelets

malignancies. Features characteristic of these children by comparison with other causes of limp or joint pain are shown in Table 24.1.12. This pain is generally more severe and unremitting, and the debility more extreme, than in children with juvenile idiopathic arthritis. Blood films must always be carefully analysed for the three cell lines (red cells, white cells and platelets). Minor degrees of anaemia or thrombocytopenia are common early features. ESR is elevated out of proportion to the degree of 'arthritic' manifestations.[51] Malignancies presenting in this fashion include leukaemia and neuroblastoma.

Tip

- Beware the child who is carried into the examination room.

OTHER IMPORTANT SUB-ACUTE PAEDIATRIC MUSCULOSKELETAL PRESENTATIONS

Apophysisitis: Osgood–Schlatter and Sever's diseases

These disorders are the result of chronic micro-avulsion injury at the apophyseal insertion sites of the major leg-muscle groups. Commonest sites are the tibial tuberosity (quadriceps via patellar tendon: Osgood–Schlatter disease) and the calcaneal apophysis (calf muscle via Achilles tendon: Sever disease). In Osgood–Schlatter disease, the child or adolescent typically presents during the growth spurt with a story of pain getting up from sitting or going up stairs, and has

tenderness localised to the tibial tuberosity and some localised swelling, with an otherwise normal joint examination. In Sever disease there is pain on walking or running, and heel tenderness. X-ray may show fragmentation of the apophysis and soft-tissue swelling. However, this is primarily a clinical diagnosis (and fragmentation may be a normal radiological variant in developing apophyses). Treatment includes rest, non-steroidal anti-inflammatory medication, and orthopaedic referral for persistent disability.

Torticollis

The infant presenting with torticollis, without specific trauma or abnormal neurology, is most likely to have congenital muscular torticollis ('sternomastoid tumour'). Theories of pathogenesis include in-utero crowding and compartment syndrome. Characteristic features include:

- Onset from birth, often brought to parents' attention by new observer.
- 'Cock-robin' appearance (head tilt on involved side with contralateral chin rotation) with range of motion limited by the affected sternomastoid tightness.
- Normal neurology, behaviour, and occipito-frontal circumference.
- Firm painless swelling within the sternomastoid muscle opposite the chin in 20% of cases.
- Mild facial hemi-hypertrophy.

Hips should always be checked, as up to 20% may have developmental dysplasia.[52,53] Infants with this characteristic constellation of features should be referred for physiotherapy and follow-up.

Other causes of torticollis in the paediatric period include vertebral anomalies such as Kippel–Feil syndrome and neurological disorders including brain and spinal-cord tumours and ocular dysfunction. Causes of acute torticollis in children with previously normal neck posture and motion include atlanto–axial rotary subluxation, a reaction to other acute head or neck pathologies, such as lymphadenopathy or retropharyngeal abscess, and short-term muscle spasm in association with respiratory-tract disorders or minor trauma. Features suggestive of significant underlying pathology and need for radiological and specialist referral include:

- Other congenital or orthopaedic anomaly.
- Abnormality of neurological or ophthalmological assessment.
- Symptoms suggestive of intracranial pathology, e.g. headache, vomiting, irritability.
- Atypical musculoskeletal examination, e.g. unlimited range of motion (visual disorder) or persistent or fixed torticollis.

Bone tumours

Osteosarcoma and osteogenic sarcoma are uncommon but serious causes of recent onset limb pain or limp in the paediatric population. Characteristic features include:

- Osteosarcoma – bone destruction and infiltration.
- Osteogenic sarcoma (Ewing tumour) – perisosteal new bone formation, 'sunray' and 'onion-skin' appearance.

Differential diagnosis includes neuroblastoma and osteomyelitis. These children should be referred for urgent orthopaedic review and investigation.

Osteoid osteoma is an occasional cause of leg pain, particularly nocturnal. X-rays show an area of periosteal thickening and new bone formation around a central radiolucency.

Simple and aneurysmal bone cysts may also be seen, either as incidental findings or in the setting of pathological fracture. All of these can be referred to the orthopaedic unit for further evaluation.

Vertebrospinal inflammation

While uncommon, vertebrospinal inflammatory and infectious problems are characterised by delay in diagnosis and diagnostic confusion.[54] These children may present with back or abdominal pain, or with altered gait or neurological dysfunction. In discitis and vertebral osteomyelitis there will be point tenderness over a spinous process, particularly to percussion, and localised scoliosis or muscle spasm. Fever and constitutional symptoms are variable. Inflammatory markers are characteristically elevated. X-ray may show muscle spasm or soft-tissue oedema, or abnormal intervertebral disc space. Bone scans are helpful to localise an abnormality where examination findings are equivocal. Definitive diagnosis and evaluation are best made by magnetic resonance imaging (MRI). Treatment with bed-rest and intravenous antibiotics is usual, although isolated discitis may respond better to steroid treatment

REFERENCES

1. Mater Children's Hospital Paediatric Orthopaedic Working Group 1999 EDIS data. Brisbane, Australia
2. Kocher MS, Zurakowski D, Kasser JR 1999 Differentiating between septic arthritis and transient synovitis of the hip in children: An evidence based clinical prediction algorithm. Harvard Journal of Bone and Joint Surgery 81(12): 1662–1669
3. Jaramillo D, Treves ST, Kasser JR et al 1995 Osteomyelitis and septic arthritis in children: Appropriate use of imaging to guide treatment. Australian Journal of Rheumatology 165: 399–403
4. Beach R 2000 Minimally invasive approach to management of irritable hip in children. Lancet 355: 1202–1203
5. Kallio MJT, Unkila-Kallio L et al 1997 Serum CRP, ESR and WCC on septic arthritis of children. CH Helsinki. Paediatric Infectious Diseases Journal 16(4): 411–413
6. Klein DM, Barbera C et al 1997 Sensitivity of objective parameters in the diagnosis of paediatric septic hips. Clinical Orthopaedics & Related Research 338: 153–159
7. Eich GF, Superti-Furga A et al 1999 The painful hip: Evaluation of criteria for clinical decision-making. European Journal of Paediatrics 158: 923–928
8. Wall EJ 1998 Childhood osteomyelitis and septic arthritis. Current Opinion in Paediatrics: Orthopaedics 10: 73–76
9. Ng T 1997 ESR, plasma viscosity and CRP in clinical practice. British Journal of Hospital Medicine 58(10): 521–523
10. Peltola H, Kallio-Unkila L, Kallio MJT & the Finnish Study Group 1997 Simplified treatment of acute staphylococcal osteomyelitis of childhood. Paediatrics 99: 846–850
11. Skinner J, Glancy S, Beattie TF, Hendry GM 2002 Transient synovitis: Is there a need to aspirate hip joint effusions? European Journal of Emergency Medicine 9(1): 15–18
12. Fink AM, Bermann L, Edwards D, Jacobson SK 1995 The irritable hip: Immediate ultrasound guided aspiration and prevention of hospital admission. Archives of Diseases in Childhood 72(2): 110–113
13. Boutin RD, Brossmann J, Sartoris DJ, Reilly D, Resnick D 1998 Update on imaging of orthopedic infections. Orthopedic Clinics of North America 29(1): 41–66
14. White PM, Boyd J, Beattie TF, Hurst M, Hendry GM 2001 Magnetic resonance imaging as the primary imaging modality in children presenting with acute non-traumatic hip pain. Emergency Medicine Journal 18(1): 25–29
15. Kermond S, Fink M, Kerr G, Carlin J, Barnett P 2002 A randomized clinical trial: Should the child

16. Morrissey RT, Weinstein SL 2001 Lovell and Winter's paediatric orthopaedics, 5th edn. Lippincott Williams and Wilkins, Philadelphia, Vol 1 959–960
17. Goldenberg DL 1993 Bacterial arthritis. In: Kelley WN, Harris ED, Ruddy S, Sledge CB (eds) Textbook of rheumatology, 4th edn. WB Saunders, Philadelphia, PA 1449–1466
18. Goldenberg DL, Reed JI 1985 Bacterial arthritis. New England Journal of Medicine 312: 764–771
19. Trobs RB, Moritz RP, Huppertz HI et al 1999 Changing pattern of osteomyelitis in infants and children. Leipzig Paediatric Surgery International 15: 363–372
20. Girschick HJ, Krauspe R, Tschammler A et al 1998 Chronic recurrent osteomyelitis with clavicular involvement in children: Diagnostic value of different imaging techniques and therapy with non-steroidal anti-inflammatory drugs. European journal of Paediatrics 157: 28–33
21. Martin JC, Desoya R, O'Sullivan MM et al 1996 Chronic recurrent multifocal osteomyelitis: Spinal involvement and radiological appearances. British journal of Rheumatology 35: 1019–1021
22. Graham HK 2003 Acute septic arthritis of the hip in children in northern Australia. Australian and New Zealand Journal of Surgery 73: 91 [commentary]
23. Brooks GF, Pons VG 1994 Septic arthritis. In: Hoeprich PD, Jordan MC, Ronald AR (eds) Infectious diseases, 5th edn. JB Lippincott, Philadelphia, PA, 1382–1389
24. Oliver G 1996 Tuberculosis notifications in Australia, 1994. Communicable Disease Intelligence 20(5): 108–115
25. Weinstein SL, Buckwalter JA (eds) 1994 Turek's orthopedics, 5th edn. JB Lippincott, Philadelphia, PA, 127–150
26. Clinician's Knowledge Network 2003 Skin, muscle and bone infections. In: Therapeutic guidelines: Antibiotics Therapeutic Guidelines Limited: Antibiotic (2003) Accessed through Clinician's Knowledge Network http://ckn.health.qld.gov.au
27. Turnidge JD, Bell JM 2000 Methicillin-resistant *Staphylococcus aureus* evolution in Australia over 35 years. Microbial Drug Resistance 6(3): 223–229
28. Syrogiannopoulos GA, Nelson JD 1998 Duration of antimicrobial therapy for acute suppurative osteoarticular infections. Lancet 1: 37–40
29. Robben SG, Lequin MH, Diepstraten AF et al 2000 Doppler sonography of the anterior ascending cervical arteries of the hip: Evaluation of healthy and painful hips in children. American Journal of Roentgenology 174(6): 1629–1634
30. Hresko MT, McDougall PA, Gorlin JB et al 2002 Prospective re-evaluation of the association between thrombotic diathesis and Legg-Calve-Perthes disease. Journal of Bone and Joint Surgery 84(9): 1613–1618
31. Kealey WD, Moore AJ, Cook S, Cosgrove AP 2000 Deprivation, urbanisation and Perthes' disease in Northern Ireland. Journal of Bone and Joint Surgery 82(2): 167–171
32. Vila-Verde VM, da Silva KC 2001 Bone-age delay in Perthes disease and transient synovitis of the hip. Clinical Orthopaedics and Related Research 385: 118–123
33. Mata SG, Aicua EA, Ovejero AH, Grande MM 2000 Legg-Calve-Perthes disease and passive smoking. Journal of Pediatric Orthopedics 20(3): 326–330
34. Keenan WN, Clegg J 1996 Perthes' disease after 'irritable hip': Delayed bone age shows the hip is a 'marked man'. Journal of Pediatric Orthopedics 16(1): 20–23
35. Robben SG, Meradji M, Diepstraten AF, Hop WC 1998 US of the painful hip in childhood: Diagnostic value of cartilage thickening and muscle atrophy in the detection of Perthes disease. Radiology 208(1): 35–42
36. Wingstrand H 1999 Significance of synovitis in Legg-Calve-Perthes disease. Journal of Pediatric Orthopedics. Part B 8(3): 156–160

37. Lahdes-Vasama T, Lamminen A, Merikanto J, Marttinen E 1997 The value of MRI in early Perthes' disease: An MRI study with a 2-year follow-up. Paediatric Radiology 27(6): 517–522
38. Kallio PE, Lequesne GW, Paterson DC, Foster BK, Jones JR 1991 Ultrasonography in slipped capital femoral epiphysis. Diagnosis and assessment of severity. Journal of Bone and Joint Surgery Britain 73(6): 884–889
39. Ankarath S, Ng AB, Giannoudis PV, Scott BW 2002 Delay in diagnosis of slipped upper femoral epiphysis. Journal of the Royal Society of Medicine 95(7): 356–358
40. Petty RE, Southwood TR, Baum J et al 1998 Revision of the proposed classification criteria for juvenile idiopathic arthritis: Durban 1997 Journal of Rheumatology 25: 1991
41. Wright DA 2001 Juvenile idiopathic arthritis. In: Morrissey RT, Weinstein SL (eds) Lovell and Winter's paediatric orthopedics, Vol. 1, 427–457, 5th edn. Lippincott Williams and Wilkins, Philadelphia
42. Schneider R, Laxer RM 1998 Systemic onset juvenile rheumatoid arthritis. Baillière's Clinical Rheumatology 12: 245

43. Bloom BJ, Tucker LB, Miller LC et al 1998 Fibrin D dimer as a marker of disease activity in systemic onset juvenile rheumatoid arthritis. Journal of Rheumatology 25: 1620
44. Stephan JL, Kone-Paut I, Galambrun C, Mouy R, Bader-Meunier B, Prieur AM 2001 Reactive haemophagocytic syndrome in children with inflammatory disorders. A retrospective study of 24 patients. Rheumatology (Oxford) 40(11): 1285–1292
45. Isaacs D 2001 Serum sickness-like reaction to cefaclor. Journal of Paediatrics and Child Health 37(3): 298–299
46. Joubert GI, Hadad K, Matsui D et al 1999 Selection of treatment of cefaclor-associated urticarial, serum sickness-like reactions and erythema multiforme by emergency paediatricians: Lack of a uniform standard of care. Canadian Journal of Clinical Pharmacology 6(4): 197–201
47. Lehman TJ, Edelheit BS 2001 Clinical trials for post-streptococcal reactive arthritis. Current Rheumatology Reports 3(5): 363–364
48. Bont L, Brus F, Dijkman-Neerincx RH et al 1998 The clinical spectrum of post-streptococcal

syndromes with arthritis in children. Clinical and Experimental Rheumatology 16(6): 750–752
49. Franks C 2002 Who is at risk of contracting acute rheumatic fever in Australia? Aboriginal and Islander Health Worker Journal 26(2): 23–32
50. Sano H, Izumida M, Shimizu H, Ogawa Y 2002 Risk factors of renal involvement and significant proteinuria in Henoch–Schönlein purpura. European Journal of Paediatrics 161(4): 196–201
51. Cabral DA, Tucker LB 1999 Malignancies in children who initially present with rheumatic complaints. Journal of Paediatrics 134: 153
52. Walsh JJ, Morrissy RT 1998 Torticollis and hip dislocation. Journal of Pediatric Orthopedics 18: 219
53. Cheng JCY, Au AWY 1994 Infantile torticollis: A review of 624 cases. Journal of Paediatrics 14: 802
54. Fernandez M, Carrol CL, Baker CJ 2000 Discitis and vertebral osteomyelitis in children: An 18-year review. Paediatrics 105(6): 1299–1304
55. Carty H, Brunelle F, Shaw D, Kendall B 1994 Imaging children, Vol. 2. Churchill Livingstone, Edinburgh

24.2 FRACTURES AND DISLOCATIONS

ROBYN BRADY • TERRY MCGUIRE

Essentials

1 Fractures are common in childhood, due to high-level motor activity, developing co-ordination, and the mechanical properties of the growing skeleton. However, compared to adult mechanisms, the majority are relatively low-force injuries.

2 The patterns of bony disruption are completely different from adult fracture patterns and include buckle fractures and growth-plate injuries. Bony disruption/deformity is more common than ligamentous disruption ('sprains' are uncommon).

3 Displaced fractures are a common and highly traumatic event for children and rapid attention to physical and psychological distress can minimise the effects of this trauma.

4 Certain missed fractures have a high propensity for serious long-term functional morbidity and must be actively sought/excluded. These include elbow injuries, such as lateral condylar and Monteggia-type fractures, and slipped upper femoral epiphysis (SUFE).

FRACTURE PATTERNS IN CHILDHOOD

In the previous chapter the impact of development (behavioural and physiological) on musculoskeletal pathology was broadly outlined (see Table 24.1.1).

With respect to injury, this means different points of cleavage or deformation from a given injury mechanism, and an extra anatomical structure (the physis) to consider when analysing the effects of trauma and the future outcome of a given disruption.

Fig. 24.2.1 shows the frequency of common fractures presenting to a children's ED. Within different age subgroups, the distribution varies thus:

- Infants/toddlers – higher proportions femur and skull fractures.
- Primary school – higher proportion of elbow-region fractures, especially supra-condylar.
- Adolescents – transition to adult pattern with ligamentous injuries, e.g. elbow dislocations, complex ankle fractures; higher force knee and forearm injuries.

The majority of ED fracture presentations occur at the distal radius and ulna. This is one of the top ten ED diagnoses for children in Australia. Many displaced forearm fractures can be reduced under sedation by emergency staff with appropriate training and follow-up, making this a most valuable area of expertise.

Paediatric limb fractures, depending on the angle of force to which they have been subjected, can occur to shaft, metaphysis, or physeal region. The different quality of developing bone means that even injuries to shaft and metaphysis tend to have different patterns of deformation,

ORTHOPAEDICS AND RHEUMATOLOGY

including 'torus' or buckle injuries, bowing, and greenstick fractures. The importance of this awareness for the emergency physician is best illustrated by the Monteggia equivalent injury in which 'shortening' from proximal radial dislocation is 'matched' by ulnar bowing. The resultant injury has no radiologically obvious 'fracture' in the traditional sense but has serious consequences if not recognised and reduced (see Fig. 24.2.2).

The Salter–Harris classification (Fig. 24.2.3) remains the most useful way of describing the pattern of cleavage with respect to the physis. In reality, types 1 and 5 represent mechanical force patterns (separation and compression) rather than a radiological pattern as, unless there is lateral translation or neighbouring bony or soft-tissue deformation, the physis may appear radiologically normal in these injuries. Examples of Salter–Harris type 1 injuries with lateral shift include the so-called 'slipped distal radial epiphysis' (see Fig. 24.2.4). The disorder of slipped upper femoral epiphysis (SUFE) has been discussed in Chapter 24.1 as, although minor trauma may precipitate an acute slippage, the cleavage is due to an abnormal physeal predisposition.

Salter–Harris type 2 injuries are the most common physeal injury pattern seen, the metaphyseal corner fragment ranging

in size from a barely visible fragment to an extensive triangle. Injuries through the epiphysis itself, Salter–Harris types 3 and 4, are more worrying in their prognosis because of the articular and growth-plate damage that is usually present. The classical example of a Salter–Harris type 4 injury is the Tillaux fracture (Fig. 24.2.5).

Table 24.2.1 shows some examples of the corresponding injury occurring in adults and children for a given mechanism. This table illustrates the maxim that children tend to fracture rather than 'sprain', as the physis is the weakest point of the musculoskeletal continuum. In

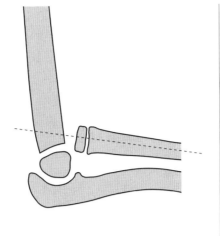

Fig. 24.2.2 Monteggia fracture-dislocation. Demonstration of the abnormal radio-capitellar relationship (see Fig. 24.2.8 for contrast). Drawing by Terry McGuire.

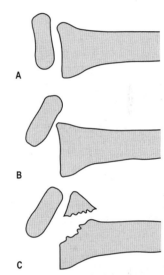

Fig. 24.2.4 Common distal radial epiphyseal fractures. (*A*) Partial slipped distal radial epiphysis (Salter–Harris 1) with 10% translation; (*B*) slipped distal radial epiphysis (Salter-Harris 1) with 50% translation and probable intact dorsal periosteal sleeve; (*C*) Salter–Harris 2 fracture of distal radius with metaphyseal fragment angulated to 45 degrees and 50% translation of epiphyseal plate. Drawing by Terry McGuire.

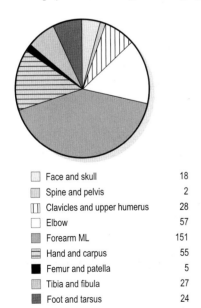

☐ Face and skull	18
☐ Spine and pelvis	2
☐ Clavicles and upper humerus	28
☐ Elbow	57
☐ Forearm ML	151
☐ Hand and carpus	55
■ Femur and patella	5
☐ Tibia and fibula	27
☐ Foot and tarsus	24

Fig. 24.2.1 Frequency of fracture types at Mater Children's Hospital ED.

Fig. 24.2.3 Salter–Harris classification of epiphyseal fractures. Drawing by Terry McGuire.

some cases, this is to the child's advantage, as the cellular architects of bone development contribute to rapid healing and extensive remodelling. A midshaft femoral fracture, for example, will heal in 2–3 weeks in an infant, whereas the same disruption will take 12 weeks to union in a teenager.

Fig. 24.2.5   Tillaux fracture (Salter–Harris 3). Early fusion of the medial distal tibial physis and relative superior strength of the distal tibiofibular ligament causes shearing force to separate the central physeal region and travel along the lateral distal tibial physis, sometimes a metaphyseal fragment is also cleaved (Salter–Harris 4).

INITIAL ASSESSMENT AND MANAGEMENT

The initial assessment of the paediatric isolated limb injury (fracture/dislocation) is shown in Table 24.2.2 and the neurovascular assessment in Table 24.2.3. Limb injury must always be considered in the broader context of trauma. Primary and secondary survey, however brief and targeted, should always be carried out bearing in mind the described injury mechanism and child's complaints of pain, so that any associated injuries, e.g. to head, abdomen, or spine, may be recognised and evaluated early. An efficient early assessment should be able to establish mechanism, possible other sites of injury, probable fracture type, presence or absence of compound features or neurovascular impairment, and organise pain relief, fasting, radiology, splintage, and antibiotics if required, within a brief period.

Fracture descriptions to the orthopaedic team should start with the child's age, mechanism, and clinical findings, and proceed to the part of bone, type of fracture, and extent of angulation and or displacement and associated findings. Clinical findings must always be kept paramount. Skin breach must be actively sought and described. Prominently placed photographic displays of common paediatric fractures may aid description.

The possibility of non-accidental injury must be borne in mind with all injuries in the pre-verbal child. Many departments have pre-formatted injury history sheets for this age group, to ensure that adequate detail is obtained at the initial consultation. Sketching the proposed injury scenario can often aid in obtaining details of environmental factors and the responses of those present. It has been shown that the amount of detail in an injury history, and the use of a proforma to prompt history acquisition, leads to an increased ability to discriminate between accidental and non-accidental injury.[1] Features suggestive of non-accidental injury are shown in Table 24.2.4, and child abuse is discussed in more detail in Chapter 18.2. As a minimum, all fractures occurring in children under twelve months should be discussed with a paediatrician or child-protection specialist.

The following sections describe the mechanism, recognition, and ED treatment of individual fractures.

Table 24.2.1   Examples of paediatric vs. adult outcomes of common fall mechanisms (different paediatric injuries occur at different ages depending on planes of weakness)

Mechanism	Adult injury	Paediatric injury
Fall onto point of shoulder	AC separation	Lateral clavicular fracture
Shoulder extension/compression	Shoulder dislocation	Proximal humeral fracture
Fall on hand, elbow hyperextension	Elbow dislocation	Supracondylar/condylar fractures
Wrist hyperextension/compression	Scaphoid fracture	Distal forearm fracture
Fall onto hand	Colles fracture	Midshaft, metaphyseal, or epiphyseal fracture
Thumb abduction 1	Bennet's fracture	Metaphyseal fracture base first metacarpal
Thumb abduction 2	Gamekeepers thumb (UCL)	Salter–Harris type 3 proximal phalanx thumb
Rotation of knee on lower leg	ACL, cartilage tear	Tibial spine fracture
Valgus/varus knee stress	Ligament, cartilage tear	Distal femoral physeal separation
Forceful jump (quadriceps)	Ligament tear	Tibial tubercle fracture
Forceful jump (calf)	Achilles tendon tear	Calcaneal avulsion fracture
Rotation of tibia on calcaneus	Ankle sprains, Potts fractures	Tibial spiral fracture, Tillaux fracture, triplane fracture
Inversion ankle	Talofibular ligament tear	Salter–Harris type 1 distal fibula

ORTHOPAEDICS AND RHEUMATOLOGY

Table 24.2.2   Initial assessment and management of traumatic limb deformity

1. **Rapport**: establish rapport and explain procedures
2. **Mechanism and associated dangers**: rapidly ascertain mechanism and ensure primary survey stability and allergy potential
3. **Pain management**: where there is a greater than 90% likelihood of initial IV success, insert a small IV cannula into the opposite hand and titrate morphine 0.05 mg kg^{-1} until pain relieved (appropriate monitoring should be in place). When no parent is present the risks of medication must be weighed against the potential benefit and attempts made to contact someone familiar with serious allergies or other medical problems. Other means of rapid pain relief include inhaled penthrane or NO_2 and intranasal fentanyl
4. **Assess for site of anatomical disruption**: look at and gently palpate the injured limb to estimate probable anatomical site of disruption, e.g. lateral elbow, mid-shaft forearm, etc. (comparison with other limb is often helpful)
5. **Check for associated neurovascular dysfunction**: (see Table 24.2.3), document and notify deficits immediately
6. **Check for any evidence of an open wound**: if this is. present, cover with a sterile dressing and commence appropriate antibiotics IV, e.g. cephalothin 50 mg kg^{-1} and notify orthopaedic team immediately
7. **Immobilise limb**: provide appropriate splintage (we use a POP slab for distal fractures, leaving radial artery palpable, and a fibreglass slab for elbow injuries, less radiological artefact)
8. **Keep stomach empty**: identify time of last ingestion and inform patient and parent about fasting
9. **Organise appropriate radiology**
10. **Discuss clinical and radiological findings with orthopaedic team**

Table 24.2 3   Presence/absence of associated neurovascular injury

- Radial a:
  Pulse, cf. other side
  Hand perfusion/capillary refill, cf. other side
- Brachial a:
  Spasm or intimal shear in supracondylar injuries
- Radial n:
  Sensation dorsum hand, *action = dorsiflex wrist, extend fingers* (displaced humeral shaft injury)
- Median n:
  Sensation thenar eminence, *action = opposition, flexion IP thumb* (supracondylar # or elbow dislocation)
- Ulnar n:
  Sensation hypothenar eminence, *action = abduction, adduction fingers* (elbow dislocation, supracondylar #)
- Posterior interosseous n:
  Branch of radial n, *action = finger extension*, e.g. (Monteggia #/dislocation)

UPPER LIMB AND SHOULDER GIRDLE INJURIES

Midshaft clavicular fractures

These may occur at any age from a fall onto the shoulder, are usually greenstick in nature and heal well in a sling or figure-of-eight bandaging. A fall onto the point of the shoulder, such as would cause an acromio-clavicular disruption in an adult, may cause a *lateral clavicular fracture-separation*. Treatment is by sling or shoulder immobilisation followed by graduated exercises.

The *neonatal shoulder* may come to medical attention due to asymmetrical arm movement or swelling. Causes include birth injury with clavicular fracture or brachial plexus injury, proximal humeral physeal separation, and joint or bone infection. Senior orthopaedic involvement is essential for the diagnosis, and non-accidental injury must be considered.

Shoulder dislocation

This is uncommon under ten. The adolescent anterior dislocation can be reduced by traction in the prone position or by gentle arm traction to a seated child against counter-traction with a sheeted thorax.

Proximal humerus

These fractures vary from minor buckling at the proximal metaphysis, to proximal humeral epiphyseal Salter–Harris type 2 fracture-separations (see Fig. 24.2.6). Because of the universal motion at the glenohumeral joint and the remodelling potential of children, a remarkable range of initial traumatic deformity is acceptable in children prior to physeal closure (age 14–16) including complete displacement and up to 60 degrees of angulation.[2]

Midshaft fractures

These are less common and sometimes the result of blunt or non-accidental trauma. Check and document radial nerve function, and immobilise with a U-slab.

Injuries to the elbow region

The elbow region accounts for 10% of all paediatric fractures. Supracondylar fractures make up 75% of these, and lateral condylar fractures 17%. Missed or inadequately treated paediatric elbow injuries figure prominently in orthopaedic litigation series.[3] Post-traumatic elbow effusion in childhood without a radiologically apparent fracture line most commonly represents a minimally displaced supracondylar fracture. These must be immobilised by collar and cuff to avoid any potential extension from further falls, and followed up in a fracture clinic within the window of manipulation opportunity, i.e. one week. It is sometimes useful to start with the examination findings in the normal elbow, as outlined in Table 24.2.5 (see also Figs 24.2.7 and 24.2.8). The first point in itself will define an anatomically intact elbow, while the other points help the physician to narrow down the type of abnormality where the first point is abnormal.

Supracondylar fracture

Supracondylar injuries occur in the young school-age child as a result of a fall on the outstretched hand, transmitted through elbow hyperextension to the narrow region between olecranon and coronoid fossae. Degrees of rotation of the distal region

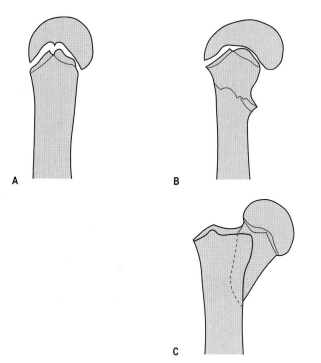

Fig. 24.2.6 Proximal humeral fractures. (*A*) Normal undulating physeal line (not a fracture); (*B*) greenstick metaphyseal fracture; (*C*) severely angulated and displaced Salter-Harris 2 fracture at the proximal humeral epiphysis. Due to the universal motion of the shoulder joint, this fracture will still unite and remodel completely with conservative treatment. Drawing by Terry McGuire, courtesy of PaEDpac;

Table 24.2.4   Features suggestive of possible non-accidental injury
Fractures
• Proximal humeral or humeral shaft fractures under three years
• Fractures with a shearing or distracting mechanism
• Corner or 'bucket-handle' metaphyseal injuries
• Femoral fractures in infants
• Rib fractures
• Complex skull fractures
• Multiple fractures, especially different ages
Presentation features
• Delayed presentation
• Different care-giver
• Unwitnessed injury
• Recurrent fractures
• Unexplained soft-tissue markings
• Unexplained tension/anxiety
Assessment
• Draw diagram of injury history as described by witness
• Examine child all over and plot weight
• Ascertain any previous history of burns or fractures
• Is the developmental level compatible with the explanation?
• **Is the history adequate to explain the injury?**
Rule of thumb
• Infants within view, toddlers within earshot, unless asleep, i.e. injuries to preschool children are usually seen or heard
Refer
• All fractures in children under twelve months, and all fractures in children under four years in which there is an inadequate or questionable mechanism, should be discussed with a child-protection specialist. In the interim, supportive and non-judgemental care for child and care-giver must be maintained

Table 24.2.5   Requirements for 'elbow clearance'
The normal paediatric elbow must have
• Full extension, supination and pronation
• No swelling or significant focal bony tenderness
• No abnormal anterior or posterior fat-pad sign
• Normally placed and age-appropriate ossification centres (see Fig. 24.2.7)
• An intact radio-capitellar relationship (see Fig. 24.2.8)

relative to the humerus are common, depending on the degree of pronation/supination at the time of fall (see Fig. 24.2.9).

Grade 1 – undisplaced supracondylar fracture

This is the presumptive diagnosis with elbow effusions that are tender bilaterally and have no ulnar or radial dislocations or significant displacement/angulation. The fracture line through the bone between olecranon and coronoid fossae may be seen on the AP view or recognised as a disruption to the normal 'teardrop' between the opposing fossae on the lateral humeral view, but its absence should not prevent the immobilisation of these elbow effusions until early orthopaedic review.

Grade 2 – posterior angulation with probable intact periosteal hinge

In this situation it is important to check for associated injury. Use the 'anterior humeral line' as a guide to the probability of posterior angulation (see Fig. 24.2.10), and consult orthopaedics about all injuries. These require manipulation for all but minor degrees of angulation. Remember that remodelling may correct some loss of flexion or extension but will not correct rotation or varus/valgus deformity.

Grade 3 – grossly displaced/rotated

Check for open injury or neurovascular compromise. Brachial artery spasm or kinking is common with this injury, and the gross associated swelling may predispose to compartment syndrome. Radial

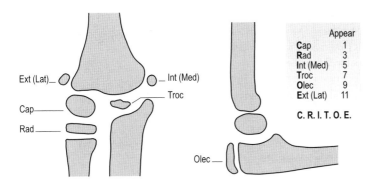

Fig. 24.2.7 CRITOE. The approximate order of appearance of the six elbow ossification centres according to the CRITOE mnemonic. Drawing by Terry McGuire, courtesy of PaEDpac.

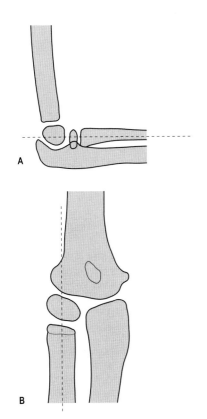

Fig. 24.2.8 The normal capitello-radial head relationship. Drawing by Terry McGuire, courtesy of PaEDpac.

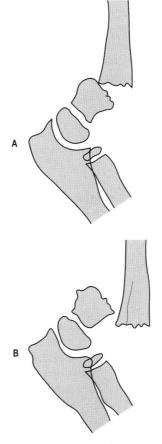

Fig. 24.2.9 Supracondylar fractures. (*A*) Grade 2, approximately 45 degrees dorsal angulation but probable intact dorsal periosteal 'hinge'; (*B*) grade 3, complete displacement, often co-existent rotation and/or neurovascular impairment. Drawing by Terry McGuire, courtesy of PaEDpac.

Fig. 24.2.10 The anterior humeral line rule for subtle supracondylar fractures. A line passed along the anterior humeral cortex on a lateral elbow radiograph should bisect the anterior and middle thirds of the capitellum. If it passes anterior to the capitellum, there is at least 20 degrees dorsal angulation of the distal humerus. Drawing by Terry McGuire, courtesy of PaEDpac.

pulse and hand perfusion should be continuously reassessed. Immediate orthopaedic notification is required.

If orthopaedic help is not available within one hour of the onset of poor hand perfusion, attempt gentle traction and reduction under anaesthesia, e.g. ketamine, aiming for the position with best hand perfusion.

Median or radial nerve injury may also occur (usually as praxis), and require orthopaedic evaluation. Ulnar nerve injury is most commonly reported as an iatrogenic injury following internal fixation.

Intercondylar (T-condylar) fracture

This is a variant of the supracondylar fracture resulting from axial impaction and intra-articular separation of capitellum and trochlea, as well as proximal disruption of the medial and lateral distal humeral columns. Treatment is by internal fixation, with or without open reduction.

Lateral condyle

This fracture results from a varus force on the supinated forearm, avulsing the condyle (see Figs 24.2.11 and 24.2.12). There is clinical swelling and tenderness, which is maximal over the lateral condyle. It is usually a Salter–Harris type 4 fracture, but the late appearance of the trochlear and lateral epicondylar ossification centres mean that the true structural disruption is not demonstrated by radiology, and therefore not appreciated by emergency staff, particularly in the

Fig. 24.2.11   Subtle lateral condylar fracture in a toddler. Note only two ossification centres (capitellum and radial head) and thin rim of metaphysis shorn away with capitellum. Greater angulation/displacement of metaphyseal fragment may be shown on lateral view. Drawing by Terry McGuire, courtesy of PaEDpac.

Fig. 24.2.12   Displaced and rotated lateral condylar fracture (Milch type I). Long-term complications may ensue if not surgically fixed. Drawing by Terry McGuire, courtesy of PaEDpac.

younger child. The varus angulating force characteristically causes disruption commencing above the lateral condyle, passing to a varying extent along the physis, and in complete disruptions exiting either lateral (in the majority of cases; Milch

type 1), or medial (Milch type 2) to the capitellar-trochlear groove. If uncorrected, the former will result in valgus deformity (and possible delayed ulnar nerve palsy), while the latter creates ulnar instability and may result in a gunstock deformity if not recognised and stabilised.

Bony displacement is often best seen on the lateral X-ray.

The clinical significance of this fracture means that:

❶ Any lateral condyle fracture with a greater than 2 mm separation of fracture segments is likely to require internal fixation.

❷ All young children with major elbow deformity/swelling as a result of injury should be assessed early by experienced orthopaedic personnel. Ultrasound, MRI, and arthrography may all have a role to play in determining the line of injury and consequent best means of fixation. Within the ED, an internal oblique radiograph can be helpful.

The elbow may be supported in a backslab while awaiting orthopaedic review.

Medial epicondylar avulsion

This may occur in association with other disruptions, e.g. elbow dislocation, or as a discrete event (Fig. 24.2.13). The medial epicondyle is the origin of the common flexor tendon, and ossifies at approximately age six. It will generally reunite readily with the humerus if it lies within 5 mm, unless there is interposing tissue. Occasionally, particularly when the avulsion has occurred in association with a posterior elbow dislocation, the epicondyle and its attachments may become lodged within the elbow joint and must be removed and repositioned as an open procedure. Ulnar nerve injury is a common association. This circumstance is one of the main practical uses of knowledge of elbow ossification centres (see Fig. 24.2.7). These must be systematically reviewed on every elbow X-ray so that missing or misplaced opacities may be identified.

Pulled elbow

Children from age six months presenting with acute disuse of one arm, which they hold in a semi-flexed and pronated pos-

A

B

Fig. 24.2.13   Medial epicondylar avulsion. (*A*) The opacity below the humerus is the avulsed medial epicondyle, which should be sitting more proximal and medial. There should not be a trochlear opacity without a medial epicondylar ossification centre (see Fig. 24.2.7). (*B*) Lateral view shows opacity 'between' capitellum and olecranon, possibly intra-articular. Drawing by Terry McGuire, courtesy of PaEDpac.

ture, can be presumed to have pulled elbow (radial head subluxation; RHS) if there is point tenderness at the radial head and no elbow effusion. After a brief explanation, these children should be held firmly by a parent while the forearm is firmly and fully supinated in extension. It is helpful for the doctor to cradle the elbow in the outer hand with the thumb over the radial head while their inner arm rotates. Success is usually denoted by a palpable click, visible momentary pain, and a return to functional use of the arm within fifteen minutes. If the procedure is not successful, hyper-pronation should be attempted, with the same set-up. This combination of techniques should elicit success in >90% of cases of radial head subluxation.[4] X-ray should be obtained in any child with other points of focal tenderness, an elbow effusion, or a failure of reduction at two attempts. Providing the X-ray shows no fracture or effusion, a further manipulation may be attempted after which the arm should be supported in a sling with review at 24 hours. Although some children sustain recurrent RHS, it rarely if ever requires operative intervention.

Elbow dislocation

Appearing first in adolescence, this injury, the result of a fall on to the hand with partially flexed elbow, is uncommon in young children (who sustain supracondylar fractures instead). The majority dislocate posteriorly, tearing joint capsule, and stretching soft tissues. The displacement may cause fracture to the coronoid process of the ulna or radial neck, or the medial epicondyle may be avulsed. Neuropraxis of median or ulnar nerves may occur.

The dislocation should be suspected clinically. After assessing for associated injuries, it should be reduced in the ED, generally under ketamine anaesthesia (see Fig. 24.2.14). Gentle downwards pressure can be applied to the supinated proximal forearm, with extension of the elbow to about 135 degrees, against counter-traction to distal humerus. Full extension

should be avoided as it may cause further damage to ulnar nerve. If there is difficulty in resiting the olecranon, there may be soft tissue inter-position and orthopaedic help should be sought. The reduced elbow should be held in flexion with a posterior splint for two weeks, with orthopaedic follow-up.

Proximal radial and ulnar fractures

Olecranon fractures

These may occur in older children as: (1) avulsion (flexion) fractures (generally requiring internal fixation); (2) extension fractures with intra-articular opening (may be stable in flexion); or (3) comminuted fractures from a direct blow to the elbow. Clinical correlation must be sought in diagnosing olecranon fractures as the ossification centre, which appears around ten years and may be bipartite or fragmentary in appearance, is easily mistaken for a fracture.

Radial neck fractures

These are relatively common injuries in the paediatric population. The radial head itself is largely cartilaginous and rarely injured. Injuries range from subtle torus-type 'beaking' of the neck, which is best seen on the lateral side on the lateral projection, to displaced Salter–Harris type 1 or 2 fractures. Suspicion of an isolated injury may be made by the presence of localised tenderness at the radial head.

Neurovascular injury, particularly to posterior inter-osseous nerve, should always be sought. Undisplaced fractures may be immobilised in a collar and cuff.

Monteggia fracture dislocation

The peak incidence of this injury complex is in the 4–10 age group. Although classically radio-capitellar disruption accompanies an angulated or shortened ulnar fracture, the displacement may occur in association with any displacement to the radio-ulnar loop. Because of the significant complications of a missed radio-capitellar disruption, this lesion must be actively clinically and radiologically sought in any child with a forearm fracture and elbow swelling. Many units adopt a rule of always X-raying the elbow of any child with forearm or wrist injury, unless the elbow has been specifically clinically cleared (see Table 24.2.5).

The classical (Type 1) Monteggia lesion involves an angulated apex-volar ulnar shaft fracture and anterior displacement of the radial head (see Fig. 24.2.2). Variants include lateral radial head displacement, often in association with proximal ulnar fractures (Type 3), 'Monteggia equivalent' fractures including proximal radial fracture/dislocation, and others. A bowing deformity may be the only evidence of fracture. Orthopaedic manipulation of the ulnar fracture generally is accompanied by reduction of the radial head dislocation.

Midshaft radial and ulnar fractures

These injuries fall into two broad groups: (1) common low-energy greenstick fractures as a common consequence of falls in childhood; and (2) higher-energy complete fractures, which may be difficult to reduce, requiring internal fixation in 5–10% of cases. In the former group, with the exception of bowing fractures (which generally require general anaesthetic/ orthopaedic reduction, as prolonged corrective force is necessary) ED reduction may be possible thus:

- Apex volar – pronate forearm and apply wrist traction and volar pressure.

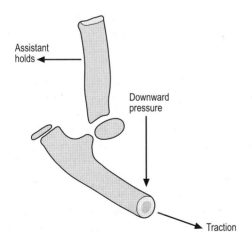

Fig. 24.2.14   Reduction of elbow dislocation. Bring arm in full supination to approximately 20 degrees from full extension, and provide simultaneous downwards traction and downwards pressure over the proximal forearm to lever the coronoid process back under the distal humerus.

- Apex dorsum – supinate forearm and apply wrist traction and dorsal pressure.

Although these fractures may be simple to relocate under anaesthesia, e.g. ketamine, their inherent instability makes expert three-point moulding essential. Therefore, manipulation should not be attempted unless such expertise is available, and follow-up within the period of potential remanipulation (e.g. one week) is advisable.

Distal radial and ulnar fractures

These common injuries may be metaphyseal or epiphyseal in nature. Dorsal angulation occurs in 80% of cases, but radial or volar angulation/displacement of the distal fragments may also occur. Regarding management, the following guidelines apply:

- Simple *torus (buckle) fractures* with no periosteal or cortical breach, which represent plastic deformation only, may be placed in a forearm splint or brace for comfort and referred for follow-up in 1–2 weeks.[5]
- *Undisplaced greenstick fractures*, in which a cortex or periosteum has been breached, have inherent instability and the potential for further deformation. These should be managed in a well-moulded (three-point fixation) full-arm plaster in neutral position,[6] and reviewed within one week.
- *Angulated or displaced greenstick fractures* of the distal forearm generally require reduction if the angulation is greater than 20 degrees, although remodelling potential varies with the age of the child and the distance of the fracture from the physis. Closed reduction may be performed in the ED if staffing and expertise permits.

Again, attention must be paid to ensure that a well-moulded plaster will maintain reduction, and follow-up orthopaedic review should be early enough to detect this and remanipulate if necessary. Early orthopaedic referral should occur for angulated isolated radial fractures and for fractures of radius and ulna with complete displacement and shortening,

as a significant proportion of these manipulations will be problematic or require internal fixation.[7]

Distal radial epiphyseal fractures

These can generally be treated by manipulation and closed reduction in the same way as metaphyseal fractures. There is a low incidence of subsequent premature physeal closure or other physeal disruption. This risk is greatest following multiple or delayed reduction attempts, or compressive injuries, or distal physeal separation of the ulna.[2]

Carpal injuries

Because of the flexibility of the paediatric wrist and the plastic properties of pre-ossified bone, carpal injuries are rare in children under ten years. Scaphoid injuries are rare under eight years and are generally over-diagnosed in children in the ED setting.[8] Of those fractures that do occur, 65% are distal pole and non-union is rare because of the different mechanical and vascular properties of immature bone. Provisional immobilisation when scaphoid views are negative is suggested only if:

- The child is adolescent (ten years and over).
- The injury involved high-velocity force, especially kickback.
- There is single-point tenderness and swelling in anatomical snuffbox.
- There is pain to compression along first metacarpal ray.

Suspected fractures should be managed with scaphoid plaster and orthopaedic follow-up as usual. It is noted with interest that of eighteen children aged 8–15 who underwent MRI for localised scaphoid pain after trauma, six had fractures, seven had evidence of extensor tenosynovitis and four showed marrow oedema that did not progress to fracture.

Metacarpal fractures

Crush injuries to metacarpal bones may occur, and adolescence sees an increase in fractures of the head of the fifth metacarpal, as in adults, although the intact distal metacarpal physis will allow some remodelling to correct flexion loss. Pen-

etrating trauma, tendon damage, open injuries and neurovascular impairment must be identified and referred. Multiple fractures may create an unstable hand plate. Finger flexion should be observed for possible associated rotational malalignment, which is not acceptable.

Thumb fractures

Forced thumb abduction, e.g. from fall onto the splayed hand, can cause avulsion of part of the proximal thumb physis (a Salter–Harris type 3 injury instead of the adult ulnar collateral ligament tear), or a metaphyseal fracture of the base of the first metacarpal. The intra-articular Salter–Harris type 3 avulsion injury should be internally fixed. However, in the latter injury, because of the universal motion of the first carpo-metacarpal joint, significant angulation and displacement will remodel if the child is under ten years, and the child may have the fracture immobilised in a scaphoid type plaster, elevated, and be referred for early orthopaedic (next-day) consultation.

Fingertip injuries

These injuries to young children are extremely common from inadvertent closure in doors or gates, especially in cooler climates where greater micro-environment control is required. Injuries include partial or complete amputation, nail-plate injuries, and distal phalangeal fractures.

The classical crush injury includes a distal phalangeal tuft fracture and a partial amputation anteriorly through the nail bed, with intact volar soft tissue attachments and vascular integrity. Tip salvage is usual. However, without meticulous repair to the nail-bed laceration nail deformities are common.

Tip amputations distal to the terminal phalanx may often heal by secondary intent, because of the excellent vascular supply in childhood. More proximal injuries require assessment of nail-bed integrity, the possibility of soft-tissue (e.g. nail-bed) interposition within an angulated/displaced fracture, or other indications for reconstructive procedures. Simple procedures may be performed in the ED under ketamine anaesthesia or sedation and ring block.

LOWER LIMB AND PELVIS INJURIES

Pelvic fractures

These injuries are less common in paediatric than adult trauma. Avulsion injuries in athletic adolescents may occur. The implications for blood loss and uro-genital injury of unstable pelvic fractures in children are similar to those in adulthood. The bladder is an intra-abdominal organ in infants.

Hip dislocation

This is uncommon in childhood, occurring either with low force as a result of increased ligamentous laxity, or in the high-force mechanisms more typical of adult hip dislocation. The sequel of avascular necrosis is less common, occurring in approximately 5% of cases.[2] Reduction, by gentle closed longitudinal traction against a fixed pelvis, should be performed within six hours. Particular care must be taken in the adolescent in whom an occult physeal injury may be displaced.

Femoral fractures

Although comprising less than 5% of paediatric fracture presentations to the ED, the infant or child presenting with a femoral fracture presents particular challenges to the emergency physician because of:

- The frequent association with major trauma and other unstable injuries.
- The high level of pain and emotional distress for the child and the family, particularly in the setting of road trauma.
- The need for procedural skills, such as femoral nerve block, and the application of traction splinting, such as the Thomas splint.
- The possibility of non-accidental injury (may be as high as 60–80% under twelve months[9]).

The simultaneous management of all these challenging priorities is a good test of the mature, multidimensional emergency physician.

As has been mentioned earlier, all limb fractures should be initially approached with rapid primary and secondary survey while the integrity of airways breathing, circulation, conscious state and spinal column are assessed, mechanism ascertained, and areas of tenderness identified. An IV cannula should be inserted immediately, under nitrous oxide or intra-nasal fentanyl if necessary. Early attention to issues of pain and anxiety have been shown to reduce the stress and pain of later procedures. Femoral nerve block should be inserted early with Thomas splint following in a timely fashion.

Not all femoral fractures are the result of major trauma. In the newly ambulant child, the torsion resulting from a change of forward momentum with the foot fixed at an angle may produce a spiral mid-shaft fracture. Mechanisms in abusive injury include forced external rotation or abduction, e.g. from nappy change position, or direct blows.

Types of femoral fracture in children, and their orthopaedic implications, are as follows:

- Proximal femoral fractures include transepiphyseal, transcervical, basicervical, and intertrochanteric fractures. Avascular necrosis and physeal growth arrest are significant potential complications of higher fractures, and early notification and reduction are urgent.
- Slipped upper femoral epiphysis is discussed in Chapter 24.1.
- In femoral shaft fractures definitive orthopaedic management depends on the degree of precipitating force, associated injuries, the age of the child, home circumstances, and the institution. Low-force injuries in young children may be treated by closed reduction and early hip spica casting. Options in older children, in whom healing is not as rapid, include skeletal traction with a distal femoral pin (avoiding the possibility of proximal tibial physeal disruption), flexible inter-medullary fixation from a distal femoral metaphyseal entry point, plating, and external fixation.

Injuries about the knee

Distal femoral physeal separation
These injuries result from high-force trauma to the knee. Any of the Salter-Harris pattern injuries may occur. Undisplaced injuries may be managed by cast immobilisation. Orthopaedic consultation is imperative because of:

- The possibility of co-existent intra-articular ligament disruption.
- The need for perfect articular surface realignment.
- The possibility of subsequent asymmetrical physeal arrest.

Tibial spine injury

Because of the mechanical properties of developing bone, twisting injuries to the paediatric knee result in avulsion of the tibial attachment of the anterior cruciate ligament (see Fig. 24.2.15). The child

Fig. 24.2.15 Lateral and AP views of the paediatric knee with an avulsed tibial spine. Due to the intact anterior cruciate ligament, the tibial spine fracture (shaded) may be hinged posteriorly, opening anteriorly on knee flexion.

presents non-weight bearing, with a large effusion and joint-line tenderness. Although AP X-ray may be deceptive, lateral projections show a characteristic beak-like appearance of the superior surface of the tibial plateau, with posterior hinging. Orthopaedic management involves an assessment, generally under anaesthetic, of the reducibility of the avulsed spine and the likelihood of, e.g., meniscal interposition. Treatment options include immobilisation in extension or partial flexion, and internal fixation. Some degree of subsequent instability and loss of extension may follow.

Avulsion of tibial tubercle

This adolescent injury represents avulsion of the insertion site of the patellar tendon, usually as a result of forceful quadriceps contraction against resistance. Displaced injuries require internal fixation and immobilisation.

Patellar dislocation

This injury occurs most commonly in adolescents with an excessive Q-angle (the complementary angle to the vastus lateralis/patellar tendon vectors) or hypermobility. The usual pattern is of lateral dislocation following a twist, e.g. during a fall. Most reduce spontaneously or during transport; extension of the knee may be facilitated in the prone position to relax hamstring muscles. A sky-line view should be obtained for best visualisation of osteochondral fragments from the medial patella. The knee should be placed in a Richards-type splint and the child referred for physiotherapy and orthopaedic follow-up. Chronic dislocation occurs in approximately 1:6 cases.

Patellar fractures

These are less common in children than in adults. Osteochondral avulsions may occur with dislocation. Displaced fractures, with tense haemarthroses and lack of full knee extension, should be referred to the orthopaedic team. The patellar sleeve fracture may be radiographically occult as it represents separation of the cartilaginous distal patella from the ossification centre. Findings will include patella alta and excessive anterior tenderness and swelling.

Bipartite patella (secondary ossification centre) is a common radiographic normal variant.

Lower leg fractures

Lower leg fractures are common in childhood. Factors to be considered in their assessment include:

- Age.
- Mechanism (low- or high-force, type of injury, e.g. valgus/rotation).
- Degree of angulation or displacement.
- Associated soft-tissue damage or other injuries.
- Involvement of physes.
- Integrity of fibula.

Compound injuries and those with physeal involvement or significant angulation or displacement should be referred for in-patient orthopaedic evaluation. Proximal tibial epiphyseal injury may be complicated by vascular compromise, as with adult knee dislocation. Varus or valgus deformity, particularly at the proximal tibia, may progress. Stable, undisplaced or minimally displaced oblique or spiral shaft fractures of the tibia may be placed in a well-moulded above-knee cast with the knee flexed to 90 degrees and the ankle in 15 degrees of plantar flexion.[10] Admission is not required if swelling is minimal, mechanism is clear, and parents are sensible.

The so-called toddler fracture is an undisplaced tibial shaft fracture that occurs as a result of a rotational shearing force in the newly ambulant child. Presentation is with non-weight bearing or limp

and the differential includes other pathologies, e.g. irritable or septic hip. Tenderness should be localised to the tibial shaft but initial radiology may be normal. If this diagnosis is suspected in a well child with normal joint examination, POP immobilisation and orthopaedic follow-up with repeat X-ray at ten days or nuclear bone scan may be helpful.

Ankle fractures

As with adults, inversion, eversion and twisting mechanisms may cause a variety of injury patterns at the ankle depending on age, degree of force, and mechanism. Ankle injuries requiring same-day orthopaedic consultation include:

- Open injuries.
- Unstable injuries or ankles with extensive bilateral tenderness and swelling, suggesting possible mortice instability.
- Displaced or angulated distal tibial fractures.
- Salter–Harris type 3 and 4 injuries.
- Triplane and Tillaux fractures.

Tillaux fracture   This is a Salter–Harris type 3 fracture at the distal tibial physis, occurring in adolescence after partial closure of the medial growth plate (see Fig. 24.2.5). External rotation of the foot and ankle causes avulsion of the anterolateral portion of the distal tibial physis by its attachment to the fibula (anterior tibiofibular ligament). The diagnosis should be suspected in a non-weight-bearing adolescent with signifi-

---

CONTROVERSIES

❶ Controversy exists surrounding boundary issues between emergency medicine and orthopaedics. Who performs which reduction should be determined by consideration of safe, effective resource use between emergency and orthopaedic services.

❷ Maintenance of supracondylar humeral fracture reductions is controversial, with some opting for transcutaneous Kwires and others collar and cuff.

❸ The optimal position for forearm fractures post-reduction (neutral vs. pronation/supination) has not been determined.

❹ Treatment of buckle fractures of the distal radius is somewhat controversial, although most would favour a splint as opposed to long arm POP.

cant anterolateral ankle swelling and tenderness. Oblique ankle views or CT assessment may be required to detail alignment.

Triplane fracture This also occurs in the adolescent with external rotation injury, but the fracture line also tears off a section of posterior tibial metaphysis, which is clearly visible on the lateral radiograph.

Both of these transitional fractures may be complicated by subsequent joint incongruity or growth disturbance.

Inversion injuries

Carefully assess point of maximal tenderness. A point of maximal tenderness over the physis may represent a Salter–Harris type 1 separation of the distal fibular physis and should be cast immobilised for 2–3 weeks until stable. Bony injury may also occur at the base of the 5th metatarsal. Radiographically this is shown by an avulsion fracture line at right angles to the metatarsal bones (the normal apophyseal plate runs parallel). Although the Ottawa ankle rules have not been specifically validated in children, the requirement for further assessment of an injury involving extensive swelling, bony tenderness, or inability to weight bear seems appropriate.

FURTHER READING

1. Donald T 1994 Physical abuse in children. Medical Observer CME 1–4 14 October
2. Morrisey RT, Weinstein SL 2001 Lovell and Winter's pediatric orthopedics, 5th edn. Lippincott Williams and Wilkins, Philadelphia
3. United Medical Protection, personal correspondence 2003 Orthopaedic claims under 16 years over the period 1985–2002

4. Davidson JS, Brown DJ, Barnes S, treatment for torus fractures of the Journal of Bone and Joint Surgery Br
5. Boyer BA, Overton B, Scrader W, Ru 2002 Position of immobilisation for p forearm fractures. Journal of Paediatric Orthopaedics 22(2): 185–187
6. Gibbons CL, Woods DA, Pailthorpe C, C J, Warlock I et al 1994 The management of isolated distal radius fractures in children. Journal of Paediatric Orthopaedics 14(2): 207–210
7. Gillon H 2001 Scaphoid injuries in children. Accident and Emergency Nursing 9: 249–256
8. Thomas SA, Rosenfield NS, Leventhal JM, Markowitz RI 1991 Long-bone fractures in young children: Distinguishing accidental injuries from child abuse. Paediatrics 88(3): 471–476
9. Yang J, Letts R 1997 Isolated fractures of the tibia with intact fibula in children: A review of 95 patients. Journal of Paediatric Orthopaedics 17: 347–351
10. Mater Children's Hospital 2002 Unpublished data from the emergency department information systems (EDIS) exit diagnosis database for the period September-November
11. Beaty JH, Kasser JR (eds) 2001 Rockwood and Wilkins' fractures in children, 5th edn. Lippincott Williams & Wilkins, Philadelphia

ORTHOPAEDICS AND RHEUMATOLOGY

24.3 SPINAL INJURY

ED OAKLEY

Essentials

1 Spine injury is often associated with other severe injury.

2 Upper cervical spine injuries are more common in children.

3 Adequate immobilisation of the entire spine is needed.

4 Clinical evaluation of the cervical spine can only occur in a child who is conscious, able to communicate and free from any other significant injuries.

5 The cervical spine can be cleared on clinical findings alone in specific circumstances.

6 A good quality three-view series of the cervical spine (lateral, AP and odontoid view) is adequate to assess the bony structures.

7 Clinical findings should be considered when clearing the cervical spine radiographically.

8 Thoracic and lumbar spine injury is strongly associated with spinal cord injury.

9 Patients with spinal injury have a high incidence of fractures at another level.

10 Spinal cord injury may cause hypotension and relative bradycardia.

11 Spinal immobilisation can cause complications especially in the patient with spinal cord injury.

12 Spinal cord injury may occur without radiographic abnormality.

INTRODUCTION

Injuries to the spine and spinal cord are less common in children than adults. The injuries have different distributions and frequency in different aged children – dependant upon the developmental anatomical and physiological differences with age. Children account for up to 10% of all spinal injuries, but the mortality among spine-injured children is higher than in adults, with estimates ranging from 25–30%, with death most often due to associated injuries to other organs – especially the brain.[1]

The incidence of spinal cord injury amongst spine-injured children is probably about 1%.[1,2] In neurologically impaired survivors the injuries are most commonly at the C1–C2 level, or in the lower cervical or thoracic spine.[1] The common causes of spine and spinal cord injuries in children are motor vehicle crashes, falls, diving accidents, sports injuries and, occasionally, non-accidental injury.[1,3,4]

The majority of injuries in children occur in the cervical spine. In children under eight most (about 80%) occur in the C1–C3 region, whereas after eight years of age the incidence is similar to that in adults with the majority in the lower three cervical vertebrae.[2,5] The thoracolumbar junction is the most commonly injured area outside the cervical spine, with the thoracic and lumbar spines having roughly equal incidence of about 25%. There is an increased incidence of neurologic injury in fractures of the thoracolumbar junction. The relatively high incidence of injuries in this region is due to the large range of motion and the changing orientation of the facet joints.[1,6] Approximately 30% of patients with spinal cord injury have fractures at more than one spinal level. A majority of these are in contiguous vertebral segments, but 5–15% may be in different regions.[6]

DEVELOPMENTAL ANATOMY AND PHYSIOLOGY

There are a number of injury patterns of the spine – and especially the cervical spine – that are unique to children. In order to understand the differences between adult and paediatric spine injuries knowledge of the developmental anatomy of the spine is essential.

The large amount of cartilage present in the paediatric cervical spine can make radiographic evaluation difficult. This is especially true in the first few years of life, and in the upper cervical vertebrae.

The *atlas* ossifies from three ossification centres: two ossification centres of the lateral masses and one ossification centre for the body. The ossification centre for the body does not ossify until about one year of age. The posterior arches fuse by three or four years of age, while the synchondrosis between the lateral masses and the body fuses at approximately seven years of age.[3,5]

The *axis* ossifies from seven ossification centres. The five primary ossification centres are two for the lateral masses, two for the odontoid (which are usually fused at birth but occasionally persist as a dens bicornis), and one for the body. The odontoid is separated from the body by a synchondrosis, which fuses between three and six years old. The two secondary ossification centres are the tip of the odontoid process (which appears at about three years of age and is usually fused by twelve years of age), and the inferior ring apophysis (which, like other ring apophyses, generally ossifies after eight years of age and fuses in the early twenties).[3,5]

The remainder of the cervical vertebrae each contain three primary ossification centres – one for the body and one for the two neural arches – and two secondary ossification centres – the ring apophyses. The neural arches fuse posteriorly by the age of three, and anteriorly the three ossification centres fuse between three and six years of age. Importantly the vertebral bodies are wedge shaped until the age of seven when they begin to square off.[3,4]

The thoracic and lumbar spines develop in a similar way with secondary ossification centres for the spinous process and the transverse processes added. By the time the child is eight to ten years of age the spine has reached near adult size.[3,4]

There are a number of other differences of importance for the spine. The fulcrum of movement of the neck is located at C2–C3 in the infant, at C3–C4 by the age of six, and by the age of eight the fulcrum is at C5–C6, as it is in the adult. There is a relatively large head and weak neck muscles; laxity of the ligaments and joint capsule; and relatively horizontal positioning of the facet joints with underdevelopment of the uncinate processes.[1,3,4] All these features increase the risk of injury to the child's spine.

INITIAL ASSESSMENT

All patients with significant trauma should be assumed to have a spine or spinal cord injury and appropriate precautions must be taken to prevent further exacerbating any possible injury. The initial assessment of patients with potential spine or spinal cord injury should be directed at the airway, breathing and circulation, in line with trauma resuscitation guidelines (see Chapter 2). The patient should be stabilised and a thorough secondary survey performed. At this point all possible spine and spinal cord injuries should be identified. The lateral cervical spine X-ray will be done at this stage in patients with major trauma. Thorough radiological assessment of the injuries should be completed once resuscitation and stabilisation and the secondary survey have all been accomplished.

A thorough history of mechanism of injury, previous spinal injury, other illnesses – particularly respiratory illness (acute or chronic), cardiac illness, or bone disorders - medication and allergies is needed to determine the patient's pre-morbid physiological status.

SPINAL IMMOBILISATION

Spinal immobilisation is currently a controversial issue – especially in young children. A balance must be found that will diminish the risk of further injury to the child's spine, but not interfere with the assessment, or the normal physiologic functions, of the child. Traditionally the spine has been immobilised in a rigid cervical collar with a head immobiliser and straps, and a spine board to which the patient is strapped, thus providing adequate control of the entire spine (see Table 24.3.1).[3,7,8]

There are a number of potential problems with this immobilisation (see Table 24.3.2). Cervical collars are not made to fit infants and alternative immobilisation is needed. An ill-fitting collar may cause the chin to become trapped under the chin support and may cause airway obstruction. The young child may become distressed from being rigidly immobilised making further as-sessment difficult, and potentially raising intracranial pressure. Rigid immobilisation in a collar and head immobiliser on a spinal board has also been shown to decrease tidal volume and respiratory excursion.[9] In addition, because the young child's head is disproportionately large the neck is flexed when immobilised on a standard spinal board. This causes flexion of the cervical spine, which may cause movement at the site of injury. To prevent this a spinal board with a recess for the head or padding that elevates the torso is needed for children less than eight years old (Fig. 24.3.1).[10–12]

Table 24.3.1 Indications for initial immobilisation of the spine

- Level of consciousness
- Inability to give history of pain
- Neck or back pain
- Neurologic signs or symptoms
- Multiple system trauma
- History of significant trauma
  Fall from height > 3 metres
  Pedestrian or cyclist hit by car
  Unrestrained passenger in motor vehicle crash diving accident
- History of spinal abnormality

Table 24.3.2 Problems associated with spinal immobilisation in children

- Incorrectly fitted cervical-spine collar causing distraction of the spine or allowing movement
- Flexion of the spine in children under eight years of age
- Reduction in tidal volume and limitation of respiratory effort
- Airway obstruction
- Increased intracranial pressure
- Discomfort
- Distress and anxiety
- Pressure sores

A number of different cervical collars are available and satisfactory to use. The clinician must be familiar with the method of sizing and applying the collar available, as an incorrect fit will allow too much movement of the collar if too small, or will produce a distraction of any existing injury if too large.

For children who have less major trauma but are at risk of spinal injury a degree of judgement is needed by the clinician as to the level of immobilisation that is appropriate. However, in all patients with multiple or significant other injuries full immobilisation is still recommended.

The back is examined by log rolling the child. This requires at least three people in the smallest of children, and up to five in larger patients. The child is freed from the head immobiliser and any strapping to the spinal board removed. One person must stabilise the cervical spine by supporting the head and neck in the neutral position throughout movement. No traction should be applied to the neck. The other team members control the shoulders, hips and legs, and one person must be free to inspect and palpate the back. The back is inspected for bruises, abrasions, wounds or deformity of the spine. The spinous processes are palpated for tenderness. The back of the neck and head and the buttocks and anus should be inspected. A rectal examination is not mandated in all children.

To limit discomfort and the likelihood of pressure sores a child should be kept on the spinal board for the shortest possible time. Once resuscitation and urgent procedures and investigations are completed the board should be removed. This is especially important in patients with suspected spinal cord injury.[13]

CERVICAL SPINE INJURIES

As the cervical spine is the most common region injured and accounts for the majority of spinal cord injuries a thorough knowledge of injuries in this region and the appropriate assessment of the spine both clinically and radiographically is man-

Fig. 24.3.1   Effects of spine-board on cervical spine position in children. Child immobilised on a standard backboard (A), and on backboards modified with an occipital recess (B) and a mattress pad (C).
Modified from Herzenberg et al 1989 Emergency transport and positioning of young children who may have an injury of the cervical spine: The standard backboard may be hazardous. Journal of Bone & Joint Surgery 71(1): 15–22.

Table 24.3.3 A classification of spine injuries

Mechanism of injury	Stability
Flexion	
Flexion teardrop fracture	Very unstable
Bilateral facet joint dislocation	Unstable
Atlanto-occipital dislocation	Unstable
Displaced odontoid fracture	Unstable
Anterior subluxation	Unstable
Anterior wedge fracture	Stable
Clay Shoveller's fracture	Very stable
Extension	
Atlantoaxial dislocation	Very unstable
Hangman's fracture C2	Unstable
Extension teardrop fracture	Unstable (in extension)
Rotation	
Rotary atlanto-axial dislocation	Unstable
Rotary atlanto-axial subluxation	Stable
Unilateral facet dislocation	Stable
Vertical compression	
Jefferson fracture (burst # C1)	Very unstable
Burst fracture vertebral body	Stable

Source: Modified from Rosen P et al 1997 Emergency Medicine, 4th edn. Mosby, St. Louis, Missouri, USA.

datory. In children younger than eight years of age the majority (but not all) injuries occur above the fourth cervical vertebra. After eight the pattern of injury is similar to that seen in adults (the majority of injuries below C4).[2,14]

Mechanisms of injury

The mechanism of injury is an important historical factor, as it will determine the type and possible instability of the underlying injury (see Table 24.3.3).

Flexion

The most common mechanism of injury seen is hyperflexion. This type of injury produces a compressive force on the anterior segment of the vertebra – leading to a compression fracture or teardrop fracture. The posterior elements of the spine are distracted with ligamentous injury, dislocations, or avulsion fractures of the spinous processes. These injuries can be stable (such as the anterior wedge compression fracture or the clay shoveller's fracture) or unstable (such as a bilateral facet joint dislocation).

Extension

Hyperextension injuries produce distracting forces anteriorly, while compressing the posterior vertebral structures. Most extension injuries are unstable, and buckling of the ligamentum flavum into the posterior of the spinal canal can cause a central or posterior spinal cord syndrome.

Rotation

In the cervical spine isolated rotary injuries are uncommon. Subluxation can be spontaneous or follow minor or major trauma. It is generally a stable injury. However, if there is dislocation of the facet joints of C1/C2 the lesion is unstable.

Vertical compression

These injuries are due to axial compression of the cervical spine. This can produce a burst fracture of any vertebra, with a lesion at C1 being most unstable. Spinal cord involvement is from a retropulsed fragment of bone or intervertebral disc.

In many instances not one but a combination of these mechanisms of injury is involved, producing more than one type of injury.

Clinical Assessment

After immobilisation and resuscitation of the injured child and as part of the secondary survey the neck should be examined. This is done to look for neck abrasions and signs of injury to other structures in the neck as well as to examine the cervical spine. The decision to evaluate the cervical spine for injury should only be made in children who are conscious and alert, who are not drug or alcohol affected, and who do not have other injuries that are painful or distracting enough to make assessment of neck pain difficult.[2,14,15]

The cervical collar should be removed while another person holds the head in-line. No traction should be applied to the neck. The cervical spine is palpated for tenderness over the spinous processes. If there is tenderness over a specific region the collar should be reapplied and the spine evaluated with X-ray. If there is no tenderness (or only soft tissue tenderness) the child should be allowed to gently move the head from side to side. If this produces pain posteriorly in the neck the collar should be reapplied and the spine X-rayed. If there is no pain on movement the collar and cervical spine protection can be removed.[2,14,15]

Young children represent a difficult subgroup. They are preverbal and cannot follow commands or communicate easily. If palpation of the posterior cervical spine does not cause distress the neck should be let free, if the child spontaneously moves the neck without discomfort the neck can be cleared. In this author's experience no young child with a neck fracture will spontaneously move its neck without discomfort.

Radiographic images

Radiological evaluation is required for all children who do not meet all the criteria for clinical clearance of the cervical spine. As part of the secondary survey in major trauma patients the cross-table lateral cervical spine X-ray would have been performed. This is a guide to the presence of serious cervical spine trauma only and cannot be used to exclude cervical spine injury.[2,14] All patients who require radiologic evaluation require a full cervical spine series.

The cervical spine series consists of a lateral film, an anterior-posterior film and an odontoid view. Using these three views all abnormal cervical spines will be detected, allowing further investigation to fully delineate the individual injuries.[2,5] All seven vertebrae must be included in the lateral view along with the cervico-thoracic junction. If this is not visible gentle traction should be applied to the arms and the film repeated, or a swimmer's view (transaxillary) should be obtained. Oblique views of the cervical spine may also be of assistance, especially if the cervico-thoracic junction is difficult to visualise. Oblique views, however, do not provide any more information regarding the likelihood of injury than the standard three views.[2,5,14]

In young children getting cooperation for the odontoid (open mouth) view is difficult. It has been shown that this view can be excluded in children under five years of age with little likelihood of missing a fracture.[16,17]

Other specialised radiological investigations have been used to evaluate cervical spine injuries:

Flexion and extension   Lateral cervical spine radiographs have been used to assess the spine for ligamentous injury. The suggested indications have been symptomatic patients with normal plain X-rays, or the unconscious patient with normal X-rays and or CT scans. These images have become popular in assessing adult patients but investigations to date have consistently failed to show a benefit over other imaging, with a significant number of studies limited by inadequate motion in the acute setting.[18] Most paediatric cervical-spine guidelines do not call for the routine use of these views.

Computerised tomography   CT of the cervical spine is common. There have been a number of indications for routine CT suggested with the most widely accepted being for further evaluation and elucidation of fractures identified, or to view areas not seen adequately on the initial cervical spine series.[14] Other suggested indications are for the assessment of the unconscious patient with normal initial radiographs, and for patients having a CT of the brain. Proponents of CT suggest scanning the entire spine in both of these instances and clearing the

spine if scans are normal (or progressing to flexion-extension views).[14,19] Another group suggests just scanning the upper three cervical vertebrae in children under eight as most injuries occur in this region.[20] There are no studies that have systematically evaluated the role of CT in the evaluation of paediatric cervical spine injuries. The CT does not see ligamentous structures well and will miss many ligamentous injuries and a significant proportion of injuries in children less than eight years of age will involve ligamentous structures.[14,21]

Magnetic resonance imaging   MRI is the imaging method of choice for assessing ligamentous injuries and for spinal cord injuries. MRI will visualise most ligamentous injuries and all spinal cord injuries. In many instances MRI will alter the specifics of surgical management in those who require surgical stabilisation. MRI provides prognostic information in children with spinal cord injury.[14,21]

Radiographic evaluation

Once the X-rays have been obtained care needs to be taken to interpret the images accurately and correlate the findings with the history and physical examination. Due to the physiologic differences described above, a number of normal radiological findings in children are significantly different from those in adults. The common findings that cause concern are: pseudo-subluxation of C2 on C3 (seen in up to 25% of children); exaggerated atlanto-dens distance (seen in 20% of children under eight years of age); and radiolucent synchondrosis between the odontoid and C2 (seen in all children under four and in 50% of those under ten years of age). Other normal findings that can be misinterpreted include a variable anterior soft tissue width – altering with head positioning and crying – the anterior ring apophyses of the vertebral bodies, and the anterior wedging of the vertebral bodies (especially C3).[14,22,23] All of these normal findings can be mistaken for acute traumatic injuries in children following trauma.

Evaluation of the lateral cervical spine radiograph begins with assessment of the

Fig. 24.3.2   Cervical spine lines.
*Lateral cervical spine. (A) Anterior vertebral bodies; (B) posterior vertebral bodies and anterior spinal canal; (C) spinolamial line and posterior spinal canal; (D) spinous process tips C2-C7; (E) odontoid process of dens of C2; (F) anterior arch of C1; (G) predental space between posterior surface of anterior arch of C1 and anterior surface of odontoid process.
Modified from Barkin et al 1994 Emergency Pediatrics, 4th edn. Mosby, St. Louis, Missouri, USA.*

four lines – corresponding to the anterior vertebral bodies, the posterior vertebral bodies, the spinolaminar line, and the tips of the spinous processes. All four of these lines should follow a smooth, even contour (see Fig. 24.3.2). The articular facets should be parallel, the intervertebral disc spaces, at the posterior margin of the vertebral bodies, should be similar, and the distances between spinous processes should show no significant widening (fanning). Review of the soft tissue shadow should show a retropharyngeal space of not more than one half the AP diameter of the vertebral body at C2 and no wider than the full width of the vertebral body at C6. As mentioned, this may be difficult to interpret in the crying child.[1,3,14]

Assessment of these areas of possible abnormality has been made easier by the formulation of a series of normal measurements. For the atlanto-axial relationship (C1–C2) a measurement of the distance

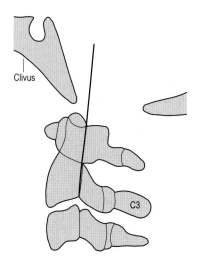

Fig. 24.3.3 Posterior axial line for identification of occipito-axial dislocation.

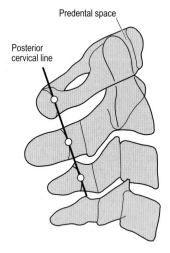

Fig. 24.3.4 Posterior cervical (Swischuk) line.

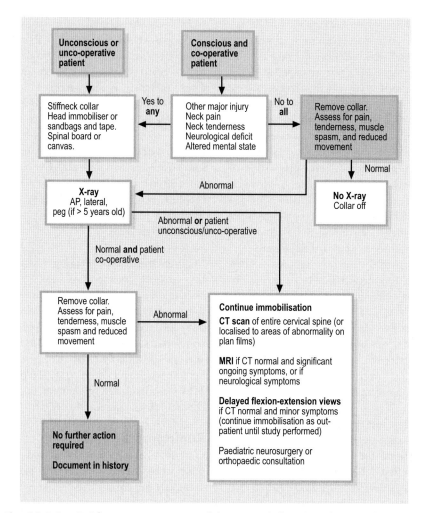

Fig. 24.3.5 Guide to management of the potentially injured cervical spine.

(on the lateral film) from the posterior border of the anterior arch of C1 to the anterior margin of the odontoid should be less than 5 mm in children under eight years of age, and ≤3 mm in older children and adults. To assess the relationship of the basion of the skull to the atlas the most reliable measurement in children is Harris's posterior axial line (see Fig. 24.3.3), which should lie within 12 mm of the basion of the skull.

The subluxation of C2 on C3 and C3 on C4 consistently causes difficulty in interpretation of paediatric cervical spine films. Swischuk's line (posterior cervical line), which joins the spinolaminar line of C1 to that of C3, allows assessment of

the likelihood of the subluxation being physiological (see Fig. 24.3.4). The spinolaminar junction of C2 should lie within 2 mm of this line. If the distance is greater than 2 mm a fracture or pathological subluxation is likely.

Cervical spine clearance guidelines

With the knowledge of mechanism of injury, immobilisation needed, clinical examination, and radiographic interpretation it is possible to devise guidelines (see Fig. 24.3.5) that allow safe and effective management of the potentially injured cervical spine while minimising the investigations needed. The guideline should include the following points:

• All patients with a significant mechanism of injury, altered conscious state, or

neurological symptoms, or who cannot be assessed should be immobilised.
• If on assessment the patient is alert, not drug affected, has no other major injuries, has no posterior cervical tenderness, has no posterior cervical pain on movement, and has no neurological signs the immobilisation can safely be removed and no further investigations are needed. If these criteria are not all satisfied or assessment is incomplete immobilisation should be maintained and a three-view plain X-ray series performed.[15]
• If the X-rays are normal the patient should be re-examined. If the patient has a normal examination the immobilisation can be removed. If there is still significant pain or tenderness a CT scan of the entire spine should be performed. If this is

normal and the patient alert and co-operative immobilisation should be kept in place and flexion and extension views performed 3–7 days later, once the muscle spasm has resolved. If the patient is significantly unwell, or has multiple trauma, MRI scanning should be considered. Consultation with a paediatric orthopaedic surgeon or neurosurgeon is recommended.

Atlantoaxial rotary subluxation

Fixed rotary subluxation at the atlanto-axial joint is more common during childhood than adulthood. It can present after minor trauma, in conjunction with an upper respiratory tract infection, and often no inciting cause is found. The clinical picture is that of the head turned to one side and held in the 'cock-robin' position. The child is unable to turn its head past the midline, and attempts to move the head often cause pain. The spasm of the sternocleidomastoid (SCM) muscle is on the side to which the head is turned (ipsilateral side), as the muscle is trying to right the head. In contrast in a wry neck the SCM spasm is on the side opposite to which the head is turned (contralateral side), with the spasm causing the head turning.[1,14]

Plain radiographs may be diagnostic revealing the lateral mass of C1 rotated anterior to the odontoid on the lateral view, or rotation of the spinous processes to the ipsilateral side on the AP view. If clinical examination and plain radiographs cannot confirm the diagnosis CT imaging should be considered.[1,14]

Rotary subluxation of short duration will often spontaneously reduce, those that do not or that have been present for a longer duration (days) may need traction or manipulation to reduce. Post-reduction immobilisation is needed to maintain reduction and the duration of immobilisation should vary according to the duration of subluxation.[1,14,24]

THORACIC AND LUMBAR SPINE INJURIES

Fractures of the thoracic spine account for 25–30% of spine injury in children while lumbar fractures account for 20–25%. Injuries to the thoracic spine and the thoracolumbar junction have a higher incidence of spinal cord injury, with neurologic deficit seen in up to 40% of cases.[1,6] The high incidence of cord injury is related to the relatively large size of the spinal cord in the thoracic region, the inherent stability of the thoracic spine requiring larger forces to cause bony injury. Multiple level injuries are seen in 30–40% of children with thoracic or lumbar spine fractures.[4,6] Fractures of the lower thoracic and upper lumbar spine have associated small bowel and visceral injury in up to 50% of cases.[1] Road traffic accidents and falls account for most of the injuries, but non-accidental injuries in these regions do occur.

Mechanism of injury

Injuries to the thoracic and lumbar spine are flexion/extension or vertical compression injuries, often a combination of these is present, and also a degree of distraction is not uncommon.

A number of bony injuries are caused by these mechanisms. Compression of the vertebral body with anterior wedging is the most common. However, a degree of anterior wedging is normal in children. Burst fractures where there is disruption of the endplates and herniation of the disc into the vertebral body. Retropulsed fragments can cause spinal cord injury. The 'seat-belt' fracture – associated with the lap-only seat belt – is a hyperflexion and distraction injury most commonly seen at the thoracolumbar junction, and is frequently associated with visceral or mesenteric injury. The posterior bony or ligamentous elements are disrupted and the fracture line extends horizontally into the vertebral body or through the intervertebral disc.[1,4,6,25]

Clinical assessment

As with all trauma patients, assessment of the spine should take place in the secondary survey after the airway, breathing and circulation have been assessed and stabilised. A history of mechanism of injury is important in identifying the risk of thoracic or lumbar spine injury. The presence of pain in the back makes injury more likely, but absence of pain does not exclude injury. Clinical examination should focus on tenderness and signs of bruising or deformity over the spine. This is assessed by log rolling the patient while spinal immobilisation is still in place. A search for signs of spinal cord or cauda equina lesions should also be made.

Any patient who has pain or tenderness over the spine should have the spine evaluated by radiography. Patients without pain or tenderness who have altered conscious state or other significant injuries are at risk of having thoracic or lumbar spine injuries missed (as they are for cervical spine injuries).[26] As multi-level injuries are common any child with a proven cervical spine fracture or spinal cord injury should have the entire spine imaged with plain radiographs (see Fig. 24.3.5).

Radiographic evaluation

After clinical evaluation, radiographs should be taken on any child who is at risk of having a thoracic or lumbar spine injury (Table 24.3.4). The standard views for both areas are the anterior-posterior radiograph and the lateral film. In the thoracic region the radiographs need to be overexposed compared to a normal chest X-ray to allow adequate views of the spine. The shoulders often obscure the upper thoracic spine and a swimmer's view may be needed to visualise the first two thoracic vertebrae.

The films should be evaluated by following the anterior and posterior vertebral body lines and the spinolaminar line on the lateral view. These three lines should have a parallel course. The height of each vertebral body should be assessed anteriorly and posteriorly, and a difference of more than about 3 mm treated as pathologic. On the AP view the para-

Table 24.3.4 Indications for thoracolumbar spine X-rays

- Pain in the thoracic or lumbar region
- Tenderness of the spine in the thoracic or lumbar region
- Significant bruising or deformity of the spine
- Altered conscious state
- Proven fracture in another region of the spine

spinal lines should be closely inspected to detect evidence of paraspinal haematoma. The posterior elements should be visible through the vertebral body and should be in alignment. Each vertebra should be inspected, an apparent empty or invisible vertebral body indicates a fracture dislocation with distraction.[1,25]

There are a number of features on the radiographs that indicate an unstable fracture: vertebral body collapse with widening of the pedicles; greater than 33% compromise of the spinal canal by retropulsed fragments of the lamina, pedicles or body; translocation of more than 2.5 mm between vertebral bodies in any direction; bilateral facet joint dislocation; or greater than 50% anterior compression of the vertebral body associated with widening of the interspinous space.[25]

While most thoracic and lumbar spine fractures are diagnosed on the initial plain radiographs, these films often do not provide enough information on the extent of the injury and a CT scan of the region is usually obtained to elucidate the full extent of the injury. MRI will be needed to visualise all ligamentous and spinal cord involvement.

Some fractures in the thoracic region can be difficult to see on plain films, especially if there were technical difficulties in obtaining the films in multiply injured patients. A number of secondary signs of thoracic spine injury exist and can help make the diagnosis. A paravertebral haematoma can usually be seen at the site of injury, blood in the pleural space may be seen as a pleural cap, and widening of the mediastinum may be present. Unfortunately these signs cannot differentiate a thoracic spine injury from an aortic arch injury.[6]

Management

Management must start with care of the airway, breathing and circulation. Only once these areas have been stabilised should management of the spine proceed. However, while the patient is being stabilised the spine should be maintained in alignment and the patient moved by log rolling. A thorough assessment and investigation of the abdomen and chest is mandatory for all patients with sig-

nificant thoracic and upper lumbar spine injuries, and injuries to the pelvis must not be forgotten with lumbar spine injuries. As many of these injuries are associated with intra-abdominal injuries an ileus is common and nasogastric or orogastric tube should be inserted. Consultation with a paediatric orthopaedic surgeon or neurosurgeon should be sought for the definitive care of the injury. Surgical stabilisation is usually required for unstable fractures and those fractures associated with neurological injury.[4,6,25]

SPINAL CORD INJURY

The goal of management of injury to the spinal cord or cauda equina is to minimise the resulting neurologic deficit. This commences with adequate immobilisation of the spine and complete and thorough investigation to detail the anatomy of the injury.[27]

Spinal cord injury should be suspected in any child who has multi-system trauma, minor trauma associated with spinal pain, sensory or motor symptoms, and any patient with altered consciousness. The patient must be adequately immobilised, such as on a spinal board with a cervical collar and head immobiliser (see section on spinal immobilization, p. 640), and any assessment of the back or patient movement accomplished by log rolling. Up to 50% of patients with spinal cord injury will have at least moderate head injury.[27]

Spinal cord injury syndromes

A number of patterns of neurologic deficit are seen in patients with spinal cord injury, with the deficit dependant on the portion of the spinal cord damaged. Neurogenic shock – the manifestations of loss of sympathetic output to the cardiovascular system – is seen immediately after complete cord injury at the level of T6 or above. This should not be confused with spinal shock, which is the reversible dysfunction of the spinal cord associated with injury. It is likened to a concussion of the cord without permanent damage. It may exist alone or in combination with permanent cord injury. Its resolution is responsible for the im-

provement in neurologic function seen in the first few days post-injury.[27]

The distinction between a complete injury and a partial injury – with preservation of some motor or sensory function below the lesion – is vital for prognosis. Many patients with partial injury will regain much or all of the neurologic function. A partial cord injury may occur at any region and with any mechanism of injury.

Complete cord injury is usually seen in injuries of the thoracic spine and thoracolumbar junction. The spinal cord is large in relation to the size of the spinal canal at this level. Complete cord injuries that remain at 24 hours rarely regain any significant function. Cauda equine lesions – injuries at or below L2 – involve the peripheral nerves rather than the spinal cord and can show significant recovery of lower limb and sphincter function even weeks after the injury.[27]

Central cord syndrome is usually seen in hyperextension injury resulting in herniation of the intervertebral disc into the spinal cord. The resulting injury causes a motor deficit that is greater in the arms than legs and most extensive in the small muscles of the hand. The sensory deficit is variable. Brown-Sequard syndrome – hemisection of the cord – causes a contralateral loss of pain and temperature sensation and an ipsilateral motor paralysis and loss of proprioception below the level of injury. Approximately two-thirds of those with central cord syndrome and one-third with Brown–Sequard syndrome will recover.[27]

Clinical assessment

Initial steps in the management of a patient with a suspected spinal cord lesion are the assessment and resuscitation of the airway, breathing and circulation. The most immediate threats to life and spinal cord function of patients with spinal cord injury remain hypoxia and hypotension. Spinal cord lesions in the upper cervical spine may impair respiratory function and require early intubation and mechanical ventilation. The unstable cervical spine must be maintained in alignment without traction during treatment of the airway. The loss of sympathetic vasomotor tone after cervical spinal cord injury will result in vasodilatation, venodilatation, and reduced venous return to the heart causing hypotension. There should be an associated relative bradycardia for age and existing blood pressure, which will help distinguish this response from haemorrhagic shock.[27]

Initial fluid resuscitation with 10–20 mL kg^{-1} should adequately replace the relative hypovolaemia. However, if hypotension persists measurement of central venous pressure (CVP) may be needed to guide fluid replacement. Excessive fluid replacement that pushes central venous and pulmonary artery pressures above the normal range will result in pulmonary oedema. Treatment with a vasoconstrictor, such as metaraminol, may be useful for the patient who has adequate CVP and remains hypotensive. In patients who are also significantly bradycardic inotropic agents, such as dopamine or adrenaline (epinephrine), may be useful. Patients requiring more than 40 mL kg^{-1} of fluid replacement and having a low CVP must be assumed to have other injuries causing blood loss.

Examination of the neurologic impairment is done as part of the secondary survey. A thorough examination of the motor function of the limbs and assessment of reflexes should be performed and a level of sensory deficit sought. Knowledge of the dermatomes and myotomes will allow determination of the level of neurological injury.

Radiographic evaluation

In all patients with suspected spinal cord injury the spine should be X-rayed. The radiographs should include the entire spine as multiple levels of injury are common. Once the patient is stabilised further investigation of the lesion should follow. The bony injuries should be investigated as discussed above. Investigation of the cord itself will require MRI. MRI should be performed as soon as possible after identification of a spinal cord injury, as it will allow identification of remedial intraspinal problems in patients with a partial neurologic deficit. The appearance of the spinal cord on MRI also allows prediction of neurological outcome. Cord transection and major hae-

morrhage have a poor outcome, minor haemorrhage and oedema have a moderate to good outcome, and a normal MRI is associated with complete recovery.[1]

Treatment

Most of the treatment available for spinal cord injuries is supportive. The breathing and circulation must be supported as needed. As there will be a neurogenic bladder, catheterisation is necessary, and a nasogastric tube is needed to treat the gastric and bowel stasis that ensues. For transport anti-emetic is useful to prevent vomiting and spine movement or airway compromise. Subcutaneous low-molecular-weight heparin should be instigated once the patient is stable to prevent deep venous thrombosis.[28]

Specific treatment of the spinal cord lesion is controversial. Four substances have been studied in prospective, randomised trials – methylprednisolone, tirilazad, naloxone and GM-1 ganglioside. All studies to date have excluded children under thirteen years of age. Tirilazad and naloxone have failed to show any benefit in trials to date. There is conflicting evidence regarding the benefits of methylprednisolone and documented evidence that its use increases the risk of bacterial infection. It is recommended that it be used with knowledge of the risks and possible benefits.[28] The current regimens for use are seen in Table 24.3.5. GM-1 ganglioside has yet to be shown to offer significant benefit in spinal cord injury, and is not recommended for routine use.

Once the patient has been stabilised and investigated, transfer to a spinal-cord-injury unit should be expedited. These units and associated intensive-care units are geared to manage the cardio-respiratory compromise that may occur

in the ensuing weeks, the psychosexual issues that accompany spinal cord injury, the urological problems, and the potential for skin breakdown that are exaggerated in these patients.

SCIWORA

Spinal cord injury without radiographic abnormality (SCIWORA) is defined as objective signs of myelopathy as a result of trauma with no evidence of fracture or ligamentous instability on plain X-rays or tomography.[29] SCIWORA is most frequently seen in younger children (especially < 8 years of age), and in injuries of the cervical spine. Postulated causes include ligamentous laxity and bony immaturity allowing excessive, transient movement during trauma causing distraction or compression of the spinal cord, or cord ischaemia due to vascular injury or hypoperfusion. The incidence reported in children is 1–10% of all spinal cord injuries.[1,30,31]

Younger children tend to have more profound neurological injury, and hence less long-term improvement.[31] A number of children will present with minor neurological injury and progress to complete or partial spinal cord injury. The incidence of this delayed presentation of the serious symptoms is 5–50%. The delay to presentation of full symptoms has been as long as four days.[1,31] Because of these presentations, all children with history of neurologic symptoms of any neurologic deficit should be treated as patients with potential spinal cord injuries.

After the primary, resuscitation and secondary survey and radiographic evaluation any patient with any neurologic

Table 24.3.5	Methylprednisolone administration in spinal cord injury		
	Time after injury		
	0–3 hours	*3–8 hours*	*> 8 hours*
Initial IV dose	30 mg kg^{-1} (over 15 minutes)	30 mg kg^{-1} (over 15 minutes)	Not recommended
Maintenance IV dose	5.4 mg kg^{-1} h^{-1}	5.4 mg kg^{-1} h^{-1}	
Duration	24 hours	48 hours	

CONTROVERSIES

❶ The clinical assessment of the preverbal child.

❷ How to adequately immobilise the cervical spine of a child less than two years of age.

❸ The use of flexion and extension films in the acute situation.

❹ The role of routine CT of the cervical spine in major trauma.

❺ Timing of removal of spinal immobilisation in the unconscious child.

❻ The role of methyl prednisolone in spinal cord injury.

deficit should remain immobilised until all bony, ligamentous and spinal cord injury is excluded or treated. Further investigation with a CT scan focused at the level of symptoms and possibly MRI to view the cord should be performed. Delayed flexion and extension radiographs can be used to determine ligamentous stability of the cervical spine. MRI provides the same prognostic information in SCIWORA injuries as in other spinal cord injuries.

REFERENCES

1. Roche C, Carty H 2001 Spinal trauma in children. Pediatric Radiology 31(10): 677–700
2. Viccellio P et al 2001 A prospective multicentre study of cervical spine injury in children. Paediatrics 108(2): e20
3. Dormans JP 2002 Evaluation of children with suspected cervical spine injury. Instructional Course Lectures 51: 401–410
4. Reynolds R 2000 Pediatric spinal injury. Current Opinion in Paediatrics 12(1): 67–71
5. Jaffe DM et al 1987 Developing a clinical algorithm for early management of cervical spine injury in child trauma victims. Annals of Emergency Medicine 16(3): 270–276
6. Brandser EA, el-Khoury GY 1997 Thoracic and lumbar spine trauma. Radiologic Clinics of North America 35(3): 533–557
7. Jaffe DM 2002 Evaluation of children for cervical spine injuries. In: Strange GR (ed) Paediatric emergency medicine: A comprehensive study guide. McGraw-Hill, Columbus, Ohio, USA
8. Woodward G 2000 Neck trauma. In: Fleisher G, Ludwig S (eds) Textbook of paediatric emergency medicine. Lippincott Williams & Wilkins, Philadelphia
9. Schafermeyer RW et al 1991 Respiratory effects of spinal immobilisation in children. Annals of Emergency Medicine 20: 1017-1019
10. Herzenberg JE et al 1989 Emergency transport and positioning of young children who have an injury of the cervical spine. The standard backboard may be hazardous. Journal of Bone & Joint Surgery – American 71(1): 15–22
11. Treloar DJ, Nypaver M 1997 Angulation of the pediatric cervical spine with and without cervical collar. Pediatric Emergency Care 13(1): 5–8
12. Curran C et al 1995 Pediatric cervical-spine immobilization: Achieving neutral position? Journal of Trauma 39(4): 729–732
13. Quigley S, Curley M 1996 Skin integrity in the pediatric population: Preventing and managing pressure ulcers. Journal of the Society of Paediatric Nurses 1(1): 7–18
14. Anonymous 2002 Management of pediatric cervical spine and spinal cord injuries. Neurosurgery 50(3 Suppl): S85–S99
15. Hoffman JR et al 2000 Validity of a set of clinical criteria to rule out injury to the cervical spine in patients with blunt trauma. New England Journal of Medicine 343: 94–99
16. Buhs C et al 2000 The paediatric trauma C-spine: Is the odontoid view necessary? Journal of Paediatric Surgery 35: 994–997
17. Swischuk LE, John SD, Hendrick EP 2000 Is the open-mouth odontoid view necessary in children under 5 years? Paediatric Radiology 30: 186-189
18. Insko E et al 2002 Utility of flexion and extension radiographs of the cervical spine in the acute evaluation of blunt trauma. Journal of Trauma 53: 426–429
19. Berne JD et al 1999 Value of complete cervical helical computed tomographic scanning in identifying cervical spine injury in the unevaluable blunt trauma patient with multiple injuries: A prospective study. Journal of Trauma-Injury Infection & Critical Care 47(5): 896–902 [discussion 902–903]
20. Browne GJ, Cocks AJ, McCaskill ME 2001 Current trends in the management of major paediatric trauma. Emergency Medicine (Fremantle WA) 13(4): 418–425
21. Holmes J et al 2002 Variability in computed tomography and magnetic resonance imaging in patients with cervical spine injuries. Journal of Trauma 53: 524–530
22. Swischuk L 1984 The cervical spine in childhood. Current Problems in Diagnostic Radiology 13: 1–26
23. Kriss VM, Kriss TC 1996 Imaging of the cervical spine in infants. Paediatric Emergency Care 13(1): 44–49
24. Subach BR et al 1998 Current management of pediatric atlantoaxial rotatory subluxation. Spine 23(20): 2174–2179
25. Clark P, Letts M 2001 Trauma to the thoracic and lumbar spine in the adolescent. Canadian Journal of Surgery 44(5): 337–345
26. Meek S 1998 Lesson of the week: Fractures of the thoracolumbar spine in major trauma patients. British Medical Journal 317(7170): 1442–1443 [comment]
27. Chiles BW, Cooper PR 1996 Acute spinal injury. New England Journal of Medicine 334(8): 514–520
28. Anonymous 2002 Pharmacological therapy after acute cervical spinal cord injury. Neurosurgery 50(3 Suppl): S63–S72
29. Pang D, Wilberger J 1982 Spinal cord injury without radiographic abnormalities in children. Journal of Neurosurgery 57: 114–129
30. Anonymous 2002 Spinal cord injury without radiographic abnormality. Neurosurgery 50(3 Suppl): S100–S104
31. Pang D, Pollack I 1989 Spinal cord injury without radiographic abnormality in children - the SCIWORA syndrome. Journal of Trauma 29(5): 654–664

24.4 RISK MANAGEMENT IN ACUTE PAEDIATRIC ORTHOPAEDICS

ROBYN BRADY

Essentials

1 Inadequate identification and management of unstable or displaced injuries such as lateral condylar elbow fractures, Monteggia fracture dislocations, and slipped upper femoral epiphysis (SUFE), can cause serious long-term deformity and malfunction.

2 Immobilisation complications, from skin ulceration to compartment syndromes, demand scrupulous departmental risk management protocols, as they often relate to 'weakest link' situations.

3 The importance of adequate initial clinical evaluation and follow-up of patient or clinician concerns cannot be over-stressed.

4 A variety of departmental risk-management strategies provide a safety net for doctor and patient.

INTRODUCTION

Emergency is a high-litigation area of medical practice and orthopaedic adverse outcomes (especially missed fractures) make up a high proportion of successful claims. Many factors intrinsic to emergency medicine contribute to this danger, including high staff turnover, 24-hour practice with multiple hand-overs, wide-ranging procedural demands, and work-load flux.

Just as many of the problems are systemic, so too are many of the solutions. Adverse outcomes can occur when the clinical problems discussed in this section are not recognised or dealt with ad-equately, and there are clear ED systemic interventions that can minimise their occurrence.

ADVERSE EVENTS IN PAEDIATRIC ACUTE ORTHOPAEDICS

Non-identification or delayed identification

'Missed fractures' is the adverse event most commonly associated with ED litigation, accounting for approximately half of ED negligence claims in Great Britain and Australia.[1] Articles auditing the correlation of ED doctor X-ray analysis with radiologist reporting in recent years show that 1–2% of these reports have a discrepant concordance significant enough to alter management[2–6] although in many series there were no long-term adverse events detailed. Fractures can be missed because of primary assessment failure (failure of thorough history or examination, therefore failure to X-ray), which will not be demonstrated by the above. X-rays may be inadequate in coverage or resolution, the abnormality may be missed by the ED physician(s), or by radiologists, this too tends not to show in reported series, which presume radiology reports to be the gold standard, and there may be breakdown between radiologist reporting and ED physician notification and recall of patient. All such oversights have been specifically associated with adverse outcomes[7] and the physician responsibility for follow-up and communication, which extends to ensuring that a booked follow-up does actually occur, must not be overlooked.

Common or serious acute paediatric orthopaedic adverse events are shown in Table 24.4.1.

Regarding missed displaced fractures and dislocations, the following points must be made:

❶ These anatomical distortions should all be clinically apparent to patient and physician. In fact in a series of 80 injuries with delayed identification,[5] there were comments about pain, swelling or loss of function documented in more than 60% of cases, which had not been acted upon. In 20% of cases the doctor was alerted to the possible problem by the patient or his/her relatives.

❷ Fractures about the joint are at disproportionately high risk both for being missed and for adverse events. Although most series of fractures missed in the ED include a large array of different sites (45 fractures at 15 sites and 69 fractures at 27 sites[5] in two series not exclusive paediatric), knee injuries (tibial spine and plateau) were disproportionately represented in the former (nine fractures compared with only one missed scaphoid fracture), and elbow injuries are disproportionately represented in paediatric adverse events. However, in all the significant paediatric elbow injuries listed as potentially missed (unstable supra-condylar fracture, lateral condyle fracture, Monteggia fracture-dislocation and a trapped medial epicondyle, e.g. after elbow dislocation), elbow examination is grossly abnormal including an effusion and a limitation of range of motion. Although the radiological Monteggia fracture-dislocation continues to be regularly missed by the untrained X-ray viewer, the clinical elbow abnormality should not have been. Some X-ray misinterpretations occur (and the few radiologist errors probably all occur) because the clinician reviewing the X-ray was not the one who assessed the patient, a trap for the supervisory system which has evolved in most

Table 24.4.1 Adverse events in acute paediatric orthopaedics

Missed displaced fracture/dislocations
- Elbow
  Supra-condylar fractures
  Lateral condyle fractures
  Monteggia fracture dislocations
  Medial epicondylar joint entrapment
- Knee
  Tibial spine
- Phalangeal fractures with angulation
- Hip
  Slipped upper femoral epiphysis (SUFE)
- Open injuries
- Fracture complications, e.g. compartment syndrome, neurovascular compromise
- High-risk patients
  Multi-trauma, multiple disability

Missed undisplaced fractures
- Buckle fractures
  Proximal humerus
  Radial neck
  Distal radius and ulna
  Distal femur
- Toddler's fracture (tibial stress fracture)

Delayed identification of
- Septic arthritis
- Osteomyelitis
- Leukaemia/other neoplastic infiltration
- Congenital serious orthopaedic disorder, e.g. CDH, spinal problems

Procedural problems
- POP-related injuries
- Loss of position post-manipulation
- Mal-union
- Anaesthetic adverse events

Table 24.4.2 Risk management strategies: acute paediatric orthopaedics

1. Training
   - Independent learning multi-media programs, e.g. for plastering, fracture identification
   - Ticketing by plaster technician or senior staff prior to procedure or POP
   - On-line clinical management guides, e.g. PaEDpac
   - Tutorials by orthopaedic and radiology personnel
   - Teaching of clinical caveats, e.g. re joints (see text)
2. Departmental information systems
   - Textbooks, PaEDpac etc
   - Availability of resource books, e.g. Keats, McRae, Gill, Swischuck, PF
   - POP wall charts
   - Paediatric fracture identification photo-chart
   - Information-technology adjuncts built into ED information software
   - Automated prompts for particular presentations, e.g.
   Injury under two
   Multi-trauma
   X-ray requests (require documentation of associated films)
   Need for registrar review with infant or LMO letter or triage category < 4
   - Links to discharge information and advice, e.g.
   Wound care
   POP management
   Post-sedation advice
   - Automated communications
   Fax advice to registered LMO
3. Departmental audit
   - Results audit (X-ray) and follow-up system
   - ED-orthopaedic weekly case-review including ED manipulations
   - Audit of in-department anaesthetics
   - Audit of triage category 1 and ICU admissions to identify retrospective problems with ED management and delayed diagnoses
4. Supervision policy
   - Automated review request as above
   - Extended-hour consultant presence
5. Procedural policies
   - What can be done: when, where and by whom?
   - Two doctor rule for procedures with IV sedation
   - Specifically designed documentation forms, including nursing observations

Australian urban EDs. Therefore all doctors need to be reminded that lack of clinical joint integrity (effusion, asymmetry cf. the other side, reduced range of movement) is an indication for early orthopaedic review even if the X-ray appears normal.

❸ Two special categories of high-risk patients deserve mention. The first is multi-trauma patients,[7,8] due to several factors including urgency of other clinical problems, the possibility of an altered or distracted conscious state, and hand-over problems. The second group of note is children with complex medical conditions including autistic spectrum disorders, due to difficulties in patient communication, occasional pre-existing anatomical abnormalities, varying pain thresholds, and a need to establish base-line 'normal'. Both of these categories of patient require senior medical involvement, careful and often repeated systematic assessment and documentation.

Problems relating to ED interventions fall into a separate category, and increase proportionally with the number and types of procedural activity undertaken in a department, which varies widely in Australia, particularly for the paediatric population. Strategies to minimise these problems are now so well described in the risk-management literature that any department planning to change procedural practice would do well to set out within these guidelines (Table 24.4.2).

Plaster of Paris (POP) immobilisation and its attendant problems continue to be the bane of ED directors: too soft; too tight; too cylindrical; inadequately immobilising; excessively immobilising; etc. At the serious end of the spectrum is the possibility of compartment syndrome, more frequent findings of adverse outcomes are skin loss, due to internally protruding plaster shelves, or incompetent plaster saw use. Departments performing manipulations must be equipped and staffed to monitor their patients for anaesthetic adverse events, and must balance the need to avoid a tight POP with the need to maintain reduction through appropriately positioned moulding. The restriction of paediatric ED orthopaedic manipulations to experienced medical personnel, and next day follow-up, will minimise problems.

REFERENCES

1. Gwynne A, Barber P et al 1997 A review of 105 negligence claims against accident and emergency departments. Journal of Accident and Emergency Medicine 14: 243–245

ORTHOPAEDICS AND RHEUMATOLOGY

2. Klein EJ, Koenig M et al 1999 Discordant radiograph interpretation between emergency physicians and radiologists in a paediatric emergency department. Paediatric Emergency Care 4: 245–8

3. Walsh-Kelly CM, Hennes HM et al 1997 False-positive preliminary radiograph interpretations in a pediatric emergency department: Clinical and economic impact. American Journal of Emergency Medicine 4: 354–356

4. Simon HK, Khan NS et al 1996 Paediatric emergency physician interpretation of plain radiographs: Is routine review by a radiologist necessary and cost-effective? Annals of Emergency Medicine 27(3): 295–298

5. Kremli MK 1996 Missed musculoskeletal injuries in a university hospital in Riyadh: Types of missed injuries and responsible factors. Injury 27(7): 503–506

6. Cameron MG 1994 Missed fractures in the emergency department. Emergency Medicine 6(1): 37–39

7. Alpers A 2002 Key legal principles for hospitalists. Disease Monitor 48(4): 197–206

8. Connors JM, Ruddy RM et al 2001 Delayed diagnosis in paediatric blunt trauma. Paediatric Emergency Care 17(1): 1–4

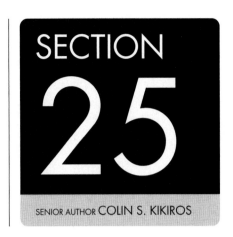

SECTION
25

SENIOR AUTHOR COLIN S. KIKIROS

MALE GENITALIA

25.1 THE ACUTE SCROTUM

COLIN S. KIKIROS

ESSENTIALS

1 A paediatric surgeon or urologist should be contacted to assess an acute scrotum so as not to miss a testicular torsion.

2 The testicles must always be examined when boys present with abdominal pain.

3 Testicular torsion is a condition requiring urgent surgery.

4 Colour Doppler ultrasound examination and nuclear scans of the testicle may be helpful, but should not be relied upon, in the diagnosis of testicular torsion. When in doubt, exploration of the testicle is by far the safest treatment.

INTRODUCTION

The acute scrotum is defined as a painful and/or enlarged scrotum and may be acute or subacute in onset. The origin of the pathology may be from the testis, the groin or the scrotal skin. In a younger child the pain will cause the child to be unsettled with crying, and it may be intractable. In an older child the reluctance to ambulate may be a predominate feature. In addition, referred pain from a sore testis may present as abdominal pain. Therefore, in patients presenting with abdominal (especially lower-abdominal) pain one must examine the inguinal scrotal region so as not to overlook torsion of a testicle.

The diffuse vasculitis of Henoch–Schönlein purpura may affect the testis and/or scrotum. Usually other manifestations of the condition such as a skin rash or haematuria are present. A radionuclide scan may assist in differentiating this condition from torsion of the testicle.

TORSION OF A TESTICULAR OR EPIDIDYMAL APPENDAGE

Appendages of the testis and epididymis occur in 90% of testicles. Torsion of these appendages is the most common cause of testicular pain. The most common age of presentation is at the onset of puberty and this is thought to be due to the release of oestrogens and androgens from the male adrenal gland stimulating the appendages and causing them to enlarge. As the appendages are on a narrow stalk they have a tendency to twist.[1] Oedema of the appendages may also occur following trauma to the testis. Onset of the pain is usually gradual and the child is often able to ambulate without difficulty. Redness and swelling of the scrotum are also mild in the first 24 hours but may increase to an alarming degree in the following days and appearances can then be similar to those of testicular torsion. The scrotal swelling is often due to a small secondary hydrocele. The testis is usually normally aligned and in normal position in the scrotum. Tenderness is maximal at the upper pole of the testis (where the appendage is located) and a blue dot may be seen through the skin at the upper pole consistent with an infarcted appendage.

TORSION OF THE TESTIS

This is an acute emergency and is due, in most situations, to medial rotation of the spermatic cord. However, in one third of cases the testis rotates in a lateral direction.[2] The torsion usually occurs spontaneously. However, sometimes it can follow direct trauma to the testis. The pain is likely to be acute and severe and may be associated with nausea or vomiting. The older child is often reluctant to ambulate. Often there is a history of previous short-lived pain in a testis

consistent with intermittent episodes of spontaneously resolving torsion. The testis is usually enlarged and in a high position in the scrotum or even in the groin. It is not usually in its normal lie and there is much redness and swelling of the scrotal skin. Usually a secondary hydrocele is present. The contralateral testicle may lie in a bell-clapper fashion owing to the insertion of the epididymis in the central part of the testicle and this in turn predisposes the testicle to undergo torsion. The child should be taken to the operating theatre urgently, even if the child is not adequately fasted, as prolonged obstruction of the testicular vessels may lead to partial or complete atrophy of the testicle. Therefore nuclear scans and colour Doppler ultrasound should be avoided if the diagnosis is clear, as these investigations may result in unnecessary delay and they are not reliable. False negatives and false positives have been reported with both modalities.[3] Colour Doppler ultrasonography may be misleading as intra-testicular flow may be seen even in testicles that have undergone torsion. Visualisation of a twist in the cord is more reliable.[4] Survival of the testicle will depend on the number of twists that the spermatic cord has undergone along with the length of time that the cord has been twisted with the prognosis being excellent for those undergoing surgery within six hours of the onset of symptoms.[5,6]

EPIDIDYMO-ORCHITIS

Infection or inflammation may affect the epididymis or the testis. Infections in the epididymis may arise from retrograde flow along the vas deferens or lymphatics from urinary tract infections, or from the blood stream. Inflammation of the testis may arise from conditions such as mumps. The epididymis is tender and swollen and the testis also may be tender. The testis is of normal lie and in a normal position in the scrotum. A raised interleukin-6 level may be clinically helpful in assisting the diagnosis of epididymitis.[7] Once the diagnosis has been confirmed the child's urine should be sent for analysis and he should then be commenced on antibiotics. Enteric organisms are the usual cause of the urinary tract infection.[8] Once the condition has resolved renal ultrasound and micturating cysto-urethrogram should be performed as the urine infection may have resulted from an abnormality in the urinary tract, such as posterior urethral valves.[9]

IDIOPATHIC SCROTAL OEDEMA

The cause of this condition is unknown. The child presents with scrotal discomfort, oedema and erythema of one side of the scrotum, which may spread to affect the entire scrotum, the penis and inguinal and perineal regions. The testis is not swollen and is normally aligned and the tenderness arises from the palpably thickened scrotal wall. Occasionally eosinophilia may occur and characteristically ultrasound examination shows marked thickening of the scrotal wall, increased peri-testicular blood flow and a mild reactive hydrocele.[10] The condition resolves in 1–4 days and no treatment, apart from pain relief, is required.

TESTICULAR TUMOURS

Primary or secondary (leukaemia for example) tumours may cause the testicle to enlarge and become painful. The onset is usually gradual and the pain more chronic. However, tumours may present acutely when they have been subjected to trauma. The testicle may become extremely large, although the scrotal skin is not usually erythematous. Ultrasound and full blood picture may aid in the diagnosis. Paediatric surgeons and oncologists are predominantly required in managing these patients.[11]

IRREDUCIBLE INGUINAL HERNIA

Segments of intestine may on occasions descend into a hernia sac in the scrotum and become irreducible. Acute pain may be felt in the scrotum and also in the groin (see Chapter 7.12 on herniae).

RUPTURE OF THE TESTIS

This is usually the result of trauma. The testis becomes enlarged and painful and there is associated bruising and frequently an associated hydrocele. Ultrasound examination often reveals irregularity of the testicular outline and intra-testicular haematoma.[12] The patient should be referred to a surgeon for exploration and repair of the testicle.

ACUTE HYDROCELE

A patent processus vaginalis may allow intraperitoneal fluid to flow into the space around the testicle in the scrotum. Often the amount of fluid is minimal and the patient does not present acutely. Occasionally, however, intercurrent illnesses, such as gastroenteritis and upper respiratory tract infections, may result in an increase in volume of the peritoneal fluid. This leads to an increase in the amount of fluid around the testis and the patient may present to the ED with a large scrotal swelling. The testis in this situation is not painful and one can determine that the swelling does not extend into the groin. Ultrasound examination is useful in confirming the diagnosis and unnecessary surgery can be avoided.

REFERENCES

1. Samnakay N, Cohen RJ, Orford J, King PA, Davies RJ 2003 Androgen and oestrogen receptor status of the human appendix testis. Pediatric Surgery International 19: 520–524
2. Sessions AE, Rabinowitz R, Hulbert WC, Goldstein MM, Mevorach TA 2003 Testicular torsion: Direction, degree, duration and disinformation. Journal of Urology 169: 663–665
3. Nussbaum Blask AR, Bulas D, Shalaby-Rana E, Rushton G, Shao C, Majd M 2002 Color Doppler sonography and scintigraphy of the testis: A prospective, comparative analysis in children with acute scrotal pain. Pediatric Emergency Care 18: 67–71
4. Arce JD, Cortes M, Vargas JC 2002 Sonographic diagnosis of acute spermatic cord torsion. Rotation of the cord: A key to the diagnosis. Pediatric Radiology 32: 485–491
5. Dunne PJ, O'Loughlin BS 2000 Testicular torsion: Time is the enemy. Australian & New Zealand Journal of Surgery 70: 441–442 [comment]
6. Rampaul MS, Hosking SW 1998 Testicular torsion: Most delay occurs outside the hospital. Annals of the Royal College of Surgeons of England 80: 169–172
7. Rivers KK, Rivers EP, Stricker HJ, Lewis J, Urrunaga J, Karriem V 2000 The clinical utility of serologic markers in the evaluation of the acute scrotum. Academic Emergency Medicine 7: 1069–1072
8. McAndrew HF, Pemberton R, Kikiros CS, Gollow I 2002 The incidence and investigation of acute scrotal problems in children. Pediatric Surgery International 18: 435–437
9. Ng JW, Chan AY, Kong CK, Wong MK 1996 Posterior urethral valves presenting as acute epididymo-orchitis: A case report and follow-up study. Australian & New Zealand Journal of Surgery 66: 129–130
10. Klin B, Lotan G, Efrati Y, Zlotkevich L, Strauss S 2002 Acute idiopathic scrotal edema in children – revisited. Journal of Pediatric Surgery 37: 1200–1202
11. Nichols CR 1998 Testicular cancer. Current problems in Cancer 22: 187–274
12. Micallef M, Ahmad I, Ramesh N, Hurley M, McInerney D 2001 Ultrasound features of blunt testicular injury. Injury 32: 23–26

25.2 ACUTE PROBLEMS OF THE PENIS AND FORESKIN

COLIN S. KIKIROS

ESSENTIALS

1 Urinary retention may arise from phimosis or balanitis and requires urgent urinary diversion or circumcision.

2 Priapism is an acute emergency and requires urgent treatment.

INTRODUCTION

Currently, approximately 90% of young males in Australia are not circumcised. This compares to a generation ago, when the majority of males were circumcised, often in the neonatal period. As a result problems with the foreskin are increasing and patients are often referred to the ED for treatment.

Parents are often unsure of the correct management of the foreskin. In most cases the foreskin should be left alone until the age of five or six and then should be retracted gently to clean the under surface of the foreskin and the glans. If the foreskin cannot be retracted easily, the use of a mild steroid ointment for a short period may correct the phimosis. If this is not successful, circumcision may be required.

PHIMOSIS OF THE FORESKIN

In this condition the foreskin cannot be easily retracted and in the more severe cases the outflow of urine is significantly obstructed. Ballooning of the foreskin may occur with micturition when the urine flow into the foreskin space is greater than the flow exiting out of the foreskin. Urinary tract infections,[1] dysuria and possibly urinary retention may develop.[2]

A sample of urine and swabs from the foreskin should be obtained and the patient should be commenced on intravenous or oral antibiotics. In cases of urinary retention, urinary diversion may be required. For example, a suprapubic catheter may need to be inserted under general anaesthesia. Alternatively, urgent circumcision can treat the condition.[2]

In mild cases of phimosis, the application of half-strength Betnovate® ointment to the tip of the foreskin for six weeks has a reported success of 75–88%.[2,3]

BALANITIS

This condition usually arises when phimosis of the foreskin is present and infection has occurred in the space under the foreskin. Bacteria, often enteral or cutaneous in origin, migrate into this space and as they cannot be washed away, infection results. This is frequently a subacute or chronic condition, but on occasions can be acute.

Again a sample of urine and swabs of the foreskin should be obtained and the patient should be commenced on IV or oral antibiotics. The condition usually subsides within a few days. However, in the long term, circumcision may be required.[4]

Balanitis xerotica obliterans, also called lichen sclerosus et atrophicus, is thought to be an autoimmune condition affecting the foreskin and glans. It leads to irreversible phimosis of the foreskin and presents with inability to retract the foreskin and varying degrees of urinary obstruction. It is best treated with circumcision as studies using topical steroid treatment have failed to show any permanent improvement.[5,6]

PARAPHIMOSIS

On occasions the foreskin may be tight but the child, or parent, may have attempted to retract it and not returned it to its normal position. Oedema of the foreskin distal to the tight ring can develop and the foreskin can become painfully swollen and difficult to reduce.

The foreskin is more easily reduced the sooner that the patient is treated.[7] The patient should be given appropriate analgesia and gentle digital pressure should be used on the foreskin through saline-soaked gauze. Once some of the oedema has been dispersed the foreskin should be gently replaced in its normal position. If this is not possible the child will need to be seen by a paediatric surgeon, who may attempt the same procedure. If this again fails the foreskin should be reduced under a general anaesthetic. Some surgeons favour circumcision whilst the child is anaesthetised so as to avoid another anaesthetic in the future.

Alternative methods described to reduce the paraphimosis are the use of hyaluronidase[8] and puncture technique[9] whereby the oedematous foreskin is punctured in several places with an 18-gauge hypodermic needle to evacuate the oedema so as to allow for easy reduction of the foreskin.

PRIAPISM

This is an acute emergency. Low-flow priapism is due to obstruction of venous outflow from the penis. It may occur spontaneously or it can be secondary to medication, sickle cell disease or leukaemia. Uncontrolled arterial inflow, usually caused by direct trauma to the penis or perineum, results in high-flow priapism. Both types of priapism result in a painful, sustained erection. Urgent referral to a paediatric surgeon or urologist is required for immediate treatment or surgery. In the meantime, perineal compression should be attempted as it may successfully reverse high-flow priapism.[10]

If this fails, colour Doppler ultrasonography of the corpora cavernosa can reveal a blood leak. Bilateral internal pudendal arteriography and embolisation can then follow.[11,12] Intracavernous injections of etilefrine can be effective in reducing priapism in children with acute sickle-cell crisis.[13] Failure to resolve the condition in a timely manner may result in permanent inability to have erections and/or penile fibrosis.[14]

REFERENCES

1. Hiraoka M, Tsukahara H, Ohshima Y, Mayumi M 2002 Meatus tightly covered by the prepuce is associated with urinary tract infection. Pediatrics International 44: 658–662
2. Ashfield JE, Nickel KR, Siemens DR, MacNeily AE, Nickel JC 2003 Treatment of phimosis with topical steroids in 194 children. Journal of Urology 169: 1106–1108
3. Kikiros CS, Beasley SW, Woodward AA 1993 The response of phimosis to local steroid application. Pediatric Surgery International 8: 329–333
4. Escala JM, Rickwood AM 1989 Balanitis. British Journal of Urology 63: 196–197
5. Webster TM, Leonard MP 2002 Topical steroid therapy for phimosis. Canadian Journal of Urology 9: 1492–1495
6. Meuli M, Briner J, Hanimann B, Sacher P 1994 Lichen sclerosus et atrophicus causing phimosis in boys: A prospective study with 5 year followup after complete circumcision. Journal of Urology 152: 987–989
7. Choe JM 2000 Paraphimosis: Current treatment options. American Family Physician 62: 2623–2628
8. Devries CR, Miller AK, Packer MG 1997 Reduction of paraphimosis with hyaluronidase. Urology 48: 464–465
9. Fuenfer MM, Najmaldin A 1994 Emergency reduction of paraphimosis. European Journal of Pediatric Surgery 4: 370–371
10. Hatzichristou D, Salpiggidis G, Hatzimouratidis K, Apostolidis A, Tzortzis V, Bekos A, Saripoulos D 2002 Management strategy for arterial priapism: Therapeutic dilemmas. Journal of Urology 168: 2074–2077
11. Volkmer BG, Nesslauer T, Kraemer SC, Goerich J, Basche S, Gottfried HW 2001 Prepubertal high flow priapism: Incidence, diagnosis and treatment. Journal of Urology 166: 1018–1022
12. Shankar KR, Babar S, Rowlands P, Jones MO 2000 Posttraumatic high-flow priapism: Treatment with selective embolisation. Pediatric Surgery International 16: 454–456
13. Gbadoe AD, Atakouma Y, Kusiaku K, Assimadi JK 2001 Management of sickle cell priapism with etilefrine. Archives of Disease in Childhood 85: 52–53
14. El-Bahnasawy MS, Dawood A, Farouk A 2002 Low-flow priapism: Risk factors for erectile dysfunction. BJU International 89: 285–290

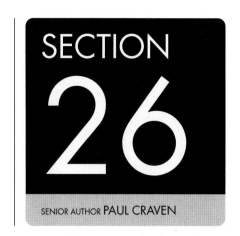

SECTION

26

SENIOR AUTHOR PAUL CRAVEN

ACUTE NEONATAL PROBLEMS

26.1 ACUTE NEONATAL EMERGENCIES

PAUL CRAVEN • ELLY MARILLIER

ESSENTIALS

1 Early recognition, appropriate treatment and referral for definitive care is the key to good outcome in the sick neonate. Recognising the signs of respiratory distress in infants allows for appropriate acute management in the ED.

2 Ensuring appropriate resuscitation equipment is available for the newborn infant, with a knowledge of drug doses is essential to appropriately manage acute respiratory arrest.

3 In the crying neonate, determine whether this presentation is part of a recurrent stereotypical pattern in an otherwise well infant, or a single acute episode. A careful history and examination will often lead to an appropriate diagnosis. Screening tests, with the exception of urine culture, have little utility. Review carefully, the carer's coping and supports and organise appropriate follow-up.

4 Recognition of peripheral versus central cyanosis in a newborn infant is essential as central cyanosis requires urgent evaluation. Respiratory and cardiac causes of cyanosis must be differentiated. Despite the majority of causes being cardiorespiratory it is important to recognise the other subtle causes of cyanosis that can affect this age group.

5 Neonatal seizures are relatively common and generally reactive in nature, and thus should not be labelled as neonatal epilepsy. Their presence is often a sign of neurological dysfunction and this should be fully investigated. The majority of neonatal seizures occur in the early neonatal period (day 1–7 of life). Neonatal seizures are subtle, they may be missed and are sometimes hard to differentiate from more benign movement disorders.

6 Persistent vomiting if found in the neonate requires full investigation. Bilious vomiting in the neonate is a surgical emergency until otherwise proven.

7 Sepsis remains the most common cause for the collapsed neonate in the emergency department.

8 In the collapsed newborn consider sepsis first then look for clues of other rarer underlying disorders if poor clinical response to treatment.

9 The key to resuscitation of the newborn is adequate ventilation.

NEONATAL EMERGENCIES

Studies have indicated that shorter post-partum hospital stays have resulted in an increased attendance at the emergency department (ED) of newborn infants and those in the first month of life. The common presenting symptoms and signs were jaundice, poor feeding, breathing difficulties and irritability.

The underlying common pathologies were found to be physiological jaundice, feeding problems and suspected sepsis.

Maternal experience, social support, early postnatal discharge and perinatal instruction influenced presentation to the ED.

THE INFANT WITH BREATHING DIFFICULTY

Respiratory emergencies are some of the commonest conditions presenting in the neonatal period. The increased work of breathing is manifested as:

- Tachypnoea (RR > 60 breaths per minute).
- Intercostal and subcostal recession (excessive use of accessory muscles of respiration).
- Flaring of the alae nares (accessory muscles of respiration).
- Grunting (forced glottic closure to create end positive pressure).
- Cyanosis (> 5 g L^{-1} of desaturated haemoglobin).
- Apnoea (a pause in breathing of > 20 seconds or less associated with bradycardia).
- Tracheal tug.

The causes of respiratory distress are varied and are summarised in Table 26.1.1. They can be broadly divided into primary respiratory and non-respiratory causes. Primary respiratory pathology is a direct result of upper, lower or mixed airway pathology.

This section will discuss:

- Emergencies of the upper airway.
- Emergencies of the lung parenchyma.

- Non-pulmonary causes affecting the lung parenchyma.
- The at-risk neonate.

UPPER AIRWAY OBSTRUCTION

Causes

Of all cases of upper airway obstruction presenting in the neonatal period 60% are congenital and 40% are acquired. Causes of upper airway obstruction include choanal atresia, Pierre Robin sequence, laryngomalacia, vocal cord anomalies and tracheomalacia. There are many rare causes.

Clinical features

Stridor is the classical presenting sign of upper airway obstruction and is a rare phenomenon in the neonatal period. Stridor is an indication of partial obstruction of the large diameter airways, from either an intrinsic developmental defect or from secondary compression and distortion. Stridor is the inspiratory noise that indicates this obstruction and

early referral to an ear, nose and throat specialist is essential. In addition to the stridor, infants often have an associated degree of respiratory distress, but may have a normal or hyper-expanded chest radiograph.

Investigations

These will be guided by the history and examination findings. Infants with severe stridor and respiratory distress should be urgently transported to a tertiary care centre, where adequate intensive-care support is available from qualified personnel. Intubation may be required and this can prove an extremely difficult procedure in this setting. Imaging studies, including plain radiographs, CT and MRI, are useful in specific clinical situations, based on the possible differential diagnosis. Other diagnostic techniques employed include barium swallow and laryngobronchoesophagoscopy (LBO).

Management

The management of upper airway obstruction requires the expertise of an ear, nose and throat specialist, and can range from

conservative management, in laryngomalacia, ensuring adequate growth and development, to the requirement for a tracheotomy in bilateral vocal cord paralysis.

RESPIRATORY DISTRESS ATTRIBUTED TO LUNG PARENCHYMA PATHOLOGY

Causes

Respiratory distress secondary to lower respiratory tract involvement may be a significant feature of either congenital or acquired parenchymal lung disease.

Acquired conditions likely to present in the ED include pneumonia, either viral or bacterial. The commonest viral presentation being bronchiolitis secondary to respiratory syncytial virus. Other parenchymal diseases include pulmonary oedema, due to either an underlying pulmonary or a cardiac anomaly.

Associated with underlying parenchymal anomalies the risks of pneumothorax are increased, once again exacerbating the respiratory distress.

Congenital anomalies that may present include cystic malformations of the lung, lobar emphysema or pleural effusions secondary to an underlying lymphatic pathology.

The causes of respiratory failure may be divided into two forms, common and uncommon:

Common
- Respiratory distress syndrome: Hyaline membrane disease Transient tachypnoea of the newborn.
- Meconium aspiration.
- Pneumonia/sepsis.
- Drug-induced respiratory depression.
- Bronchiolitis.
- Bronchopulmonary disease.
- Congestive heart failure.

Uncommon
- Diaphragmatic hernia.
- Congenital airway abnormalities, such as choanal atresia.
- Pulmonary hypoplasia.

Table 26.1.1 General causes of respiratory distress

General causes of respiratory distress	Specific conditions
Respiratory disorders	Hyaline membrane disease Congenital pneumonia Meconium aspiration syndrome Transient tachypnoea of the newborn Pneumothorax Hydro/haemothorax
Upper airway abnormalities	Laryngomalacia Micrognathia Vocal cord anomalies
Cardiac anomalies	Heart failure Myocarditis Pericardial effusion Transposition of the great arteries
Structural abnormalities	Diaphragmatic hernia Congenital cystic lesions Diaphragmatic paralysis
Chest deformities	Arthrogryposis Thoracic dystrophy
Haematologic causes	Anaemia
CNS lesions	Infection
Metabolic conditions	Metabolic acidosis

- Cystic adenomatoid malformation.
- Pulmonary haemorrhage.

Clinical features

History

In respiratory distress attributed to parenchymal involvement a clinical history is essential to elucidate potential predisposing factors. Of the causes of parenchymal disease presenting to the ED, pneumonia and extra-pulmonary cardiac failure are the two most common causes. These can often be differentiated by clinical history.

Bacterial pneumonia in the first few days of life may be impossible to distinguish from hyaline membrane disease or transient tachypnoea of the newborn. Therefore, respiratory distress in newborns generally should be treated as bacterial pneumonia until proven otherwise. When associated with chorioamnionitis, it is caused most commonly by *Escherichia coli* or by Group B streptococci (GBS). However, *Haemophilus influenzae*, *Streptococcus pneumoniae* (pneumococcus), Group D streptococci, *Listeria*, and anaerobes have also been described as pathogens in this setting. Infants infected with these organisms are often preterm and have very early onset of respiratory distress. Of note, infants may also develop bacterial pneumonia transnatally in the absence of maternal chorioamnionitis. Here, the causative organism is likely to be GBS, and the onset of symptoms tends to occur 12–24 hours after birth.

Neonatal pneumonia can be either congenital or acquired. Congenital pneumonia commences before birth and the most common infecting organisms include Group B *Streptococcus* and *E. coli*. Despite the majority of infants being unwell at birth some infants do acquire these infections after birth and present with similar signs and symptoms of respiratory distress, poor feeding, fever and apnoea. The clinical history should focus on the maternal Group B *Streptococcus* carriage in pregnancy, length of rupture of membranes, maternal antibiotic therapy during labour and maternal fever. Acquired neonatal pneumonias are commonly viral, with respiratory syncytial virus, adenovirus and parainfluenza virus all commonly identified. A history of affected family members gives some indication of this potential.

Any infant with underlying lung pathology is at risk of air leak, and any sudden decompensation in an infant with respiratory distress should lead one to consider this diagnosis. In addition, air leak can be a spontaneous phenomenon with no identified cause.

Non-infectious causes of acquired respiratory distress include any conditions in which there is an abnormally high or low blood flow to the lungs, an increased demand for oxygen, or a decreased number of red blood cells.

The commonest non-pulmonary cause of respiratory distress seen in the ED is that of pulmonary oedema, secondary to congenital heart disease.

Congenital heart disease is one of the commonest malformations, with an incidence of 0.6%. Although 30–60% of congenital heart disease is identified antenatally, this still leaves a large percentage presenting in the postnatal period. Cyanotic lesions generally present early but neonates with ductal-dependent systemic circulations are often well in the early neonatal period and collapse around day four of life. Closure of the ductus, with associated systemic collapse is one of the commonest presentations to the ED with severe respiratory distress.

Factors in the history pointing towards congenital heart disease being the cause of collapse include a family history, syndromic malformations and associated abnormalities.

In addition to predisposing factors, a history of poor feeding often predates the collapse.

Other causes of respiratory distress presenting in the ED are:

- Inborn errors of metabolism, with associated acidosis.
- Central nervous system anomalies.
- Non-accidental injury.

Examination

Infants with disease affecting the lung parenchyma, either primary respiratory or cardiac, generally present with the classical examination findings of respiratory distress, notably: recession of the intercostal and subcostal spaces; nasal flaring; tachypnoea (> 60 bpm); and expiratory grunting.

Nasal flaring is a result of the alae nasi being the first muscles to be activated during inspiration and they aim to decrease airway resistance. The recession of the inter and subcostal spaces is a result of the compliance of the chest wall being reduced in neonates. During inspiration the pleural pressure is reduced, but in neonates with parenchymal lung disease this needs to be reduced more than normal and thus the consequences are that the compliant chest wall may cave in as a result of these more negative pressures. The recession in conjunction with the abdominal protuberance associated with diaphragmatic descent give the characteristic seesaw pattern of neonatal respiratory distress.

Infants with respiratory infections may present in a very similar manner to those with cardiac anomalies. Specific findings for infants with pneumonia may be the presence of fever or temperature instability, feed intolerance and rhinorrhoea.[7]

If there is a suggestion of pulmonary air leak, the clinical signs are specific. There will be reduced air entry on the side of the leak, with a reduction in chest movement on that side. Percussion should be hyper-resonant and if the air leak is under tension there may be associated displacement of the trachea and apex beat to the contralateral side.

If a primary respiratory cause cannot be identified, non-respiratory causes should be sought. Signs indicative of congenital heart disease may include weak femoral pulses, an active praecordial impulse and a cardiac murmur.

The classical cardiac lesions presenting with respiratory distress in the neonatal period include:

❶ Left to right shunting lesions (ventriculoseptal defects; VSD). Typically large VSDs present between weeks two and four of life after the pulmonary pressures have reduced and this allows increased left to right flow with resultant pulmonary oedema.

❷ Ductal-dependent obstructive left ventricle conditions (hypoplastic left heart, critical aortic stenosis and coarctation of the aorta). Once the ductus arteriosus closes around week one of life, the systemic circulation is no longer maintained. Infants present shocked, pale and with severe respiratory distress. Specifically they have weak pulses and invariably a large liver.

With other causes of respiratory distress there may be features consistent with specific diagnoses. Metabolic conditions are often associated with hepatosplenomegaly, coma, hypoglycaemia and jaundice. CNS lesions may have seizures associated.

Investigations

Any infant in the first month of life with respiratory distress should be observed and monitored closely. This includes pulse rate, oxygen saturation, respiratory rate, temperature, blood pressure and capillary refill time.

The normal heart rate for a neonate in the first month of life is 120–160 bpm. Some newborn infants, however, have a resting heart rate below 90 bpm. Respiratory distress is generally associated with respiratory rate greater than 60 breaths per minute. Fever, as a sign of sepsis is variable.

Plain radiographs of the chest are useful, but do not generally differentiate the various causes of distress. Sepsis and cardiac failure both demonstrate increased interstitial markings. In cardiac failure fluid more specifically radiates into the interstitium from the hilum and in severe cases may be associated with an effusion. Again, in cardiac disease the size of the cardiac shadow may be increased. A cardiac silhouette greater than 60% of the transthoracic diameter is indicative of cardiac disease and needs to be investigated further, by means of an electrocardiogram and echocardiogram, and referral to a cardiologist.

The chest radiograph of an infant with pneumonia may show lobar or diffuse interstitial changes. Chest radiographs of infants who have bacterial pneumonia may exhibit a diffuse reticular nodular appearance but, in contrast to hyaline membrane disease, they tend to show normal or increased lung volumes with possible focal or coarse densities. There may also be pleural effusions, particularly with GBS pneumonia. In the newborn who has bacterial pneumonia, blood cultures obtained before the initiation of antibiotics commonly grow the offending organism. Cultures of urine and cerebrospinal fluid should be obtained at the time of the blood culture. If the diagnosis is viral, mucus plugging, with over-aeration and hyper-expansion may be characteristic. Although tension pneumothorax should be a clinical diagnosis, the plain radiograph is good at demonstrating small pneumothoraces. An anterior pneumothorax may be subtle and easily missed by the unwary.

Laboratory investigations, including full blood count, CRP and blood cultures, are useful adjuncts to the diagnosis. The white cell count may show a leucocytosis with associated left shift or, more commonly, may show a consumptive picture with neutropenia and associated thrombocytopenia in the septic infant. The C-reactive protein (CRP) is another marker of infection, but appears more useful in monitoring response to treatment of infection rather than in its diagnosis.

If a viral respiratory tract infection is suspected then a nasopharyngeal sample viewed with electron microscopy for respiratory viruses may reveal the common causes of bronchiolitis.

Arterial blood gas analysis or indirect transcutaneous monitoring may reveal arterial hypoxaemia and hypercarbia. The degree of hypoxaemia and acidosis will be a guide to the need for respiratory positive pressure support. In addition to diagnosing the severity of the respiratory acidosis an arterial blood gas may also reveal a metabolic acidosis, making inborn errors of metabolism a potential differential diagnosis of the respiratory distress.

Management

A neonate with respiratory distress needs to be observed closely. Evaluation of airway, breathing and circulation are imperative as outlined in the resuscitation guidelines devised by the International Liaison Committee on Resuscitation (ILCOR).

If sepsis is suspected then intravenous antibiotics should be commenced, to cover both Gram-positive and Gram-negative bacteria and an evaluation made of the need for both fluid and inotropic support. Empiric treatment should be initiated as soon as possible with ampicillin $100 \text{ mg kg}^{-1} \text{ d}^{-1}$ divided every twelve hours (infants < 1.2 kg) or every eight hours (infants > 1.2 kg) and cefotaxime $100 \text{ mg kg}^{-1} \text{ d}^{-1}$ divided every twelve hours or $150 \text{ mg kg}^{-1} \text{ d}^{-1}$ divided every eight hours (infants > 1.2 kg and > 7 days old). Gentamicin is an alternative treatment, particularly when there is no evidence of meningitis. Treatment should be continued for at least ten days, although 14–21 days may be required, particularly for Gram-negative infections.

Viral infections are treated conservatively by respiratory and circulatory support as required. An unusual or unresponsive neonatal presentation of pneumonia warrants further evaluation. The maternal history may offer important clues. Neonatal pneumonia involving cytomegalovirus (CMV) or other viruses may be transmitted transplacentally. CMV pneumonia usually does not require treatment in the otherwise healthy infant. However, neonatal respiratory distress in the setting of perinatal exposure to herpes simplex virus, particularly if there is primary maternal genital infection, warrants treatment with aciclovir 30 mg kg^{-1} per day divided every eight hours for 14–21 days until all cultures are negative. *Ureaplasma urealyticum* is another important organism that can lead to chronic lung disease. Treatment of *Ureaplasma* infection in the newborn should include erythromycin $50 \text{ mg kg}^{-1} \text{ d}^{-1}$ divided every six hours.

If the cause of the respiratory distress is believed to be cardiac then once again supporting the airway, breathing and circulation is imperative. Added caution with fluid resuscitation should be considered so as not to exacerbate the cardiac failure. Use of prostaglandin E2 allows reopening of the ductus and increased systemic circulation. This is a temporising measure prior to the definitive surgery the infant may require.

Management of a pneumothorax requires either acute drainage with needle thoracocentesis, in the presence of a tension pneumothorax, or intercostal catheter insertion followed by appropriate underwater drainage. A repeat chest X-ray (CXR) to ensure adequate lung expansion is required prior to the removal of the chest drain.

THE CRYING INFANT

Crying is an important method of communication for infants. Carers are usually able to identify and manage the cause (e.g. hunger, discomfort) and console the infant. Medical advice is sought if the crying is felt to be unusually intense or persistent or the infant is unable to be consoled by the usual methods. 'Normal crying' was defined in Brazelton's 1962 study of 80 infants of American families selected to have minimal psychological stressors. There was a peak of crying to a median of $2\frac{3}{4}$ hours per day by six weeks, with a wide variation, and a decrease thereafter. The classification of crying as normal or excessive is highly subjective and will vary according to infant, carer and situational factors. All three areas need to be assessed in this type of presentation.

Either a single episode of or recurrence of a pattern of excessive crying may precipitate ED presentation.

RECURRENT CRYING – COLIC

History and examination
Recurrent excessive crying in an otherwise healthy infant is often termed colic. This diagnosis can only be made if the pattern is recurrent and stereotypical and a careful history, examination and period of follow-up have ruled out other important causes. The definition of colic varies but it is frequently arbitrarily defined as a total of more than three hours per day of irritability, fussing and crying on at least three days a week for at least three weeks. This pattern typically occurs in the afternoon or evening ceasing by three to four months of age.

Management
Current specific dietary, drug and behavioural strategies meet with limited success. Cows' milk protein intolerance, however, may have a role in a small proportion of infants. The positive effects of changing from cows' milk-based formula to casein hydrolysate formula have been noted to diminish with time suggesting that colic is not related to allergy. A trial of hydrolysate may be appropriate in a formula-fed baby but its long-term use is likely to be unnecessary. It is notable that soy protein formulas may have similar adverse effects to those of cows' milk formulas. Behavioural interventions, including advice to reduce stimulation in combination with permission to leave the infant when the crying was no longer tolerable was effective when compared to a non-specific empathic interview. Reduction of stimulation advice includes avoiding excessive patting, winding, lifting, vigorous jiggling and loud noises or toys. Carers were advised not to intervene in the early part of sleep when the infant may appear restless and also given an assurance that a certain amount of crying is normal. It is important to remember that even if behavioural interventions do not change the infant's temperament, they may well alter the impact colic has on the carer and on carer–infant interactions.

Carers very reasonably assume that there must be something wrong either with the child or their parenting for an infant to cry frequently and excessively. Much reassurance that the child is healthy can be gained from witnessing the conduct of a complete history and thorough examination. Similarly an explanation that this is a common problem that does not reflect on their parenting, that some babies may be assisted by some simple behavioural techniques and that the carers will be supported by appropriate referral will also reduce anxiety considerably.

ACUTE CRYING
Causes
The causes of a single episode of excessive crying in an infant are vast. In an afebrile infant without a cause apparent to the carer, a careful history has been shown to provide clues to the final diagnosis in 20% of cases. Physical examination was revealing in more than 50% and a period of follow-up often useful in patients where the diagnosis was still in question.

Clinical features
History
History includes the timing and amount of crying, duration of behaviour, measures taken to resolve the situation, specific carer concerns, the carer's response to crying, expectations and experience, specific social difficulties (including substance abuse), contact with child health nurse or other medical supports. A thoughtful review of the carer's supports and coping is essential.

Also important are details of pregnancy, labour and neonatal difficulties, feeding activities including volumes of feed (considerations include under- and overfeeding), dietary changes, past medical history, vomiting (gastrointestinal reflux, gastroenteritis, sepsis, meningitis). Consider changes in stools (constipation, gastroenteritis, bleeding anal fissure, intussusception), type of feeding (breast or bottle), type of milk, drug exposure, recent immunisation, fever, respiratory symptoms, rash, contacts with infectious illness and growth history.

Examination
A complete set of vital signs is essential including oxygen saturation (tachypnoea with pneumonia, sepsis or metabolic acidosis, tachycardia with supraventricular tachycardia, sepsis or dehydration, desaturation with pneumonia or bronchiolitis). Examination should include tone and activity, alertness/conscious state (meningitis, encephalitis, sepsis, metabolic crisis, hypoglycaemia, electrolyte disturbance), perfusion, hydration, fontanelle (bulging with infection or trauma,

sunken in poor feeding and dehydration), assessment of chest for respiratory distress, (pneumonia, bronchiolitis, metabolic acidosis, cardiac failure). An abdominal examination (herniae, testicular torsion, evidence of surgical abdomen), cardio-vascular examination (murmurs, femoral pulses, cardiac ischaemia due to aberrant coronary vessels is a reported but extremely rare cause), ears (otitis media), and oropharynx (herpes stomatitis, tonsillitis, upper respiratory tract infection).

Several additional manoeuvres may also assist:

- Rectal examination (constipation, intussusception, anal fissure).
- Fluorescein staining of cornea (corneal abrasion).
- Palpation of long bones (fractures, osteomyelitis).
- Eversion of eyelids (foreign bodies).
- Inspection of skin beneath clothing (bruising).
- Retinal examination (shaken baby syndrome).
- Close attention to digits and penis (hair tourniquet).

Investigations

Investigations should be guided by initial clinical assessment. Screening investigations with the exception of urine analysis and culture have little utility.

Disposition

The diagnosis of serious medical conditions during the initial clinical assessment will clearly indicate admission. Admission should also be considered in those cases where the clinical assessment is normal but the child continues to cry excessively in the ED beyond the time of the initial assessment. Persistent crying in these circumstances may be an indicator of serious illness.

Occasionally it may be necessary to admit an infant with colic or minor medical problem to allow recovery of a sleep-deprived or poorly supported carer.[9] The involvement of social work services is appropriate under circumstances where the family or child is considered at risk. Serious injury to children by non-accidental shaking injury is preceded by other episodes of abuse or neglect in over 70% of cases. Admission and social work assessment is always warranted if non-accidental injury or neglect is suspected.

Ensure appropriate follow-up is organised for infants discharged from the ED – particularly where the diagnosis is not yet clear or where excessive crying is likely to be recurrent.

THE BLUE INFANT

Neonatal cyanosis is a result of deoxygenated blood in the systemic circulation. It is defined by an arterial saturation less than 90% and an arterial partial pressure of oxygen less than 60 mmHg.

History, examination and simple investigations available in the ED should be able to distinguish the cause of the cyanosis and this will predict the management of this condition.

Causes

Babies can be peripherally blue or centrally blue and this is important in differentiating the cause of the cyanosis. Peripheral cyanosis, affecting the hands and feet, known as acrocyanosis is a normal phenomenon that generally clears within 1–2 days and needs no treatment. Central cyanosis, evidenced by cyanosis of the gums and mucous membranes is generally pathological and needs urgent evaluation if presenting in the ED. Babies can be centrally cyanosed for many reasons including heart disease, lung or other breathing problems, being cold, or having seizures. Not all children who turn blue have a heart problem. A thorough history, examination and simple investigations will be able to differentiate these causes of central cyanosis.

Non-respiratory causes of cyanosis

- Cardiac defects:
  Decreased pulmonary blood flow
  Admixture lesions
  Congestive heart failure (pulmonary congestion).
- Primary pulmonary hypertension of the newborn.

- Central nervous system disease:
  Intracranial haemorrhage
  Maternal sedative administration
  Meningitis.
- Methaemoglobinaemia.
- Hypoglycaemia.
- Sepsis.
- Cold.

Clinical features

History

Once cyanosis has been diagnosed in an infant presenting to the ED, the most important step is to differentiate between pulmonary and cardiac causes of cyanosis.

Pulmonary causes of cyanosis include pneumonia, both bacterial and viral, pneumothorax, pleural effusions and airway anomalies. If the cause of the cyanosis is felt to be pulmonary the infant will generally have a history of worsening respiratory distress, this interferes with the infants ability to feed successfully. The history may be indicative of an infective cause, with rhinorrhoea, fever, cough, poor feeding and worsening recession of the inter- and subcostal spaces. In addition there may be a history of other affected family members and respiratory infections are generally more prominent in the winter months especially associated with epidemics of bronchiolitis.

Infants with cardiac causes of cyanosis may have no preceding history and generally breathe normally. A detailed antenatal history, including results of antenatal ultrasound scans, will be important. In addition, the timing of the cyanosis may also give a clue to the diagnosis with ductal-dependent cardiac lesions generally worsening when the ductus arteriosus shuts around day three or four of life. Although congenital heart disease is generally divided into cyanotic and acyanotic, those lesions generally classified as acyanotic but ductal dependent can present with severe respiratory distress and a degree of cyanosis.

Again, a family history of congenital heart disease will also heighten one's suspicion of cyanotic congenital heart disease.

In addition to congenital heart disease and pulmonary causes an infant may present cyanosed because they have neurological depression or seizures. A history of the infant's general activity, tone and feeding patterns will be helpful. Infants with neurological depression may be hypotonic, have poor feeding with associated failure to thrive and may indeed have seizure activity.

Once again, if seizures are suspected then a detailed family history may indicate a genetic syndrome as the cause of the seizures. A thorough history of the pregnancy and delivery are also important to rule out other causes of seizures. If no antenatal or perinatal risk factors are identified then a history indicating neonatal sepsis is imperative and also a detailed account of maternal substance abuse may indicate drug withdrawal as the cause of the seizures.

Examination

Once a detailed history has been taken to elicit possible causes of cyanosis then the infant should be examined carefully.

Infants with respiratory causes for cyanosis will generally have signs of distress, namely tachypnoea, recession of the intercostal and subcostal spaces, tracheal tug, nasal flaring and expiratory grunting. As to the precise respiratory cause of this distress, septic infants often have an associated tachycardia and may have temperature instability. They may have poor capillary return and may also have associated apnoeas, a pause in breathing of greater than twenty seconds or a pause in breathing less than twenty seconds but associated with bradycardia. Infants who are septic and cyanosed may have localised respiratory infections, such as viral bronchiolitis or may be septicaemic.

A cyanosed infant with little or no respiratory distress is more likely to have congenital heart disease. The commonest lesions presenting with cyanosis in the neonatal period are: transposition of the great arteries; total anomalous pulmonary venous return; pulmonary atresia with an intact ventricular septum; severe pulmonary stenosis; and severe tetralogy of Fallot.

Examination of a cyanosed infant with suspected cardiac disease might reveal dysmorphic features suggesting a syndromic association with congenital heart disease. Auscultation of the lung fields and precordium may reveal evidence of pulmonary oedema and murmurs, and an abdominal examination may reveal hepatomegaly.

To differentiate an infant with noncardiopulmonary causes for the cyanosis, the examination would need to concentrate on the neurological system of the infant. Tone, movements and reflexes will all give important information as to the neurological status. Examination for dysmorphic features and examination of the fundi and skin may add important information as to the cause of the seizures. In the neonatal period, important causes of seizures would include hypoxia, hypoglycaemia and biochemical anomalies, narcotic withdrawal and structural brain abnormalities.

Investigations

To differentiate the various causes of cyanosis in the neonatal period a full set of observations should be performed. Oxygen saturations should be performed initially in room air to serve as a baseline. Subsequent oxygen measures should be performed in 100% oxygen, achieved by means of a headbox sealed over the babies head and neck. The so-called hyperoxia test helps to differentiate cyanotic heart disease from other causes of neonatal cyanosis. Infants with neurological or pulmonary causes of the cyanosis will demonstrate substantial increases in the arterial blood saturation, while infants with cyanotic congenital heart disease will show minimal elevation. As well as oxygen saturation changes the difference should be confirmed with arterial blood gas analysis of arterial oxygen partial pressures. A partial pressure < 100 mmHg is more indicative of cardiac disease than one > 100 mmHg, which is more likely to suggest pulmonary or neurological causes for the cyanosis.

Once arterial oxygen saturations and blood gas analysis have been performed the infant should have a chest radiogram. Abnormalities of the lung fields may suggest a primary pulmonary cause for the cyanosis or a cardiac cause if the changes are suggestive of pulmonary oedema with increased vascular markings.

Assessing the cardiothoracic diameter and shape of the cardiac shadow may give some clues to a cardiac cause of the cyanosis. A typical boot-shaped heart is classically described in tetralogy of Fallot and an egg on a string appearance is described in transposition of the great arteries. Generally differentiating the cardiac causes of cyanosis is difficult and requires an echocardiogram. Additional investigations that may be useful in the diagnosis of neonatal cyanosis include a full blood count to reveal polycythaemia and a raised or depressed white blood cell count, blood cultures and a nasopharyngeal aspirate.

In addition to blood gas analysis to indicate fixed or variable hypoxia, the carbon dioxide will generally be raised in respiratory pathologies contributing to the cyanosis but may be normal in cardiac disease.

An ECG may help differentiate cardiac disease, but the gold standard investigation to help differentiate cardiac causes of cyanosis from non-cardiac causes will be an echocardiogram combined with colour Doppler flow mapping and pulsed-wave Doppler studies. The echocardiogram should be performed as a matter of urgency in such situations to allow appropriate management of congenital heart disease. Echocardiography can be easily performed by a paediatric cardiologist in the ED.

Management

Any neonate that presents with cyanosis should be appropriately resuscitated as outlined in the guidelines devised by the International Liaison Committee on Resuscitation (ILCOR).

Once the presence of cyanosis is determined from the physical examination of the infant, its degree of severity should be documented immediately by oximetry and confirmed by arterial blood gas and pH determinations. Arterial blood gases and pH should be determined with the patient breathing room air (if clinically stable) and following the breathing of 100% oxygen for 5–10 minutes. If the oxygen tension rises to exceed 150 mmHg, cyanotic congenital heart disease can be excluded, although little or no change in oxygen tension strongly suggests that such a defect is the cause of the cyanosis. The gold standard for immediately ruling out non-cardiac causes of cyanosis and establishing the diagnosis of cyanotic congenital heart disease remains echocardiography. The cyanosis that results from pulmonary disease usually resolves partially, if not completely, following the administration of oxygen. Such treatment should not produce similar results in patients who have non-respiratory cyanosis. Here the cause must be determined to achieve a successful outcome.

All neonates should initially receive oxygen until a definitive diagnosis has been made. If the diagnosis is pulmonary then the addition of oxygen should resolve the cyanosis. If the respiratory distress is severe, additional support by means of positive end expiratory pressure or positive pressure ventilation may be required. If an infant requires intubation then a person skilled in this procedure should be asked to attend the ED. Following institution of airway support the infant requires intensive-care admission. Once the airway and breathing have been supported then appropriate assessment and management of the circulation is essential. In any infant with a pulmonary cause for the cyanosis the potential for sepsis should be evaluated and treated with intravenous antibiotics.

The laboratory evaluation of most neonates who are cyanosed includes a haematocrit and haemoglobin determination, white blood cell count, differential count, blood glucose determination, and a chest radiograph. If a cardiac aetiology is likely, echocardiography is essential. In selected cases, cardiac catheterisation and angiocardiography may be necessary to define the cardiac anatomy more precisely. Electrocardiography should be performed if clinical findings suggest a tachyarrhythmia. If a central nervous system aetiology is suspected, appropriate scans and drug levels should be considered. The presence of methaemoglobin may be detected by placing a few drops of the patient's blood on filter paper and comparing it with normal blood. Methaemoglobin will produce a chocolate-brown colour.

Seizures that result in cyanosis should be managed according to the results of initial investigations. Hypoglycaemia should be managed with a 5 mL kg^{-1} bolus of 10% dextrose, followed by an infusion of dextrose. Hypocalcaemia should be managed with intravenous calcium and other electrolyte imbalances should be corrected before trying to control the seizure. Once treatable causes of neonatal seizures have been identified and treated then appropriate anticonvulsant therapy should be administered. Phenobarbital or phenytoin are first-line anticonvulsants used in the neonatal period.

In any infant with seizures in the first month of life sepsis should be thoroughly investigated with both blood culture and cerebrospinal fluid cultures for both bacteria and viruses. Treatment with antibiotics and antiviral medications should be considered if there are any risk factors, symptoms or signs of sepsis.

Of all of the above aetiologies, the most common cause of cyanosis in the neonate is a cyanotic congenital heart defect. In many such infants, pulmonary blood flow depends primarily or entirely upon the patency of the ductus arteriosus. If congenital heart disease is suspected from the hyperoxia test, chest radiograph, ECG or echocardiogram then referral should be made to a paediatric cardiologist. A discussion should take place as to whether prostaglandin E1 should be commenced to either open or maintain the patency of the ductus arteriosus. This will allow mixing of deoxygenated and oxygenated blood, increasing the oxygen saturations of the infant. A dose of 0.05–0.1 μg kg^{-1} min^{-1} IV is generally recommended, remembering that the most serious side effects of this drug are hypoventilation and apnoea.

Once a diagnosis of congenital heart disease has been made then ongoing management by a paediatric cardiologist is essential. Transfer to a paediatric cardiology centre should be organised and the infant should be fully monitored prior to transfer, including pre- and post-ductal saturations, respiratory rate, temperature, pulse, ECG monitoring and blood pressure. Transport should be provided by a team expert in neonatal resuscitation.

THE INFANT WITH POSSIBLE SEIZURES

Although the incidence of seizures is higher in the first four weeks of life than in any other age group, the actual incidence cannot be delineated because of the large number of subtle presentations. The seizures that do present to the ED generally do so in the early neonatal period (days 1–7) and it is essential to recognise these for two reasons:

❶ They may represent the manifestation of serious underlying disease that needs treating.

❷ If unrecognised, and thus untreated, seizures may be prolonged and cause brain damage.

Seizures in the neonatal period are a result of an excessive depolarisation of neurones from many different causes. Disturbances of electrolytes (sodium, calcium, and magnesium) and an imbalance of excitatory and inhibitory amino acids have been identified as predisposing to neonatal seizure activity. It is important to identify the cause of the seizures, as many of them are easily treatable, because if missed there may be major long-term consequences.

Causes of neonatal seizures

- Hypoxia: hypoxic ischaemic encephalopathy.
- Intracranial haemorrhage: primary subarachnoid, periventricular/intraventricular, subdural.
- Electrolyte imbalance: hypoglycaemia, hypocalcaemia, hypomagnesaemia, hyponatraemia.
- Metabolic: amino acidopathies, organic acidopathies, hyperammonaemia, pyridoxine deficiency.
- Intracranial infections: bacterial and viral.
- Developmental defects: neuromigrational disorders.
- Drug withdrawal: opiates or maternal benzodiazepine abuse.
- Familial.

Clinical features

History

The clinical history will provide essential clues to the cause of the seizures. A thorough history of the pregnancy, labour and delivery should be established as well as a detailed family history of seizures.

A perinatal history of maternal fever, prolonged rupture of membranes, low vaginal swab positive for Group B *Streptococcus* and associated fetal distress may be clues to an infective cause of the seizures. In addition, a history of poor Apgar scores and the need for resuscitation at birth may indicate a perinatal asphyxial event.

If a perinatal cause for the seizures is not identified in the history then a postpartum cause needs to be considered. A history of maternal substance abuse may indicate seizures secondary to neonatal abstinence syndrome and a family history of seizures are suggestive of a genetic cause for the seizures.

Poor understanding of the nutritional requirements of the newborn and excessive weight loss may indicate an electrolyte imbalance as the cause of the seizures. Hypoglycaemia and hypocalcaemia may both present with a preceding history of jitteriness.

In addition to the history of the actual cause of the seizures it is also important to get a realistic picture as to the nature of the seizures. Although most neonatal seizures are partial, they can be generalised, and there are many other presenting signs of neonatal seizure activity including: jitteriness; cyanosis; apnoea; tachycardia; lethargy; and collapse.

Examination

Any infant that has presented with seizures or potential seizures needs a thorough examination. The anterior fontanelle should be soft and non-bulging in the neonatal period. A tense fontanelle is suggestive of raised intracranial pressure. This may result from an intracranial bleed or excessive swelling secondary to neonatal meningitis. If a bleed is suspected this may be idiopathic, secondary to a bleeding tendency or a result of non-accidental injury. If a bleeding tendency is suspected other bruising or other bleeding diatheses may be identified and the stool and urine should both be examined for the presence of blood. The head should be measured and the head circumference should be plotted on a centile chart to compare with the initial centile that the head circumference lay on initially. This will indicate if there is progressive hydrocephalus. Once the fontanelle has been examined the rest of the nervous system should be assessed. Tone and reflexes should be elicited to indicate any CNS involvement. The eyes should be examined for retinal haemorrhages and signs that the intracerebral injury could be deliberate. Severe hydrocephalus associated with seizures may be associated with a downward deviation of the eyes.

Considering the multitude of causes of neonatal seizures there will be many potential physical signs that can be elicited. Signs of infection, either congenital or acquired, may include a petechial rash and hepatosplenomegaly, or in neonatal meningitis they may be associated with severe septic shock.

It is important to recognise that a lethargic infant may be dehydrated and suffering from the effects of an electrolyte imbalance. In addition, an infant with metabolic derangements may also present shocked, acidotic and with seizures. The metabolic derangements may have a characteristic odour that, if identified, may lead to a rapid diagnosis of the seizures.

Although there are many causes of seizures in the neonatal period, the diagnosis is only made when adequate investigations are performed. A paediatric neurologist may be involved in more intractable forms of seizure.

Investigations

Any neonate presenting to the ED with possible seizures needs prompt investigation. A first line would be to perform a full set of clinical observations, including oxygen saturations and ECG. Once the airway and breathing have been assessed, then a blood sugar should be performed, and serum taken for calcium, magnesium and sodium levels.

In any infant, sepsis should be high on the list of differential diagnoses and thorough investigation should be performed. This should include full blood count, blood cultures and, importantly, a lumbar puncture. The cerebrospinal fluid should be examined for evidence of both bacterial and viral infections. If viral infection is suspected then polymerase chain reaction should be performed for herpes simplex virus. Glucose and protein performed on the CSF also help guide the differential diagnosis. If a congenital infection is possible, either the mother is non-immune or has risk factors for the possible development of rubella, cytomegalovirus or toxoplasmosis in pregnancy, then a TORCH screen should be performed.

In addition to biochemical and infective profiles, a metabolic screen should be performed on fresh urine collected from the infant, and certain inborn errors of metabolism can be eliminated by chasing the newborn screening test performed on all newborn infants between days three and five of life.

Once basic blood, urine and CSF tests have been collected, a cerebral ultrasound scan should be organised. This allows both sagittal and coronal views of the brain through the anterior and posterior fontanelle. This simple bedside test will demonstrate intracerebral haemorrhage and may demonstrate certain changes typical of congenital infections. If there is ongoing suspicion of intracerebral pathology an MRI or CT scan may be required. At this stage the infant would require admission and ongoing investigation in hospital.

Once a neonate is admitted to hospital with seizures, further investigations may involve an EEG, with video telemetry to differentiate a true seizure from other common diagnoses.

Differential diagnoses

As neonatal seizures can present with such a complex array of symptoms and signs, the list of differential diagnoses is great. Some of the commoner differential diagnoses include benign neonatal sleep myoclonus, gastro-oesophageal reflux, anoxia and neonatal jitters.

Management

Any neonate presenting with a potential seizure needs urgent management. Phenobarbital remains the standard first-line treatment for neonatal seizures worldwide but is ineffective in many neonates. Second-line anticonvulsant regimens vary widely but usually involve the benzodiazepines (diazepam, clonazepam, lorazepam, midazolam), phenytoin, or paraldehyde.

Acute treatment

- Ensure respiration. Endotracheal intubation and respiratory support are often required due to the limited respiratory reserves of the neonate. This should be considered early as the rapid correction of hypoxia aids in limiting seizure time.
- Ensure cardiac support.
- If hypoglycaemic: glucose 10% solution: 2 mL kg^{-1} IV followed by continuous infusion at $5–7 \text{ mg kg}^{-1} \text{ min}^{-1}$.
- Other specific treatments (as indicated): calcium gluconate 5% solution 4 mL kg^{-1} IV; magnesium sulfate 50% solution 0.2 mL kg^{-1} IM; pyridoxine 50–100 mg IV.
- Symptomatic treatment: phenobarbital loading dose 20 mg kg^{-1} IV; additional doses 5 mg kg^{-1} IV (10–15 minutes) to maximum of 20 mg kg^{-1}; phenytoin 20 mg kg^{-1} ($1 \text{ mg kg}^{-1} \text{ min}^{-1}$).

The most important determinant of prognosis is the underlying aetiology. Thus, infants who have cerebral dysgenesis have uniformly poor outcomes, and 50–100% of those who have moderate or severe hypoxic-ischaemic encephalopathy develop sequelae. In contrast, infants who have transient metabolic derangements and are treated promptly or who have only subarachnoid haemorrhage usually have a good outcome. Intracranial infection and inborn errors of metabolism are associated with a variable prognosis.

THE VOMITING INFANT

True vomiting in babies is best divided into two broad categories: non-bilious and bilious. Bilious vomiting occurs when bile is purged along with the gastric contents. Although some small intestinal reflux into the stomach is common with all vomiting, in non-bilious vomiting, antegrade intestinal flow is preserved, and the majority of the bile drains into the more distal portions of the intestine. If an obstruction is present, non-bilious vomiting implies that the obstruction is proximal to the ampulla of Vater. Conditions leading to bilious vomiting involve either a disorder of motility or physical blockage to this antegrade flow of proximal intestinal contents distal to the ligament of Treitz.

NON-BILIOUS VOMITING

Gastro-oesophageal reflux (GOR), although not true vomiting, is frequently included in discussions of vomiting but really only occurs as a result of failed normal oesophageal function. Normally, the lower oesophageal sphincter (LES) relaxes with swallowing and propagation of oesophageal peristalsis, allowing a food bolus to enter the stomach. Its basal contraction prevents food from re-entering the oesophagus from the stomach. Transient relaxation of the LES predisposes to GOR and is the major mechanism in infants who have GOR. The LES is aided by surrounding structures, especially the crural diaphragm, and disruption of these structures, as with a hiatal hernia, contributes to the GOR in some patients. Nicotine, alcohol, caffeine, and some medications can increase relaxation of the LES, contributing to GOR in some individuals. GOR also is distinguished from true vomiting by its symptoms – the emesis of GOR is effortless and generally not associated with retching or autonomic symptoms.

Both inborn errors of metabolism and endocrine disorders can cause vomiting in neonates. The physician should consider glycogen storage disease II (Pompe disease), galactosaemia, urea cycle defects, phenylketonuria, Zellweger disease, adrenal leukodystrophy and carnitine deficiency syndromes in the sick vomiting neonate. The inborn errors of metabolism generally present in early infancy, and the vomiting is associated with symptoms of lethargy, hypo- or hypertonia, seizures, or coma. The constellation of symptoms is similar to that seen in sepsis, necessitating a high index of suspicion in the evaluation of these patients. The presence or absence of metabolic acidosis, hypoglycaemia, hyperammonaemia, or ketosis and a family history that includes possible consanguinity can help to determine the diagnosis.

Vomiting occurs in any neurological condition that involves increased intracranial pressure (ICP), such as hydrocephalus, congenital malformation, intracranial haemorrhage or mass lesion and infection. Additionally, babies who have seizures, autonomic disorders (Riley–Day syndrome), and conditions affecting the floor of the fourth ventricle without increased ICP frequently have their condition worsened by vomiting.

The anatomic and, thus, the generally surgical causes of non-bilious vomiting are those that affect the intestinal tract proximal to the point of bilious drainage (ampulla of Vater), which is proximal to the ligament of Treitz. These include oesophageal/gastric atresia, duplication/diverticulum/choledochal cyst, pyloric stenosis and web. Any infant who exhibits persistent non-bilious vomiting, with or without feeding, in the immediate newborn period must be suspected of having an intestinal atresia or a luminally obstructing lesion (pyloric stenosis, luminal band, web) proximal to the point of bile drainage (ampulla of Vater). An easy and rapid test to evaluate possible oesophageal atresia is the ability to pass a nasogastric tube easily into the stomach. After the tube has been passed, it is important to obtain a radiograph to assure that the tube is in the stomach and not coiled in an atretic oesophagus. Any resistance to passage of the tube is an indication for evaluation by contrast radiograph for an obstruction. If an obstruction is present, naso-oesophageal tube drainage is important to prevent aspiration of pooled oesophageal secretions. Contrast studies are the standard for the diagnosis of these conditions.

BILIOUS VOMITING

Although not absolute, anatomic conditions causing luminal obstruction distal to the ligament of Treitz usually cause bilious vomiting. Bilious vomiting is an ominous sign that mandates immediate evaluation. Conditions to be considered in the vomiting baby include intestinal atresia and stenosis, malrotation with or without volvulus and intestinal duplication. In the neonate intestinal atresias and stenosis and malrotation with or without volvulus need to be ruled out immediately. Also, malrotation with volvulus is a surgical emergency that is diagnosed relatively easily by gastrointestinal contrast study. It is more common in older children.

Management

Any infant who is seriously ill with vomiting requires immediate resuscitation and admission to hospital. In many cases aggressive fluid management in addition to resuscitation following ILCOR recommendations will need to be implemented without delay.

In the case of the infant with nonbilious vomiting early consultation with a paediatrician should occur as in many cases further evaluation may be necessary. Where an underlying metabolic or endocrine disorder was considered in the differential diagnosis, stabilisation should occur as outlined above with particular attention to any underlying metabolic and electrolyte derangement. Early consultation with a special unit with experience in the care of these rare metabolic conditions should occur as soon as the diagnosis entertained. Stable infants with vomiting that is not serious and who are otherwise well, such as those with GOR, can be discharged from the ED, provided that suitable follow-up and family support have been organised.

For those infants with bilious vomiting an underlying surgical disorder must be considered until otherwise proven. Early consultation with a paediatric surgeon is mandatory in every case. If the infant is seriously ill, then resuscitation should commence immediately following ILCOR recommendations with a particular focus on maintaining circulation and fluid status in addition to correcting underlying metabolic and electrolyte derangements. After the diagnosis has been established radiographically, the gastrointestinal tract should be decompressed with a nasogastric tube, the infant kept nil by mouth and supported with intravenous fluids until definitive surgical intervention can be undertaken.

THE COLLAPSED INFANT

Occasionally, a young infant will be brought to the ED because they just don't look right to the parents. Even inexperienced parents whose first baby is just a few weeks old may notice when their child is unusually sleepy, fussy, or not eating as well as usual. To the physician in the ED, such an infant may appear quite ill, with pallor, cyanosis, or ashen in colour. The infant may be irritable or lethargic, with or without fever. In addition there may be tachypnoea or tachycardia and/or hypotension, and other signs of poor perfusion may also be apparent.

The most common entities to be considered include bacterial infection and viral syndromes. There are a number of other disorders that are uncommon, but demand diagnostic consideration because they are potentially life threatening, yet treatable (Table 26.1.2).

An infant who is critically ill in the first month of life should initially be presumed to have sepsis and empiric antibiotics commenced. As *Escherichia coli*, Group B streptococci (GBS), *Listeria*, and other anaerobes are the most likely causative organisms, a combination of ampicillin 200 mg kg^{-1} d^{-1} and gentamicin 7 mg kg^{-1} d^{-1} in divided doses is a reasonable starting point. In the case of suspected meningitis the addition of cefotaxime 200 mg kg^{-1} d^{-1} in divided doses may also be considered. This is a life-threatening situation, the airway, breathing, and circulation should be restored, vascular access obtained and supportive care commenced. The approach to the collapsed infant is presented in Figure 26.1.1.

Table 26.1.2 Differential diagnosis of the collapsed infant

1. Infectious diseases
   - Bacterial sepsis
   - Meningitis
   - Urinary tract infection
   - Virus infection
   - Congenital syphilis
2. Cardiac disease
   - Congenital heart disease
   - Paroxysmal arterial tachycardia
   - Myocardial infarction due to anomalous coronary vessels
   - Pericarditis
   - Myocarditis
3. Endocrine disorders
   - Congenital adrenal hyperplasia
4. Metabolic disorders
   - Hyponatraemia
   - Hypernatraemia
   - Inborn errors of metabolism
   - Hypoglycaemia
   - Drug toxicity
5. Haematologic disorders
   - Severe anaemia
   - Methaemoglobinaemia
6. Gastrointestinal disorders
   - Gastroenteritis with dehydration
   - Pyloric stenosis
   - Intussusception
7. Neurological disease
   - Infant botulism
   - Child-abuse intracranial bleed

SEPSIS

Sepsis should always be considered when confronted with an ill-appearing infant. The signs and symptoms of sepsis may be quite subtle. The history may vary, and some infants may seem to be ill for several days, while others deteriorate rapidly. Any one or a combination of symptoms, such as lethargy, irritability, diarrhoea, vomiting, anorexia, or fever may be a manifestation of sepsis. Fever is a very unreliable finding in the septic infant as most septic infants will be hypothermic. The septic infant is often pale, ashen, or even cyanotic, with the skin often cool and mottled owing to poor perfusion. The infant may seem lethargic, obtunded, or quite irritable. If there is marked tachycardia (heart rate approaching 200 bpm) together with tachypnoea (respiratory rate > 50 min^{-1}), this may herald a rapid collapse. Disseminated intravascular coagulopathy may develop manifest as scattered petechiae or purpura, suggesting a less than favourable

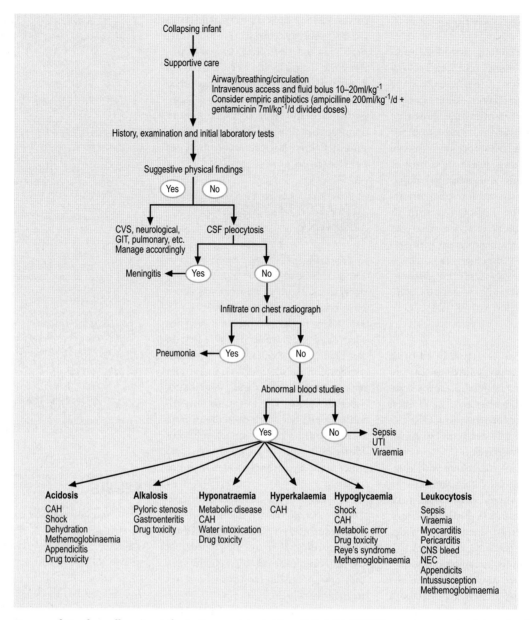

Fig. 26.1.1 Approach to the collapsing infant. (Source: Adapted from Selbst SM 1985 The septic-appearing infant. Paediatric Emergency Care 3: 160–167.)

outcome. If meningitis is present there may be a bulging or tense fontanelle with a high-pitched cry. If the infection has localised elsewhere, there may be otitis media, abdominal rigidity, joint swelling or tenderness in one extremity, or possibly chest findings, such as crackles. The disease may progress rapidly with the infant developing hypotension and/or frank shock.

A high index of suspicion is need, although the laboratory may be helpful in suggesting a diagnosis of sepsis, defini-

tive cultures require time for processing. A complete blood count may reveal a leukocytosis or left shift although this is often unreliable in infants. A coagulation profile may show evidence of disseminated intravascular coagulopathy, and blood chemistries may reveal hypoglycaemia or metabolic acidosis. Aspiration and Gram stain of urine, joint fluid, and spinal fluid, or pus from the middle ear may reveal the offending organism. Similarly, a chest X-ray may show a lobar infiltrate if pneumonia is present. A Gram stain of a pet-

echial scraping should be considered as this will often reveal the responsible organism.

VIRAL INFECTIONS

Overwhelming viral infections must be considered in the unwell-looking infant. Enteroviral infections in neonates commonly present as a sepsis-like illness. Respiratory distress will be present in all of these infants, and haemorrhagic manifestations, including gastrointestinal bleeding or bleeding into the skin, may be seen. Seizures often occur as well as icterus, splenomegaly, congestive heart failure and abdominal distension. Mortality rates for enteroviral infections in neonates are quite high. Epidemics of respiratory syncytial virus (RSV) occur in the winter, and infants may present with apnoea or respiratory distress with cyanosis. Those born prematurely, or with previous respiratory disorders, are especially susceptible to apnoea. These infants often appear septic. However, a knowledge of illness in the community and a predominance of respiratory signs may lead one to suspect RSV bronchiolitis. A rapid slide test for RSV will quickly be diagnostic. The chest X-ray shows diffuse patchy infiltrates and possibly lobar atelectasis.

CARDIAC DISEASE

When confronted with an unwell infant, cardiac disease should be considered. An infant with a ventriculoseptal defect, valvular insufficiency or stenosis, hypoplastic left heart syndrome, or coarctation of the aorta may present with congestive heart failure. The infant may arrive collapsed with clinical findings that are quite similar to those of sepsis. A chronic history of poor growth and poor feeding may suggest heart disease. The presence of a cardiac murmur is very suggestive that a structural lesion needs to be considered. The presence of a gallop rhythm, hepatomegaly, neck vein distension, and peripheral oedema should lead to the early consideration of primary cardiac pathology. Crackles, wheezing and intercostal retractions are non-specific findings that commonly present in either heart failure or pneumonia. A chest X-ray is the most useful investigation and will often show cardiac enlargement, pulmonary vascular engorgement or interstitial pulmonary oedema. This must be distinguished from the lobar infiltrates seen in pneumonia. An electrocardiogram (ECG) may be helpful in revealing certain congenital heart lesions, in particular in hypoplastic left heart syndrome where the ECG invariably shows right

axis deviation, with right atrial and ventricular enlargement. If primary cardiac pathology is considered an early consultation with a paediatric cardiologist should occur, as an urgent echocardiogram will be essential in making the definitive diagnosis. Another important cause of the collapsed infant to consider is a tight coarctation of the aorta. In this situation the commencement of prostaglandin E2 may be life saving, stabilising the infant so that urgent transfer to a tertiary centre can take place for definitive diagnosis and operative care.

Rarely, an infant with anomalous or obstructed coronary arteries will develop a myocardial infarction and appear initially as a collapsing septic infant. Such infants present with dyspnoea, cyanosis, vomiting, pallor, and general signs of cardiac heart failure. These infants may also have cardiomegaly on chest X-ray, and ECG changes of T-wave inversion and deep Q waves in leads I and AVL. There is a high level of urgency in transferring these infant to a tertiary centre where definitive investigation and specialist intensive care can be commenced.

An arrhythmia may cause an infant to appear quite ill. An infant with supraventricular tachycardia often presents with findings quite similar to those of a septic infant. This arrhythmia is most commonly idiopathic or may be associated with CHD drugs, fever, or infection. Infants with SVT often go unrecognised at home for days, initially only exhibiting poor feeding, fussiness, and rapid breathing. If untreated the infants will develop congestive heart failure often presenting in a collapsed state, with a heart rate in excess of 300 bpm. The ECG will show regular atrial and ventricular beats with 1:1 conduction and the chest X-ray may show cardiomegaly and pulmonary congestion. Management should begin with simple manoeuvres such as dunking the infant's face in a cold water/ice bath, if this is ineffective adenosine intravenously in increments of 50 μg kg^{-1} every two minutes until tachycardia resolves (maximum 4 mg). In those rare situations where there is no response to therapy, and the infant remains in heart failure, cardioversion should be considered.

Additional cardiac pathologies to be considered include myocarditis and pericarditis. Such infections are now most commonly due to *Staphylococcus aureus* and coxsackie B virus. These are often fulminant infections, and the baby with such a condition will appear critically ill. A complete physical examination may help to distinguish these conditions from other diagnoses in that signs of heart failure may be seen. Pericarditis may produce distant heart sounds together with a friction rub. Laboratory tests may be helpful, since a chest X-ray will show cardiomegaly and a suggestion of effusion if pericarditis is present. The ECG will show generalised T-wave inversion and low voltage QRS complexes, especially if pericardial fluid is present. Also, ST-T-wave abnormalities may be seen. The echocardiogram will confirm the presence or absence of a pericardial effusion.

ENDOCRINE DISORDERS

Infants with congenital adrenal hyperplasia (CAH) may present with a history of vomiting, lethargy, or irritability. On arrival, signs of marked dehydration may be present, with tachycardia and possibly hypothermia. A history of poor feeding from birth and symptoms that have progressed over a few days may distinguish this condition from sepsis. The physical examination can establish the diagnosis in females if ambiguous genitalia are noted. Metabolic disturbance is common with marked hyponatraemia with severe hyperkalaemia. Other non-specific laboratory findings include hypoglycaemia, acidosis, and peaked T waves or arrhythmias on the ECG. The finding of elevated urinary excretion of seventeen ketosteroids confirms the diagnosis. The infant should be referred to a tertiary centre where management will commence with steroid replacement tailored to the infant's underlying needs.

METABOLIC DISORDERS

Metabolic disorders may result from prolonged diarrhoea or vomiting producing dehydration, electrolyte disturbances, and acid–base abnormalities so that an infant will appear quite ill. These infants may have marked hyponatraemia, appear extremely lethargic, with slow respirations, hypothermia, and possibly seizures. Likewise, dehydrated infants with hypernatraemia may be lethargic or irritable with muscle weakness, seizures, or coma. Those infants with persistent vomiting may have hypochloraemic alkalosis with hypokalaemia, and they may appear weak or have cardiac dysfunction. Rare inborn errors of metabolism may produce vomiting in young infants who will then present with lethargy, seizures, or coma caused by metabolic acidosis, hyperammonaemia. or hypoglycaemia. It is thus essential to evaluate the electrolytes and blood sugar in young infants with significant symptoms of gastroenteritis, lethargy, or irritability and coma.

HAEMATOLOGIC DISORDERS

Any infant with severe anaemia or blood loss can look quite ill. In addition to anaemia, disorders of haemoglobin, such as methaemoglobinaemia can produce a toxic-appearing infant. This condition was reported when the local anaesthetic agent prilocaine was used in penile blocks for circumcision, (methaemoglobinaemia is a well-known adverse effect of excessive doses of this local anaesthetic). These infants may present with cyanosis, poor feeding, vomiting, diarrhoea, lethargy, hypothermia, tachycardia, tachypnoea, hypotension and severe acidosis. They appear mottled, cyanotic, or ashen, and oxygen administration does not affect the cyanosis. The diagnosis will be confirmed by a methaemoglobin level and if elevated to 65% (normal 0–2%) the infant should be transferred to intensive care and treatment with methylene blue considered.

GASTROINTESTINAL DISORDERS

Gastroenteritis even without electrolyte disturbances, can lead to severe dehydration in the infant with little reserve.

Bacterial infections like *Salmonella* and *Campylobacter* and even viral agents need to be considered. A stool smear that shows polymorphonuclear leukocytes is suggestive of bacterial infection.

Pyloric stenosis is most commonly seen in male infants 4–6 weeks of age and may cause severe vomiting with significant dehydration and lethargy without fever. A careful history reveals vomiting to be the predominant feature of the illness, and there may be a positive family history for pyloric stenosis. The physical examination may reveal an abdominal mass, or 'olive', in up to 50% of cases, this strongly suggests the diagnosis of pyloric stenosis. Electrolytes typically show hypochloraemia and hypokalaemia, and alkalosis is prominent. An abdominal ultrasound gives a definitive diagnosis in the majority of cases.

While intussusception is rare in infants less than five months old, some young infants may present with vomiting, fever, or signs of abdominal pain (legs drawn up, irritability). The infant may appear to have spasms of pain during which he/she is quite fretful. This can be followed by apathy and listlessness. Diarrhoea is a late sign as is the typical 'redcurrant jelly' stool. An abdominal mass may be palpated, however the diagnosis can be made using ultrasound. A plain film of the abdomen will show evidence of small bowel obstruction.

Several other unusual but important gastrointestinal disorders have to be considered in infants. Necrotising enterocolitis occurs in premature infants in the first few weeks of life and can also occur in term infants, usually within the first ten days of life. A history of an anoxic episode at birth, or other neonatal stresses, may suggest necrotising enterocolitis. These infants are quite ill with lethargy, irritability, and anorexia, as well as distended abdomen and bloody stools. Abdomen radiographs may be very helpful and usually show pneumatosis cystoides intestinalis because of gas in the intestinal wall. Neonatal appendicitis is a rare event, but several cases have been reported to closely mimic sepsis. The mortality for this disorder is close to 80%, and perforation obviously worsens

the prognosis. Thus, rapid diagnosis is essential. The most common presenting signs include irritability, vomiting, and abdominal distension on examination. There may also be hypothermia, ashen colour, and shock as the condition progresses. There may also be oedema of the abdominal wall, localised to the right flank, and possibly erythema of the skin in that area as well. The white blood cell count may be quite elevated with a left shift, and there may be a metabolic acidosis present, as well as disseminated intravascular coagulation. Abdominal radiographs may show a paucity of gas in the right lower quadrant, evidence of free peritoneal fluid, or an abnormally thickened right abdominal wall owing to oedema. Other unusual gastrointestinal emergencies to consider include volvulus, perforation due to trauma from enemas or thermometers, and Hirschsprung's enterocolitis.

NEUROLOGICAL DISEASE

The infant with infant botulism (*Clostridium botulinum*) may present with similar symptoms to an infant with collapse or sepsis. An infant with botulism will often be quite lethargic upon presentation to the ED, with a weak cry and possibly signs of dehydration. These infants are usually afebrile. If constipation has preceded the acute illness, botulism should be seriously considered. In Australia the disease is most commonly associated with the ingestion of honey. The parents may note a more gradual progression of this illness. Infants with botulism are notably hypotonic, hyporeflexic, and may have increased secretions due to bulbar muscle weakness. Also, the presence of a facial droop, ophthalmoplegia, and decreased gag reflex are consistent with botulism, while they remain unusual findings for a septic infant. A stool specimen to identify toxins of *Clostridium botulinum* may be diagnostic but requires considerable time for identification. Management is with good supportive care, an antitoxin exist but it is not readily available.

Intracranial haemorrhage secondary to non-accidental injury must be considered in the evaluation of the very ill infant. The history may or may not be helpful in establishing a diagnosis. The infant may appear gravely ill with apnoea, bradycardia, hypothermia, and bradypnea. Careful physical examination may suggest abuse rather than any other diagnosis. The head circumference is often above the 90th percentile, the fontanelle may be full or bulging and retinal haemorrhages are found. A computer-assisted tomography scan will usually demonstrate a small posterior, interhemispheric subdural haematoma. Referral to the appropriate authority for further investigation and ongoing management is now legally mandatory and a key component of the infant's acute care.

RESUSCITATION OF THE NEWBORN INFANT

The following is based on the ILCOR recommendations for newborn infants. Resuscitation of the newborn infant presents its own set of challenges. The transition from placental gas exchange in a liquid-filled intrauterine environment to spontaneous breathing of air requires dramatic physiological changes in the infant within the first minutes to hours after birth. Up to 10% of all newborn infants may require some degree of active resuscitation at birth. In most cases the need for resuscitation of the newborn infant can be predicted. However in the ED such circumstances may arise suddenly and may occur in facilities that do not routinely provide neonatal intensive care. With adequate anticipation, it is possible to optimise the delivery setting with appropriately prepared equipment and trained personnel who are capable of functioning as a team during neonatal resuscitation.

Neonatal resuscitation can be divided into four actions: (1) basic steps, which include rapid assessment and stabilisation; (2) ventilation; (3) chest compressions; and (4) administration of medications or fluids. Tracheal intubation may be required during any of these steps. All newborn infants require rapid assessment, including

examination for the presence of meconium in the amniotic fluid or on the skin; evaluation of breathing, muscle tone, and colour, and classification of gestational age as term or preterm. Newborn infants with a normal rapid assessment require only routine care (warmth, clearing the airway, drying). All others receive the initial steps, including warmth, clearing the airway, drying, positioning, stimulation to initiate or improve respirations, and oxygen as necessary. Subsequent evaluation and intervention are based on a triad of characteristics: (1) respirations; (2) heart rate; and (3) colour. Most newborn infants require only the basic steps, but for those who require further intervention, the most crucial action is establishment of adequate ventilation. Only a very small percentage will need chest compressions and medications.

EVALUATION OF THE NEWBORN

Determination of the need for resuscitative efforts should begin immediately after birth and proceed throughout the resuscitation process. An initial complex of signs (meconium in the amniotic fluid or on the skin, cry or respirations, muscle tone, colour, term or preterm gestation) should be evaluated rapidly and simultaneously by visual inspection. Actions are dictated by integrated evaluation rather than by evaluation of a single vital sign, followed by action on the result, and then evaluation of the next sign (sequential action). Evaluation and intervention for the newly born are often simultaneous processes, especially when more than one trained provider is present. To enhance educational retention, this process is often taught as a sequence of distinct steps. The appropriate response to abnormal findings also depends on the time elapsed since birth and how the infant has responded to previous resuscitative interventions.

Most newborn infants will respond to the stimulation of the extrauterine environment with strong inspiratory efforts, a vigorous cry, and movement of all extremities. If these responses are intact, colour improves steadily from cyanotic

or dusky to pink, and heart rate can be assumed to be adequate. The infant who responds vigorously to the extrauterine environment and who is term can remain with the mother to receive routine care (warmth, clearing the airway, drying). Indications for further assessment under a radiant warmer and possible intervention include: meconium in the amniotic fluid or on the skin, absent or weak responses, persistent cyanosis and preterm birth.

Further assessment of the newly born infant is based on the triad of respiration, heart rate, and colour. After initial respiratory efforts, the newly born infant should be able to establish regular respirations sufficient to improve colour and maintain a heart rate > 100 bpm. Gasping and apnoea are signs that indicate the need for assisted ventilation. Heart rate should be consistently > 100 bpm in an uncompromised newly born infant. An increasing or decreasing heart rate also can provide evidence of improvement or deterioration. An uncompromised newly born infant will be able to maintain a pink colour of the mucous membranes without supplemental oxygen. Pallor may be a sign of decreased cardiac output, severe anaemia, hypovolaemia, hypothermia, or acidosis.

BASIC STEPS

Preventing heat loss in the newborn is vital because cold stress can increase oxygen consumption and impede effective resuscitation. Placing the infant under a radiant warmer, rapidly drying the skin, removing wet linen immediately, and wrapping the infant in warm blankets will reduce heat loss. The infant's airway is cleared by positioning of the infant and removal of secretions by suctioning if needed. If respiratory efforts are present but not producing effective tidal ventilation, often the airway is obstructed. Immediate efforts must be made to correct over-extension or flexion or to remove secretions. Aggressive pharyngeal suction can cause laryngeal spasm and vagal bradycardia and delay the onset of spontaneous breathing. In the absence of meconium or blood, limit mechanical suction with a catheter in depth and duration. Negative pressure of the suction apparatus should not exceed 100 mmHg (13.3 kPa or 136 cmH$_2$O). If copious secretions are present, the infant's head may be turned to the side, and suctioning may help clear the airway. Maintaining proper head position may be helpful in up to 12% of deliveries.

SUCTIONING

If time permits, the person assisting delivery of the infant should suction the infant's nose and mouth with a bulb syringe after delivery of the shoulders but before delivery of the chest. Healthy, vigorous, newly born infants generally do not require suctioning after delivery. Secretions may be wiped from the nose and mouth with gauze or a towel. If suctioning is necessary, clear secretions first from the mouth and then the nose with a bulb syringe or suction catheter (8F or 10F). Aggressive pharyngeal suction can cause laryngeal spasm and vagal bradycardia and delay the onset of spontaneous breathing. In the absence of meconium or blood, limit mechanical suction with a catheter in depth and duration. Negative pressure of the suction apparatus should not exceed 100 mmHg (13.3 kPa or 136 cmH$_2$O). If copious secretions are present, the infant's head may be turned to the side, and suctioning may help clear the airway.

CLEARING THE AIRWAY OF MECONIUM

Approximately 12% of deliveries are complicated by the presence of meconium in the amniotic fluid. When the amniotic fluid is meconium-stained, suction the mouth, pharynx, and nose as soon as the head is delivered (intrapartum suctioning) regardless of whether the meconium is thin or thick using a large-bore suction catheter. Thorough suctioning of the nose, mouth, and posterior pharynx before delivery of the body appears to decrease the risk of meconium-aspiration syndrome. Nevertheless, a significant

number (20–30%) of meconium-stained infants will have meconium in the trachea despite such suctioning and in the absence of spontaneous respirations. This suggests the occurrence of in-utero aspiration and the need for tracheal suctioning after delivery in *depressed* infants. If the fluid contains meconium and the infant has absent or depressed respirations, decreased muscle tone, or heart rate < 100 bpm, perform direct laryngoscopy immediately after birth for suctioning of residual meconium from the hypopharynx (under direct vision) and intubation/suction of the trachea. Tracheal suctioning of the vigorous infant with meconium-stained fluid does not improve outcome. Accomplish tracheal suctioning by applying suction directly to a tracheal tube as it is withdrawn from the airway. Repeat intubation and suctioning until little additional meconium is recovered or until the heart rate indicates that resuscitation must proceed without delay. If the infant's heart rate or respiration is severely depressed, it may be necessary to institute positive-pressure ventilation despite the presence of some meconium in the airway. Delay gastric suctioning to prevent aspiration of swallowed meconium until initial resuscitation is complete. Meconium-stained infants who develop apnoea or respiratory distress should receive tracheal suctioning before positive-pressure ventilation, even if they are initially vigorous.

Drying and suctioning produce enough stimulation to initiate effective respirations in most newborn infants. Tactile stimulation may initiate spontaneous respirations in newly born infants who are experiencing primary apnoea. If these efforts do not result in prompt onset of effective ventilation, discontinue them because the infant is in secondary apnoea and positive-pressure ventilation will be required. Hypoxia is nearly always present in a newborn infant that requires resuscitation. Therefore, if cyanosis, bradycardia, or other signs of distress are noted in a breathing newborn during stabilisation, administration of 100% oxygen is indicated while determining the need for additional intervention. Free-flow oxygen can be delivered through a

face mask and flow-inflating bag, an oxygen mask, or a hand cupped around oxygen tubing. The oxygen source should deliver at least 5 L min^{-1}, and the oxygen should be held close to the face to maximise the inhaled concentration. Many self-inflating bags will not passively deliver sufficient oxygen flow (i.e. when not being squeezed). The goal of supplemental oxygen use should be normoxia. Sufficient oxygen should be administered to achieve pink colour in the mucous membranes. If cyanosis returns when supplemental oxygen is withdrawn, post-resuscitation care should include monitoring of administered oxygen concentration and arterial oxygen saturation.

VENTILATION

The key to successful neonatal resuscitation is establishment of adequate ventilation. Reversal of hypoxia, acidosis, and bradycardia depends on adequate inflation of fluid-filled lungs with air or oxygen. Most newborn infants who require positive-pressure ventilation can be adequately ventilated with a bag and mask. Indications for positive-pressure ventilation include apnoea or gasping respirations, heart rate < 100 bpm, and persistent central cyanosis despite 100% oxygen. Resuscitation bags used for neonates should be no larger than 750 ml and preferably self-inflating.

Although the pressure required for establishment of air breathing is variable and unpredictable, higher inflation pressures (30–40 cmH$_2$O or higher) and longer inflation times may be required for the first several breaths than for subsequent breaths. Visible chest expansion is a more reliable sign of appropriate inflation pressures than any specific manometer reading. The assisted ventilation rate should be 40–60 breaths per minute (30 breaths per minute when chest compressions are also being delivered). Signs of adequate ventilation include bilateral expansion of the lungs, as assessed by chest wall movement and breath sounds, and improvement in heart rate and colour. If ventilation is inadequate, check the seal between mask and face, clear any airway obstruction (adjust head position, clear secretions, open the infant's mouth), and finally increase inflation pressure. Prolonged bag-mask ventilation may produce gastric inflation and this should be relieved by insertion of an orogastric tube. If such manoeuvres do not result in adequate ventilation, endotracheal intubation should follow.

After thirty seconds of adequate ventilation with 100% oxygen, spontaneous breathing and heart rate should be checked. If spontaneous respirations are present and the heart rate is ≥ 100 bpm, positive-pressure ventilation may be gradually reduced and discontinued. Gentle tactile stimulation may help maintain and improve spontaneous respirations while free-flow oxygen is administered. If spontaneous respirations are inadequate, or if heart rate remains below 100 bpm, assisted ventilation must continue with bag and mask or tracheal tube. If the heart rate is < 60 bpm, continue assisted ventilation, begin chest compressions, and consider endotracheal intubation.

ENDOTRACHEAL INTUBATION

Endotracheal intubation may be indicated at several points during neonatal resuscitation: when tracheal suctioning for meconium is required; if bag-mask ventilation is ineffective or prolonged; when chest compressions are performed; when tracheal administration of medications is desired; or during special resuscitation circumstances, such as congenital diaphragmatic hernia or extremely low birth weight. The timing of endotracheal intubation may also depend on the skill and experience of the resuscitator. Perform endotracheal intubation orally, using a laryngoscope with a straight blade (size 0 for premature infants, size 1 for term infants). Insert the tip of the laryngoscope into the vallecula or onto the epiglottis and elevate gently to reveal the vocal cords. Cricoid pressure may be helpful. Insert the tube to an appropriate depth through the vocal cords as indicated by the vocal cord guide line and check its position by the centimetre

marking at the upper lip. Record and maintain this depth of insertion. Variation in head position will alter the depth of insertion and may predispose to unintentional extubation or endobronchial intubation.

After endotracheal intubation, confirm the position of the tube by the following: observing symmetrical chest-wall motion; listening for equal breath sounds, especially in the axillae, and for absence of breath sounds over the stomach; confirming the absence of gastric inflation; watching for a fog of moisture in the tube during exhalation and noting improvement in heart rate, colour, and activity of the infant.

CHEST COMPRESSIONS

Asphyxia causes peripheral vasoconstriction, tissue hypoxia, acidosis, poor myocardial contractility, bradycardia, and eventually cardiac arrest. Establishment of adequate ventilation and oxygenation will restore vital signs in the vast majority of newly born infants. Initiate chest compressions if there is a heart rate < 60 bpm, even if ventilation is adequate on 100% oxygen for thirty seconds. Because chest compressions may diminish the effectiveness of ventilation, do not initiate them until lung inflation and ventilation have been established. Provision of chest compressions is likely to compete with provision of effective ventilation. Coordinate compressions and ventilations to avoid simultaneous delivery. There should be a 3:1 ratio of compressions to ventilations, with 90 compressions and 30 breaths to achieve approximately 120 events per minute. Reassess the heart rate approximately every thirty seconds. Continue chest compressions until the spontaneous heart rate is ≥ 60 bpm.

DRUGS

Drugs are rarely indicated in resuscitation of the newborn infant. Bradycardia in the newly born infant is usually the result of inadequate lung inflation or profound hypoxia, and adequate ventilation is the most important step in

correcting bradycardia. Administer medications if, despite adequate ventilation with 100% oxygen and chest compressions, the heart rate remains < 60 bpm. Medications and fluids are easily administered via a peripheral intravenous cannula or umbilical venous catheter, the intraosseous route in less commonly needed in neonates.

Administration of adrenaline (epinephrine) is indicated when the heart rate remains < 60 bpm after a minimum of thirty seconds of adequate ventilation and chest compressions. Adrenaline is particularly indicated in the presence of asystole. The recommended intravenous or endotracheal dose is 0.1–0.3 mL kg^{-1} of a 1:10 000 solution (0.01–0.03 mg kg^{-1}), repeated every 3–5 minutes as indicated. Higher doses have been associated with exaggerated hypertension but lower cardiac output in animals. The sequence of hypotension followed by hypertension possibly increases the risk of intracranial haemorrhage, especially in preterm infants.

Volume expanders may be necessary to resuscitate a newly born infant who is hypovolaemic. Suspect hypovolaemia in any infant who fails to respond to resuscitation. Consider volume expansion when there has been suspected blood loss or the infant appears to be in shock (pale, poor perfusion, weak pulse) and has not responded adequately to other resuscitative measures. The fluid of choice for volume expansion is an isotonic crystalloid solution such as normal saline or Ringer's lactate. Administration of O-negative red blood cells may be indicated for replacement of large-volume blood loss. The initial dose of volume expander is 10 mL kg^{-1} given by slow intravenous push over 5–10 minutes. The dose may be repeated after further clinical assessment and observation of response. Higher bolus volumes have been recommended for resuscitation of older infants. However, volume overload or complications such as intracranial haemorrhage may result from inappropriate intravascular volume expansion in asphyxiated newly born infants as well as in preterm infants.

Use of sodium bicarbonate is discouraged during brief CPR. If it is used during prolonged arrests unresponsive to other therapy, it should be given only after establishment of adequate ventilation and circulation. Later use of bicarbonate for treatment of persistent metabolic acidosis or hyperkalaemia should be directed by arterial blood gas levels or serum chemistries, among other evaluations. A dose of 1–2 mEq kg^{-1} of a 0.5 mEq mL^{-1} solution may be given by slow intravenous push (over at least two minutes) after adequate ventilation and perfusion have been established.

Naloxone hydrochloride is a narcotic antagonist without respiratory-depressant activity. It is specifically indicated for reversal of respiratory depression in a newly born infant whose mother received narcotics within four hours of delivery. Always establish and maintain adequate ventilation before administration of naloxone. Do not administer naloxone to newly born infants whose mothers are suspected of having recently abused narcotic drugs because it may precipitate abrupt withdrawal signs in such infants. The recommended dose of naloxone is 0.1 mg kg^{-1} of a 0.4 mg mL^{-1} or 1.0 mg ml^{-1} solution given intravenously, endotracheally, or – if perfusion is adequate – intramuscularly or subcutaneously. Because the duration of action of narcotics may exceed that of naloxone, continued monitoring of respiratory function is essential, and repeated naloxone doses may be necessary to prevent recurrent apnoea.

FURTHER READING

Alexander R, Crabbe L, Sato Y et al 1990 Serial abuse in children who are shaken. American Journal of Diseases in Childhood 144: 58–60

Brazelton TB 1962 Crying in infancy. Paediatrics 29: 579–88

Carey WB 1994 The effectiveness of parent counseling in managing colic. Paediatrics 94(3): 333–334

Forsyth BWC 1989 Colic and the effect of changing formulas: A double blind, multiple-crossover study. Journal of Paediatrics 115: 521–526

Holzki J, Laschat M, Stratmann C 1998 Stridor in the neonate and infant. Implications for the paediatric anaesthetist. Prospective description of 155 patients with congenital and acquired stridor in early infancy. Paediatric Anaesthesia 8(3): 221–227

ILCOR 1999 International Liaison Committee on Resuscitation (ILCOR). Advisory statement: Resuscitation of the newly born infant. Paediatrics103: 56

Illingworth RS 1954 Three month's colic. Archives of Diseases in Childhood 145: 165–174

Lucassen PLBJ, Assendelft WJJ, Gubbels JW et al 1998 Effectiveness of treatments for infantile colic: Systemic review. British Medical Journal 316: 1563–1569

McKenzie S 1991 Troublesome crying in infants: Effect of advice to reduce stimulation. Archives of Diseases in Childhood 66: 1416-1420

Millar KR, Gloor JE, Wellington N, Joubert G 2000 Early neonatal presentations to the paediatric ED. Paediatric Emergency Care 16(3): 145–150

Poole SR 1991 The infant with acute, unexplained, excessive crying. Paediatrics 88(3): 450–455

Selbst SM 1985 The septic-appearing infant. Paediatric Emergency Care 3: 160–167

Singer JI, Rosenberg NM 1992 A fatal case of colic. Paediatric Emergency Care 8(3): 171–172

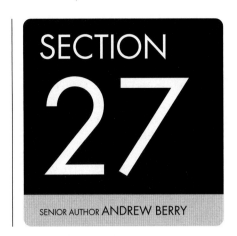

SENIOR AUTHOR ANDREW BERRY

TRANSPORT AND RETRIEVAL

27.1 EMERGENCY MEDICAL TRANSPORT AND RETRIEVAL

ANDREW BERRY

ESSENTIALS

1 Children are different from adults and have different needs during medical retrieval. Early consultation with clinicians skilled in paediatric critical care is encouraged. Their advice can assist in making a diagnosis, determining treatment and the urgency for transfer.

2 Careful stabilisation of the child pre-transfer achieves the best clinical outcome. Stabilisation is undertaken immediately by staff at the referring hospital often under the supervision of medical experts through the use of teleconferencing.

3 The transport network has the responsibility for the organisation of a clinical escort, retrieval transfer and type of vehicle. The centralisation of the retrieval network ensures this occurs in a rapid and seamless manner.

4 The medical retrieval team is especially equipped and trained to handle all situations that may be encountered during patient transfer and hence are the preferred clinical escort.

5 The key to good patient outcome throughout this process remains effective communication.

INTRODUCTION

This chapter addresses the secondary transportation of patients. Primary transport is beyond the scope of this chapter. In particular, the role of 'medical retrieval' is discussed. Most medical retrieval transports of children require an emergency response because the problem is time-critical.

It is often said that children are not small adults and in several important respects their physiology, pathophysiology and behaviour are different from adults. In patient transport, not only are these differences relevant, but the organisation of critical care services and hospital networks is also different. There is a more centralised organisation of specialist and intensive medical care for children than adults and this has implications for their transport and how transport systems are delivered.

REGIONALISATION

Different hospitals within a region offer differing levels of care for children. There are broadly three levels of care for children: (1) basic; (2) specialist; and (3) tertiary. In Australia and New Zealand, intensive or critical care tends to be centralised to a few tertiary hospitals. (There are twenty-two neonatal ICUs in Australia and six in New Zealand. There are seven full-time paediatric ICUs in Australia and one in New Zealand. Some adult units have a specialist interest in paediatric ICU as well.) This principle is based on evidence that a 'centralised' approach produces better outcomes than having a larger number of hospitals in a region each doing a small amount of critical care.[1,2] As a result:

- Most newborns likely to need critical care are delivered in tertiary perinatal centres where neonatal intensive care is available on site and from birth. Progressive improvements are being achieved in selecting more and more high-risk pregnancies for a more appropriate place of birth.
- Newborns with major surgical conditions or complex medical problems requiring intensive care are treated in children's hospitals.
- Infants and children requiring major surgery or intensive care are treated in children's hospitals.

Basic hospitals admit children with non-life-threatening illnesses. Regional and urban hospitals with specialist paediatric services take care of children with significant illness but not those needing intensive care. Children who need intensive care will usually require a medical retrieval team to move them safely to a tertiary hospital. Other children admitted to rural or basic hospitals with less-critical conditions may be appropriate for transfer and admission to a regional specialist hospital.

WHAT'S DIFFERENT ABOUT CHILDREN?

This general question is addressed in other chapters. However, from a transport point of view, the type of illness or injury and the process by which a clinical diagnosis is reached are often different in children. For instance, some conditions, such as bronchiolitis, are not only largely unique to children, but manifest in quite different ways from adults. In the first few months of life, presentation with 'apnoea' along with a history of close-family upper respiratory infection suggests this diagnosis even though there may be no signs of respiratory distress or problem with gas exchange. Making this diagnosis is often possible 'over the phone' by means of clinicians who are experienced in paediatric critical care offering advice. Assessing conscious state in a young child with a head injury requires knowledge of developmental milestones. A baby presenting unexpectedly at one week of age with 'shock' is more likely to have a congenital heart lesion, such as left heart obstruction, than more traditional causes of shock. These and other examples require patient transfer decisions to be made by clinicians aware of these differences and skilled in eliciting information that will clarify the situation.

REFERRING A PATIENT TO ANOTHER HOSPITAL

Referring doctor/hospital → Referral doctor/hospital

Referring a patient for a higher level of care involves a dialogue between clinicians. For emergency transfers this generally involves a telephone call to a selected *referral* hospital or physician. The referrer usually makes this selection on the basis that the referral clinician has the skills and resources to deal with the problem and is geographically proximate. Although a simple and intuitive relationship, the referral of a critical-care patient can be confounded by resource and logistic issues with the potential to prevent or impair an appropriate and constructive clinical discussion. The process of telephone triage (teletriage) is a skill requiring careful listening and intelligent questioning. It is not learnt overnight. Clinical discussion should precede and determine the logistics of transport, not the other way around.

This referral dialogue is complicated by the process of deciding what level of care the patient requires and therefore whether or not to call a regional or tertiary hospital. Some regional specialist or major urban hospitals offer tertiary-level care, such as adult intensive care, or are designated trauma centres. Although they may treat adults with the same condition, they don't cater for children with a similar level of injury or illness and definitive care of a child, such as surgery, involves transferring the child to a children's hospital. Although emergency departments and surgical facilities may be quite sophisticated, the post-acute care facilities available within those hospitals (paediatric wards) are generally not suitable places for continuing care. Decisions about how these children move and whether transport should be to a regional

hospital or a tertiary hospital can be difficult. Sometimes a discussion with both will help determine the best plan. Moreover, the appropriate place of care and the best transport solution will be different from those required by adults.

The relationships between the three levels of care are shown diagrammatically in Fig. 27.1.1.

A dialogue with one referral hospital option may recommend that the other is a more appropriate destination. Unfortunately, a series of discussions with different referral hospitals can be time-consuming and may interfere with direct patient care.

Various means have been introduced to streamline this process. In some referral hospitals, there is often a designated person available to take such calls. Occasionally, a specific telephone number in the referral hospital is advertised for that purpose. However, if that number takes the referrer down a one-way path (e.g. to a personal cellular phone), he or she may need to make other calls or await a 'call-back'. Now that hospital voice-response systems with menus designed for the public and long queues awaiting an operator have become common, simply calling the switchboard of a hospital no longer provides 'direct' access for the referring doctor.

In an ideal world the referring doctor would make just one call. After all, the clinical problem, which by definition exceeds them and/or their hospital, often requires their full attention. Subverting their clinical activities to make several (or many) phone calls can significantly compromise patient care and out-

come. As referral hospitals become busier and/or more efficient, the availability of resources to care for the patient can dominate the referral process. Too often, the question of whether a 'Bed' (defined as: Space + Equipment + Nurses + Doctors + Other Resources) is available intrudes on the referral call and can interrupt the conversation with an invitation to 'try elsewhere'. Whenever the clinical referral process becomes a question of 'bed-finding', many referring doctors respond by delegating the task to others. Such staff won't necessarily have any clinical knowledge of the patient or the problem requiring transfer. Some referral hospitals have similarly delegated the process of 'bed-locating' to managers whose focus is on managing the 'bed' resource rather than entering into a clinical discussion about the patient. This combination results in lost opportunities for clinical decisions that can change the course of events independently of the transport process. For instance, an incorrect diagnosis or treatment may be recognised and corrected as the result of a clinical discussion. Having discussed the patient, an alternative referral hospital may be recommended on 'clinical' grounds. Such a conversation is possible, regardless of bed availability.

In some regions, where there are several referral hospitals serving the same referring hospitals, a single point of contact is provided for transport of a critical-care patient. In most cases, however, such 'single number' systems are designed to facilitate the logistics of transport and the clinical referral process requires a separate, additional phone call. Translated simply this amounts to: 'find the bed and we'll arrange transport'. An integrated approach is possible, where the same number is used not only as a clinical conduit into the referral hospital 'system' but also to activate the logistics of transport.[3]

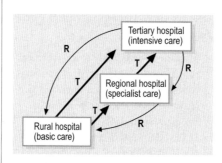

Fig. 27.1.1   The relationship between the three levels of care.

WHICH PATIENTS?

Selecting patients for retrieval depends on the threshold for referral in each hospital. The important point is that discussing the possibility of transfer should be part of a clinical consultation. The following list suggests conditions that should prompt that discussion with a paediatric ICU or retrieval service:

❶ Head injury (symptomatic).
❷ Altered level of consciousness (for any reason).
❸ Hypoxia despite oxygen therapy.
❹ High oxygen requirement.
❺ Respiratory failure (e.g. bronchiolitis, severe asthma, apnoea).
❻ Upper airway obstruction.
❼ Near drowning (especially with neurological depression or respiratory symptoms).
❽ Ingestion with risk of circulatory, airway or neurological compromise.
❾ Envenomation.
❿ Burns:
  • >10%
  • Encircling the neck or involving the airway, face, hands, feet, perineum, or inner joint surfaces
  • Associated other significant injury
  • Electrical or chemical burns.
⓫ Seizures (with persisting neurological depression).
⓬ Major trauma (including spinal injury)
⓭ Metabolic disturbance, e.g.
  • Diabetic ketoacidosis
  • Acidaemia
  • Severe biochemical abnormality.
⓮ Heart failure or arrhythmia (symptomatic).
⓯ Shock (requiring treatment with volume replacement or inotropes), e.g.
  • Blood or fluid loss
  • Dehydration
  • Septicaemia.
⓰ Other causes of neurological depression:
  • CNS infection
  • Acute life-threatening episode.
⓱ Any condition with the potential for sudden cardiovascular or neurological deterioration.

Adapting such a list may be helpful in determining the local policy. If in doubt, *consult*.

WHO WILL MOVE THE PATIENT AND HOW?

After an appropriate clinical discussion, the question of how the patient should be moved can be addressed. This can be straightforward or complex, depending on circumstances. The transfer of any patient from referring hospital to referral hospital can be accomplished in several ways. In a *patient transfer*, an escort transports the patient and then returns (in Fig. 27.1.1, T followed by R). In a *retrieval transfer*, the dispatch of a team (response) is followed by patient transport (R followed by T).

Decisions need to be made about three main topics:

❶ Clinical escort.
  a. Patient transfer:
    • Ambulance officer (various levels may be available)
    • Nurse
    • Doctor.
  b. Retrieval transfer:
    • Flight nurse or flight paramedic
    • Doctor (medical retrieval)
    • Other.
❷ Degree of urgency.
  a. Urgent (immediate response).
  b. Emergency (specify expectation of response).
  c. Time window (before a particular time).
  d. Elective.
❸ Type of vehicle.
  a. Surface (road, boat, train, etc.).
  b. Air:
    • Rotary wing
    • Fixed wing.

A patient transfer is one in which the skill level of the escort is below or at that of the referring hospital. That is, the patient can be escorted by ambulance personnel (*ambulance transfer*). Alternatively, staff from the referring hospital may accompany the patient (*medical or nursing transfer*). In theory these options offer a more rapid process, although review of actual experience often shows that time benefits can be overrated. Using local resources on an ad hoc basis is often slower to mobilise than anticipated. A

doctor or nurse from the referring hospital may well offer an adequate level of care but the implications for that hospital during their absence may include a significant staffing reduction for that hospital. The smaller the hospital, the greater the impact that this will have on local cover and, since distances tend to be greater for smaller hospitals, the longer this impact will last. A hospital clinician who, having cared for the patient for some time already, then leaves town escorting a patient may experience significant fatigue. There may be problems finding transport back.

On the other hand, the level of care available to the patient should not regress during the transport process. Indeed, care should increase at each stage of the patient's progress through the system. If the patient's condition is unstable, it may be better to continue treatment in the referring hospital and await the arrival of a retrieval team.

In the retrieval transfer, options for clinical escort include a flight nurse or paramedic attached to an air ambulance service. Exact team composition will vary according to local practice and the regulations governing the skills and certification required for administration of specific treatments and drugs.

Doctors participate in medical retrieval teams in Europe, South Africa and Australasia but less so in North America. Most doctors are tasked from the referral hospital but others are attached as a regional or state-wide retrieval service.

The principle of medical retrieval is to bring the required critical care skills to the patient from an ICU setting and initiate that care prior to transport. In a randomised trial, medical retrieval has been shown to offer significant benefits to preterm infants in terms of mortality and morbidity.[4] However, evidence is not so strong in older age groups. Medical retrieval offers a higher level of care both during transport and, importantly, prior to travel. Patients can be stabilised prior to transport using skills and equipment not normally available in the referring hospital. This approach is preferable to hurriedly rushing from A to B with the patient in an unstable condition (the 'mercy dash') and risking en-route deterioration. To the extent that the arrival of the retrieval team in the referring hospital represents the patient's 'arrival' in intensive care, the patient should not suffer any time penalty from using the 'retrieval' rather than the 'transfer' strategy.

The exceptions are conditions requiring a procedure or an investigation that a retrieval team cannot supply. In children, the proportion of situations where this is the case appears to be smaller than in adults. Examples include head injury requiring urgent neurosurgery, some cases of penetrating trauma, volvulus with ischaemia and transposition of the great arteries with intact septum.

On the other hand, there is the additional time awaiting the arrival of the 'retrieval team'. It is often tempting to say, 'we could have been there by now!' However, young children and newborns travel poorly if inadequately stabilised and the lost ground may never be regained.

Assessing the level of urgency requires assessment of how quickly skills or intervention are required in the referring hospital and also how quickly the patient needs definite care in a referral hospital. In most cases, the operational response in reaching the patient is more relevant.

DEGREES OF URGENCY

Urgent The patient is in extremis, or is deteriorating, or needs immediate, time-critical therapy.

Emergency The patient has a serious condition and the treatment required is not possible in the referring hospital.

Time window The patient needs to be at the destination by a certain time - there is a latest time by which the transfer should be concluded.

Elective The timing of transfer is discretionary – hours or days.

The factors determining how quickly a team can be at the bedside include:

❶ Geographical distance.
❷ Modes of transport available.

❸ Functional distance:
  • Team availability
  • Vehicle availability
  • Accessibility
  • Number of vehicle changes.

Looking at a map to judge the time to reach the patient may be misleading. When alternative modes of transport are available, fixed wing is roughly twice the speed of helicopter and helicopter twice the speed of surface transport by road. However, the process of activating a helicopter or plane with a team on board can mean the overall response time is double or triple the flight time. The response time also includes components of travel after the flight, which may involve ground transport. The more vehicle changes that are required, the greater the overall time. Each vehicle change adds significantly to the total time. Traditionally, arbitrary distance arcs are specified to help in selecting between road, helicopter and fixed wing options. However, the cut-over from one mode of transport to another in any particular system of retrieval needs to be determined around functional distance rather than geographical distance.

No matter how fast a vehicle travels the availability of a suitable vehicle and/ or team may delay departure. Therefore deployment by road may sometimes result in a more rapid response time than by air. For a particular referring hospital, the choice of appropriate vehicle (road, helicopter or fixed wing) may differ from time to time.

Good data about actual response times involved in previous cases can inform the decision-making process. Such information is much more useful than simple speed versus distance graphs.

In some cases, the choice of vehicle for the patient transport phase is different from that selected for team mobilisation. If, for instance, a helicopter could not respond because of availability or weather and the retrieval was launched by road, it may be possible, and clinically appropriate, as the weather improves, to use a helicopter for the next 'leg'. When stabilisation times are significant, the use of different vehicles for the outbound and inbound legs of a retrieval may make better use of those vehicles without impairing the clinical process.

WHILE WAITING

The clinical discussion with the referral hospital should include specifics of the actual condition of the patient, their current treatment and a clearly communicated plan of management. Depending on the confidence of the referring doctor about these issues, this discussion may require more or less input from the referral doctor. Telephone advice is always valuable. Such consultation is even more relevant when distance and the time taken to reach definitive care increases. The expertise of specialists in paediatric ICU, ED, surgery, burns, neonatology, and other paediatric disciplines, as well as toxicology and envenomation experts, is available by telephone through regional, state and national networks.

STABILISATION

Stabilisation is intended to reduce the risk of 'en route' deterioration, improve tolerance of transport and increase the safety of the process.

All patients should receive a certain amount of stabilisation prior to transport, whether their departure is imminent (as is generally the goal if a local escort is planned) or delayed until a retrieval team has arrived to transport them.

Transport medicine is not so much about how a patient is managed in a mobile setting but how to prepare for the transport process. Stabilisation involves 'packaging' the patient so that basic physiology is controlled, with airway, breathing and circulation supported. The threshold for intervening in each of these areas is reduced for patients being moved. A successful stabilisation is one in which the risk of an unplanned intervention being necessary en route is reduced to a negligible level. Rigorous attention is required to the patency and security of the artificial airway and vascular lines. These lines and other connections to the patient, such as non-invasive monitoring probes, ECG leads, transducers and drains, should be positioned in such a way that there is no physical force causing either traction or torsion. Despite firm fixation, these forces will cause dislodgement in transit.

PRINCIPLES OF MEDICAL RETRIEVAL

The 'stay and play' approach is the default for children and 'wrap and run' the exception. The 'golden hour' philosophy can be mistakenly applied to paediatric patients. It relies on battlefield experience and the principle that the outcome depends on the patient being on the operating table in less than an hour from injury. This principle evolved from management of penetrating trauma in military personnel during the Vietnam war and is rarely relevant to critically ill or injured children – particularly when the have already presented to a health facility and some or all of that 'hour' has already gone. It is tempting for rescue retrieval services, who normally deal with adults, to take this approach with children and arrive with a patient who then needs post-transport resuscitation.

Improvements in the responsiveness of retrieval teams have shortened the 'R' phase. This is gradually eroding the reflex tendency to 'wrap and run' with the patient in the hope that their condition will survive a 'mercy dash'. Such improvements are occurring through use of dedicated retrieval teams, on-site staffing and more readily available and/or faster forms of transport. Additional strategies include pre-alerting of the system during the pre-hospital phase of a major case, encouraging earlier referral by the referring hospital and more streamlined processes occurring in parallel rather than in series.

COMPARING ADULT PRACTICE

In recent years medical retrieval services for adults have developed and are now found in both metropolitan and regional centres. It is important that paediatric clinicians have input into decisions made about any older children whom these services might plan to transport. Many older children may be appropriately moved by an adult team. Good communication between the clinical players is essential; particularly if the referring hospital calls the regional hospital that has an adult retrieval capability and it seems clear that the child is likely to need a higher level of care. In some rural emergencies, a joint response to the primary hospital by both a regional service and a specialist paediatric retrieval team may be appropriate. After such a joint response, the optimum destination for the patient can be determined (regional hospital or specialist children's hospital).

Medical retrieval teams that mostly deal with adults are often inclined to be fairly aggressive in controlling the airway. Unnecessary intubation and mechanical ventilation only complicates the post-transport management in the ICU and a little more time spent in assessment and stabilisation of, for instance, seizure disorder may obviate this intervention.

ACCOMPANYING PARENTS?

Parents will often wish to remain with their child. Sometimes the presence of a parent may be therapeutic if it has a calming affect on an otherwise distressed child. The child who is aware but has significant upper airway obstruction or respiratory failure is a good example. In other cases the parent may not be required to make the child's transport safe but it seems unreasonable not to make provision for a parent to travel in the ambulance or aircraft, where possible. Vehicle specifications should allow for a parent to be accommodated in paediatric medical retrievals. Should a parent be unwell themselves (e.g. a post-natal mother after an operative delivery or a parent injured in a multiple trauma case), their medical needs cannot reasonable be catered for by a medical retrieval team whose focus is on the child. Clinicians making decisions about moving these parents should judge the risks and safety of their transfer independently of the child and, if it is appropriate to move them, a suitable escort should be provided.

PREVENTION

The retrieval process is not an end in itself. If possible, patients should not be allowed to reach a level of clinical severity needing intensive care. Some of this involves general preventative strategies in health care and injury prevention. Those patients that do come to intensive care should, where possible, present directly to the appropriate facility. Of course, geography makes this goal unachievable in many cases. However, processes that seek to have the pre-hospital response deliver the patient to the right hospital, bypassing less-well-equipped hospitals, are becoming more sophisticated. Trends towards greater centralisation in health-care organisation make this goal harder to achieve and the retrieval process is likely to be more frequently applied in the future. A summary of preventative strategies includes:

❶ Reduce the need.
   a. Injury prevention and immunisation programs, better interval care of recurrent severe conditions, such as asthma.
   b. Recognise the fetus at-risk of needing ICU or urgent surgery or other intervention.
   c. Plan for high-risk births to occur in a tertiary perinatal centre (major surgical and cardiac conditions).
   d. Facilitate emergency transfer of women when that will result in the birth occurring in the appropriate hospital – in particular, in preterm labour.
❷ Assist and support all participants and players (including remote, rural, regional and metropolitan hospitals) with resources, education and support to optimise the care of seriously ill or injured patients at every stage of the process.
❸ Conduct quality activities – including audit, incident monitoring, case review.
❹ Amelioration:
   a. Telemedicine – improve the referral process by adding images to enhance simple telephone conversations.

b. Improved data interfaces between hospital systems to increase the information flow between referring hospital, retrieval team and referral hospital.

EXPECTATIONS AND ROLES

What are the expectations of those participating in the retrieval process? There are four key players:

❶ The referring clinician.
❷ The receiving clinician.
❸ The transport service.
❹ The transport clinician.

An organised and streamlined interaction between these components is required for the best results. What follows is a summary of the expectations, roles and responsibilities of each of them.

The referring clinician

- Expects to make just one phone call to initiate the process.
- Focuses on the basic principles:
  Airway, breathing, circulation, for a child
  'Warm, pink and sweet', for a newborn.
- Provides basic details of history, assessment, examination and interventions.
- Nominates a preferred destination, based on clinical need, proximity, family, etc.

The receiving clinician

- Offers telephone advice about management.
- Elicits appropriate additional information from the referrer.
- Assumes some responsibility for the patient and the solution of their problem.
- Accepts the transfer or ensures that an appropriate alternative is arranged.
- Ensures that others within the tertiary hospital are informed and involved.
- Is available to advise the referrer and/or transport team about further management.
- Reviews professional and service practice in quality activities.

The transport service

- Assesses the level of clinical care required to transport the patient.
- Selects the most appropriate (based on clinical skills) and best available (most timely) team to treat and escort the patient.
- Chooses the most appropriate transport vehicle (road or air; rotary or fixed wing) through liaison with ambulance and other vehicle providers.
- Offers a link between the referring clinician and receiving physician. This is particularly relevant when there are several potential destination units.

The transport clinician

- Participates in, or is informed about, prior clinical discussions about the patient.
- Prepares for the obvious and considers the not-so-obvious possibilities while outbound to the patient.
- Assesses the patient at 'first look' and acts according to clinical need.
- May re-triage the patient to a different level of care and/or initiate an alternative transport plan.
- Chooses between rapid-sequence and full stabilisation retrieval.
- Stabilises the patient.
- Communicates with receiving clinician(s), as appropriate.

WHAT EQUIPMENT?

Medical equipment used for patients in transport needs to be adequate to the task, robust and capable of operating at all stages of the process. It should be secured in the vehicle according to the applicable safety standards for that vehicle. A monitor or ventilator attached to an IV pole by friction nut or lying in the bed near the patient is not safely restrained in a moving vehicle.

Power requirements of the equipment and battery capacities should be thoroughly understood. Electrically powered devices should be able to utilise external power, where possible.

Medical oxygen and medical air should be available to supply constant flows or drive mechanical ventilators. Some ventilators do not require a supply of medical air.

Most modern monitors designed for transport are appropriate for children if they have suitable transducers for age for oxygen saturation monitoring, appropriate algorithms for non-invasive blood pressure measurement and selectable respiratory waveforms. Monitoring of temperature, blood pressure (nIBP and IBP), oxygen saturation, ECG and end-tidal CO_2 should be available. For the newborn, skin surface oxygen and CO_2 tension is often added.

Infusion pumps are no longer age-specific and most are capable of driving fluids at accurate low rates suitable for young children.

There are many mechanical ventilators designed for adults that are also suitable for children over the weight of about 20 kg. There are also ventilators suitable for newborns and infants up to about 5 kg. However, the patient weighing 5–20 kg presents some difficulties and a suitable transport ventilator may be hard to find.

Defibrillation equipment suitable for children should be available in the referring hospital and, in selected cases, to the team in transit. The requirement for cardioversion is quite rare in childhood and the need can *usually* be anticipated.

A portable point of care testing unit for blood gas analysis and basic chemistry is particularly useful. Even in referring hospitals with such facilities, the improved turn-around time to obtain a result may utilise the team's time far more efficiently.

Stretchers are not normally designed for young children and it is necessary to rely on paediatric immobilisation systems or restraint systems that interface between the patient and an 'adult' stretcher. Spinal immobilisation requires an age-appropriate spinal board and careful selection of cervical collars – particularly in smaller children and infants.

All equipment should be tested for electromagnetic interference and radiation. That is, their susceptibility to external radiofrequency interference as well as their ability to adversely affect aircraft navigation systems. Specific items of transport equipment have been certified for use in aircraft.

The pack carried by teams should include basic and advanced life-support equipment. For inter-facility transports, some reliance on referring hospital equipment is reasonable. However, for any foreseeable need during transport itself, self-reliance is essential. On the other hand, carrying too many items or too many of a particular item can be a disadvantage. It is not possible to cater for absolutely every contingency and a 'reasonable' inventory is the product of common sense and experience.

WHICH VEHICLE?

The most frequently available transport vehicles include road ambulances, fixed-wing planes and helicopters. The choice of vehicle depends on the nature of the distance and the total time involved in the outward and return journeys and the requirements of the patient's illness or injury. Other considerations may include availability of airports or helipads for aircraft, and weather conditions.

Remember it is not the vehicle per se that is important to the patient – it is the maximisation of available treatment, in the least time reasonably possible, and movement to the tertiary centre in a careful, safe and controlled manner.

Each vehicle type has advantages and disadvantages.

Road vehicles

These are relatively slow, and are even slower if the patient cannot tolerate much movement and the driver travels cautiously to compensate. The driver can stop if required by the team, allowing the team to re-evaluate the situation and possibly perform a procedure, such as suction, intubation or chest-tube insertion.

Road vehicles are at the mercy of road congestion – even if use is made of warning devices such as lights and sirens to expedite progress.

Most road ambulance vehicles are constructed on a rigid chassis and have relatively stiff suspension. A fully configured ambulance is quite heavy, with handling and ride quality akin to a truck. For a patient with a painful injury or dis-

ease process, a road journey on anything worse than ideal road surfaces can be a very painful one. Patients with unstable cardiorespiratory status often tolerate poor road surfaces badly and need more aggressive support and/or increase sedation, analgesia or muscle relaxation to improve the situation.

Road transfers generally involve less handling, since the patient is loaded and unloaded only once. The exception is that some ambulance services conduct long-distance road trips using multiple road crews in relay.

Helicopters

These are fast and travel point to point. They generally offer a smooth trip although turbulence can have an impact on the patient as well as the team. The efficiency of a helicopter is highly dependent on whether they can offer 'door to door' service. If a road ambulance is required to provide transport between landing site and hospital, their efficiency is compromised. Even short trips by road to the helipad add substantially to the time factor. The handling of the stretcher and patient from one vehicle to another is more important that the actual road distance.

Helicopters expose the patient to the effects of altitude. The amplitude and frequency of airframe vibration in helicopters vary according to type of blade system and the number of blades in the main rotor. Most patients seem to tolerate higher frequencies associated with multi-blade aircraft better than two-bladed machines. Anecdotal experience is that newborns with persistent pulmonary hypertension actually improve as a result of these vibrations. These observations have not been tested.

Fixed-wing aircraft

These offer speed and, if pressurised, can fly higher at levels less exposed to weather and turbulence. Pressurisation systems are not designed to make patient transport easier for medical retrieval teams. They are intended to provide physiologically tolerable conditions for healthy passengers at altitudes that would not normally be comfortable. Think of it as being at the elevation of Mount Everest (29 035 ft) but

in a cabin pressure altitude (CPA), effectively no higher than Mount Kosciusko (7310 ft). Healthy passengers travel reasonably comfortably at altitudes up to about 10 000 ft.

Patients at increased altitude can find their problems with oxygen delivery exacerbated and trapped internal fluids (gases and liquids) subject to expansion according to Boyle's law. A patient with marginal oxygenation may not tolerate a substantial altitude and trapped gases in the gut, pleural space or pericardium should be vented to atmosphere prior to flight. Otherwise, ground transport or transport by fixed-wing aircraft pressurised at or close to sea level should be used. Not all fixed-wing aircraft can pressurise the cabin to sea level equivalence – at least not without operating at a significantly lower actual altitude. Aircraft pressurisation cannot be activated on the ground, even if the airport is quite high and the patient might benefit from 'descending' to denser air. In a flight originating from an airport at a significant elevation and intending to land at sea level or at a significantly lower elevation, the pilot can dial up the destination altitude quite soon after take off. This strategy can be quite helpful in a marginal patient.

Weather factors

Both helicopters and fixed-wing aircraft are subject to weather limitations. Operated under visual flight rules (VFR), either type of aircraft can be mobilised quite quickly by day. A brief assessment of the weather is adequate and, if suitable for flight, the aircraft can be airborne within minutes. The pilot navigates by visual reference to the ground and recognisable landmarks. Short-range helicopter operations are particularly suitable for this kind of operation.

At night and in poor weather, instrument flight rules (IFR) operations are generally used. A totally different approach to the planning and conduct of the flight is required. For most of the flight the pilot cannot assume that anything outside is visible and all navigation and descent to land at the destination relies on the instruments in front of him.

The weather conditions at the departure point, en route and at the destination must all be assessed. Not only must the pilot be able to take off visually, but the in-flight conditions must be compatible with the aircraft's capabilities. If the expected weather conditions at the destination fall below specified minima, an alternative landing site with better weather conditions must be within range. The logical algorithms by which such assessments are made are unambiguous, quantifiable and not open to subjectivity. The process of IFR planning leads the pilot to give either a 'go' or 'no go' decision. The planning process might be quite complex and at least thirty minutes may be required to reach a conclusion about the flight's feasibility. A decision to go may not guarantee arrival at the intended destination. It simply says that the flight to reach that location can be attempted safely in the knowledge that landing at an alternative location (including the departure point) is factored in.

As an oversimplification, modern fixed-wing aircraft are able to operate in most weather conditions. Helicopters cannot fly in cloud that is close to freezing point or in severe turbulence. Neither type of aircraft can operate through contiguous lines of thunderstorm activity or when fog is present for take off or landing.

COMMUNICATIONS

The process of discussing a referral and triaging the optimal transport solution relies on good communication. Earlier, reference has been made to easy access to the key personnel in the referral hospital. Subsequently, the lines of communication need to be maintained so that any change in the patient's condition or further advice sought about management can be conveyed effectively. During transport, transfer and retrieval teams should have the ability to call and be called at any phase of the process. Relaying messages through non-clinical radio operators is not sufficient. The communication devices should allow duplex (two-way simultaneous communications akin to a telephone call or face-to-face communi-cation) for conversational dialogue between clinicians. Where conventional radios are used, a lack of familiarity with their simplex mode of operation, where a press-to-talk switch is required, can lead to information being missed because both parties talk simultaneously.

Wireless technology now makes communication more ubiquitous than ever. Cellular phones and/or satellite phones can be installed in road vehicles and aircraft used for patient transport. Performance depends on the type of technology employed and the coverage offered by the network. GSM digital phones are not designed to be used in the air and are almost useless for aero-medical work. CDMA digital phones work well in aircraft and offer wide coverage and good noise suppression. Satellite phones require careful installation, especially in helicopters where the aerial should not be mounted beneath the rotor hub. When installed they can be quite effective although call rates and voice delay make them less desirable than terrestrial systems. These systems are now ready to carry data as well as voice. Some services are working at creating a 'paperless' environment for the retrieval team using electronic devices to enter patient-care information.

MEDICAL CONTROL

Most medical retrieval teams operate under clinical policies and procedures determined in advance. Such 'off-line' control of the team's practice should be supplemented by 'on-line' control as required. That is, the team should be able to seek advice and guidance at any stage of the process by a telephone conversation in real time with a senior clinician at consultant level. It is helpful if the advice of several senior clinicians is available in a conference call whenever there are multidisciplinary management issues.

It seems ironic that once a patient is in a major institution, many levels of medical control are applied to their care. Prior to that and at the phase of their disease process when the information was leanest and the greatest uncertainty applied, the responsibility for medical care is traditionally delegated to a quite junior medical or paramedical level.

SOME DEFINITIONS

Common expressions
- CPA: cabin pressure altitude.
- IFR: instrument flight rules.
- VFR: visual flight rules.
- Referring: doctor or hospital with the patient needing transfer.
- Referral: doctor or hospital receiving the call & possibly accepting transfer.

Process
- Response time: launch time + outbound leg + circulation (time spent moving from one vehicle to the next or from the last vehicle to the bedside).
- Scene time: stabilisation time + circulation.
- Inbound leg: time travelling toward the destination hospital + circulation.
- Re-positioning leg: time taken to return from the destination to base.
- Mission time: response + scene + inbound + outbound + re-positioning.
- Restoration time: time reconfiguring equipment and restocking the kit.

INFORMATION SYSTEMS

Data about patients being transported are supplied from telephone conversations in the referral process and paper records travelling with the patient or transmitted by fax. In an acute-care setting, many of the details required to assist the consultative process have yet to be committed to paper, either during pre-hospital care or in the referring hospital. Furthermore, electronic data systems developed to support pre-hospital care, EDs and neonatal nurseries are generally not designed to 'talk' with the next party in the chain. As a result, each party collects the same information and records it again. This process is inefficient and also liable to error, duplication and doubt. A challenge yet to be met is to develop a 'daisy-chain' between information systems, which allows previous information to be automatically accessible to the next "player" in the process. From pre-hospital to referring hospital to medical retrieval team to referral hospital, each field of information should only be collected once. It should then be accessible to and shared with subsequent carers. Ultimately, this chain should link back to the referring hospital, completing a circular pathway that ensures outcome and feedback is provided to the original carers.

QUALITY

The search for improvement applies to patient transport as much as any other area of care. Given the multiple participants and complex and variable scenarios, a robust and thorough process of quality assurance is essential.

The medical retrieval process cannot stand alone from referring and referral hospital practice. In practice, conducting routine case debriefs, morbidity and mortality meetings and open-case presentations should include as many players as possible. To permit full participation, retrieval teams need to consider holding these activities both in referring hospitals and referral hospitals. The informal contact accompanying these quality activities breaks down barriers, increases mutual respect and facilitates telephone communication about real patients in the future.

It is also recommended that retrieval teams contribute to anonymous incident monitoring systems (AIMS). Such tools help to quantify adverse events.

SUMMARY

- Be available.
- Teletriage intelligently.
- Respond rapidly as appropriate.
- Stabilise fully ('stay and play' rather than 'wrap and run').
- Transport carefully.
- Provide feedback to clients.
- Monitor and review practice.

REFERENCES

1. Pearson GA et al 1997 Should paediatric intensive care be centralised? Trent versus Victoria. Lancet 349: 1213–1217
2. Lewis FR 1991 Improved outcomes from tertiary center pediatric intensive care: A statewide comparison of tertiary and non-tertiary care facilities. Critical Care Medicine 19(2): 150–159
3. NSW Emergency Transport Service, Australia. www.nets.org.au
4. Chance GW, Matthew JD, Gash J, et al 1978 Neonatal transport: A controlled study of skilled assistance. Mortality and morbidity of neonates < 1.5 kg birth weight. Journal of Pediatrics 93(4): 662–666

Index